CURRENT THERAPY OF INFECTIOUS DISEASE

SECOND EDITION

CURRENT THERAPY OF INFECTIOUS DISEASE

SECOND EDITION

Edited by

David Schlossberg, M.D., F.A.C.P.
Director, Medical Services
Merck & Co., Inc.
West Point, Pennsylvania;
Professor of Medicine
Temple University School of Medicine,
Professor of Medicine
Jefferson Medical College
Thomas Jefferson University
Philadelphia, Pennsylvania

With 88 illustrations

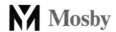 Mosby

A Harcourt Health Sciences Company

St. Louis   London   Philadelphia   Sydney   Toronto

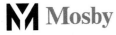

Mosby

A Harcourt Health Sciences Company

Senior Medical Editor: Richard Zorab
Associate Developmental Editor: Jennifer Shreiner
Project Manager: Carol Sullivan Weis
Project Editor: Florence Achenbach
Designer: Mark A. Oberkrom

Mosby, Inc.
A Harcourt Health Sciences Company
11830 Westline Industrial Drive
St. Louis, Missouri 63146

Printed in the United States of America

Library of Congress Cataloging-in-Publication Data

Current therapy of infectious disease / edited by David Schlossberg.—2nd ed.
   p. ; cm.
   Includes bibliographical references and index.
   ISBN 0-323-00907-7
   1. Communicable diseases. 2. Anti-infective agents. I. Schlossberg,
David.
   [DNLM: 1. Communicable Diseases—therapy. WC 100 C9769 2000]
   RC111.S35 2000
   615.5'8—dc21
                                                                00-057854

00 01 02 03 04 GW/MVY 9 8 7 6 5 4 3 2 1

Contributors

Mujahed Abbas, M.D.
Assistant Professor
Texas Technical University Health Sciences Center,
Staff Member
Medical Center Hospital,
Odessa Regional Hospital,
Odessa, Texas;
Memorial Hospital and Medical Center,
Westwood Hospital,
Midland, Texas
Sepsis and Septic Shock

Elias Abrutyn, M.D.
Professor of Medicine and Public Health
Interim Chairman, Department of Medicine
MCP Hahnemann University
Philadelphia, Pennsylvania
Urinary Tract Infection

Rima Abu-Nader, M.D.
Fellow, Division of Infectious Diseases
Mayo Clinic
Rochester, Minnesota
Infection in Transplant Patients

David W.K. Acheson, M.D.
New England Medical Center;
Associate Professor of Medicine
Tufts University:
Boston, Massachusetts
Campylobacter
Shigella

Alexander Ackley, Jr., M.D.
Hospital Epidemiologist
Chairman, Department of Quality Improvement
Princeton Hospital
Princeton, New Jersey;
Professor of Clinical Medicine, Division of Infectious
Diseases
UMDNJ, Robert Wood Johnson Medical School
New Brunswick, New Jersey
Polyarthritis and Fever

Karim A. Adal, M.D.
Staff Physician
Department of Infectious Diseases
Cleveland Clinic Foundation
Cleveland, Ohio
Cellulitis and Erysipelas

Adaora A. Adimora, M.D., M.P.H.
Assistant Professor of Medicine
University of North Carolina School of Medicine
Chapel Hill, North Carolina
Syphilis and Other Treponematoses

N. Franklin Adkinson, Jr., M.D.
Program Director
Graduate Training Program in Clinical Investigation
Training Program Director of Allergy and Clinical
Immunology;
Professor of Medicine
Johns Hopkins University School of Medicine
Baltimore, Maryland
Hypersensitivity to Antibiotics

Claude Afif, M.D.
Fellow, University of Texas
MD Anderson Cancer Center
Houston, Texas
Intravascular Catheter–Related Infections

Daniel M. Albert, M.D., M.S.
University of Wisconsin Hospital and Clinics
F.A. Davis Professor and Chair
Lorenz E. Zimmerman Professor
University of Wisconsin Medical School;
Madison, Wisconsin
Retinitis

Phillip B. Amidon, M.D., F.A.C.P.
Chief, Gastroenterology
Veterans Administration Medical Center
Togus, Maine
Whipple's Disease and Sprue

V.T. Andriole, M.D.
Professor of Medicine
Yale University School of Medicine
New Haven, Connecticut
Focal Renal Infections and Papillary Necrosis

Julie Antique, M.D.
Fellow, Division of Infectious Diseases
SUNY at Stony Brook
Stony Brook, New York
Toxoplasma

Donald Armstrong, A.B., M.D.
Consultant in Infectious Disease
Memorial Sloan-Kettering Cancer Center;
Professor of Medicine
Cornell University Medical College
New York, New York
Infections in Patients with Neoplastic Disease

Stephen Ash, F.R.C.P., M.B., B.S., B.Sc.
Consultant Physician
Ealing Hospital;
Honorary Clinical Senior Lecturer
Imperial College
London, United Kingdom
Deep Soft-Tissue Infection: Fasciitis and Myositis

Aris P. Assimacopoulos, M.D.
Private Practice
St. Paul Infectious Disease Associates
St. Paul, Minnesota;
Clinical Professor of Family Practice and
Community Health
University of Minnesota Medical School
Minneapolis, Minnesota
*Staphylococcal and Streptococcal Toxic Shock
and Kawasaki Syndromes*

Alfred E. Bacon, III, M.D., F.A.C.P.
Associate Program Director
Department of Medicine
Christiana Health Care Services;
Clinical Assistant Professor of Medicine
Jefferson Medical College
Wilmington, Delaware
Chlamydia psittaci (Psittacosis)

Robert S. Baltimore, M.D.
Associate Director of Hospital Epidemiology
Yale New Haven Hospital;
Professor of Pediatrics and Epidemiology
Yale University School of Medicine
New Haven, Connecticut
Neonatal Infection

John G. Banwell, M.D., F.A.C.P.
Consultant
Gastroenterology Medical and Regional Office Center
Department of Veterans Affairs
Togus, Maine
Whipple's Disease and Sprue

Jamie S. Barkin, M.D.
Chief, Division of Gastroenterology
Mount Sinai Medical Center;
Professor of Medicine
University of Miami;
Miami Beach, Florida
Infectious Complications in Acute Pancreatitis

Fred F. Barrett, M.D.
Medical Director
Le Bonheur Children's Medical Center;
Professor of Pediatrics
University of Tennessee, Memphis:
Memphis, Tennessee
Cerebrospinal Fluid Shunt Infection

Michele Barry, M.D., F.A.C.P.
Chief, Generalist Firm
Internal Medicine
Yale New Haven Hospital;
Professor of Medicine and Public Health
Director, Office International Health
Yale University School of Medicine
New Haven, Connecticut
Viral Hemorrhagic Fever

John G. Bartlett, M.D.
Chief, Infectious Diseases
Johns Hopkins Hospital;
Professor of Medicine
Johns Hopkins University School of Medicine
Baltimore, Maryland
Antibiotic-Associated Diarrhea

Joseph H. Bates, B.S., M.D., M.S.
Deputy State Health Officer
Arkansas Department of Health;
Staff Physician
University of Arkansas for Medical Sciences
Central Arkansas Veterans Health Care System;
Professor of Medicine and Microbiology
University of Arkansas for Medical Sciences
Little Rock, Arkansas
Community-Acquired Pneumonia

Jules Baum, M.D.
Boston Eye Associates
Chestnut Hill, Massachusetts
Keratitis

Robert T. Bechtel, M.D.
Chief, Department of Ophthalmology
Altoona Hospital
Altoona, Pennsylvania
Retinitis

Susan E. Beekmann, R.N., M.P.H.
Nurse Epidemiologist
University of Iowa College of Medicine
Iowa City, Iowa

Vascular Infection

Irmgard Behlau, M.D.
Staff Physician
Division of Infectious Diseases
Mount Auburn Hospital
Cambridge, Massachusetts;
Research Assistant Professor
Molecular Biology and Microbiology
Tufts University School of Medicine
Boston, Massachusetts

Croup, Epiglottis, and Laryngitis

Romelle Belmonte, M.D.
Fellow, Infectious Diseases
Hartford Hospital
Hartford, Connecticut

Clostridia

Joseph R. Berger, M.D.
Professor and Chairman, Department of Neurology
University of Kentucky College of Medicine
Lexington, Kentucky

Progressive Multifocal Leukoencephalopathy

Richard E. Berger, M.D.
Professor
University of Washington School of Medicine
Department of Urology
Seattle, Washington

Epididymo-orchitis

Maye Berroya, M.D.
Attending Physician
Paintsville Medical Care
Paintsville, Kentucky

Toxoplasma

Mitchell A. Blass, M.D.
Fellow, Infectious Disease
Emory University School of Medicine
Atlanta, Georgia

Nonsurgical Antimicrobial Prophylaxis

Charles D. Bluestone, M.D.
Director, Department of Pediatric Otolaryngology
Children's Hospital of Pittsburgh,
Eberly Professor of Pediatric Otolaryngology
University of Pittsburgh School of Medicine
Pittsburgh, Pennsylvania

Sinusitis

Fernando Borrego, M.D.
Clinical Researcher
Division of Infectious Diseases
Department of Medicine
Mount Sinai Medical Center;
Fellow
Division of Infectious Diseases
Department of Medicine
Mount Sinai School of Medicine
New York, New York

Aseptic Meningitis Syndrome

William R. Bowie, M.D., F.R.C.P.C.
Professor of Medicine
Division of Infectious Diseases
University of British Columbia
Vancouver, British Columbia
Canada

Urethritis and Dysuria

Suzanne F. Bradley, M.D.
Associate Professor of Internal Medicine
University of Michigan Medical School;
Veterans Affairs Medical Center
Ann Arbor, Michigan

Staphylococcus

Roy D. Brod, M.D.
Chief, Division of Ophthalmology
Lancaster General Hospital
Lancaster, Pennsylvania;
Dean, State University School of Medicine
Hershey Medical Center
Hershey, Pennsylvania

Endophthalmitis

Itzhak Brook, M.D.
Attending, Infectious Diseases
Georgetown University Hospital
Washington, DC;
Naval Hospital
Bethesda, Maryland;
Professor, Pediatrics
Georgetown University School of Medicine
Washington, DC

Pharyngotonsillitis

Arthur E. Brown, M.D.
Attending Physician, Infectious Disease Service
Memorial Sloan-Kettering Cancer Center;
Attending Pediatrician
New York Presbyterian Hospital;
Visiting Associate Physician
The Rockefeller University Hospital;
Professor of Clinical Medicine and Clinical Pediatrics
Weill Medical College of Cornell University:
New York, New York

Hospital-Acquired Fever

John D. Brownlee, M.D.
Trauma Fellow
Metro Health Medical Center;
Case Western Reserve University
Cleveland, Ohio

Trauma-Related Infection

Stefan Bughi, M.D.
Physician Specialist
Rancho Los Amigos National Rehabilitation Center
Downey, California;
Assistant Professor of Clinical Medicine
Keck School of Medicine at University of California
Los Angeles, California

Diabetes and Infection

Martha I. Buitrago, M.D.
Director, HIV Services
Fair Haven Community Health Center;
Clinical Instructor
Department of Medicine—AIDS Program
Yale University School of Medicine
New Haven, Connecticut

Fever and Lymphadenopathy

Joseph J. Burrascano, Jr., B.A., M.D.
Attending Physician
Southampton Hospital
Southampton, New York

Borreliosis

Thomas Butler, M.D.
Chief of Infectious Diseases
University Medical Center;
Professor of Internal Medicine and Microbiology
Texas Technical University Health Sciences Center
Lubbock, Texas

Enterobacteriaceae

Christopher H. Cabell, M.D.
Fellow, Division of Cardiology
Duke University Medical Center
Durham, North Carolina

HACEK

Christopher F. Carpenter, M.D.
Senior Fellow, Division of Infectious Diseases
Johns Hopkins University School of Medicine
Baltimore, Maryland

Candidiasis

Carlos Carrillo, M.D.
Principal Professor of Medicine
Universidad Peruana Cayetano Heredia
Lima, Peru

Brucellosis

Feng-Yee Chang M.D., D.M.S.
Chief, Division of Infectious Diseases and Tropical
Medicine
Department of International Medicine
Tri-Service General Hospital;
Associate Professor of Medicine
National Defense Medical Center
Taipei, Taiwan

Haemophilus

Sanford Chodosh, M.D.
Chief of Staff
Veteran's Affairs Outpatient Clinic;
Associate Professor of Medicine
Boston University School of Medicine
Boston, Massachusetts

Acute and Chronic Bronchitis

Shurjeel Choudhri, B.Sc., M.D., F.R.C.P.C.
Director of HIV Services
St. Boniface General Hospital;
Assistant Professor, Departments of Medical
Microbiology and Internal Medicine
University of Manitoba Faculty of Medicine
Winnipeg, Manitoba
Canada

Genital Ulcer Adenopathy Syndrome

Mashiul H. Chowdhury, M.D.
Fellow
Division of Infectious Diseases
Medical College of Pennsylvania/Hahnemann
University
Philadelphia, Pennsylvania

*Endocarditis of Natural and Prosthetic Valves:
Treatment and Prophylaxis*

C. Glenn Cobbs, A.B., M.D.
Professor Emeritus
University of Alabama School of Medicine
Birmingham, Alabama

Bartonellosis (Carrión's Disease)

Clay J. Cockerell, M.D.
Medical Director
University of Texas Southwestern Medical Center
Dallas, Texas

Leprosy

Carlo Contoreggi, M.D.
Clinical Chief, Brain Imaging Branch
Intramural Research Program
National Institute on Drug Abuse
National Institutes of Health
Johns Hopkins Medical Institutions
Departments of Medicine and Radiology
Baltimore, Maryland

Infectious Complications in the Injection Drug User

Roberto Baun Corales, D.O.
Chief Fellow, Department of Infectious Disease
The Cleveland Clinic Foundation
Cleveland, Ohio

Miscellaneous Gram-Positive Organisms

J. Thomas Cross, Jr., M.D., M.P.H.
Associate Professor, Departments of Internal Medicine
and Pediatrics
LSU Health Sciences Center
Shreveport, Louisiana

Tick-Borne Disease

Kent Crossley, M.D.
Associate Chief of Staff for Education
Minneapolis Veterans Affairs Medical Center;
Professor of Medicine and Pharmacy
University of Minnesota
Minneapolis, Minnesota

Infections in the Elderly

Burke A. Cunha, M.D.
Chief, Infectious Diseases Division
Winthrop-University Hospital
Mineola, New York;
Professor of Medicine
State University of New York School of Medicine
Stony Brook, New York

Fever of Unknown Origin
Nosocomial Pneumonias

Scott F. Davies, M.D.
Division Chief of Pulmonary and
Critical Care Medicine
Hennepin County Medical Center;
Professor
University of Minnesota Medical School
Minneapolis, Minnesota

Mucormycosis (Zygomycosis)

Charles Davis, M.D.
Assistant Professor of Medicine
Institute of Human Virology
University of Maryland
Baltimore, Maryland

Meningococcus and Miscellaneous Neisseriae

Andrew J. Deck, M.D.
Resident Physician
University of Washington School of Medicine
Department of Urology
Seattle, Washington

Epididymo-orchitis

George S. Deepe, Jr., M.D.
Attending Physician
University Hospital;
Staff Physician
University of Cincinnati Medical Center;
Consulting Physician
Jewish Hospital;
Russell Morgan Professor of Medicine
Director, Infectious Disease Division
University of Cincinnati Medical Center
Cincinnati, Ohio

Nocardia

E. Patchen Dellinger, M.D.
Vice Chairman, Department of Surgery
Chief, Division of General Surgery
Associate Medical Director
University of Washington Medical Center;
Professor of Surgery
University of Washington
Seattle, Washington

Postoperative Wound Infections

L.M. Dembry, M.D.
Associate Professor of Medicine and Epidemiology
Yale University School of Medicine
New Haven, Connecticut

Focal Renal Infections and Papillary Necrosis

Stanley C. Deresinski, M.D.
Associate Chief, Infectious Disease
Santa Clara Valley Medical Center
San Jose, California;
Clinical Professor of Medicine
Division of Infectious Diseases and
Geographic Medicine
Stanford University
Stanford, California

Coccidioidomycosis

Lisa L. Dever, M.D.
Chief, Infectious Diseases Clinic
Veteran's Affairs New Jersey Health Care System
East Orange, New Jersey;
Associate Professor
Department of Medicine
UMDNJ, New Jersey Medical School
Newark, New Jersey

Lung Abscess

Catherine Diamond M.D., M.P.H.
Assistant Clinical Professor
University of California Irvine Medical Center;
Assistant Clinical Professor, College of Medicine
University of California, Irvine
Orange, California

Myocarditis

James D. Dick, Ph.D.
Associate Professor, Pathology, Molecular
Microbiology and Immunology
Johns Hopkins University, School of Medicine
Baltimore, Maryland

Infection in the Neutropenic Patient

Gordon Dickinson, M.D.
Chief, Infectious Diseases
Miami VA Medical Center;
Professor
Chief, Infectious Disease
University of Miami School of Medicine
Miami, Florida

Infected Implants

Mark J. DiNubile, M.D.
Associate Professor of Medicine
University of Medicine and Dentistry of New Jersey
Robert Wood Johnson Medical School
Camden, New Jersey

*The Diagnosis and Management of Spinal Epidural
Abscess*

Bradley N. Doebbeling, M.D., M.Sc.
Medical Center Epidemiologist and Staff Physician
Veteran's Affairs Medical Center;
Staff Physician and Consultant, Department of
Internal Medicine
University of Iowa Health Care;
Associate Professor, Department of Internal Medicine
University of Iowa College of Medicine;
Department of Epidemiology
University of Iowa College of Public Health:
Iowa City, Iowa

Percutaneous Injury: Risks and Management

Herbert L. DuPont, M.D.
Chief, Internal Medicine Service
St. Luke's Episcopal Hospital;
Mary W. Kelsey Professor of Medical Science
The University of Texas–Houston School of Public
Health and Medical School
Houston, Texas

Travelers' Diarrhea

Asim K. Dutt, M.D.
Chief, Medical Service
Alvin C. York Veterans Administrative Medical Center
Murfreesboro, Tennessee;
Professor and Vice Chairman
Department of Medicine
Meharry Medical College
Nashville, Tennessee

Tuberculosis

Molly E. Eaton, M.D.
Assistant Professor of Medicine
Division of Infectious Diseases
Department of Medicine
Emory University School of Medicine
Atlanta, Georgia

Pasteurella multocida

Rebecca Edge Martin, M.D.
Staff Physician
Central Arkansas Veterans' Healthcare System;
Associate Professor of Medicine
Division of Infectious Diseases
University of Arkansas for Medical Sciences
Little Rock, Arkansas

Community-Acquired Pneumonia

Lawrence J. Eron, M.D.
Director, Ambulatory Treatment Center
Kaiser Moanalua Medical Center;
Clinical Associate Professor of Medicine
John A. Burns School of Medicine
University of Hawaii
Honolulu, Hawaii

Papillomavirus

Janine Evans, M.D.
Associate Professor of Medicine
Yale University School of Medicine
West Haven, Connecticut
Lyme Disease

Sebastian Faro, M.D., Ph.D.
John M. Simpson Professor and Chair
Department of Obstetrics and Gynecology
Rush Medical College
Chicago, Illinois
Vaginitis and Cervicitis

Michael J.G. Farthing, M.D., F.R.C.P.
Professor of Gastroenterology
St. Bartholomew's and the Royal London School
of Medicine and Dentistry
London, United Kingdom
Intestinal Protozoa

Henry M. Feder, Jr., M.D.
University of Connecticut Health Center
Farmington, Connecticut
Classic Viral Exanthems

Thomas M. File, Jr., M.S., M.D.
Chief, Infectious Disease Service
Summa Health System
Akron, Ohio;
Professor of Internal Medicine
Northeastern Ohio Universities College of Medicine
Roots Town, Ohio
Atypical Pneumonia

Sydney M. Finegold, M.D.
Staff Physician
Infectious Diseases Section
Veteran's Affairs Center West Los Angeles;
Professor of Medicine
Professor of Microbiology and Molecular Genetics
University of California Los Angeles School
of Medicine
Los Angeles, California
Anaerobic Infections

Evelyn J. Fisher, M.D.
Associate Professor of Medicine
Division of Infectious Diseases
Medical College of Virginia at Virginia
Commonwealth University
Richmond, Virginia
*The Prophylaxis of Opportunistic Infections
in HIV Disease*

Neil Fishman, M.D.
Director, Antimicrobial Management Program
Hospital of the University of Pennsylvania;
Assistant Professor of Medicine
University of Pennsylvania School of Medicine
Philadelphia, Pennsylvania
Influenza

Thomas A. Fleisher, M.D.
Chief, Clinical Pathology Department
Warren G. Magnuson Clinical Center
National Institutes of Health
Bethesda, Maryland
Evaluation of Suspected Immunodeficiency

Harry W. Flynn, Jr., M.D.
Professor of Ophthalmology
Department of Ophthalmology
Bascom Palmer Eye Institute;
University of Miami
School of Medicine
Miami, Florida
Endophthalmitis

Gerald Friedland, M.D.
Director, AIDS Program
Professor of Medicine and Epidemiology
and Public Health
Yale School of Medicine
Yale–New Haven Hospital
New Haven, Connecticut
Fever and Lymphadenopathy

Harvey M. Friedman, M.D.
Professor of Medicine
Chief of Infectious Disease
University of Pennsylvania
Philadelphia, Pennsylvania
Influenza

Thomas R. Gadacz, M.D., F.A.C.S.
Professor and Chairman, Department of Surgery
Medical College of Georgia;
Augusta, Georgia
Splenic Abscess

Nelson M. Gantz, M.D., F.A.C.P.
Chairman, Department of Medicine
Chief, Section of Infectious Diseases
Pinnacle Health System
Harrisburg, Pennsylvania;
Clinical Professor of Medicine
MCP Hahnemann University
Philadelphia, Pennsylvania
Mediastinitis

Michael J. Gehman, D.O.
Division of Infectious Diseases
MCP Hahnemann University
Philadelphia, Pennsylvania

Moraxella (Branhamella)

Jeffrey A. Gelfand, M.D.
New England Medical Center
Boston, Massachusetts

Babesiosis

Martha J. Gentry-Nielsen, Ph.D.
Associate Professor of Medicine, Medical
Microbiology and Immunology
Creighton University School of Medicine
University of Nebraska College of Medicine
Omaha, Nebraska

Infection in the Alcoholic

Gary Gitnick, M.D.
Professor of Medicine
Chief, Division of Digestive Diseases
UCLA School of Medicine
Los Angeles, California

Chronic Hepatitis

Aaron E. Glatt, M.D., F.A.C.P., F.C.C.P., F.I.D.S.A.
Director, Graduate Medical Education
Chief, Infectious Diseases and Infection Control
The Catholic Medical Centers of Brooklyn and Queens
New York, New York;
Professor of Clinical Medicine
Albert Einstein College of Medicine
Bronx, New York

HIV Infection: Initial Evaluation and Monitoring

Richard Gleckman, M.D.
Chairman, Department of Medicine
Chief, Infectious Disease Divisions
St. Joseph's Hospital and Medical Center
Paterson, New Jersey;
Clinical Professor of Medicine
Mount Sinai School of Medicine
New York, New York

Principles of Antibiotic Therapy

Mitchell Goldman, M.D.
Director, Immunocompromised Infectious Disease
Indiana University Medical Center;
Associate Professor
Indiana University School of Medicine
Division of Infectious Diseases
Indianapolis, Indiana

Histoplasmosis

Ellie J.C. Goldstein, M.D.
Director
R.M. Alden Research Laboratory
Santa Monica–University of California Los Angeles
Medical Center;
Clinical Professor of Medicine
University of California, Los Angeles School
of Medicine
Santa Monica, California

Human and Animal Bites

Jeffrey A. Goldstein, M.D.
Mount Sinai Medical Center;
Senior GI Fellow
University of Miami
Miami, Florida

Infectious Complications in Acute Pancreatitis

Harumi Gomi, M.D.
Infectious Disease Fellow
Memorial Hermann Hospital and LBJ General Hospital;
Infectious Disease Fellow
The University of Texas–Houston Medical School
Houston, Texas

Travelers' Diarrhea

Ramya Gopinath, M.B., B.S., F.R.C.P.(C), A.B.I.M.
Visiting Associate
Helminth Immunology Section
Laboratory of Parasitic Diseases
National Institutes of Health
Bethesda, Maryland

Intestinal Roundworms

Eduardo Gotuzzo, M.D., F.A.C.P.
Chief of Infectious Diseases and Tropical Medicine
Hospital Nacioma Cayetan Heredis;
Principal Professor of Medicine
Universidad Perusis Cayetano Heredis
Lima, Peru

Brucellosis

Jeremy D. Gradon, M.D., F.A.C.P.
Attending Physician, Division of Infectious Diseases
Department of Medicine
Mount Sinai Hospital;
Associate Professor of Medicine
Johns Hopkins University School of Medicine
Baltimore, Maryland

Deep Neck Infection

David Y. Graham, M.D.
Chief, Gastroenterology
Veteran's Affairs Medical Center;
Professor of Medicine and Molecular Biology
and Microbiology
Baylor College of Medicine
Houston, Texas
Helicobacter pylori

Jennifer Rubin Grandis, M.D., F.A.C.S.
Program Leader, Head and Neck Cancer
University of Pittsburgh Cancer Institute;
Associate Professor
University of Pittsburgh School of Medicine
Pittsburgh, Pennsylvania
Dental Infection and Its Consequences

Jane M. Grant-Kels, M.D.
Department of Dermatology
University of Connecticut Health Center
University of Connecticut Medical School
Farmington, Connecticut
Classic Viral Exanthems

J. Thomas Grayston, M.D.
Professor
Department of Epidemiology
School of Public Health & Community Medicine
University of Washington
Seattle, Washington
Chlamydia pneumoniae (TWAR)

Ruth M. Greenblatt, M.D.
Professor of Clinical Medicine, Epidemiology
and Biostatistics
University of California, San Francisco
San Francisco, California
Human Herpesvirus 6, 7, 8

Ronald A. Greenfield, M.D.
Staff Physician
Oklahoma City Veteran's Affairs Medical Center;
Professor of Medicine
Chief, Infectious Diseases Section
University of Oklahoma Health Sciences Center
Oklahoma City, Oklahoma
Sporotrichosis

Donald L. Greer, Ph.D.
Director, TB/Mycology Laboratory
Charity Hospital;
Professor
LSU Medical Center
New Orleans, Louisiana
Miscellaneous Fungi and Algae

David W. Gregory, M.D.
Associate Chief of Staff
Veterans Affairs Medical Center;
Associate Professor of Medicine
Division of Infectious Diseases
Vanderbilt University School of Medicine
Nashville, Tennessee
Pseudomonas

Diane Griffin, M.D.
Acute Viral Encephalitis

Arnold W. Gurevitch, M.D.
Professor and Chief
Division of Dermatology
Keck School of Medicine, University
of Southern California
Los Angeles, California
Superficial Fungal Infection of Skin and Nails

Alejandra Gurtman, M.D.
Attending Physician
Mount Sinai Medical Center;
Assistant Professor of Medicine
Division of Infectious Diseases
Department of Medicine
Mount Sinai School of Medicine
New York, New York
Aseptic Meningitis Syndrome

Ray Y. Hachem, M.D.
Research Investigator
University of Texas
MD Anderson Cancer Center
Houston, Texas
Infection of the Salivary and Lacrimal Glands

Lisa Haglund, M.D.
Medical Director
Hamilton County;
Tuberculosis Control
Staff Physician
University Hospital, Inc.;
Associate Professor of Clinical Medicine
University of Cincinnati School of Medicine
Cincinnati, Ohio
Nocardia

W. Lee Hand, M.D.
Assistant Dean for Research
Professor of Internal Medicine
Texas Technical University Health Science Center
El Paso, Texas
Erysipelothrix

Shahbaz Hasan, M.B., B.S., M.D.
Staff Physician
Veteran Affairs North Texas Health Care System;
Assistant Professor of Medicine, Department of
Internal Medicine, General Medicine Section
University of Texas Southwestern Medical School
Dallas, Texas

Infection of Native and Prosthetic Joints

David K. Henderson, M.D.
Deputy Director for Clinical Care
Warren G. Magnuson Clinical Center
National Institutes of Health
Bethesda, Maryland

Vascular Infection

H. Franklin Herlong, M.D.
Associate Professor of Medicine
Associate Dean for Student Affairs
John Hopkins School of Medicine
Baltimore, Maryland

Pyogenic Liver Abscess

Hoi Ho, M.D.
Professor of Internal Medicine
Texas Tech University Health Sciences Center
El Paso, Texas

Erysipelothrix

Craig J. Hoesley, M.D.
Assistant Professor of Medicine
University of Alabama at Birmingham
Birmingham, Alabama

Bartonellosis (Carrión's Disease)

Charles H. Hoke, Jr., M.D.
Attending Physician
Walter Reed Army Medical Center
Washington, DC

Dengue and Related Syndromes

James Wm. C. Holmes, M.D.†
Diverticulitis

Paul D. Holtom, M.D.
Associate Professor of Clinical Medicine
and Orthopaedics
University of Southern California
Los Angeles, California

Rickettsial Infections

Richard B. Hornick, M.D.
Assistant Director, Internal Medicine
Residency Program
Orlando Regional Healthcare System
Orlando, Florida;
Adjunct Clinical Professor of Medicine
University of Florida
Gainesville, Florida

Tularemia

Thomas R. Howdieshell, M.D., F.A.C.S., F.C.C.P.
Associate Professor of Surgery
Trauma/Surgical Critical Care
Medical College of Georgia
Augusta, Georgia

Splenic Abscess

Walter T. Hughes, M.D.
Professor of Pediatric and Preventive Medicine
University of Tennessee College of Medicine;
Former Member, St. Jude Children's Research Hospital
Memphis, Tennessee

Pneumocystis carinii

Christopher D. Huston, M.D.
Howard Hughes Postdoctoral Fellow
Division of Infectious Diseases
University of Virginia School of Medicine
Charlottesville, Virginia

Leptospirosis

Steven Huy-Han, M.D.
Assistant Clinical Professor of Medicine
UCLA School of Medicine
Los Angeles, California

Acute Viral Hepatitis

Robert A. Hyndiuk, M.D.
Professor Emeritus
Medical College of Wisconsin
Department of Ophthalmology;
Eye Institute
Elm Grove, Wisconsin

Conjunctivitis

Newton E. Hyslop, Jr., M.D.
Chief, Infectious Diseases Section
Tulane Medical Director, Infectious Diseases
Isolation Service
Charity Hospital;
Professor of Medicine
Tulane University School of Medicine
Division of Infectious Diseases
New Orleans, Louisiana

Myelitis and Peripheral Neuropathy

†Deceased.

Roger T. Inouye, M.D.
Instructor, Department of Medicine
Harvard University School of Medicine
Beth Israel Deaconess Medical Center
Boston, Massachusetts

Acute Viral Encephalitis

Raul E. Isturiz, M.D.
Chief, Infectious Diseases
Centro Medico Docente La Trinidad;
Consultant in Infectious Diseases
Centro Medico de Caracas
Caracas, Venezuela

Pregnancy and the Puerperium: Infectious Risks

Lisa A. Jackson, M.D., M.P.H.
Assistant Investigator
Center for Health Studies
Group Health Cooperative;
Assistant Professor
Department of Epidemiology
School of Public Health & Community Medicine
University of Washington
Seattle, Washington

Chlamydia pneumoniae (TWAR)

Richard F. Jacobs, M.D., F.A.A.P.
Horace C. Cabe Professor of Pediatrics
Chief, Pediatric Infectious Disease
University of Arkansas for Medical Sciences and
Arkansas Children's Hospital
Little Rock, Arkansas

Tick-Borne Disease

**D. Geraint James, M.D., F.R.C.P., F.A.C.P.,
F.R.C.O.P.H.**
Professor of Medicine
Royal Free Hospital
London, England
United Kingdom

Iritis

William R. Jarvis, M.D.
Investigation and Prevention Branch
Hospital Infections Program
Centers for Disease Control and Prevention
Atlanta, Georgia

Transfusion-Related Infection

D. Rohan Jeyarajah, M.D.
General Surgeon
Zale-Lipshy University Hospital;
Assistant Professor, Department of Surgery
University of Texas Southwestern Medical Center
Dallas, Texas

Biliary Infection: Cholecystitis and Cholangitis

Waldemar G. Johanson, Jr., M.D., M.P.H.
Professor and Chairman, Department of Medicine
University of Medicine and Dentistry of New Jersey
New Jersey Medical School
Newark, New Jersey

Lung Abscess

Malcom John, M.D., M.P.H.
Postdoctoral Fellow, Infectious Diseases Division
University of California, San Francisco
San Francisco, California

Human Herpesvirus 6, 7, 8

Jonas T. Johnson, M.D., F.A.C.S.
Vice Chairman, Department of Otolaryngology
Director, Otolaryngology Residency Training Program
University of Pittsburgh, Eye and Ear Institute;
Professor, Departments of Otolaryngology and
Radiation Oncology
University of Pittsburgh School of Medicine
Pittsburgh, Pennsylvania

Dental Infection and Its Consequences

Royce H. Johnson, M.D.
Chair, Department of Medicine
Chief, Infectious Disease
Kern Medical Center
Bakersfield, California;
Professor of Medicine
University of California Los Angeles
Los Angeles, California

Yersinia

James F. Jones, M.D.
Senior Staff Physician
National Jewish Medical and Research Center;
Professor of Pediatrics
University of Colorado School of Medicine
Denver, Colorado

Chronic Fatigue Syndrome

Ronald N. Jones, M.D.
Director
CAST Laboratories;
Professor of Pathology
University of Iowa College of Medicine
Iowa City, Iowa

Enterococcus

Elaine C. Jong, M.D.
Co-Director, Travel and Tropical Medicine Service
V.W. Medical Center;
Clinical Professor of Medicine
University of Washington
Seattle, Washington

Immunizations

Niranjan Kanesa-thasan
Staff Physician, Pediatrics
Walter Reed Army Medical Center
Washington, DC;
Adjunct Assistant Professor, Preventive Medicine
and Biometrics
Uniformed Services University of the Health Sciences
Bethesda, Maryland
Dengue and Related Syndromes

Judith E. Karp, M.D.
Professor of Medicine and Oncology
University of Maryland school of Medicine
Baltimore, Maryland
Infection in the Neutropenic Patient

William N. Katkov, M.D.
Assistant Clinical Professor of Medicine
UCLA School of Medicine
Los Angeles, California
Chronic Hepatitis

Carol A. Kauffman, M.D.
Chief, Infectious Diseases Section
Veterans Affairs Ann Arbor Healthcare System;
Professor of Internal Medicine
University of Michigan Medical School
Ann Arbor, Michigan
Staphylococcus

Paul Kelly, M.D., M.R.C.P.
Senior Lecturer
Digestive Diseases Research Center
St. Bartholomew's and the Royal London School of
Medicine and Dentistry
London, United Kingdom
Intestinal Protozoa

Jay S. Keystone, M.D., F.R.C.P.C.
Staff Physician, Tropical Disease Unit
Toronto General Hospital;
Professor of Medicine
University of Toronto
Toronto, Ontario
Canada
Advice for Travelers
Intestinal Roundworms

Dina B. KiaNoury, M.D.
Fellow, Division of Pulmonary/Critical Care
Department of Medicine
Georgetown University Medical Center
Washington, DC
Nontuberculous Mycobacteria

David W. Kimberlin, M.D.
Assistant Professor of Pediatrics
University of Alabama at Birmingham
The Children's Hospital
Birmingham, Alabama
Herpes Simplex Viruses

Natalie C. Klein, M.D., Ph.D.
Associate Director, Infectious Disease Division
Winthrop-University Hospital
Mineola, New York;
Assistant Professor of Medicine
State University of New York School of Medicine
Stony Brook, New York
Fever of Unknown Origin

Oksana M. Korzeniowski, M.D.
Professor of Medicine
Division of Infectious Diseases
Medical College of Pennsylvania/Hahnemann
University
Philadelphia, Pennsylvania
Endocarditis of Natural and Prosthetic Valves:
Treatment and Prophylaxis

Frederick Koster, M.D.
Professor of Internal Medicine and Biology
University of New Mexico School of Medicine
Albuquerque, New Mexico
Hantavirus Cardiopulmonary Syndrome

Phyllis E. Kozarsky, M.D.
Associate Professor of Medicine
Emory University School of Medicine;
Associate Professor of International Health
Emory University School of Public Health
Atlanta, Georgia
Advice for Travelers
Malaria—Treatment and Prophylaxis

William L. Krinsky, M.D., Ph.D.
Associate Clinical Professor of Epidemiology
Yale University School of Medicine
Department of Epidemiology and Public Health
New Haven, Connecticut
Lice, Scabies, and Myiasis

Sampath Kumar, M.B.B.S., M.D.
Clinical Instructor
Division of Infectious Diseases
Rush University
Rush Presbyterian St. Lukes Medical Center
Chicago, Illinois
Miscellaneous Gram-Negative Organisms

John S. Lambert, M.D.
HIV and Opportunistic Infections Clinical
Development Branch
Glaxo-Wellcome
London, United Kingdom;
University of Maryland at Baltimore
Institute of Human Virology
Baltimore, Maryland
Infectious Complications in the Injection Drug User

Susan M. Lareau, B.S.
Student, School of Medicine
University of Virginia School of Medicine
Charlottesville, Virginia
*Miscellaneous Tissue Protozoa: Trypanosomiasis
and Leishmaniasis*

William J. Ledger, A.B., M.D.
Professor, Obstetrics and Gynecology
Weill Medical College of Cornell University
New York, New York
Pelvic Inflammatory Disease

Jenny K. Lee, M.D.
Clinical Instructor
Northwestern University Medical School
Department of Infectious Diseases
Chicago, Illinois
Corticosteroids, Cytotoxic Agents, and Infection

John M. Leedom, M.D.
Chief, Division of Infectious Diseases
LAC and University of Southern California
Medical Center;
Professor of Medicine
University of Southern California:
Los Angeles, California
Rickettsial Infections

A. Martin Lerner, M.D.
Attending Physician
William Beaumont Hospital
Royal Oak, Michigan;
Clinical Professor of Medicine
Wayne State University School of Medicine
Detroit, Michigan
Pericarditis

Matthew E. Levison, M.D.
Chief, Division of Infectious Diseases
Medical College of Pennsylvania Hospital;
Professor of Medicine and Public Health
MCP Hahnemann University
Philadelphia, Pennsylvania
Peritonitis

Stuart M. Levitz, M.D.
Attending Physician, Department of Medicine
Boston Medical Center;
Professor of Medicine and Microbiology
Boston University School of Medicine
Boston, Massachusetts
Aspergillosis

Howard Levy, M.D., M.B., B.Ch., Ph.D.
Director of Critical Care
University Hospital, Department of Internal Medicine;
Professor of Medicine
University of New Mexico Health Sciences Center
Albuquerque, New Mexico
Hantavirus Pulmonary Syndrome

Daniel P. Lew, M.D.
Head, Infectious Diseases Division
Geneva University Hospital;
Professor of Medicine
Geneva Medical School University Hospital
Geneva, Switzerland
Acute and Chronic Osteomyelitis

Poh-Lian Lim, M.D., M.P.H.T.M.
Active Medical Staff
Overlake Hospital;
Medical Staff
Vencor Hospital
Seattle, Washington
Myelitis and Peripheral Neuropathy

Neil S. Lipman, V.M.D.
Director and Professor of Veterinary Medicine in
Pathology
Research Animal Resource Center
Weill Medical College of Cornell University and the
Memorial Sloan-Kettering Cancer Center
New York, New York
Rat-Bite Fevers

Pamela A. Lipsett, M.D.
Co-Director, Surgical Intensive Care Unit
Johns Hopkins Hospital;
Associate Professor, Surgery, Anesthesia,
Critical Care, Nursing
Johns Hopkins University
Baltimore, Maryland
Psoas Abscess

Tze Shien Lo, M.D.
Fellow, Infectious Disease
University of Utah
Department of Internal Medicine
Salt Lake City, Utah
AIDS: Therapy for Opportunistic Infections

Sarah S. Long, M.D.
Chief, Section of Infectious Diseases
St. Christopher's Hospital for Children;
Professor of Pediatrics
MCP Hahnemann University School of Medicine
Philadelphia, Pennsylvania
Bordetella

Bennett Lorber, M.D., D.Sc. (Hon)
Chief, Section of Infectious Diseases
Temple University Hospital;
Thomas M. Durant Professor of Medicine
Temple University School of Medicine
Philadelphia, Pennsylvania
Listeria

Benjamin J. Luft, M.D.
Edmund D. Pellegrino Professor
Chairman, Department of Medicine
State University of New York at Stony Brook
Stony Brook, New York
Toxoplasma

Rodger D. MacArthur, M.D.
Attending Physician
Detroit Medical Center;
Associate Professor of Medicine
Wayne State University
Detroit, Michigan
Sepsis and Septic Shock

Karl Madaras-Kelly, Pharm.D.
Clinical Pharmacist
Veterans Affairs Medical Center
Boise, Idaho;
Assistant Professor
College of Pharmacology
Idaho State University
Rocatello, Idaho
Streptococcus Groups A, B, C, D, and G

Janine Maenza, M.D.
Acting Assistant Professor of Medicine
University of Washington
Seattle, Washington
Candidiasis

Joanne T. Maffei, M.D.
Department of Medicine
Section of Infectious Diseases
Louisiana State University Health Science Center
New Orleans, Louisiana
Skin Ulcer and Pyoderma

James H. Maguire, M.D.
Clinical Director, Division of Infectious Disease
Brigham and Women's Hospital;
Associate Professor of Medicine
Harvard Medical School;
Associate Professor in the Department of Immunology
and Infectious Diseases
Harvard School of Public Health
Boston, Massachusetts
Schistosomes and Other Trematodes

Mark A. Malangoni, M.D.
Chairperson, Department of Surgery
Metro Health Medical Center;
Professor and Vice Chairman
Case Western Reserve University:
Cleveland, Ohio
Trauma-Related Infection

Stephen E. Malawista, M.D.
Professor of Medicine
Yale School of Medicine
New Haven, Connecticut
Lyme Disease

Andrew M. Margileth, M.D.
Director, Pediatric Dermatology Clinic
Backus Children's Hospital
Memorial Health, Mercer University Clinical Center;
Clinical Professor of Pediatrics
Mercer University School Medicine
Savannah, Georgia
Cat-Scratch Disease

Peter R. Mariuz, M.D.
Attending Physician
Strong Memorial Hospital;
Associate Professor of Medicine
University of Rochester School of Medicine
Rochester, New York
Dialysis-Related Infection

Paul Martin, M.D.
Associate Professor of Medicine
Director, Hepatology
Division of Digestive Diseases and Dumont-UCLA
Liver Transplant Program
UCLA Medical Center
Los Angeles, California
Acute Viral Hepatitis

C. Hewitt McCuller, Jr., M.D.
Staff Pulmonologist
Director, MICU
Overton Brooks VA Medical Center;
Assistant Professor of Medicine
Pulmonary and Critical Care Medicine
LSU Center for Health Sciences
Shreveport, Louisiana
Aspiration Pneumonia

Joseph E. McDade, Ph.D.
Deputy Director
National Center for Infectious Diseases
Centers for Disease Control and Prevention
Atlanta, Georgia
Ehrlichiosis

John E. McGowan, Jr., M.D.
Professor of Epidemiology
Rollins School of Public Health of Emory University
Atlanta, Georgia
Prevention of Nosocomial Infection in Staff and Patients

J. Anthony Mebane, P.A.
Internal Medicine
Veterans Affairs Medical Center
Boise, Idaho
Streptococcus Groups A, B, C, D, and G

Jeffrey L. Meier, M.D.
Assistant Professor, Division of Infectious Diseases
Department of Internal Medicine
The University of Iowa College of Medicine
Iowa City, Iowa
*Epstein-Barr Virus and Other Causes of the Infectious
Mononucleosis Syndrome
Cytomegalovirus*

Barbara Menzies, M.D.
Assistant Professor of Medicine
Division of Infectious Diseases
Vanderbilt University School of Medicine
Nashville, Tennessee
Pseudomonas

William G. Merz, Ph.D.
Director, Mycology, Mycobateriology and Molecular
Epiosmiology Labs
The Johns Hopkins Hospital
Baltimore, Maryland
Infection in the Neutropenic Patient

Burt R. Meyers, M.D.
Attending Physician, Division of Infectious Disease,
Department of Medicine
The Mount Sinai Medical Center;
Professor of Medicine, Division of Infectious Diseases,
Department of Medicine
Mount Sinai School of Medicine
New York, New York
Aseptic Meningitis Syndrome

T. Erik Michaelson, M.D.
Fellow in Infectious Diseases
Robert Wood Medical School
Camden, New Jersey
*The Diagnosis and Management
of Spinal Epidural Abscess*

Abdolghader Molavi, M.D.
Professor of Medicine
MCP Hahnemann University
Philadelphia, Pennsylvania
Moraxella (Branhamella)

Thomas A. Moore, M.D.
Clinical Assistant Professor
Department of Internal Medicine
University of Kansas School of Medicine
Wichita, Kansas
Tissue Nematodes

Douglas R. Morgan, M.D., M.P.H.
Gastroenterology
Wake Area Health Education Center
Wake Medical Center;
Clinical Associate Professor
University of North Carolina at Chapel Hill
Chapel Hill, North Carolina
Gastroenteritis

Maurice A. Mufson, M.D., M.A.C.P.
Active Medical Staff
Cabell Huntington Hospital;
Active Medical Staff
St. Mary's Hospital;
Professor and Chairman, Department of Medicine
Professor, Department of Microbiology
Marshall University School of Medicine
Huntington, West Virginia
Pneumococcus

Lütfiye Mülazimoglu
Associate Professor of Infectious Diseases and
Clinical Microbiology
Marmara University School of Medicine, Infectious
Disease Section
Istanbul, Turkey
Legionellosis

Jorge Murillo, M.D.
Faculty Member, Infectious Diseases Division
Consultant, Microbiology and Infectious Diseases
Hospital Vargas and Hospital Privado Centro Medico
de Caracas
Caracas, Venezuela
Pregnancy and the Puerperium: Infectious Risks

Robert L. Murphy, M.D.
Professor
Northwestern University Medical School
Chicago, Illinois
Corticosteroids, Cytotoxic Agents, and Infection

Sharat Narayanan, M.D.
Infectious Disease Fellow
Washington Hospital Center
Washington, DC
Principles of Antibiotic Therapy

Theodore E. Nash, M.D.
Head, Gastrointestinal Parasites Section
Laboratory of Parasitic Diseases
National Institutes of Health
Bethesda, Maryland
Tissue Nematodes

Judith L. Nerad, M.D., M.S.
Attending Physician, Division of Infectious Diseases
Cook County Hospital;
Assistant Professor of Medicine
Rush Medical College
Chicago, Illinois
Miscellaneous Gram-Negative Organisms

Ronald Lee Nichols, M.D.
William Henderson Professor of Surgery
Professor of Microbiology and Immunology
Tulane University School of Medicine
Department of Surgery
New Orleans, Louisiana
Diverticulitis

Lindsay E. Nicolle, M.D., F.R.C.P.C.
H.E. Sellers Professor and Head
Department of Internal Medicine
University of Manitoba
Winnipeg, Manitoba
Canada
Infections Associated with Urinary Catheters

Zhannat Z. Nurgalieva, M.D.
Instructor of Medicine
Kazsk State University;
Fellow, Gastroenterology
Baylor College of Medicine
Houston, Texas
Helicobacter pylori

Judith A. O'Donnell, M.D.
Attending Physician, Division of Infectious Disease
Medical College of Pennsylvania Hospital;
Assistant Professor of Medicine and Public Health
MCP Hahnemann School of Medicine
Philadelphia, Pennsylvania
Urinary Tract Infection

James G. Olson, Ph.D.
Supervisory Research Biologist
National Institute of Public Health, Cambodia
Phnom Penh, Cambodia
Ehrlichiosis

Robert L. Owen, M.D.
Environmental Health Physician
Gastrointestinal Infectious Disease Consultant
Veteran's Affairs Medical Center;
Professor of Medicine, Epidemiology, and Biostatistics
University of California San Francisco
San Francisco, California
Gastroenteritis

Frank J. Palella, Jr., M.D.
Assistant Professor of Medicine
Northwestern University Medical School
Chicago, Illinois
HIV Infection: Antiretroviral Therapy

George A. Pankey, B.S., M.S., M.D.
Director, Infectious Disease Research
Alton Ochsner Medical Foundation;
Clinical Professor of Medicine
Tulane and Louisiana State University Schools
of Medicine
New Orleans, Louisiana
Miscellaneous Fungi and Algae

Peter G. Pappas, M.D.
Associate Professor of Medicine
Department of Medicine
Division of Infectious Diseases
University of Alabama at Birmingham
Birmingham, Alabama

Blastomycosis

Richard H. Parker, M.D.
Chairman, Department of Medicine
Providence Hospital;
Associate Professor of Medicine
Howard University College of Medicine:
Washington, DC

Bursitis

Thomas F. Patterson, M.D., F.A.C.P.
Associate Professor
University of Texas Health Science Center
at San Antonio
San Antonio, Texas

Antifungal Therapy

Andrew T. Pavia, M.D.
Director for Clinical Research
AIDS Center;
Associate Professor of Pediatrics and Medicine
University of Utah School of Medicine
Salt Lake City, Utah

Food Poisoning

Zbigniew S. Pawlowski, M.D.
Clinic of Parasitic and Tropical Diseases
University of Medical Sciences
Poznan, Poland

Tapeworms (Cestodes)

Carlos V. Paya, M.D., Ph.D.
Professor of Medicine and Immunology
Division of Infectious Disease
Mayo Clinic
Rochester, Minnesota

Infection in Transplant Patients

Richard D. Pearson, M.D.
Professor of Medicine and Pathology
Division of Geographic and International Medicine
Departments of Medicine and Pathology
Charlottesville, Virginia

*Miscellaneous Tissue Protozoa: Trypanosomiasis
and Leishmaniasis*

R. Stokes Peebles, Jr., M.D.
Assistant Professor of Medicine
Division of Allergy, Pulmonary and Critical Medicine
Vanderbilt University School of Medicine
Nashville, Tennessee

Hypersensitivity to Antibiotics

Rosalie Pepe, M.D.
Head, Infectious Disease Section
Episcopal Hospital;
Clinical Assistant Professor
Temple University School of Medicine
Philadelphia, Pennsylvania

Antimicrobial Agent Tables

Sofia Perea, Pharm.D., Ph.D.
Postdoctoral Fellow
University of Texas Health Science Center
at San Antonio
San Antonio, Texas

Antifungal Therapy

William A. Petri, Jr., M.D., Ph.D.
Attending Physician
University of Virginia Hospital;
Professor, Departments of Medicine, Microbiology
and Pathology
University of Virginia School of Medicine
Charlottesville, Virginia

Leptospirosis

John P. Phair, M.D.
Professor of Medicine
Director, Comprehensive AIDS Center
Northwestern University Medical School;
Director, Division of Infectious Disease
Northwestern Memorial Hospital
Chicago, Illinois

HIV Infection: Antiretroviral Therapy

Robert S. Pinals, M.D.
Chairman, Department of Medicine
The Medical Center at Princeton
Princeton, New Jersey;
Professor of Medicine and Vice-Chairman,
Department of Medicine
UMDNJ, Robert Wood Johnson Medical School
New Brunswick, New Jersey

Polyarthritis and Fever

Roger J. Pomerantz, M.D.
Professor of Medicine and Director, Division
of Infectious Diseases
Jefferson Medical College of Thomas
Jefferson University
Philadelphia, Pennsylvania
Antiviral Therapy

Debra Poutsiaka, M.D.
Babesiosis

William G. Powderly, M.D.
Chief, Division of Infectious Diseases
Barnes Jewish Hospital;
Professor of Medicine
Washington University School of Medicine
St. Louis, Missouri
Cryptococcus

John H. Powers, M.D.
Infectious Diseases Attending
National Institute of Allergy and Infectious Diseases
National Institutes of Health
Bethesda, Maryland
Gonococcus-Neisseria Gonorrhoeae

Laurel C. Preheim, M.D.
Professor of Medicine, Microbiology,
and Immunology
Creighton University School of Medicine
University of Nebraska College of Medicine
Omaha, Nebraska
Infection in the Alcoholic

Thomas C. Quinn, M.D.
Senior Investigator
National Institute of Allergy and Infectious Diseases
Bethesda, Maryland;
Professor of Medicine
Johns Hopkins University School of Medicine
Baltimore, Maryland
Sexually Transmitted Enteric Infections

Richard Quintiliani, M.D.
Director, Anti-Infective Research and
Pharmacoeconomic Studies
Hartford Hospital;
Professor of Medicine
University of Connecticut School of Medicine;
Clinical Professor of Pharmacology
University of Connecticut School of Pharmacy
Hartford, Connecticut
Clostridia

Isaam Raad, M.D.
Deputy Chairman, Department of Internal
Medicine Specialties
Chief, Section of Infection Control
The University of Texas
MD Anderson Cancer Center;
Professor of Medicine
The University of Texas
MD Anderson Cancer Center:
Houston, Texas
Infection of the Salivary and Lacrimal Glands
Intravascular Catheter–Related Infections

Ahmed S. Rabbat, M.D.
Senior Fellow, Division of Infectious Diseases
Catholic Medical Center of Brooklyn and Queens
Jamaica, New York
HIV Infection: Initial Evaluation and Monitoring

Sanjay Ram, M.D.
Attending Physician, Department of Medicine
Boston Medical Center;
Assistant Professor of Medicine
Boston University School of Medicine
Boston, Massachusetts
Aspergillosis

Carlos R. Ramírez-Ramírez, M.D.
Infectious Diseases Fellow
San Juan Veteran's Affairs Medical Center
San Juan, Puerto Rico;
Instructor in Medicine
University of Puerto Rico School of Medicine
Rio Piedras, Puerto Rico
Corynebacteria

Carlos H. Ramírez-Ronda, M.D.
Chief, Department of Medicine
Director, Infectious Diseases Division
San Juan Veteran's Affairs Medical Center
San Juan, Puerto Rico;
Professor of Medicine
University of Puerto Rico School of Medicine
Rio Piedras, Puerto Rico
Corynebacteria

Jean-Pierre Raufman, M.D.
Chief, Digestive Disease and Nutrition
McClellan Memorial Veteran's Affairs Hospital;
Jerome S. Levy Professor of Internal Medicine
Director, Division of Gastroenterology
Little Rock, Arkansas
Esophageal Infections

S. Frank Redo, B.S., M.D.
Emeritus Chief Division of Pediatric Surgery
The New York Hospital;
Emeritus Professor of Surgery
Weill Medical College of Cornell University
New York, New York

Acute Appendicitis

Robert V. Rege, B.S., M.D.
Chief of Surgery
Zale-Lipshy University Hospital;
Professor, Department of Surgery
Chairman, Division of GI/Endocrine Surgery
University of Texas Southwestern Medical Center
Dallas, Texas

Biliary Infection: Cholecystitis and Cholangitis

Michael F. Rein, M.D.
Professor of Medicine
University of Virginia
Charlottesville, Virginia

Gonococcus-Neisseria Gonorrhoeae

Vivian E. Rexroad, Pharm.D.
Investigational Drug Service
Johns Hopkins Hospital
Johns Hopkins Medical Institutions
Baltimore, Maryland

Infectious Complications in the Injection Drug User

Bruce S. Ribner, M.D., M.P.H.
Hospital Epidemiologist
Ralph H. Johnson VAMC;
Hospital Epidemiologist
Medical University Hospital;
Associate Professor of Medicine
Medical University of South Carolina:
Charleston, South Carolina

Salmonella

Gilberto Rodriguez, M.D.
Assistant Professor of Medicine
University of Miami School of Medicine
Miami, Florida

Infected Implants

Allan Ronald, M.D., F.R.C.P.C.
Consultant, Infectious Diseases
St. Boniface Hospital;
Professor Emeritus
University of Manitoba
Winnipeg, Manitoba
Canada

Genital Ulcer Adenopathy Syndrome

Harry Rosado-Santos, M.D.
Assistant Professor
University of Utah School of Medicine
Department of Internal Medicine
Division of Infectious Disease
Salt Lake City, Utah

AIDS: Therapy for Opportunistic Infections

Virginia R. Roth, M.D., F.R.C.P.(C), D.T.M. & H.
Epidemic Intelligence Service Officer
Centers for Disease Control and Prevention Hospital
Infections Program
Atlanta, Georgia

Transfusion-Related Infection

Thomas A. Russo, M.D., C.M.
Staff Physician
Veteran's Affairs Medical Center;
Staff Physician
Erie County Medical Center;
Assistant Professor of Medicine,
Department of Medicine
Division of Infectious Diseases
State University of New York at Buffalo
School of Medicine and Biomedical Sciences
Buffalo, New York

Actinomycosis

William A. Rutala, Ph.D., M.P.H.
Director, Hospital Epidemiology and
Occupational Health
University of North Carolina Health Care System;
Professor of Medicine
University of North Carolina School of Medicine
Chapel Hill, North Carolina

Systemic Infection from Animals

Carole A. Sable, M.D.
Director of Clinical Research, Infectious Disease
Merck Research Laboratories
West Point, Pennsylvania

Intracranial Suppuration

Merle A. Sande, M.D.
Professor and Chairman
University of Utah School of Medicine
Department of Internal Medicine
Salt Lake City, Utah

AIDS: Therapy for Opportunistic Infections

Francisco L. Sapico, M.D.
Chief, Division of Infectious Diseases
Rancho Los Amigos National Rehabilitation Center
Downey, California;
Professor of Medicine
Keck School of Medicine at University
of Southern California
Los Angeles, California
Diabetes and Infection

Clarence B. Sarkodee-Adoo, M.D.
Hematologist and Oncologist
Associate Fellowship Program Director
Greenebaum Cancer Center;
Assistant Professor of Medicine
University of Maryland, School of Medicine:
Baltimore, Maryland
Infection in the Neutropenic Patient

George A. Sarosi, M.D.
Chief, Medical Service
Roudebush VA Medical Center;
Professor of Medicine
Indiana University School of Medicine
Indianapolis, Indiana
Histoplasmosis

Patrick M. Schlievert, Ph.D.
University of Minnesota
Medical School
Minneapolis, Minnesota
*Staphylococcal and Streptococcal Toxic Shock
and Kawasaki Syndromes*

Steven K. Schmitt, M.D.
Staff Physician
Cleveland Clinic Foundation
Cleveland, Ohio
Miscellaneous Gram-Positive Organisms

Keith W. Schumann, M.D.
Department of Dermatology
Cleveland Clinic Foundation
Cleveland, Ohio
Cellulitis and Erysipelas

William A. Schwartzman, M.D.
Assistant Professor of Medicine
UCLA San Fernando Valley Program;
Clinical Sciences Director
UCLA Integrated Program in Infectious Diseases
and Microbial Pathogenesis;
Acting Chief, Section of Infectious Diseases
Sepulveda VA Medical Center
Sepulveda, California
Bartonella (Rochalimaea) Infection

E. Nan Scott, Ph.D.
Associate Professor of Research Medicine, Retired
University of Oklahoma Health Science Center
Oklahoma City, Oklahoma
Sporotrichosis

John W. Sensakovic, M.D., Ph.D.
Corporate Director of Medical Education
Saint Michael's Medical Center
Newark, New Jersey;
Professor of Medicine and Infectious Diseases
Seton Hall University School of Graduate
Medical Education
South Orange, New Jersey
Fever and Rash

Daniel J. Sexton, M.D.
Director, Infection Control Unit
Duke University Medical Center;
Professor of Medicine
Duke University School of Medicine
Durham, North Carolina
HACEK

Dennis J. Shale, M.D., F.R.C.P.
David Davies Chair, Respiratory and
Communicable Diseases
Honorary Consultant Physician
University Hospital of Wales and Landough Hospital
NHS Trust
Penarth, South Glamorgan, United Kingdom;
University of Wales College of Medicine
Cardiff, United Kingdom
Empyema and Bronchopleural Fistula

Andrew M. Shapiro, M.D.
Department of Surgery
Hershey Medical Center;
Assistant Professor
Penn State University College of Medicine
Hershey, Pennsylvania
Sinusitis

Robert H. Shapiro, M.D.
Resident Physician
University of Washington Medical Center
School of Medicine
Department of Urology
Seattle, Washington
Epididymo-orchitis

Geetika Sharma, M.D.
Private Practice
McAllen, Texas
Rabies

Bhavna P. Sheth, M.D.
Assistant Professor of Ophthalmology
Section of Comprehensive Ophthalmology
The Eye Institute/Medical College of Wisconsin
Milwaukee, Wisconsin
Conjunctivitis

Jeffrey L. Silber, M.D.
Director, Clinical Research
Merck Research Laboratories
Merck & Co., Inc.
West Point, Pennsylvania
The Diagnosis and Management of Spinal Epidural Abscess

Upinder Singh, M.D.
Postdoctoral Fellow
Department of Microbiology and Immunology
Stanford University
Stanford, California
Infectious Polymyositis

Linda A. Slavoski, M.D.
Wyoming Valley Infectious Diseases Associates
WVHCS Mercy Hospital
Wilkes Barre, Pennsylvania
Peritonitis

James W. Smith, M.D.
Staff Physician
Veterans Affairs North Texas Health Care System;
Professor of Medicine, Department of Internal
Medicine, Infectious Diseases Section
University of Texas Southwestern Medical School
Dallas, Texas
Infection of Native and Prosthetic Joints

Leon G. Smith, B.A., M.D.
Chief of Infectious Disease
St. Michael's Hospital;
Chairman of Medicine, Seton Hall
Post Graduate School of Medicine
Newark, New Jersey
Fever and Rash

Jack D. Sobel, M.D.
Chief, Division of Infectious Diseases
Detroit Medical Center;
Professor of Medicine
Wayne State University School of Medicine
Detroit, Michigan
Candiduria

Joseph Solomkin, M.D.
Professor of Surgery
University of Cincinnati College of Medicine
Department of Surgery
Cincinnati, Ohio
Surgical Prophylaxis

Samuel L. Stanley, Jr., M.D.
Attending Physician
Chief Medical Consultant
Barnes Jewish Hospital;
Professor, Division of Infectious Diseases,
Department of Medicine
Washington University School of Medicine
St. Louis, Missouri
Extraintestinal Amoebic Infection

William W. Stead, MD
Ex-Director, Tuberculosis Program
Arkansas Department of Health;
Professor of Medicine Emeritus
University of Arkansas College of Medicine
Little Rock, Arkansas
Tuberculosis

Barbara W. Stechenberg, M.D.
Vice Chairman and Director of Pediatric
Infectious Diseases
Baystate Medical Center
Springfield, Massachusetts;
Professor of Pediatrics
Tufts University School of Medicine
Boston, Massachusetts
Poststreptococcal Immunologic Complications

James M. Steckelberg, M.D.
Consultant, Division of Infectious Diseases
Mayo Clinic and Foundation;
Professor of Medicine
Mayo Medical School
Rochester, Minnesota
Pacemaker and Defibrillator Infections

Roy T. Steigbigel, M.D.
Attending Physician
University Hospital at Stony Brook;
Professor of Medicine, Molecular Genetics
and Microbiology, Pathology, and
Pharmacological Sciences
Vice Chair, Department of Medicine
State University of New York
Stony Brook, New York
Dialysis-Related Infection

James P. Steinberg, M.D., F.A.C.P.
Chief of Infectious Diseases
Associate Chief of Medicine
Crawford Long Hospital of Emory University;
Associate Professor of Medicine
Division of Infectious Diseases
Emory University School of Medicine
Atlanta, Georgia

Nonsurgical Antimicrobial Prophylaxis

David S. Stephens, M.D.
Professor of Medicine and Microbiology
and Immunology
Director, Division of Infectious Diseases
Executive Vice Chair, Department of Medicine
Emory University School of Medicine
Atlanta, Georgia

Pasteurella multocida

Dennis L. Stevens, Ph.D., M.D.
Chief, Infectious Disease Section
Veterans Affairs Medical Center
Boise, Idaho;
Professor of Medicine
University of Washington School of Medicine
Seattle, Washington

Streptococcus Groups A, B, C, D, and G

J.B. Stricker, D.O.
Bellmead Medical Director of Laboratories
Hewitt Medical Director of Laboratories
Scott and White Clinic;
Plasma Donor Center Physician
Alpha Therapeutic Corporation
Hewitt, Texas;
Assistant Clinical Instructor in Pathology and
Laboratory Medicine
Texas A&M University College of Medicine
College Station, Texas

Leprosy

Harris R. Stutman, M.D.
Former Director, Pediatric Infectious Disease
Memorial Children's Hospital
Long Beach, California;
Former Associate Professor of Pediatrics
University of California Irvine
Irvine, California

Otitis Media and Externa

Sankar Swaminathan, M.S., M.D.
Associate Professor
UF Shands Cancer Center
University of Florida;
Associate Professor
Division of Infectious Diseases
Department of Internal Medicine
Gainesville, Florida

Antiviral Therapy

James S. Tan, M.D.
Professor and Vice Chairman of Internal Medicine
Head, Infectious Disease Section
Northeastern Ohio Universities College of Medicine
Rootstown, Ohio;
Chairman, Department of Medicine
Summa Health System
Akron, Ohio

Atypical Pneumonia

Woraphot Tantisiriwat, M.D.
Clinical Instructor
Vajira Hospital Campus;
Clinical Instructor
Faculty of Medicine
Srinakarinwirot University
Bangkok, Thailand

Cryptococcus

Maureen R. Tierney, M.D., M.Sc.
Clinical Associate
Massachusetts General Hospital;
Assistant Professor of Medicine
Harvard Medical School
Boston, Massachusetts

Croup, Epiglottis, and Laryngitis

Jeremiah G. Tilles, M.D.
Chief, Division of Infectious Diseases
UCI Medical Center
Orange, California;
Professor of Medicine
Professor of Microbiology and Molecular Genetics
University of California, Irvine
Irvine, California

Myocarditis

Lisa S. Tkatch, M.D., F.A.C.P.
Teaching Faculty, Infectious Diseases
Pinnacle Health Hospitals;
Clinical Assistant Professor of Medicine
MCP Hahnemann University
Harrisburg, Pennsylvania

Mediastinitis

Kenneth J. Tomecki, M.D.
Department of Dermatology
Cleveland Clinic Foundation
Cleveland, Ohio

Cellulitis and Erysipelas

Edmund C. Tramont, M.D.
Associate Director and Professor
Institute of Human Virology
University of Maryland Biotechnology Institute
University of Maryland School of Medicine
Baltimore, Maryland

Meningococcus and Miscellaneous Neisseriae

Donald D. Trunkey, M.D.
Professor and Chairman, Department of Surgery
Oregon Health Sciences University
Portland, Oregon

Abdominal Abscess

Allan R. Tunkel, M.D., Ph.D.
Associate Chair for Education
Director, Internal Medicine Residency Program;
Professor of Medicine
MCP Hahnemann University
Philadelphia, Pennsylvania

Bacterial Meningitis

Rajiv R. Varma, M.D.
Director, Hepatology Unit
Medical College of Wisconsin
Froedtert Memorial Lutheran Hospital
Milwaukee, Wisconsin

Reye's Syndrome

Boris Velimirovic, M.D., D.P.T.H.
Director Emeritus Institute of Social Medicine
Oesterreich, Austria

Anthrax and Other Bacillus Species

Stacey R. Vlahakis, M.D.
Fellow, Infectious Diseases
Mayo Clinic Foundation
Rochester, Minnesota

Pacemaker and Defibrillator Infections

Duc J. Vugia, M.D., M.P.H.
Chief, Disease Investigations and Surveillance Branch,
Division of Communicable Disease Control
California Department of Health Services
Berkeley, California;
Clinical Assistant Professor of Medicine
University of California at San Francisco School
of Medicine
San Francisco, California

Vibrios

Kenneth F. Wagner, D.O.
Attending Physician and Infectious Disease Consultant
Department of Medicine
National Naval Medical Center;
Associate Professor, Department of Medicine
Uniformed Services University of the Health Sciences
F. Edward Hèbert School of Medicine
Bethesda, Maryland

Mycetoma (Madura Foot)

Ken B. Waites, M.D.
Director of Clinical Microbiology
University of Alabama Hospitals and Clinics;
Professor of Pathology, Microbiology, and Physical
Medicine and Rehabilitation
University of Alabama at Birmingham Schools
of Medicine and Dentistry
Birmingham, Alabama

Mycoplasma

Francis A. Waldvogel, M.D.
Head, Department of Medicine
Geneva University Hospital;
Professor of Medicine
Geneva Medical School
Geneva, Switzerland

Acute and Chronic Osteomyelitis

Chatrchai Watanakunakorn, M.D., F.A.C.P., F.C.C.P.
Director, Infectious Disease
St. Elizabeth Health Center
Youngstown, Ohio;
Professor of Internal Medicine
Northeastern Ohio Universities College of Medicine
Rootstown, Ohio

Viridans Streptococci

David J. Weber, M.D., M.H.A., M.P.H.
Medical Director, Hospital Epidemiology and
Occupational Health
University of North Carolina Health Care System;
Professor of Medicine, Pediatrics and Epidemiology
University of North Carolina Schools of Medicine and
Public Health
Chapel Hill, North Carolina

Systemic Infection from Animals

Hannah M. Wexler, M.D.
Director, Wadsworth Anaerobe Laboratory
Greater Los Angeles VA Medical Center;
Adjunct Professor of Medicine
UCLA School of Medicine
Los Angeles, California

Anaerobic Infections

Richard J. Whitley, M.D.
Loeb Eminent Scholar Chair in Pediatrics
Professor of Pediatrics, Microbiology, and Medicine
University of Alabama at Birmingham
The Children's Hospital
Birmingham, Alabama
Herpes Simplex Viruses

Lucy E. Wilson, M.D., Sc.M.
Fellow in Infectious Diseases
Johns Hospital University
Baltimore, Maryland
Viral Hemorrhagic Fever

Mary E. Wilson, M.D.
Chief, Infectious Diseases
Director, Travel Resource Center
Mount Auburn Hospital
Cambridge, Massachusetts;
Associate Professor of Medicine
Harvard Medical School
Associate Professor of Population and
International Health
Harvard School of Public Health
Boston, Massachusetts
Recreational Water Exposure

Brian Wispelwey, M.S., M.D.
Associate Professor of Medicine
Director, Infectious Diseases Clinic
University of Virginia Health Sciences Center
Charlottesville, Virginia
Intracranial Suppuration

Martin S. Wolfe, M.D., F.A.C.P.
Tropical Medicine Consultant
Department of State;
Clinical Professor of Medicine
George Washington University Medical School:
Washington, DC
Fever in the Returning Traveler

Henry Yeager, Jr., M.D.
Professor, Division of Pulmonary/Critical Care
Department of Medicine
Georgetown University Medical Center
Washington, DC
Nontuberculous Mycobacteria

Neal S. Young, M.D.
Chief, Hematology Branch
National Heart, Lung, and Blood Institute
National Institutes of Health
Bethesda, Maryland
Acute and Chronic Parvovirus Infection

Victor L. Yu, M.D.
Chief, Infectious Disease Section
Veteran's Affairs Medical Center;
Professor of Medicine
University of Pittsburgh School of Medicine
Pittsburgh, Pennsylvania
Haemophilus
Legionellosis

Qian Yun Xie, M.D.
Assistant Professor, Division of Gastroenterology
University of Arkansas for Medical Sciences
Little Rock, Arkansas
Esophageal Infections

Roger W. Yurt, M.D.
Director, Burn Center and Trauma Center
The New York Hospital;
Professor and Vice-Chairman, Department of Surgery
Cornell University Medical College
New York, New York
Infection in the Burn-Injured Patient

John A. Zaia, M.D.
Professor
Director, Department of Virology
City of Hope National Medical Center
Duarte, California
Varicella-Zoster Virus

Jonathan M. Zenilman, M.D.
Associate Professor
Johns Hopkins University School of Medicine
Baltimore, Maryland
Prostatitis

This book is dedicated to Dr. Daniel L. Scharf—esteemed friend, respected colleague, unofficial family member, and all-around mensch.

Preface

The gratifying response to *Current Therapy of Infectious Disease* has encouraged this new edition. The entire text has been updated, and we have added completely new chapters on Hantavirus, Psoas Abscess, Splenic Abscess, Infectious Polymyositis, Babesiosis, Infectious Esophagitis, Transplant-Related Infection, Cytomegalovirus, and Herpesvirus 6, 7, and 8. In addition, the individual chapter updates include such timely clinical issues as drug-drug interactions, bioterrorism, the present status of microbial resistance, antimicrobial prophylaxis, and current recommendations for vaccination. Important new antibacterial and antiviral drugs (including recently developed antiretroviral agents) have been added, both in individual chapters and in the comprehensive Antimicrobial Tables. New illustrations, diagrams, and algorithms complement this new edition.

The book continues its overall clinical orientation. Information is organized by syndrome and by organism, covering clinical presentation, diagnosis and relevant differential diagnosis, specific therapeutic recommendations, and suggested readings at the end of each chapter. We hope this practical, clinically oriented approach to infectious diseases continues to provide a concise yet authoritative resource for the busy clinician.

Many thanks to our expert contributors and to our superb editorial and production staff, particularly Richard Zorab, Elizabeth Corra, Sharyl Wolf, Wendy Buckwalter, Amanda Starr, Jennifer Shreiner, Claire Powell, Lynne Gery, and Suzanne Copple.

David Schlossberg, M.D.

Preface to the First Edition

The goal of *Current Therapy of Infectious Disease* is a brief but authoritative consultation for the busy clinician. We hope this text will bridge the gap between larger encyclopedic textbooks on the one hand and the convenient pocket handbooks on the other. Thus, we have tried to make it convenient, user-friendly, and practical.

Although emphasis is on therapy, pertinent information is provided regarding pathophysiology, clinical and laboratory diagnosis, and differential diagnosis. Therapeutic recommendations are specific, and suggested readings are provided at the end of each chapter for readers who would like to pursue topics in greater detail.

The book is divided into six parts. Part I lists clinical presentations both by organ system (for example, eye, skin, respiratory, cardiovascular) and by environmental clues such as travel and animal exposure. Part II discusses patient presentations in the immunocompromised or otherwise susceptible host. Thus, this section includes AIDS, iatrogenic immunosuppression, diabetes, drug abuse, alcoholism, dialysis, malignancy, and other settings that render a patient vulnerable to infection. Part III deals with nosocomial infections, ranging from needlestick injury to blood transfusion, and Part IV covers prevention of infection, including concepts of prophylaxis, advice for travelers, and immunization. Part V is organism related and lists specific infections due to bacteria, viruses, spirochetes, rickettsia, mycoplasmas, parasites, and fungi. In Part VI general therapeutic considerations are arranged in chapters on principles of antibiotic therapy, antifungal therapy, antiviral therapy and antibiotic allergy and skin testing. Finally, comprehensive antimicrobial agent tables are provided with dosage, costs, toxicity, and practical pharmacokinetic data.

Many thanks are due to our army of contributors and to the editorial and production staff, particularly Carey Conover and Mike Ederer, and especially Lynne Gery, whose unflagging optimism, encouragement, and professionalism were indispensable.

David Schlossberg, M.D.

Contents

SPECIFIC PATHOGENS AND INFECTIONS

Bacteria

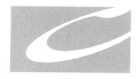

CLINICAL PRESENTATION

GENERALIZED SYMPTOMATOLOGY

FEVER OF UNKNOWN ORIGIN

Natalie C. Klein
Burke A. Cunha

The classic definition of fever of unknown origin (FUO) was originally formulated by Petersdorf and Beeson in 1961 as an illness characterized by fever greater than 38° C (100.4° F), lasting more than 3 weeks without a diagnosis after 1 week of investigation in a hospital. This classic definition of FUO remains useful with some modifications because of the increase in outpatient workups with noninvasive diagnostic methods (Table 1). An updated definition of *classical FUO* no longer requires 1 week of hospital investigation, but instead, 3 days of investigation of the source of the fever either in the hospital or as an outpatient. In addition to the classical FUO, several patient subsets with prolonged fevers have also been termed FUO (e.g., nosocomial FUO, neutropenic FUO, and human immunodeficiency virus [HIV] FUO). Nosocomial FUO describes hospitalized patients with fever who had no infection on admission, in whom the cause of fever is obscure after 3 days of investigation. Neutropenic FUO refers to patients with 500 neutrophils/mm³ or more who have persistent unexplained fever after 3 days of investigation. HIV/acquired immunodeficiency syndrome (AIDS) FUO are fevers 38.0° C [100.4° F] or greater lasting for more than 4 weeks in an outpatient or more than 3 days in hospitalized HIV/AIDS patients. These patient subsets may be approached diagnostically/therapeutically as FUO or prolonged fevers in special populations (Table 2).

■ FUO

The three major causes of classical FUOs in adults are infections, neoplasms, and collagen-vascular disease, which account for about 70% of FUOs. Infections were the most common cause of FUO in the original Petersdorf and Beeson series in 1961, whereas neoplasms are presently the most common cause of FUO in adults. Other causes of recurrent FUO include drug fever, granulomatous hepatitis, pulmonary embolism, inflammatory bowel disease, sarcoidosis, familial Mediterranean fever, and factitious fever. A small number of FUOs remain undiagnosed even after thorough investigation.

Diagnostic Approach to FUO

The approach to the patient with classical FUO should begin with a history and physical examination to exclude common causes of fever (e.g., phlebitis, abscesses, endocarditis, or drug fever). A patient should be questioned about travel, animal exposure, tick bites, and occupational exposures. Physical examination should focus on heart murmurs, lymphadenopathy, hepatosplenomegaly, and an eye examination. Repeated physical examinations are often necessary because new physical findings may appear in the course of the disease.

Much can be learned from basic laboratory tests (differential white blood cell [WBC] counts, erythrocyte sedimentation rate, liver function tests, and urinalysis). Often, important diagnostic clues are overlooked with these tests. Laboratory tests should include cultures of blood, urine, sputum, stool, pleural and peritoneal fluid, if present, and cerebrospinal fluid if indicated. Biopsies of enlarged lymph nodes, liver, bone marrow, and any skin nodules if present should be considered. Direct examination of the blood smear should be performed to exclude a diagnosis of malaria, relapsing fever, and trypanosomiasis if the patient has a travel or transfusion history. An intermediate purified protein derivative (PPD) test along with an anergy panel should be performed. Serum samples should be obtained from the patient and a portion frozen for subsequent viral titers. Serologic tests should be guided by physical, laboratory, and historical clues, and they should not be ordered blindly. Computed tomography (CT) or magnetic resonance imaging (MRI) scan of abdomen/pelvis and radionuclide scans, gallium citrate, or indium-III are useful. Echocardiography should be performed if endocarditis is suspected. Advances in diagnostic radiology have markedly reduced the need for exploratory laparotomy in patients with FUO. Diagnostic laparotomy should be reserved for biopsying abnormalities localized on scans that are not approachable

Table 1   Causes of Classical FUO (Percentage)

INFECTIONS, 31%-40%
Extrapulmonary tuberculosis
Intraabdominal/pelvic abscess
Endocarditis
Liver-biliary tract infection
Chronic Pyelonephritis
Chronic Osteomyelitis
Chronic Sinusitis
Brucellosis
Whipple's disease
NEOPLASM, 20%-31%
Non-Hodgkin's lymphoma
Hodgkin's disease
Metastastes tumor to liver
Hepatoma
Hypernephroma
Atrial myxoma
COLLAGEN-VASCULAR DISEASE, 9%-15%
Rheumatic fever
Still's disease
Systemic lupus erythematosus
Temporal arteritis
Polyarteritis nodosa
Wegener's granulomatosis
Rheumatoid arthritis
Polymyalgia rheumatica
Vasculitis
MISCELLANEOUS, 9%-23%
Drug fever
Periodic fever
Granulomatous hepatitis
Pulmonary embolus
Familial Mediterranean fever
Inflammatory bowel disease (regional ileitis)
Factitious fever
Sarcoidosis
Thyroiditis
Laennec's cirrhosis
UNDIAGNOSED, 5%-22%

From Cunha BA: *Infect Dis Clin North Am* 10:111, 1996.

Table 2   Categories of FUOs

FUO
Fever ≥38.0° C (100.4° F) on several occasions
Fever of >3 weeks' duration
Diagnosis uncertain despite appropriate investigations, after at least 3 outpatient visits or at least 3 days in hospital
NOSOCOMIAL FUO
Fever ≥38.0° C (100.4° F) on several occasions in a hospitalized patient receiving acute care
Infection not present or incubating on admission
Diagnosis uncertain after 3 days despite appropriate investigation, including at least 2 days' incubation or microbiologic cultures
NEUTROPENIC FUO
Fever ≥38.0° C (100.4° F) on several occasions
Patient has <500/mm³ in peripheral blood expected to fall <500/mm³ within 1 or 2 days
Diagnosis uncertain after 3 days despite appropriate investigation, including at least 2 days' incubation of microbiologic cultures
HIV-ASSOCIATED FUO
Fever ≥38.0° C (100.4° F) on several occasions
Confirmed positive serology for HIV infection
Fever of >4 weeks' duration for outpatients or >3 days' duration in hospital
Diagnosis uncertain after 3 days despite appropriate investigation, including at least 2 days' incubation of microbiologic cultures

From Durack DT, et al: Fever of unknown origin—reexamined and redefined. In Remington JS, Swartz MN, eds: *Current clinical topics in infectious diseases,* Boston, 1991, Blackwell Scientific.
AIDS, Acquired immunodeficiency syndrome; *HIV,* human immunodeficiency virus.

by percutaneous route, or as a final step in the workup of a patient with FUO in whom an abdominal process is strongly suspected.

Management of FUO

The use of empiric therapy for the patient with classical FUO should be discouraged. Repeated testing of the patient with monitoring of temperature and pulse patterns without antipyretics is helpful diagnostically and as a guide to efficacy of therapy. The empiric use of antibiotics that could partially treat or mask an occult infection should be avoided. However, if after careful and thorough investigation, a definitive diagnosis cannot be made, a therapeutic trial with antibiotics or antiinflammatory agents may be indicated if clinical suspicion of a particular diagnosis is high.

In patients with granulomatous hepatitis, a short course of antituberculous therapy should be initiated. If fevers are unresponsive to antituberculous medication, a trial of steroids should be tried. In a patient in whom a neoplastic disease is suspected, an empiric trial of naproxen (Naprosyn) or indomethacin (Indocin) is diagnostic and therapeutic. In a patient in whom mycobacterial disease is strongly suspected, an empiric trial of antituberculous therapy for several weeks may cause defervescence of fever. Finally, a patient with suspected culture-negative endocarditis should receive a course of empiric antibiotics, usually a combination of penicillin with gentamicin.

■ FUO IN HOSPITALIZED PATIENTS

Hospitalized patients with prolonged fevers are often elderly; have major underlying medical problems such as diabetes, heart disease, chronic lung disease, or cancer, or have undergone recent surgery; and are often hospitalized in intensive care units. Management includes a thorough review of culture results, appropriate radiologic procedures such as CT scan of abdomen/pelvis, sinus films, hepatitis serology, echocardiography of the heart, or bronchoscopy with biopsy and/or brushing for lung infiltrates. Etiologies of obscure fever are often infectious and include candidiasis, hepatitis, acalculous cholecystitis, *Clostridium difficile* colitis, septic thrombophlebitis, sinusitis, or drug fever.

■ FUOs IN NEUTROPENIA

Prolonged fevers in neutropenic patients are most commonly caused by bacteremias, mucositis, perianal infection, central-line infections, or candidemia. Empiric, broad-spectrum antimicrobial therapy should be started in neutropenic patients with fever. Monotherapy (e.g., cefepime, meropenem) or combination (e.g., cefepime plus aminoglycosides or aztreonam, piperacillin, levofloxacin) with an antipseudomonal antibiotic is the preferred approach. Anti-*Staphylococcus aureus* and anti-*Bacteroides fragilis* coverage is unnecessary. *S. aureus* is only a pathogen in patients with central intravenous line infection, and catheter removal rather than antistaphylococcus antibiotics is the proper approach. If fever persists or increases after about 2 weeks of anti-*Pseudomonus aeruginosa* therapy, empiric antifungal therapy with fluconazole-amphotericin B may be started.

■ FUOs IN HIV/AIDS

The major causes of FUO in HIV/AIDS patients are disseminated *Mycobacterium tuberculosis*, *Mycobacterium avium-intracellulare* (MAI), disseminated leishmaniasis, cytomegalovirus, *Pneumocystis carinii* pneumonia (PCP), lymphoma, and drug fever. Patients with CD_4 counts of 100/mm^3 or greater in advanced HIV/AIDS are at high risk of opportunistic disease (Table 3). Usually there is no need for immediate empiric antimicrobial therapy unless the patient has a neutrophil count of 500 µl or less. The distribution of pathogens relates to geographic areas. The pathogens presently as FUOs in HIV/AIDS patients are directly related to the depression in the CD_4 count. Interestingly, PCP presents with prolonged fevers without pulmonary infiltrates in advanced HIV rather than as community-acquired pneumonia (CAP) in early HIV.

Table 3   Prolonged Fevers/FUO in HIV/AIDS Patients*

WORLDWIDE EXPERIENCE	UNITED STATES EXPERIENCE
MOST COMMON	
Mycobacterium tuberculosis (TB)	*Mycobacterium avium-intracellulare* (MAI)
Leishmaniasis	*Pneumocystic carinii* pneumonia (PCP)
Histoplasmosis	Cytomegalovirus
Hepatitis	
COMMON	
Lymphomas	*Mycobacterium tuberculosis*
Drug fevers	Lymphomas
	Drug fevers

From Armstrong NS, Katz JT, Kazanjian PH: *Clin Infect Dis* 28:341, 1999.
HIV, Human immunodeficiency virus; *AIDS,* acquired immunodeficiency syndrome.
*FUOs usually occur advanced disease with ≤100 CD_4 counts.

Suggested Reading

Armstrong WS, Katz JT, Kazanjian PH: Human immunodeficiency virus-associated fever of unknown origin: a study of 70 patients in the United States and review, *Clin Infect Dis* 28:341, 1999.

Chang JC, Gross HM: Utility of naproxen in the differential diagnosis of fever of undetermined origin in patients with cancer, *Am J Med* 76:597, 1984.

Cunha BA: Fever of unknown origin in the elderly—a commentary, *Infect Dis Clin Pract* 2:380, 1993.

Cunha BA: Fever of unknown origin, *Infect Dis Clin North Am* 10:111, 1996.

Durack DT, Street AC: Fever of unknown origin—re-examined and redefined. In Remington J, Swartz M, eds: *Current clinical topics of infectious diseases,* St Louis, 1991, Mosby.

Larson EB, Featherstone HJ, Petersdorf RG: Fever of undetermined origin: diagnosis and follow up of 105 cases 1970-1980, *Medicine* 61:269, 1982.

Petersdorf RG, Beeson PB: Fever of unexplained origin: report on 100 cases, *Medicine* 40:1, 1961.

SEPSIS AND SEPTIC SHOCK

Rodger D. MacArthur
Mujahed Abbas

Sepsis is the systemic response to infection. Septic shock occurs when there is significant hypotension in the presence of sepsis. These and other related terms and diagnostic criteria developed at a consensus conference sponsored jointly by the American College of Chest Physicians and the Society for Critical Care Medicine in August 1991 are listed in Tables 1 and 2. The consensus conference recommended against using the term *septicemia* because it is ambiguous and used too often to imply bacteremia.

The clinical manifestations of the sepsis syndrome are caused by the body's inflammatory response to toxins and other components of microorganisms. For example, infusion of endotoxin into humans is sufficient to initiate the cascade of inflammatory mediators seen in sepsis. Endotoxin is the lipoidal acylated glucosamine disaccharide core of the cell wall of many aerobic gram-negative bacteria. Known as *lipid A*, this moiety exhibits all of the hemodynamic and inflammatory characteristics associated with endotoxicity. Lipid A is highly conserved among the *Enterobacteriaceae* and to a lesser extent among the *Pseudomonadaceae*. Anaerobic gram-negative bacteria, such as *Bacteroides fragilis*, lack lipid A, perhaps explaining why sepsis is not commonly seen when infection is caused solely by this anaerobe.

Table 1   Sepsis-Related Terminology and Definitions

Infection	A microbial phenomenon characterized by an inflammatory response to the presence of microorganisms or the invasions of normally sterile host tissue by those organisms
Bacteremia	The presence of viable bacteria in the blood
SIRS	The systemic inflammatory response to a variety of severe clinical insults, including infection, pancreatitis, ischemia, multiple trauma and tissue injury, hemorrhagic shock, immune-mediated organ injury, and exogenous administration of inflammatory mediators, such as tumor necrosis factor alpha (TNF-α) and other cytokines
Sepsis	The systemic response to infection; this response is identical to SIRS, except that it must result from infection
Septic Shock	Sepsis with hypotension (systolic blood pressure <90 mm Hg, or a reduction of >40 mm Hg from baseline) despite adequate fluid resuscitation, in conjunction with organ dysfunction and perfusion abnormalities (e.g., lactic acidosis, oliguria, obtundation), in the absence of other known causes for the abnormalities
MODS	Multiple organ dysfunction syndrome; the presence of altered organ function in an acutely ill patient such that homeostasis cannot be maintained without intervention; primary multiple organ dysfunction syndrome is the direct result of a well-defined insult in which organ dysfunction occurs early and can be directly attributable to the insult itself; secondary multiple organ dysfunction syndrome develops as a consequence of a host response and is identified within the context of SIRS

SIRS, Systemic inflammatory response syndrome; *MODS,* Multiple organ dysfunction syndrome.

Table 2   Numeric Criteria for SIRS

Two or more of the following must be present:
   Temperature >38° C (100.4° F) or <36° C (96.8° F)
   Heart rate >90 beats/min
   Respiratory rate >20 breaths/min or $Paco_2$ <32 mm Hg
   White blood cells >12,000 cells/μl or <4000 cells/μl or >10% immature (band) forms

Note: These changes should represent acute alterations from baseline in the absence of other known causes for the abnormalities.
SIRS, Systemic inflammatory response syndrome.

Cytokines and other immune modulators that are released in response to lipid A and other bacterial products mediate the clinical manifestations of sepsis. Interleukin (IL)-1 and other interleukins, tumor necrosis factor alpha (TNF-α), interferon gamma, and several colony-stimulating factors are produced rapidly (minutes to hours) after the interaction of monocytes and macrophages with lipid A. Although the effects of TNF-α appear to be central to the pathophysiology of sepsis, many other immune modulators

interact with TNF-α, host defense mechanisms, and bacterial pathogens in complex ways.

The sepsis cascade can be simplified by dividing it into at least five components with complex feedback loops among these components. The process starts with the release of intracellular or extracellular bacterial activators, such as lipid A in gram-negative sepsis and peptidoglycan, teichoic acid, or toxic shock syndrome toxin-1 (TSST-1) in gram-positive sepsis. The second event is the activation of macrophages by the bacterial products. This activation leads to the third component of sepsis, which consists of the release of the highly active molecules (e.g., cytokines) that have many potent biologic effects. The most important and best studied cytokine is TNF-α. IL-1 is another cytokine that is released early in the sepsis cascade, with effects similar to TNF-α. The release of TNF-α and IL-1 leads to the fourth component in the sepsis cascade, which includes the release of stress hormones, other cytokines (e.g., IL-2, IL-6, IL-8, IL-10), and other inflammatory mediators of sepsis (e.g., nitric oxide, the lipooxygenase and cyclooxygenase metabolites, platelet activation factor, interferon gamma). All of these immune modulators interact in a complex fashion to effect, in the fifth stage, the various observable changes to multiple organ systems (e.g., vascular endothelium, myocardial cells, pulmonary alveolar cells, liver cells). The result is the clinical picture of sepsis and the development of multiorgan system failure. Table 3 lists some of the important biologic and clinical manifestations of the sepsis syndrome.

There are several points to be made based on our understanding of sepsis: (1) It is essential to contain and eliminate the infection source with all possible measures (e.g., antibiotics, surgical or tube drainage of pus). (2) After the sepsis cascade has been activated, the clinical outcome of the patient may depend not only on effective antiinfective therapy but also on the ability to control the vigorous inflammatory response that led to the manifestations of sepsis. Elevations of many of the cytokines have been correlated with poor outcome among persons with sepsis. Greatly elevated levels of IL-6, in particular, have been shown in multiple studies to be correlated with decreased likelihood of survival.

There are no U.S. Food and Drug Administration (FDA)-approved therapies available at this time to achieve immune modulation. A trial of methylprednisolone for severe sepsis and septic shock, published in 1987, failed to demonstrate any efficacy of that agent. Multiple large, well-controlled trials have failed to demonstate any efficacy of monoclonal antibodies directed against lipid A, other components of the gram-negative bacterial cell wall, and TNF-α. Still, the trials of similar monoclonal antibodies continue, with the results of one large trial (2600 persons) of the efficacy of a monoclonal anti–TNF-α antibody reportedly showing efficacy in persons with elevated levels of IL-6.

Historically, antibiotic recommendations for therapy of sepsis and septic shock were based primarily on coverage of gram-negative organisms. However, sepsis caused by gram-positive organisms is clinically identical to sepsis caused by gram-negative organisms. Although the incidence of gram-negative nosocomial bacteremias has not decreased in recent years and *Escherichia coli* has remained the most common pathogen isolated in nosocomial infections, *Staphylococcus*

Table 3 Selected Biologic and Clinical Manifestations Seen in the Sepsis Syndrome

SUBSTANCE	SELECTED BIOLOGIC MANIFESTATIONS	SELECTED CLINICAL MANIFESTATIONS
Endotoxin	Activation of macrophages Release of TNF-α Release of IL-1	Clinical effect is mediated by the release of TNF-α and the other mediators
TNF-α	↑ IL-1 ↑ IL-6 ↑ IL-8 ↑ Nitric oxide (NO) ↑ Myocardial depressant factor Activate arachidonic metabolism PMN activation	Fever ↑ Catabolic state Microthrombi Mental status changes ↑ Cortisol level
IL-1	Virtually identical to TNF-α effects, except less effect on PMN function and chemotaxsis	Same as TNF-α
Nitric oxide	↓ Myocardial performance ↓ Vascular smooth muscle tone	↓ Tissue oxygen supply Hypotension Ileus and abdominal distension Hypoxemia from increased shunting
Thromboxanes	High levels suppress TH1 T-cell function Platelet and PMN aggregation Increased PMN adhesiveness Vasoconstriction of regional blood vessels Enhanced capillary permeability Increased airway resistance	Regional hypoperfusion ARDS Pulmonary shunting Edema Wheezing
Prostaglandins	Vasodilation (PGI₂, PGE₁) Vasoconstriction (PGF₂) Antiaggregatory effects on platelets Enhanced capillary permeability	Hypotension ↑ Systemic and pulmonary shunting Arterial hypoxemia ↑ Edema

TNF-α, Tumor necrosis factor alpha; *IL,* interleukin; *PMN,* polymorphonuclear cells; *TH1,* T-helper cell; *ARDS,* adult respiratory distress syndrome; *PGI,* prostaglandin I; *PGE,* prostaglandin E; *PGF,* prostaglandin F.

epidermidis has become the most common cause of nosocomial bacteremias, followed by *Staphylococcus aureus,* enterococci, and *Candida* species. Infections caused by vancomycin-resistant enterococci (VRE), particularly *Enterococcus faecium,* and infections caused by non-*albicans Candida* species have become increasingly common in the last several years. Gram-negative bacteria such as *Pseudomonas aeruginosa, Enterobacter* species, and *Acinetobacter* species also are increasingly likely to be resistant to multiple antibiotics.

The diagnosis of sepsis should be considered when a patient meets the numeric criteria for systemic inflammatory response syndrome (SIRS) (see Table 2). Unfortunately, there currently are no bedside tests available to differentiate quickly and reliably infectious causes of SIRS from noninfectious causes. Furthermore, the mortality from septic shock or sepsis with multiple organ dysfunction syndrome (MODS) is between 25% and 45%. Consequently, prompt empiric administration of antibiotics is appropriate in most situations. However, every attempt should be made to determine the source, microbiology, and pathophysiology of the infection because this knowledge will guide the optimal management. Often, various underlying risk factors predispose individuals to infection with specific organisms. Some of these conditions and associated pathogens are listed in Table 4.

A thorough history and physical examination are crucial to the diagnosis of sepsis; their importance cannot be overemphasized. Multiple cultures from multiple sites need to be

Table 4 Special Circumstances in Septic Patients

CIRCUMSTANCE	POSSIBLE PATHOGENS
Splenectomy (traumatic or functional)	*Streptococcus pneumoniae,* *Hemophilus influenzae,* *Neisseria meningitidis*
Neutropenia (<500 neutrophils/μl)	Gram-negatives, including *Pseudomonas aeruginosa,* gram-positives, including *Staphylococcus aureus* Fungi, especially *Candida* species
Hypogammaglobulinemia (e.g., CLL)	*Streptococcus pneumoniae,* *Escherichia coli*
Burns	*Staphylococcus aureus* (methicillin resistant), *Pseudomonas aeruginosa,* resistant gram-negatives
AIDS	*Pseudomonas aeruginosa* (if neutropenic), *Staphylococcus aureus, Pneumocystis carinii* (pneumonia)
Intravascular devices	*Staphylococcus aureus, Staphylococcus epidermidis*
Nosocomial infections	*Staphylococcus aureus* (methicillin resistant), *Enterococcus* species, resistant gram-negatives, *Candida* species

CLL, Chronic lymphocytic leukemia; *AIDS,* acquired immunodeficiency syndrome.

obtained when infection is suspected. All culture material needs to be delivered promptly to the microbiology laboratory. Gram stains should be made and read as soon as possible on all specimens submitted for culture. Ideally, cultures should be obtained before the initiation of antibiotics. However, the administration of antibiotics should not be delayed by more than 10 to 20 minutes for patients who are clinically or hemodynamically unstable.

Two sets of blood cultures, drawn from different sites, should be obtained from all patients suspected of being septic. Each blood culture set consists of one aerobic and one anaerobic bottle. At least 10 ml of blood needs to be injected into each bottle. If an indwelling venous or arterial catheter is present, it is important to obtain additional cultures through each port of the device.

Sputum for culture can be spontaneously expectorated, induced with 3% saline, or obtained by nasotracheal, endotracheal, or transtracheal techniques. Specimens should have fewer than 25 squamous epithelial cells per low-power (100×) microscopic field to decrease the chance that the specimen is contaminated with upper airway flora.

Urine should be obtained for culture when possible. Clean-catch or straight-catheterization specimens are preferred. Urine that has been present in a closed collection system for more than 1 hour should not be sent for culture. If necessary, urine can be obtained directly from the catheter tubing or bladder (suprapubic aspiration) using a syringe and a small-gauge needle. It is important to remember that many bacteriuric patients, especially those with indwelling urinary catheters, may be septic from another source. Although the presence of more than 100,000 bacteria on culture suggests infection, this criterion has been validated only for ambulatory young adults with gram-negative bacillary organisms.

Cultures from other sites should be obtained if clinically indicated. Computed tomography (CT) scans of the abdomen and sinuses often reveal previously overlooked fluid collections that may be accessible by needle aspiration. All patients with diarrhea should have stool sent for a cytotoxic assay for *Clostridium difficile* toxin A and B. Ultrasonography is useful for detecting ascites and biliary, hepatic, and pancreatic pathologic conditions. A portable (bedside) ultrasound can be obtained for critically ill patients who are too unstable to be transported to the radiology department. A lumbar puncture for cell count, protein, glucose, bacterial antigens, Gram stain, and culture should be performed on any septic patient with unexplained altered mentation.

Antibiotics form the cornerstone of therapy for sepsis. Although it is difficult to prove, most authorities believe that outcome is improved in septic patients if the diagnosis is suspected early and appropriate antibiotics are started without delay. In addition, appropriate surgical intervention often is as important as the initial choice of antibiotics. Our recommendation for empiric antibiotic therapy is outlined in Figure 1 and Table 5. A few principles are worth emphasizing: (1) Antipseudomonal agents should be used for empiric therapy for nosocomial infection. (2) Antibiotic dosages should be optimized for the site of infection, usually requiring the highest allowable dosage adjusted for organ dysfunction. Intravenously administered antibiotics often result in higher serum and tissue levels than orally adminis-

tered antibiotics. The oral route of antibiotic administration should not be used for persons in whom gut absorption is compromised. (3) Community-acquired infections are likely to be caused by organisms different from those encountered in the hospital. For example, *P. aeruginosa* is unlikely to be encountered in community-acquired infections; therefore antipseudomonal coverage is not warranted routinely. On the other hand, *Streptococcus pneumoniae* is one of the most common causes of community-acquired sepsis. This organism needs to be covered adequately, something that may not be accomplished with the use of many of the antipseudomonal antibiotics currently available. (4) Aminoglycosides offer rapid killing of gram-negative aerobic bacteria in a dose-dependent fashion, whereas toxicity depends on the time that serum levels are above the toxicity threshold. The risk of nephrotoxicity and ototoxicity, the poor penetration of aminoglycosides into abscesses and lung parenchyma, and the lack of data to indicate that the addition of aminoglycosides affects the outcome in septic patients call for the judicious use of aminoglycosides. Our current recommendations for the use of aminoglycosides are as follows: (1) Large single daily doses (e.g., 5 mg/kg of tobramycin daily) in patients who are hemodynamically unstable, (2) small doses (e.g., 1 to 1.5 mg/kg of tobramycin every 8 hours) when used for synergy against streptococcal and enterococcal infections, (3) in the first few days to provide empiric coverage for aerobic gram-negative bacteria.

The choice of the specific antibiotic agent depends on multiple factors. Table 6 lists some of the factors that affect the choice of antibiotics beyond what is outlined in the algorithm and in Table 5.

Despite the increase in the incidence of nosocomial beta-lactam–resistant gram-positive organisms, the Centers for Disease Control and Prevention (CDC) recommends against the routine empiric use of vancomycin. The rationale for this recommendation is to decrease the likelihood of emergence of VRE infections. Routine use of antifungal therapy also is not recommended in patients with sepsis, unless a fungus has been isolated in the bloodstream or in a sterile tissue (excluding sites with drainage tubes). The presence of macronodular skin lesions shown on biopsy to be consistent with candidal infection or the presence of candida endophthalmitis is synonymous with dissemination. Because only a fraction of patients with systemic candidiasis will have positive blood cultures, a number of schemes have been developed to stratify the risk for systemic fungal infection in hospitalized patients. In general, when *Candida* species are isolated from three or more nonblood sites, the risk of subsequent infection of the blood by these fungi increases. Determining when to initiate therapy in such situations typically depends on evaluating the total clinical picture. In any case, the efficacy of the azole antifungals (e.g., fluconazole), with their associated favorable toxicity profiles, has made the empiric use of antifungal therapy much more acceptable.

The duration of antibiotic therapy depends on the clinical response and, occasionally, the infecting pathogen. A "typical" course of antibiotics is given for 7 to 14 days. A good rule of thumb is to administer the antibiotics for 3 days beyond the point at which the patient becomes afebrile or

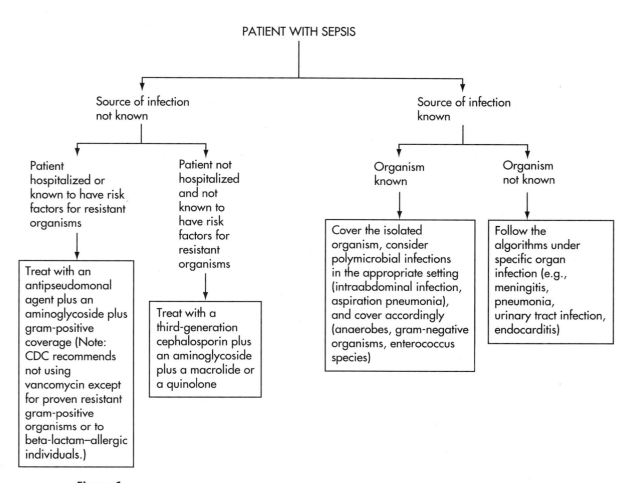

Figure 1
Algorithm for antibiotic coverage in patients with sepsis.

has normalization of laboratory values. There are some important exceptions: (1) Neutropenic (absolute neutrophil count <500 cells/μl) patients should receive 14 days of antibiotic therapy. This therapeutic approach is a compromise between stopping antibiotics shortly after the patient becomes afebrile and continuing the antibiotics for the entire duration of neutropenia. If a previously febrile neutropenic patient becomes afebrile and is no longer neutropenic, a shorter course of antibiotic therapy can be considered. (2) Patients with *S. aureus* pneumonia or bacteremia should receive at least 14 days of antibiotics. If the patient has responded rapidly to antibiotics, the last several days of therapy can be given via the oral route. (3) Patients with *Pneumocystis carinii* pneumonia should receive 14 to 21 days of therapy.

Antibiotic decisions should be reevaluated at least daily. Changes need to be considered as culture and sensitivity results become available or as the clinical course dictates. In addition, a patient who has not responded to therapy or who has relapsed after an initial improvement needs to be reevaluated thoroughly. Additional diagnostic studies may be indicated, and repeat cultures should be obtained to search for new or resistant pathogens.

The persistently febrile neutropenic patient represents an especially challenging problem. Intravenous amphotericin

B, at a dosage of 0.5 to 0.6 mg/kg/day, should be started if fever persists despite broad-spectrum antibiotic coverage for more than 5 to 7 days. A number of amphotericin B lipid formulations have become available that may decrease the number and severity of side effects, but these approaches have not been compared with standard amphotericin B infusions in large clinical trials. Although the optimal duration of therapy is unknown, it is prudent to continue antifungal therapy at least as long as neutropenia exists, or to a minimum total dose of 500 mg. Fluconazole has been shown to be at least as good as amphotericin B in nonneutropenic patients.

Poor decisions about antibiotic use have immediate and future negative consequences. Long-term antibiotic use will not protect patients from infection; rather, patients will become infected with resistant organisms. The best practical way to avoid widespread resistance problems is to continuously reevaluate the need for antibiotic therapy. In addition, side effects, such as rashes and *C. difficile* diarrhea, are much more common after long courses of multiple antibiotics.

Sepsis is a systemic disease, and proper management requires diligent attention to supportive care, particularly in the presence of multiorgan dysfunction. There has been considerable controversy about the extent to which organ perfusion is to be optimized. Our recommendation is to aim

Table 5   Recommended Initial[a] Antibiotic Regimens for Septic Patients with Normal Renal Function

CLINICAL SITUATION	REGIMEN
Empiric coverage	Either imipenem,[b] 500 mg IV q6h, or trovafloxacin,[c] 300 mg IV q24h, with or without tobramycin,[d,e] 5 mg/kg IV q24h
Community-acquired pneumonia[f,g]	Ceftriaxone, 1 g IV q12h, with or without azithromycin, 500 mg IV or PO q24h
Community-acquired urosepsis	Ciprofloxacin, 400 mg IV q12h, with or without ampicillin, 2 g IV q4h
Nosocomial infections *or*	Piperacillin/tazobactam,[i] 3.375 g IV q4-6h, or ceftazidime, 2 g IV q8h, *or*
Neutropenia[h]	Imipenem,[b] 500 mg IV q6h, or ciprofloxacin, 400 mg IV q12h, or trovafloxacin,[c] 300 mg IV q24h, each with or without tobramycin,[d,e] 5 mg/kg IV q24h
HIV+ with pneumonia[j]	Trimethoprim-sulfamethoxazole, 5 mg/kg IV q6h, or pentamidine, 4 mg/kg IV q24h, either with ceftriaxone, 1 g IV q12h, and with or without azithromycin, 500 mg IV or PO q24h; add prednisone (or equivalent), 40 mg PO q12h, for room air P_{O_2} <70 mm Hg

HIV, Human immunodeficiency virus.

[a]Antibiotics should be adjusted according to the microbiologic results.

[b]Imipenem dosage should be adjusted according to weight, age, and creatinine clearance.

[c]Benefits of drug must outweigh risks of hepatotoxicity.

[d]Amikacin at 15 to 20 mg/kg/day can be substituted for tobramycin at institutions with significant bacterial resistance rates to tobramycin.

[e]Aminoglycosides should be used in patients with hemodynamic instability because of their rapid killing of bacteria and broad spectrum of activity against aerobic gram-negative organisms. Single daily dosing is recommended when feasible.

[f]May use vancomycin instead of ceftriaxone for beta-lactam–allergic patients with *Streptococcus pneumoniae* or *Staphylococcus aureus* or if the infection is caused by resistant organisms.

[g]Levofloxacin or trovafloxacin could be used for initial therapy of community-acquired pneumonia.

[h]Imipenem and ceftazidime are the preferred agents in neutropenic patients.

Meropenem may be substituted for imipenem, particularly in the elderly, patients with renal failure, patients with seizure disorders, or patients with central nervous system infections.

[i]Must dose every 4 hr if covering *Pseudomonas aeruginosa* infections. Other appropriate antipseudomonal agents are meropenem and cefepime.

[j]Use the above recommendations for HIV-positive patients with CD4+ cell counts <200 cell/mm^3; otherwise, cover the same as in community-acquired pneumonia without HIV. If Gram stain reveals gram-negative rods, antibiotics appropriate for *Pseudomonas aeruginosa* must be added.

Table 6   Factors That May Affect the Choice of Antibiotics in Sepsis

FACTOR AFFECTING THE CHOICE OF ANTIBIOTIC	LESS FAVORABLE ANTIBIOTIC CHOICE	MORE APPROPRIATE ANTIBIOTIC CHOICE
Antibiotic penetration into infected site		
Pyelonephritis	Trovafloxacin	Ciprofloxacin
Biliary infection	Penicillin	Ciprofloxacin, trovafloxacin
Central nervous system infection	Imipenem, quinolones	Meropenem, third-generation cephalosporins
Underlying medical problems that affect antibiotic metabolism or safety		
Renal dysfunction	Imipenem, trimethoprim-sulfamethoxazole	Trovafloxacin, meropenem
Hepatic dysfunction	Trovafloxacin	
Seizure disorder	Imipenem	Meropenem
Identification of the organism		
Enterobacter species	Cephalosporins, penicillins	Carbapenems, trimethoprim-sulfamethoxazole
Staphylococcus aureus	Quinolones	Nafcillin, vancomycin
Enterococci	Quinolones, cephalosporins, trimethoprim-sulfamethoxazole	Ampicillin, piperacillin, imipenem, vancomycin
Allergies	Avoid the offending agent	Use a different class of antibiotic if the allergy is significant
Hemodynamically unstable patient	Avoid bacteriostatic agents	Use bacteriocidal agent; consider aminoglycosides

---

Table 7   General Principles in the Management of Sepsis

1. Control the infection:
   Provide appropriate antibiotics (see Tables and Figure 1).
   Initiate surgical or invasive management of the infection if appropriate (drain any abscesses, correct a perforated viscous, remove infected device if appropriate).
2. Optimize tissue perfusion and oxygenation:
   Optimize arterial oxygen saturation.
   Optimize fluid status (crystalloids are preferred).
   Optimize cardiac output and oxygen delivery (note that supernormal values have not been proven to be beneficial and may be harmful).
   Transfuse blood only if patient is symptomatic and hemoglobin is <8 g/dl.
3. Consider active nutritional support:
   If the patient has malnutrition or is expected to be without nutrition for more than 3 days.
   Gut feeding is preferable to parenteral feeding.
4. Optimal management of organ failure:
   Use PEEP and low tidal volume in the management of ARDS complicating sepsis.
   Norepinephrine may improve visceral perfusion.
   Consider the use of gastric tonometry to evaluate visceral organ perfusion.
5. Prevent nosocomial complications:
   DVT prophylaxis.
   Stress ulcer prophylaxis.
   Judicious use of antibiotics to avoid nosocomial infections by resistant organisms.

PEEP, Positive end-expiratory pressure; *ARDS,* adult respiratory distress syndrome; *DVT,* deep venous thrombosis.

to achieve normal perfusion parameters. Supernormal perfusion is not warranted and may be harmful. It also has been suggested that the manner in which organ failure is managed could affect the outcome and that supportive therapy may have a negative or a positive effect on the process of sepsis.

For example, there is increasing evidence that the approach used to mechanically ventilate patients with adult respiratory distress syndrome (ARDS) may affect outcome. Table 7 describes some of the current recommendations in regard to supportive care in patients with sepsis.

The sepsis syndrome is incredibly complex, involving many mediators that we are just starting to appreciate. Better identification of the subset of patients likely to benefit from these products is necessary, as are rapid diagnostic assays for endotoxin, TNF, and various cytokines. A clinical trial currently is under way to demonstrate the clinical utility of bedside testing for IL-6 levels. For now, we must continue with our attempts to improve patient survival by aggressively diagnosing the cause of sepsis and treating the manifestations of the syndrome with antibiotics, source control, and supportive therapy.

Suggested Reading

Bone RC, et al: Sepsis syndrome: a valid clinical entity, *Crit Care Med* 17:389, 1989.

Fein AM, et al: *Sepsis and multiorgan failure,* Baltimore, 1997, Williams & Wilkins.

MacArthur RD, Bone RC: Sepsis, SIRS, and septic shock. In Bone RC, ed: *Pulmonary and critical care medicine,* ed 4, vol 3, St Louis, 1997, Mosby.

Marik PE, Varon J: The hemodynamic derangements in sepsis: implications for treatment strategies, *Chest* 114:854, 1998.

Natanson C, et al: Selected treatment strategies for septic shock based on proposed mechanisms of pathogenesis, *Ann Intern Med* 120:771, 1994.

Wheeler AP, Bernard GR: Treating patients with severe sepsis, *N Engl J Med* 340:207, 1999.

Young LS: Sepsis syndrome. In Mandell GL, Bennett JE, Dolin R, eds: *Principles and practice of infectious diseases,* ed 4, New York, 1995, Churchill Livingstone.

CHRONIC FATIGUE SYNDROME

James F. Jones

■ CFS AND INFECTION

In the early to mid-1980s, several reports described patients with chronic illnesses that resembled infectious mononucleosis (IM). The illnesses consisted of an acute onset of malaise, pharyngitis, lymph node pain or swelling, myalgia, arthralgia, sleep disturbances, headaches, cognitive problems, and aggravation of symptoms after engaging in physical activity. Patients were also characterized as being moody or depressed, particularly by friends and family. This clinical picture and its duration of months to years were clinically compatible with previous reports of protracted or reactivated IM (and of course the myriad infections that produce "mononucleosis").

The attribution of the illnesses to Epstein-Barr virus (EBV) was based primarily on the presence of either antibodies to the viral capsid antigen (VCA) of the IgM class, persistent "high" anti–early antigen (EA) antibodies, or low to absent levels of anti-EBNA antibodies. The methodology used to detect these antibodies was the immunofluorescence techinque described by the Henles and their group. Serologic profiles developed by these investigators also were used as the basis of comparison in the attempts to distinguish past versus chronic or active infections. The other principle that impacted on the recent rebirth of evaluation of these patients was the perception that altered immunity was responsible for the prolonged infection.

The experience of Holmes et al. from the Centers for Disease Control and Prevention (CDC), while studying a cluster of illness in the Lake Tahoe area, suggested that reliance on serologic methodologies could not identify EBV or other viruses as the cause of such chronic illnesses. Their experience was echoed by a number of investigators who evaluated EBV serologic responses and found them to be nondiagnostic.

The number of patients that began to be considered as having such an illness, regardless of its origin, led to preparation of a research definition that included the main symptoms expressed by these patients. Because a common problem was debilitating fatigue and it appeared that no specific infection nor specific disease in general was responsible for the illnesses being described, the name *chronic fatigue syndrome* was agreed on by the majority of the international group that prepared the definition. Critical components of the definition were that it attempted to quantify the illness and that it contained physical examination findings. Noticeably absent from the definition was a requirement for laboratory abnormalities. The presence of a variety of underlying medical and psychiatric diseases precluded patients from being placed in this diagnostic category.

The first definition did allow identification of patients in the United States. Different definitions were developed in Great Britain and Australia. Each definition allowed detection of patients throughout the world. Once evaluated, even though the number of patients fulfilling the 1988 definition in various studies were not large, concern arose that the large numbers of symptoms might allow inclusion of persons with somatoform disorders and thus dilute the population base for future studies or miss important psychiatric disorders. It was also determined that the inclusion of quantitative elements was not helpful and that reduction of the number of certain symptoms did not decrease the ability of the investigators to identify individuals identified using the longer version.

Thus a revised, clinically simplified definition was published in 1994 (Table 1). Although it removed the problems described in the aforementioned definition by including a smaller number of symptoms, it has allowed identification of larger numbers of patients. This definition also has a component of idiopathic chronic fatigue, where patients are fatigued for the same length of time as those with chronic fatigue syndrome, but who did not fit the other criteria. Although less stringent on the clinical side, the research component was enhanced in terms of patient subgrouping and specific criteria for analysis.

From a public health viewpoint, the complete 1994 definition allows application of a standard instrument to address the presence of fatigue and fatigue-associated illnesses associated with considerable morbidity in the population at large. Unlike the first definition, it does not attempt to define or divine a disease.

Two additional points that influence the study of these patients are the presence of a symptom complex that contains the hallmark symptoms of an infectious disease and the high percentages of patients (67%) presenting to community-based clinics with a precipitating "viral illness." These observations influenced past, and continue to impact present, evaluations of these patients at both the clinical and research levels.

■ PROPOSED INFECTIOUS AGENTS

A wide variety of infectious agents have been proposed to be "the" causative agents of chronic fatigue syndrome. A list of such agents includes enteroviruses, several herpes viruses

---

Table 1 1994 Research Definition of Chronic Fatigue Syndrome

PRIMARY CRITERIA
Fatigue >6 mo and absence of other disease process to explain fatigue

SECONDARY CRITERIA (4 OF 8)
Sore throat, lymph nodes, myalgia, arthralgia
Headache, cognitive problems, sleep disturbance, and aggravation of symptoms with activity

From Fukuda K, et al, and the International Chronic Fatigue Syndrome Study Group: The chronic fatigue syndrome: a comprehensive approach to its definition and study, *Ann Intern Med* 121:953, 1994.

(particularly EBV and human herpes virus 6—HHV 6), parvovirus B19, Inoue-Melnik virus, retroviruses, *Borrelia burgdorferi*, parasites, hepatitis viruses, *Mycoplasma* species, and yeast. Serious attempts to evaluate chronic infections have relied on cultures, serology, antigen and/or nucleic acid detection in tissue and serum or plasma by use of monoclonal antibodies and detection of DNA and RNA by Southern blots, Northern blots, dot blot, polymerase chain reaction, and in situ hybridization techniques.

Most of the serious studies find exposure to the agent in question in the respective study, and its presence by one or more of the aforementioned methods in patients with the syndrome, in greater numbers than healthy individuals. In no study, however, has a cause-and-effect relationship between an infectious agent and chronic fatigue syndrome been established. In some of the studies, a few patients appear to have an active disease. Establishment of the diagnosis of an active infection with agents that cause latent or persistent infections in the population at large is fraught with difficulty. In fact, if a patient is shown to have an active infection, should he or she not be considered as having an infectious disease that was difficult to identify or has not completely resolved rather than having chronic fatigue syndrome caused by that agent?

■ IMMUNOLOGY

Since the studies in the early 1980s queried whether the immune systems of their participants were normal, there has been a continuing effort to attribute the syndrome to either immune deficits or to "immune dysfunction." As with the reports that attempted to identify causative agents, some of the studies that evaluated immune system components and function found peculiarities in the parameters that were addressed. Again, most of the findings were based on numerical differences between healthy control subjects and patients with chronic fatigue syndrome. It is important to note that the patient values were usually, if not always, within the normal range for the laboratory in question, but mean patient values varied from mean control subject values.

■ KOCH-EVANS POSTULATES?

Establishment of an infectious cause for specific agents has historically required fulfillment of this series of universally accepted requirements that rely on qualities of the infectious agent and the immune response to it. None of the studies to date achieve these aims. Two critical components are often overlooked: (1) the need for the illness in question to make biologic and epidemiologic sense and (2) the role of the genetic response of the subject in question in the production of the illness. An example of questioning whether a set of observations makes biologic and epidemiologic sense is whether low natural killer (NK) numbers or faulty NK cell function contributes to the syndrome. This cell is associated with a variety of immune functions, including initial response to virus infection and production of interferon gamma. The patients that have been well documented to

have serious deficits in these categories either have other types of true infections or they are very rare. Because the immune system has many layers and backup systems are present to control most infections, other explanations should be sought to explain the symptoms described by these patients. One such avenue is the apparent high incidence of expression of the atopic phenotype in patients with chronic fatigue syndrome. An overlap in symptoms between infection and allergy contributes to a possible role for this immune state in playing a role in chronic fatigue syndrome.

■ EVALUATION OF SYMPTOMS

The symptoms described by the patients consist of those observed in most human illness. They are shared in both medical and psychiatric diseases. They are the complaints made by people who cannot function properly. The same complaints are registered by subjects under evaluation for chronic infection or for chronic fatigue syndrome (Table 2). The symptoms are learned from the first infectious illness that a human can remember. In the context of illness altering behavior, the symptoms of systemic infection are protective for the ill animal in that it forces it to rest and to seek isolation so that stored energy can be used to produce proteins required to fight off the infection. The changes in physical behavior are accompanied by alterations in mood that prevent socialization and spread of infection. These behavioral changes are produced by the host. They are the result of physiologic changes brought on by cytokines and other mediators of inflammation. Interestingly, the same or similar changes in these mediators are brought on by exercise above baseline activity. The same symptoms are also seen in patients with depression. In each of these situations, innate responses appear to be marshaled to protect the host. Therefore it is intuitive to consider that when physiologic function is impaired, humans fall back on patterns of altered behavior that have been protective in their past experiences.

Table 2 Ranking of Symptoms in Studies of Chronic Fatigue Syndrome versus Chronic Infection	
CDC SURVEILLANCE DATA	**CHRONIC EBV STUDY—1987**
Neuropsychologic	Fatigue
Fever/chills	Headache
Sore throat	Difficulty concentrating (neurologic)
Myalgia	Depression (neurologic)
Sleep disturbances	Sore throat
Weakness	Muscle/pain
Lymph node swelling	Arthraigia
Postexertion fatigue	Dizziness (neuropsychologic)
Arthraigia	Mood swings (neuropsychologic)
Headache	Sleep disturbances
	Heat/cold

CDC, Centers for Disease Control and Prevention; *EBV,* Epstein-Barr virus.

■ EVALUATION OF THE PATIENT

Alterations in virtually any organ system will produce the symptoms included in the definition. It is critical to address when, where, and how the symptoms are produced to consider chronic fatigue syndrome as a working diagnosis. The most productive method of obtaining the required information is to ask the patient to describe his or her problems and to pursue how these complaints affect the patient's day-to-day functioning. Asking the patient to fill out lists that are designed to identify chronic fatigue syndrome per se is not in the patient's best interest. Fulfillment of the definition requires efforts to identify disease processes that would explain the symptom pattern.

If the problem occurs only at work or in a specific season of the year, chronic fatigue syndrome may not be the appropriate diagnosis. The symptom pattern described by the patient should accompany the fatigue both in duration and magnitude. Efforts should be made to discern the meaning of the term *fatigue* in each patient. To some individuals *fatigue* means lethargy, and to others it means malaise (feeling tired and sick). The inclusion of sleep problems in the definition leads to identification of many patients with sleep disorders because the consequences of nonrestorative sleep are the symptoms of this syndrome.

■ USE OF THE LABORATORY

Standard screening tests include a complete blood count (CBC) and differential, blood chemistries, urinalysis, thyroid function, antinuclear antibodies (ANA), and rheumatoid factor. Positive results in any of these areas suggest that further evaluation should be performed before considering chronic fatigue syndrome as a diagnosis. If the history is strongly suggestive of the syndrome following an acute infection, instead of looking for all of the possible infectious agents that are potential causes of prolonged illness, it appears clinically prudent to check for evidence of systemic inflammation as a clue to the presence of an infectious or other inflammatory processes. A low sedimentation rate does not exclude an active process. Performance of a C-reactive protein and a serum protein electrophoresis, along with serum IgG, IgA, and IgM, will often identify such an ongoing illness. Appropriate studies directed at specific diseases can then follow.

As stated in the 1994 definition, there is no clinical role for random performance of specific serologic testing, lymphocyte enumeration/functional testing, or brain imaging of any type.

■ DIFFERENTIAL DIAGNOSES

The illnesses that have been identified in patients referred for evaluation for chronic fatigue syndrome include all diagnostic categories in medicine and psychiatry. The most common problems in which mediators of inflammation play a role include sinusitis, autoimmune diseases, and inadequately treated or resolving infections. Infectious diseases that have been identified include parvovirus B19, *B. burgdorfii*, herpes viruses, group A beta-hemolytic streptococci, adenoviruses, and enteroviruses. Other diseases include hypothyroidism, Hashimoto's thyroiditis, cardiovascular diseases, autonomic nervous system dysfunction, psychologic and psychiatric diseases, and very often, sleep disorders.

■ THERAPY

The diagnostic process is the most important therapeutic component for evaluating patients under consideration for chronic fatigue syndrome. As emphasized in the 1994 definition, one of two major criteria is the exclusion of other illnesses. Occasionally, patients are prematurely diagnosed with chronic fatigue syndrome when another process is obvious, or patients receive an appropriate working diagnosis of chronic fatigue syndrome, but there is failure to follow the patient and pursue evolving diseases. If chronic fatigue syndrome is the diagnosis, the patient must be informed that the illness is multifactorial and that there is no specific therapy. It is important for the patient to learn to adapt to his or her current situation and not expect immediate return to the premorbid state. Most longitudinal studies have shown that resolution of the syndrome occurs within 2 years when the illness has been triggered by an infection. Although the condition is aggravated by physical activity that is greater than usual for the patient, some level of activity is usually helpful. The approach that is most beneficial is low-level, nonaerobic exercise in which the patient stops his or her activity before becoming tired. If the patient can follow this course, he or she can gradually increase personal productive activity level.

The course of action just described is an informal approach to cognitive-behavioral therapy where the patient in essence learns about his or her illness and alters behavior with the goal of improvement of functional capacity and quality of life. In some cases, advancement to this endpoint is hastened by the use of symptomatic pharmacologic therapy. The medications that are in greatest use include tricyclic antidepressants, sleep-inducing compounds, nonsteroidal antiinflammatory agents, analgesics per se, anxiolytics, and serotonin reuptake inhibitors. The use and success of these agents in alleviating symptoms in patients with chronic fatigue syndrome does not mean that a psychiatric origin is present in a given patient. In fact, most of these medications have multiple pharmacologic effects that might influence patients' symptoms. For example, it is of interest that tricyclic antidepressants have remarkable antihistaminic activity, antiinflammatory activity, and hypnotic effect, and through their inhibition of norepinephrine reuptake, have a potentially positive effect on the autonomic nervous system. Because there appears to be no single process that is responsible for the production of the syndrome, it is unlikely that a single regimen will suffice for all patients. Likewise, the concept that "enhancement of immunity" by the use of vitamins, minerals, herbs, and other supplements has not been established in formal trials.

Each component of the patient's illness may require specific therapy. If sinusitis is present, it may need both acute and chronic therapy. If sleep problems are present and a trial of medication to assist in relieving insomnia is not helpful after a few weeks, formal evaluation of the sleep problems is mandatory. As with most symptoms of chronic fatigue syndrome, medications are not curative.

Suggested Reading

Fukuda K, et al, and the International Chronic Fatigue Syndrome Study Group: The chronic fatigue syndrome: a comprehensive approach to its definition and study, *Ann Intern Med* 121:953, 1994.

Jones JF: Chronic fatigue syndrome. In Rakel RE, ed: *Conn's current therapy,* Philadelphia, 1999, WB Saunders.

Mawle A, Reyes M, Schmid DS: Is chronic fatigue syndrome an infectious disease? *Infect Agents Dis* 2:333, 1994.

White T, et al: Incidence, risk and prognosis of acute and chronic fatigue syndromes and psychiatric disorders after glandular fever, *Psychiatry* 173:475, 1998.

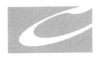

PHARYNGOTONSILLITIS

Itzhak Brook

Pharyngotonsillitis (PT) is characterized by the presence of increased redness and finding of an exudate, ulceration, or a membrane covering the tonsils. Because the pharynx is served by lymphoid tissues of the Waldeyer ring, an infection can spread to various parts of the ring, such as the nasopharynx, uvula, soft palate, tonsils, adenoids, and the cervical lymph glands. Based on the extent of the infection, the infection can be described as pharyngitis, tonsillitis, tonsillopharyngitis, or nasopharyngitis. The duration of any of these illnesses can be acute, subacute, chronic, or recurrent.

■ CAUSES

The diagnosis of PT generally requires the consideration of group A beta-hemolytic streptococci (GABHS) infection. However, numerous other bacteria, viruses, and other infections and noninfectious causes should be considered. Recognition of the cause and choice of appropriate therapy are of utmost importance in ensuring rapid recovery and preventing complications.

Table 1 lists the different causative agents and their characteristic clinical features. The occurrence of a certain etiologic agent depends on numerous variables, including environmental conditions (season, geographic, location, exposure) and individual variables (age, host resistance, immunity). The most prevalent causes of PT are GABHS and viruses. However, the exact cause generally is not determined, and the role of some potential pathogens is uncertain.

Studies suggest that interactions between various organisms, including GABHS, other aerobic and anaerobic bacteria, and viruses, may occur during PT. Some of these interactions may be synergistic (i.e., between Epstein-Barr virus [EBV] and anaerobic bacteria), thus enhancing the virulence of some pathogens, whereas others may be antagonistic (i.e., between GABHS and certain "interfering" alpha-hemolytic streptococci). Furthermore, beta-lactamase–producing bacteria can protect themselves as well as other bacteria from beta-lactam antibiotics.

Aerobic Bacteria

Because of the potential of serious suppurative and nonsuppurative sequellae, GABHS are the best known cause of sore throat. Occasionally, groups B, C, and G beta-hemolytic streptococci are responsible. Streptococcal tonsillitis can be serious because it may lead to rheumatic fever and because of the increased virulence of GABHS. An increased number of cases of sepsis and toxic shock syndrome resulting from streptococci have been observed in the past decade. The clinical presentation of PT caused by all types of streptococci generally is identical and is characterized by exudation, petechiae, and follicles. GABHS PT occurs mainly in children 5 to 15 years of age during winter and early spring (in temperate climates). The isolation rate of non-GABHS is higher in adults than in children.

GABHS can be involved in suppurative complications of tonsillitis, such as peritonsillar and retropharyngeal abscesses and cervical lymphadenitis.

Streptococcus pneumoniae also can be involved in PT that can either subside or spread to other sites. *Corynebacterium diphtheriae* and *Corynebacterium (Arcanobacterium) hemolyticum* cause an early exudative PT with grayish-green thick membranes that may be difficult to dislodge and that often leaves a bleeding surface when torn off. The infection can spread to the throat, palate, and larynx. *C. (Arcanobacterium) hemolyticum* produces a lethal systemic exotoxin. *C. (Arcanobacterium) hemolyticum* was reported to be a major cause of PT in the United Kingdom and Scandinavia and is common in teenagers and young adults; about half of patients with PT have a scarlatiniform rash.

Neisseria gonorrheae is common in homosexual men and can be detected in adolescents with pharyngitis. The infection often is asymptomatic but may result in bacteremia and can persist after treatment. *Neisseria meningitidis* can cause symptomatic or asymptomatic PT that may be a prodrome for septicemia or meningitis.

Nontypable *Haemophilus influenzae* and *Haemophilus parainfluenzae* can be recovered from inflamed tonsils. These organisms can cause invasive disease in infants and the elderly, as well as acute epiglotitis, otitis media, and sinusitis.

Staphylococcus aureus in PT often is recovered from chronically inflamed tonsils and peritonsillar abscesses. It can produce the enzyme beta-lactamase, which may interfere with the eradication of GABHS.

Rare causes of PT are *Francisella tularemia, Treponema pallidum, Mycobacterium* species, and *Toxoplasma gondii.*

Mycoplasma

Mycoplasma pneumoniae and *Mycoplasma hominis* also can cause PT, usually as a manifestation of a generalized infection. The prevalence of *Mycoplasma* infection increases with age.

Anaerobic Bacteria

The anaerobic species that have been implicated in PT are *Actinomyces* species, *Fusobacterium* species, and pigmented

Prevotella and *Porphyromonas* species. Anaerobes' role is supported by their predominance in tonsillar or retropharyngeal abscesses and in Vincent's angina (*Fusobacterium* species and spirochetes). Furthermore, patients with non-GABHS tonsillitis (i.e., infectious mononucleosis) respond to antibiotics directed against anaerobes; in addition, elevated serum levels of antibodies to *Prevotella intermedia* and *Fusobacterium nucleatum* were found in patients with acute and recurrent non-GABHS tonsollitis, peritonsillar cellulitis, and abscess.

Viruses and Chlamydia

Viruses known to cause PT are as follows: *adenovirus, coxsackie A,* parainfluenza, *enteroviruses, EBV, herpes simplex, respiratory syncytial virus* [RSV]*, influenza A and B, parainfluenza, enterovirus,* and *cytomegalovirus. Chlamydia pneumoniae* may cause PT, often accompanying pneumonia or bronchitis.

■ CLINICAL FINDINGS

PT generally has a sudden onset, with fever and sore throat, nausea, vomiting, headache, and rarely, abdominal pain. At an early stage, redness of throat and tonsils is observed, and the cervical lymph glands become enlarged. The clinical manifestations may vary by causative agent (see Table 1), but they are rarely specific. Erythema is common to most agents; however, the occurrence of ulceration, petechiae, exudation, or follicles varies. The common features include the following: exudative pharyngitis, palatal petichieae, red beefy uvuyla, and scarlatiniform rash, in GABHS infection; ulcerative lesions in enteroviruses; and membranous pharyngitis in *C. diphtheriae.* Petechiae often can be seen in GABHS, EBV, measles, and rubella infections.

Viral disease generally is self-limited and lasts 4 to 10 days. Viral disease generally is associated with conjunctivitis, cough, hoarseness, coryza, anterior stomatitis, discrete ulceration, diarrhea, and viral exanthema. The most unique features of anaerobic tonsillitis or PT are enlargement and ulceration of the tonsils associated with fetid or foul odor and the presence of fusiform bacilli, spirochetes, and other organisms on Gram stain.

■ DIAGNOSIS

Throat culture obtained by throat swab of both tonsilar surfaces and the posterior pharyngeal wall, plated on sheep blood agar media, is the standard. Incubation in anaerobic condition and use of selective media can increase the recovery rate. A single throat culture has the sensitivity of 90% to 95% in detection of GABHS in the pharynx. False-negative results can occur in patients who received antibiotics. Throat cultures generally identify GABHS by direct growth on a blood agar plate that may take 24 to 48 hours. Reexamination of plates at 48 hours is advisable. Using a bacitracin disk provides presumptive identification. Attempts to identify beta-hemolytic streptococci, other than group A, may be worthwhile in older individuals. Commercial kits containing group-specific antisera are available for identifying the specific streptococcal group.

Table 1 Infectious Agents of Pharyngotonsillitis	CLINICAL LESIONS	CLINICAL FREQUENCY
BACTERIA		
Aerobic		
Groups A, B, C, and G streptococci	F, Er, Ex, P	A
Streptococcus pneumoniae	E	C
Staphylococcus aureus	F, ER, Ex	C
Neisseria gonorrhoeae	Er, Ex	C
Neisseria meningitidis	Er, Ex	C
Corynebacerium diphtheriae	Er, Ex	C
Cornebacterium hemolyticum	Er, Ex	C
Arcanobacterium hemolyticum	Er, Ex	C
Bordetella pertussis	Er, Er	C
Haemophilus influenzae	Er, Ex	C
Haemophilus parainfluenzae	Er, Ex	C
Salmonella typhi	Er	C
Francisella tularensis	Er, Ex	C
Yersinia sp. (*pestis, enterocolitica, pseudotuberculosis*)	Er	C
Treponema pallidum	F, Er	C
Mycobacterium sp.	Er	C
Anaerobic		
Peptostreptococcus sp.	Er, E	C
Actinomyces sp.	Er, U	C
Pigmented *Prevotella* and *Porphyromonas* spp.	Er, Ex, U	B
Bacteroides sp.	Er, Ex, U	C
MYCOPLASMA		
Mycoplasma pneumoniae	F, Er, Ex	B
Mycoplasma hominis	Er, Ex	C
VIRUSES AND CHLAMYDIA		
Adenovirus	F, Er, Ex	A
Enteroviruses (polio, echovirus, coxsackievirus)	Er, Ex, U	A
Parainfluenzae 1-4	Er	A
Epstein-Barr	F, Er, Ex	B
Herpes simplex	Er, Ex, U	C
Respiratory syncytial	Er	C
Influenzae A and B	Er	A
Cytomegalovirus	Er	C
Reovirus	Er	C
Measles	Er, P	C
Rubella	P	C
Rhinovirus	Er	C
Chalmydia psittaci	Er	C
Chalmydia pneumoniae	Er	C
FUNGI		
Candida sp.	Er, Ex	B
PARASITES		
Toxoplasma gondi	Er	C
RICKETTSIA		
Coxiella burnetii	Er	C

F, Follicular; *Er,* erythematous; *Ex,* exudative; *P,* petechial; *A,* most frequent (more than 66% of cases); *B,* frequent (between 66% and 33% of cases); *C,* uncommon (less than 33% of cases).

The presence of more than 10 colonies of GABHS per blood agar plate is considered to represent a true infection rather than colonization. However, using the number of colonies of GABHS in the plate as an indicator for the presence of true infection is difficult to implement because there is overlap between carriers and infected individuals. Repeated testing for GABHS at the end of therapy generally is not recommended in asymptomatic individuals.

A rise in ASO streptococcal antibodies titer after 3 to 6 weeks can provide retrospective evidence for GABHS infection and can assist in differentiating between the carrier state. Determining the ASO titers is indicated when the occurrence of GABHS infection must be proven.

Rapid antigen detection tests (RADT) for GABHS that take 10 to 60 minutes are available. They are more expensive than the routine culture, but they allow immediate administration of therapy and reduction of morbidity. However, these tests are associated with false-negative results 5% to 15% of the time. Therefore it is recommended that a bacterial culture be performed when the RADT is negative.

Other pathogens should be identified in specific situations when no GABHS is found or when a search for other organisms is warranted. Because many of the other potential pathogens are part of the normal pharyngeal flora, interpretation of the data is difficult.

Attempts to identify corynebacteria should be made whenever a membrane is present in the throat. Cultures should be obtained from beneath the membrane using a special moisture-reducing transport media. A Loeffler slant, a tellurite plate, and a blood agar plate should be inoculated. Identification by fluorescent antibody technique is possible.

Viral cultures or rapid tests for some viruses (i.e., RSV) are available. A heterophile slide test or other rapid tests for infectious mononucleosis can provide a specific diagnosis.

■ THERAPY

The goals of therapy of GABHS PT are to prevent suppurative and nonsuppurative complications, alleviate symptoms, and reduce infectivity. Therapy is indicated in those with symptomatic PT in whom the organisms were recovered or detected by RADT. The physician can start therapy in patients whom he or she has a high clinical suspicion of infection, but therapy should be discontinued if GABHS is not recovered.

Many antibiotics are available for the treatment of GABHS PT. However, the recommended optimal treatment for GABHS infection is penicillin administered three times a day for 10 days (Table 2). Oral penicillin VK is used more often than intramuscular (IM) benzathine penicillin G. However, IM penicillin can be given as initial therapy in patients who cannot tolerate oral medication or to ensure patient compliance. An alternative medication is amoxicillin, which is just as active against GABHS but has a more reliable absorption. In addition, blood levels are higher, the plasma half-life is longer, and protein binding is lower, giving it theoretical advantages. Furthermore, oral amoxicillin has a better patient compliance rate (because it has a better taste). However, amoxicillin should not be used in patients suspected of having infectious mononucleosis because it can produce a skin rash.

Alternative agents for the treatment of acute GABHS tonsillitis are the macrolides. However, the current resistance of GABHS to macrolides in the United States is 5% to 10%, and in countries where their use was extensive,

Table 2 Daily Dose of Oral Antibiotics for 10-Day Treatment of Acute GABHS Pharyngotonsillitis

GENERIC NAME	DOSAGE (IN mg)		FREQUENCY
	PEDIATRIC (mg/kg/day)	ADULT	
Penicillin V	25-50	250	q6-8h
Amoxicillin	40	250	q8h
Cephalexin*	25-50	250	q6-8h
Cefadroxil*	30	1000	q12h
Cefaclor*	40	250	q8h
Cefdinir	14	600	q24h
Cefuroxime-axetil*	30	250	q12h
Cefpodoxime-proxetil*	30	500	q12h
Cefprozil*	30	250	q12h
Azithromycin†	12	250‡	q24h
Clarithromycin	7.5	250	q12h
Cefixime	8	400	q24h
Ceftibuten	9	400	q24h
Erythromycin estolate	40	250	q8-12h
Amoxicillin-calvulanate§	45	875	q12h
Clindamycin§	20-30	150	q6-8h

*Effective also against aerobic BLPB.
†Duration of therapy, 5 days.
‡First-day dose is 500 mg.
§Effective also against aerobic and anaerobic beta-lactamase–producing bacteria.

GABHS resistance to these agents reached up to 70%. Therefore it is advisable to limit their use to patients who have a true allergy to penicillins. Compliance with the newer macrolides (clarithromycin and azithromycin) is better compared with that of erythromycin because of their longer half-life and the reduced adverse gastrointestinal side effects.

The success rate of treatment of acute GABHS tonsillitis was consistently found to be higher with cephalosporins than with penicillin. The cephalosporins' increased efficacy may be the result of their activity against aerobic beta-lactamase–producing bacteria (BLPB) such as *S. aureus* and *Haemophilus* species. Another possible reason is that the nonpathogenic alpha-hemolytic streptococci, which compete with GABHS and help eliminate them, are more resistant to cephalosporins than to penicillin. These streptococci therefore are more likely to survive cephalosporin therapy.

The length of therapy of acute tonsillitis with medication other than penicillin has not been determined by large comparative controlled studies. However, certain new agents have been administered in shorter courses of 5 days or more. Until a large number of comparative studies are done, it is safe to use the same length of therapy used with penicillin—10 days (Tables 2 and 3). Early initiation of antimicrobial therapy results in faster resolution of signs and symptoms. However, spontaneous disappearance of fever and other symptoms generally occurs within 3 to 4 days, even without antimicrobials. Furthermore, acute rheumatic fever can be prevented even when therapy is postponed up to 9 days.

Prevention of recurrent tonsillitis caused by GABHS by prophylactic administration of daily oral or monthly benzathine penicillin should be attempted in patients who had rheumatic fever. American Heart Committee guidelines on the prevention of rheumatic fever should be followed, and if any family members are carrying GABHS, the disease should be eradicated and the carrier state monitored. Clindamycin is the most effective agent in the treatment of the carrier state.

When *C. diphtheriae* infection is suspected, erythromycin is the drug of choice; penicillin and rifampin are alternatives. Supportive therapy of PT includes antipyretics and analgesics, such as aspirin or acetaminophen, and attention to proper hydration.

Recurrent and Chronic Tonsillitis

Recent studies document penicillin bacteriologic failure rates in the treatment of GABHS. PT can reach up to 25% and is even higher in retreatment. Although about half of the patients who harbor GABHS after therapy may be carriers, the rest may still show signs of infection and represent true clinical failure. The increased treatment failure rates necessitated the consideration of alternative therapies for patients who failed penicillin therapy.

Penicillin failure in eradicating GABHS tonsillitis has several explanations (Table 4). These explanations include noncompliance with the 10-day course of therapy, carrier state, reinfection, bacterial interference, bacterial internalization, and penicillin tolerance. One explanation is that repeated penicillin administration results in a shift in the oral microflora with selection of beta-lactamase–producing strains of *S. aureus*, *Haemophilus* species, *Moraxella catarrhalis*, *Fusobacterium* species, pigmented *Prevotella* and *Porphyromonas* species, and *Bacteroides* species.

It is possible that beta-lactamase–producing bacteria (BLPB) can protect the GABHS from penicillin by inactivating the antibiotic. Such organisms in a localized soft tissue infection may degrade penicillin in the area of the infection, protecting not only themselves but also penicillin-susceptible pathogens such as GABHS. Thus penicillin therapy directed against a susceptible pathogen can be rendered ineffective.

An increase in in vitro and in vivo resistance of GABHS to penicillin was observed when GABHS was inoculated with beta-lactamase–producing *S. aureus*, *Haemophilus* species, and pigmented *Prevotella* and *Porphyromonas* species *Bacteroides* species protected a penicillin-sensitive GABHS from penicillin therapy in mice. Both clindamycin and the combination of penicillin and clavulanic acid (a beta-lactamase inhibitor), which are active against both GABHS and BLPB, eradicated the infection.

Several clinical studies demonstrated the superiority of lincomycin, clindamycin, and amoxicillin-clavulanic acid over penicillin. These antimicrobial agents are effective against aerobic and anaerobic BLPB and GABHS in eradicating recurrent tonsillar infection. However, no studies showed them to be superior to penicillin in the treatment of acute tonsillitis. Other drugs that also may be effective in the

---

Table 3 Oral Antimicrobials in the Treatment of GABHS Tonsillitis

ACUTE	RECURRENT/ CHRONIC	CARRIER STATE
FIRST LINE		
Penicillin (amoxicillin)	Clindamycin Amoxicillin-clavulanate	Clindamycin
SECOND LINE		
Cephalosporins* Clindamycin Amoxicillin-clavulanate Macrolides†	Metronidazole and macrolide Penicillin and rifampin	Penicillin and rifampin

NOTE: For dosages and length of therapy, see Table 2.
*All generations.
†GAS may be resistant.

Table 4 Possible Reasons for Antibiotic Failure or Relapse in GABHS Tonsillitis

Presence of beta-lactamase–producing oral microflora
Resistance (i.e., erythromycin) or tolerance (i.e., penicillin) to antibiotic
Inadequate bacterial interference or production of bacteriocins by oral flora (generally by alpha-hemolytic streptococci)
Bacterial internalization
Inappropriate dose, duration of therapy, or choice of antibiotic
Poor compliance with taking medication
Reacquisition from close contact, or fomite (i.e., toothbrush)
Carrier state, not disease

therapy of recurrent or chronic tonsillitis are penicillin plus rifampin and a macrolide (e.g., erythromycin) plus metronidazole (see Table 3). Referral of a patient for tonsillectomy should be considered only after these medical therapeutic modalities have failed.

Suggested Reading

Bisno AL, et al: Diagnosis and management of group A streptococcal pharyngitis: a practice guideline. Infectious Diseases Society of America, *Clin Infect Dis* 25:574, 1997.

Brook I: The role of beta-lactamase-producing bacteria in the persistence of streptococcal tonsillar infection, *Rev Infect Dis* 6:601, 1984.

Brook I: Treatment of recurrent tonsillitis, penicillin vs. amoxicillin plus clavulanic-potassium, *J Antimicrob Chemother* 24:221, 1989.

Brook I, Foote PA Jr, Slote J: Immune response to *Fusobacterium nucleatum*, *Prevotella intermedia* and other anaerobes in children with acute tonsillitis, *J Antimicrob Chemother* 39:763, 1997.

Brook I, Gober AE: Persistence of group A beta-hemolytic streptococci in toothbrushes and removable orthodontic appliances following treatment of pharyngotonsillitis, *Arch Otolaryngol Head Neck Surg* 124:993, 1998.

Brook I, Yocum P, Friedman EM: Aerobic and anaerobic bacteria in tonsils of children with recurrent tonsillitis, *Ann Otol Rhinol Laryngol* 90:261, 1981.

Dajani AS, et al: Prevention of bacterial endocarditis: recommendations by the American Heart Association, *Clin Infect Dis* 25:1448, 1997.

Pichichero ME, Cohen R: Shortened course of antibiotic therapy for acute otitis media, sinusitis and tonsillopharyngitis, *Pediatr Infect Dis J* 16:680, 1997.

Roos K, Grahm E, Holm SE: Evaluation of beta-lactamase activity and microbial interference in treatment of acute streptococcal tonsillitis, *Scand J Infect Dis* 18:313, 1986.

Shulman ST: Value of new rapid tests for the diagnosis of group A streptococcal pharyngitis, *Pediatr Infect Dis J* 14:923-4, 1995.

OTITIS MEDIA AND EXTERNA

Harris R. Stutman

■ OTITIS MEDIA

Otitis media (OM) is the most common infection for which infants and children seek medical care. In 1990, more than 24 million such visits were reported at a cost of more than $2 billion in the United States. Almost 25% of prescriptions written for antimicrobial agents are for the treatment of acute OM. More than 50% of all children have at least one episode of OM in the first year of life; nearly all have an episode by age 7. In most of the 25% to 30% who have three or more episodes, fluid persists in the middle ear space for weeks to months after an acute episode. This distinction between acute otitis media (AOM) and otitis media with effusion (OME), defined as middle ear fluid without signs or symptoms of acute infection, is important. Although recurrent acute episodes are common in children with OME, more important are studies suggesting that speech, language, and cognitive abilities may be affected by persistent middle ear effusion.

The age of peak incidence for AOM is 6 to 15 months. The age at which the first episode occurs appears to be an important predictor of recurrent episodes. Children whose first episode occurs before 6 months of age are three times as likely to have more than three episodes before the second birthday than other children. Gender, ethnicity, familial crowding, lack of breast-feeding, day care, and exposure to smoking have also been shown to be important risk factors for early and recurrent episodes of AOM. Boys, whites, native Americans, and those with a sibling history of recurrent OM appear most at risk. Breast-feeding appears to be a significant protective factor.

Microbiology

Bacteria are isolated from the middle ear fluid in 70% to 90% of children with acute symptomatic disease, depending on the technical rigor used. The distribution of pathogens has changed little over the past 25 years. Although resistance patterns have changed dramatically, the most common pathogen is consistently *Streptococcus pneumoniae* (30% to 50%), followed by nontypable *Haemophilus influenzae* (15% to 30%) and *Moraxella catarrhalis* (5% to 20%). Although several studies have suggested that patients with pneumococcal otitis may have more severe symptoms and higher fever, it is typically difficult to distinguish among these pathogens by clinical presentation. Less common pathogens include *Streptococcus pyogenes*, *Staphylococcus aureus,* and *Staphylococcus epidermidis*. Gram-negative bacilli and group B streptococcus are occasional pathogens in children younger than 3 months of age. Anaerobic bacteria are very rare in AOM. Respiratory syncytial virus and other respiratory viruses are found in 15% to 20% of middle ear fluid (MEF) aspirates, but in only one third of these cases are independent of bacterial pathogens. Hence they are usually considered predisposing, or copathogens.

Diagnosis

The diagnosis of AOM is based on the clinical findings of an inflamed tympanic membrane (TM) with a purulent middle ear effusion and associated symptoms, including otalgia, fever, and irritability. Progression from the "predisposing" upper respiratory infection (URI) to AOM occurs within 5 days in 50% of cases but may be delayed 7 to 14 days in up to 40% of other URI cases. The typical progression is from an erythematous TM to one that is opaque, then full or bulging as MEF accumulates. Pneumatic otoscopy is indispensable for distinguishing the position (neutral, retracted, bulging) and mobility of the TM. Tympanometry is often useful in confirming the findings on pneumatic otoscopy. This technique assesses TM compliance and middle ear pressure gradients. An abnormal tympanogram suggesting middle ear effusion or lack of compliance is strongly predictive of OM, although some children with abnormal tympanograms do not have OM. Tympanocentesis usually is not required to make a diagnosis of AOM. However, it is useful in establishing microbial etiology in patients with (1) serious illness or toxicity, (2) unsatisfactory response to initial attempts at empiric therapy, (3) immunodeficiency or of neonatal age, or (4) a serious suppurative complication such as mastoiditis or brain abscess.

Therapy

Because most episodes of AOM are associated with bacterial, as opposed to viral, pathogens, antimicrobial therapy is the mainstay of treatment when active management is chosen. Not only has there been a decrease in the frequency of suppurative complications with the advent of antimicrobial therapy, but all evidence indicates that effective antimicrobial therapy eradicates bacteria in MEF. Meta-analysis of available studies shows that the spontaneous rate of resolution of initial episodes of AOM can be as high as 80%, but antimicrobial therapy is still associated with an increase of 13% or more in the resolution rate. Because the characteristics of patients who might respond to shortened or no therapy are not defined, as are the characteristics of those patients who may develop serious suppurative complications, and antibiotics are generally well tolerated, nontreatment of diagnosed AOM cannot be recommended at present. A number of studies have shown that among the common pathogens, S. pneumoniae is more likely to persist in MEF when placebo or ineffective therapy is given, compared with H. influenzae and M. catarrhalis. This strongly suggests that antimicrobial therapy, when given, should be primarily directed at S. pneumoniae (and has led some to suggest that this organism alone should be the target of antibiotic selection). Furthermore, the apparent fact that many ear infections caused by H. influenzae and M. catarrhalis resolve spontaneously leads many to conclude that the approach to unresponsive infections should specifically

focus on enhancing the antipneumococcal coverage. This analysis has been further complicated by the rapid development of drug-resistant S. pneumoniae during the 1990s. Penicillin resistance in pneumococci was initially described in the 1970s but remained a rare phenomenon until recently. Over the past decade, drug-resistant S. pneumoniae (DRSP) has become a common epidemiologic event, approaching 50% of isolates in some studies, with half of these representing high-level resistance.

To try to reach consensus on therapy in this era of increasing DRSP, a working group was convened by the U.S. Centers for Disease Control and Prevention, and their recommendations have been widely publicized. Based on the factors just discussed, and the antimicrobial agents available for use in the management of AOM (Table 1), an approach has been developed. These agents and their activity against S. pneumoniae of varying susceptibility, as well as H. influenzae and M. catarrhalis, are summarized in Table 2. According to these susceptibility patterns in the United States, amoxicillin remains the drug of choice for initial episodes of OM. However, a number of studies have demonstrated that increased dosages of this drug are well tolerated and need to be given to achieve MEF levels consistent with bacterial eradication and clinical response for DRSP. Although traditional dosing (40 mg/kg) may be appropriate in some locations where pneumococcal resistance is low, in most areas these data are not readily available and the high-dose regimen (80 to 90 mg/kg) is recommended. Other studies confirm that amoxicillin can be given in two daily doses (rather than the three doses previously recommended), providing more convenient therapy.

Patients who have received antibiotics in the previous month are more likely to have other resistant bacteria present in MEF, particularly beta-lactamase–producing H. influenzae and M. catarrhalis, and in these cases, alternatives to high-dose amoxicillin are preferred. These include amoxicillin-clavulanate, at the same high dosage of amoxicillin, or cefuroxime axetil. These drugs should be considered for the initial treatment of particularly toxic-appearing or immunocompromised patients, typically pending the results of bacterial culture of MEF and other body fluids. Other agents that might be considered in this circumstance,

Table 1   Antibiotics Useful in the Management of Acute Otitis Media in Children (United States, 1999)

ANTIBIOTIC	DAILY DOSAGE (mg/kg/day)	DOSES PER DAY	ADVERSE EFFECTS
Amoxicillin	80–90	2	
Amoxicillin-clavulanate (new formulation)	80–90 (amoxicillin) (14:1 ratio)	2	Diarrhea, vomiting
Cefuroxime axetil	30	2	
Ceftriaxone (IM)	50	1	
Cefprozil	30	2	
Cefpodoxime	10	2	
Cefixime	8	1	Diarrhea
Ceftibuten	15	1	Diarrhea
Erythromycin-sulfasoxazole	50	3	Vomiting
TMP-SMX	8 (as TMP)	2	Rash, hematologic disorders
Clarithromycin	15	2	

TMP-SMX, Trimethoprim-sulfamethoxazole.

Table 2 Activity of Antimicrobial Agents Against Middle Ear Pathogens

ANTIBIOTIC	PENICILLIN-SUSCEPTIBLE STREPTOCOCCUS PNEUMONIAE	PENICILLIN-INTERMEDIATE S. PNEUMONIAE	PENICILLIN-RESISTANT S. PNEUMONIAE	HAEMOPHILUS INFLUENZAE	MORAXELLA CATARRHALIS
Amoxicillin (high dose)	++	++	+	+	−
Amoxillin-clavulanate	++	++	+	++	++
Cefuroxime	++	++	+/−	+	++
Ceftriaxone	++	++	+	++	++
Cefprozil	++	++	+/−	+	+
Cefixime	+	−	−	++	++
Ceftibuten	+	−	−	++	++
Clindamycin	++	++	++	−	−
Erythromycin-sulfasoxazole	++	+	+/−	++	+
TMP-sulfamethoxazole	++	+	−	++	++

++, Always effective; +, often effective; +/−, occasionally effective.

or when the patient has recently received antibiotic therapy, include cefprozil, cefpodoxime, and intramuscular ceftriaxone. Trimethoprim-sulfamethoxazole and macrolide regimens have also been common choices when amoxicillin cannot or should not be given. However, the cross-resistance between these agents and beta-lactams against DRSP is substantial, and macrolide-resistant *H. influenzae* is also increasingly common. Therefore these drugs have a diminished role in the management of AOM compared with previous assessments.

With effective antimicrobial therapy, the patient should show clinical improvement within 48 to 72 hours. If symptoms persist or progress, the patient should be evaluated for contiguous or disseminated infection, such as mastoiditis or meningitis. The patient originally treated with high-dose amoxicillin and with no evidence of suppurative extension should be given alternative therapy directed against the possibility of resistant bacteria, primarily DRSP. In this analysis, intramuscular ceftriaxone has become a popular alternative to oral regimens such as amoxicillin-clavulanate or cefuroxime axetil. It is given in a single dose of 50 mg/kg and is associated with effective levels of antibiotic in MEF for up to 7 days after the injection. Clinical experience with this regimen is limited, and at least one study has suggested that a three-dose course may be superior to the one-dose regimen. However, this option should be given serious consideration in ill-appearing patients, those having difficulty with oral intake, or those at high risk for resistant organisms because of recent antibiotic exposure. Clindamycin, a drug with high activity against DRSP, might also be considered, but its lack of efficacy against *H. influenzae* and *M. catarrhalis* is a concern if these organisms have not been ruled out. Similarly, the extended-spectrum oral cephalosporins (cefixime, ceftibuten, cefprozil, cefpodoxime) can be considered for the patient failing initial therapy, but their general lack of activity against DRSP and staphylococci is probably even more of a concern. If signs and symptoms persist during or after a second empiric selection, a more precise microbiologic assessment based on MEF obtained at

tympanocentesis can be invaluable, especially in toxic-appearing children. This procedure can identify unsuspected bacterial or viral pathogens and unusual resistance patterns, enabling the clinician to pinpoint additional antimicrobial selections. Tympanocentesis or myringotomy can also be therapeutic, with the resolution of accumulations of MEF resulting from mechanical obstruction or excessively purulent secretion.

The standard duration of oral therapy for AOM remains 10 days, although several studies have appeared suggesting that results with 5- to 7-day courses of amoxicillin or cephalosporin-containing regimens may be similar to that seen with the traditional duration. However, until these results have been confirmed in a number of settings, it appears premature to adopt this shorted duration. Although the risk of recurrent AOM is increased in children with persistent effusion, the use of antibiotics to treat asymptomatic patients with effusion is not recommended. Most such effusions clear without therapy, and the widespread use of antibiotics for this common indication may result in additional adverse effects, as well as contribute to the further emergence of bacterial resistance.

There is no evidence that antihistamines, decongestants, or steroids are useful in the management of AOM. Similarly, there is little evidence that decongestants or antihistamines are useful for OME. The role of oral steroids in OME is controversial. In some studies, children with OME had a better short-term response rate to prednisone than placebo, but the relapse rate was higher in the steroid group. Nevertheless, prednisone, 1 mg/kg/day in two divided doses, combined with antibiotic therapy should be considered before considering otolaryngologic referral. When OME persists for 3 months or longer despite medical therapy and tincture of time, surgical evaluation should be considered. This typically consists of myringotomy with tympanostomy tube insertion. However, adenoidectomy and other procedures to control regional infection may be considered in selected children. Tympanostomy tubes are not without risk; cholesteatoma or persistent perforation occasionally occurs, but there is evidence that their use results in better hearing, at least in the short term.

Children who are otitis prone and at risk for multiple episodes of AOM during the first 3 to 5 years of life typically have their first episodes during the first year of life. Children with frequent episodes of AOM should be evaluated carefully for predisposing factors such as allergy, sinusitis, submucous cleft palate, adenoidal hypertrophy, and immunologic deficiency, including human immunodeficiency virus (HIV). Antimicrobial prophylaxis may significantly reduce the number of recurrences in children without remediable factors. Amoxicillin, 20 mg/kg, and trimethoprim-sulfamothoxazole, 75 mg/kg, have been shown to be effective for this indication when given as a single bedtime dose. Prophylaxis generally should be given during the period of highest incidence of upper respiratory tract infection, winter and early spring. In most studies these agents have resulted in 60% to 75% decreases in the number of AOM episodes. If recurrent episodes continue while the patient is on prophylactic therapy, otolaryngologic referral for consideration of tympanostomy tube placement is appropriate. In one study, 46% of children with tubes remained free of AOM over 6 months, compared with only 5% of controls. The efficacy appears confined to the period that the tubes are in place, however, and tympanostomy tubes can have long-term morbidities. Adenoidectomy should be considered for patients with recurrent otitis media who have failed both antimicrobial and tympanostomy tube therapy and who have a significant degree of adenoidal obstruction of the nasopharynx.

Other complications of OM include local suppurative spread such as mastoiditis, brain abscess, and meningitis, and chronic OM with hearing loss and persistent foul-smelling otorrhea. Chronic OM is typically caused by *Pseudomonas aeruginosa* with or without *S. aureus*. These patients are best managed with instillation of an otic antibiotic suspension, daily suctioning and debridement until the canal is dry, and systemic antibiotic treatment directed against the common pathogens. Subsequent sequelae may require a more aggressive approach, including exploratory tympanostomy, ossiculoplasty, or tympanoplasty.

■ OTITIS EXTERNA

Acute otitis externa (swimmer's ear) is the most common infectious disease of the external ear. It usually follows prolonged exposure of the ear canal to moisture, with maceration leading to secondary bacterial infection. The most common pathogen is *P. aeruginosa*, although other gram-negative bacilli, such as *Escherichia coli* and *Proteus*, are occasional pathogens and gram-positive cocci, including *S. aureus*, are not uncommon. Chronic otitis externa is usually secondary to a persistent suppurative condition of the middle ear following TM perforation and chronic drainage. The flora is similar in the acute and chronic conditions.

In the earliest phases of otitis externa, the canal is edematous and symptoms are limited to otorrhea. Later, pruritus and otalgia may be noted, and the ear drainage may progress from clear to purulent. Finally, the canal may be filled with purulent debris, leading to diminished hearing. Tenderness

of the earlobe and severe pain noted with earlobe traction are common at this point. In addition to the common inflammatory condition, foreign bodies in the ear canal, AOM with perforation, malignant otitis externa, and mastoiditis should be considered.

Therapy

Therapy for acute otitis externa centers on thorough drying and debridement of the external canal, with a topical antibiotic solution used to help eliminate the secondary bacterial pathogens. In minor infections the ear canal is easily rinsed with Burow's solution and dried with cotton-tipped swabs. The patient should avoid getting water into the ear canal during treatment. Ear plugs or cotton pledgets can be used during showers and shampooing, although these should be removed as soon as possible. Swimming should be avoided, even with ear plugs. In more serious infections, purulent material may obstruct an edematous ear canal and should be removed with gentle irrigation and suctioning. If the TM is not perforated, a warmed saline or 2% acetic acid solution may be useful in removing debris. This may be followed with a gentle rinse with a vinegar–isopropyl alcohol solution followed by drying with cotton-tipped swabs or a hair dryer. This procedure of suctioning and irrigation should probably be repeated daily or every other day until the inflammation remits. The 2% acetic acid solution is usually all that is necessary to provide appropriate antibacterial activity, although a variety of pharmaceutical agents (colistin, gentamicin, and others) are available. When the TM is perforated, acetic acid solutions are not well tolerated and are best replaced by commercially available solutions such as neomycin-polymyxin B-hydrocortisone. If there is cellulitis, consider adding an oral antistaphylococcal agent to the regimen.

If otic drops are to be effective, they must be instilled appropriately. Generally, this is best accomplished by having the patient lie with the affected ear up and the canal straightened with gentle tugging of the earlobe. After the drops are instilled, the patient should remain in this position for at least 1 full minute. If the drops do not easily flow down the canal because of edema or inflammation, a cotton wick can be used. The wick should be inserted about 1 cm into the canal and the drops put on it. The medication swells the wick, ensuring that the drops remain in the canal until they can diffuse down the inflamed lumen. Drops are typically used three or four times a day until the inflammation has resolved, generally about 7 days. If pain is severe, systemic analgesics should be used. Acetaminophen or ibuprofen is usually sufficient, although codeine occasionally is necessary.

If infection is severe or associated with a chronic draining middle ear infection, consultation with an otolaryngologist is appropriate. After cultures are obtained for specific microbiologic diagnosis, daily irrigation and debridement are needed. Patients typically should be started on systemic therapy effective against *Pseudomonas* because this is the pathogen most commonly involved. Several investigators have suggested that *S. aureus* is frequent enough to be included in the initial regimen, but I have not found that routinely necessary unless culture results suggest it. Intravenous ceftazidime with or without gentamicin or tobramycin is an appropriate initial regimen. In malignant otitis externa, the infection invades cartilage and bone and may cause neurologic complications such as seventh nerve palsy, meningitis, and brain abscess. It is typically seen in elderly diabetic patients, and diagnosis is best established by computed tomography or magnetic resonance imaging. Treatment requires surgical debridement as well as systemic antibiotics. The causative agent is almost always *Pseudomonas*. (See also the chapters *Pseudomonas* and *Diabetes and Infection*.)

If cellulitis is present or the results of initial cultures document *S. aureus*, nafcillin or cefazolin should be added. For reasons that are not entirely clear, some patients are prone to recurrent external otitis, usually associated with swimming. These patients should avoid prolonged stays in the water under any circumstances, although dermatologic conditions such as eczema and seborrhea may also be considered. In patients who cannot avoid the water, such as competitive swimmers, recurrent otitis externa usually can be prevented by the instillation of a 2% acetic acid solution into the ear canals after swimming and at bedtime.

Suggested Reading

Carlin S, Marchant CD, Shurin PA: Host factors on early therapeutic response in acute otitis media: does symptomatic response correlate with bacterial outcome? *J Pediatr* 18:178, 1991.

Dowell SF, et al: Acute otitis media: management and surveillance in an era of pneumococcal resistance—a report from the DRSP Therapeutic Working Group, *Pediatr Infect Dis J* 18:1, 1999.

Klein JO: Otitis media, *Clin Infect Dis* 19:823, 1994.

Marchant CD, et al: Measuring the comparative efficacy of antibacterial agents for otitis media: the "Pollyanna phenomenon," *J Pediatr* 120:72, 1992.

Rosenfeld RM, et al: Clinical efficacy of antimicrobial drugs to acute otitis media: metaanalysis of 5400 children from 33 randomized trials, *J Pediatr* 124:355, 1994.

Teele DW, et al: Epidemiology of otitis media during the first 7 years of life in children in greater Boston: a prospective cohort study, *J Infect Dis* 160:83, 1989.

SINUSITIS

Andrew M. Shapiro
Charles D. Bluestone

Sinusitis is one of the most commonly recognized diseases in clinical practice, yet definitive diagnostic criteria remain elusive and the optimal therapy is ill defined. The cost of medical and surgical therapy demand a rational approach to this disease. Most patients with acute sinusitis recover without any therapy. Furthermore, the problem of antimicrobial resistance is fueled, in part, by the liberal treatment of routine upper respiratory infections with antimicrobials. The clinician should strive to develop a rational, individualized approach to the patient with sinusitis.

■ SINUS ANATOMY

The paired ethmoid and maxillary sinuses are present at birth, whereas the frontal and sphenoid sinuses appear in early childhood. The sinuses continue to grow into early adult life. The maxillary and anterior ethmoid sinuses drain in a nondependent fashion into the *middle meatus*, lateral to the middle turbinate. The tiny recesses within this *ostiomeatal complex* are the key to normal sinus function and have gradually shifted attention away from the historical dominance of the more easily accessed maxillary sinuses.

■ PATHOGENESIS

Most inflammatory diseases of the nasal mucosa, including viral upper respiratory infections, are associated with an inflammatory response within the paranasal sinuses as well—hence the term *rhinosinusitis*. The normal state of health within the paranasal sinuses depends on maintenance of the mucociliary clearance system. Any process that results in obstruction of the sinus ostia, thickening of nasal secretions, or disturbance of ciliary function will result in overgrowth of pathogens and to the clinical entity of sinusitis (Table 1). Rarely, direct inoculation of bacteria into the sinus (dental disorders, swimming) may result in sinusitis as well.

The bacteriology of sinusitis in both children and adults has been demonstrated in a number of studies through maxillary sinus aspiration or direct culture of the ethmoid sinuses (Table 2). The most common organisms in acute sinusitis remain *Streptococcus pneumoniae*, *Haemophilus influenzae*, and *Moraxella catarrhalis*. The spectrum of organisms widens in chronic sinusitis to include anaerobic bacteria, *Staphylococcus aureus*, and gram-negative organisms. Obviously, the explosive growth of antimicrobial resistance must be considered in the treatment of all patients with sinusitis.

■ DIAGNOSIS

The diagnosis of sinusitis is based on a constellation of historical and physical findings, supported by radiologic imaging and, in selected cases, aspiration of sinus contents. It is often difficult to distinguish between viral upper respiratory infections and acute sinusitis. The most common symptoms—purulent rhinorrhea, nasal congestion, cough,

Table 1   Predisposing Conditions

OBSTRUCTION OF SINUS OSTIA
Nasal septal deviation
Concha bullosa
Hypoplastic maxillary sinus
Polyps
Nasal foreign body
Mucosal edema (e.g., rhinitis)
Nasogastric/nasotracheal tubes
THICKENING OF SECRETIONS
Allergic rhinitis
Viral upper respiratory infection
Cystic fibrosis
CILIARY DYSFUNCTION
Viral upper respiratory dysfunction
Ciliary dyskinesia
OTHER
Immunodeficiency

Table 2   Causative Organisms of Sinusitis

	PERCENTAGE OF ADULT CASES BY SINUS ASPIRATE	
	ACUTE	CHRONIC
BACTERIA		
Streptococcus pneumoniae	40	7
Haeomophilus influenzae	30	10
Moraxella catarrhalis	7	—
Anaerobic bacteria	8	50-100
Staphylococcus aureus	3	17
Streptococcus pyogenes	3	—
Alpha-hemolytic streptococci	3	15
Gram-negative bacteria	—	5
VIRUSES		
Rhinovirus		
Influenza virus		
Parainfluenzia virus		
Adenovirus		

From Evans FO, et al: Sinusitis of the maxillary antrum, *N Engl J Med* 293:735, 1975.

and headache—may be manifestations of a wide variety of nasal disorders. Localized pain involving a sinus or maxillary tooth are more specific indicators but are less commonly encountered. The duration and severity of these signs and symptoms are often the most important clues. The presence of a high fever in conjunction with nasal drainage or progression of symptoms beyond 7 to 10 days may be highly suggestive of acute sinusitis.

Physical examination should include anterior rhinoscopy, which can be accomplished with an otoscope before and after decongestion of the nasal mucosa. One should focus on the middle meatus for edema or purulent drainage, a relatively specific sign of sinusitis. Septal deviation, nasal polyps, and the appearance of the nasal mucosa should be noted. Nasal endoscopy allows a more detailed examination of the middle meatus and nasal airway. Palpation of the sinuses may identify localized tenderness, a fairly reliable localizing clinical indicator. Transillumination may be helpful in adults when either normal or completely absent, but is unreliable in children or in the examination of the ethmoid and sphenoid sinuses.

Plain sinus films may help confirm the diagnosis when acute maxillary sinusitis is suspected, but they are often superfluous. These studies are less reliable in the ethmoid or frontal sinuses, particularly in children. In contrast, the clinical suspicion of chronic sinusitis should routinely be confirmed with computed tomography (CT) scans, which can display subtle pathologic changes within the paranasal sinuses and ostiomeatal complex. Generally, CT scans should be obtained when the patient is not acutely ill and after an appropriate course of therapy. Within this context, this study is considered the gold standard in the evaluation of the sinusitis patient.

■ THERAPY

The treatment of acute sinusitis should be directed at improvement of sinus ventilation and appropriate antimicrobial therapy. Topical decongestants, such as oxymetazolone, reduce mucosal edema and provide relief of nasal obstruction. There is evidence that they may also reduce ciliary beat frequency, but short-term use is unlikely to be detrimental in acute sinusitis. Systemic decongestants and mucolytic agents may facilitate clearance of secretions. There is scant evidence of a role for histamine in acute sinusitis. Thus antihistamines, which tend to thicken secretions and impair drainage, have little role in acute sinusitis.

Antimicrobial therapy for uncomplicated acute sinusitis may be initiated on an empiric basis with an oral agent effective against the common causative organisms. A variety of appropriate antimicrobials are available (Table 3), but studies demonstrating clear advantages of any particular drug are lacking. Many of these agents are not approved by the U.S. Food and Drug Administration (FDA) for sinusitis because of the difficulty in obtaining bacteriologic cure data. Considerable controversy surrounds the appropriate duration of therapy—regimens from 3 days to 3 weeks have been proposed. Most patients would probably recover from acute sinusitis with no therapy. It seems reasonable to use a relatively narrow-spectrum, first-line agent for the patient suffering from an occasional episode of sinusitis. Initial treatment failure, defined as the persistence of symptoms for more than 72 hours after initiation of therapy, can be managed with a diagnostic (and potentially therapeutic) maxillary aspiration or lavage, or by a change to one of the more expensive, broader-spectrum second-line antimicrobials.

Chronic sinusitis has been arbitrarily defined as sinusitis that persists for more than 90 days. It is a common misconception that pathologic changes within the mucosa are irreversible in this setting. In fact, medical therapy directed at the cause of the inflammation is often very helpful in addressing symptoms and pathologic changes. Saline irrigations, topical steroids, systemic antihistamines/decongestants, and allergy therapy should be attempted. Antimicrobial therapy consisting of 3 to 4 weeks of second-line

Table 3 Antimicrobial Therapy

FIRST LINE
Amoxicillin
Trimethoprim-sulfamethoxazole
SECOND LINE
Amoxicillin-clavulanate
Azithromycin
Cefpodoxime proxetil
Ceftibuten
Cefuroxime axetil
Ceprozil
Clarithromycin
Clindamycin
Levofloxacin
Loracarbef

agents may be effective when shorter courses have failed to provide resolution.

An otolaryngologist should evaluate patients with chronic or recurrent sinusitis who fail to respond to these measures. A thorough search for anatomic and physiologic risk factors may define a correctable source for persistent problems. Last, surgery of the paranasal sinuses may be considered. Contemporary approaches to sinus surgery emphasize the restoration of drainage and ventilation through a conservative approach to the sinus ostia, and in particular the ostiomeatal complex. Outcome studies suggest very significant improvement in quality of life scores, and patient satisfaction in most studies exceeds 80%.

■ FUNGAL SINUSITIS

Fungal infections of the sinus constitute a wide spectrum of diseases. *Invasive fungal sinusitis* occurs in the immunocompromised patient, who is typically affected by poorly controlled diabetes, transplant immunosuppression, or hematologic malignancies. The causative organisms are usually *Rhizopus* or *Aspergillis*. Affected patients develop sinus tenderness and fever, and examination reveals progressive edema followed by necrosis of the nasal mucosa. These infections are associated with high mortality and require aggressive therapy. Reversal of the immunocompromised state is ideal, but unfortunately difficult. Surgical debridement to remove necrotic material in conjunction with high-dose amphotericin B is the treatment of choice. A rare, more indolent, form of chronic invasive sinusitis may be seen in immunocompetent patients.

Allergic fungal sinusitis typically is seen in atopic patients predisposed to the development of nasal polyps. The diagnosis can be established by identification of allergic mucin with Charcot-Leyden crystals, eosinophils, and chronic inflammatory cells. Treatment with topical and systemic steroids, antifungal therapy, and conservative surgical debridement can provide significant symptom relief and cure.

Mycetoma, or fungus balls, usually are isolated to a single sinus and may be indistinguishable from routine chronic sinusitis. Treatment is conservative surgery, without the need for additional medical therapy.

■ COMPLICATIONS

Complications usually occur in the setting of acute sinusitis. Infections of the frontal sinus may spread through vascular channels or preformed pathways into the intracranial space, leading to meningitis or intracranial abscesses. Orbital infections, ranging from preseptal cellulitis, to orbital abscess, to cavernous sinus thrombosis may result from ethmoid sinusitis. Treatment consists of high-dose intravenous antibiotic therapy, ideally directed at organisms obtained from culture of the sinuses or abscess. Surgery is usually required to provide drainage of the intracranial or orbital abscess, as well as the affected sinus.

Suggested Reading

Kennedy DW: Prognostic factors, outcomes, and staging in ethmoid sinus surgery, *Laryngoscope* 102:1, 1992.

Williams JW, et al: Clinical evaluation for sinusitis, *Ann Intern Med* 117:705, 1992.

Winther B, Gwaltney JM: Therapeutic approach to sinusitis: anti-infectious therapy as the baseline of management, *Otolaryngol Head Neck Surg* 103(suppl):876, 1990.

DENTAL INFECTION AND ITS CONSEQUENCES

Jennifer Rubin Grandis
Jonas T. Johnson

■ ANATOMY

It is helpful when discussing the manifestations and treatment of odontogenic infections to have an understanding of the fascial spaces surrounding maxillomandibular dentition. Although both maxillary and mandibular teeth can become infected, infections of mandibular dentition are more common. Anatomic spaces involved by maxillary infections include the canine and buccal spaces, with the orbit and cavernous sinus less commonly affected. If untreated, odontogenic infections tend to erode through the thinnest, closest cortical plate. The thinner bone in the maxilla is on the labial-buccal side, the palatal cortex being thicker. The canine space is that region between the anterior surface of the maxilla and the levator labii superioris. Infection of this fascial space usually results from maxillary canine tooth infection. The buccal space is located between the buccinator muscle and the skin and superficial fascia. Infections of this space usually results from maxillary molar processes with the premolars as the rare culprits. Orbital cellulitis or cavernous sinus thrombosis are unusual but serious manifestations of maxillary infection. Under such circumstances, the infection most likely spreads both by direct extension as well as hematogenously.

In the mandible, the thinnest region is on the lingual aspect around the molars and the buccal aspect anteriorly. The primary mandibular spaces include the submental, sublingual, and submandibular fascial spaces. The submental space is that area between the anterior belly of the digastric muscle, the mylohyoid muscle, and the skin. Infection here usually results from the mandibular incisors. Medially, the sublingual and submandibular spaces are typically affected by the mandibular molars. Whether the infection is in the sublingual or submandibular space is determined by the relationship between the area of perforation and the mylohyoid attachment. Specifically, if the apex of the offending tooth is superior to that of the mylohyoid (e.g., premolars, first molar, and occasionally the second molar), the sublingual space is affected; if the infection is inferior (e.g., third molar and occasionally the second molar), the submandibular space is involved. Multiple fascial spaces can be infected simultaneously. For example, the sublingual space lies between the oral mucosa and the mylohyoid and communicates along the posterior bounder of the mylohyoid muscle with the submandibular space. When infection involves the primary mandibular spaces bilaterally it is known as Ludwig's angina.

Odontogenic infection can extend beyond the mandibu-lar spaces to the neck to involve the cervical fascial spaces. The secondary mandibular spaces include the pterygomandibular, masseteric, and temporal spaces. These fascial spaces become infected as the result of secondary spread from more anterior spaces, including the buccal, sublingual, and submandibular spaces. The pterygomandibular space lies between the medial aspect of the mandible and the medial pterygoid muscle. The masseteric space is that area between the lateral mandible and the masseter muscle, and the temporal space is superior and posterior to the pterygomandibular and masseteric spaces. Infection of these areas almost uniformly produces trismus resulting from inflammation of the muscles of mastication.

Infection in these spaces may progress to the deep neck spaces, which include the lateral pharyngeal (parapharyngeal) space, the retropharyngeal space, and the prevertebral space. Infections of these spaces are discussed in detail in the chapter *Deep Neck Infection*. One should keep in mind, however, that up to 30% of deep neck infections may result from odontogenic processes. These so-called deep neck infections may spread distally into the mediastinum.

■ PATHOPHYSIOLOGY

Odontogenic infections and their complications may be encountered by any clinician who treats diseases of the mouth and throat. Most infections are minor and self-limited, confined to the offending tooth and its apex. Under certain circumstances, however, the infectious process may break through the bony, muscular, fascial, and mucosal barriers and spread to contiguous spaces, resulting in soft tissue infections.

Typically, infections originate within the dental pulp, periodontal tissue, or pericoronal tissue from a carious tooth. This results in bacterial invasion and a local inflammatory response, which includes vasodilation and edema leading to increased pressure, which exacerbates the pain and decreases the blood supply. This sequence of events only serves to further the periapical necrosis, with subsequent bacterial invasion into bone and erosion of the bony cortex into surrounding soft tissues. The spreading infection can result in a chronic sinus tract or, under the appropriate circumstances (e.g., perforation of the cortical bone above the muscular attachment), a fascial space collection.

The microbiology of odontogenic infection reflects the normal endogenous oral cavity flora. A large number of bacteria are contained in the mouth, particularly around the dental crevices. These bacteria are primarily anaerobic (species such as *Bacteroides melaninogenicus*, *Fusobacterium nucleatum*, *Peptococcus,* and *Peptostreptococcus*), although gram-positive aerobic organisms (primarily *Streptococci*) are found as well. Infections that result from the spread of these organisms into surrounding soft-tissue spaces are often polymicrobial (e.g., more than one organism may be cultured).

■ DIAGNOSIS

Odontogenic infections commonly present with pain and swelling around the infected tooth (Figure 1). As the infec-

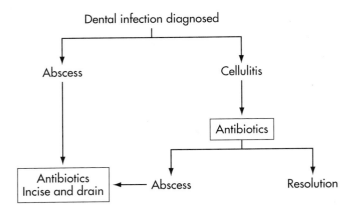

Figure 1
Diagnosis and progression of dental infection.

Table 1   Emergency Considerations
Presence of subcutaneous air
Consider necrotizing fasciitis
Ludwig's angina—progressive severe soft-tissue edema
Consider tracheotomy

tion progresses, a sinus tract may develop as detected by drainage and usually decreased discomfort. If the infection spreads into the surrounding soft tissues and fascial spaces, the signs and symptoms may become systemic and include fever, leukocytosis, and dehydration. It should be noted that with the spread of the infection, local signs and symptoms of odontogenic infection may diminish and the origin of the space infection may seem remote or obscure.

Signs and symptoms of fascial space involvement include swelling of the region (e.g., face, lateral neck), trismus, dysphagia, and airway compromise. To assess the airway for impending compromise, one should note tongue mobility, floor of mouth edema, uvular deviation, and lateral pharyngeal swelling. The presentation of infection of the floor of mouth, or Ludwig's angina, deserves special mention. Patients may develop this widespread fascial space infection as a result of second or third molar infection or wide spread periodontal disease. Cellulitis of the floor of mouth rapidly becomes a spreading, gangrenous process producing elevation and displacement of the tongue and brawny induration of the entire submandibular region. Airway compromise can occur precipitously (Table 1), hence appropriate precautions should be undertaken.

■ THERAPY

Initial evaluation should seek to determine the site and nature of the infectious process. Palpable fluctuation usually indicates abscess. Abscesses located under thick muscles may not be palpable. Under these circumstances, computed tomography (CT) may be invaluable. If abscess is diagnosed, treatment is surgical for drainage.

It is often not difficult to obtain material for Gram stain and culture. One approach is needle aspiration. However, precautions should be taken to obtain the material in a sterile fashion, process it under anaerobic conditions, and make an effort to evaluate the Gram stain before starting antibiotics. The administration of antibiotics is necessary under most circumstances to control the infection. Antibiotics should be administered before surgical drainage or if the process is determined to be in the cellulitic phase. The choice of antimicrobial agent(s) sometimes must be made empirically. In addition, the general condition of the host (e.g., dehydration, predisposing conditions such as diabetes mellitus and immunocompromise) must be taken into consideration when devising a treatment plan. The presence of palpable subcutaneous air or air on radiographs is an indication of infection by gas-forming organisms and is a hallmark of necrotizing fascitis, a surgical emergency.

Choosing an effective antibiotic for an odontogenic infection depends on the ability of the clinician to correctly predict the offending organism(s). As noted, these infections are nearly always polymicrobial and caused by endogenous oral cavity flora. Monotherapy is generally preferable because of the reduced cost, fewer potential side effects, and greater ease of administration. The antibiotic should have activity against oral anaerobes and *Streptococci*.

Penicillin G, once a first choice for odontogenic infection, is rarely used for serious infection because of the rising incidence of penicillin-resistant *Streptococci* in the community as well as the frequency of beta-lactamase–producing *Bacteroides* species (estimated to be greater than 30%). Clindamycin is an effective agent in this setting. Much has been written about metronidazole in the treatment of odontogenic infections. One must keep in mind, however, that although effective against oral anaerobes, this agent has no activity against aerobic organisms and must be used in combination with another antimicrobial. If one chooses a cephalosporin, it should be noted that the higher "generations" tend to sacrifice gram-positive aerobic activity for gram-negative efficacy. First-generation agents, such as cefazolin and cefoxitin, are likely more effective than other, broader-spectrum drugs. Antibiotics should be administered parenterally in the perioperative period (e.g., 24 to 48 hours), but once the drainage catheters are removed and the patient is ready for discharge, the oral route of administration is adequate. Decisions regarding the duration of antimicrobial administration are made empirically, but a 2-week course usually is adequate.

Evacuation of the purulent collection is the standard of care for odontogenic infections. If the process is cellulitis that has not proceeded to abscess, administration of antibiotics may result in resolution. However, the patient must be followed closely and surgery undertaken if abscess ensues. Surgery may entail a minor procedure, such as drainage of a periapical abscess, or extensive debridements of adjacent fascial compartments in the case of necrotizing fasciitis.

The route of drainage should be evaluated on an individual basis. General principles to be followed include stabilization of the airway, protection of vital structures, adequate visualization at the time of drainage, copious irrigation of the abscess cavity with antibiotic-containing solution, and postoperative drainage of the wound. Canine and isolated sublingual space infections can usually be drained transorally. Buccal space infections can be drained transorally or extraorally with care taken to identify Stenson's duct and the buccal branch of the facial nerve. The submental space is best approached extraorally via an incision that parallels the inferior border of the mandibular symphysis. Buccal, submandibular, masseteric, pterygomandibular, and sublingual spaces can all be drained extraorally via a horizontal incision parallel to the inferior angle of the mandible.

Drainage catheters are generally used when a transcutaneous route is used and should be left in place until wound drainage has essentially ceased (<10 ml in 24 hours). In our experience, the catheters do not serve as a route for infection (i.e., to draw bacteria inward). In all cases, special attention should be paid to the status of the airway. In Ludwig's angina, urgent tracheotomy is usually required. Other, less-rapidly progressing maxillomandibular space infections can usually be managed with careful endotracheal intubation. If the airway compromise continues in the postoperative period, the patient should remain intubated or an elective tracheotomy should be performed.

If necrotizing fasciitis is diagnosed based on identification of subcutaneous air or recognition of tissue necrosis at the time of drainage, the wound must be opened widely, necrotic tissue debrided, and the wound packed open for observation and potential further debridement. Hyperbaric oxygen administration may be beneficial in this circumstance.

The successful treatment of these infections depends on a combination of accurate diagnosis and institution of appropriate therapy in a timely fashion. Adjunctive laboratory and radiographic tests may confirm the diagnosis and help plan the drainage procedure, but a thorough history and physical examination often provides the clinician with sufficient information.

Suggested Reading

Bridgeman A, Weisenfeld D, Newland S: Anatomical considerations in the diagnosis and management of acute maxillofacial bacterial infections, *Aust Dent J* 41:238, 1996.

Gill Y, Scully C: Orofacial odontogenic infections: review of microbiology and current treatment, *Oral Surg Oral Med Oral Pathol* 70:155, 1990.

Krishnan V, Johnson JV, Helfrick JF: Management of maxillofacial infections: a review of 50 cases, *J Oral Maxillofac Surg* 51:868, 1993.

Langford FP, et al: Treatment of cervical necrotizing fasciitis with hyperbaric oxygen therapy, *Otolaryngol Head Neck Surg* 112:274, 1995.

Mandel L: Diagnosing protracted submasseteric abscess: the role of computed tomography, *J Am Dent Assoc* 127:1646, 1996.

Peterson LJ: Contemporary management of deep infections of the neck, *J Oral Maxillofac Surg* 51:226, 1993.

INFECTION OF THE SALIVARY AND LACRIMAL GLANDS

Ray Y. Hachem
Issam Raad

Sialadenitis, an infection of the salivary glands, is a relatively common disease. Sialadenitis can be acute, subacute, or chronic in nature, and it can be of bacterial or viral origin. Bacterial infections may reach the salivary gland tissue mostly via the ductal system, whereas viral infections invade the salivary glands via the bloodstream. The incidence of bacterial sialadenitis is in direct relation to factors such as old age, nutritional and health status, trauma, anatomic abnormalities, and use of drugs that decrease the salivary flow. Several etiologic predisposing local and systemic generalized factors play an important role in the development and course of sialadenitis (Table 1).

Table 1   Etiologic Classification of Sialadenitis
ACUTE BACTERIAL SIALADENITIS
Acute purulent parotitis
Acute postoperative parotitis
Acute bacterial submandibular sialadenitis
CHRONIC BACTERIAL SIALADENITIS
Chronic recurrent parotitis
Chronic sclerosing sialadenitis of submandibular gland
Obstructive sialadenitis
VIRAL SIALADENITIS
Parotitis epidemica (mumps)
Cytomegalovirus infection (salivary gland viral disease)
Other types (coxsackievirus, infectious mononucleosis, measles, encephalomyocarditis [EMC] virus, Echovirus)
GRANULOMATOUS SIALADENITIS
Giant cell sialadenitis
Tuberculosis

■ ACUTE BACTERIAL SIALADENITIS

Acute bacterial sialadenitis, also called *suppurative sialadenitis,* mainly affects the parotid and submandibular glands. Sialadenitis of the intraoral and sublingual glands is rare. This may be because the serous saliva produced by the parotid gland has less bacteriostatic activity or because of a secretory disorder that changes the amount and chemical composition of saliva, including most of the protein, mucins, and electrolytes. Primary acute bacterial parotitis (ABP) has been reported mainly in elderly patients with dehydration, malnutrition, liver cirrhosis, or diabetes mellitus. Acute parotitis has only occasionally been observed in premature infants. The use of antisialanogic drugs, the most common being diuretics, has been associated with acute bacterial sialadenitis. Acute postoperative parotitis as a special type of acute purulent parotitis is observed particularly after a major abdominal operation accompanied by large fluid losses and reduction of salivary secretions.

Pathogenic organisms are mostly *Staphylococcus aureus*, followed by group A streptococcus and *Streptococcus viridans*. Strict anaerobes such as *Fusobacterium nucleatum* and *Peptostreptococcus anaerobius* also may play a role. Recent reports show an increasing incidence of gram-negative rods, especially in seriously ill patients, who tend to be colonized by these bacteria. Clinically, the patient experiences an intense radiating pain in the affected side of the face. General malaise and fever with erythema and swelling are common. Some patients complain of limited movement of the mandible and difficulty in swallowing. In some cases disturbance of the facial nerve may be noticed. Sometimes, a toxic state of mental obtundation occurs. In this situation aggressive treatment is required because the mortality rate is high. The diagnosis of sialadenitis is based on the clinical presentation, Gram stain, and culture of the purulent material from Stensen's duct. Laboratory findings commonly include marked leukocytosis, with a shift to left. A plain film of the parotid gland may be useful to detect stones; however, this is not a common situation in parotitis. The use of sialography is discouraged because of the often painful swelling. Treatment of ABP consist of (1) eliminating the cause (e.g., a mucous plug) by using adequate hydration to increase the salivary flow and (2) using systemic antibiotics that cover gram-positive cocci, spirochetes, and mouth anaerobes while awaiting the results of Gram stain and cultures. In cases involving abscess formation, incision and drainage are indicated. Drainage is done by surgical exposure of the gland and penetration of the capsule by blunt probing. A semisynthetic antistaphylococcal penicillin such as nafcillin usually is adequate as initial empiric treatment; first-generation cephalosporins are good alternatives. Quinolones and third-generation cephalosporins may be added, especially in the seriously ill hospitalized patient in whom infection with gram-negative rods is increasing (Table 2). Adjuvant treatment should include optimal oral hygiene, discontinuation of anticholinergic drugs that reduce salivary flow or increase the viscosity of the saliva, and use of sialagogic agents such as lemon juice. Irradiation of the glands is no longer recommended. Needle aspiration of the gland is not indicated because it is a blind procedure that endangers the facial nerve and does not provide adequate drainage.

Acute bacterial submandibular sialadenitis (ABSS), unlike ABP, often is associated with obstruction of Wharton's duct by stones or structures. Predisposition to stone formation in the submandibular gland is caused by the alkalinity, calcium concentrations in its secretions, and anatomic factors such as the length and tortuosity of Wharton's duct. Medical treatment is the same as that for ABP. If ductal calculi are present, excision is the only effective treatment. Excision can be done by ductal dilation or sialolithotomy depending on the location. Repeated ductal stone formation may cause chronic submandibular infection, in which case surgical excision of the gland is indicated.

Subacute necrotizing sialadenitis (SANS) is a recently described inflammatory disease of unknown origin. It usually affects the palatal salivary glands. Clinically, the patient has pain, swelling, or both. The main etiologic factor seems to be infarction of the salivary gland by ischemic injury as a result of surgery or trauma. Nevertheless, it remains possible that SANS is part of necrotizing sialometaphasia.

■ CHRONIC BACTERIAL SIALADENITIS

Chronic bacterial sialadenitis, also called *recurrent bacterial sialadenitis,* involves the parotid or submandibular glands. Chronic (adult) parotitis can follow a subclinical course. The infection usually occurs via the excretory duct. Inflammation of the oral mucosa and a decreased salivary flow may lead to an ascending or retrograde infection in the major salivary glands. This chronic infection sometimes is associated with Sjögren's syndrome, in which case manifestations of xerostomia and systemic autoimmune disease are present.

Table 2 Treatment of Sialadenitis		
	ANTIBIOTIC TREATMENT	**SURGICAL TREATMENT**
Acute bacterial sialadenitis	· Susceptible gm+: penicillinase-resistant penicillin or first-generation cephalosporin · Resistant gm+ (MRSA, *S. pneumoniae*): vancomycin · Gm−: third-generation cephalosporin, quinolone · Anaerobes: metronidazole or clindamycin	Parotid drainage may be needed; silolithectomy in submandibular infection
Chronic bacterial sialadenitis	Same as above	Gland extirpation usually required
Viral sialadenitis	None; symptomatic treatment	None
Granulomatous sialadenitis	Directed to specific cause	Rarely needed

Gm+, Gram positive; *gm−,* gram negative; *MRSA,* multiresistant *Staphylococcus aureus.*

Chronic juvenile recurrent parotitis is a combination of a congenital malformation of a portion of the salivary ducts and infections ascending from the mouth following dehydration in children. Boys are affected more often than girls. The clinical course is characterized by recurrent episodes of acute sialadenitis of either the parotid or submandibular glands. Although the inflammation may occur bilaterally, the symptoms of a painful swelling are often unilateral. In cases involving swelling in the parotid glands area, salivary gland neoplasm should be considered, as well as sialadenitis and lymphadenopathies, which may be caused by variety of diseases, including cat-scratch disease, toxoplasmosis, and neoplasm. As in acute parotitis, culturing of the saliva is recommended. Several studies have identified *S. viridans* as the most common causative organism followed, by *Staphylococcus aureus*, *Streptococcus pneumoniae*, and mixed aerobic-anaerobe oral flora. Involvement of a specific microorganism, such as *Mycobacterium tuberculosis* or actinomyces, is rare.

Sialography, which involves the retrograde injection of a radiopaque dye into the main excretory duct, is the most important tool in establishing a diagnosis of chronic parotitis. In addition to plain radiographs, computed tomography (CT) sialography may provide additional and more detailed information. Scintigraphy is considered a useful diagnostic aid in chronic recurrent parotitis, especially in patients in whom sialography cannot be performed. Ultrasound examination is not very useful in detecting chronic inflammation. Laboratory data commonly show a persistent elevation of the erythrocyte sedimentation rate. Histologically, in chronic parotitis the parenchymal structures may largely be replaced by fibrosis and fat. The ducts often are dilated and surrounded by a dense lymphocytic infiltrate. Initial treatment should be conservative; patients with chronic parotitis should be instructed to massage the involved gland carefully in a dorsoventral direction four to six times a day and to eat sour foods to stimulate parotic secretion. Systemic antibiotic irrigation and proper oral hygiene have been advocated as effective treatment. Despite medical treatment, some patients require surgical management. Submandibular sialadenitis usually presents earlier, is secondary to calculi, and requires early intervention. Parotidectomy with facial nerve dissection is preferred.

CHRONIC SCLEROSING SIALADENITIS

Chronic sclerosing sialadenitis of the submandibular gland is a chronic inflammatory process that produces a firm, swollen submandibular area that is difficult to distinguish from a tumor. In 50% of the cases, it is associated with sialolithiasis and is most commonly seen in the elderly. The inflammatory process can be focal or a diffuse lymphocytic infiltrate with varying degrees of intensity.

OBSTRUCTIVE SIALADENITIS

Obstructive sialadenitis is the most common type of sialadenitis. Of the cases, 37% are localized in the submandibular gland, 30% in the salivary glands, and 20% in the parotid gland. The remaining 13% are in the sublingual glands. Two distinguishing factors play a role in the pathogenesis of obstructive sialadenitis. One is a mechanical obstruction, including a salivary cyst and tumor or a lesion of the oral mucosa. The other is a disturbance of the secretory changes in electrolyte concentration, leading to the development of a viscous secretory product.

VIRAL SIALADENITIS

Viral infection of the salivary glands is a common condition, mainly affecting the parotid glands. Mumps, a paramyxovirus, is by far the most common virus producing clinically significant parotitis. This disease is contagious and is transmitted by droplets of saliva. Mumps is predominantly a childhood disease and is more common in boys than in girls. Young adults also may be affected and have a more aggressive clinical course. Mumps often is preceded by a viral infection in the oral cavity or the nose, leading to viremia and hematogenous infection of the salivary glands. Apart from the major salivary glands, the testes, meninges, pancreas, and mammary glands may become involved. The incubation period is approximately 3 weeks, followed by 1 to 2 days of fever, chills, headache, and jaw pain with chewing. Rapid and painful swelling of the parotid gland follows. The submandibular glands also may become involved. In 30% to 40% of infected patients, no clinical symptoms have been noticed. The virus can be isolated from the saliva during the first week of the clinical manifestation of the disease. During this period, leukopenia with relative lymphocytosis and elevation of serum analyses is observed. Serologic diagnosis can be made using a complement-binding reaction or a fourfold increase in antibody titer, usually at the end of the second week. With the exception of vaccination, no effective treatment for mumps is available. Cytomegalovirus (CMV) sialadenitis is rare and usually presents as painful salivary gland and swelling. The diagnosis typically is based on an elevated complement fixation titer of antibodies to CMV, a positive CMV titer, and detection of CMV in the salivary gland. Other viruses that produce sialadenitis are coxsackievirus, measles, echovirus, influenza A, parainfluenza, and Epstein-Barr virus. Most of these viral infections are self-limiting and produce lifelong immunity.

GRANULOMATOUS SIALADENITIS

A rare condition, granulomatous sialadenitis is most often secondary to regional lymph node involvement rather than involvement of the gland parenchyma itself. Granulomatous giant cell sialadenitis is mostly localized in the submandibular gland. The inflammatory reaction is caused by obstruction of the ducts and development of granulomas with multinuclear foreign body giant cells. Tuberculosis is the most common type of granuloma and starts mostly from the parotid and submandibular lymph nodes. Clinically, there is a firm, nontender swelling of the gland that resembles a tumor more than parotitis. Most patients have simultaneous pulmonary tuberculosis. The diagnosis may be established by acid-fast bacilli (AFB) smear and culture of the salivary gland drainage if present. Tissue biopsy with culture may be necessary to make the diagnosis.

Treatment, as in other forms of extrapulmonary tuberculosis, consists of a three- to four-drug regimen that usually includes isoniazid, rifampin, ethambutol, and pyrazinamide. The duration of therapy depends on the clinical response but usually is 6 to 9 months. Surgical excision of salivary tissue is rarely needed. Atypical *Mycobacterium* infection most often affects children and usually presents as facial or cervical masses that may drain spontaneously. As in tuberculosis, the diagnosis is based on AFB smears and cultures. Chemotherapy should be based on the kind of atypical *Mycobacterium* isolated and the susceptibility pattern. Actinomycosis usually is caused by *Actinomyces israelii*, which can be part of the oral flora, particularly in patients with dental caries. It may present as acute suppurative parotitis or have a more chronic course. The diagnosis is based on smears and cultures of draining material or tissue biopsy. Surgical drainage and high dosages of penicillin for a prolonged period are indicated.

Other agents that have been reported to cause granulomatous sialadenitis include syphilis, tularemia, toxoplasmosis, cat-scratch disease, blastomycosis, and coccidioidomycosis. Xanthogranulomatous sialadenitis of the parotid gland presenting as B-cell lymphoma has also been reported.

■ LACRIMAL SYSTEM INFECTION

Infection of the lacrimal system includes three types: (1) canaliculitis, (2) dacryocystitis, and (3) dacryoadenitis.

Canaliculitis

Canaliculitis is inflammation of the canaliculi that leads to obstruction of the lumen. It presents clinically as conjunctivitis and is associated with excessive tears. *Staphylococcus* and *Actinomycosis* species and *Arachnia propionica* are commonly implicated. Other organisms less frequently causing canaliculitis include *Fusobacterium, Enterobacter cloacae,* nocardia, *Candida albicans,* and aspergillus. Viruses like herpes also can be involved. The diagnosis is based on isolation of the organism from the lacrimal passage and fluroescein to see the patency of the duct lumen. Treatment consists of topical antibiotics. Eyedrops with penicillin or macrolides may be used (see Table 2).

Dacryocystitis

Dacryocystitis is a common infection of the lacrimal sac. It can be either an acute or chronic infection. Dacryocystitis often occurs in children as a complication of congenital or acquired nasolacrimal proximal or distal duct obstruction of the drainage system. In the neonate period it often results from dacryocele and presents as a duct cyst. In older infants and children, nasolacrimal duct obstruction may occur as a consequence of ethmoidal sinusitis or facial fracture. Clinically, it presents with epiphora (i.e., excessive tearing) and an acute onset of suppuration associated with cellulitis of the tissue surrounding the lacrimal sac. The most common organisms isolated in the acute stage are *S. aureus, S. pneumoniae,* gram-negative rods (*P. aeruginosa, Haemophilus influenzae*) and rarely *Sternotrophomonas maltophilia,* in which case quinolones are recommended for the treatment of chronic dacryocystitis. *S. pneumoniae* is by far the most common organism responsible for dacryocystitis. The diagnosis can be made by isolation of the organism or radiographically by dacryocystography, CT, or scintigraphy. Treatment consists of hot compresses applied to the affected area and systemic antibiotics based on Gram stain and cultures results. Surgical intervention is indicated for an abscess or when the symptoms do not resolve with medical therapy (Table 3).

Dacryoadenitis

Dacryadenitis is inflammation of the lacrimal gland. It usually is present as localized tenderness and swelling of the eyelid. Acute bacterial infections can be caused by pyogenic bacteria such as *S. aureus* and streptococci. Viral infections with mumps and infectious mononucleosis are most often implicated as causes. Clinically, patients with acute dacryoadenitis complain of severe pain in the lacrimal gland region, edema, and redness and swelling, whereas in chronic dacryoadenitis, only minimal eyelid edema and mild tenderness can be observed. Chronic infection of the lacrimal gland can be associated with various infectious and noninfectious causes. Tuberculosis, syphilis, leprosy, and schistosomiasis have been reported. Management of dacryoadenitis includes symptomatic treatment with local hot compresses or systemic antibiotics when bacteria are the cause. If symptoms persist or an orbital abscess develops, surgical drainage is necessary.

Table 3 Treatment of Lacrimal System Infection

	ANTIBIOTIC TREATMENT	SURGICAL TREATMENT
Canaliculits	Topical antibiotic drop plus antibiotic irrigation of canaliculi (penicillin G) plus oral penicillin V or macrolides	None
Acute dacrocystitis		
Neonatal (duct cyst)	Topical antibiotic drops or IV plus oral cephalosporin antibiotic	Duct-probing nasal endoscopy
Preseptal cellulitis	IV antibiotics	Duct probing
Trauma	IV antibiotics	Dacryocystorhicostomy nasolacrimal intubation
Chronic dacryocystitis	IV antibiotics	Endoscopic intranasal, dacryocystorhinostomy
Acute dacryoadenitis	Systemic antibiotics	Incision and drainage if spontaneous resolution does not occur
Chronic dacryoadenitis	Directed toward specific cause	Rarely required

IV, Intravenous.

Suggested Reading

Aetological and histological classification of sialadenitis, *Pathologica* 89:7, 1997.

Batsakis JG: Granulomatous sialadenitis, *Ann Otol Rhinol Laryngol* 100:166, 1991.

Campolattaro BN, Lueder GT, Tychsen L: Spectrum of pediatric dacryocystitis: medical and surgical management of 54 cases, *J Pediatr Ophthal Strabismus* 34:143, 1997.

Goldberg MH: Infections of the salivary glands. In Topazian RG, Goldberg MH, eds. *Oral and maxillofacial infection,* Philadelphia, 1994, WB Saunders.

Johnson A: Inflammatory conditions of the major salivary glands, *Ear Nose Throat* 68:94, 1989.

Newel FW: The lacrimal system. In Newell FW, ed. *Ophthalmology principles and concepts,* St Louis, 1992, Mosby.

Raad II, Sabbagh MF, Caranasos GJ. Acute bacterial sialadenitis: a study of 29 cases and review, *Rev Infect Dis* 12:591, 1990.

DEEP NECK INFECTIONS

Jeremy D. Gradon

Infections of the various anatomic spaces of the deep neck structures are uncommon. However, when they occur they often do so in hosts with underlying immunocompromising conditions such as diabetes mellitus or neutropenia. An odontogenic source of these infections is the most common etiology. These infections often are life-threatening and require prompt recognition and an organized, well-coordinated multidisciplinary management plan to maximize the likelihood of successful clinical outcome. In general, computed tomography (CT) scanning of the neck is an excellent diagnostic modality and is critical in the diagnosis and management of these infections. As a general caveat, these patients are so critically ill that when they go for radiologic studies they must be accompanied by a physician at all times in case of acute clinical deterioration or airway compromise.

Most of these infections are polymicrobial, reflecting the flora of the oral cavity from which most of the infecting organisms arise. Anaerobic bacteria inhabit the gingival crevice at a concentration of more than 10^{11} organisms per milliliter. The commonly encountered pathogens are outlined in Table 1.

Table 1 Pathogens Encountered in Deep Neck Space Infections	
COMMON	**RARE**
Viridans and other streptococci	*Moraxella*
Staphylococcus aureus and coagulase-negative species	*Haemophilus* sp.
Bacteroides sp.	*Pseudomonas* sp.
Prevotella sp.	*Actinomyces* sp.

■ RELEVANT ANATOMY OF THE DEEP NECK SPACES

To understand the clinical course and appropriate management of deep neck space infections, the clinician must have at least a rudimentary grasp of the relevant anatomy. This knowledge provides a basis for understanding the potential complications and routes of spread of these infections. The deep neck spaces are anatomically distinct but can connect, allowing spread of infection. The important areas are as follows:

· The submandibular space
· The lateral pharyngeal spaces—anterior and posterior
· The retropharynx—retropharyngeal space, the "danger" space, and the prevertebral space

Submandibular Space Infections ("Ludwig's Angina")

Infections of the submandibular space originate most often by spread from the lower molar teeth and are more common in persons with diabetes, lupus, or neutropenia. Patients experience the acute onset of fever, mouth pain, drooling of oral secretions, brawny edema of the submandibular soft tissues, and stiff neck (Figure 1). Patients may progress to develop sudden airway obstruction from upward and backward displacement of the tongue or tracheal compression from surrounding edema. Management is outlined in Table 2, and complications are listed in Table 3.

Lateral Pharyngeal Space Infections

Infection of the lateral pharyngeal spaces may occur as a secondary complication of submandibular space infections or complicate dental, salivary gland, local lymph node, or retropharyngeal space infections. In inner-city areas, intravenous drug use with insertion of nonsterile needles into the lateral pharyngeal space (attempting to access the jugular vein) is the most common cause. Overall, lateral pharyngeal abscess is the most common of the deep neck space infections. Patients have neck pain, fever, and rigors. Trismus occurs if the anterior compartment of this space is involved. Infection of the posterior compartment is not associated with trismus or obvious externally visible neck swelling. Complications of lateral pharyngeal space infection are

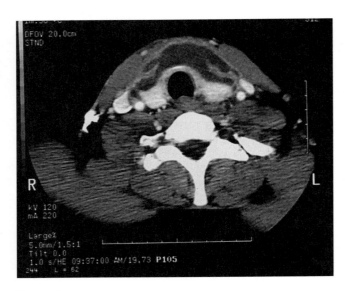

Figure 1
CT scan of the neck in Ludwig's angina showing multiple low-density lesions with rimlike enhancement in the sub-mandibular region, more prominent on the right than on the left side.

Table 2   Management of Deep Neck Space Infections

· Computed tomography scan of mouth/neck/mediastinum (with medical supervision throughout) to evaluate for drain-able collections, airway impingement, major vascular occlu-sions, mediastinal involvement
· Protection of airway—otolaryngology evaluation essential
· Dental evaluation for odontogenic source of infection
· Correction of the underlying medical problems—maximize glycemic control, treat neutropenia
· Intravenous antibiotics (for at least 7 days or until stable based on clinical course):

Penicillin G 3 million units IV q4h, *plus* metronidazole 500 mg IVPB q6h

or

Ampicillin-sulbactam 3 g IV q6h (*plus* gentamicin 1.5 mg/kg q8h if immunocompromised)

or

Ticarcillin-clavulanate 3.1 g IV q6h (*plus* gentamicin 1.5 mg/kg q8h if immunocompromised)

or

Imipenem-cilastatin 500 mg IV q6h
Clindamycin 600 mg IV q8h, *plus* gentamicin 1.5 mg/kg q8h

IV, Intravenously; *IVPB*, intravenous piggyback.

---

listed in Table 3. Management of lateral pharyngeal space infections is outlined in Table 2.

Retropharyngeal Space Infections (Retropharyngeal, "Danger," and Prevertebral Space Infections)
Retropharyngeal Space
Patients have fever, sore throat, dysphagia, toxicity, and neck stiffness. Intraoral examination often will demonstrate bulg-ing or swelling of the posterior pharyngeal soft tissues.

Table 3   Complications of Deep Neck Space Infections

DEEP NECK SPACE	COMPLICATIONS
Submandibular space	Acute airway obstruction
	Aspiration pneumonia
	Tongue necrosis
	Carotid artery erosion
	Jugular vein thrombosis
	Spread to the lateral pharyngeal space
Lateral pharyngeal space	
Anterior	Spread of infection to the parotid gland
Posterior	Carotid artery erosion
	Suppurative jugular vein thrombosis
	Cranial nerve palsies (IX-XII)
Retropharyngeal space	Respiratory distress
	Decompression into posterior oral cavity
Danger space	Spread of infection to the mediastinum
	Spread of infection to the pleural space
Prevertebral space	Spread of infection along vertebral column
	Cervical vertebral osteomyelitis
Lemierre syndrome	Jugular venous thrombosis
	Septic pulmonary emboli
	Dyspnea (from edema of epiglottis/larynx)

Table 4   Management of Lemierre Syndrome

· Intravenous antibiotics (for at least 7 days or longer based on clinical course):

Ampicillin-sulbactam 3 g IV q6h

or

Clindamycin 600 mg IV q8h

or

Metronidazole 500 mg IV q6h

· Drainage of metastatic abscesses (other than septic pulmanry emboli)
· Rarely: ligation and resection of the infected vein (for unre-lenting sepsis)
· No clear role for anticoagulation

Respiratory distress may occur if the swelling impinges on the supraglottic area.

"Danger" Space
The "danger" space is an anatomic potential space that connects the deep neck with the mediastinum. The anterior mediastinum is reached via the pretracheal fascia to the parietal pericardium and the posterior mediastinum via the danger space from the retropharyngeal area. These connec-tions may result in one of the most feared complications of deep neck infections, namely, spread of infection to the mediastinum with the development of acute mediastinitis. Conversely, postoperative mediastinal infections may track up to the retropharyngeal space and present as an apparent primary neck problem.

Prevertebral Space

This fascial plane runs from the base of the skull to the coccyx along the anterior borders of the vertebrae. Thus infection in this space may potentially spread from the retropharyngeal area along the whole length of the vertebral column. The management of retropharyngeal space infections is outlined in Table 2, and complications are listed in Table 3.

■ LEMIERRE SYNDROME

Lemierre syndrome is the eponym describing jugular vein septic thrombophlebitis. This infection usually is anaerobic, most commonly caused by *Fusobacterium necrophorum.*

Patients have fever, systemic toxicity, and tenderness to palpation along the angle of the jaw and the sternocleidomastoid muscle. Trismus is not a feature. Complications of this infection include persistent bacteremia and cavitating septic pulmonary emboli. The management of Lemierre syndrome is outlined in Table 4.

Suggested Reading

Chen MK, et al: Predisposing factors of life-threatening deep neck infection: logistic regression analysis of 214 cases, *J Otolaryngol* 27:141, 1998.

el-Sayed Y, Dousary S: Deep neck space abscesses, *J Otolaryngol* 25:277, 1996.

Gidley PW, Ghorayeb BY, Stiernberg CM: Contemporary management of deep neck space infections, *Otolaryngol Head Neck Surg* 116:16, 1997.

Gradon JD: Space-occupying and life-threatening infections of the head, neck and thorax, *Infect Dis Clin North Am* 10:857, 1996.

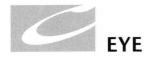

CONJUNCTIVITIS

Bhavna P. Sheth
Robert A. Hyndiuk

Infection of the conjunctiva is a common cause of red eyes. Although most cases resolve without sequelae, infections such as *Neisseria gonorrhoeae,* herpes simplex virus, keratoconjunctivitis, and trachoma can result in significant loss of vision.

Common symptoms of conjunctivitis, depending on the causative agent, include redness, discharge, tearing, foreign body sensation, and transient blurring of vision with blinking. Symptoms such as vision loss, marked pain, and photophobia suggest a more severe disease process such as glaucoma, iritis, or keratitis (Table 1). Clinical findings may include conjunctival follicles, papillae, and/or preauricular adenopathy.

Gram stain and culture aid in identifying the causative agent and its susceptibility to antibiotics but are not essential in most cases of mild conjunctivitis. They are mandatory in hyperacute conjunctivitis and neonatal conjunctivitis to evaluate for *N. gonorrhoeae.*

Even though most cases of conjunctivitis are self-limited, antibiotic therapy for bacterial conjunctivitis is suggested to reduce the risk of complications, recurrence, and transmission to other individuals.

■ BACTERIAL CONJUNCTIVITIS

Bacterial conjunctivitis may be subdivided into hyperacute, acute, and chronic cases.

Hyperacute Bacterial Conjunctivitis

Hyperacute purulent conjunctivitis is usually caused by the *Neisseria* species. *N. gonorrhoeae* most commonly occurs in sexually active young adults. The usual mode of transmission is by autoinoculation from infected genitalia. Signs include unilateral or bilateral marked conjunctival redness, chemosis, purulent discharge, and preauricular adenopathy. *N. gonorrhoeae* is one of the few bacteria that cause preau-

Table 1 Red Eye: Differential Features

	CONJUNCTIVITIS			KERATITIS		IRITIS	GLAUCOMA (ACUTE)
	BACTERIAL	VIRAL	ALLERGIC	BACTERIAL	VIRAL		
Blurred vision	0	0	0	+++	0 to ++	+ to ++	++ to +++
Pain	0	0	0	++	0 to +	++	++ to +++
Photophobia	0	0	0	++	++	+++	+ to ++
Discharge	Purulent + to +++	Watery + to ++	White, ropy +	Purulent +++	Watery +	0	0
Injection	+++	++	+	+++	+	0 to + (limbal)	+ to ++ (limbal)
Corneal haze	0	0	0	+++	+ to ++	0	+ to +++
Ciliary flush	0	0	0	+++	+	+++ to +++	+ to ++
Pupil	Normal	Normal	Normal	Normal or miotic (iritis)	Normal	Miotic	Mid-dilated Nonreactive
Pressure	Normal	Normal	Normal	Normal	Normal	Normal, low or high	High
Preauricular nodes	Rare	Usual	0	0	0	0	0
Smear	Bacteria PMNs	Lymphs	Eosinophil	Bacteria PMNs	0	0	0
Therapy	Antibiotics	Nonspecific	Nonspecific	Antibiotics	Antivirals (if herpes)	Cycloplegia Topical steroids	Medical or surgical

+, Mild; ++, moderate; +++, severe; *PMNs,* polymorphonucleocytes.

ricular adenopathy. This infection is rapidly progressive, with potential for severe ocular destruction resulting from the bacteria's capability of invading intact conjunctival and corneal epithelium and causing severe corneal ulcers and vision loss. A Gram stain to identify intracellular gram-negative diplococci and a culture are necessary in all suspected cases. Systemic treatment with adjunctive topical treatment is required for gonococcal conjunctivitis (Table 2). Also, frequent topical irrigation with saline is recommended. Affected patients are commonly coinfected with chlamydia and require treatment with oral tetracycline, erythromycin, or doxycycline for a week.

Neisseria meningitidis is a rare cause of hyperacute conjunctivitis. Clinical features are similar to those described for gonococcal conjunctivitis, except *N. meningitidis* tends to affect younger individuals. Although primary meningococcal infection of the conjunctiva can occur, the conjunctivitis is more commonly seen secondary to meningococcal septicemia. Systemic treatment, as outlined for gonococcal conjunctivitis, is required to prevent dissemination.

Acute Bacterial Conjunctivitis

Acute bacterial conjunctivitis is characterized by an abrupt onset of conjunctival hyperemia, mild to moderate mucopurulent discharge, and mild foreign body sensation. The disease lasts less than 3 to 4 weeks. Common causative agents include *Streptococcus pneumoniae*, *Haemophilus* species, and *Staphylococcus aureus*.

S. pneumoniae causes a bilateral, self-limited conjunctivitis with small petechial subconjunctival hemorrhages. Infections tend to occur in epidemics in temperate climates. *Haemophilus influenzae* produces a similar acute catarrhal conjunctivitis and is a common cause of infection in children. Systemic symptoms, including fever, otitis media, and upper respiratory infection, may also be present. The Koch-Weeks bacillus, a subtype (aegyptius) of *H. influenzae*, also causes an acute mucopurulent conjunctivitis. In contrast to *S. pneumoniae*, the Koch-Weeks bacillus produces epidemics in warm climates. *S. aureus* is the predominant pathogen implicated in both acute and chronic conjunctivitis in adults.

Treatment of routine acute bacterial conjunctivitis with topical antibiotics, such as bacitracin, erythromycin, combinations of neomycin and polymyxin, or trimethoprim-polymyxin four times a day for 7 days is appropriate. With *H. influenzae* infections, systemic antibiotics should be added if systemic symptoms or otitis media is present. Aminoglycosides, gentamicin and tobramycin, and the topical fluoroquinolones ciprofloxacin and ofloxacin are also effective against most pathogens, but their use is often reserved for treatment of severe or resistant conjunctivitis.

Chronic Bacterial Conjunctivitis

Chronic bacterial conjunctivitis is often associated with adjacent lid disease and lasts longer than 3 to 4 weeks. Chronic *S. aureus* conjunctivitis can accompany simultaneous lid infection (blepharitis). Symptoms include conjunctival injection and papillae, mild foreign body sensation, mild mucoid discharge, and eyelid crusting. *Moraxella lacunata* can also produce chronic conjunctivitis in association with angular blepharitis involving the lateral canthal region of the eyelid. Treatment of these chronic infections consists of nightly application of bacitracin, erythromycin, or trimethoprim-polymyxin ointment, as well as lid hygiene.

■ CHLAMYDIAL CONJUNCTIVITIS

Trachoma

Chlamydia trachomatis (serotype A to C) is the most common cause of infectious blindness in the world. Sporadic cases are seen in various parts of the United States. It is characterized by conjunctival follicles of the superior tarsus that cicatrize to produce a thickened and scarred superior tarsus. The scarring may cause the eyelashes to turn inward and rub against the eye (trichiasis). Corneal involvement with vascularization and opacification may occur later in the course of the disease. Treatment consists of either topical erythromycin or tetracycline ointment or oral tetracycline (Table 3).

Adult Chlamydial Conjunctivitis

Adult chlamydial conjunctivitis is a sexually transmitted disease caused by *C. trachomatis* serotype D to K. Affected individuals usually have concurrent genital infection, which can be asymptomatic. Ocular infection usually results from autoinoculation with genital secretions; rarely, transmission may occur from unchlorinated swimming pools. Symptoms include tearing, foreign body sensation, photophobia, and lid edema. Conjunctival follicles of the lower lid with a preauricular node are present. Corneal involvement may also occur. Treatment of adult infection is with oral tetracycline, doxycycline, or erythromycin for 3 weeks (see Table 3).

Table 2   Treatment of Gonococcal Conjunctivitis

IN ADULTS
  A. Without septicemia
     Ceftriaxone 1 g IM × 1 dose
     Frequent topical saline irrigation
     Bacitracin ointment q2h × 2 days, then 5 times a day until
        resolution
  B. With septicemia
     Ceftriaxone 1 g IM or IV q12-24h for at least 3 days
     Frequent topical saline irrigation
     Bacitracin ointment q2h × 2 days then 5 times a day until
        resolution
  C. With corneal ulcer
     Ceftriaxone 1 g IM or IV q12-24h for at least 3 days
     Frequent topical saline irrigation
     Ciprofloxacin or ofloxacin drops q5min for 30 min (load);
        then q15min for 6 hours; then q30min around the clock
        for 1 to 2 days; then hourly with morning and evening
        load until resolved (5-7 days)

IN CHILDREN
  Ceftriaxone, 25-50 mg/kg/day IV or IM qd × 7 days
  Cefotaxime, 25 mg/kg IV or IM q12h × 7 days
  Penicillin G, 100,000 U/kg/day q12h × 7 days
     (susceptible strains)

PLUS
  Erythromycin ointment qh × 24 hours then 4 to 8 times a
  day × 10 days

Table 3   Treatment of Chlamydial Conjunctivitis

TRACHOMA
Erythromycin or tetracycline ointment bid for 2 mo
Tetracycline, 1.5 mg PO qd for 3 wk
ADULT INCLUSION CONJUNCTIVITIS
Tetracycline, 500 mg PO qid for 3 wk
Doxycycline, 100 mg PO bid for 3 wk
Erythromycin, 500 mg PO for 3 wk
Azithromycin, 1 g PO for one dose
NEONATAL INCLUSION CONJUNCTIVITIS
Erythromycin or sulfacetamide ointment qid for a minimum
  of 3 wk, plus erythromycin oral syrup at 40 mg/kg/day in
  4 divided doses for 2-3 wk

Affected patients may need further evaluation and treatment of concurrent genital infection.

Neonatal Inclusion Conjunctivitis

Neonatal inclusion conjunctivitis, also caused by *C. trachomatis* serotype D to K, is discussed later in this chapter.

■ VIRAL CONJUNCTIVITIS

The adenovirus is a common cause of sporadic or epidemic follicular conjunctivitis. It is characterized by unilateral or bilateral conjunctival hyperemia, tearing, irritation, follicles, and tender preauricular nodes. Pharyngoconjunctivitis caused by adenovirus types 3 and 7 is a self-limited conjunctivitis associated with fever and pharyngitis. Epidemic keratoconjunctivitis, caused by adenovirus types 8 and 19, is extremely contagious and is transmitted via direct contact, hand-to-eye contact, or contaminated water (e.g., swimming pools). Affected patients may also have corneal epithelial or subepithelial infiltrates, which are usually self-limited but may persist for months to years, impairing the vision. Patients are infectious for up to 2 weeks after the start of symptoms. Treatment is supportive, with cool compresses and artificial tears for comfort.

Molluscum contagiosum produces a chronic, toxic follicular conjunctivitis that results from the release of viral particles from an eyelid lesion. The lesion typically appears as a pearly white raised nodule with an umbilicated center. Treatment consists of removal of the nodule's central core, incision of the nodule to produce bleeding, or complete excision of the nodule.

Primary infection with type 1 herpes simplex virus (HSV) occurs in children and young adults and typically produces a unilateral follicular conjunctivitis with eyelid vesicles and a tender preauricular node. A severe keratitis may also be present. Recurrent HSV infection usually manifests with corneal disease, which may threaten the vision. Treatment of HSV requires antiviral agents. Details on HSV keratitis can be found in the chapter *Keratitis*.

Enterovirus 70 and Coxsackievirus A24 can produce a highly contagious, acute hemorrhagic conjunctivitis. Clinical signs include follicular conjunctivitis with subconjunctival hemorrhages, transient epithelial keratitis, and a preauricular node. The condition is usually self-limited, and treatment is supportive.

■ NEONATAL CONJUNCTIVITIS

Important infectious agents that cause conjunctivitis during the first month of life include *N. gonorrhoeae, C. trachomatis, S. aureus, S. pneumoniae, Haemophilus* species, and *Pseudomonas*. The causative agent cannot be reliably identified by clinical manifestations alone. Thus appropriate Gram or Giemsa stains and culture are mandatory.

Both *N. gonorrhoeae* and *Chlamydia* are sexually transmitted pathogens that infect the newborn during passage through the birth canal. *N. gonorrhoeae* produces a bilateral, hyperacute conjunctivitis 1 to 13 days after birth with features similar to those affecting adults. Treatment includes frequent ocular irrigation and topical erythromycin ointment. Systemic treatment recommendations for neonates are listed in Table 2.

Neonatal inclusion conjunctivitis resulting from chlamydial infection presents 5 to 14 days after birth with lid swelling, conjunctival hyperemia with a possible pseudomembrane, and watery to mucopurulent discharge. Associated pneumonia and otitis media may also be present. Topical erythromycin or sulfacetamide ointment along with oral erythromycin syrup for 2 to 3 weeks is necessary (see Table 3).

Other bacterial causes of neonatal conjunctivitis, which are usually nosocomial, may be treated with topical erythromycin, sulfacetamide, or gentamicin drops, depending on the infection.

Prophylaxis of neonatal conjunctivitis with erythromycin ointment, tetracycline ointment, or silver nitrate 1% aqueous solution is recommended for every neonate within 1 hour of delivery. Silver nitrate solution is not effective against chlamydia and can cause a chemical conjunctivitis. Thus the other two agents may be preferred.

■ CONJUNCTIVITIS MEDICAMENTOSA

Conjunctivitis medicamentosa is associated with the overuse of vasoconstricting drops. It is analogous to rhinitis medicamentosa, the well-recognized condition of chronic nasal congestion associated with the overuse of vasoconstricting nose drops. Vasoconstricting eyedrops, available over the counter, increase conjunctival injection and often a rebound hyperemia that persists despite discontinuation of eyedrops. Vasoconstrictor eyedrops should be discontinued in favor of more appropriate treatment of the underlying condition.

Suggested Reading

Jackson WB: Differentiating conjunctivitis of diverse origins, *Surv Ophthalmol* 38(suppl):91, 1993.

Spector SL, Raizman MB: Conjunctivitis medicamentosa, *J Allergy Clin Immunol* 94:134, 1994.

Tabbara KF, Hyndiuk RA, eds: *Infections of the eye*, ed 2, Boston, 1995, Little, Brown.

World Health Organization: *Conjunctivitis of the newborn: prevention and treatment at the primary health care level*, Geneva, 1986, World Health Organization.

KERATITIS

Jules Baum

Corneal infections are often sight-threatening, and the accompanying inflammation can induce metalloproteinase activity, which can thin and perforate a cornea. Because identification of the specific pathogen requires clinical expertise in addition to laboratory data and a manipulation of the therapeutic regimen based on evolving signs, many ophthalmologists in the United States refer patients with microbial keratitis other than that caused by herpes simplex virus (HSV) epithelial infection to specialists in cornea and external disease. Thus the role of the nonophthalmic infectious disease expert lies mainly in helping the ophthalmologist identify the pathogen and select an appropriate antimicrobial regimen. This chapter addresses HSV and varicella-zoster (VZ) keratitis and bacterial, fungal, and acanthamoeba infections of the cornea. As a general rule topical drug delivery is the most effective treatment of microbial keratitis.

■ MICROBIOLOGIC DIAGNOSIS

A kit for the collection of corneal microbiologic specimens should include a platinum (Kimura) spatula, an alcohol lamp, sterile calcium alginate swabs, proparacaine 0.5% topical anesthetic, glass slides, 95% methanol to fix specimens, a Coplin jar, and various media. Commonly used media include blood and chocolate agar for aerobic bacteria, PRAS Brucella blood agar plate enriched with vitamin K and hemin for anaerobes, Sabouraud dextrose agar for fungi, and a nonnutrient agar plate overlaid with *Escherichia coli* for acanthamoeba. Most corneal fungal infections are caused by species associated with filament production, and cyclohexamide, commonly added to media used for fungal growth, inhibits growth of such species. Stains used to examine corneal scrapings obtained with a platinum spatula include Gram, Giemsa, methenamine silver for fungi, and two fluorescent stains, calcofluor white for detection of acanthamoebal cysts and acridine orange, which stains bacteria, fungi, and acanthamoebal cysts. Both HSV and VZ may be elucidated by immunofluorescence of cells reacted with specific viral monoclonal antigen and by polymerase chain reaction (PCR) amplification and Southern blot analysis for specific viral genomic sequences. HSV may also be cultured. Culture of VZ is difficult and seldom performed.

■ VIRAL KERATITIS

Herpes Simplex Keratitis

HSV keratitis, characteristically type 1, typically is seen in adults as a uniocular condition and is classified as either epithelial or stromal disease, although there is often overlap.

When seen in infants and children, the infection commonly involves the eyelids and conjunctiva.

In epithelial infection, one or more characteristic dendritic figures are seen following staining with fluorescein after the onset of pain and photophobia. Treatment consists of trifluorothymidine eyedrops, one drop every hour, nine times a day initially, then reduced to five times a day after several days. With this regimen, more than 95% of dendritic ulcers are cured in less than 2 weeks. Vidarabine ointment is also available and may be used initially five times a day. Topical acyclovir is unavailable in the United States. The use of a topical corticosteroid is proscribed when the disease is purely epithelial and the corneal stroma is unaffected.

Stromal disease manifests with a thickened edematous cornea, but opaque focal infiltrates, scarring, and neovascularization can occur. Treatment usually entails the use of both a topical antiviral agent and a topical corticosteroid over months. Use of a topical prophylactic antibiotic to prevent secondary bacterial infection is indicated when the corticosteroid is instilled frequently. The addition of oral acyclovir to the topical regimen has been shown to reduce the severity of the stromal disease and the frequency of recurrence. The latter was true as long as treatment (400 mg twice daily) was maintained.

Varicella-Zoster Keratitis

The cornea is the ocular tissue most often affected in herpes zoster ophthalmicus (trigeminal nerve involvement). Oral acyclovir, 800 mg five times a day for 7 days, is effective therapy, provided the drug is started within 3 days of the appearance of skin lesions. Famciclovir, a prodrug of penciclovir, is now commercially available. The recommended oral dosage is 500 mg three times a day for 7 days. If therapy is delayed or ineffective, neurotrophic keratitis, a dry eye, stromal infiltration, thinning, and perforation may result. There is no consensus regarding the use of topical corticosteroid or the effectiveness of oral cimetidine in reducing pain. Ancillary therapy often includes tear supplements, punctal occlusion to preserve tears, partial eyelid patching, and tarsorrhaphy.

■ BACTERIAL KERATITIS

Bacterial keratitis is the most likely of all microbial infections to scar the cornea rapidly and permanently. Prompt recognition and appropriate therapy minimize loss of vision. Species most often involved include staphylococci (most common), streptococci (*S. pneumoniae*, alpha-, beta-nonhemolytic), *Listeria*, *Bacillus cereus*, *Pseudomonas*, *Acinetobacter*, Enterobacteriaceae, *Neisseria*, *Haemophilus*, *Moraxella*, *Mycobacterium* (especially *M. fortuitum* and *M. chelonei*), *Nocardia*, and some anaerobes (*P. acnes*, *Actinomyces*, *Peptococcus*, and *Peptostreptococcus*). Wearing soft contact lenses overnight is a strong risk factor for the development of *Pseudomonas* keratitis. Infection with this organism, if untreated, can thin and perforate a cornea within several days. Symptoms of bacterial keratitis, which are characteristically severe, include decreased vision, pain, photophobia, and tearing. Typical are a red eye, a focal cloudy cornea, a whitish infiltrate, possibly a hypopyon, and a miotic pupil.

Standard therapy in the recent past involved the use of fortified antibiotic eyedrops compounded from products formulated for parenteral use. Some still initiate therapy with a single antibiotic selected on the basis of Gram stain identification; others administer two antibiotics that best cover the spectrum of potential pathogens (because there is a relatively poor correlation between the results of Gram stain and culture). However most ophthalmologists at present begin therapy with a commercially available topical fluoroquinolone, one drop every 15 to 60 minutes around the clock, in many instances forgoing laboratory identification of the pathogen. With the introduction of commercially available fluoroquinolone eyedrops, which generally are effective against most strains commonly encountered except some streptococci, and with recent reports suggesting similar clinical outcomes with and without the use of laboratory data, standard therapy has undergone reexamination.

For almost two decades I used cefazolin, 50 mg/ml, and either gentamicin or tobramycin, 14 mg/ml, as initial therapy. More recently I have used vancomycin, 50 mg/ml, in place of cefazolin. Based on the work of others, I suggest ceftazidime, 50 mg/ml as an alternative to the aminoglycoside. However, when *Pseudomonas* is the suspected pathogen, tobramycin and either piperacillin or ticarcillin, 6 to 12 mg/ml, serve as initial therapy. Eyedrops are instilled every 15 to 60 minutes around the clock for the first 24 to 72 hours, allowing at least a 5-minute interval between two antibiotics to avoid a washout effect. Frequency of instillation is reduced over several weeks. A change in initial therapy may be considered after several days if antibiotic resistance is demonstrated and the clinical condition worsens. Resistance alone is insufficient reason to alter therapy because corneal concentrations of drug reach much higher levels than those safely achievable in blood.

■ FUNGAL KERATITIS

Fungal keratitis, most common in warm climates and rural areas often is associated with corneal trauma, typically botanic. Most infections are caused by filamentous species. In the United States *Aspergillus* is probably the pathogen most commonly encountered, occurring in both the North and the South. However, the most common agent seen in the South is *Fusarium solani*, whereas in the North keratitis caused by *Candida* is more common, especially in patients who are immunosuppressed and whose corneas are dry, hypaesthetic, or overexposed. *Curvularia*, *Acromonium*, and *Alternaria* are other species less commonly seen. The typical corneal infiltrate develops more slowly than one of bacterial origin and may be seen in association with smaller satellite lesions. Symptoms typically are less severe than those resulting from bacterial infection. When possible, the pathogen should be identified before treatment is started.

Most ophthalmologists begin therapy with natamycin 5% suspension eyedrops, the only commercially available antifungal ocular product in the United States. However, instillation of amphotericin B 0.05% to 0.15% eyedrops may be preferable because natamycin penetrates corneal tissue poorly and *Fusarium* may reside in deep stroma, especially when treatment is delayed. In addition, amphotericin B is the drug of choice for *Candida* keratitis and, in many instances, is effective in treating infections caused by *Aspergillus*. Clotrimazole 1% dermatologic lotion or vaginal cream, miconazole as a topical preparation (Monistat) or fabricated from the intravenous product, and oral preparations of ketoconazole, fluconazole, and itraconazole are also used in the treatment of this disease with varying degrees of success. Flucytosine, given orally or as a 1% eyedrop, may be effective as alternative therapy for candidal infection but should not be used as the sole agent because resistance to flucytosine develops rapidly. Initially, antifungal eyedrops are instilled every 2 to 3 hours while the patient is awake and then are slowly reduced according to the clinical response. Ointments may be applied less frequently. Therapy is maintained over many weeks.

■ ACANTHAMOEBA KERATITIS

The corneal infection, *Acanthamoeba* keratitis, first documented in 1973, is uncommon, and its incidence seems to have been decreasing since its two main risk factors, trauma and soft contact lens wear, were recognized. The infection, which starts insidiously in the corneal epithelium, progresses to involve the stroma in 1 to 3 weeks. Severe pain, out of proportion to the signs, is the rule. Keratitis resulting from HSV is the entity with which this infection is most likely to be confused. Following laboratory identification of the organism with calcaflor staining and culture, therapy, until recently, consisted of alternately administering propamadine isethionate 0.1% and neomycin 5% eyedrops or the commercially available neomycin-gramicidin-polymyxin product on a long-term basis, for some months to a year. Eyedrops are administered initially every hour for the first week and then slowly tapered. Two newer agents, polyhexamethylene biguanide (PHMB) 0.02% and chlorhexidine 0.02% eyedrops, have been shown to be possibly more effective than other therapy. Unlike other agents used to treat this infection, PHMP is cysticidal at low concentrations. It is sold in the United States as Bacquicil, a swimming pool disinfectant. Because topical antiamoebic therapy is not very effective, therapy at present is to use two or, more commonly, three agents simultaneously. (See also the chapter *Extraintestinal Amoebic Infection.*)

Suggested Reading

Krachmer JH, Mannis MJ, Holland EJ, eds: vol II, Cornea, *Cornea and external disease: clinical diagnosis and management,* vol II, Cornea, St Louis, 1997, Mosby.

Pavan-Langston D: Viral infections of the cornea and external eye. In Albert D, Jakobiec F: *Principles and practice of ophthalmology,* ed 2, Philadelphia, Saunders (in press).

Tabbara KF, Hyndiuk RA, eds: *Infections of the eye,* ed 2, Boston, 1995, Little, Brown.

Tasman W, Jaeger EA, eds: *Duane's clinical ophthalmology,* vol 4, External diseases, diseases of the uvea, Philadelphia, 1999, Lippincott Williams & Wilkins.

IRITIS

D. Geraint James

The uveal tract is a continuous vascular structure consisting of the iris, ciliary body, and choroid. It is convenient, if somewhat artificial, to subdivide inflammation of the uveal tract into anterior uveitis (iritis and iridocyclitis) and posterior uveitis (choroiditis and choroidoretinitis). Exogenous uveitis may follow injury or surgery to the eye or may have a local intraocular cause, which usually is obvious from history or examination. Endogenous uveitis may be regarded as a symptom of some widespread infection or multisystem disorder.

■ PRESENTATION

Iritis may have an acute explosive or a chronic insidious onset. Acute iritis is characterized by abrupt onset of pain, photophobia, and blurring of vision. There is circumcorneal infection, which should not be confused with conjunctivitis. There is a ciliary flush, but the pupil is not stuck down. Inflammatory cells (keratic precipitates) are seen on the back of the cornea, or they may settle into a sterile abscess, or hypopyon, in the anterior chamber.

Chronic iritis has an insidious onset. The pupil is small and sluggish, and it may be irregular because of adhesions between the iris and lens (posterior synechiae). The patient

may have had previous attacks and be able to anticipate a recurrence. The cause is rarely evident by examination of the eye alone. General examination of the patient is essential, as is slit-lamp examination of the eye (Figure 1). From this multisystem approach emerge several patterns of uveitis.

■ PATTERNS OF UVEITIS

Distinctive patterns of multisystem iritis permit more efficient investigation and treatment (Table 1).

■ SARCOID UVEITIS

Sarcoid uveitis is most common in women of childbearing age. The clinical diagnosis becomes obvious if there are associated skin lesions and an abnormal chest radiograph (Figure 2). The diagnosis is confirmed by histology of skin, lung, or liver. Transbronchial biopsy by fiberoptic bronchoscopy is a fruitful source of sarcoid tissue. The course may be acute or chronic (Table 2).

■ BEHÇET'S DISEASE

Behçet's disease is diagnosed at the bedside. There are no definitive laboratory tests. The diagnosis is evident when iritis is associated with orogenital mucocutaneous ulceration, dermatographia, polyarthritis, erythema nodosum, thrombophlebitis, and neurologic and cardiac abnormalities; the pathology is that of vasculitis. It may mimic sarcoidosis, causing diagnostic confusion; it is important to distinguish the two disorders because the management is different (Table 3). Behçet's disease is underdiagnosed,

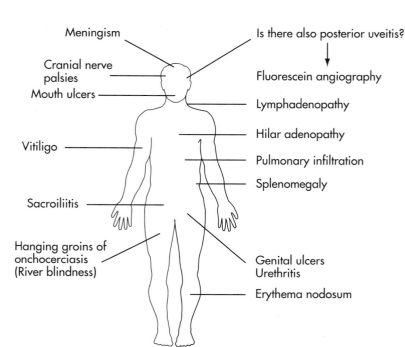

Figure 1
Clinical examination of a patient with uveitis.

Table 1   Patterns of Multisystem Iritis

SYSTEM	DISORDER	OTHER FEATURES	USEFUL INVESTIGATION
Pulmonary	Sarcoidosis	Lacrimals, skin	Chest x-ray study
	Tuberculosis	Fever, lassitude	Chest x-ray study, tuberculin test
	Churg-Strauss	Asthma	Eosinophilia
Renal	Wegener's granulomatosis	Scleritis, nasopharyngeal and renal involvement	ANCA, chest x-ray studies, kidney biopsy
	Interstitial nephritis	Pars planitis	Kidney biopsy
Autoimmune and rheumatic	Behçet's disease	Orogenital ulceration, erythema nodosum	Bedside clinical diagnosis
	Stevens-Johnson syndrome	Erythema multiforme, mucosal ulceration	Cold agglutinins, mycoplasma serology
	Juvenile rheumatoid arthritis	Polyarthritis	X-ray study of joints
	Ankylosing spondylitis	Apical fibrosis of lungs	X-ray studies, HLA-B27
	Reiter's syndrome	Urethritis, aoritis, arthritis	X-ray studies, HLA-B27
	Polychondritis	Floppy pinna, aortic aneurysm	Biopsy of cartilage
Infections	Leprosy	Thickened nerves, anesthetic plaques	Biopsy of skin, nose
	Onchocerca	Posterior uveitis	Skin biopsy
	Syphilis	Secondary stage rash; lymph nodes	Treponema antibody
	AIDS	Multisystem involvement	Specific antibody
	Herpes	Vesicles at tip of nose	Virus isolation, cell inclusions
	Lyme borreliosis	Facial nerve palsy, erythema chronicum migrans	Specific antibody
Intestinal	Chronic inflammatory bowel disease	Colitis	Sigmoidoscopy and biopsy
Vascular	Fuchs' heterochromic cyclitis	Moth-eaten depigmented iris	Slit-lamp examination

ANCA, Antineutrophil cytoplasmic antibody; *AIDS,* acquired immunodeficiency syndrome.

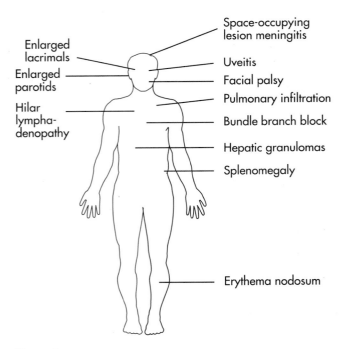

Figure 2
Clinical examination of a patient with sarcoidosis.

and sadly, the road to blindness is recognized too late. The more numerous the physical signs, the more confident the diagnosis of Behçet's disease. A personal points scoring system allows a confident diagnosis with 14 points or more (Table 4). This points scheme helps differenti-ate it from sarcoidosis, the seronegative arthritides, multiple sclerosis, inflammatory bowel disease, Stevens-Johnson syndrome, or other vasculitides.

Behçet's disease has an interesting geographic prevalence, predominating between latitudes 30° and 45° north in what was known as the old Silk Route or what is now called the Karakoram Highway. It is seen most often in Japan, China, India, Pakistan, Iran, Turkey, Greece, Cyprus, and other eastern Mediterranean areas. A background genetic factor may be associated with HLA Bw51.

■ HLA-B27 ANTERIOR UVEITIS

HLA-B27 anterior uveitis usually is severe, unilateral, and recurrent in young adults. It is often caused by ankylosing spondylitis, particularly in men. These patients or their families may also be identified because of accompanying peripheral arthritis, chronic inflammatory bowel disease, or psoriasis (Table 5). Infection with *Yersinia enterocolitica,* *Salmonella,* or *Mycoplasma* may trigger iritis, seronegative arthropathy, or erythema nodosum. A careful family history may be most rewarding.

■ HERPES

Herpes zoster ophthalmicus results from involvement of the ophthalmic branch of the trigeminal nerve. Jonathan Hutchinson suggested that vesicles on the tip of the nose indicated involvement of the nasociliary branch and therefore ocular inflammation caused by the ciliary branch. The

Table 2 Differences between Acute and Chronic Iridocyclitis Caused by Sarcoidosis

ANTERIOR UVEITIS	ACUTE	CHRONIC
Onset	Abrupt	Insidious
Decade of onset	20-35	35-50
Course	Transient	Persistent
Signs	Ciliary congestion, turbid aqueous keratic precipitates	Fatty nodules, synechiae
Sequelae	Rare	Lens opacities, glaucoma, cataract, blindness
Chest radiograph	Hilar adenopathy	Pulmonary fibrosis
Skin lesions	Erythema nodosum	Lupus pernio
Bone cysts	No	Yes
Response to corticosteroids	Good	Poor
Alternative treatment	Indomethacin	Chloroquine, methotrexate

earlier the diagnosis is made, the more useful intravenous acyclovir or famcyclovir. The classical lesion of herpes simplex is dendritic keratitis, but the iris also may be involved.

■ JUVENILE RHEUMATOID ARTHRITIS (STILL'S DISEASE)

Iritis may be associated with rheumatoid arthritis in children, particularly in girls. It may be acute febrile, polyarticular, or monoarticular. Iritis is most commonly found in children with only a few joints affected. Slit-lamp examination of the eye must be undertaken in all children with chronic arthritis. There is a strong association with antinuclear factor.

■ BLAU'S SYNDROME

Edward Blau is a Wisconsin pediatrician who described a granulomatous disease of the eyes, skin, and joints resembling childhood sarcoidosis. The histology may be indistinguishable, so pediatricians should be aware of this multisystem granulomatosis mimicking sarcoidosis. Granulomatous anterior and posterior uveitis are observed in both disorders, and exacerbations of the skin disease may be associated with increased activity of the iritis in both. A major difference is that there is no lung involvement in Blau's syndrome (Table 6).

■ THERAPY

The immediate treatment is to reduce the inflammation and prevent adhesions within the eye. The pupil is dilated to prevent adhesions between the iris and lens. Inflammatory cells may block the trabecular meshwork and cause a rise of the intraocular pressure, so antiglaucoma treatment must

Table 3 Comparison of Behçet's Disease and Sarcoidosis

FEATURES	BEHÇET'S DISEASE	SARCOIDOSIS
Uveitis		
Anterior	+	+
Posterior	+	+
Polyarthritis	+	+
Papilledema	+	+
Retinal vasculitis	+	+
Meningitis	+	+
Facial nerve palsy	−	+
Cardiac	+	+
Orogenital ulceration	+	−
Lymphadenopathy	−	+
Erythema nodosum	+	+
Dermatographia	+	−
Skin lesions	Pyoderma	Plaques
Bone cysts	−	+
Chest radiographs	Venous occlusion Aneurysms	Lymphadenopathy Pulmonary infiltration
Negative tuberculin	No	Yes
Positive Kveim	No	Yes
Hypercalcemia	−	+
Angiotensin-convertase	Normal	Elevated
HLA	B51 DrW52	B8/B13/A1,Cw7 DR3
Treatments		
Steroids	+	+
Cyclosporin	+	±
Azathioprine	+	+
Colchicine	+	−

Table 4 Points Scoring System for the Clinical Diagnosis of Behçet's Disease

FEATURE	POINTS
Oral ulceration	4
Genital ulceration	4
Ocular inflammation	4
Retinal vasculitis	2
Erythema nodosum	2
Joints	2
Central nervous system	2
Cardiovascular	2
Gastrointestinal	2
Kidney	1
Lung	1
Dermatographia	1
Confident diagnosis	**>14**

also be considered. Thus the mainstays of treatment are topical and possibly oral corticosteroids together with local cyclopentolate (mydriatic) eyedrops. Steroid eyedrops are applied frequently throughout the day and reinforced with a steroid eye ointment at night. If no substantial and contin-

Table 5	Seronegative HLA-B27 Arthropathy
Psoriatic	
Reiter's syndrome	
Ankylosing spondylitis	
Crohn regional enteritis	
Ulcerative colitis	
Behçet's disease	
Whipple's disease	

Table 6	Blau's Syndrome
Children	
Anterior and posterior uveitis	
Arthritis	
Flexion contracture of joints	
Butterfly rash of face	
Red papules	
Normal chest radiograph	
Granulomatous histology	
Hypergammaglobulinemia	
Autosomal-dominant transmission	

Table 7   Iritis Treatment to Combine with Steroid Therapy

IRITIS	TREATMENT
Sarcoidosis	Nonsteroidal antiinflammatory agents, hydroxychloroquine, methotrexate
Tuberculosis	Isoniazid, rifampicin, pyrazinamide
Behçet's syndrome	Cyclosporin, azathioprine, colchicine, interferon
Wegener's granulomatosis	Cyclophosphamide, staphylococcal nasal carriage
Leprosy	BCG, ofloxin, rifampicin, dapsone, clofazimine, interferon
Onchocerciasis (river blindness)	Thiabendazole, diethylcarbamazine, suramin
Syphilis	Penicillin
Herpes	Acyclovir, famcyclovir
Inflammatory bowel disease	Sulfasalazine, metronidazol, azathioprine, cyclosporin
	Tumor necrosis factor antibody

BCG, Bacille Calmette Guerin.

uing improvement is seen after 1 week, the concentration of corticosteroid in the anterior segment of the eye may be increased by a local subconjunctival injection of cortisone or by oral steroid therapy. If ophthalmoscopy reveals posterior uveitis in addition to the anterior uveitis, oral steroids are indicated.

Local steroid therapy must be monitored carefully by intraocular pressure levels because topical steroids may provoke rises or even precipitate secondary glaucoma. This is not a particular hazard of oral steroids. High intraocular pressure necessitates switching from topical to oral steroids and giving timolol eyedrops to reduce the pressure to normal. In addition to steroid therapy, there may be specific therapy for the various associated disorders (Table 7).

Suggested Reading

James DG: A comparison of Blau's syndrome and sarcoidosis, *Sarcoidosis* 11:100-101, 1994.

James DG, Friedmann AI, Graham E: Uveitis: a series of 368 patients, *Trans Ophthalm Soc UK* 96:108-112, 1976.

James DG, Jones Williams W: Sarcoidosis and other granulomatous disorders, Philadelphia, 1985, WB Saunders.

James DG, Zumla A: *The granulomatous disorders,* Cambridge, 1999, University Press.

Wechsler B, Godeau P: Behçet's disease. In *Proceedings of the Sixth International Conference,* New York, 1993, Excerpta Medica.

RETINITIS

Daniel M. Albert
Robert T. Bechtel

■ CYTOMEGALOVIRUS RETINITIS

Cytomegalovirus (CMV) retinitis is the most common and clinically significant opportunistic ocular infection seen in patients with acquired immune deficiency syndrome (AIDS). CMV retinitis is a late complication of AIDS, with most cases occurring in individuals with T4 cell counts less than 0.1×10^9/L. CMV retinitis occurs in approximately 30% of patients with AIDS and fulfills the Centers for Disease Control and Prevention (CDC) criteria for the diagnosis of AIDS.

The presentation of CMV retinitis may be unilateral or bilateral. The onset is insidious, and symptoms may include blurred vision, floaters, visual field defects, or other nonspecific visual complaints. Clinically, the initial lesions of CMV retinitis may appear as cotton-wool spots. Gradually, the lesions enlarge to become a confluent area of full-thickness retinal necrosis with a yellow-white granular appearance and associated retinal hemorrhages, which has been likened to a "pizza pie" appearance. Vitreous inflammation is minimal or absent. Visual loss may be profound if the macula or optic nerve is involved. Without treatment, CMV retinitis will become bilateral in 80% of cases and eventually results in blindness from retinal atrophy, retinal detachment, or optic nerve involvement.

In patients known to have human immunodeficiency virus (HIV) or to be immunosuppressed, the diagnosis of CMV retinitis is based on clinical examination and confirmed by positive blood cultures for CMV. In individuals not known to be HIV-positive, the diagnosis is suspected based on clinical appearance and an investigation of immune status is required.

In an effort to halt the progression and improve visual outcome, CMV retinitis requires treatment with one of three currently available virostatic agents: ganciclovir, foscarnet, or cidofovir (Table 1). The choice of the antiviral agent and its route of delivery should be based on the location and extent of the infection, potential side effects, and the effectiveness of prior treatments.

Ganciclovir, an inhibitor of CMV DNA-polymerase, may be administered intravenously, orally, or intravitreally. Intravenous (IV) ganciclovir should be used as induction therapy for 14 to 21 days, followed by maintenance therapy by either an IV or oral route. Because ganciclovir is virostatic, maintenance therapy is required indefinitely. The dosage of ganciclovir requires reduction in patients with impaired renal function. The most common side effect of ganciclovir is neutropenia, which arises in 20% to 40% of patients and is reversible upon discontinuation of the drug. Because ganci-

clovir and zidovudine may result in granulocytopenia, the concomitant use of these two agents may result in pronounced bone marrow suppression.

The use of a sustained-release ganciclovir implant placed directly into the vitreous cavity of the eye protects against reactivation of CMV retinitis for up to 7 months. The intravitreal implant reduces intraocular recurrence of CMV retinitis and systemic side effects of ganciclovir, but it is not protective against involvement of the fellow eye or systemic CMV infection. Adverse effects associated with the ganciclovir implant include decreased vision in the postoperative period and an increased risk of retinal detachment.

Foscarnet, an inhibitor of DNA-polymerase and reverse transcriptase, is administered intravenously for 14 to 21 days as induction therapy, followed by maintenance therapy indefinitely. The most common side effect of foscarnet is nephrotoxicity, which occurs in 25% of patients and is reversible with early cessation of the drug. Because foscarnet undergoes renal elimination and is nephrotoxic, careful monitoring of renal function is necessary.

Cidofovir, the newest agent available for the treatment of CMV retinitis, acts by inhibiting CMV DNA-polymerase. Cidofovir has an advantage over ganciclovir and foscarnet in that it may be administered intravenously much less frequently, once weekly as induction for 2 weeks and once every 2 weeks for maintenance therapy thereafter. Nephrotoxicity is the most common dose-limiting side effect, which may be reduced with the concurrent administration of oral probenecid and IV hydration.

Initial response to antiviral therapy occurs 1 to 2 weeks after the initiation of the induction regimen and is evident by termination of the growth of the retinal lesions and gradual atrophy of the involved retina. Patients should undergo funduscopic examination by an ophthalmologist every 2 to 3 weeks to monitor the effectiveness of antiviral therapy. Recurrence of CMV retinitis, which may occur in 30% to 50% of patients receiving maintenance doses of systemic antiviral therapy, requires reinduction for 2 weeks followed by indefinite maintenance therapy.

■ OCULAR TOXOPLASMOSIS

Ocular toxoplasmosis, which accounts for 30% to 50% of all cases of posterior uveitis, is caused by the obligate intracellular parasite *Toxoplasma gondii*. Infection may be congenital through transplacental transmission or acquired through contact with cat excreta or by ingestion of oocysts from undercooked meat. Most cases of ocular toxoplasmosis occur as a result of reactivation of congenital ocular lesions.

Symptoms of active infection include blurred vision and vitreous floaters. Most commonly, ocular toxoplasmosis presents as a white-yellow area of focal necrotizing retinitis adjacent to an old atrophic chorioretinal scar. Vitreous inflammation typically is present over the area of active retinitis, and granulomatous iridocyclitis or optic nerve swelling may be present.

Not all active retinal lesions require treatment when present in immunocompetent individuals. Small peripheral lesions, which often are self-limited and not visually threatening, can be observed. Without treatment, active lesions

Table 1   Therapy for Retinitis

	AGENT	REGIMEN	SIDE EFFECTS
CMV retinitis	Ganciclovir	Induction of 5 mg/kg IV every 12 hours for 14 to 21 days, then 5 mg/kg/day IV 7 days per week or 6 mg/kg 5 days per week 1000 mg PO three times daily as maintenance therapy	Granulocytopenia Thrombocytopenia Anemia
	Foscarnet	Induction of 60 mg/kg IV every 8 hours for 14 to 21 days, then 90 to 120 mg/kg/day IV	Nephrotoxicity Electrolyte imbalance Seizures/headache
	Cidofovir	Induction of 3 to 5 mg/kg IV once per week for 2 weeks, then 3 mg/kg IV every 2 weeks as maintenance	Nephrotoxicity Neutropenia Uveitis
Ocular toxoplasmosis	Pyrimethamine	75 mg PO, then 25 mg PO daily for 4 to 6 weeks	Anemia Thrombocytopenia Leukopenia
	Sulfadiazine	2 g PO, then 1 g PO four times daily for 4 to 6 weeks	Stevens-Johnson syndrome Hypersensitivity reaction Crystalluria
	Clindamycin	300 mg PO four times daily for 4 to 6 weeks	Diarrhea Pseudomembranous colitis
Acute retinal necrosis	Acyclovir	500 mg/m^2 IV every 8 hours for 7 to 10 days, the 800 mg PO five times daily for 6 to 12 weeks	Localized phlebitis Elevated serum creatinine

CMV, Cytomegalovirus; *IV*, intravenously; *PO*, orally.

heal in 2 to 4 months. Medical therapy is indicated when the toxoplasma lesions involve or threaten the macula or optic nerve or when visually disabling vitreous inflammation is present.

The goal of treatment for ocular toxoplasmosis is to halt the infectious process and reduce scarring of the retina and vitreous. Traditional therapy consists of the concurrent use of two folate antagonists: sulfadiazine and pyrimethamine. Sulfadiazine is administered as a loading dose of 2 g orally, followed by 1 g four times daily for 4 to 6 weeks. Pyrimethamine is given as a loading dose of 75 mg followed by 25 mg orally per day for a similar duration. Pyrimethamine requires weekly complete blood counts and may be administered with leucovorin calcium, 5 mg orally twice weekly, to reduce the incidence of bone marrow suppression. Clindamycin, 300 mg orally four times daily for 4 to 6 weeks, has been suggested in combination with sulfadiazine and pyrimethamine for severe ocular toxoplasmosis infections.

Systemic corticosteroids should be administered when inflammation from the active toxoplasmosis lesions threaten the macula or optic nerve and when severe vitreous inflammation is present. Corticosteroids should never be used in the treatment of ocular toxoplasmosis without the concurrent use of antibiotic agents. Prednisone at a dosage of 60 to 80 mg/day is administered during the first week of treatment and rapidly tapered based on clinical response and patient tolerance.

■ ACUTE RETINAL NECROSIS SYNDROME

The acute retinal necrosis syndrome (ARN) is characterized by a triad of clinical findings that have been associated with infection by the varicella-zoster virus (VZV), or less commonly, the herpes simplex virus (HSV). This triad consists of peripheral retinal necrosis, vitreous inflammation, and retinal vasculitis. Although initially described only in immunocompetent patients, recent cases have been reported in immunosuppressed individuals, including those with AIDS.

Clinically, ARN presents as confluent areas of white retinal necrosis in the far periphery, which may spread rapidly within days. In addition, moderate to severe vitreous inflammation and vasculitis with narrowing of the retinal arterioles is seen. Anterior granulomatous uveitis, optic nerve swelling, and macular edema may be associated findings. As many as 75% of patients with ARN may develop retinal breaks and subsequent rhegmatogenous retinal detachments.

The onset of ARN typically is unilateral, although bilateral involvement may occur in up to 30% of patients within several weeks of onset. The active phase of inflammation generally lasts several weeks and is followed by a convalescent phase when vitreous fibrosis results in the highest incidence of retinal detachment.

Because of the association with VZV and HSV, treatment of ARN consists of antiviral agents and antiinflammatory agents to reduce the complications associated with intraocular inflammation. Acyclovir at a dosage of 1500 mg/m^2/day IV is administered in three divided doses daily for 7 to 10 days. Dosages as high as 1500 mg IV every 8 hours may be necessary in immunosuppressed patients. IV therapy is followed by oral acyclovir, 800 mg five times daily for 6 to 12 weeks, to reduce bilateral involvement. Ganciclovir, which has activity against VZV and HSV, may be used in patients in whom acyclovir has failed. Systemic and periocular corticosteroids may be administered to reduce intraocular inflammation, but only concomitant with antiviral therapy.

Suggested Reading

Blumenkranz MS, et al: Treatment of acute retinal necrosis syndrome with intravenous acyclovir, *Ophthalmology* 93:296-300, 1986.

Duker JS, Blumenkranz MS: Diagnosis and management of acute retinal necrosis syndrome, *Survey Ophthalmol* 35:327-343, 1991.

Hardy W: Management strategies for patients with cytomegalovirus retinitis, *J Acq Imm Def Syn* 14:S7-S14, 1997.

Jabs DA, Enger C, Bartlett JG: Cytomegalovirus retinitis and acquired immunodeficiency syndrome, *Arch Ophthalmol* 107:75-80, 1989.

Lakhanpal V, Schocket SS, Nirankari VS: Clindamycin in the treatment of toxoplasmic retinochoroiditis, *Am J Ophthalmol* 95:605-613, 1983.

Tamesis RR, Foster CS: Toxoplasmosis. In Albert DM, Jakobiec FA, eds: *Principles and practice of ophthalmology,* vol 2, Philadelphia, 1994, WB Saunders.

ENDOPHTHALMITIS

Roy D. Brod
Harry W. Flynn, Jr.

Endophthalmitis is a vision-threatening inflammation of the inner eye fluids and tissues. Infectious endophthalmitis results from either exogenous or endogenous entry of microbes into the eye. In reported clinical series, exogenous endophthalmitis is much more common than endogenous (or metastatic) endophthalmitis. By far, the most common cause of exogenous infection is intraocular surgery. Because cataract surgery is the most commonly performed type of intraocular surgery, it accounts for the greatest number of exogenous endophthalmitis cases. Exogenous endophthalmitis can also occur after other types of intraocular surgery, including secondary lens implantation, glaucoma filtering surgery, vitrectomy surgery, and corneal transplantation. Organisms may also enter the eye during penetrating trauma and contiguous spread into the eye from an infected corneal ulcer. Gram-positive bacteria are the most common cause of exogenous endophthalmitis.

■ INCIDENCE

A retrospective nosocomial survey of postoperative endophthalmitis cases from the University of Miami (Bascom-Palmer Eye Institute) over a 10-year period (1984 to 1994) demonstrated the incidence of nosocomial endophthalmitis after cataract surgery to be 0.09%. Endophthalmitis occurs after penetrating trauma in 3% to 30% of patients depending on the nature of the injury. The rate of development of *Candida* endogenous endophthalmitis in patients with documented candidemia has been reported to range from 2.8% to 45%.

■ CLINICAL FEATURES

Exogenous endophthalmitis can be classified into the following general categories: (1) acute-onset postoperative endophthalmitis, (2) delayed-onset postoperative endophthalmitis, (3) conjunctival filtering bleb-associated endophthalmitis, (4) posttraumatic endophthalmitis, (5) endogenous (metastatic), or (6) endophthalmitis associated with microbial keratitis (corneal ulcer) (Table 1). Each category has characteristic clinical features and often predictable causative organisms.

Most cases of acute-onset postoperative endophthalmitis present within 3 to 7 days of intraocular surgery (Figure 1). Symptoms may start as early as 12 hours after the surgery. The classic symptoms include visual loss and ocular pain in 75% of cases. The loss of vision is typically profound and is reduced out of proportion to the usual postoperative course. The presenting signs often include lid edema, conjunctival injection and swelling, conjunctival discharge, corneal edema, anterior chamber inflammation, fibrin formation, and vitreous inflammatory response. In most cases, a layer of inflammatory cells (hypopyon) can be visualized in the inferior portion of the anterior chamber. Redness and purulent discharge from the conjunctiva and lid margins are also commonly seen. A severe intraocular inflammatory response will often obscure a view of the posterior pole and may cause loss of the red reflex. In these cases, echographic examination of the eye may be useful in ruling out posterior segment complications, such as retinal detachment or retained lens fragments.

In the Endophthalmitis Vitrectomy Study (EVS), the coagulase-negative staphylococci were the most commonly cultured organisms (68% of the 291 patients with confirmed growth). Other gram-positive organisms were cultured in 22% of patients and included *Streptococcus* and *Staphylococcus aureus*. Gram-negative organisms were isolated in 6% of the cases in the EVS and more than one species was confirmed in 4% of cases. Fortunately, the coagulase-negative staphylococci are one of the least virulent causes of acute-onset postoperative endophthalmitis. *S. aureus,* streptococcus species and the gram-negative organisms usually produce a rapidly progressive and fulminant inflammation that often leads to severe vision loss.

Another subgroup of postoperative endophthalmitis is the delayed-onset category (Figure 2). These patients present 6 weeks or more after intraocular surgery with a slowly progressive, often milder inflammatory response. The inflammation can be isolated to the anterior segment or involve both the anterior segment and vitreous. The intraocular inflammation may respond initially to topical steroid therapy but usually recurs as the topical steroids are tapered. A common cause of delayed-onset postoperative

Table 1 Endophthalmitis Categories

Acute-onset postoperative
Delayed-onset postoperative
Conjunctival filtering bleb-associated
Posttraumatic
Endogenous (metastatic)
Endophthalmitis associated with microbial keratitis

endophthalmitis is *Propionibacterium acnes.* This is a ubiquitous, gram-positive, non–spore-forming pleomorphic bacillus. Clinical features of intraocular infection caused by this organism include granulomatous inflammation with large keratic precipitates (clumps of inflammatory cells) on the corneal endothelium. A characteristic diagnostic feature is the presence of a white intracapsular plaque, which has been shown to consist of organisms mixed with residual lens

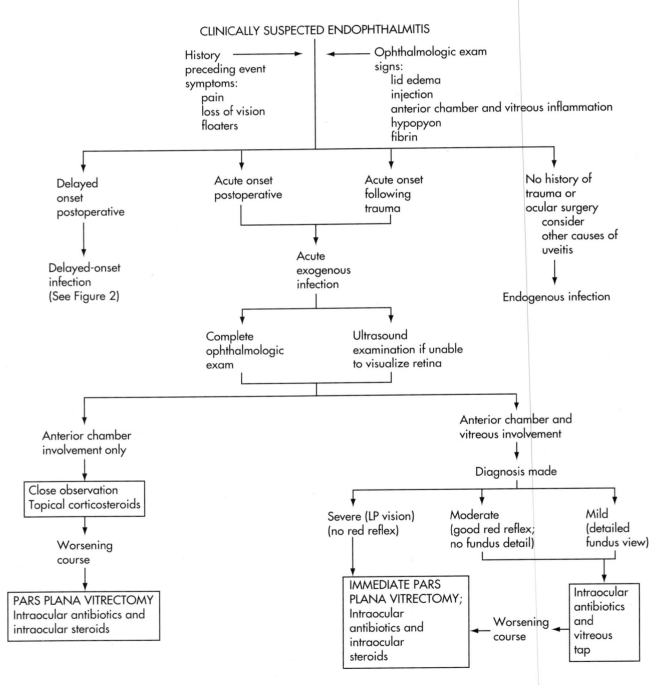

Figure 1
Algorithm for the management of acute-onset endophthalmitis.

cortex. Because *P. acnes* is a slow-growing anaerobic organism, it is important for the microbiology laboratory to be instructed to keep these anaerobic cultures for at least 2 weeks. Other organisms responsible for delayed-onset postoperative endophthalmitis include *Candida, Staphylococcus epidermidis,* and *Corynebacterium* species.

Delayed-onset endophthalmitis associated with conjunctival filtering blebs may present months or years after glaucoma filtering surgery. The organisms enter the eye directly through the thin wall of the conjunctival bleb. The presenting symptoms and signs are similar to acute-onset postoperative endophthalmitis. Streptococcal species are the most common organisms isolated. *Hemophilus influenzae* is also a common cause of this category of endophthalmitis. Because these organisms are generally more virulent than those causing acute-onset postoperative endophthalmitis, the visual outcomes are worse. Optic nerve damage from the preexisting glaucoma may also be a factor in the poor visual

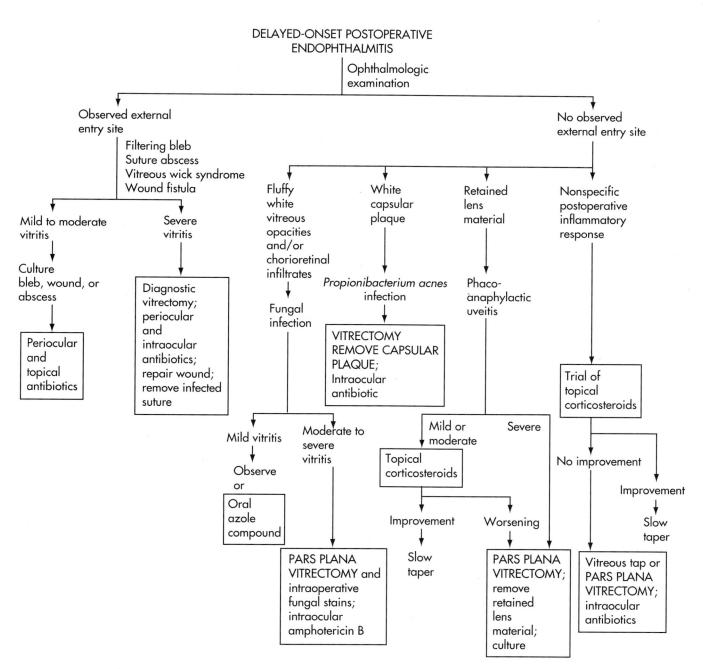

Figure 2
Algorithm for the management of delayed-onset endophthalmitis.

outcome. Fewer than half of the eyes achieve 20/400 or better vision. The treatment is similar to that for acute-onset postoperative endophthalmitis.

Endophthalmitis after penetrating trauma should be suspected when a greater-than-expected inflammatory response is observed. Because the organisms (e.g., *Bacillus* species) causing posttraumatic endophthalmitis are generally more virulent than organisms causing postoperative endophthalmitis, the final visual outcome is often poor. The incidence of endophthalmitis after open globe injuries ranges from 3% to 30% and depends on the nature of the injury. The associated trauma to the eye and the frequent delay in diagnosis also contribute to a poor visual prognosis. A high index of suspicion and early diagnosis are important because even traumatized eyes infected with virulent organisms can sometimes be salvaged when treatment is initiated promptly. Prophylactic antibiotic treatment for high-risk injuries (rural setting, injuries involving vegetable matter or soil, contaminated eating utensils, retained foreign bodies) should be administered. The management of posttraumatic endophthalmitis is similar to that for other endophthalmitis categories and often includes vitrectomy and intravitreal, subconjunctival, and topical antibiotics and steroids.

Endogenous endophthalmitis results from hematogenous spread of organisms to the eye. Fungi are a more common cause than bacteria, and *Candida albicans* is the most common fungus isolated. The second most commonly encountered fungus is *Aspergillus* species. *Streptococcus* species, *S. aureus,* and *Bacillus* species are the most common cause of endogenous bacterial endophthalmitis. These patients are often debilitated or immunocompromised with indwelling catheters, although endogenous endophthalmitis can occur in drug abusers and rarely in otherwise healthy patients. The infection may be caused by a transient bacteremia or fungemia, in which case blood cultures may be negative. Sepsis with deep-organ involvement may also be present. When the source of infection is not apparent, a systemic workup is indicated.

Endophthalmitis can occur from direct spread of organisms into the eye from an infected corneal ulcer. Factors predisposing to the development of endophthalmitis associated with microbial keratitis include corticosteroid use, systemic immune dysfunction, and local ocular factors. Visual outcomes are poor because of the unusual and virulent nature of the infecting organisms.

■ DIAGNOSIS

Two important factors in the diagnosis of endophthalmitis include the clinical recognition and microbiologic confirmation. Endophthalmitis should be suspected in any eye that has a marked inflammatory response out of proportion to that usually seen in the usual clinical course. Because of the potential for significant visual loss, diagnostic tests usually are performed concurrently with treatment.

The clinical diagnosis is confirmed by obtaining aqueous and vitreous specimens. Although vitreous specimens are more likely to yield a positive culture than simultaneously acquired aqueous specimens, both are important because either one can be positive without the other. Aqueous cultures are obtained by needle aspiration. Vitreous cultures

can be obtained using needle aspiration or using an automated vitrectomy instrument that simultaneously cuts and aspirates the vitreous. Vitreous obtained by needle aspiration can be inoculated directly onto appropriate culture media, including chocolate agar, 5% blood sheep agar, thioglycollate broth, or Sabouraud agar. A specimen obtained during vitrectomy can be concentrated by filtration through a 0.45-micron filter, which is then placed on culture media. An alternative method for processing the vitrectomy specimen involves inoculating approximately 10 ml of the diluted vitrectomy specimen into standard blood culture bottles. This culture technique has been shown to yield a similar rate of culture positivity when compared with the traditional membrane filter technique. Gram stains are usually performed on aqueous and vitreous samples. In suspected fungal cases, additional information may be obtained using the Giemsa, Gomori's methenamine silver, and periodic acid–Schiff stains.

■ TREATMENT

Endophthalmitis can lead to rapid intraocular tissue destruction and irreparable damage. It is inappropriate to wait for culture results before implementing therapy. In addition, the clinical features of the endophthalmitis may not always be accurate in predicting the exact causative organism. For this reason, empiric broad-spectrum antibiotic therapy is initiated immediately. The mainstay of treatment for bacterial endophthalmitis is intraocular antibiotic therapy. The unique properties of the eye, including the fact that it is an enclosed cavity as well as the presence of a blood ocular barrier, make intraocular injection of antibiotic an ideal way of achieving rapid and high antibiotic concentrations within the eye. Subconjunctival and topical antibiotics are also recommended (Table 2).

Systemic antibiotics traditionally have been used to supplement intravitreal antibiotic injections in the management of endophthalmitis. The rationale for using systemic antibiotics is based on the fact that they can maintain adequate intraocular antibiotic levels at a time when the intravitreally

Table 2 Treatment for Acute-Onset Postoperative Endophthalmitis		
ROUTE	**DRUG**	**DOSAGE**
Intravitreal	Vancomycin	1.0 mg/0.1 ml
	Ceftazidime or amikacin	2.25 mg/0.1 ml 0.4 mg/0.1 ml
	Dexamethasone	0.4 mg/0.1 ml
Subconjunctival	Vancomycin	25 mg/0.5 ml
	Ceftazidime	100 mg/0.5 ml
	Dexamethasone	10-24 mg/1.0 ml
Topical	Vancomycin and ceftazidime	50 mg/ml 100 mg/ml
	Steroids and cycloplegics	
Systemic (for more severe cases)	Vancomycin and Ceftazidime (or ciprofloxacin, 750 mg PO q12h)	1.0 g IV q12h 1.0 g IV q12h

administered antibiotic levels are declining. However, cases of successful endophthalmitis treatment without the use of systemic antibiotics have been reported. The EVS randomized patients to receive intravenous ceftazidime and amikacin versus no systemic antibiotic therapy, but all patients received intravitreal antibiotics. The results of that study demonstrated that there was no beneficial effect on final visual outcome or media clarity when these systemic antibiotics were used.

Because much of the intraocular tissue destruction during endophthalmitis results from the inflammatory response, it is important to reduce intraocular inflammation as quickly as possible. Up to 1.2 mg of dexamethasone has been shown to be nontoxic when injected intravitreally in

human eyes. We recommend an intravitreal injection of dexamethasone (0.4 mg in 0.1 ml) at the time of initial treatment. Although both animal studies and small retrospective clinical trials have shown improved endophthalmitis treatment results when intravitreal steroids were combined with intravitreal antibiotic injection, definitive proof of the value of intravitreal steroids is not available. The EVS protocol did not use intravitreal steroids, but EVS patients were placed on prednisone (60 mg) for 5 to 10 days. In addition to intravitreal dexamethasone, we also recommend a 10- to 24-mg subconjunctival injection of dexamethasone at the time of initial treatment.

Vitrectomy surgery (Figures 1, 2, and 3) traditionally has been recommended for more severe cases of endophthalmi-

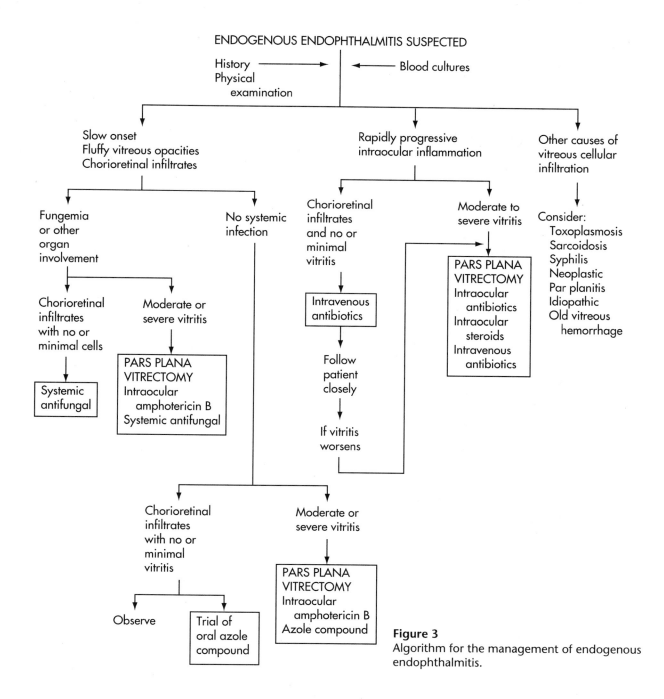

Figure 3
Algorithm for the management of endogenous endophthalmitis.

tis (e.g., initial visual acuity of light perception only, rapid onset within 2 days of surgery, more severe intraocular inflammation). Theoretic advantages of vitrectomy include the rapid removal of infecting organisms and intraocular toxins, removal of vitreous opacities and membranes that may lead to traction retinal detachment, and more rapid clearing of the vitreous cavity. Vitrectomy also allows for collection of a greater volume of material for culture and the potential for enhanced distribution of intravitreal antibiotics. In both animal models of infectious endophthalmitis and in some retrospective studies, eyes treated with vitrectomy combined with intravitreal antibiotics had better results than eyes treated with intravitreal antibiotics alone, but in the EVS, outcomes were equal.

The management of endogenous fungal endophthalmitis depends on the specific fungus isolated and the severity of infection (see Figure 3). When a diagnosis of endogenous fungal endophthalmitis is suspected, evidence for other organ involvement must be obtained. This usually should be done in cooperation with an internist or infectious disease subspecialist. The use and type of systemic antifungal therapy will depend on the presence or absence of systemic fungal infection. In suspected endogenous *Candida* endophthalmitis cases, the management approach is tailored to the clinical situation. When the infection is limited to the choroid and retina, systemic therapy alone may be adequate. Fluconazole has generally replaced amphotericin B as the systemic drug of choice for treating susceptible *Candida* endophthalmitis not associated with significant systemic involvement. Fluconazole is less toxic than amphotericin B and has better intraocular penetration. When moderate to severe vitreous involvement is present, a pars plana vitrectomy and intravitreal injection of amphotericin B (5 to 10 μg) is usually recommended. Intravitreal steroids may be injected simultaneously with intravitreal amphotericin.

Endogenous *Aspergillus* endophthalmitis occurs more often in immunocompromised patients, patients with *Aspergillus* endocarditis or pulmonary disease, or patients with a history of intravenous drug abuse. This organism has a propensity to involve the macular area, resulting in macular abscess and a layering of white blood cells under the retina or internal limiting membrane. When endogenous *Aspergillus* endophthalmitis is suspected, a comprehensive systemic evaluation is indicated, looking for other organ involvement. A combination of local ocular therapy and systemic antifungal therapy (amphotericin B or itraconazole) is often recommended for treatment of this virulent organism.

■ PREVENTION

Because the ocular surface and adnexa are the primary sources of bacteria in exogenous endophthalmitis cases, the best way to theoretically reduce the rates of postoperative endophthalmitis is by minimizing the ocular surface flora. The administration of a topical 5% povidone-iodine solution to the conjunctival surface significantly reduces the conjunctival bacterial colony count. Reduction of conjunctival organisms may also be enhanced with the addition of 3 days of topically applied, broad-spectrum antibiotics. Additional preventive measures include covering the eyelashes completely with a sterile plastic drape and using a meticulous surgical technique, including careful wound closure and aseptic technique. Minimizing excessive pooling of fluid around the wound may also be helpful.

The role of prophylactic antibiotics added to the irrigating solution during surgery is controversial and has not been proven to reduce the incidence of postoperative endophthalmitis. In the EVS, 10 enrolled patients had a history of receiving intraocular antibiotics in the irrigating fluid during cataract surgery. In addition, the potential for intraocular toxicity and development of resistant organisms limit the potential value of this method of prophylaxis. Postoperative periocular antibiotic injections are commonly used but again are unproven in reducing the incidence of postoperative endophthalmitis.

Suggested Reading

Aaberg TM Jr, et al: Nosocomial acute-onset postoperative endophthalmitis survey, *Ophthalmology* 105:1004, 1998.

American Academy of Ophthalmology: *Basic and clinical science course, section 9: intraocular inflammation and uveitis, 1999-2000,* San Francisco, American Academy of Ophthalmology.

Endophthalmitis Vitrectomy Study Group: Results of the Endophthalmitis Vitrectomy Study: a randomized trial of immediate vitrectomy and of intravenous antibiotics for the treatment of postoperative bacterial endophthalmitis, *Arch Ophthalmol* 113:1479, 1995.

Essman TF, et al: Treatment outcomes in a 10-year study of endogenous fungal endophthalmitis, *Ophthal Surg Lasers* 28:185, 1997.

Flynn HW Jr, et al: Endophthalmitis management. In Tasman W, Jaeger E, eds: *Duane's clinical ophthalmology,* vol 6, Philadelphia, 1994, Lippincott.

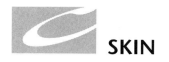

SKIN

FEVER AND RASH

John W. Sensakovic
Leon G. Smith

The approach to the patient presenting with fever and rash is one of the most challenging clinical syndromes in infectious disease. When faced with the patient with fever and rash, the physician must be acutely aware of those several very serious infections that are commonly fulminant and that can be rapidly fatal. Thus the physician must quickly address a series of important issues simultaneously (Table 1). These include the question of contagious potential to the medical staff, the need for rapid resuscitation in those patients who can present in shock, the rapid recognition of and therapeutic intervention for those infections that tend to be fulminant, and the need for a thorough evaluation and workup for the extensive list of diagnostic possibilities that can present with fever and rash.

■ EMERGENT CONDITIONS PRESENTING WITH FEVER AND RASH

Rapid recognition and therapeutic intervention are essential in certain diseases presenting with fever and rash to minimize as much as possible the associated morbidity and mortality. The major conditions involved include meningococcemia, Rocky Mountain spotted fever, staphylococcal toxic shock syndrome, streptococcal toxic shocklike syndrome, bacteremia or endocarditis with septic emboli, and the rapidly spreading cellulitidies (Tables 2 and 3). All of

Table 1   Major Issues in Patients with Fever and Rash
Contagious potential
Resuscitation
Rapid therapy
Diagnostic evaluation
Clinical setting
Severity of illness
Nature of rash
Petechial
Cellulitic
Vessiculobullous
Maculopapular

these conditions can present with fever and rash in a fulminant, rapidly progressive form, requiring expedient therapeutic intervention, often on an empiric basis, before confirmation of the diagnosis, if the associated mortality rates are to be minimized.

Generally, the most serious and rapidly progressive of these are associated with a petechial rash. These 1- to 2-mm purple lesions do not blanch with pressure, often coalesce to form larger ecchymotic areas, and usually are in the presence of leucocytosis and thrombocytopenia. Meningococcemia, Rocky Mountain spotted fever, and bacteremia/endocarditis with septic emboli are perhaps the most notable. However, other causes include gonococcemia, typhus and rat-bite fever; viral infection, including dengue, hepatitis B, rubella, and Epstein-Barr virus [EBV]; and noninfectious causes, including thrombotic thrombocytopenic purpura, Henoch-Schönlein purpura, vasculitis, and scurvy.

Rapidly progressive diseases with erythematous rash include staphylococcal toxic shock syndrome and streptococcal toxic shocklike syndrome, as well as the rapidly progressive cellulidities, which often have a vesicobullous component. Viral infections often present with fever and erythematous rash, and vessiculobullous lesions can be caused by herpes simplex virus, varicella-zoster virus, Rickettsialpox, and contact dermatitis.

Maculopapular rashes, palpable lesions with erythema, occur in a wide variety of conditions. Although some can be serious, they generally do not present in fulminant fashion. These include syphilis, typhoid fever, mycoplasma, Lyme disease, many rickettsial diseases, numerous viral infections, and noninfectious causes, including erythema multiforme, systemic lupus erythematosus, serum sickness, Sweet's syndrome, and allergic reactions.

■ MENINGOCOCCEMIA

Of all the diseases presenting with fever and rash, meningococcemia is the one most likely to be rapidly fatal without early recognition and treatment. The ominous palpable purpura in an acutely ill, febrile patient characteristically suggests this disease. Other features that may be helpful in earlier diagnosis include sore throat, fever, muscle tenderness, and headache in the presence of significant leucocytosis and thrombocytopenia. The illness tends to occur in late winter and early spring and is well known to occur under crowded living conditions. The initial rash may be maculopapular, with the earliest petechial lesions occurring over pressure points such as the small of the back, and can easily be overlooked. The rash can progress rapidly over a few hours to the more classic, petechial form with peripheral acrocyanosis. Management requires immediate recognition, vigorous fluid replacement, and rapid therapy with aqueous

Table 2 Approach to Seriously Ill Patients with Fever and Rash

CLUES	DISEASE	DIAGNOSIS	THERAPY
Multiple purpuric lesions Earliest lesions small of back Rapid progression over hours	Meningococcemia	Gram stain of pustules Blood cultures	Aqueous penicillin, 3,000,000 U/kg/day up to 24 million ×5-7 days IV Vigorous fluid support Steroids—controversial IV gamma globulin—controversial
Tick exposure headache, fever, rash 2nd-6th day Wrists, ankles, progressing to palms, soles, trunk	Rocky Mountain spotted fever	DFA of skin biopsy Serology (CF)	Vibramycin, 100 mg bid ×7 days PO Vigorous fluid support
Fever, rash, hypotension, menstruating female using tampons Surgical wound or skin infection	Toxic shock syndrome	Isolation of phage group I staphylococci	Vigorous fluid replacement Remove tampon Drain focus Nafcillin 2 g IV q4h ×10 days
Fever, rash, hypotension, rapid onset of organ dysfunction	Group A streptococcal toxic shocklike syndrome	Evidence of group A streptococcal infection	Vigorous fluid replacement Ceftriaxone 2 g IV q12h + clindamycin, 900 mg IV q8h
Elderly or immunocompromised patient Several lesions, macular to necrotic pustules	Bacteremia with septic emboli	Gram stain of pustules Blood cultures Gram stain of buffy coat	Nafcillin IV, 2 g IV 4h and gentamicin IV, 5 mg/kg/day ×14 days (longer if endocarditis)
Painful spreading lesions Local trauma	Rapidly spreading cellulitis	Clinical	Antimicrobials Surgical consultation if suspect necrosis or deeper extension

Table 3 Characteristics of Serious Rashes

Onset with or after fever
Petechial lesions
Rapid spread
Purpuric lesions
Palmar/plantar involvement

penicillin, 12 to 24 million units daily intravenously (IV). Patients presenting with signs of adrenal insufficiency also require steroid replacement. The use of gamma globulin and the routine use of corticosteroids are controversial. For more details of therapy, see *Meningococcus and Miscellaneous Neisseria.*

■ ROCKY MOUNTAIN SPOTTED FEVER

Rocky Mountain spotted fever can also present with fever and petechial rash in an acutely ill patient, yet is different from meningococcemia in several respects. The illness begins with fever and severe headache, occurs between May and September in temperate-zone states, and there is a history of tick exposure in 75% of the cases. The rash appears several days into the illness, begins as a maculopapular rash on wrists and ankles, and progresses to a petechial form and spreads to palms, soles, and trunk. A leukocytosis with thrombocytopenia are commonly present.

Therapy is with doxycycline, 100 mg every 12 hours, and must be instituted early on a presumptive basis, before serologic confirmation, if mortality is to be significantly reduced. Alternative therapy is with chloramphenicol, 50 mg/kg/day IV. In institutions where available, immunofluorescence staining of a skin biopsy specimen of the rash can yield a rapid diagnosis. A review from Duke University Medical Center cited 10 cases of illness without rash or with fleeting atypical skin eruptions, emphasizing the need for a high index of suspicion in acutely ill patients.

■ TOXIC SHOCK SYNDROME

Toxic shock syndrome caused by the pyrogenic exotoxin of phage group 1 *Staphylococcus aureus* classically presented in a young menstruating female using a tampon. However, cases have also occurred as a result of nonvaginal foci of staphylococcal infection, including surgical wound infections and infectious endocarditis. The rash tends to be diffuse and scarlatiniform in character, with associated conjunctival hyperemia and a "strawberry tongue." The rash is associated with fever, hypotension, and evidence of multisystem derangement. Therapy requires vigorous fluid replacement, removal of the infected tampon or drainage of an identified infected focus, and nafcillin or oxacillin at 8 to 12 g/day. Some experts also recommend vaginal lavage with a betadine solution as a local antibacterial agent as well as for removal of any nonabsorbed exotoxin.

Another staphylococcal disease, staphylococcal scalded skin syndrome, can be seen in young children infected with a staphylococcal strain producing epidermolysin A or B. The result is a superficial sloughing of the skin with a painful erythema. Nikolsky's sign, "onion skin" peeling of the skin with gentle pressure, is seen.

A somewhat similar, noninfectious entity, toxic epidermal necrolysis, is seen in adults. This typically is drug induced, and the sloughing of the skin occurs deeper, at the epidermal-dermal junction.

■ GROUP A STREPTOCOCCAL TOXIC SHOCKLIKE SYNDROME

The changing epidemiology of group A streptococcal infections has been recognized as a resurgence in rheumatic fever and an increase in the frequency of invasive infections and bacteremia. In addition, the group A streptococcal toxic shocklike syndrome has been recently defined by its characteristic early onset of shock and multiorgan failure in the presence of group A streptococcal infection, often with a generalized erythematous rash that may desquamate. Most of the isolates produce pyrogenic exotoxin A, and some cases have been associated with necrotic soft-tissue infections.

Septic Emboli
The diagnosis of septic emboli associated with bacterial bloodstream infection must be considered in any seriously ill patient with fever and rash. Such infections most commonly present in elderly or immunocompromised patients. Solitary or widely scattered purplish lesions, nonblanching and often with necrotic centers, suggest the diagnosis. The lesions often involve the digits. Ecthyma gangrenosum is one such lesion seen with *Pseudomonas aeruginosa* bacteremia. Such lesions are also seen most often in *S. aureus* bacteremia, *Candida albicans* fungemia, and infectious endocarditis. Gram stain of aspirates from the skin lesions and of the buffy coat of the blood can be rapidly diagnostic; blood cultures are confirmatory. Presumptive therapy should be with nafcillin and gentamicin pending cultural confirmation. In institutions where methicillin-resistant *S. aureus* is a problem, a regimen of vancomycin, 1 g IV every 12 hours, and ceftazidime, 1 g IV every 8 hours, is recommended.

Rapidly Spreading Cellulitis
The various types of rapidly spreading cellulitis associated with fever and rash are not difficult to recognize in most instances because of the painful spreading inflammatory lesion on the skin. The diagnostic difficulty involves differentiating the various types of rapidly spreading cellulitis based on probable causative organism or organisms and whether infection is confined to the surface or extends to deeper structures, including fascia and muscle. With deep extension, case adequate surgical debridement is essential, along with appropriate antibiotic therapy. "Flesh-eating" necrotizing fasciitis from group A streptococcus can be difficult to diagnose and is increasing in frequency.

■ OTHER CONDITIONS

Most diseases associated with fever and rash are less rapidly progressive than those previously discussed. They mainly include viral exanthems, drug eruptions, and vasculitis. Several characteristics of the rash suggest the more serious conditions (see Table 3). Viral exanthems are most often maculopapular and blanch with pressure. The patients appear less toxic; the complete blood count (CBC) and sedimentation rate often suggest a nonbacterial origin; and oral lesions (enanthema) are common. Drug eruptions range from maculopapular to petechial to vesiculobullous and can have mucous membrane involvement, as in Stevens-Johnson syndrome. A history of drug exposure is important. Patients often are not toxic in proportion to the fever; there is often a pulse-temperature discrepancy; and an associated eosinophilia, transaminitis, or nephritis can sometimes be found. Vasculitis of the skin is often suspected because of the nonblanching, often petechial rash with associated findings of multisystem involvement, but diagnosis usually requires skin biopsy along with serologic diagnostic testing.

Several other specific entities are commonly seen with fever and rash. Erythema nodosum lesions are painful, tender, reddish-brown nodules, mainly on the shins, seen in a variety of infectious diseases (tuberculosis, histoplasmosis, coccidioidomycosis, *Yersinia,* beta-hemolytic streptococcal infection), and they may be drug induced (sulfa, penicillin, oral contraceptives). Erythema multiforme characteristically presents as target lesions, often on the palms, but can become vesiculobullous. They are seen in a variety of infections (herpes, *Mycoplasma*) and drug reactions (penicillin, sulfa, phenytoin).

Although a wide variety of diagnostic tests and procedures can be helpful in the workup of the patient presenting with fever and rash, none of these is as important as a careful history and physical examination.

Suggested Reading

Drage L: Life-threatening rashes: dermatologic signs of four infectious diseases, *Mayo Clin Proc* 74:68, 1999.

Kingston M, Mackey D: Skin clues in the diagnosis of life-threatening infections, *Rev Infect Dis* 8:1, 1986.

Oblinger M, Sande M: Fever and rash. In Stein JH, ed: *Internal medicine,* Boston, 1983, Little, Brown.

Schlossberg D: Fever and rash, *Infect Dis Clin North Am* 10:101, 1996.

The Working Group on Severe Streptococcal Infections: Defining the group A streptococcal toxic shock syndrome, *JAMA* January 269:390, 1993.

STAPHYLOCOCCAL AND STREPTOCOCCAL TOXIC SHOCK AND KAWASAKI SYNDROMES

Aris P. Assimacopoulos
Patrick M. Schlievert

■ TOXIC SHOCK SYNDROME

Staphylococcal and streptococcal toxic shock syndromes (TSS) are acute-onset multiorgan illnesses defined by the criteria listed in Tables 1 and 2. Staphylococcal TSS is caused by *Staphylococcus aureus* strains that make pyrogenic toxin superantigens (PTSAgs); coagulase-negative strains do not make the causative toxins. Streptococcal TSS is caused mainly by toxin-producing group A strains but occasionally by groups B, C, F, and G strains. Several subsets of staphylococcal TSS exist, with two major categories being menstrual and nonmenstrual.

Menstrual TSS, which occurs within a day or two of and during menstruation, primarily has been associated with use of certain tampons, notably those of high absorbency, and is associated with production of TSS toxin-1 (TSST-1) by the causative bacterium. Three theories have been proposed to explain the role of tampons in menstrual TSS: (1) tampons introduce oxygen, which is required for production of TSST-1, into the vagina; (2) tampons bind magnesium, which alters growth kinetics of *S. aureus* and thus alters the time when TSST-1 is made; and (3) pluronic L-92, a surfactant present in the Rely tampon, which was highly associated with TSS, amplifies production of TSST-1. Certain other surfactants may have similar effects.

Nonmenstrual TSS occurs in both males and females, adults and children, and it is associated with *S. aureus* strains that make TSST-1 or staphylococcal enterotoxins, notably enterotoxin serotypes B and C. The illness occurs in association with nearly any kind of staphylococcal infection, but major forms have been identified: postsurgical, influenza associated, RED syndrome, and occasionally with use of contraceptive diaphragms. Postsurgical TSS is often associated with *S. aureus* infections that do not result in pyogenic responses, and thus the source of infection may be difficult to find. Influenza TSS may occur as a consequence of influenza or parainfluenza damage to the respiratory tract epithelium and superinfection with toxin-producing *S. aureus.* This illness is highly fatal in children. RED syndrome is a recalcitrant erythematous desquamating disorder in patients with acquired immunodeficiency syndrome (AIDS) that may last 70 days or more or until the patient succumbs. Finally, nonmenstrual TSS associated with use of diaphragms may be similar to menstrual TSS, although the reason for the association is unclear.

Table 1 Diagnostic Criteria for Staphylococcal Toxic Shock Syndrome

1. Temperature greater than 38.8° C
2. Systolic blood pressure ≤90 mm Hg for adults, less than the 5th percentile for children, or greater than a 15 mm Hg orthostatic drop in diastolic blood pressure or orthostatic dizziness/syncope
3. Diffuse macular rash with subsequent desquamation
4. Three of the following organ systems involved:
   Liver: bilirubin, AST, ALT more than twice the upper normal limit
   Blood: platelets <100,000/mm^3
   Renal: BUN or creatinine more twice the upper normal limit or pyuria without urinary tract infection
   Mucous membranes: hyperemia of the vagina, oropharynx, or conjunctivae
   Gastrointestinal: diarrhea or vomiting
   Muscular: myalgias or CPK more than twice the normal upper limit
   Central nervous system: disorientation or lowered level of consciousness in the absence of hypotension, fever, or focal neurologic deficits
5. Negative serologies for measles, leptospirosis, and Rocky Mountain spotted fever. Blood or CSF cultures negative for organisms other than *Staphylococcus aureus*

AST, Aspartate transaminase; *ALT,* alanine aminotransferase; *BUN,* blood urea nitrogen; *CPK,* creatine phosphokinase; *CSF,* cerebrospinal fluid.

Table 2 Diagnostic Criteria for Streptococcal Toxic Shock Syndrome

1. Isolation of group A streptococci:
   From a sterile site for a *definite* case
   From a nonsterile site for a *probable* case
2. Clinical criteria:
   Hypotension *and* two of the following:

Renal dysfunction	Coagulopathy
Liver involvement	ARDS
Erythematous macular rash	Soft-tissue necrosis

ARDS, Adult respiratory distress syndrome.

Streptococcal TSS primarily is associated with group A streptococcal infections, particularly M types 1 and 3. The illness may or may not be associated with necrotizing fasciitis and myositis. Occasionally, streptococcal TSS is caused by other groups of streptococci, primarily groups B, C, and G.

Group A streptococcal strains that cause TSS produce streptococcal pyrogenic exotoxins. The major association has been with SPE serotype A, but other members of the family may also contribute significantly. Non–group A streptococci associated with TSS also make PTSAgs, only one of which has been characterized—that made by some group B strains.

Major risk factors for development of streptococcal TSS include chickenpox in children, penetrating and nonpenetrating wounds, use of nonsteroidal antiinflammatory agents, and pregnancy.

Table 3   Clinical Criteria for Kawasaki Syndrome*

1. Fever, usually of at least 5 days' duration
2. Four of five of the following:
  Extremity changes, induration, edema, erythema
  Oropharyngeal and lip changes, strawberry tongue
    cracked lips
  Cervical lymphadenopathy: at least one node >1.5 cm
  Injected conjunctivae
  Rash, erythematous and polymorphous
3. Other diseases excluded

*Strict fulfillment is not always necessary; see Suggested Reading.

■ KAWASAKI SYNDROME

Kawasaki syndrome (KS) is an acute multisystem vasculitis that occurs primarily in children younger than 4 years of age (Table 3). KS shares many features with scarlet fever and TSS, except that hypotension is absent; KS is a leading cause of acquired heart disease in this age group. Coronary artery abnormalities, including aneurysms, develop in 15% to 25% of patients.

The causative agent of KS remains unclear, but studies suggest that *S. aureus* and streptococcal PTSAgs may have important causal roles in many cases.

■ THERAPY

Staphylococcal Toxic Shock Syndrome
Differential Diagnosis

- Viral disease, including measles, rubella, and parvovirus B19
- Spotted fever group rickettsiae
- Leptospirosis
- Drug reactions, including Stevens-Johnson syndrome
- Collagen-vascular diseases, including systemic lupus erythematosus and Still's disease
- Scarlet and rheumatic fever
- Syphilis
- Typhoid fever

Initial Evaluation
Possible sources of infection must be identified. The physician should perform a vaginal examination, remove any tampon, and culture for *S. aureus*. Any wound packing should be removed.

Supportive Care
Supportive care is of primary importance. Patients often require large amounts of intravenous fluids, vasopressors, and management of associated problems such as acute renal failure, adult respiratory distress syndrome, disseminated intravascular coagulation, or myocardial suppression.

Antibiotics
Antistaphylococcal therapy decreases the risk of recurrence. One of the antistaphylococcal penicillins such as nafcillin (adults: 2 g intravenously [IV] q4h; children: 150 mg/kg/day IV q6h) is an appropriate choice. For penicillin-allergic

patients, cefazolin (adults: 1 to 2 g IV q8h; children: 50 to 100 mg/kg/day IV q8h) or vancomycin (adults: 1 g IV q12h; children 40 mg/kg/day IV q6h) can be used. Some support the use of clindamycin (adults: 900 mg IV q8h; children: 40 mg/kg/day IV q6-8h) or other protein synthesis inhibiting antibiotics because experimental data suggest that it inhibits toxin production. Dosage adjustments for renal failure may be required.

Surgical Intervention
Any obvious source of infection should be drained, and a low threshold for exploring possible sites, even if they lack signs of significant inflammation, must be maintained.

Prevention
Up to 30% recurrence has been suggested. A course of rifampin is sometimes given in hopes of eliminating colonization. Avoidance of further tampon use is prudent after menstrual TSS.

Other Therapeutic Issues
Although no controlled trials have been conducted, intravenous immunoglobulin (IVIG) and steroids have been used in the treatment of TSS. Although these may not be warranted in a patient with "mild" TSS, which responds rapidly to therapy, in the critically ill patient, the benefits probably outweigh the risks.

Streptococcal Toxic Shock Syndrome (STSS) and Myositis
Differential Diagnosis

The differential diagnosis is mentioned in the preceding section. Consider myositis in any patient who has severe local pain, especially in an extremity, and a paucity of other findings. Because early intervention is lifesaving, it is most important to maintain a very high index of suspicion. An elevated creatinine, elevated creatine kinase (CK), or significant bandemia should suggest the diagnosis but can be absent in atypical cases.

Initial Evaluation
The physician should look for a skin or soft tissue focus. Any painful or tender areas must be attended to, even in the absence of inflammatory signs. The physician should unpack and inspect any wounds. There may be no obvious site of infection. Because early surgical intervention is extremely important, it is imperative to identify any focus quickly. Magnetic resonance imaging (MRI) has been used to identify deep soft-tissue infections and may be helpful in revealing necrosis of tissue and guiding surgical intervention (see Suggested Reading).

Supportive Care
Patients often require large amounts of intravenous fluids, vasopressors, and management of associated problems such as acute renal failure, adult respiratory distress syndrome, disseminated intravascular coagulation, or myocardial suppression.

Antibiotics
For group A streptococci (GAS), treatment includes a combination of a beta-lactam and protein synthesis inhibitor:

penicillin (adults: 4 mU IV q4h; children: 250,000 U/kg/day IV q4h) or ceftriaxone (adults: 2 g IV q24h; children: 50 to 75 mg/kg/day IV q12-24h) in combination with clindamycin (adults: 900 mg IV q8h; children: 40 mg/kg/day IV q6-8h) or erythromycin (adults: 1 g IV q6h; children: 20 to 40 mg/kg/day IV q6h).

Surgical Intervention

Any obvious source of infection should be drained, and a low threshold to explore other sites must be maintained, remembering that expected signs of inflammation may be absent in streptococcal myositis. Radionuclide white blood cell (WBC) scanning has been used to identify undrained foci of necrotizing fasciitis in a nonresponding patient (see Suggested Reading).

Prevention

Appropriate cleansing of any wounds is important. There is no controlled experience with antibiotic prophylaxis. As expected, anecdotal experience indicates that close contacts of an index case of STSS may carry toxin-producing streptococci in the nasopharynx. There are no data on the beneficial or adverse effects of prophylactic treatment in these patients. Group A streptococci can also colonize the skin, vagina, and anus.

Other Therapeutic Issues

IVIG has been used. Although no controlled trials have been conducted, anecdotal experience indicates that there may be some benefit. It may act to neutralize toxins elaborated by the streptococci or to decrease endogenous mediators of sepsis. Steroids have also been used in extremely ill patients and may be of benefit. In the critically ill patient, the possible benefits of IVIG and steroids are probably worth any potential risk.

Kawasaki Syndrome
Differential Diagnosis

- Viral exanthemata, especially measles
- Scarlet fever
- Drug reactions, Stevens-Johnson syndrome, erythema multiforme
- Spotted fever group rickettsiosis
- Toxic shock syndrome
- Staphylococcal scalded skin syndrome
- Juvenile rheumatoid arthritis
- Leptospirosis
- Mercury poisoning

Initial Evaluation

The physician must try to exclude other diagnostic possibilities. Measles and scarlet fever present the most common diagnostic dilemma. The physician should bear in mind that KS may be atypical or incomplete in presentation. It is important to identify and refer any patient with possible atypical presentation because he or she may be at higher risk for coronary artery lesions (CALs). Treatment should be rendered within 10 days for proven benefit.

Supportive Care

Cardiorespiratory monitoring, close clinical observation, and maintaining attention to fluid balance are required.

Aspirin

High dosages of aspirin (80 to 100 mg/kg/day in four divided doses) should be given until the fever is gone; then the patient should be maintained on low dosages (3 to 5 mg/kg/day [maximum, 80 mg/day] in one dose) for 6 to 8 weeks or until the platelet count and sedimentation rate are normal. Monitoring of serum salicylate levels in nonresponders should be considered. Some prefer high dosages until day 14. Coronary artery abnormalities necessitate longer therapy. Influenza or varicella exposure may prompt discontinuation of aspirin therapy for up to 14 days because of the risk of Reye's syndrome. Dipyridamole (4 to 9 mg/kg/day in two or three divided doses) may substitute during this time in high-risk patients. The patient should get an influenza vaccination yearly while taking aspirin.

Intravenous Immunoglobulin

The physician should administer 2 g/kg of IVIG over 12 hours. This has a more rapid effect than the alternative regimen of 400 mg/kg/day for 4 days. Measles, mumps, and rubella vaccines should be delayed for 5 to 11 months after IVIG administration unless the patient is at high risk. If so, the vaccination can be given on schedule and repeated 11 months later.

Monitoring for Cardiac Complications

Inpatient and outpatient serial examinations are important. An electrocardiogram and cardiac echocardiogram should be obtained early and repeated at 3 and 8 weeks. A cardiology consultation should be considered. Stress testing and coronary angiography have value in specific clinical situations. The patient with CALs requires more intensive monitoring.

Evaluation of Therapy

Ten percent of patients may not respond. If fever or signs of inflammation persist or recur, the physician should consider retreatment with IVIG (1 to 2 g/kg over 10 to 12 hours). Pulsed doses of corticosteroids have been used in nonresponders with success despite initial reports that corticosteroids may increase the risk for CALS.

Long-Term Management

Physical activity should be restricted for 6 to 8 weeks. The frequency of follow-up is determined on an individual basis. It is possible to identify a group of low-risk patients who may not require intensive follow-up. Complicated management issues, such as use of warfarin, calcium channel blockers, and angiography, are beyond the scope of this text. The reader is referred to several excellent reviews of KS found in the Suggested Reading section.

Other Issues. Antibiotics are not routinely used. Pentoxifylline has been tried experimentally but is not of any proven benefit.

Suggested Reading

Barry W, et al: Intravenous immunoglobulin therapy for toxic shock syndrome, *JAMA* 267:3315, 1992.

Beiser AS, et al: A predictive instrument for coronary artery aneurysms in Kawasaki disease, *Am J Cardiol* 81:1116, 1998.

Brothers TE, et al: Magnetic resonance imaging differentiates between necrotizing and non-necrotizing fasciitis of the lower extremity, *J Am Coll Surg* 187(4):416, 1998.

Lee BE, Robinson JL: The use of technetium-99m-labeled white blood cell scan in the management of a case of group A streptococcus necrotizing fasciitis with polymyositis, *Clin Infect Dis* 28:153, 1999.

Mason WH, Takahashi M: Kawasaki syndrome, *Clin Infect Dis* 28:169, 1999.

Peter G, ed: Report of the Committee on Infectious Diseases of the American Academy of Pediatrics, Elk Grove, IL, 1997, Red Book, p 316.

Rowley AH: Controversies in Kawasaki syndrome, *Adv Pediatr Infect Dis* 13:127, 1998.

Rowley AH, Shulman ST: Kawasaki syndrome, *Clin Microb Rev* 11(3):405, 1998.

Stevens DL: The toxic shock syndromes, *Infect Dis Clin North Am* 10(4): 727, 1996.

Todd JK: Therapy of toxic shock syndrome, *Drugs* 39:856, 1990.

Wright DA, et al: Treatment of immune globulin-resistant Kawasaki disease with pulsed doses of corticosteroids, *J Pediatr* 128:146, 1996.

CLASSIC VIRAL EXANTHEMS

Henry M. Feder, Jr.
Jane M. Grant-Kels

During the early 1900s, six common childhood exanthematous infections were defined by the numbers 1 through 6. The etiologic agents of these infections were unknown. Over the next century, the etiologies of these exanthems were defined, and four of the six were demonstrated to be caused by viruses (Table 1). The first exanthem was caused by the measles virus, the third by the rubella virus, the second and fourth by bacterial toxins, the fifth by parvovirus, and the sixth by human herpesvirus-6.

In developed countries where most children have received measles and rubella vaccinations, other viral exanthems are often confused with breakthrough measles or rubella. For example, in a study of 2299 Finnish children with exanthems thought to be measles or rubella, only 6% actually had measles or rubella. When acute and convalescent serologies were performed, other diagnoses, including parvovirus (20%), enterovirus (9%), adenovirus (4%), and human herpesvirus (4%), were defined.

Table 1	Classic Exanthems of Childhood	
ORDER	**EXANTHEMS**	**AGENT**
First	Rubeola or measles	Measles virus
Second	Scarlet fever	Streptococcal toxin
Third	Rubella or German measles	Rubella virus
Fourth	Filatow-Dukes' disease*	Streptococcal or staphylococcal toxin
Fifth	Erythema infectiosum	Parvovirus
Sixth	Exanthem subitum or roseola	Human herpesvirus-6

*Not a separate exanthem but a variant of scarlet fever or a variant of toxin-producing staphylococcal disease.

This chapter discusses the classic childhood viral exanthems: measles (rubeola), German measles (rubella), and exanthem subitum (roseola). Parvovirus infection is discussed in the chapter *Acute and Chronic Parvovirus Infection.*

■ RUBEOLA

Rubeola (measles) is caused by an RNA virus with one antigenic type and is classified as a paramyxovirus. The licensure of both a live attenuated and killed measles vaccine in 1963 resulted in a 98% diminution in incidence rates. The killed vaccine proved problematic, and only the live vaccine has remained available since 1967. Most cases of measles occur in the fall, winter, or spring, with the highest number of cases occurring in early spring. The measles virus is disseminated by tiny respiratory droplets and, like chickenpox, can be spread through the air without direct contact. If a patient is hospitalized, airborne precautions are indicated for 4 days after the onset of rash. However, if the patient is immunosuppressed, airborne precautions are required until the illness resolves. Measles and chickenpox are two of the most contagious common infectious diseases. The measles virus is labile and survives only a short time on fomites. The highest rates of transmission occur in the home, day-care centers, nursery schools, primary and secondary schools, and colleges and universities. School outbreaks can occur despite greater than 95% immunity among students. Most cases of measles occur after face-to-face contact. Thus, when a physician suspects measles, a defined or potential exposure should be identified.

Clinical and Laboratory Diagnosis

Measles demonstrates a characteristic clinical presentation, which makes the diagnosis straightforward. The incubation period is 10 to 12 days. There is a prodrome of low-grade fever, malaise, and headache. This is followed or accompanied by cough, coryza, and conjunctivitis. During the prodrome, Koplik spots, the enanthem of measles, appear on the buccal mucosa. Koplik spots are punctate white spots (like grains of sand) on erythematous bases. As the infection evolves, the number of Koplik spots increases and they appear as salt on a red background. They begin to resolve at the onset of rash. After about 4 days of increasing prodromal symptoms, the patient develops high fever (103° to 105° F) and rash. The rash begins as erythematous macules and papules at the hairline, on the forehead, behind the ears, and on the upper neck. This characteristic morbiliform rash occurs in almost 100% of normal individuals. The rash spreads to the trunk and extremities over the next 3 days. This erythematous rash blanches on pressure and may coalesce, and when it resolves, it may leave brownish staining that results from capillary hemorrhage. The characteristic morbiliform rash may not occur in up to 30% of patients who are immunosuppressed. When present, the high fever and rash persist for 2 to 4 days. When the rash fades, the coryza and conjunctivitis clear, but the cough may persist for another 5 days. A patient is contagious from the onset of the prodrome until approximately 5 days after the onset of the rash.

The most common complications of measles are secondary bacterial infections, including pneumonia and otitis media. The risk of complications is highest for infants younger than 1 year of age. A rare complication is postinfectious encephalomyelitis. This is a demyelinating disease that occurs in 1 per 1000 measles cases and has a mortality rate of 10% to 20%. Clinically, it begins with vomiting, then obtundation and seizures develop. Measles has a mortality rate of less than 0.1% in normal patients; however, this increases to up to 50% with immunosuppression.

Measles can be confirmed by viral cultures of the nasopharynx, conjunctiva, blood, or urine. However, culture is technically difficult and not readily available. Sera may be obtained for measles antibody determinations both at the onset of the rash and 2 to 4 weeks later. A fourfold or greater increase of measles antibody is diagnostic. Finally, a measles-specific IgM antibody test is also available. This IgM antibody is detectable from about 7 to 30 days after the onset of the rash. Immunity after measles infection is lifelong, and a second attack is very rare.

Treatment and Prevention

Treatment of measles is usually symptomatic—acetaminophen or a nonsteroidal antiinflammatory drug (NSAID) is used for pain and fever. There are data to suggest that oral vitamin A supplementation lessens morbidity and mortality in malnourished patients. The dose is 100,000 IU in a single oral dose for infants younger than 1 year of age and 200,000 IU for patients older than 1 year. For reasons that are not defined, malnourished patients may suffer acute vitamin A deficiency when infected with measles. Vitamin A is necessary for the maintenance of epithelial cell integrity and for normal immune function. Vitamin A supplementation for measles infection is recommended in patients who are malnourished and in immigrants from countries where malnourishment (and a high measles mortality rate, 1% or higher) is common. Because measles may be complicated by secondary bacterial infection, prophylactic antibodies are sometimes prescribed, although not generally recommended. The most common bacterial complication is pneumonia caused by *Streptococcus pneumoniae*, *Hemophilus influenzae*, or *Staphylococcus aureus*.

Measles virus is susceptible in vitro to the antiviral agent ribavirin. However, ribavirin has not been studied in vivo for the treatment of measles. There are anecdotal reports of successful use of intravenous and/or aerosolized ribavirin to treat severely ill, immunosuppressed patients with measles.

Table 2   Contraindications for Measles Vaccine
Pregnancy
Immunodeficiency or immunocompromise except for human immunodeficiency virus infection
History of anaphylaxis to eggs
History of anaphylaxis to neomycin

Live measles vaccine is routinely recommended at ages 12 to 15 months. The efficacy of this vaccine is hindered by passive maternal antibody, which is no longer present by 12 months. If the mother is immune via natural infection, not immunization, then maternal antibody can persist in the infant until 15 months. A measles booster is recommended at 5 to 12 years of age. Unimmunized children and adults should be given two measles doses at least 1 month apart. After exposure to measles, in an unimmunized person, measles vaccine may be efficacious if given within 72 hours of exposure. Measles vaccine should be administered to patients with human immunodeficiency virus (HIV) because of the potentially devastating outcome of measles in this group. Because measles inoculation is a live vaccine, it is not recommended for immunosuppressed patients (see Table 2 for contraindications for measles vaccine).

Patients traveling to foreign countries should be immune to measles. For infants traveling to developing countries where measles is endemic, the measles vaccine can be given as early as 6 months of age.

Immunoglobulin (IG) may prevent or reduce the severity of measles if given within 6 days of an unimmunized patient's exposure. The recommended dose is 0.25 ml/kg given intramuscularly (0.50 ml/kg for immunocompromised patients) with a maximum dose of 15 ml. IG is also recommended for HIV-positive patients who are exposed to measles even if they have been previously immunized.

■ RUBELLA

Rubella is a togavirus with a single strand of RNA at its core. Rubella vaccine is a live attenuated virus that was licensed in 1969. Before the rubella vaccine, the major danger posed by rubella virus was the specter of infection during pregnancy, which could cause congenital rubella syndrome in the newborn. Before the vaccine was available, thousands of cases of congenital rubella were reported each year in the United States. The vaccine was very successful. From 1985 through 1996, 122 cases of congenital rubella were reported to the National Congenital Rubella Syndrome Registry in this country. The number of cases has been decreasing from 1992 until the present. Indigenous rubella and congenital rubella syndrome may be eliminated from the United States during the next decade. Congenital rubella has now become the unfortunate, preventable result of failing to immunize women of childbearing potential.

Clinical and Laboratory Diagnosis

Rubella infection in infants and children is usually mild, and up to 50% of infections in children are asymptomatic. A prodrome characterized by tender postauricular, posterior cervical, and suboccipital adenopathy with malaise is common among adolescents and adults with rubella. The adenopathy may persist for weeks. The rubella exanthem begins on the face, neck, and scalp and spreads downward. The rash may be associated with fever, headache, myalgias, and arthralgias. The rash consists of pink macules and papules that range in diameter from 1 to 4 mm. The exanthem fades as it spreads; thus it may be absent on the face when it is prominent on the trunk. The enanthem, Forchheimer's sign, occurs in 20% of patients and is characterized as petechiae or red spots on the soft palate. It occurs during the prodrome or at the onset of the enanthem. Rubella is most commonly seen during late winter and early spring.

Rubella is spread by small droplets from the respiratory mucosa. Patients are contagious for a few days before, until up to 7 days after, the onset of rash. Prolonged exposure usually is necessary for transmission of rubella. The incubation period is 14 to 21 days.

Complications of rubella are unusual. The most common complication is arthritis, which occurs almost exclusively in females and has an increasing incidence with advanced age. Rare complications include thrombocytopenia and encephalitis. The most devastating complication is congenital rubella syndrome. The frequency of congenital rubella is 50% if rubella infection occurs during the first 12 weeks of pregnancy. This incidence diminishes to 25% for infections occurring from 13 to 24 weeks. Congenital rubella syndrome is rare if maternal infection occurs after 24 weeks' gestation. Congenital rubella syndrome is commonly characterized by deafness, congenital cataracts, and patent ductus arteriosus. Severe involvement is often fatal, and infection involves many organs, including the skin (described as a blueberry muffin because of bluish areas of extramedullary hematopoesis).

Rubella can be diagnosed by the typical exanthem and the associated adenopathy. Posterior auricular adenopathy is suggestive of rubella. Rubella virus can be isolated from nasal secretions, but most laboratories do not have the proper reagents needed for isolation. Acute and convalescent (2 to 4 weeks after rash) serology should show a fourfold or greater rise in rubella antibodies. A rubella-specific IgM antibody test is also available. The IgM antibody persists for several months after acute infection.

Treatment and Prevention

Typical rubella infection is mild and requires no therapy. The occasional patient with severe arthralgias or arthritis should respond to therapy with NSAIDs. Arthralgias and arthritis are much more common in females. The routine administration of IG after exposure is not recommended. However, if a pregnant patient is exposed to rubella in early pregnancy and termination of the pregnancy is not an option, the administration of IG can be considered. Limited data suggest that IG may decrease the manifestations of clinical rubella, but this does not guarantee a diminution in the incidence or severity of congenital rubella.

Rubella vaccine should be given with measles and mumps vaccines (MMR) in the same two-dose schedule: the first dose at 12 to 15 months and the second at 5 to 12 years of age. Contraindications for rubella vaccine are listed in Table 3. Because rubella is a live vaccine and can potentially

Table 3   Contraindications for Rubella Vaccine
Pregnancy
Immunodeficiency or immunocompromise except human immunodeficiency virus infection
Immunoglobulin in the last 3 months

infect the fetus, it should not be given during pregnancy, although the risk of fetal infection is low. In a study of 226 susceptible women who were inadvertently immunized with rubella vaccine during the first trimester, there were no congenital abnormalities in the offspring and two offspring showed asymptomatic infection. This benign outcome may reflect the fact that this is an attenuated viral vaccine.

■ ROSEOLA

Roseola, or exanthem subitum, is the sixth of the classic exanthems and is caused by human herpesvirus-6 (HHV-6). This is a herpesvirus, and after the initial infection, the virus becomes latent. At birth, passively acquired HHV-6 antibody usually is present in the newborn. This protects the infant until about 6 months of age. From 6 to 24 months of age, about 80% of infants become infected with HHV-6. Most cases of roseola occur in the spring and early fall. The mode of transmission is unknown. It is unusual to demonstrate roseola spreading from one infant to another. After acute infection, HHV-6 can often be isolated from saliva. Saliva transmission from an asymptomatic contact to a susceptible infant may be the common route of transmission. HHV-6 can also be isolated from both peripheral blood lymphocytes and cerebrospinal fluid.

HHV-6 is a herpesvirus distinct from herpes simplex 1 and 2, varicella-zoster virus, cytomegalovirus, and Epstein-Barr virus. HHV-6 was first isolated in 1986. This was followed by the isolation of human herpesvirus-7 (which may also cause roseola) in 1990 and the subsequent isolation of human herpesvirus-8 (the cause of Kaposi's sarcoma) in 1994. HHV-6 may be divided into two major groups: variants A and B. Primary infection may be associated with roseola and is caused by variant B strains. In addition to causing roseola, HHV-6 causes a febrile illness without rash, a febrile illness with lymphadenopathy, gastroenteritis, upper respiratory infection, and inflamed ear drums; see the chapter *Human Herpesvirus 6, 7, 8.*

Clinical and Laboratory Diagnosis

The incubation period of roseola is 7 to 15 days, and the disease has no prodrome. Clinical illness begins with a high fever (102° to 105° F). Febrile seizures can occur. Roseola accounts for 10% of visits to the emergency room for infants younger than 2 years old. In addition, roseola accounts for 33% of febrile and recurrent febrile seizures seen in emergency rooms. The fever typically lasts 3 days. Classically, when the fever resolves, the exanthem appears. The exanthem may also begin before the fever resolves. The exanthem is characterized by discrete, pale, pink macules, varying in size from 1 to 5 mm in diameter. Around each lesion, there is a pale areola. The rash commonly begins on the trunk, on the neck, and behind the ears and spreads to the proximal extremities. The rash may become confluent. It rarely involves the face or distal extremities. The rash usually lasts for 2 to 48 hours. Before the rash appears, an enanthem of erythematous macules may be present on the soft palate.

Acute HHV-6 infection may be diagnosed by a specific IgM antibody. This IgM antibody peaks 7 to 14 days after the onset of illness and becomes undetectable in several weeks. Specific IgG antibody develops 2 to 4 weeks after the onset of illness and may remain detectable indefinitely. Also, the IgG antibody may intermittently rise and fall, especially in association with cytomegalovirus or Epstein-Barr virus infections. In research laboratories, HHV-6 can be cultured from mononuclear cells and detected by polymerase chain reaction (PCR).

Treatment and Prevention

At present, no treatment or prevention strategies are available for HHV-6 infection (except for the posttransplant patient; see the chapter *Human Herpesvirus 6, 7, 8*). However, because HHV-6 is a common cause for febrile seizures in infants between 6 months and 2 years of age, an immunization would be valuable. Finally, it is not known how HHV-6 is spread. Thus there are no recommendations for isolation of infected hosts either in or out of the hospital.

Suggested Reading

American Academy of Pediatrics, Peter G, ed: *1997 Red Book: Report of the Committee on Infectious Diseases,* ed 24, Elk Grove Village, IL, 1997, American Academy of Pediatrics.

Bialecki C, Feder HM Jr, Grant-Kels JM: The six classic childhood exanthems: a review and update, *J Am Acad Dermatol* 21:891, 1989.

Davidkin I, et al: Etiology of measles and rubella-like illnesses in measles, mumps and rubella-vaccinated children, *J Infect Dis* 178:1567, 1998.

Hall CB, et al: Human herpesvirus-6 infection in children, *N Engl J Med* 331:432, 1994.

Hussey G: Managing measles, *Br Med J* 314:316, 1997.

Kaplan LJ, et al: Severe measles in immunocompromised patients, *JAMA* 267:1237, 1992.

Schluter WW, et al: Changing epidemiology of congenital rubella syndrome in the United States, *J Infect Dis* 178:636, 1998.

SKIN ULCER AND PYODERMA

Joanne T. Maffei

Skin lesions are important clues to systemic diseases, and conversely, host factors make patients susceptible to skin infections caused by certain organisms. The skin has a limited response to insults from the microbial world, forming vesicles and pustules that eventually rupture and leave exposed dermis. Accurate diagnosis and appropriate treatment depend on a detailed history that includes systemic complaints, history of exposure and travel, and the initial appearance of the skin lesions. Sound diagnosis of difficult cases also depends on appropriate cultures and histopathology. When possible, cultures should be obtained by aspirating pus or blister fluid from under intact skin; cultures from ulcerated skin are less reliable because of colonization by nonpathogenic skin flora. A Gram stain and routine culture should be done first; if the ulcer persists despite a course of antibiotics, a skin biopsy with histopathology and cultures for routine agents, acid-fast organisms, and fungal pathogens is appropriate. If the lesion has multiple thin-walled vesicles with interspersed shallow ulcers and crusts or is on a mucous membrane, a direct fluorescent antibody test (DFA) or Tzanck smear for herpes and viral culture should be considered.

Most superficial skin infections and ulcers can be treated empirically according to the typical clinical presentation of the lesions. A workup is required for lesions that do not respond to routine therapy, that are rapidly progressive, or that occur in an immunocompromised host.

■ SKIN ULCERS

Skin ulcers are superficial defects in the tissues of the epidermis and dermis, with surrounding inflammation. Infection, collagen-vascular diseases, and malignancy can cause cutaneous ulcerations. Information on host factors, exposure history, and the clinical course of the lesions is critical to narrowing the differential diagnosis. The lesion's anatomic location also may offer clues to the cause. Facial ulcers may be caused by syphilis, herpes, or blastomycosis, whereas ulcers of the arms or hands may be caused by sporotrichosis, nocardia, atypical mycobacteria, herpetic whitlow, or cutaneous anthrax. Ulcers in the groin or perineum may result from sexually transmitted diseases such as syphilis, chancroid, and herpes, as well as from Behçet's disease or fixed drug eruption.

Ulcers on the lower extremities result from venous insufficiency in 70% to 90% of cases and occur below the knee but never on the bottom of the foot. The patient with venous stasis ulcers has good peripheral pulses and no peripheral neuropathy. Ulcers in patients with poor peripheral pulses or sensory loss must be investigated further because venous stasis is not the cause. Any ulcer on the leg that does not respond to treatment for venous stasis ulcers should be investigated further by biopsy and culture, as

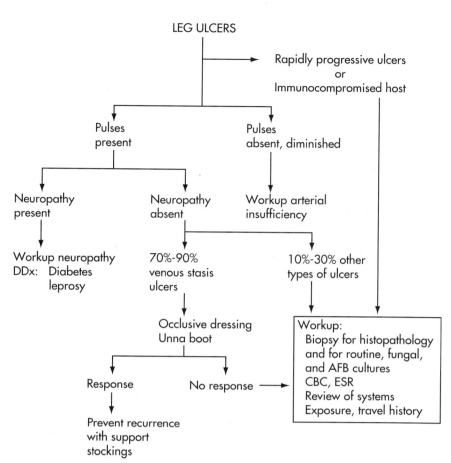

Figure 1
Algorithm for the evaluation of leg ulcers. *DDX*, Differential diagnosis; *CBC*, complete blood count; *ESR*, erythrocyte sedimentation rate; *AFB*, acid-fast bacilli.

should any ulcer that is rapidly progressive or appears on an immunocompromised host. Figure 1 outlines the steps in evaluating and treating leg ulcers.

A history of an unusual occupation, hobby, or exposure can suggest causes of skin ulcers, such as tularemia in rabbit hunters, *Mycobacterium marinum* in aquarium enthusiasts, and leishmaniasis in travelers to endemic areas of Central and South America. Host factors also may predispose individuals to any of several types of ulcers. Patients with malignancies can be at risk for ecthyma gangrenosum caused by *Pseudomonas aeruginosa* or dense neutrophilic infiltration of the dermis that is noninfectious but that responds to steroids (Sweet's syndrome, discussed later). Ecthyma gangrenosum caused by *P. aeruginosa* is a rapidly progressive (12 to 24 hours), necrotic ulceration with hemorrhagic bullae and skin sloughing in the setting of gram-negative sepsis and neutropenia. Empiric agents for ecthyma gangrenosum should include tobramycin plus piperacillin, ceftazidime, or imipenem.

Treatment of skin ulcers depends on the cause of the lesion. For venous stasis ulcers, local care with occlusive dressings on the wounds and compression bandages to aid venous return is necessary. If cellulitis or folliculitis is present, antibiotics to cover *Staphylococcus aureus* should be administered. After the ulcer has healed, compression stockings should be worn to prevent new ulcers. Therapy for

other types of ulcers should address their cause; Table 1 outlines the clinical presentation and epidemiology of infectious ulcers.

Noninfectious Ulcers

Noninfectious causes of cutaneous ulcers include drug reactions, collagen-vascular diseases, and malignancy. Drugs reported to cause ulcerations include methotrexate, etretinate, and warfarin. Wegener's granulomatosis, a systemic disease with involvement of the respiratory tract and kidneys, can form necrotizing ulcerations of the skin. Biopsy of these lesions may be positive for leukocytoclastic vasculitis, granuloma, and inflammatory infiltrates. Serology for IgG antibodies against neutrophilic cytoplasmic components (c-ANCA) are highly specific for Wegener's granulomatosis. Treatment includes prednisone, cyclophosphamide, or nonsteroidal antiinflammatory agents. Behçet's disease is another systemic condition that involves recurrent oral and genital aphthous ulcerations, arthritis, and uveitis; in some cases it attacks the central nervous system. Treatment is prednisone, chlorambucil, azathioprine, or cyclophosphamide. Malignancy should always be considered as a possible cause of ulcers that have not responded to antimicrobial therapy because basal cell carcinoma, hematologic malignancies, and metastatic cancers may form skin ulcers.

Table 1   Clinical Presentation of Skin Ulcers Caused by Infectious Agents

CAUSE	LABORATORY WORKUP	EPIDEMIOLOGY	CLINICAL CLUES TO DIAGNOSIS
BACTERIAL	Routine culture and Gram stain		
Bacillus anthracis (anthrax)	Gram+ rod	Wool handler; Western Asia, West Africa	Lesions on face and arms; painless papule develops into vesicle that dries, forming black eschar that then separates from the base to form an ulcer with marked surrounding gelatinous edema; LN common
Corynebacterium diphtheriae (diphtheria)	Gram+ rod	Tropical climates; rare in the United States	Ulcer with sharp margins and clean base; preexisting skin lesions may become infected
Francisella tularensis (tularemia)	Gram− coccobacillus, serology	Rabbit hunter	Systemic febrile illness; tender ulcer with painful LN
Nocardia brasiliensis	Branching, beaded Gram+ rod, modified AFB+	Soil exposure	Ulcer with purulent drainage, nodular lymphangitis
Pseudomonas aeruginosa (ecthyma gangrenosum)	Gram− rod, may have associated bacteremia	Neutropenic or immunocompromised patients	Rapidly progressive eruption from papules to hemorrhagic vesicles or bullae that undergo central necrosis and ulceration
Polymicrobial	Mixed Gram+ and Gram−	Debilitated, immunocompromised, diabetic	Pressure sores, decubitus ulcers, foot ulcers
Yersinia pestis (plague)	Gram− coccobacillus, serology	Rodent zoonosis transmitted to humans via fleas; Far East, India, Africa, Central and South America	Bubonic plague with classic inguinal painful LN; may have skin lesions on lower extremities; pustule, papule, vesicle, or eschar may occur at inoculation site
SPIROCHETES			
Treponema pallidum (syphilis)	Serology	Sexually transmitted disease	Tertiary syphilis; nodular, ulceronodular, gummas; punched-out ulcer with gummy discharge
FUNGAL	Fungal smear, culture		
Blastomyces dermatitidis	Fungal smear, culture, broad-based budding yeast, dimorphic fungus	Sugar cane worker, HIV positive, immunocompromised; North America, Africa	Subcutaneous nodule that enlarges and ulcerates, forming a crusted, verrucous plaque; may resemble squamous cell carcinoma
Coccidioides immitis	Fungal smear, culture, dimorphic fungus, serology	Soil exposure, HIV positive; Southwestern United States, Northern Mexico, Central and South America	Usually single nodule or plaque; may form pustules, subcutaneous nodules, or abscesses
Cryptococcus neoformans	Fungal smear, India ink, culture, encapsulated yeast, mucicarmine+ capsule, cryptococcal antigen	Exposure to pigeons, soil exposure, HIV positive, immunocompromised	Papule with crust resembling molluscum contagiosum; also forms ulcers on skin, mouth, and genitalia
Histoplasma capsulatum	Fungal smear, culture, dimorphic fungus, histoplasma antigen	Bats, birds, and soil exposure; HIV positive, immunocompromised; Eastern and Central United States in Ohio/Mississippi River valleys, Central and South America, West Indies	Papule with crust resembling molluscum contagiosum; ulcerative plaques, and oral ulcerations

Table 1   Clinical Presentation of Skin Ulcers Caused by Infectious Agents—cont'd

CAUSE	LABORATORY WORKUP	EPIDEMIOLOGY	CLINICAL CLUES TO DIAGNOSIS
Sporothrix schenckii	Fungal smear, culture, dimorphic fungus	Rose gardening, soil exposure	Papule or pustule at inoculation site develops into subcutaneous nodules or ragged-edged ulcer with proximal nodular lymphangitis; usually on upper extremities
MYCOBACTERIAL	AFB smear, culture		
Mycobacterium marinum	AFB smear, culture	Aquarium enthusiasts	Ulcer with thin seropurulent drainage, nodular lymphangitis
Mycobacterium ulcerans (Buruli ulcer)	AFB smear, culture	Africa, Australia, South East Asia, South America, North America (Mexico)	Subcutaneous nodule that ulcerates with extensive scarring and contracture formation
Mycobacterium avium complex	AFB smear, culture	HIV positive, immunocompromised; soil, water	Multiple subcutaneous nodules or ulcers; may be associated with cervical lymphadenitis drainage to skin, or direct innoculation
Mycobacterium haemophilum	AFB smear, culture; requires iron-supplemented culture medium and incubation at 30°-32° C	Australia, United States, Canada, France; HIV positive, transplantation	Papules develop into pustules that form deep ulcers, usually on extremities overlying joints; may have septic arthritis +/− osteomyelitis, may have LN
Mycobacterium tuberculosis	AFB smear, culture; also PPD helpful if positive	Worldwide	Nodules or ulcers, especially in HIV-positive patients
VIRAL			
Herpes simplex	DFA, viral culture, Tzanck prep	Sexually transmitted disease	Oral, perineal, genital ulcers; whitlow on hands; lesions with thin-walled vesicles; shallow painful ulcers
PARASITIC			
Leishmaniasis	Punch biopsy of skin for culture, histopathology, and touch prep using Wright's and Giemsa stains to look for amastigotes at base of lesion; +/− serology	Sandfly bites	Papule at the site of insect bite enlarges to form a nodule, which then develops into a punched-out ulcer; may have associated LN; nodules rarely form without ulceration
Old World Leishmaniasis L. aethiopica L. major L. tropica		Mediterranean, Middle East, Africa, Southern Asia, India	
New World Leishmaniasis L. braziliensis complex L. mexicana complex		Latin America, Central and South America	

LN, Lymphadenopathy; *AFB,* acid-fast bacilli; *HIV,* human immunodeficiency virus; *PPD,* purified protein derivative; *DFA,* direct fluorescent antibodies.

■ PYODERMA

Pyoderma is a general term used to describe superficial disruption of the skin with pus formation in response to a bacterial infection. Generally caused by a single organism, pyoderma can be primary or secondary. Similar lesions can be produced by neutrophilic dermatoses such as pyoderma gangrenosum and Sweet's syndrome. Table 2 outlines the clinical presentation of pyoderma and suggested treatment.

Primary Pyoderma

Primary pyoderma is an infection of previously healthy skin, usually caused by *S. aureus* or *Streptococcus pyogenes.*

Impetigo

Impetigo is a superficial infection of the skin involving only the epidermis. Impetigo is highly contagious and usually occurs in young children following minor skin trauma. Nonbullous impetigo, the classic honey-colored crusts on the face or extremities, is caused by *S. pyogenes* or *S. aureus;* toxin-producing strains of *S. aureus* cause bullous impetigo (varnishlike crust). Treatment of bullous and nonbullous impetigo requires coverage of methicillin-sensitive *S. aureus* (MSSA): dicloxacillin, 500 mg orally every 6 hours, or first-generation cephalosporins such as cephalexin, 500 mg orally every 6 hours for 7 days. The oral cephalosporins cefixime, ceftibuten, and cefetamet pivoxil have no activity against MSSA. For penicillin-allergic patients, clindamycin, 150 to 300 mg orally every 6 hours, or clarithromycin, 500 mg orally every 12 hours, is appropriate. Topical mupirocin applied to the lesion three times daily is an equally effective alternative to systemic therapy.

Ecthyma

Ecthyma is impetigo that extends through the epidermis, forming shallow ulcers with crusts. It occurs in immunocompromised patients and is caused by *S. pyogenes* or *S. aureus.* Gram stain and culture of the lesion must be performed to rule out ecthyma gangrenosum, which is caused by *P. aeruginosa* sepsis or methicillin-resistant *S. aureus* (MRSA). Treatment of ecthyma caused by streptococci or staphylococci is the same as that for impetigo, but duration of therapy may be longer. Unlike impetigo, ecthyma may heal with scarring.

Folliculitis

Folliculitis is an inflammation of the hair follicles, usually caused by *S. aureus.* Topical therapy with mupirocin three times daily for 7 days is usually adequate. If the infection does not respond, oral therapy with agents used for impetigo should be adequate. Lesions that do not respond to antistaphylococcal antibiotics should be cultured because they may be caused by MRSA or other pathogens. Therapy should be tailored to antimicrobial sensitivities. On rare occasions, gram-negative organisms cause folliculitis, typically in association with either superinfection in patients taking long-term antibiotics for acne vulgaris or hot-tub bathing. Gram-negative folliculitis in acne patients is caused by *Klebsiella, Enterobacter,* and *Proteus* species and usually occurs on the face. Treatment depends on susceptibilities, but ampicillin-clavulanic acid or trimethoprim-sulfamethoxazole may be used empirically. Hot-tub folliculitis caused by *P. aeruginosa* is usually self-limiting in a normal host, and no action is necessary beyond decontaminating the water and ensuring proper chlorination.

Furuncles and Carbuncles

Furuncles are skin abscesses caused by *S. aureus;* they may begin as folliculitis that extends into the surrounding dermis and subcutaneous tissue. Carbuncles comprise several furuncles that coalesce to form loculated abscesses with draining pus. Treatment of furuncles and carbuncles includes antistaphylococcal antibiotics along with careful incision and drainage of the abscess. Some patients with recurrent furuncles and carbuncles may require elimination of nasal *S. aureus* carriage with nasal applications of mupirocin daily for 1 week each month, or rifampin, 600 mg orally daily for 1 week each month. Bathing with antibacterial soap also helps decrease *S. aureus* carriage.

Secondary Pyoderma

Secondary pyoderma is a bacterial superinfection of skin previously disrupted by trauma, surgery, or chronic skin conditions such as eczema or psoriasis. The usual organism is *S. aureus,* which can be methicillin resistant if the lesions are nosocomial or if the patient has been receiving chronic antibiotic therapy. Treatment for serious wound infections is intravenous nafcillin or oxacillin. Mild to moderate infections can be treated with oral dicloxacillin or cephalexin. If the lesion does not respond, culturing should be considered; if it is methicillin resistant, treatment is intravenous vancomycin or in some cases trimethoprim-sulfamethoxazole, depending on sensitivities. Secondary pyoderma caused by pressure sores and diabetic foot ulcers is usually polymicrobial and requires broad-spectrum therapy with piperacillin-tazobactam, imipenem, or a combination of ciprofloxacin and clindamycin. Table 2 summarizes the suggested therapy for pyoderma.

Neutrophilic Dermatoses

Pyoderma caused by neutrophilic infiltrates usually is associated with underlying disease such as cancer or inflammatory bowel disease (IBD). The main entities are pyoderma gangrenosum and Sweet's syndrome.

Pyoderma Gangrenosum

The diagnosis of pyoderma gangrenosum is clinical. The lesion begins as a small erythematous papule, rapidly progressing to tender pustules that undergo central necrosis and ulceration. The border of the ulcers are ragged, violaceous, and surrounded by erythema. Distinguishing characteristics include severe pain at the ulcer site, lesions at the site of minor trauma, parchment scarring, and associated systemic diseases such as IBD, rheumatologic diseases, or malignancy. Biopsy of the lesions is done mainly to exclude infection because histopathologic findings are nonspecific. Central necrosis and lymphocytic and neutrophilic infiltrates with or without vasculitic changes are seen on histopathology of pyoderma gangrenosum lesions; lymphocytes and plasma cells around vessels are common findings. Pyoderma gangrenosum usually occurs on the lower extremities over bony prominences, where repeated trauma aggravates the condi-

Table 2 Clinical Presentation and Therapy of Pyoderma

TYPE OF DISEASE	DISTINGUISHING FEATURES	CAUSATIVE ORGANISM	TREATMENT
PRIMARY PYODERMA			
Impetigo			Dicloxacillin, 500 mg PO q6h
			or
			Cephalexin, 500 mg PO q6h (*not cefixime*)
			or
			Clindamycin, 150-300 mg PO q6h
			or
			Ampicillin-clavulanic acid, 875 mg PO q12h
			or
Nonbullous impetigo	Superficial honey-colored crusts	*Streptococcus pyogens, Staphylococcus aureus*	Azithromycin, 250 mg PO qd
			or
Bullous impetigo	Thin vesicles and bullae, when ruptured produce varnishlike crust	Toxin-producing strains of *S. aureus*	Clarithromycin, 500 mg PO bid
			or
			Mupirocin topically tid
			For MRSA:
			Minocycline, 100 mg PO bid
			or
			Trimethoprim-sulfamethoxazole (TMP-SMX), one double-strength (TMP 160 mg) PO bid
Ecthyma	Ulcer with crust	*Streptococcus pyogenes, S. aureus*	Treat as impetigo with oral agents, may need longer duration of therapy
Folliculitis	Hair follicle with pustules, erythema	*S. aureus*	*Topical:*
			Clindamycin
			or
			Erythromycin
			or
			Mupirocin topically tid
			or
			Benzoyl peroxide lotion
			Unresponsive:
			Treat as impetigo
Gram-negative folliculitis	Usually on face in patients with acne vulgaris on chronic suppressive antibiotic therapy	*Klebsiella, Enterobacter, Proteus* species	Ampicillin-clavulanic acid, 875 mg PO q12h
			or
			TMP-SMX, one double-strength (TMP 160 mg) PO bid
Hot-tub folliculitis	Pustules and vesicles on an erythematous base in bathing-suit distribution	*Pseudomonas aeruginosa*	Self-limited in normal hosts; decontaminate and chlorinate hot tub
Furuncle/carbuncle	Abscess formation in dermis, subcutaneous tissue that may coalesce and drain; if cellulitis or sepsis associated, needs intravenous antibiotics; patients may have recurrences; suggest culture to rule out MRSA or gram-negative organisms	*S. aureus*	Careful incision and drainage; antistaphylococcal antibiotics including the following: Dicloxacillin, 500 mg PO q6h
			or
			Cephalexin, 500 mg PO q6h
			If associated with cellulitis or sepsis:
			Nafcillin **or** oxacillin, 2 g IV q6h,
			or
			Cefazolin, 1-2 g IV q8h
			If recurrent, eradicate nasal carriage of *S. aureus* by:
			Mupirocin (topical 2%) intranasally bid ×5 days
			or
			Rifampin 600 mg PO qd plus either dicloxacillin 500 mg PO qid ×10 days *or* TMP-SMX one double-strength tab PO bid ×10 days

Table 2 Clinical Presentation and Therapy of Pyoderma—cont'd

TYPE OF DISEASE	DISTINGUISHING FEATURES	CAUSATIVE ORGANISM	TREATMENT
Neutrophilic Pyoderma gangrenosum	Rapidly progressive painful ulcers, ragged violaceous edges with necrotic centers, usually on lower legs; underlying IBD, malignancy, arthritis, monoclonal gammopathy; *Biopsy:* PMN, lymphocytic infiltration, +/− vasculitis	No organisms seen, culture negative	Prednisone, 1 mg/kg/day PO or Sulfasalazine, 1-4 g PO qd (for patients with IBD) or Dapsone, 100-200 PO qd (contraindicated in G6PD-deficient patients) or Clofazimine, 200-400 mg PO qd or Minocycline, 100 mg PO bid Mild cases: intralesional triamcinolone Severe cases: immunosuppressive agents have been tried such as azathioprine, cyclosporin
Sweet's syndrome	Fever, neutrophilia, prompt response to steriods, painful erythematous plaques that may form bullae and ulcerate; located on head, neck, arms; 20% have associated malignancy, usually AML, elevated sedimentation rate *Biopsy:* dense PMN infiltration of the dermis, no vasculitis	No organisms seen, culture negative	Prednisone, 1 mg/kg/day, slow taper over 4-6 wks; dramatic response If steroids contraindicated, may use cyclosporin, clofazimine, indomethacin, dapsone, or colchicine
SECONDARY PYODERMA	Preexisting lesions of dermatitis such as eczema, psoriasis, or surgical/traumatic wounds		Based on culture data

AML, Acute myelogenous leukemia; *G6PD,* glucose-6-phosphate dehydrogenase; *IBD,* inflammatory bowel disease; *MRSA,* methicillin-resistant *S. aureus*; *PMN,* polymorphonuclear leukocytes.

tion (pathergy); its cause is unknown. Treatment includes prednisone, 1 mg/kg by mouth daily; in patients with underlying IBD, sulfasalazine, 1 to 4 g by mouth daily, is recommended. In difficult cases, dapsone, 100 to 200 mg by mouth daily (dapsone is contraindicated in G6PD-deficient patients), or clofazimine, 200 to 400 mg by mouth daily, should be administered. Cyclosporin, minocycline, azathioprine, colchicine, topical 4% cromolyn sodium, and many other drugs have been used to treat pyoderma gangrenosum; response to therapy varies.

Sweet's Syndrome
Sweet's syndrome is an acute febrile neutrophilic dermatosis that may be idiopathic or associated with a malignancy. Lesions are painful erythematous plaques usually on the upper extremities, head, and neck. These lesions are classically associated with fever and neutrophilia, but some patients have myalgia, arthralgia, proteinuria, and conjunctivitis. Nearly all patients with Sweet's syndrome have an elevated erythrocyte sedimentation rate. Dense neutrophilic infiltration of the dermis without vasculitis is the classic

finding on biopsy, and it is important to exclude bacteria, mycobacteria, and fungi because steroids are the appropriate therapy for Sweet's syndrome. The response to prednisone, 1 mg/kg/day, is dramatic; constitutional symptoms improve within hours, and skin lesions improve over 1 to 2 days. Steroids should be tapered slowly over 4 to 6 weeks. If steroids are contraindicated, alternative treatments include clofazimine, dapsone, and indomethacin.

Herpetic Whitlow
Herpetic whitlow, a herpes simplex infection of the pulp of the finger, may occur in anyone who has mucocutaneous herpes or who comes in contact with herpetic lesions (i.e., health care workers). The initial lesion is a tender vesicle filled with turbid fluid. Lesions may be multiple and may ulcerate and become secondarily infected, developing purulent drainage. Axillary and epitrochlear lymphadenopathy with erythema of the proximal forearm also may occur. Diagnosis can be made by aspirating a vesicle and sending the fluid for viral culture, doing a Tzanck test, or performing a direct fluorescent antibody (DFA) test on the blister

fluid. Treatment includes acyclovir, and surgery should be avoided. Some lesions may be superinfected, so clinicians should consider coverage for *S. aureus* with clindamycin, 300 mg orally every 6 hours, if the lesion does not respond to acyclovir therapy alone.

Suggested Reading

Burton CS III: Treatment of leg ulcers, *Dermatol Clin* 11:315, 1993.

Cohen PR, Talpaz M, Kuzrock R: Malignancy-associated Sweet's syndrome: review of the world literature, *J Clin Oncol* 6:1887, 1988.

Feingold DS: Staphylococcal and streptococcal pyodermas, *Semin Dermatol* 12:331, 1993.

Fitzgerald RL, McBurney EI, Nesbitt Jr LT: Sweet's syndrome, *Int J Dermatol* 35:9, 1996.

Fitzpatrick TB, et al: *Color atlas and synopsis of clinical dermatology common and serious diseases*, ed 3, New York, 1997, McGraw-Hill.

Kostman JR, DiNubile MJ: Nodular lymphangitis: a distinctive but often unrecognized syndrome, *Ann Intern Med* 118:883, 1993.

Myskowski PL, White MH, Ahkami R: Fungal disease in the immunocompromised host, *Dermatol Clin* 15:295, 1997.

Powell FC, Su WPD, Perry HO: Pyoderma gangrenosum: classification and management, *J Am Acad Dermatol* 34:395, 1996.

Sadick NS: Current aspects of bacterial infections of the skin, *Dermatol Clin* 15:341, 1997.

Sanders CV, Nesbitt LT, eds: *The skin in infectious disease*, Baltimore, 1995, Williams & Wilkins.

Shelley WB, Shelley ED: *Advanced dermatologic diagnosis*, Philadelphia, 1992, WB Saunders.

CELLULITIS AND ERYSIPELAS

Keith W. Schumann
Karim A. Adal
Kenneth J. Tomecki

Soft-tissue infections (STIs), or cellulitides, are common infections that vary widely in severity. Erysipelas is a superficial STI; cellulitis is a deeper infection that extends into the dermis and subcutaneous tissues.

■ ERYSIPELAS

Epidemiology and Clinical Manifestations

Erysipelas is a superficial STI with lymphatic involvement. The most common sites of predilection are the thighs and legs; the more classic facial disease is now uncommon (5% to 20% of patients). Young, elderly, and immunocompromised patients are particularly susceptible to infection. Predisposing factors include venous insufficiency, diabetes mellitus, alcoholism, chronic lymphatic obstruction, and any epidermal defect that limits barrier function (e.g., stasis ulcers, puncture wounds). Because erysipelas itself produces lymphatic obstruction, it tends to recur in areas of earlier infection in approximately 30% of cases.

Clinically, erysipelas is a tender, sharply demarcated, bright red edematous plaque. Fever, chills, and malaise may occur, and leukocytosis is common. Complications are uncommon but may include bacteremia (5% of patients), subcutaneous abscess formation, "toxic-strep" syndrome, as well as cellulitis and necrotizing fasciitis when disease extends deeply.

The most common cause of erysipelas is group A beta-hemolytic streptococci (GAS), less so groups B, C, and G. Other causative agents are rare but may include *Staphylococcus aureus*, *Pneumococcus* species, *Klebsiella pneumoniae*, *Yersinia enterocolitica*, and *Haemophilus influenzae*. Group B streptococcus is a common cause of erysipelas in newborns.

Clinical presentation establishes the diagnosis. Bacteriologic tests, predicated on swabs from a local portal of entry, for Gram stain and culture, are not necessary on a routine basis. Unfortunately, the injection-reaspiration method of tissue fluid collection has little value. If done, nonbacteriostatic saline should be injected into the advancing border, followed by aspiration of tissue fluid. Tissue culture, via skin biopsy (punch biopsy with specimen in nonbacteriostatic saline) may help confirm the diagnosis. Blood cultures are positive in 5% of patients.

Therapy

Therapy begins with local measures and correction of any predisposing factors: immobilization and elevation of the affected area, if possible, to reduce edema; application of cool compresses to offset discomfort; and debridement of bullae, if present. Systemic antimicrobial therapy is essential (Table 1), and treatment regimens vary widely in the literature. Empiric therapy for mild erysipelas should target *Streptococcus pyogenes* (GAS), which continues to be susceptible to beta-lactam antimicrobials, specifically penicillin. Macrolides such as erythromycin are an option for penicillin-allergic patients, as are cephalosporins if such an allergy is mild. Cross-reactions between penicillin and cephalosporins occur in about 5% of patients.

Outpatient therapy is reasonable for clinically mild cases in healthy patients. Hospitalization for intravenous antimicrobial therapy and supportive care is warranted for patients with facial disease and/or extensive disease, especially those with underlying medical illness such as diabetes. Therapy should be intravenous aqueous penicillin G (600,000 to 2 million units every 6 hours) or intravenous vancomycin (1 g every 12 hours in adults; 10 mg/kg every 6 hours in children), with dosing based on renal function. If streptococcal

Table 1 Oral Antimicrobial Therapy for Erysipelas

MEDICATION	ADULT DOSAGE	PEDIATRIC DOSAGE
Penicillin V	250-500 mg qid	25-50 mg/kg/day in 3 to 4 divided doses
Erythromycin	250-500 mg qid	30-50 mg/kg/day in 4 divided doses
Cephalexin	250-500 mg qid	25-50 mg/kg/day in 4 divided doses
Clarithromycin	500 mg bid	7.5 mg/kg bid

Note: duration of therapy is 10 days.

toxins are present with severe or extensive disease, the treatment of choice is clindamycin (600 to 900 mg IV every 8 hours in adults; 20 to 40 mg/kg/day IV divided every 8 hours in children), either alone or in addition to penicillin. Clindamycin inhibits synthesis of bacterial toxins; as such, it is more efficacious than penicillin alone in such cases. If penicillin therapy fails, streptococci may not be the causative organism. For such patients, cultures with drug sensitivity are necessary to guide therapy.

Recurrence is common in patients with erysipelas of the legs, especially in patients with impaired circulation, such as venous insufficiency. Often associated with the pharyngeal carrier state of GAS, recurrence may necessitate continuous antimicrobial prophylaxis for such patients.

Infection of the periocular soft tissue is a special circumstance requiring ophthalmologic evaluation to differentiate preseptal STI from orbital cellulitis, a medical emergency. Computed tomographic (CT) scanning can quickly differentiate these two entities. Orbital cellulitis warrants treatment with ceftriaxone.

■ CELLULITIS

Epidemiology and Clinical Manifestations

Cellulitis is inflammation of the soft tissues, typically the result of infection. In contrast to erysipelas, cellulitis is a deeper infection of the skin extending into the subcutis. S. aureus and GAS are the most common etiologic agents of cellulitis, but other organisms, such as other bacteria, mycobacteria, fungi, and even green algae (prototheca), may produce disease. Localized necrosis may complicate cellulitis, and extensive necrosis of the skin and subcutaneous tissue is characteristic of gangrenous cellulitis (infectious gangrene), a rapidly occurring and severe infectious disease.

Cellulitis is different from erysipelas: cellulitic areas are neither raised nor sharply demarcated, but they are indurated (firm) on palpation. Typically, both erysipelas and cellulitis begin as an enlarging, edematous plaque that becomes tender, painful, and warm. Cellulitis may even begin as erysipelas. Fever, leukocytosis, lymphangitis, regional lymphadenopathy, hematogenous dissemination, focal abscess formation, and bullae may accompany cellulitis. Predisposing/host factors include lymphedema, chronic venous insufficiency, nephrotic syndrome, diabetes, and im-

munosuppression. Previous trauma and underlying skin disease such as stasis dermatitis/ulcerations and interdigital tinea pedis may predispose patients to cellulitis. Facial cellulitis may follow nasopharyngeal colonization with GAS.

Microbiology

A variety of organisms can produce cellulitis, some of which are associated with particular environments. S. aureus, a common cause of cellulitis, is the most common cause of wound infections, especially postoperative wound infections, which typically arise rapidly within 1 to 2 days of a procedure. Several strains of S. aureus produce toxins responsible for clinical disease, namely staphylococcal scalded skin syndrome, toxic shock syndrome, and staphylococcal scarlet fever. GAS, another common cause of cellulitis, is the main pathogen of perianal cellulitis in children, characterized by perianal erythema, pruritus, and pain on defecation. The perianal skin becomes edematous, painful, and fragile, and stools are often blood streaked. GAS STI may lead to nonsuppurative complications such as acute glomerulonephritis and streptococcal toxic shocklike syndrome. In contrast, rheumatic fever typically follows pharyngitis, not STI. Group B streptococcus colonizes the perineum and may produce STI in this location; groups C and G streptococci may do the same. Streptococcus pneumoniae and gram-negative bacilli, including Escherichia coli, rarely causes cellulitis. Since the advent of the polysaccharide vaccine, H. influenzae is now an uncommon cause of facial cellulitis.

Aqueous-related pathogens (e.g., Pseudomonas aeruginosa, Aeromonas species, Stenotrophomonas maltophilia, and Vibrio species) can cause cellulitis. P. aeruginosa causes ecthyma gangrenosum (EG), a necrotizing STI characterized by an erythematous, painful plaque or vesicle that quickly enlarges and undergoes central necrosis. EG commonly occurs as a nosocomial infection in immunocompromised hosts. Most cases are a primary skin infection, but STI may follow P. aeruginosa bacteremia. STI with Aeromonas hydrophila follow injury in a freshwater environment, less often the therapeutic use of leeches. Vibrio species, particularly V. vulnificus, can cause STI and sepsis, especially in patients with cirrhosis and diabetes mellitus. Naturally found in the marine environment, Vibrio can be inoculated directly into a superficial wound or spread to the skin via metastatic infection (bacteremia). For this reason, patients with cirrhosis and diabetes mellitus should not eat raw seafood.

Soil-related pathogens, specifically Clostridium species and Cryptococcus neoformans, can cause cellulitis. Clostridium species cause crepitant anaerobic cellulitis and myonecrosis (gas gangrene), which occur in the setting of trauma followed by contamination of the site with soil or other foreign material that contains spores. C. neoformans cellulitis occurs most often in immunocompromised individuals. Infection follows dissemination of the yeast to the skin from a primary pulmonary focus of infection, with development of well-demarcated vesiculobullous erythematous plaques.

Animal-related pathogens can cause cellulitis. Erysipelothrix rhusiopathiae causes STI in food handlers (poultry, meat, shellfish, and saltwater fish), typically tender, sharply demarcated, bright red to purplish plaques (usually on the hands). Streptococcus iniae is a fish pathogen that can cause hand cellulitis and bacteremia in fish handlers. Pasteurella

Table 2   Additional Gangrenous Cellulitides (Broad Classification)

TYPE	PREDISPOSING FACTORS	CLINICAL FINDINGS	SYSTEMIC TOXICITY	USUAL ETIOLOGIC AGENT	ANTIMICROBIAL THERAPY
Streptococcal gangrene	Epithelial injury secondary to trauma or surgery	Overlying skin becomes dusky blue; ± bullae; rapid progression to necrosis; although initially severely painful, involved area may become anesthetic	Marked	Group A streptococcus	Penicillin G
Mixed flora gangrene*	Trauma, surgery (especially abdominal), draining sinus, perirectal abscess, decubitus ulcer, intestinal perforation, diabetes mellitus, alcoholism, intravenous drug abuse	Often indistinguishable from streptococcal gangrene; crepitus often present, especially in patients with diabetes mellitus	Marked	Anaerobes (e.g., *Peptostreptococcus, Bacteroides*) plus at least one facultative species (e.g., non–group A streptococcus, *Enterobacter, Proteus*)	Imipenem-cilastatin Ticarcillin-clavulanate Ampicillin-sulbactam
Clostridial cellulitis	Trauma, with dirty or inadequately debrided wound	Crepitus; thin dark gray-brown foul serous discharge; from clostridial myonecrosis (gas gangrene) by relatively little local pain, edema, or toxemia	Minimal	*C. perfringens*	Penicillin G

*Subtypes include Fournier's gangrene, involving the scrotum and penis, and Meleney's gangrene, which typically follow abdominal surgery.

multocida STI occur after dog or cat bites and scratches; they may even follow wound licking by cats, less commonly by dogs.

Infectious gangrene follows thrombosis or occlusion of dermal and subcutaneous blood vessels. Such gangrene occurs with EG and with STI caused by *Vibrio* species, *A. hydrophila, C. neoformans,* and *Clostridium.* For further characterization of clostridial cellulitis and other gangrenous cellulitides (streptococcal gangrene and mixed flora gangrene), see Table 2.

Diagnosis

Convincing clinical disease should suggest the diagnosis, but a positive culture is confirmatory. Unfortunately, cultures are often negative, but exudate, erosions, ulcerations, abscesses, surgical wound, and tissue biopsy cultures have a higher yield than aspirate or blood culture. Adjunctive measures include Gram stain of aspirate or exudate, laboratory studies (CBC with differential, anti-DNase antibody, antistreptolysin titer, cryptococcal antigen, and blood cultures), and imaging studies. Conventional radiography can delineate the pockets of gas of anaerobic cellulitis, especially clostridial cellulitis. Magnetic resonance imaging (MRI) may aid in the diagnosis of STI. T_2-weighted images highlight the disease process best.

Table 3   Oral Antistaphylococcal Antibiotics

MEDICATION	ADULT DOSAGE	PEDIATRIC DOSAGE
Dicloxacillin	250-500 mg qid	12.5-25 mg/kg/day in 4 divided doses
Erythromycin	250-500 mg qid	30-50 mg/kg/day in 4 divided doses
Cephalexin	250-500 mg qid	25-50 mg/kg/day in 4 divided doses
Clindamycin	150-300 mg qid	8-16 mg/kg/day in 3-4 divided doses

Note: duration of therapy is 14 days.

Therapy

Empiric therapy of streptococcal or staphylococcal cellulitis requires an oral antistaphylococcal antibiotic (Table 3), coupled with local care, including immobilization and elevation of the involved area to reduce swelling and the use of cool compresses to reduce pain. Moist heat may help localize infection in patients with signs of fluctuance. All abscesses require drainage and culture. Afterwards, support stockings and good skin hygiene can reduce the likelihood of recurrence in patients with peripheral edema (e.g., emollients and

Table 4 Drugs of First Choice and Alternatives for Treatment of Cellulitis

ORGANISM	DRUG OF FIRST CHOICE	ALTERNATIVE DRUGS
Haemophilus influenzae	Cefotaxime or ceftriaxone	Cefuroxime, trimethoprim-sulfamethoxazole, a fluoroquinolone
Pseudomonas aeruginosa	Ceftazidime + tobramycin	Antipseudomonal penicillin or imipenem + aminoglycoside
Stenotrophommonas maltophilia	Trimethoprim-sulfamethoxazole	Ticarcillin-clavulanate
Vibrio vulnificus	A tetracycline	Cefotaxime, a fluoroquinolone
Aeromonas	A fluoroquinolone	Imipenem-trimethoprim-sulfamethoxazole
Clostridium perfringens	Penicillin G	Clindamycin, chloramphenicol, metronidazole, erythromycin
Erysipelothrix rhusiopathiae	Penicillin G	Imipenem, a fluoroquinolone
Pasteurella multocida	Penicillin or amoxicillin-clavulanate	Cefuroxime, tetracycline
Cryptococcus neoformans	Amphotericin B ± flucytosine	Fluconazole

an antifungal cream to offset the possibility of tinea pedis in patients who have had saphenous vein harvesting).

Parenteral antibiotics and hospitalization are necessary for toxic or immunocompromised patients and those with extensive disease. For severe streptococcal or staphylococcal infections, a penicillinase-resistant penicillin or first-generation cephalosporin is the therapy of choice, with vancomycin as an alternative in penicillin-allergic patients. Diabetic patients with leg ulceration and cellulitis often have a polymicrobial infection that warrants broader coverage (e.g., a cephalosporin or clindamycin plus a fluoroquinolone). See Table 4 for treatment of cellulitis caused by other pathogens.

Tissue necrosis demands hospitalization, parenteral antibiotics, and prompt surgical evaluation, including early and complete surgical debridement, extending beyond the areas of gangrene to reach healthy tissue, coupled with the release of subcutaneous compartmental pressure. Indicators of deep STI include gangrenous skin changes, severe pain or anesthetic skin, crepitus or abscess formation with multiple tracts, and a cellulitis with extensive surrounding edema or one that progresses despite antibiotics or complicates a surgical wound. Systemic signs may include confusion, tachycardia, and tachypnea (see *Deep Soft-Tissue Infection: Fasciitis and Myositis*).

Suggested Reading

Bisno AL, Stevens DL: Streptococcal infections of skin and soft tissues, *N Engl J Med* 334:240, 1996.

Chartier C, Grosshans E: Erysipelas: an update, *Int J Derm* 35:779, 1996.

Veien NK: The clinician's choice of antibiotics in the treatment of bacterial skin infection, *Br J Derm* 139:30, 1998.

DEEP SOFT-TISSUE INFECTION: FASCIITIS AND MYOSITIS

Stephen Ash

Myositis and fasciitis are uncommon infections but may be rapidly progressive, with a high rate of morbidity and mortality. The many classifications and subdivisions of fasciitis and myositis serve only a limited purpose to the clinician because most have similar causes and therapeutic strategies. Table 1 illustrates the varied nomenclature for the spectrum of deep soft-tissue infections, but for simplicity and pragmatic reasons, it is adequate to divide them into three categories: (1) necrotizing fasciitis, (2) necrotizing myositis, and (3) pyomyositis.

Most patients with one of these conditions have a predisposing underlying disorder that may require separate therapy (e.g., diabetes mellitus) (Table 2), and many cases are polymicrobial (Table 3).

■ NECROTIZING FASCIITIS

Recently, much attention has been focused on the spectrum of infections caused by group A beta-hemolytic streptococci (GAS), one manifestation of which is necrotizing fasciitis (NF). It appears that GAS, although declining as a cause of serious disease in the first three decades of the second half of the century, is now making something of a comeback. This recurrence is possibly related to two virulence factors, the M protein and pyrogenic exotoxin, which appear to be present in most GAS isolates from NF. However, it is unwise to assume that GAS is the sole cause of a case of NF because

Table 1 Deep Soft-Tissue Infections

Necrotizing fasciitis	Usually polymicrobial, restricted to fascial layers, and often associated with profound systemic upset
Necrotizing myositis	Traditionally called *gas gangrene,* classically monomicrobial (Clostridia)
Pyomyositis	Traditionally tropical but more recently recognized in temperate climates and associated with human immunodeficiency virus infection as well as intravenous drug users; commonly staphylococcal
Parasitic myositis	Usually nonsuppurating, most commonly caused by trichinosis
Synergistic gangrene	Full-thickness soft-tissue infection with necrosis, usually with less initial systemic toxicity than with necrotizing fasciitis; commonly follows surgery (Meleney's gangrene) and may preferentially affect the scrotum (Fournier's gangrene); both usually polymicrobial

Table 2 Factors Predisposing to Deep Soft-Tissue Infections

Diabetes mellitus	Trauma, insect bites
Alcoholism	Malnutrition
Recent surgery	Immunocompromise
Intraabdominal sepsis	Recent chickenpox (children)
Intravenous drug use	Old age
Obesity	

Table 3 Common Organisms Cultured from Deep Soft-Tissue Infections

Gram-positive	*Staphylococcus, Streptococcus*
Gram-negative	*Enterobacteriaceae, Pseudomonas*
Anaerobic	*Bacteroides, Clostridium* (often as sole cause)
Fungal	*Candida* (exact role is uncertain)

many cases are polymicrobial and require broad-spectrum antibiotic therapy.

The disease begins as a painful enlarging red area deep to the superficial skin, the center of which discolors as the condition spreads. As its name implies, NF infects the fascial layers of the soft tissue, the planes of which allow its rapid spread to involve large areas of a limb or the torso. The patient, usually febrile and toxic, may develop complications such as septicemia, disseminated intravascular coagulation, shock, acute renal failure, and adult respiratory distress syndrome. The diagnosis is made on clinical grounds, and therapy is started at once because morbidity and mortality are high, especially if there is a delay. The main principles of treatment consist of surgical debridement with excision of all nonviable tissue, broad-spectrum antibiotic therapy, and supportive treatment with specific treatment of any identified predisposing factors (Figure 1). Second and further surgical assessments may be necessary, and alteration of antibiotic therapy can be made once microscopy of gram-stained smears and culture reports are received. The use of hyperbaric oxygen for NF and necrotizing myositis remains controversial. If the facility is local, hyperbaric therapy may be an option, but most patients with NF are not in a safe condition to travel for it.

Several adequate antibiotic regimens can be used for initial empiric therapy of NF. One is benzylpenicillin, 2 million U IV q2h, plus nafcillin, 1 g q6h, plus metronidazole, 500 mg q6h, plus ciprofloxacin, 400 mg q12h (adult dosages). Clindamycin, 600 mg q6h, can be used for penicillin-allergic patients. Imipenem, 500 mg IV q6h, is a further alternative. Extended-spectrum antibiotics such as piperacillin-tazobactam, 4.5 g IV q8h, which cover both streptococci and staphylococci, are alternatives to benzylpenicillin plus nafcillin. Although laboratory cultures may report sensitivity to aminoglycosides, these agents generally are ineffective in anaerobic environments, and their usefulness is therefore limited. Some authorities supplement antibiotic therapy with an antifungal agent because there have been several reports of *Candida* spp. being isolated with bacteria from specimen cultures taken from NF. The addition of fluconazole, 200 mg daily, may be advisable.

■ NECROTIZING MYOSITIS

Necrotizing myositis (NM) is an infection of muscle with profound necrosis at an early stage of evolution, unlike pyomyositis in which it occurs late. Classically, this infection occurs after surgery or trauma and is caused by clostridia, with production of gas in the tissues, which may be detectable radiologically. However, other bacteria may be involved, some of which also produce gas, and it is therefore wise to use broad-spectrum antibiotics as empiric therapy. The treatment of NM, similar to that of NF, consists of surgical debridement, the same antibiotic regimens, and supportive therapy (see Figure 1).

■ PYOMYOSITIS

Traditionally, pyomyositis is a condition common in the tropics, where it presents as a tender mass, most often on the hip or thigh. Initially, the disease process is one of abscess formation with healthy surrounding muscle that may undergo necrosis late if the illness is neglected. *Staphylococcus* is the most common causative organism, but approximately 20% of cases are exceptions, especially in the rarer but increasingly well-recognized temperate zone cases. These are often associated with intravenous drug users or immunocompromised patients, particularly those infected by human immunodeficiency virus. Computed tomography of the affected part is usually most helpful. Needle aspiration

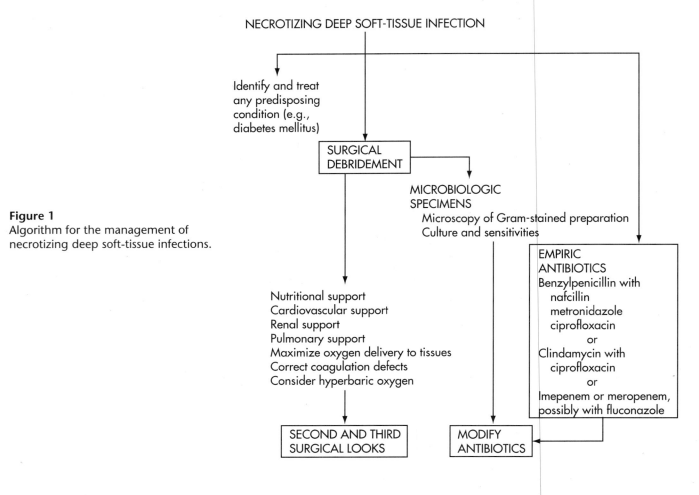

Figure 1
Algorithm for the management of necrotizing deep soft-tissue infections.

and drainage may eliminate the need for surgery. Antibiotic therapy should cover *Staphylococcus,* for example, nafcillin, 1 g IV q6h, or clindamycin, 600 mg q6h, for penicillin-allergic patients with additional agents to cover other possible organisms, for example, ciprofloxacin, 200 mg IV q12h, plus metronidazole, 500 mg IV q6h. Extended-spectrum penicillins (e.g., piperacillin-tazobactam, 4.5 g IV q8h, or imipenem, 500 mg IV q6h) also have adequate individual spectra of activity.

Suggested Reading

Ash SA: Bacterial skin and soft tissue infections. In O'Grady FW, et al, eds: *Antibiotics and chemotherapy,* ed 7, New York, 1997, Churchill Livingstone.

Lewis RT: Necrotizing soft-tissue infections, *Infect Dis Clin North Am* 6:693, 1992.

Roggiani M, Schlievert PM: Streptococcal toxic shock syndrome, including necrotizing fasciitis and myositis, *Curr Opin Infect Dis* 7:423, 1994.

Sawyer MD, Dunn DL: Deep soft tissue infections, *Curr Opin Infect Dis* 4:649, 1991.

HUMAN AND ANIMAL BITES

Ellie J.C. Goldstein

Annually, in the United States, more than 4.8 million animal and untold numbers of human bite wounds occur and account for 10,000 persons hospitalized and 1% (300,000) of all emergency department visits. Patients with bite wounds are also commonly seen as outpatients in primary care physician and specialist (orthopedics, plastic/hand surgery, infectious diseases physicians) offices. The bacteriology of these wounds is diverse and comprises oral flora organisms, both aerobic and anaerobic, of the biting animal/human, the victim's skin flora, and occasionally environmental isolates.

■ ANIMAL BITES

Microbiology
An extensive number of bacterial species are isolated from infected dog and cat bite wounds. *Pasteurella* species, especially *P. multocida* and *P. septica,* will be present in 75% and 65% of cat bite and dog bite wounds, respectively. Anaerobes will be present in 50% of dog bite wounds and 67% of cat bite wounds. Streptococci, excluding group A beta-hemolytic streptococci *(Streptococcus pyogenes)* are present in 46% of dog and cat bite wounds, whereas *Staphylococcus aureus* is present in 20% of dog bites but only 4% of cat bites. *S. pyogenes* (group A), if present, usually comes from the victim's skin because it is rarely isolated from dog oral flora. *S. aureus* is also a secondary invader originating as skin flora. *Capnocytophaga canimorsus* is an uncommon wound isolate but has been associated with bacteremia, some fatal, in asplenic and cirrhotic patients. Other veterinary species are often isolated but are difficult for the routine laboratory to identify.

■ WOUND CARE EVALUATION AND CARE

The elements of wound care are outlined in Table 1. The most important principle of immediate wound care is for the patient to wash the wound with soap and water as soon as possible after the injury. This will reduce any bacterial or viral (rabies prevention) inoculum. The addition of topical antiseptics or other remedies does not appear to affect the outcome or the incidence of infection. Washing the wound and keeping the wound clean and dry are sufficient for minor wounds. Minor injuries to compromised hosts (Table 2) can cause serious infection. Wounds that are on the hands, have associated crush injury or edema, are nearby a joint or may have penetrated a bone or a joint, and are moderately extensive should be treated aggressively. Bites, especially those around the head and neck, may

Table 1 Components of Care for Human and Animal Bites

History—Situation, pet ownership/identity
  Geographic location
Examination—Nerve function
  Tendon function
  Blood supply (pulses)
  Presence of edema, crush injury
  Proximity to joint
  Bone penetration
Diagram of wound(s)
Wound care—Irrigation
  Debridement
  Elevation
  Immobilization/exercise
Antimicrobials
  Prophylaxis, 3 to 5 days (PO)
  Therapy for established infection (PO versus IM initial dose)
  Empirical versus specific (animal specific)
Culture (if infected)
Baseline radiograph
Tetanus toxoid (0.5 ml IM) if required
Rabies prophylaxis (RIG/human diploid cell vaccine) if needed
Health department report (if required)
Decision regarding need for hospitalization

Table 2 Compromised Hosts Requiring Prophylactic Antimicrobial and Aggressive Care for Animal Bite Wounds

Local defense defects
  Preexisting edema
  Prior lymph node dissection
  Prior radiation therapy
Medications
  Steroids
  Immunosuppressives
Diseases/conditions
  Alcoholism
  Asplenia
  Cirrhosis
  Leukemia
  Lymphoma
  Mastectomy (radical or modified radical)
  Myeloma
  Neutropenia
  System lupus, erythematoses

penetrate a blood vessel and cause exsanguination. In addition, nerves and tendons may be injured or severed, and their function must always be evaluated, especially when wounds involve the hand. If edema is present, develops, or is preexisting, 24-hour-a-day elevation to reduce the edema is an important component of primary therapy. The use of slings is mandatory, and they should be worn to heart level when hand injury results in edema.

Cat scratches are more prone to infection than dog scratches, which are generally minor and rarely cause infection. Any eschar of a wound should be removed if there is more than 1 to 2 mm of erythema surrounding it or it is obviously infected. Puncture wounds are prone to infection,

Table 3 Activity of Selected Antimicrobials against Animal Bite Isolates

	PASTEURELLA MULTOCIDA	STAPHYLOCOCCUS AUREUS	STREPTOCOCCI	CAPNOCYTOPHAGA	ANAEROBES
Penicillin	+	−	+	+	V
Ampicillin	+	−	+	+	V
Amoxicillin-clavulanate	+	+	+	+	+
Ampicillin sulbactam	+	+	+	+	+
Dicloxacillin	−	+	+	−	−
Cephalexin	−	+	+	−	−
Cefuroxime	+	+	+	+	−
Cefoxitin	+	+	+	+	+
Tetracyclines	+	V	−	V	V
Fluoroquinolones	+	V	−	+	−*
Erythromycin	−	+	+	+	−
Azithromycin	+	+	+	+	−
Clarithromycin	V	+	+	+	−
Sulfa-trimethoprim	+	+	V	+	−
Clindamycin	−	+	+	−	+

+, Active; −, poor or no activity; V, variable activity against listed pathogen.
*New fluoroquinolones with anaerobic activity are under clinical development.

especially when associated with edema. They should be irrigated with sterile normal saline (no added iodine or antimicrobials) using an 18-gauge needle or catheter tip with a 20-ml syringe. The puncture is entered in the direction of injury and care taken to neither extend injury nor create a new one. This system functions as a high-pressure jet and reduces bacterial inoculum, whereas surface cleansing does not. Tears or avulsion should be copiously irrigated, any debris removed, and necrotic tissue cautiously debrided. Overly aggressive debridement can cause a defect that requires subsequent surgery.

Closure of infected wounds is contraindicated. Wounds to the head and neck seen less than 8 hours after injury may be closed if there is copious irrigation, debridement, no undue tension on the suture lines, and antimicrobials are given. The risks of closure with early presenting wounds to other parts of the body have not been studied. Approximating the edges with a tape bandage or delayed primary closure are often used.

Elevation is vital to decrease edema and prevent spread of infection and cannot be overemphasized. The failure of the patient to properly elevate the area is a common cause of therapeutic failure. In the hospital, elevation of a hand should be carried out using a 4-inch tubular stockinette, numerous safety pins, and an intravenous (IV) pole. A knot is placed at the elbow and the forearm placed between two layers of uncut stockinette held together by strategically placed safety pins.

If a tetanus booster has not been given within 10 years, 0.5 ml of tetanus toxoid should be given intramuscularly. Rabies prophylaxis will depend on local patterns of infection, and the local department of health should be consulted (refer to the chapter *Rabies* for details of Rabies prophylaxis).

Antimicrobial Selection

The empirical selection of antimicrobials should take into account the microbiology of these wounds. Fortunately, most dog and cat bite isolates are susceptible to penicillin and ampicillin. Antimicrobial selections are outlined in Table 3. Of note is the relatively poor activity of cephalexin, cefaclor, cephadroxil, and erythromycin against *P. multocida*. Patients who present more than 24 hours after injury without clinical signs of infection rarely require antibiotics. Patients who present for care less than 8 hours after injury and without signs of established infection should be given prophylactic antibiotics for 3 to 5 days if they have moderate to severe wounds; have had a prior splenectomy or have splenic dysfunction; are immunocompromised; have cirrhosis or severe liver dysfunction; have multiple puncture wounds, especially to the hands; have wounds over a bone or joint; or have developed edema or have preexisting edema or crush injury. Unreliable patients should also be managed more aggressively and may require intramuscular (IM) antimicrobials and/or inpatient observation. Follow-up should be in 24 to 48 hours, and the patient should be instructed to call before that if the condition worsens. The most common complications are septic arthritis, osteomyelitis, and residual joint stiffness.

Patients who present with established infection should receive proper wound care with irrigation, cautious debridement, tetanus and rabies evaluation, and courses of antibiotics. The decision to hospitalize a patient should follow the items in Table 4. The course for antimicrobial therapy for cellulitis is 7 to 14 days; for septic arthritis, 3 to 4 weeks; and for osteomyelitis, 4 to 6 weeks. Abscesses should be drained, and wounds should be cultured. Therapeutic failure of outpatient therapy, including those listed in Table 5, should lead to consideration of hospitalization.

Table 4 Criteria for Hospitalization of an Animal Bite Patient

Fever (>38° C [100.5° F])
Sepsis
Compromised host (see Table 1)
Advance of cellulitis
Patient noncompliance
Acute septic arthritis
Acute osteomyelitis
Severe crush injury
Tendon/nerve injury or severance
Tenosynovitis

Table 5 Causes of Therapeutic Failure for Animal Bite Wound Infections

Incorrect antimicrobial selection
Short antimicrobial duration
Insufficient antimicrobial dosage
Resistant isolates
Failure to elevate
Failure to recognize joint/bone involvement
Unrecognized abscess

Table 6 Activity of Selected Antimicrobials against Human Bite Wound Isolates

	EIKENELLA CORRODENS	STAPHYLOCOCCUS AUREUS	STREPTOCOCCI	HAEMOPHILUS SPECIES	ANAEROBES
Penicillin	+	−	+	−	−
Ampicillin	+	−	+	V	−
Amoxicillin-clavulanate	+	+	+	+	+
Ampicillin sulbactam	+	+	+	+	+
Dicloxacillin	−	+	+	−	−
Cephalexin	−	+	+	−	−
Cefuroxime	+	+	+	+	−
Cefoxitin	+	+	+	+	+
Tetracyclines	+	V	−	V	V
Fluoroquinolones	+	V	−	+	−*
Erythromycin	−	+	+	V/−	−
Azithromycin	+	+	+	+	−
Clarithromycin	V	+	+	+	−
Sulfa-trimethoprim	+	+	V	+	−
Clindamycin	−	+	+	−	+

+, Activity; −, poor or no activity; *V,* variable activity against listed pathogen.
*New fluoroquinolones with anaerobic activity are under clinical development.

■ HUMAN BITES

Human bites are either occlusional, where the teeth bite directly into flesh, or clenched-fist (closed-fist) injuries. Most occur during fights, and the patient often has a delayed presentation. They tend to be more severe than other animal bites but are managed similarly.

Occlusional bites may be to any part of the body and include "love nips." Bites to children may be the result of abuse and should be paid particular attention. Occlusional injuries to the hand are often particularly severe and result in abscess or osteomyelitis. The bacteria associated with infection include streptococci such as *viridans,* and *S. pyogenes* (group A), *S. aureus, Haemophilus* species, *Eikenella*

corrodens, and in more than 55% of cases, oral anaerobes. Antimicrobial therapy is outlined in Table 6. Of note is the poor activity of cephalexin and erythromycin against *E. corrodens* and anaerobes.

Clenched-fist injuries (CFIs) are the most severe of human bite wounds, and the patients often require hospitalization. CFIs are often complicated by septic arthritis and osteomyelitis. Their management should include an evaluation by a surgeon familiar with hands to determine whether the joint capsule was penetrated. Elevation and splinting are usually required, as are intravenous antimicrobials.

An algorithmic summary of the approach to bite wounds is presented in Figure 1.

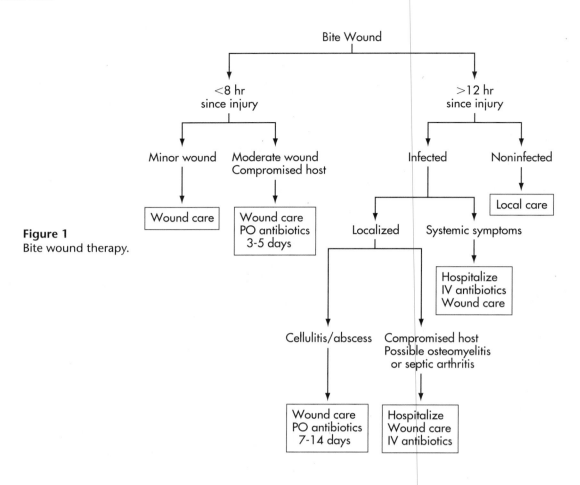

Figure 1
Bite wound therapy.

Suggested Reading

Brogan TV, et al: Severe dog bite wounds in children, *Pediatrics* 96:947, 1995.

Chuinard RG, D'Ambrosia RD: Human bite infections of the hand, *J Bone Joint Surg* 59:416, 1977.

Goldstein EJC: Bite wounds and infection, *Clin Infect Dis* 14:633, 1992.

Goldstein EJC: New horizons in the bacteriology, antimicrobial susceptibility, and therapy of animal bite wounds, *J Med Microbiol* 47:1, 1998.

Lockwood R: Dog-bite-related fatalities—United States, 1995-1996, *Morb Mort Weekly Rep* 46:463, 1997.

Talan DA, et al, and the Emergency Medicine Animal Bite Infection Study Group: The bacteriology and management of dog and cat bite wound infections presenting to Emergency Departments, *N Engl J Med* 340:85, 1999.

LICE, SCABIES, AND MYIASIS

William L. Krinsky

Louse and scabies infestations and myiasis involve parasitism by arthropods. Louse infestations and myiasis are caused by insects, and scabies is caused by mites. Diagnosis of each of these parasitic problems depends on accurate identification of the infesting arthropod. Lice and scabies mites are readily transmitted between close contacts; myiasis is not a contagious condition.

■ PEDICULOSIS CAPITIS

The most common form of louse infestation in North America is caused by the head louse, *Pediculus capitis*. The stage of the louse most commonly seen is the egg (nit). Each nit is oval, opaque, and white (about 0.8×0.3 mm) and attached individually to a single hair by the female louse. Each nit is laid about 1 mm from the scalp surface. Screening of large numbers of individuals is expedited by use of a Wood's light because nits fluoresce under ultraviolet (UV) light. Infested individuals usually first notice itching of the scalp, most often in the postauricular and occipital regions. Adult and immature lice are wingless and, like all insects, have six legs. Each leg ends in a claw used for gripping hair. The adult lice are about 2 to 3.5 mm long and are white or cream in color.

Three immature stages (nymphs) precede the formation of the adult louse. All immatures and adults require blood and, as a result of feeding, produce erythematous, papular lesions that are the cause of the pruritus. Some patients react to louse saliva with urticaria or lymphadenopathy. Erythematous lesions on the trunk, or postauricular and posterior cervical lymph node enlargement in the absence of other lymphadenopathy, should lead to suspicion of head louse infestation. Definitive diagnosis requires identification of the nits or lice. Nits are firmly attached to the hair shafts and will not readily slide off, as will most other contaminants, such as dandruff, hair casts, dried serous secretions, or dried hair spray, with which they may be confused (pseudopediculosis).

Therapy
Treatment of pediculosis capitis includes the use of one of various insecticidal shampoos or rinses (Table 1). Some preparations, such as lindane and pyrethrins, are not very effective at killing the nits; therefore permethrin, which has pediculocidal and ovicidal properties as well as low mammalian toxicity, usually is the drug of choice.

All family members and close contacts should be examined, and those with signs of infestation should be treated. Dead nits, which will eventually drop off when the hair they are attached to falls out or is cut, may be removed (with difficulty) for cosmetic purposes with a fine-toothed comb or forceps. All materials that touched the heads of infested persons, such as hats, scarves, bedding, and cushions, should be thoroughly washed in hot water or dry cleaned. Lice eggs require 6 to 10 days to hatch, and lice will not survive without blood for more than 10 days, so any infested materials kept in plastic bags for 4 weeks may be used safely. Hair grooming aids, such as brushes, combs, and curlers, should be discarded or soaked in a pediculicide for about 20 minutes or left in Lysol (2% in water) or isopropyl alcohol for about an hour and then thoroughly washed in hot, sudsy water.

■ PEDICULOSIS PUBIS (PTHIRIASIS)

Pubic louse infestation is caused by the crab louse, *Pthirus pubis,* named for its crablike appearance caused by the enlargement of the second two pairs of legs. Adult crab lice are 1 to 2 mm long and equally wide, and are gray, yellow, or brown. Extreme pruritus in the inguinal region usually is the first sign of infestation. Dried serous fluid, blood, or louse feces in the pubic hair are indicative of an infestation. Heavily infested individuals may have blue or gray macules that do not blanch under pressure. Nits usually are laid on the pubic and perianal hair, but infestations of facial hair, including eyebrows, eyelashes, mustache, and beard, may occur, as do less frequent infestations of the axilla. Transmission occurs most often during sexual contact. Definitive diagnosis requires identification of the nits or lice.

Therapy
Pubic lice are treated with insecticidal creams or shampoos applied to the inguinal region. Lindane 1% applied as a 4-minute shampoo to the infested areas generally is effective. Infestations of the eyelashes should be treated by an ophthalmologist. Conservative treatment with petrolatum (applied twice a day for 8 days), followed by mechanical removal of the nits, is most often recommended.

As in other louse infestations, all intimate contacts should be examined and treated when necessary. Undergarments and other clothing that touches infested persons should be thoroughly washed in hot water or dry cleaned. Infested materials placed in sealed plastic bags may be safely used after 1 month. Prepubertal children with pubic louse infestations of facial hair or eyelashes should be evaluated with regard to possible child abuse or sexual molestation.

■ PEDICULOSIS CORPORIS

Body louse infestation is caused by *Pediculus humanus,* a louse species virtually identical to the head louse, except that it usually is slightly larger, about 2 to 4 mm long. Body lice feed on blood but then retreat to hide in clothing, on which the nits are laid. Infestations are recognized by extreme pruritus in conjunction with observation of nits firmly attached to clothing fibers. Lice are rarely seen. The erythematous, maculopapular feeding lesions are often scratched beyond recognition, leaving only serous or bloody crusts, or secondary infection.

Table 1 Treatment for *Pediculosis capitis*

DRUG	REGIMEN	FOLLOW-UP
Permethrin (Nix)—1% creme rinse	Use after shampooing, rinsing with water and towel-drying; saturate hair and scalp; leave on for 10 minutes; work into a lather and rinse thoroughly with water.	One treatment usually is sufficient; repeat 7 days later if lice are seen.
Lindane (hexachlorocyclohexane) 1%	Apply shampoo to dry hair, work in and lather; leave on hair for 4 minutes; rinse off and towel briskly.	Second treatment may be given 7 days later.
Pyrethrins with piperonyl butoxide (A-200)	Apply shampoo to dry hair; wash out after 10 minutes.	Repeat treatment as often as needed 7-10 days later.

Therapy

Unlike the other forms of louse infestations, the lesions caused by body lice are the main focus of treatment. Antipruritics and antibiotics (for secondary infections) are used to treat the skin lesions. Louse eggs that are laid on clothing (especially in seams) may be destroyed by pressing with a hot iron. Washing clothes in hot water and dry cleaning will kill lice and nits as in the other forms of louse infestation. Infested furniture, mattresses, and box springs should be fumigated to destroy lice and nits. Infested materials sealed in plastic bags may be used safely after 4 weeks.

■ SCABIES

Scabies dermatitis is caused by the mite *Sarcoptes scabiei* and its secretions and excretions. The mites are microscopic; the adult female is the largest stage, 300 to 400 µm long. The female mites burrow into the skin and lay eggs. Skin lesions and intense pruritus are first noted 2 to 6 weeks after a person becomes infested. The most common lesions in order of frequency are papules, vesicles, crusted lesions, pustules, mite burrows, and wheals. The burrows, which have been observed in less than 25% of patients, are linear (5 to 15 mm long) or serpentine and gray, erythematous, slightly swollen, or scaly. Burrows are pathognomonic for scabies and occur most commonly in the interdigital areas, wrists, elbows, and lateral aspects of the hands, feet, and ankles. The burrows may be highlighted by applying mineral oil, ink, or tetracycline (which fluoresces under a UV lamp) and wiping off the excess that is not retained in the skin. Definitive diagnosis requires identification of the mite, which may be removed from a burrow by gently lifting the top off with a scalpel or needle and placing the debris from the burrow on a microscope slide. Observations of the material at 50× to 100× magnification can reveal living mites, ova, and mite feces. Mineral oil, immersion oil, or 10% potassium hydroxide placed on the burrow material on the slide may enhance identification of the mite.

Therapy

As in pediculosis, treatment of scabies involves use of any of various lotions or creams. The most commonly used preparations are lindane lotion, permethrin cream, and crotamiton lotion, or vanishing cream (Table 2). Permethrin, which is generally more effective than crotamiton and lacks the potential toxicity associated with lindane use, especially in infants, children, and pregnant or nursing women, is the treatment of choice for children and adults. Special effort should be made to coat the subungual areas and intertriginous spaces, such as the intergluteal cleft, with the scabieticide. Many patients, especially those with heavy mite burdens, as in crusted scabies, may continue to experience pruritus for several days after treatment. Repeat treatments should be given only if examination reveals the persistence of mites.

As in pediculosis, all close contacts should be treated. Laundering clothing and bedding in hot water or dry cleaning will destroy the mites. Suspect materials may be used safely after storage for 10 days in sealed plastic bags.

■ MYIASIS

Myiasis is the invasion of living vertebrate (including human) tissue by fly larvae. Various species of flies that normally deposit eggs or larvae on garbage, carrion, or corpses occasionally may deposit these stages on wounds or skin adjacent to draining infections. Other fly species are specifically adapted to deposit eggs that will hatch into larvae that invade intact skin or skin damaged by injury or disease. Flies in the former group are various house flies, blow flies (greenbottles and bluebottles), and flesh flies. The true myiasis-producers in the second group are bot flies and warble flies. Although bot fly and warble fly larvae usually infest nonhuman hosts, such as sheep, cattle, horses, rodents, deer, and other wild mammals, these larvae occasionally invade human tissues. Myiasis is most often cutaneous, but fly larvae may also invade the nose and throat, eye, ear, and intestinal or genitourinary tract.

Dermal myiasis, arising in intact skin and caused by the human bot fly (*Dermatobia hominis*) in Central and South America and the tumbu fly (*Cordylobia anthropophaga*) in Africa appears as a painful or itching swelling with an opening at the skin surface. Observation of the opening under low magnification will reveal the posterior end of a moving larva, on which will be two dark circular areas, the respiratory openings (spiracular plates). If the larva is left in the skin, it will continue to feed just below the skin surface for several days to weeks and eventually back out and drop to the ground to complete its development.

Table 2 Treatment for Scabies

DRUG	TREATMENT	FOLLOW-UP
Permethrin (Elimite or Acticin)—5% cream	Massage cream into skin from head to soles of feet (scalp, temples, and forehead to soles of children older than 2 months of age); wash off 8-14 hours later.	One treatment usually is curative.
Lindane (hexachlorocyclohexane) lotion 1%	Massage lotion into skin from neck down to soles of feet; wash off 8-12 hours later.	Repeat treatment may be needed 7 days later.
Crotamiton (Eurax)—10% lotion or cream	Massage into skin of whole body from chin down; may repeat application 24 hours later; bathe thoroughly 48 hours after last application.	May irritate raw or denuded skin, so close evaluation is necessary.

■ THERAPY

Myiasis of the nose and throat, eye, ear, or internal organs may require surgical intervention, or at least use of anesthetics for manual removal of the larvae with a forceps.

In dermal myiasis, early diagnosis and removal of the larva will relieve the irritation and discomfort caused by its movements and feeding under the skin. Direct removal involves application of a local anesthetic, followed by grasping the larva with a forceps and pulling with constant pressure to dislodge its hold, which may be strong because of the retrorse teeth or spines on its body. Indirect methods of removal involve application of an occlusive dressing containing petrolatum or even a piece of meat or animal fat if medical supplies are not readily available. Within a few hours, the suffocating larva will back out of the opening into the dressing or embed itself in the animal tissue. Secondary infections are rare, and little further treatment beyond local disinfection is needed. Wound myiasis, which may even occur in modern medical facilities, can be prevented by frequent changes of dressings and isolation of patients, especially immobile ones, within screened rooms.

Suggested Reading

Baird JK, Baird CR, Sabrosky CW: North American cuterebrid myiasis: Report of seventeen new infections of human beings and review of the disease, *J Am Acad Dermatol* 21:763, 1989.

Chodosh J, Clarridge J: Ophthalmomyiasis: a review with special reference to *Cochliomyia hominivorax, Clin Infect Dis* 14:444, 1992.

Peterson CM, Eichenfield LF: Scabies, *Pediatr Ann* 25(2):97, 1996.

Shorter N, et al: Furuncular cuterebrid myiasis, *J Pediatr Surg* 32:1511, 1997.

Taplin D, Meinking TL: Permethrin, *Curr Probl Dermatol* 24:255, 1996.

Vander Stichele RH, Dezeure EM, Bogaert MG: Systematic review of clinical efficacy of topical treatments for head lice, *Br Med J* 311:604, 1995.

SUPERFICIAL FUNGAL INFECTION OF SKIN AND NAILS

Arnold W. Gurevitch

■ DERMATOPHYTE INFECTIONS

Tineas are infections caused by the group of fungi called *dermatophytes.* These organisms can infect structures containing keratin, including the skin, hair, and nails. The tineas are clinically classified by the part of the body infected: tinea corporis, tinea cruris, tinea pedis, tinea manuum, tinea faciei, tinea barbae, tinea capitis, and tinea unguium (onychomycosis). The dermatophyte group consists of three fungal genera: *Trichophyton, Microsporum,* and *Epidermophyton.* A given species may cause a variety of skin lesions on different sites.

Specific Infections
Tinea Corporis

Dermatophyte infections of the glabrous (hairless) skin produce the classic ringworm picture. Although seen in any age group, tinea corporis is most common in children. Infection can be acquired from pets, humans, or the soil and may be caused by any species of dermatophytes. The most common fungi are *Microsporum canis, Trichophyton rubrum,* and *Trichophyton mentagrophytes.* The eruption begins as a small erythematous scaling patch. As the infection spreads outward, it tends to clear partially or completely in the center, producing an annular, or ringlike, lesion. The characteristic lesions are roughly circular, with a well-defined elevated erythematous scaling border. Differential diagnoses include nummular dermatitis, psoriasis, pityriasis rosea, seborrheic dermatitis, impetigo, erythema annulare centrifugum, and granuloma annulare.

Tinea Cruris

Tinea cruris is a fungal infection of the groin and inner thighs with extension to the perineum and buttocks. It is most common in warm, humid climates, and it affects men more often than women. In most cases the patient has coexisting tinea pedis, probably the source of the infection. A sharply marginated serpiginous scaling border is usually seen on the inner thighs. Central clearing is common. The scrotum and penis usually are uninvolved, and when they are infected, they have minimal scaling and erythema. Candidiasis is more common in women. It does not have a well-defined raised border, but it does have satellite papules and pustules and intense erythema. In men candidiasis often affects the scrotum and penis. Intertrigo, a dermatitis caused by local heat, moisture, and friction, is also common in this area. Other diagnostic considerations are contact dermatitis, psoriasis, seborrheic dermatitis, and erythrasma.

Tinea Pedis

Tinea pedis is the most common dermatophyte infection. Symptomatic tinea pedis affects 4% of the population. However, asymptomatic infections are found in up to 20% of those surveyed. *Trichophyton rubrum, Trichophyton interdigitale,* and *Epidermophyton floccosum* are responsible for almost all cases. The wearing of shoes, with accompanying sweating and maceration in the toe webs, is considered a major pathogenetic factor. Of the three clinical forms, the most common is intertriginous (interdigital). In this type whitish macerated scale in the web spaces between the toes is often accompanied by a foul odor. Fissuring can lead to secondary bacterial infection. An increase in bacterial flora, especially coryneforms, may play a pathogenic role as well. A second highly inflammatory form, vesiculopustular, presents with marked erythema, vesicles, pustules, erosions, fissures, and scaling. The arch of the foot is involved most often, as well as the undersurface of the toes. This variety may resolve spontaneously, only to recur. The most common form of tinea pedis is the dry, chronic, scaling type caused by *T. rubrum.* The soles are involved with extension to the sides of the feet (moccasin distribution). The nails are often involved as well. This type may be asymptomatic to pruritic. Maceration between the toes caused simply by hyperhidrosis, without infection, must be distinguished from interdigital tinea pedis. Interdigital gram-negative bacterial infections can also mimic tinea. Patients with dyshidrotic eczema and pustular psoriasis may develop plantar vesicles and pustules, respectively. Contact dermatitis and dry skin are other diagnostic considerations.

Tinea Manuum

Ringworm of the hands alone is uncommon. Tinea manuum most often accompanies tinea pedis. Scaling of the palms and fingers, especially in the creases, is the usual presentation. Much less common are vesicular lesions and involvement of the dorsal surface. In half of the cases, one hand and both feet (two foot, one hand syndrome) are involved. Differential diagnoses are much the same as with tinea pedis.

Tinea Faciei

Tinea faciei is tinea corporis of the face. It is rare, and the diagnosis is often missed. Erythema with or without scale is the usual presentation. A few small vesicles or pustules may be found. The classic ringworm appearance is not usual. Tinea faciei is often misdiagnosed as seborrheic dermatitis, photosensitivity, or rosacea.

Tinea Barbae

In contrast to tinea faciei, tinea barbae is a dermatophyte infection of the bearded area of the face and neck with invasion of fungi into the hairs. It occurs in men, most commonly farm workers. The two main causative species are *T. verrucosum* and *T. mentagrophytes.* The clinical picture can range from dry, red scaling patches to a deep pustular folliculitis with alopecia. The involved hairs are brittle, are lusterless, and pull out easily. Tinea barbae must be distinguished from bacterial folliculitis, acne, rosacea, and pseudofolliculitis barbae (ingrown hairs).

Tinea Capitis

Most cases of ringworm of the scalp and hair in the United States are caused by *Trichophyton tonsurans.* This organism does not produce the characteristic green fluorescence under Wood's light. Children are affected almost exclusively, and spread is primarily from human to human. African-American children are affected much more commonly than white children. In a recent study, almost 50% of families of an infected child had at least one other member with a positive culture. Varying combinations of erythema, scaling, and bald patches are seen. One or many infected patches may be found. In some cases, erythema and alopecia may be minimal or even absent, with severe scaling the predominant feature. Other children may show severe inflammation. *T. tonsurans* can also cause a black dot alopecia, in which black dots are produced by swollen infected hair shafts that break off at the surface of the scalp.

Occasionally, a kerion develops at the infected sites. The kerion is a boggy, nodular mass with severe follicular inflammation. The involved hairs are lost, and pustules and crusting often appear. Secondary bacterial infection may occur, but the primary pustule is a hypersensitivity reaction to the fungus. Kerions often heal with scarring and some degree of permanent alopecia. Tinea capitis may mimic psoriasis, seborrheic dermatitis, atopic dermatitis, and lupus erythematosus. However, the primary diagnostic consideration in a child with scalp scaling and no other cutaneous involvement is tinea capitis. The kerion can be confused with a bacterial folliculitis or even a carbuncle.

Tinea Unguium

Tinea unguium, nail plate invasion by a dermatophyte, is one type of onychomycosis. Onychomycosis can also be produced by other types of fungi, including *Candida albicans* and nondermatophyte molds. Only 50% of dystrophic nails are actually caused by fungi, and dermatophytes account for 90% of these cases. Some 20% of adults in the United States have onychomycosis, usually associated with chronic tinea pedis. Toenail infection is four times as common as fingernail infection. Of the several clinical patterns of onychomycosis, the most common is the distal subungual form. The fungus first causes hyperkeratosis of the nail bed under the distal aspect of the nail. This is followed by onycholysis (separation of the distal nail from the underlying bed) and thickening and distortion of the nail plate. A second clinical form, proximal white subungual, affects the cuticle and proximal nail bed with a white discoloration of the intact nail plate. This form is common in patients with human immunodeficiency virus (HIV) infection and others who are immunocompromised. In white superficial onychomycosis (the third type), fungal organisms in the nail plate produce a crumbled white surface. All three clinical patterns can ultimately lead to total nail destruction. Psoriasis in the nails may closely mimic onychomycosis, although fine pitting suggests psoriasis. Chronic eczematous eruptions and lichen planus may also produce nail dystrophy. Candidal nail infection usually begins with a paronychia, seen as erythema and swelling of the nail fold, followed by lateral onycholysis. Chronic trauma may also result in onycholysis and nail alterations that simulate onychomycosis.

Diagnosis

Definitive diagnosis of a dermatophyte infection rests with either a potassium hydroxide (KOH) preparation or a fungus culture. Scales for either technique should be taken from the active border of skin infections. Infected hairs from tinea capitis and tinea barbae can be plucked and used. Another technique in the diagnosis of tinea capitis is to rub a dry toothbrush over the area of alopecia or scale and then place the material on a slide or in a fungal medium. In tinea unguium, material should be taken from the infected nail bed (subungual debris) and the involved plate. Nail clippings can be used, especially for culture.

In a KOH preparation, the scrapings or hairs are placed on a microscopic slide and covered with a coverslip. One or two drops of 10% to 20% KOH are applied to the edges of the coverslip and allowed to run under it. The slide should be heated gently with a low flame, and then the coverslip is lightly pressed to thin the preparation. Initial examination of the field may be performed under the 10× objective. Lowering the condenser will increase the contrast and make hyphae easier to see. Hyphae will often be visible as translucent, slightly greenish rod-shaped filaments, often with branching. Areas suspicious for hyphae should be examined under the 40× objective for confirmation. It often is necessary to examine the entire specimen carefully because hyphae may be found in only one small fragment of scale. In tinea capitis and tinea barbae, chains of spores will be seen either within or surrounding the hair shaft. Interpretation of the KOH preparation requires a great deal of experience. Often, very few hyphae are present, and they are difficult to see. Artifacts are common and misleading. Lipid droplets and crystallized KOH may confuse the inexperienced observer, as will a mosaic artifact that resembles true hyphae.

Fungal culture in Sabouraud's glucose agar is the diagnostic method of choice for nail infections because hyphae are more difficult to find in KOH preparations from that site. One can also examine a nail histologically for evidence of fungi with a periodic acid–Schiff (PAS) or methenamine silver stain. A culture is often necessary in tinea capitis as well. Sabouraud's agar may be supplemented with an antibiotic (e.g., chloramphenicol) to inhibit the growth of bacteria or cycloheximide to suppress the growth of molds. Another medium, DTM, contains a color indicator that turns red in the presence of a dermatophyte. One disadvantage of the culture is the 2 to 4 weeks required to obtain growth.

Therapy

Most dermatophyte infections of limited areas of skin can be managed with topical agents. Several topical antifungals are available over the counter; others are available only by prescription. Most topical antifungal products fall into two classes: the imidazole derivatives and the allylamines. In addition, three other products are available: ciclopirox, haloprogin, and tolnaftate. The imidazoles include clotrimazole, econazole, ketoconazole, miconazole, oxiconazole, and sulconazole. Efficacy rates of these fungistatic agents are generally greater than 80%. Three allylamines, naftifine, butenafine, and terbinafine, are available, the first two by prescription; the latter is now available over the counter. These fungicidal products are effective in 90% to 100% of cases. In a recent cost analysis of topical drug regimens for dermatophyte infections, it was recommended that an inexpensive generic imidazole, such as miconazole or clotrimazole, be used first. Only patients with unresponsive infections should be treated with the higher-priced drugs. In the latter situation, the best choice may be an allylamine. The antifungal cream or solution is rubbed in well twice daily for 2 to 4 weeks, at least 1 week beyond clinical clearing. For tinea pedis and tinea cruris, I recommend use of an antifungal powder containing miconazole after each application of the cream. The dry chronic type of tinea pedis invariably recurs, and tinea cruris often recurs as well. To prevent recurrence, I suggest the regular and continued use of an antifungal powder after the course of a topical antifungal agent has been completed. Persons with recurring tinea cruris should also be advised against wearing tight undergarments. Careful drying between the toes, avoidance of occlusive footwear, and wearing cotton socks help prevent reinfection or recurrence of tinea pedis.

Extensive or resistant cases of cutaneous dermatophyte infections require systemic therapy. The five available systemic agents are griseofulvin, ketoconazole, fluconazole, itraconazole, and terbinafine. Fluconazole is not approved to treat dermatophyte infections, and itraconazole and terbinafine are approved for onychomycosis. I use ultramicrosize griseofulvin (Fulvicin PG, Gris PEG), 250 mg twice daily for 3 to 4 weeks, for the average adult. Griseofulvin is highly effective against dermatophytes and has relatively few significant side effects. Hair and nail infections require systemic therapy for effective control. For tinea capitis, my choice is ultramicrosize griseofulvin, 10 to 15 mg/kg/day, or griseofulvin microsize suspension, 15 to 20 mg/kg/day in two divided doses for 2 weeks beyond clinical clearing of the erythema or scaling. This may require 1 to 3 months of treatment. A complete blood count and liver function tests should be ordered before treatment of children with risk factors for liver diseases and when treatment extends beyond 3 months. Recently, fluconazole and itraconazole, at a dosage of 5 mg/kg body weight per day, or terbinafine, at 6 mg/kg, have been used. The course of therapy is only 1 month, but these agents are not approved for this use by the U.S. Food and Drug Administration (FDA). When treating a kerion, I use griseofulvin plus prednisone, 1 mg/kg/day, for the first 2 to 3 weeks of therapy. Topical antifungal shampoos, such as selenium sulfide or ketoconazole, may help prevent spread to other children, but they are not effective for definitive therapy. It is wise to suggest that other family members use the shampoo as well.

The treatment of tinea unguium remains difficult. Most of these patients seem to have an underlying inherited immune defect predisposing them to this infection. Therefore recurrences are common, certainly greater than 50% with toenail disease. Whether to treat and what form of therapy to use should be individualized. Factors to consider are the age and general health of the patient, compliance, cost of therapy, drug interactions, and side effects. However, it is vital to establish the diagnosis by KOH preparation, culture, or fungal stain before instituting systemic therapy.

For many years, griseofulvin was the drug of choice for fungal nail infections. Unfortunately, this drug has many drawbacks. It must be taken daily for 6 to 9 months for fingernails and 12 to 18 months for toenails. Even with this duration of treatment, only 25% of patients with toenail disease and 70% with fingernail infection are permanently cured. Most patients require 750 mg to 1 g daily to clear the infection. At that dosage, headaches and gastrointestinal disturbances are the most common side effects. A baseline complete blood count and liver panel should be obtained before beginning treatment and every 2 months thereafter. Ketoconazole has limited use in the treatment of nail infections because of the risk of hepatotoxicity. However, in the recent past, itraconazole and terbinafine have been approved for the treatment of toenail infections. They have only rarely been associated with hepatotoxicity. Itraconazole usually is given in a pulse dose of 200 mg twice daily for 1 week of each month for 2 months for fingernails and 3 months for toenails. The terbinafine regimen is 250 mg/day for 12 weeks for toenails and 6 weeks for fingernails. Itraconazole has several potential drug interactions, whereas terbinafine does not. Comparison studies suggest that terbinafine is also the more effective agent. However, a clinical cure occurs in only 75% to 80% of patients after one course. Therefore, in many patients, a second course may be required. Fluconazole, although not FDA approved for nail infections, has been used successfully at a dosage of 250 mg/week for 3 months for fingernails and 6 months for toenails. Baseline complete blood count and liver profiles, with a follow-up at 4 to 6 weeks, are recommended.

For patients unwilling or unable to take systemic medication, topical therapy may inhibit progression of nail disease. Chemical nail avulsion using a 40% urea preparation and surgical avulsion are further options. Avulsion works best in combination with either topical or systemic antifungal therapy. In addition, after control of the nail infection has been achieved, daily to weekly application of a topical antifungal agent may help prevent recurrence.

Tinea Versicolor

Tinea versicolor (TV) is a superficial fungal infection of the skin caused by *Pityrosporum ovale (Malassezia furfur)*. This yeast organism is found on the oily areas of the head and upper trunk in 95% of normal adults. An overgrowth of its hyphal form produces tinea versicolor. Because the organism is part of normal flora, it is not truly a communicable disease. Factors that promote the development of TV in-

clude high humidity and temperature, hereditary predisposition, systemic steroids, and defective cell-mediated immunity. TV is most common in tropical and subtropical climates and tends to appear during the summer, chiefly in persons with high sebum production (puberty through age 50). Recurrences are common.

The most commonly affected sites are the neck, upper trunk, and proximal extremities. However, the entire trunk, distal extremities, and face may be involved. TV begins as small, well-demarcated, finely scaling macules. The scaling can be extremely mild and subtle. Lesions are usually hypopigmented on dark or tanned skin and light pink or tan on pale skin. Some of the small macules usually coalesce into larger patches. Symptoms are often absent, and the patient seeks medical care because of the discoloration. Occasionally, mild itching occurs, especially when the patient has been sweating.

Differential diagnosis includes vitiligo, pityriasis alba, pityriasis rosea, and seborrheic dermatitis. Vitiligo is characterized by depigmentation and a lack of scaling, whereas TV is hypopigmented and finely scaling. Pityriasis alba consists of ill-defined hypopigmented dry scaling patches, often seen on the face or upper trunk of atopic children. Seborrheic dermatitis of the chest may resemble TV. Pityriasis rosea does not have coalescent large patches, and it has a distinctive Christmas tree arrangement of lesions.

Diagnosis

KOH examination of the scales is the best diagnostic procedure. Clusters of round yeast cells with short, rod-shaped hyphae (bats and balls or spaghetti and meatballs) are characteristic. The organism does not grow on routine fungal culture media. Examination with a Wood's light may give yellow to yellow-green fluorescence. However, this procedure is often negative, especially if the patient has recently showered.

Therapy

Tinea versicolor can usually be managed with topical therapy unless it is very extensive or recalcitrant. I use either 2.5% selenium sulfide (Selsun, Exsel) or 2% zinc pyrithione (DHS Zinc, Sebulon) shampoo. Ketoconazole (Nizoral) shampoo has also been reported to be effective. Although many regimens have been advocated, I instruct the patient to apply the shampoo as a lotion to the trunk, neck, upper arms, or other involved areas, leaving it on for 10 minutes before showering. This procedure is repeated nightly for 1 or 2 weeks, then weekly for 1 month. I inform patients that they may prevent recurrences by repeating the procedure monthly. Topical imidazole antifungals are also effective, but they are too expensive if the involvement is widespread. The patient should be informed that repigmentation takes place gradually over several months.

Systemic therapy may be required for widespread disease and in patients unresponsive to topical modalities. Oral ketoconazole has been most commonly used. The proposed treatment schedules vary from a single 400-mg dose to a dosage of 200 mg/day for 1 to 2 weeks. I usually recommend 400 mg/day for 3 days. Fluconazole, 400 mg repeated in 1 week, and itraconazole, 200 mg/day for 5 days, are also reported to be effective but are not approved for this use in the United States. Although recurrences are less frequent after systemic therapy, I suggest that the topical prophylactic regimen be followed every 1 to 3 months.

Suggested Reading

Epstein E: How often does oral treatment of toenail onychomycosis produce a disease-free nail? *Arch Dermatol* 134:1551, 1998.

Glyn E, Evans V, Sigurgeirsson B: Double blind, randomized study of continuous terbinafine compared with intermittent itraconazole in treatment of toenail onychomycosis, *Br Med J* 318:1031, 1999.

Katz HI: Systemic antifungal agents used to treat onychomycosis, *J Am Acad Dermatol* 38:S48, 1998.

Lange DS, et al: Ketoconazole 2% shampoo in the treatment of tinea versicolor, *J Am Acad Dermatol* 39:944, 1998.

Macura AB: Dermatophyte infections, *Int J Dermatol* 32:313, 1993.

MYCETOMA (MADURA FOOT)

Kenneth F. Wagner

$\mathbf{M}$adura foot, or mycetoma, is a chronic localized infection of the skin, subcutaneous tissue, fascia, and muscle. Tumefaction, draining sinuses, and grains that are made up of aggregates of organisms characterize it. Although it is a well-defined clinical entity, it may be caused by a wide array of bacteria and fungi.

■ EPIDEMIOLOGY

Mycetomas are seen most commonly in countries with tropical and hot temperate climates that lie between the tropics of Cancer and Capricorn. Mycetoma is relatively common in Mexico, where it is the most common manifestation of deep mycotic infection. Other locations in the Western Hemisphere where the incidence is high include Central and South America. It is an uncommon disease in the United States, where it is seen mostly in the Southeast. Other locations worldwide where mycetomas are reported with some frequency include Senegal, Sudan, Somalia, India, and Southern Asia.

Men are affected about four to five times as often as women, with the peak incidence between ages 20 and 40 years. Farmers and other rural workers who work outdoors or go barefoot are most commonly affected.

■ CAUSES

Mycetomas fall into two broad categories based on the causative organism: *actinomycetomas*, which account for 60% of all mycetomas worldwide, are caused by aerobic bacteria, including *Nocardia*, *Streptomyces*, and *Actinomadura* species (Table 1); *eumycetomas* are caused by true fungi, and many organisms have been implicated (Table 2). The distribution of agents varies with geographic location. *Nocardia brasiliensis* is the most common cause in Mexico and Central and South America, where 98% of mycetomas are actinomycotic. *Madurella mycetomatis* and *Streptomyces somaliensis* predominate in Africa and India. The most common cause of mycetoma in the United States is *Pseudallescheria boydii*.

■ PATHOGENESIS

The inciting event in a mycetoma is the traumatic inoculation of the causative agent into the skin or subcutaneous tissues of an otherwise healthy individual. This most often occurs to people who walk barefoot and receive penetrating injuries from thorn pricks, splinters, and animal and insect bites. Truncal infections develop after carrying sacks con-

Table 1	Causative Agents and Treatment of Actinomycetomas		
ORGANISM	**GRAIN COLOR**	**TREATMENT**	

Nocardia asteroides
Nocardia brasiliensis
Nocardia otitidis-caviarum
or (*Nocardia caviae*)
	White or yellow	Initial:
		    16 mg/kg/day TMP and 80 mg/kg/day SMX PO in divided doses
		    and/or dapsone, 3 mg/kg/day in divided doses
		Severe disease:
		    Add amikacin, 15 mg/kg/day × 3 wk IM or IV for 2-3 cycles with 15
		    days between cycles	

Actinomadura madurae *Actinomadura pelletieri* *Streptomyces somaliensis*	White or yellow Red Yellow	Streptomycin, 14 mg/kg/day, and TMP-SMX or dapsone at above dosages	

TMP, Trimethoprim; *SMX*, sulfamethoxazole.

taining contaminated branches, leaves, and plants without wearing protective clothing. Head and neck mycetomas may result from carrying contaminated wood bundles on the head and shoulders. The sex, occupational, and geographic predilections likely reflect greater opportunity for soil contact and predisposition to injury in these groups.

Table 2   Causative Agents of Eumycetomas

BLACK GRAIN	WHITE GRAIN
Exophiala jeanselmei	Acremonium falciforme
Leptosphaeria senegalensis	Acremonium kiliense
Leptosphaeria tompkinsii	Acremonium recifei
Madurella mycetomatis	Aspergillus flavus
Madurella grisea	Aspergillus nidulans
Pseudochaetospharanema larense	Arthrographis kalrae
Pyrenochaeta romeroi	Curvularia lunata
Pyrenochaeta mackinnonii	Cylindrocarpon destructans
	Fusarium sp.
	Neotestudina rosati
	Pseudallescheria boydii
	Trichophyton sp.
	Microsporum sp.

■ CLINICAL MANIFESTATIONS

Some 60% to 70% of mycetomas involve the lower limbs (Figures 1 and 2), but any region of the body can be affected. The most common site is the foot, followed by the hands. Other fairly common sites include the torso (Figure 3), thighs, head, neck, and buttocks.

The disease starts as a hard, usually painless, papule or subcutaneous nodule. The initial lesion progressively increases in size and forms sinuses that communicate with the surface of the skin. Granules composed of aggregates of organisms are discharged through these sinuses. As old sinuses close up and scar, new ones develop. Over time, new nodules form adjacent to the original lesion. Direct extension along fascial planes leads to deep abscesses and bony involvement. This eventuates in bone destruction and remodeling. Untreated, this process is chronic and progressive with continued cycles of swelling, suppuration, and scarring.

■ DIAGNOSIS

The combination of tumefaction and multiple sinuses that drain grain-filled serosanguinous fluid in a typical anatomic

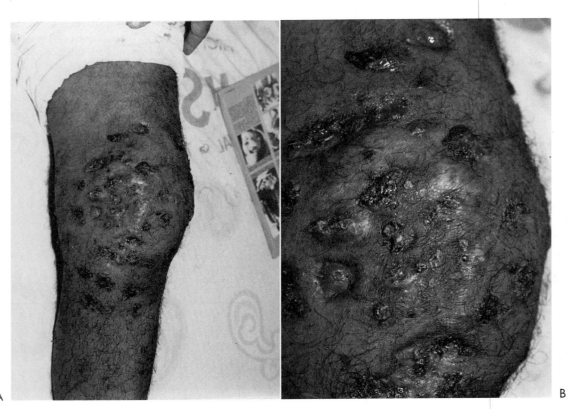

A   B

Figure 1
A and **B**, Multiple active and scarred sinus tracts of knee and lower leg in a Panamanian native with mycetoma caused by *Nocardia brasiliensis*.

location such as the foot is highly characteristic of mycetoma. After a thorough history, the initial diagnostic step should be the gross and microscopic examination of the grains. A crush preparation of the fluid in 20% KOH and a Gram stain should be performed, with organisms initially being separated by the color and size of the grains. A biopsy should be obtained for histology and culture. The grain for culture should be rinsed quickly in 70% alcohol and washed in sterile saline to eliminate fungal and bacterial contamination. Hematoxylin-eosin (H & E) stain will detect grains in tissue specimens. Tissue Gram stain, Gomori methenamine silver, and periodic acid–Schiff (PAS) stains may be helpful in identifying hyphae. Tissue cultures for primary isolation on Lowenstein-Jensen medium, 7H12B medium, and brain-heart infusion with blood agar with and without antibiotics and subculture on Sabouraud's medium usually will lead to specific identification of the causative organism. Newer molecular diagnostic and typing methods such as 16S ribosomal RNA sequencing may provide improved diagnostic identification of members of clinically significant species. Serologic testing for diagnosis and follow-up during treatment is currently not routinely used. Radiographs of the affected area should also be obtained to evaluate for bony involvement.

DIFFERENTIAL DIAGNOSIS

Actinomycosis is similar to mycetoma. It presents with sinuses that drain sulfur granules. Unlike mycetomas, which are externally induced, actinomycosis is caused by organisms that are normal flora of the oral cavity, such as *Actinomyces israelii*. The differentiation between these two processes is important because the management and prognosis for actinomycosis is significantly different from that for a mycetoma.

Other processes that can clinically mimic mycetoma are botryomycosis, cutaneous tuberculosis, and squamous cell carcinoma. Botryomycosis is a chronic bacterial infection in which the sinuses drain granules composed of clusters of bacteria. Although the most common agent is *Staphylococcus aureus*, many gram-positive and gram-negative organisms may cause this disorder. If mycetoma has invaded bone, it can be confused with chronic bacterial osteomyelitis. Again, an accurate diagnosis using Gram and acid-fast bacilli stains, cultures, and histopathology is important so that the appropriate treatment regimens can be instituted.

■ THERAPY

At all stages of disease, mycetoma could be cured by medical treatment alone or in combination with limited surgery.

Actinomycetoma

Several agents are effective in the treatment of actinomycetomas (see Table 1). The selection of medication depends on the causative agent, antimicrobial susceptibility, severity of disease, possible side effects, and cost. In the Western Hemisphere, where *Nocardia* is the major cause of mycetomas, sulfonamides are a good initial therapeutic choice. Trimethoprim with sulfamethoxazole (TMP-SMX), given orally at a dosage of 16 mg/kg/day trimethoprim and 80 mg/kg/day sulfamethoxazole, has proved to be successful in 60% to 70% of cases. Dapsone at an oral dosage of 3 mg/kg/day has also been useful either alone or in combination with TMP-SMX. These have been used for an average of 4 months to 2 years and should be continued until at least 6 months after all detectable signs of active disease have disappeared. The main side effects of sulfonamides in general include hematologic, gastrointestinal, and allergic skin reactions. The use of dapsone specifically may be limited by the development of methemoglobinemia, hemolytic anemia, and leukopenia. Therefore, when dapsone is used, close monitoring with serial complete blood counts is necessary. Resistance to TMP-SMX has been noted recently. Several newer antibiotics, including fluoroquinolones, carbapenems, broad-spectrum cephalosporins, and minocycline,

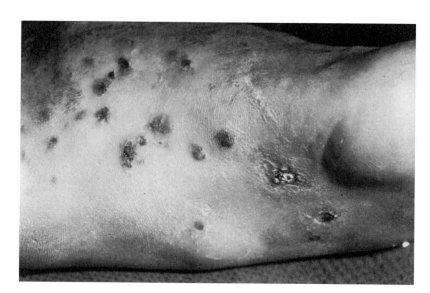

Figure 2
Mycetoma (Madura foot) caused by *Nocardia brasiliensis* in a classic location on a Panamanian patient.

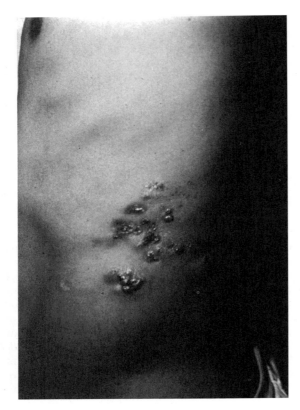

Figure 3
Truncal mycetoma demonstrating multiple tumors and sinus tracts.

have shown in vitro activity and some clinical efficacy when used alone or in combination against *Nocardia,* but their full clinical utility is yet to be determined.

Amikacin, either alone or in combination with TMP-SMX, has also been shown to be effective in the treatment of mycetoma caused by *Nocardia.* Amikacin is administered intramuscularly at a dosage of 15 mg/kg/day for 3 weeks. Two to three cycles with 15 days between each cycle are usually necessary. However, because of the associated risks of nephrotoxicity and ototoxicity, the need to follow peak and trough levels, and its cost, amikacin is best viewed as a second-line agent. It is most useful when there is resistance to prior therapy and when the extent or activity of the disease is severe and there is risk of dissemination to an adjacent organ.

In the Eastern Hemisphere, where *S. somaliensis* and *Actinomadura* are considerations, streptomycin sulfate given intramuscularly at a dosage of 14 mg/kg/day has been used. This generally is used in combination with TMP-SMX or dapsone. When streptomycin is used, the patient must be monitored for ototoxicity.

Eumycetoma

The medical management of eumycetomas is less successful and predictable than that of actinomycetomas. Small eumycetomas can be surgically excised, although recurrence may result if the lesion is incompletely excised. In more extensive lesions, surgical debulking followed by a prolonged course of an antifungal medication is likely to yield the best results. For eumycetomas, miconazole has demonstrated some effect in the past, but side effects and poor outcome limit its use. The most experience is with ketoconazole, 200 to 400 mg orally twice a day. Although many of these cases were caused by *M. mycetomatis,* successes have been seen with other fungi, including *Madurella grisea, Acremonium falciforme, Acremonium kiliense,* and *Pyrenochaeta romeroi.* However, therapeutic failures have also been noted. In vitro studies and accumulating clinical experience suggest that the newer triazole antifungal agents, especially itraconazole, may be more potent than ketoconazole against the fungi that cause eumycetomas. Itraconazole, 100 to 400 mg/day, has been successful in treating the same fungi previously treated with ketoconazole and in some instances effective in cases where ketoconazole had failed. There are also recent reports of successful treatment of eumycetomas with itraconazole for *A. nidulans, A. flavus, A. recife, A. kalrae, Fusarium,* and *P. boydii.* The new itraconazole cyclodextrin solution achieves higher serum itraconazole and hydroxy-itraconazole concentrations than the capsule formulation, which may translate into better clinical outcomes. It appears that itraconazole may be more effective than fluconazole for mycetomas. Amphotericin B and griseofulvin have been used with limited success. The use of these agents is constrained by the high minimal inhibitory concentrations for these fungi and the adverse reactions that they cause. Because of the cost and limited clinical improvement by liposomal amphotericin B preparations at dosages up to 3 mg/kg/day, these agents have minimal use for eumycetomas.

Three investigational antifungal drugs, voriconazole, SCH56592 (both triazoles), and MK-0991 (an echinocandin), seem to have in vitro activity equal to or greater than itraconazole against many of the agents that cause mycetoma. Optimal dosage and duration of therapy of these new antifungal drugs are still to be determined.

As response rates of different agents of mycetoma to the same antifungal may be different, it is at present unclear whether the newer drugs will be equally potent and have a similar range of applications as current therapy either used alone or in combination. In all cases of mycetoma, prolonged medical therapy will be necessary to accomplish a cure.

Suggested Reading

Boiron P, et al: Nocardia, nocardiosis and mycetoma, *Med Mycol* 36(suppl)1:26, 1998.

McGinnis MR: Mycetoma, *Dermatol Clin* 14(1):97, 1996.

Pfaller MA, et al: In vitro activity of two echinocandin derivatives, LY303366 and MK-0991 (L-743, 792), against clinical isolates of *Aspergillus, Fusarium, Rhizopus,* and other filamentous fungi, *Diagn Microbiol Infect Dis* 30(4):251, 1998.

Welch O: Treatment of eumycetoma and actinomycetoma, *Curr Top Med Mycol* 6:47, 1995.

Wildfeuer A, et al: In vitro evaluation of voriconazole against clinical isolates of yeasts, moulds and dermatophytes in comparison with itraconazole, ketoconazole, amphotericin B and griseofulvin, *Mycoses* 41(7-8):309, 1998.

FEVER AND LYMPHADENOPATHY

Gerald Friedland
Martha I. Buitrago

The occurrence of fever and lymphadenopathy is common in clinical practice. It is important to have a logical and systematic approach for the diagnosis and treatment of patients with this syndrome. A careful history and examination are often the key to the diagnosis.

Important elements of the history include location and duration of lymphadenopathy and the presence or absence of systemic symptoms. Additional information, such as occupational and animal exposures, geographic residence, recent travel, or high-risk behaviors, could be associated with specific disorders. For example, hunters and trappers and tularemia, residence in southern California and coccidioidomycosis, travel to Central and West Africa and African trypanosomiasis (sleeping sickness), travel to the Mediterranean and kala-azar (leishmaniasis), travel to South America and typhoid fever and American trypanosomiasis (Chagas' disease).

All lymph node areas should be evaluated. When lymph nodes are palpated, certain characteristics such as size, tenderness, consistency, whether or not nodes are matted, and location should be noted and described.

In general, a node larger than 1 cm should be considered abnormal. Pain is usually the result of an inflammatory process or suppuration but may also represent hemorrhage into the necrotic center of a malignant node. The presence or absence of tenderness does not reliably differentiate from malignant nodes. Stony hard nodes are typically a sign of cancer, usually metastatic. Very firm, rubbery nodes suggest lymphoma. Softer nodes are the result of infectious or inflammatory conditions because suppurant nodes may be fluctuant. The term *shotty* refers to small nodes that feel like buckshot under the skin, as found in the cervical nodes of children with viral illnesses.

A group of nodes that feels connected and seems to move as a unit is said to be "matted." Nodes that are matted can either be benign (e.g., tuberculosis, sarcoidosis, or lymphogranuloma venereum) or malignant (e.g., metastatic carcinoma or lymphomas). Last, the anatomic location of localized adenopathy will often be helpful narrowing the differential diagnosis.

The evaluation of a patient with fever and lymphadenopathy also requires that four questions be answered:

1. Is the adenopathy local or generalized?
2. Is the process acute or chronic?
3. Is the cause infectious or noninfectious?
4. Is there a primary peripheral lesion?

To answer the first question, a thorough physical examination of all accessible major lymph node–bearing areas should be performed. These include the nodes of the head and neck and the axillary, epitrochlear, and inguinal nodes.

Radiologic studies are necessary to define the two other clinically important major lymph node–bearing areas, the mediastinum and hilum of the lung and the retroperitoneum. The somewhat arbitrary period of 1 month separates acute from chronic lymphadenopathy in adults. In children, a period of 2 or 3 months is more reasonable. Figure 1 provides an overview of guidelines to the differential diagnosis of fever and lymphadenopathy.

◼ GENERALIZED LYMPHADENOPATHY

Generalized lymphadenopathy is present if nodes in two or more noncontiguous major lymph node–bearing areas are enlarged.

Lymphadenopathy is a common finding in persons infected with human immunodeficiency virus (HIV). This subject is addressed later in this chapter.

Acute generalized infectious lymphadenopathy, which is most often viral, is a common feature of many childhood viral infections, including rubella, measles, and varicella. Generalized lymph node enlargement may also be seen in the prodromal period of hepatitis A and B. Epstein-Barr virus (EBV), cytomegalovirus (CMV), HIV, and toxoplasmosis may all produce a mononucleosis syndrome with generalized lymphadenopathy. Bacterial pathogens are much less often the cause of generalized lymphadenopathy, which may, however, occur in relatively uncommon entities such as brucellosis and leptospirosis. In all these infections, the nodes are typically tender, discrete, firm to touch, and without fluctuance.

Acute generalized noninfectious lymphadenopathy is often caused by hypersensitivity reactions, most commonly drug induced. Sulfonamides, hydralazine, carbamazepine, and phenytoin are among the agents implicated in such reactions, which rapidly disappear with the withdrawal of the drug. Other medications that may cause lymphadenopathy include allopurinol, atenolol, captopril, quinine, primidone, and sulindac. Collagen-vascular diseases, including rheumatoid arthritis and systemic lupus erythematosus (SLE), may cause acute generalized lymphadenopathy and fever. In Kawasaki's disease (mucocutaneous lymph node syndrome), a disease of uncertain origin that affects mostly children, lymphadenopathy is present in about half of patients, is most common in the cervical nodes, and may be unilateral.

Chronic generalized infectious lymphadenopathy, less likely to be viral, suggests more serious diagnostic possibilities. Disseminated bacterial and fungal diseases, including tuberculosis, syphilis, histoplasmosis, and cryptococcosis, should be considered. In children, persistent lymphadenopathy and fever may suggest an immunodeficiency state, including chronic granulomatosis disease.

Chronic generalized noninfectious lymphadenopathy is most often neoplastic. Lymphoreticular neoplasms (Hodgkin's disease, non-Hodgkin's lymphoma, chronic

FEVER AND LYMPHADENOPATHY

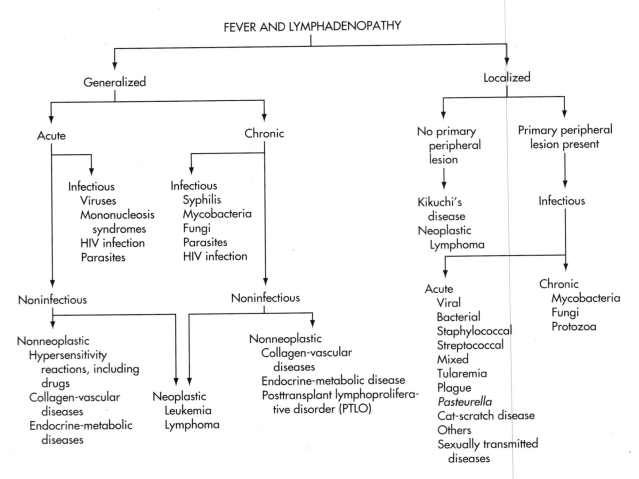

Figure 1
Algorithm for the differential diagnosis of fever and lymphadenopathy.

lymphocytic leukemia) predominate. Fever, when present, may be caused by the underlying malignant disease or by secondary infection. Nonneoplastic diseases that with variable frequency cause chronic generalized lymphadenopathy and fever include sarcoidosis, Still's disease, and hyperthyroidism. Enlarged, tender lymph nodes and low-grade fevers are common findings in patients who meet the case definition for chronic fatigue syndrome, a disorder characterized by a debilitating fatigue for which no cause has been established (see the chapter *Chronic Fatigue Syndrome*). In patients receiving immunosuppressive therapy after a solid organ or bone marrow transplant, the clinician should consider the diagnosis of posttransplant lymphoproliferative disorders (PTLDs), which are a heterogeneous group of lymphoid proliferations, most of which are of B-cell lineage and associated with EBV. These disorders can occur months to years after transplantation.

■ LOCALIZED LYMPHADENOPATHY

Lymphadenopathy is localized if not more than two contiguous lymph node groups are involved. Anatomically and clinically, the node-bearing areas are divided into five major groups: the head and neck, the axilla, the inguinal area, the mediastinal-hilar areas, and the retroperitoneal paraaortic area (Table 1). The clinician again must consider both infectious and noninfectious causes. In addition, a careful search for a primary lesion in the anatomic areas drained by the affected lymph node group will help distinguish between these categories.

Noninfectious local adenopathy is usually chronic and is not associated with a primary peripheral lesion. When fever is present, the most likely noninfectious cause is a lymphoproliferative neoplasm. Nodes that are hard, immobile, and nontender are often associated with metastatic carcinoma.

Infectious local adenopathy, usually associated with a primary peripheral lesion, requires an appreciation of the anatomic areas that each nodal area drains. The evaluation of localized lymphadenopathy should always include a thorough examination of these areas, although in some cases, the peripheral lesion will be subtle or inapparent.

Localized lymphadenopathy resulting from infections may be acute or chronic. The lymph nodes may be tender with classic signs of inflammation or may be firm and nontender. The next section discusses each nodal area separately. However, many of the diseases discussed may present in any anatomic site, and generalized adenopathy may be first or most easily recognized in a single lymph node area.

The lymph nodes of the head and neck are often collec-

Table 1   Localized Lymphadenopathy: Areas Drained and Associated Conditions

LYMPH NODE AREA	ANATOMIC AREA	AREAS DRAINED	ASSOCIATED CONDITIONS/ COMMENTS
Head and neck	Occipital and posterior auricular	Scalp, face	Local infections with skin pathogens: staphylococcus, streptococcus, acute viral illnesses Children: secondarily infected insect, tick, or spider bites, dermatophyte infections (ringworm)
	Anterior auricular	Eyelids, palpebral cunjunctivae, external auditory meatus, pinna	Conjunctivitis, oculoglandular syndrome (*Francicella tularensis*, *N. gonorrhoeae*, *B. henselae*), keratoconjunctivitis
	Tonsillar, submaxillary, submental	Pharynx, mouth, teeth, lips, tongue, cheeks	Infections of the head, neck, sinuses, ears, scalp, pharynx, teeth, and oral mucosa
	Posterior cervical	Scalp and neck, skin of arms and pectorals, thorax, cervical and axillary nodes	Mononucleosis, Kikushi's disease, tuberculosis, lymphoma, head and neck malignancy
Axillary		Upper extremity Thoracic wall, breasts, and back	Acute pyogenic infection, cat-scratch disease, brucellosis, melanoma, breast malignancy
Inguinal		Lower extremities Abdominal wall Genitalia: penis, scrotum, vulva, vagina, perineum, perianal region	Pyogenic infections of the lower extremities Sexually transmitted diseases: herpes simplex, syphilis, chancroid, lymphogranuloma venereum Pelvic and perianal malignancy
Mediastinal—hilar		Lungs, trachea, esophagus	Granulomatous disease (infectious and noninfectious), malignancies
Abdominal		Abdominal viscera	Usually granulomatous disease:
Retroperitoneal		Retroperitoneal organs: kidneys	*M. tuberculosis*, *M. avium complex*, Malignancies: lymphoma
Paraaortic		Pelvic organs	

tively called *cervical* but are more accurately divided into several anatomic and clinical areas. The occipital and posterior auricular nodes drain large areas of the scalp and face. Adenopathy of these groups may be associated with primary infectious lesions in these areas but is also a common feature of many acute viral illnesses. In children, secondarily infected insect, tick, or spider bites and ringworm (dermatophyte infection) are common ~~es~~.

The anterior auricular nod~~es~~ ~~drai~~n the eyelids, palpebral conjunctivae, external audit~~ory meatu~~s, and pinna. Conjunctivitis and anterior au~~ricular adeno~~pathy (the oculoglandular syndrome) is clas~~sically associate~~d with *Francicella tularensis* via direct inoc~~ulation of the conj~~unctival sac but may also be seen with ~~direct inoc~~ction from *Neisseria gonorrhoeae, Bartonella* ~~(cat-scr~~atch bacillus), and epidemic keratoconjunctiv~~itis~~.

The tonsillar, submaxillary, and submen~~tal nodes~~ drain the tonsils and other structures of the pharynx an~~d m~~outh, and they have great clinical significance. Enlargement of these nodes should prompt careful inspection and often palpation of the mouth, teeth, and pharynx. In addition, nodes of this group drain the external structures of the medial face, including the lips, chin, cheeks, and the medial aspects of the conjunctivae.

The posterior cervical nodes are in the occipital triangle of the neck above the inferior belly of the omohyoid muscle

and posterior to the sternomastoid muscle. They are commonly involved in the generalized lymphadenopathy of infectious mononucleosis and mononucleosis-like syndromes. Involvement of these nodes is highly unlikely in localized infections of the mouth and pharynx. Kikuchi's disease, or histiocytic necrotizing lymphadenitis, is a fairly common self-limited disorder that usually involves the cervical lymph nodes predominantly in females of Asian and Middle Eastern origin. Often, the disease is associated with fever or flulike symptoms and an elevated sedimentation rate and leukopenia. Its etiology is still obscure, but it has been associated with Kaposi's sarcoma–associated herpesvirus (KSHV-HHV8). However, because of its association with systemic lupus erythematosus (SLE) and Still's disease, it is also suspected to be autoimmune in origin. Recognition of this disease is important because it can be mistaken, by pathologists unfamiliar with the condition, for other conditions that require treatment such as malignant lymphoma and Kawasaki's disease.

The inferior deep cervical nodes lie below the level of the inferior belly of the omohyoid muscle and both posterior (the supraclavicular nodes) and anterior (the scalene nodes) to the sternomastoid muscle. Those nodes receive drainage from the scalp, the superior deep cervical nodes, the axillary nodes, and the nodes of the hilum of the lung, mediastinum, and abdominal viscera. Their enlargement may signify primary disease at any of these distant sites. Adenopathy in this area not readily palpable may be detected with the Valsalva maneuver.

Acute cervical adenopathy is most likely to be of pyogenic bacterial or viral origin. Staphylococci and streptococci predominate among bacterial agents, the former from primary skin sites and the latter from oral and dental infections. Infections of the tonsils, pharynx, and skin are the most common primary sites in children, and dental infections more commonly result in cervical adenopathy in adults. Penicillin is prescribed for oral and dental infections. A semisynthetic penicillinase-resistant penicillin is used when the primary site of infection is the skin. Ruptures of cervical nodes into their fascial spaces may require surgical drainage if there is fluctuance, impingement on vital structures, or both.

Chronic cervical adenopathy raises the possibility of granulomatous infections, particularly *Mycobacterium tuberculosis* and atypical mycobacteria, primarily *Mycobacterium avium* complex. Toxoplasmosis may cause chronic cervical lymphadenopathy, particularly involving the posterior cervical nodes.

Supraclavicular lymphadenopathy has been associated with malignancy in most patients older than 40 years of age. The left supraclavicular (Virchow's) node receives lymphatic flow from the thorax and abdomen and may signal pathology in the testes, ovaries, kidneys, pancreas, prostate, stomach, or gallbladder.

Mediastinal and hilar adenopathies are usually detected on conventional radiographs. These nodes are rarely involved in acute suppurative disease. A useful diagnostic criteria is whether the lymphadenopathy is unilateral or bilateral. Unilateral enlargement of the hilar or mediastinal lymph nodes most frequently includes granulomatous disease of both infectious and noninfectious causes (sarcoidosis) as well as neoplasms. Among granulomatous infections, *M. tuberculosis* and fungal disease, such as histoplasmosis, predominate. Bilateral hilar adenopathy is present in approximately three fourths of patients with sarcoidosis (only 10% of such patients have neoplastic disease) and in patients with SLE and other collagen-vascular disease. The diagnostic approach to patients with hilar adenopathy includes mycobacterial skin tests, sputum examination, cultures, and sputum cytology. Computed tomography (CT) is useful in assessing the size and location of the lymph nodes. Criteria for lymph node enlargement are dependent on the diameter of the node or nodes in question. A node less than 1 cm wide can usually be considered normal. In the absence of a primary diagnostic lesion, the clinician should perform a biopsy on a node larger than 1 cm wide.

Tissue for histologic examination may be obtained from inferior cervical node biopsy, transbronchial lung biopsy, mediastinoscopy, or percutaneous or surgical biopsy of hilar nodes.

The axillary nodes drain the entire upper extremity as well as the lateral parts of the chest wall, back, and the breasts. This cluster of nodes is most commonly involved in acute pyogenic infections of these drainage areas. By far, the most common organisms involved are the staphylococci and streptococci, often associated with primary areas of cellulitis, lymphangitis, or furunculosis. The extremities are often

the site of infections from organisms acquired from the environment, including zoonoses. Among the diseases and pathogens in this category are tularemia, plague, *Pasteurella multocida,* and *Erysipelothrix.*

Cat-scratch disease, which is caused by *B. henselae* (formerly *Rochalimea*), may present as lymphadenopathy and fever.

Inguinal lymphadenopathy is commonly encountered clinically. The inguinal nodes drain not only the lower extremities but also the lower abdominal wall, the genitalia, the perineum, and the perianal area. Acute pyogenic bacterial infection is most common, usually caused by the organisms enumerated in the discussion of axillary adenopathy. The drainage of the perineum and perianal area suggests that enteric aerobic gram-negative organisms and gram-positive and gram-negative anaerobic organisms may be present. Because of the drainage of the genitalia, venereal infections often involve the inguinal nodes. Those most likely to present with prominent inguinal adenopathy are syphilis, lymphogranuloma venereum, chancroid, and genital herpes simplex.

The abdominal and retroperitoneal nodes drain the abdominal viscera and retroperitoneal and pelvic organs and may receive drainage from the inguinal nodes as well. Neither the nodes nor the primary site of infection, except the testes, are directly clinically accessible, making assessment difficult. Radiologic procedures must be used for evaluation, most often CT or magnetic resonance imaging (MRI).

■ ADENOPATHY AND HIV INFECTION

Acute retroviral infection is a mononucleosis-like syndrome that occurs 2 to 10 weeks after exposure to HIV. Acute bilateral generalized lymphadenopathy, which may be accompanied by fever, maculopapular rash, headache, mucosal ulcerations, myalgias, and malaise, is a common feature of this syndrome. Sometimes, there are symptoms and signs of meningitis because HIV involves the neural tissues soon after infection. Tests for HIV antibody are negative during the early stage of primary infection, so the diagnosis is best made by testing for HIV RNA in plasma. Titers are extremely high during the initial infection and may be assayed by the reverse transcription polymerase chain reaction (PCR) method, branched DNA testing, or amplification based on nucleic acid sequence. PCR tests for HIV DNA and cocultures of circulating mononuclear cells or other tissues should also be positive during primary infection. The mean interval between the onset and resolution of symptoms during primary HIV infection is approximately 25 days.

The long period of asymptomatic infection that follows may last for years. During this time, many infected individuals exhibit persistent generalized lymphadenopathy (PGL). The nodes are typically nontender and firm to rubbery. PGL may persist for several years, into the period of early symptomatic HIV infection, which may include fevers, night sweats, weight loss, and diarrhea.

As HIV disease progresses, more severe complications, including opportunistic infections and malignancies, may develop. This period defines acquired immunodeficiency syndrome (AIDS). In contrast to earlier stages, lymphadenopathy is not a common finding in those with advanced HIV disease, and its presence suggests an infectious or neoplastic process involving the reticuloendothelial system. Of infectious causes, disseminated *M. avium* complex infection, *M. tuberculosis,* histoplasmosis, CMV infection, toxoplasmosis, syphilis, and cryptococcosis are most common. Although high-grade B-cell lymphomas are common in patients with AIDS, they are typically extranodal. Kaposi's sarcoma may involve lymph nodes, occasionally without apparent skin lesions (see the chapter *AIDS: Therapy of Opportunistic Infections*).

■ GENERAL DIAGNOSTIC APPROACHES

In most cases of infectious lymphadenopathy, clinical and laboratory findings short of biopsy often suggest the causative agent in the enlarged nodes. Some of these findings are as follows:

1. Primary site of infection (e.g., streptococcal cellulitis, staphylococcal furuncle, syphilitic chancre)
2. Associated symptoms: "B" symptoms with lymphomas, rash, serositis with systemic lupus; arthritis with Still's disease, or rheumatoid arthritis
3. Characteristic rash (e.g., rubella, rubiola, drug eruption, acute HIV infection)
4. Characteristic physical findings: splenomegaly in mononucleosis, lymphoma
5. Typical hematologic findings (e.g., eosinophilia [drug reactions], atypical lymphocytosis [mononucleosis syndromes], high erythrocyte sedimentation rate in rheumatologic diseases)
6. Skin tests (e.g., tuberculosis)
7. Serologic tests (e.g., EBV, hepatitis, syphilis, HIV, tularemia)
8. Stains and culture of material from peripheral primary lesions and pulmonary lesions (atypical mycobacteria, tuberculosis, plague)

Lymph Node Biopsy versus Fine-Needle Aspiration

The simplicity, safety, and cost-effectiveness of fine-needle aspiration (FNA) make it a useful test for the evaluation of persistent lymphadenopathy. The advent of radiologically guided FNA has made accessible the nodes of the hilum and retroperitoneum, thus avoiding extensive surgical procedures during their evaluation. The presence of a cytopathologist on site to determine the adequacy of the specimens has been shown to increase the yield of FNA considerably. However, there are limitations to the procedure.

FNA is useful in the diagnosis of benign reactive processes, certain infections, or metastatic disease, yet its accuracy in the diagnosis of lymphoma and primary malignancies remains controversial. Technical difficulties pose an obstacle for the effective differentiation of certain malignancies. Because the chemotherapeutic agents used for treatment of patients with lymphoma are selected on the basis of the specific type of lymphoma, excisional biopsy remains necessary for definitive subclassification of lymphoma in the majority of patients.

Another limitation of FNA is the frequent unavailability of sufficient material for histology, special stains, and culture, particularly when mycobacterial disease or other granulomatous infections are under consideration. These additional tests are often necessary to establish the diagnosis and select appropriate therapy. This is especially important for *M. tuberculosis* when establishing the species and resistance pattern is of critical importance.

The following general guidelines are intended to suggest to the clinician circumstances in which excisional biopsy is appropriate.

1. Undiagnosed chronic lymphadenopathy of 1 month in adults, 3 months in children
2. Localized nonsuppurative lymphadenopathy without an accessible or apparent peripheral lesion
3. Enlarging undiagnosed lymphadenopathy after 2 weeks of observation
4. Nontender, matted to hard lymphadenopathy or a high clinical suspicion of neoplastic disease
5. Radiologic findings or systemic signs and symptoms suggesting granulomatous or lymphoproliferative disease when noninvasive tests are unrevealing
6. Positive tuberculin test in absence of diagnostic pulmonary tuberculosis
7. New adenopathy in immunocompromised patients, although otherwise asymptomatic patients with HIV and PGL do not need biopsies
8. Lymphadenopathy in the setting of fever of undetermined origin
9. Persistently nondiagnostic or inconclusive FNA results

Technique

Approximately half of lymph node biopsies lead to a specific diagnosis. Careful attention to several rules maximizes the usefulness of the invasive diagnostic procedure.

1. Discuss the differential diagnosis with the surgeon, the pathologist, and the microbiology laboratory in advance of the procedure so that any special considerations (e.g., fixation, staining, special culture media) can be made known.
2. Select the best site. Avoid lymph nodes often involved in minor inflammatory processes, such as the inguinal and submandibular nodes. In the presence of generalized lymphadenopathy, the inferior or posterior cervical nodes are preferred; the second choice is the axillary nodes.
3. Remove the largest node in a cluster of enlarged nodes.
4. Remove nodes in their entirety with capsules intact. Bisect them, sending half of the specimen to the pathology laboratory and the other half to the microbiology laboratory for stains and culturing of common pathogens, mycobacteria, fungi, and other suspected organisms.
5. Request that the pathologist make additional sections of the excised tissue if the node is abnormal but not diagnostic.
6. Consider a repeat biopsy and the excision of more tissue if the node is abnormal but not diagnostic and the clinical picture is unclear.

Interpretation

Entities discussed in this chapter that have a characteristic histologic pattern and for which a specific or strongly suggestive diagnosis can be made histologically are lymphoma and other neoplasms, tuberculosis, fungal disease, sarcoidosis, toxoplasmosis, and cat-scratch disease. Most noninfectious noneoplastic disorders and most acute viral infections show nonspecific lymphadenitis or hyperplasia only. However, a significant number of patients with initially nondiagnostic lymph node biopsies and persistent lymphadenopathy will ultimately prove to have a serious underlying disease. If the biopsy is not initially diagnostic, it is essential to follow the patient carefully and to consider repeat biopsy if adenopathy persists.

Suggested Reading

Ferrer R: Lymphadenopathy: differential diagnosis and evaluation, *Am Fam Phys* 58:1313, 1998.

Quinn T: Acute primary HIV infection, *JAMA* 278:58, 1997.

Tarantino DR, et al: The role of fine needle aspiration biopsy and flow cytometry in the evaluation of persistent neck adenopathy, *Am J Surg* 176:413, 1998.

Weekly clinicopathological exercises: case 5-1997: a 24-year-old woman with cervical lymphadenopathy, fever and leukopenia, *N Engl J Med* 336:492, 1997.

Weekly clinicopathological exercises; case 5-1999: a 37-year-old man with fever and diffuse lymphadenopathy, *N Engl J Med* 340:545, 1999.

ACUTE AND CHRONIC BRONCHITIS

Sanford Chodosh

Bronchial infections with viral and bacterial microorganisms are responsible for a significant percentage of ambulatory care visits and are the principle causes of time lost from work. These infections occur in individuals with and without underlying chronic bronchial disease, each with important differences in etiology, clinical presentation, laboratory findings, and requirements for therapy.

■ ACUTE BRONCHITIS

Acute infectious bronchitis in individuals without underlying chronic lung disease is most commonly caused by viral pathogens, with a lesser contribution by *Mycoplasma, Chlamydia,* and *Legionella.* The relative frequencies of these etiologies vary with time and place and have epidemic-like characteristics in the population. The clinical presentation is usually abrupt and is characterized by the onset of cough, which may be productive of scanty sputum. There are variable associated symptoms, including coryza, sore throat, burning sensation in tracheal area, malaise, feverishness, chilliness, and other symptoms of viremia. Wheezing and dyspnea are unusual symptoms in adults but may be present in young children, in which case it can be confused with asthma. All of these symptoms are most troublesome in the first few days of the infection and should significantly improve or resolve within 1 week. Medical intervention is rarely sought or required and symptomatic therapy usually suffices. Routine laboratory studies are rarely indicated and are not likely to be useful. If the patient produces sputum, the cytologic findings are of neutrophils with swollen bronchial epithelial cells, which may demonstrate vacuolization. A Gram stain is characteristically free of bacteria. However, if symptoms worsen or persist beyond a week, a nonviral etiology should be suspected. If the Gram stain now reveals significant bacterial types morphologically consistent with *Haemophilus, Streptococcus pneumoniae* or

Moraxella, antimicrobial therapy would be appropriate. The choice of agent would be similar to what will be covered under acute exacerbations of chronic bronchitis, but the duration of therapy can be reduced. If *Mycoplasma, Chlamydia,* or *Legionella* infection were suspected, a 7-day course of a macrolide, tetracycline, or a selected quinolone would be appropriate. Experience has shown that patients who seek medical care for acute bronchitis should be suspected of having unrecognized chronic bronchial disease, which usually delays the course of resolution observed in normal individuals.

■ ACUTE BRONCHITIS ASSOCIATED WITH CHRONIC BRONCHIAL DISEASE

Exacerbations caused by bacterial bronchitis are more common and more severe in patients with chronic bronchitis and chronic bronchial asthma. Because the incidence of both diseases is common, bacterial exacerbations represent one of the most common indications for prescribing an antimicrobial agent by clinicians. Chronic bronchitis affects an estimated 15% to 25% of adults, many of whom have both acute exacerbations of chronic bronchitis (AECB) and acute bacterial exacerbations of chronic bronchitis (ABECB) over the course of their illness with the associated increased morbidity associated with such events. Besides the deleterious individual effects, the costs to society are measured in billions of dollars. Despite this, the diagnosis and therapy of such episodes are often haphazard. The pathologic and physiologic abnormalities of the bronchial system that may predispose patients with chronic bronchial disease to bacterial infection include impaired mucociliary clearance, bronchi obstructed by abnormal secretions and bronchoconstriction, and in patients with chronic bronchitis, an indolent presence of pathogenic bacteria in the bronchial epithelium as well as impaired host defenses. For example, bacterial phagocytosis and intracellular bactericidal activity by polymorphonuclear neutrophils is impaired, macrophage recruitment is decreased, and sputum immunoglobulin levels are subnormal.

Most acute bacterial exacerbations (ABE) present without an identifiable precipitating event. However, many occur following acute viral respiratory infections, excessive cigarette smoking, thickened secretions secondary to reduced humidity associated with winter heating, alcohol consumption, and anesthesia. The latter factor likely accounts for the increased frequency of postoperative bronchopulmonary infections noted in patients with underlying chronic bronchitis. All acute exacerbations of chronic bronchitis present with similar bronchopulmonary symptoms, which may include increased frequency and severity of cough, greater sputum production that is usually purulent, chest congestion, chest discomfort, increased dyspnea and wheezing, and

The views expressed in this chapter are those of the author and do not reflect the official policy or position of the Department of Veterans Affairs of the U.S. government.

scant hemoptysis. Systemic symptoms of malaise, anorexia, chilliness, or feverishness may also be present. However, shaking chills, fever, or pleuritic pain usually indicates the presence of pneumonia. Physical examination may reveal rhonchi, coarse rales, wheezes, decreased breath sounds, tachypnea, and tachycardia. Patients with chronic bronchitis who are admitted to hospital or treated in emergency rooms with compromised pulmonary function usually have had a preceding acute exacerbation.

Bacterial infection is the etiology of approximately 50% of the acute exacerbations suffered by patients with chronic bronchitis. Other common etiologies are acute viral tracheobronchitis, inhalation of toxic gases or particles (e.g., cigarette smoke), thickened secretions, inhalation of allergens, or discontinuation of background therapy. The differentiation of ABE from other types of exacerbations is only occasionally possible from history, physical examination, blood tests, urine tests, chest roentgenograph, pulmonary function tests, or the gross appearance of the sputum. Purulence of the sputum is often equated with infection. However, the characteristic yellow to green color of purulence is caused by myeloperoxidase released from polymorphonuclear neutrophils and eosinophils and reflects the stasis of secretions in the bronchial tree, which is a common factor in most types of exacerbations. Microscopic assessment of the sputum by means of a Gram stain and simple wet preparation reveal the two essential characteristics of bacterial infection: increased numbers of bacteria and increased bronchial neutrophilic inflammation. The Gram stain must have bacteria in numbers significantly above two per oil immersion field, the top level present when the patients are stable. In addition, the wet preparation of the sputum should reveal that the majority of the inflammatory cells are neutrophils. This with an associated increase of the volume of sputum expectorated reflects the outpouring of neutrophils into the bronchial lumen in response to the bacterial infection. Microscopic screening of the sputum is essential to the selection of aliquots for evaluation, which are free of oropharyngeal admixture. Much of the distrust of sputum findings commented on in the literature can be related to the failure to adhere to this simple procedure. If sputum is not selected for examination, the results will not reflect the bronchial pathology.

Table 1 details the distinguishing characteristics of the cellular population and Gram stain findings in each etiologically different type of acute exacerbations seen in chronic bronchitis or asthma. The identification of the specific etiology allows for selection of appropriate therapy and avoids the costs and adverse effects associated with the use of unnecessary medications.

Bacteriologic cultures and sensitivity testing are rarely indicated to determine treatment for ambulatory ABE. Exceptions to this rule are when gram-negative bacilli (other than *Haemophilus*-like organisms) or staphylococcal-like bacteria are noted on Gram stain. However, staphylococcal ABE are rare in ambulatory chronic bronchitis outpatients. Gram stains can provide immediate information with which to initiate therapy; waiting for cultures is not justified. In patients with chronic bronchitis, culture results from poorly selected aliquots are often falsely positive or negative and can lead to inappropriate choice of therapy.

Table 2 details the critical primary treatment modalities for the various types of acute exacerbations as well as those that are important supportive measures. Antimicrobials are not indicated for any of the AE, which are not bacterial in etiology. Their use can only add adverse side effects. A recent trend to treat all types of exacerbations empirically with both antimicrobials and corticosteroids should be discouraged. The decrease of host defenses associated with corticosteroids can be detrimental if the bacteria responsible for the ABE are not covered by the arbitrarily chosen antimicrobial.

The two main goals in the therapy of ABE are to effect a prompt resolution of the acute infection and to provide a long infection-free posttherapy period. The characteristics desirable in the chosen antimicrobial should include coverage of the major pathogens etiologic in ABE, a dosage regimen that favors compliance, and a low incidence of undesirable side effects. Educating patients at risk of developing ABE to recognize early symptoms can lead to early initiation of adequate antimicrobial therapy that decreases morbidity, unnecessary visits to emergency rooms, and expensive hospitalizations. The signs and symptoms of ABE should be significantly improved within 5 to 7 days after starting antimicrobial therapy. Patients should be reevaluated if this does not occur, and therapy may need to be modified.

Published investigations should help clinicians decide on an appropriate antimicrobial for ABECB. Unfortunately, such publications can be misleading because of poorly conceived study designs. Deficiencies that should be looked for include the use of nonbacterial AECB cases mixed in with true ABECB cases obscuring any true differences between agents, investigations specifically designed to only demonstrate equivalence between antibiotics, and the exclusion of cases with in vitro–resistant bacteria from the analysis of efficacy. These types of investigations can lead clinicians to believe that all antibiotics are equally effective. Conversely, because no advantage of any antibiotic can be demonstrated in such studies—despite marked differences noted in in vitro activities—it is easy to incorrectly conclude that antibiotic therapy is unimportant in the treatment of ABECB. In addition, when all AECB are treated as if they were ABECB, the true cause of an AECB may not be identified and the specific therapy that could benefit the patient is not used.

Carefully controlled investigations in which a bacterial etiology is an absolute prerequisite demonstrate that there may be profound differences of outcome of ABECB between antibiotics. Selection of the proper antimicrobial once bacterial infection is identified as the cause of the AECB should assume that any of the four major pathogens might be present. *Haemophilus influenzae*, *Moraxella catarrhalis*, *S. pneumoniae*, and *Haemophilus parainfluenzae* make up more than 90% of the organisms etiologic in ABECB, with a predominance of *Haemophilus* species. During the 1990s, the older antimicrobials have lost a significant degree of their original efficacy because of the increasing incidence of beta-lactamase active *M. catarrhalis* (80%) and *H. influenzae* (40%) and of penicillin-resistant *S. pneumoniae*.

The goals of therapy for ABE are the expeditious resolution of the acute infection without significant early relapses and with a long infection-free posttreatment period. Success

Table 1 Key Sputum Characteristics in the Differential Diagnosis of Acute Exacerbations of Chronic Bronchitis or Asthma

	NEUTROPHILS*,†	EOSINOPHILS*,†	TYPE OF BRONCHIAL EPITHELIAL CELLS†	BACTERIA ON GRAM STAIN‡
Acute bacterial bronchitis	Increased	No change	Pyknotic	Increased
Acute viral bronchitis	Increased	No change	Swollen	No change
Inhalation of toxic gases or particles	Increased	No change	Pyknotic	No change
Thickened secretions	No change	No change	Pyknotic	No change
Inhalation of allergens	Variable	Increased	Swollen	No change
Discontinuation of background therapy	No change	No change	Pyknotic	No change

*Percentage of all cell types and numbers excreted per day.
†As observed in wet sputum preparations.
‡Numbers per oil immersion field with 0 to 2 as the numbers seen in nonacute patients.

Table 2 Therapy for Acute Exacerbations of Chronic Bronchitis with or without Asthma

	ANTI-MICROBIAL	CORTICO-STEROIDS	HYDRATION AND HUMIDIFICATION	AVOIDANCE OF INHALED IRRITANTS	EXPECTORANT	BRONCHO-DILATOR
Acute bacterial bronchitis	1	NA	2	2	2	2
Acute viral bronchitis	NA	NA	2	2	2	2
Inhalation of toxic gases particles	NA	NA*	2	1	2	2
Thickened secretions	NA	NA	1	2	1	2
Inhalation of allergens	NA	1	2	2	2	1
Discontinuation of background therapy	NA	NA	Renew appropriate background therapy			

1, Primary or very important therapy; *2*, secondary or supportive therapy; *NA*, not applicable.
*Exception for acute inhalation of toxic materials known to cause serious acute inflammatory response.

and compliance will be facilitated by selection of an antimicrobial drug with the best antibacterial sensitivity pattern, having few adverse effects and a simple dosage regimen. A first-choice antibiotic should provide prompt resolution of the acute infection in more than 94% of patients with ABECB, have less than a 10% relapse rate in the first 2 weeks after therapy, and keep most patients infection free for at least 5 to 6 months (Table 3). Recommendations to treat ABECB in which the severity of the underlying chronic bronchitis is mild with less effective antimicrobials is not based on adequate comparison studies. Use of low dosages and short periods of treatment are also of questionable validity. The little data that exist strongly suggest that these practices lead to higher early relapses and shorter infection-free intervals. The tenacity of bacterial infection in chronic bronchitis is usually underestimated.

Prompt and adequate antimicrobial therapy will decrease the period of morbidity and the chances of progression to pneumonia and/or respiratory failure. All episodes of ABECB should be treated to achieve these positive outcomes. The vast majority of ABECB are treatable in the ambulatory setting with orally administered antimicrobials.

Table 3 Ranking Criteria for Assessing Antimicrobial Therapy in ABECB

RANKING	1	2	3	4
Positive response during therapy (% of cases)	94-100	88-93	75-87	<74
Continued positive response 2 weeks after therapy (% of cases)	83-88	72-82	61-71	<60
Duration of infection-free period in days (based on mean values)*	>200	156-200	100-150	<100
Probable sensitivity of infecting pathogens to the antimicrobial (%)	>95	85-95	75-85	<75

*These data are from double-blind and crossover studies in which the same subjects were treated with different antimicrobials for separate ABECB.

If the patient is not already receiving adequate background therapy for his or her underlying disease, these measures should be instituted concomitant with the antimicrobial therapy. Resolution of the acute bacterial exacerbation should be defined as a return to the preexacerbation level of symptoms and bronchial inflammation. Acceptance of partial improvement can lead to a protracted period of morbidity and a higher level of bronchial mucosal damage and inflammation than was present before the infection. Insufficient improvement after 7 days of therapy is an indication for reevaluation. Persistence of the original bacteria or the emergence of new bacterial types in association with continued elevation of sputum neutrophilic inflammation indicates that the antimicrobial agent needs to be changed.

Oral agents used for ABECB come from most of the major antimicrobial classes (e.g., penicillins, tetracyclines, quinolones, macrolides, cephalosporins, sulfonamides). Efficacy of representative antimicrobials can be ranked from 1 (best results) to 4 (poorest results) using the criteria noted in Table 3 for the three major clinical and bacteriologic outcomes. Treatment failures are defined as failure to respond during treatment, early relapses as recurrences within 2 weeks of stopping therapy, and the infection-free period defined from the mean values from double-blind studies as the average number of days from stopping therapy to the next ABECB. A fourth criterion relates to the current sensitivity of the common ABECB pathogens to the antimicrobial. The best choice should be an antimicrobial with four "1"s.

Table 4 details the efficacy and sensitivity patterns of antimicrobials that have been or are being commonly used to treat ABECB. Only data in which the cases evaluated had

Table 4   Oral Antimicrobials for Acute Bacterial Exacerbation in Chronic Bronchitis*†

	DOSAGE DOSE/DAY (mg)	SCHEDULE DURATION (DAYS)	RESPONSE DURING THERAPY	EARLY RELAPSE AFTER THERAPY	INFECTION-FREE INTERVAL	BACTERIAL SUSCEPTIBILITY
PENICILLINS						
Ampicillin	500 qid	14	1	1	1	4
Amoxicillin	500 tid	14	2	1	2	4
Amoxicillin-clavulanic acid	500/125 tid	14	1	2	2	2
Amoxicillin-clavulanic acid	500/125 bid	7	(2)	ND	ND	2
QUINOLONES						
Ciprofloxacin	750 bid	14	1	1	1	1
Ciprofloxacin	500 bid	14	1	2	2	2
Ofloxacin	400 bid	10	(1)	ND	ND	2
Grepafloxacin	600 qd	10	(1)	(1)	ND	1
Trovafloxacin	100 qd	10	(1)	(1)	ND	1
Trovafloxacin	100 qd	7	(2)	(2)	ND	1
Trovafloxacin	300 qd	10	(1)	(1)	ND	1
Sparfloxacin	400 qd	1				
	200 qd	9	(3)	(2)	ND	1
TETRACYCLINES						
Doxycycline	100 bid	14	1	1	2	2
Doxycycline	200 qd	1				
	100 qd	9-13	(2)	(4)	ND	2
Tetracycline	1000 qid	14	2	4	3	3
MACROLIDES						
Clarithromycin	500 bid	14	2	3	2	2
Azithromycin	500 qd	1				
	250 qd	4	(2)	ND	ND	2
Azithromycin	500 qd	3	(3)	ND	ND	2
Erythromycin	250 qid	7	(3)	(4)	ND	4
CEPHALOSPORINS						
Cefuroxime	500 bid	14	(2)	ND	(2)	2
Cefaclor	500 tid	14	4	4	4	4
Cephalexin	500 tid	14	3	4	4	4
Cefprozil	500 bid	10	(4)	ND	ND	3
SULFONAMIDES						
Trimethoprim-sulfamethoxazole	800/160 bid	14	1	2	3	3

ND, No data available.

*Ranking 1 to 4: see Table 3.

†Parallel assignment studies noted by numbers in parenthesis. All others from crossover assignment studies.

bacterial pathogens identified in double-blind designed studies are listed. Efficacy data from parallel assignment studies are noted in parentheses, whereas data from crossover assignment studies are not. Crossover study comparisons benefit from having the same host for the two separate ABECB, diminishing some of the variability related to host factors. Antimicrobials are not listed in Table 4 if they are not commonly used for ABECB, if published data do not meet the criteria of having identified pretherapy pathogens for all analyzed cases, or the study excluded cases with resistant bacteria. Many of the studies were done before 1990, so it is important to consider the current sensitivity pattern when selecting an antimicrobial. These values will likely continue to change with time and vary because of locality differences.

The once highly efficacious penicillins have lost their preeminence as the drugs of choice for treatment of ABECB because of the significant increase of beta-lactamase–active *H. influenzae* (40%) and *M. catarrhalis* (80%) and the rising incidence of penicillin-resistant *S. pneumoniae*. The rankings for ampicillin and amoxicillin (see Table 4) were established before the emergence of these factors and are included for their historical perspective. Even without current studies of these agents, the assumption should be that neither agent alone would now be as efficacious for ABECB. The addition of a beta-lactamase inhibitor (e.g., clavulanic acid) to amoxicillin or ampicillin should theoretically restore their previous efficacy for *M. catarrhalis* and *H. influenzae*, but critical studies comparing these with and without inhibitors are not available. Not all beta-lactamase subtypes are covered by the available inhibitors, suggesting that full theoretical advantage may not be realized. These inhibitors will not eliminate the problem of penicillin-resistant *S. pneumoniae*.

The fluoroquinolone class of antimicrobials has demonstrated the positive attributes that ampicillin once possessed. These are very effective against *H. influenzae* and *M. catarrhalis* and not affected by beta-lactamase activity. The relative activity against *S. pneumoniae* by the various quinolones has defined those most efficacious for ABECB. Enoxacin, lomefloxacin, and fleroxacin, with poor activity against *S. pneumoniae*, are not indicated for treatment of ABECB. Ciprofloxacin at the higher recommended dosage (750 mg twice daily) is quite effective in eradicating *S. pneumoniae* in clinical outcome studies, whereas at a lower dosage (500 mg twice daily), activity against pneumococci becomes marginal. Ofloxacin and levofloxacin appear to be only slightly less efficacious, but the published reports of these agents do not usually address relapse rates and infection-free intervals for pathogen proven cases. Despite sparfloxacin's excellent in vitro profile of bacterial susceptibility, the clinical and bacteriologic outcome studies have been less than anticipated. Interaction with other drugs and the risks of photosensitivity will also discourage common use of this drug. A number of newer quinolones, either recently approved or being studied, have in vitro profiles suggesting a greater potential against *S. pneumoniae*. However, as activity against *S. pneumoniae* improves, efficacy against organisms such as *Pseudomonas aeruginosa* generally declines. These new quinolones include grepafloxacin, trovafloxacin, moxifloxacin, and gatifloxacin. Outcome studies in ABECB with these quinolones have not evaluated all of the efficacy criteria.

Grepafloxacin and trovafloxacin appear to rank high in terms of acute response and early relapse rates. There are little or no data published on the efficacy of the other two agents in ABECB, and infection-free interval studies have not been reported. Based on the available published experience, ciprofloxacin, 750 mg twice daily, appears to be the quinolone of choice for treatment of ABECB pending definitive studies of the newer quinolones.

When quinolones are contraindicated, one of the synthetic tetracyclines can be used. Doxycycline and minocycline are comparable in efficacy, have convenient dosage schedules not dependent on food restriction, have few adverse effects to restrict compliance, and are not limited by beta-lactamase–active microorganisms. The side effects of regular tetracycline make compliance difficult and contribute to their poor efficacy. Although tetracycline-resistant *S. pneumoniae* have been reported, the clinical impact of this has not been evident in ABECB.

The newer macrolides, clarithromycin and azithromycin, are superior to erythromycin for ABECB. However, critical published data on efficacy of these two agents for ABECB are scant. Clinical and bacteriologic outcome data suggest a role as second-choice therapy for ABECB. This is primarily related to a relatively poor ability to eradicate *H. influenzae*. Although they have low degrees of toxicity, interactions with other therapeutic agents may cause some confusion regarding indications in individual patients. Macrolides have significant activity against *Chlamydia pneumoniae*, *Mycoplasma pneumoniae*, and *Legionella*, but although these pathogens are important in community-acquired pneumonia, they play a lesser role in ABECB. Erythromycin is not indicated for ABECB.

Trimethoprim-sulfamethoxazole is efficient during active treatment for ABECB, but it has a significant incidence of early relapse rate, and the infection-free interval is considerably shorter than with first-choice antibiotics. Although the low initial cost is favorable, the need to treat a new infection within 3 months is not cost-effective. There are also concerns relating to increased toxicity in older patients.

Cephalosporins have variable success in treating ABECB. The efficacy of individual cephalosporins is difficult to assess from most of the published data. Resistant bacteria are commonly excluded from analysis in these studies. The appearance of equivalence with virtually any effective or ineffective comparative antibiotic is an inevitable outcome. Of the few properly studied cephalosporins, cefuroxime compared favorably with low-dose ciprofloxacin. Well-controlled studies with older cephalosporins, such as cephalexin and cefaclor, indicate a level of ineffectiveness in all outcome criteria approaching what would be expected from placebo therapy. Results from studies with ineffective agents like these strongly support the need for effective antibiotic therapy for ABECB. If antibiotic therapy was not important, the results of even carefully designed investigations should never demonstrate any differences.

The effectiveness of even the best antimicrobial may be significantly affected by the use of an insufficient daily dose, too short a period of therapy, or both. Lower dosages often decrease the incidence of troublesome side effects, and shorter duration of therapy promotes better compliance. However, this must be balanced against a higher rate of early relapses and a more frequent occurrence of ABE in these chronically ill patients. Unfortunately, very few investigations have addressed this issue directly. Inference from a variety of studies strongly suggests that the higher recommended dosages given for at least 10 to 14 days are advantageous in treating ABECB. Examples from Table 4 support this. Ciprofloxacin, 750 mg twice daily, provides fewer relapses and a longer infection-free interval than does a dosage of 500 mg twice daily when both are given for 14 days. Azithromycin, 500 mg/day for 3 days, is not as effective during therapy as a 5-day course at a lower daily dose. Doxycycline, 100 mg twice daily, is more effective during and immediately after therapy than a lower (standard) regimen for the same duration of therapy.

When parenteral therapy is necessary in hospitalized patients, it is more important to identify the causative pathogen(s). Depending on the pathogen, ampicillin, ciprofloxacin (particularly for gram-negative infections), or doxycycline would be common choices. Trovafloxacin would be indicated if anaerobic infection is present. Multiple-drug therapy, including cephalosporins and aminoglycosides, may be necessary. Oral therapy should be considered as early as possible in these circumstances.

Antimicrobial therapy should always be accompanied by good supportive therapy. This should include the avoidance of smoking or other inhalation irritants, hydration, humidification, expectorants, bronchodilators, and adequate treatment of any associated asthma. When secretion clearance is particularly difficult, chest physiotherapy and mucolytic therapy are appropriate. Patients who have both chronic bronchitis and asthma will often note an exacerbation of asthmatic symptoms as the infection is controlled. Prompt recognition of this possibility should lead to vigorous treatment of the asthma and not be misdiagnosed as a failure of the antimicrobial. This can be easily detected by examination of the sputum, which would show a shift to a predominance of eosinophils and an absence of significant bacterial flora on Gram stain.

In summary, the first choice antimicrobials for ABECB are ciprofloxacin, 750 mg twice daily; trovafloxacin, 100 to 200 mg/day; or one of the other new quinolones when *Pseudomonas* infection is not a concern. Second-choice agents are ciprofloxacin, 500 mg twice daily; amoxicillin with clavulanic acid; and doxycycline. Other agents should be considered only when contraindications for the main antimicrobials exist.

Suggested Reading

Chodosh S: Treatment of acute exacerbations of chronic bronchitis: state of the art, *Am J Med* 91:87S, 1991.

Chodosh S: Bronchitis and asthma. In Gorbach SL, Bartlett JG, Blacklow NR, eds: *Infectious diseases*, Philadelphia, 1992, WB Saunders.

Chodosh S: Sputum production and chronic bronchitis. In Takishima T, Shimura S, eds: *Airway secretion: physiological bases for the control of mucus hypersecretion*, New York, 1994, Marcel Dekker.

CROUP, EPIGLOTTITIS, AND LARYNGITIS

Maureen R. Tierney
Irmgard Behlau

■ CROUP

Croup is a clinical syndrome characterized by a barking cough, hoarseness, inspiratory stridor, and often some degree of respiratory distress. The term *croup* is usually used to refer to acute laryngotracheitis. Other crouplike syndromes can include epiglottis, spasmodic croup, and bacterial tracheitis (Table 1). Croup is overwhelmingly a disease of children between the ages of 1 to 6 with peak incidence between 1 and 2 years. Parainfluenza 1, 2, and 3 and respiratory syncytial virus (RSV) are the most common causes, with outbreaks occurring predominantly in the winter months. Other causes include influenza and adenovirus with rare cases secondary to *Mycoplasma, C. diphtheriae,* and herpes simplex virus (HSV). In adults, the causes are also predominantly viral, including reported cases of influenza, parainfluenza, RSV, HSV, cytomegalovirus (CMV) and *Haemophilus influenzae* type b (Hib). In either children or adults, secondary bacterial infections with staphylococci, *H. influenza, Moraxella,* and *Pneumococcus* can be seen.

Croup usually follows a relatively mild upper respiratory infection. Its onset may be abrupt. Inflammation of the nasopharyngeal area moves inferiorly to the respiratory epithelium of the larynx and trachea, impairing the mobility of the vocal cords and producing hoarseness. The subglottic region in children is surrounded by a narrow firm ring of cartilage. Only a small amount of swelling will restrict air flow and produce inspiratory stridor. Epiglottitis may have a similar onset, but there is more rapid progression to a toxic state. If a foreign body is causing the obstruction, there may be a history of choking at onset and little fever. Spasmodic croup is recurrent with less fever. See Table 1 for guidelines in differentiating these conditions.

Evaluation of the child should occur in a calm manner because anxiety may worsen the respiratory compromise. Assessment of tachypnea, tachycardia, and intercostal and substernal retractions is essential. Radiologic examination may be useful when the diagnosis is in question. The classic steeple sign produced by the narrowed air column in the subglottic area is seen in approximately 50% of patients. Direct visualization of the airway can be attempted if the

Table 1 Comparison of Crouplike Syndromes

	SPASMODIC CROUP	LARYNGOTRACHEO-BRONCHITIS	BACTERIAL TRACHEITIS	EPIGLOTTITIS
Age range	6 mo-3 yr	0-5 yr (peak, 1-2 yr)	1 mo-6 yr	2-6 yr
Etiology	? Viral ? Airway reactivity	Parainfluenza Influenza Adenovirus Respiratory syncytial virus	*Staphylococcus aureus* *Haemophilus influenzae*	*H. influenzae* Group A streptococcus *Moraxella catarrhalis*
Onset	Sudden	Insidious	Slow/sudden deterioration	Sudden
Clinical manifestations	Afebrile Nontoxic Barking cough Stridor Hoarse	Low-grade fever Nontoxic Barking cough Stridor Hoarse	High fever Toxic Barking cough Stridor Hoarse	High fever Toxic Nonbarking cough Muffled voice Drooling Dysphagia Sitting, leaning forward
Endoscopic findings	Pale mucosa Subglottic swelling	Deep-red mucosa Subglottic swelling	Deep-red mucosa Copious tracheal secretions	Cherry-red epiglottis Arytenoepiglottic swelling
Complete blood count, differential	Normal	Mild leukocytosis Lymphocytosis	Normal to mild leukocytosis; marked bandemia	Marked leukocytosis Bandemia
Radiographic findings	Subglottic narrowing	Subglottic narrowing	Subglottic narrowing Irregular tracheal border	Large epiglottis Thick arytenoepiglottic folds
Therapy	Mist Calm (occasionally) Racemic epinephrine (occasionally) Steroids	Mist Calm Racemic epinephrine ? Steroids Intubation (if necessary)	Intubation Antibiotics	Intubation Antibiotics
Response	Rapid	Transient	Slow (1-2 wk)	Rapid (40 hr)
Intubation	Rare	Occasional	Usual	Usual

From Chernck V, Boat TF: *Kendig's disorders of the respiratory tract in children,* ed 6, Philadelphia, 1998, WB Saunders.

symptoms are not typical and the child is stable. If intubation appears imminent or there is a strong suspicion of epiglottitis, this may be performed under anesthesia.

Management options include humidified air, humidified oxygen, analgesics, steroids, epinephrine, heliox, and intubation. No clear data exist on the benefits of mist or humidified air; therefore the use of mist tents, which separate children from their parents and impair the observation of the child's respiratory status, are discouraged. Cool mist at home or sitting in a steamy bathroom may loosen secretions. Analgesics improve sore throat and overall comfort.

Steroids have been shown to improve status in the hospitalized child and recently in the outpatient as well. Dexamethasone in doses of 0.15 to 0.6 mg/kg has been shown to be beneficial. Oral administration is effective and preferred in children who can swallow adequately. Optimal dosing schedules have yet to be defined. It is not clear whether patients with mild disease seen in the office will benefit from steroid therapy. Nebulized budesonide, 2 mg, has been shown to be as effective as dexamethasone. The combination of oral dexamethasone and nebulized budesonide is better than either alone and will probably be used more in the future.

The use of nebulized racemic epinephrine has markedly reduced the need for intubation, even in hospitalized patients, to less than 2%. After administration, improvement will occur quickly. Symptoms can recur within 2 hours; therefore patients must be observed in the emergency room for 3 hours. Heliox, a mixture of oxygen and helium, may help reduce the need for intubation in the severely ill child by improving laminar gas flow through an obstructed airway.

If intubation is deemed necessary, an endotracheal tube one to two sizes smaller than would be used for the same-size healthy child will be needed to prevent pressure necrosis and resulting subglottic stenosis. For those children who appear toxic, antibiotic therapy similar to that recommended for epiglottis should be considered to treat the possibility of a secondary bacterial process. Table 2 outlines therapy recommendations depending on the clinical state of the patient.

■ ACUTE SUPRAGLOTTITIS (EPIGLOTTITIS)

Supraglottitis is characterized by inflammation and edema of the supraglottic structures, including the epiglottis, arytenoepiglottic folds, arytenoids, and false vocal cords; paradoxically, the epiglottis may be spared.

In children, acute supraglottitis is typically characterized by a fulminating course of severe sore throat, high fever,

Table 2 Recommended Therapy for Croup (Laryngotracheitis)

CONDITION	TREATMENT
MILD	
No stridor	Analgesics
No distress	Hydration
	Cool mist or steamy bathroom
MILD-MODERATE	
Stridor at rest	Above plus oral dexamethasone,
No retraction	0.15-0.6 mg/kg
No distress	Observe in emergency room
MODERATE	
Stridor at rest	Above plus nebulized budesonide,
Retractions	2 mg, where available and/or
No significant	dexamethasone 0.15-0.6 mg/kg
respiratory distress	If no improvement, nebulized
	racemic epinephrine (0.5 ml
	of 2.25%)
	Observe in emergency room for
	at least 3 hr
SEVERE	
Significant respiratory	Nebulized racemic epinephrine
distress	(0.5 ml of 2.25%)
Decreased air	Oral or parenteral dexamethasone
movement	or prednisolone
	Consider heliox
	Intubation if necessary

Modified from Rosekrans J: *Mayo Clin Proc* 73:1102, 1998; and Klassen TP: *Pediatr Clin North Am* 44:249, 1997.

dysphagia, drooling, low-pitched inspiratory stridor, and airway obstruction, which, if left untreated, can lead to death. The child appears toxic and prefers an airway-preserving posture—sitting upright, jaw protruding forward, while drooling. In adults, the presentation is more variable; most adults have mild illness with a prolonged prodrome. In immunocompromised patients, there may be a paucity of physical findings.

Definitive diagnosis is made by examination of the epiglottis and supraglottic structures. No attempt should be made to visualize the epiglottis in an awake child; therefore a severely ill child must be examined in the operating room at the time of control of the airway. In children, the epiglottis is typically fiery red and extremely swollen, but occasionally the major inflammation involves the ventricular bands and arytenoepiglottic folds, and the epiglottis appears relatively normal. In adults, awake indirect laryngoscopy may be performed, but only when it is possible to establish an artificial airway. In adults, the supraglottic structures may appear pale with watery edema. If indirect laryngoscopy is unavailable, lateral neck radiographs are also useful for evaluating supraglottitis, but they are not as sensitive and should never delay protecting the airway.

The epidemiology of acute supraglottitis is changing dramatically since the introduction of the Hib vaccines in the mid to late 1980s. Supraglottitis, which most commonly had affected children 2 to 7 years of age, is becoming much rarer in young children, is now a disease of older children and adults, and is increasingly being caused by other microbial pathogens. The organisms typically involved, besides Hib, are *Streptococcus pneumoniae*, *Staphylococcus aureus*, beta-hemolytic streptococci, *H. influenzae* type non-b, *H. parainfluenzae*, and in adults, *Pasteurella multocida*. There are very rare reports of children developing Hib epiglottitis despite vaccination. The role respiratory tract viruses play as primary pathogens remains unclear. There have been reports of *Herpes simplex* type 1 and varicella as primary pathogens in immunocompromised hosts.

Therapy

Treatment of acute supraglottitis is directed at establishing an airway and administering appropriate antibiotics. Children with epiglottitis should routinely have an artificial airway established; observation cannot be routinely recommended because the mortality rate is 6% to 25% and increases to 30% to 80% for those that develop obstruction. Most deaths occur within the first hours after arrival. The use of a "prophylactic airway" has reduced the mortality rate to less than 1%. The management of the airway in adult supraglottitis reflects the greater variability of clinical presentation and course. It has a range of mortality rates from 10% to 32%. Vigilant airway monitoring and continuous staging are needed for adults whose disease may progress to respiratory compromise. A formal written "acute airway obstruction protocol" should be followed. Factors associated with airway obstruction include symptomatic respiratory difficulty, stridor, drooling, shorter duration of symptoms, enlarged epiglottitis on radiograph, and *H. influenzae* bacteremia.

An endotracheal tube is preferred over a tracheotomy for the following reasons: (1) ease of removal of the tube 2 to 3 days after the edema has subsided, thereby shortening the hospital stay; (2) no surgery; and (3) mortality and complication rates equal to or lower than those for tracheotomy.

Antibiotic therapy should include coverage for *H. influenzae*, *S. pneumoniae*, group A beta-hemolytic streptococci, other streptococci, *H. parainfluenzae*, and *S. aureus*. Second- and third-generation cephalosporins are first-line agents. Pediatric dosages are intravenous cefuroxime, 150 mg/kg divided in three doses per day; cefotaxime, 150 mg/kg divided in three doses per day; or ceftriaxone, 50 mg/kg/day. The recommended adult dosages are intravenous cefuroxime, 0.75 to 1.5 g given three times per day; ceftriaxone, 2 g/day; or cefotaxime, 2 g every 4 to 8 hours. Antibiotic therapy should be continued for 10 to 14 days.

Steroids are commonly used for supraglottitis to theoretically decrease inflammation. There has been no evidence for any significant benefit, and in adults, there is no indication that steroids prevent the need for airway intervention. With epiglottitis being so uncommon and therefore all studies being small, it will be difficult to evaluate any beneficial role. The use of steroids remains controversial.

Prevention

Prophylaxis is indicated for supraglottitis secondary to Hib. Rifampin, 20 mg/kg, not to exceed 600 mg/day, for four doses is recommended for (1) all household contacts (except pregnant women) when there is a child younger than 12 months irrespective of vaccine status or there is a child younger than 4 years of age with incomplete vaccination; (2) day-care and nursery school classroom contacts (including adults) if (a) two or more cases of invasive disease have occurred within 60 days and unvaccinated or incompletely vaccinated children attend or (b) with one case and susceptible children 2 years or younger who attend for 25 hours or more per week and susceptible children should be vaccinated; if children are older than 2 years, rifampin prophylaxis need not be given irrespective of vaccination status; and (3) the patient should receive prophylaxis before discharge if treated with ampicillin or chloramphenicol to prevent reintroduction of the organism into the household. Prophylaxis is not needed for those treated with the aforementioned recommended cephalosporins because they eradicate Hib from the nasopharynx.

Since the introduction of conjugated vaccines for infants beginning at 2 months of age, the incidence of supraglottitis resulting from Hib in this age group has declined by 95%, along with other invasive forms of Hib. There have been isolated rare reports of supraglottitis in children who have been vaccinated, but in general, we are seeing a near-eradication of Hib supraglottitis in young children. Supraglottitis caused by Hib occurs now in this country primarily in undervaccinated children, infants too young to have completed the primary series of vaccinations, and older children and adults who have never been immunized.

■ LARYNGITIS

The larynx rests in the hypopharynx and consists of (1) the supraglottic larynx, which includes the laryngeal inlet formed by the epiglottis anteriorly and the arytenoepiglottic folds bilaterally merging inferiorly into false cords, and (2) the glottic larynx, which consists of the true vocal cords.

Acute laryngitis often presents with hoarseness, odynophagia, and localized pain, which may also be referred and manifest as otalgia. Obstruction of the airway is uncommon in adults but more common in young children, especially if associated with tracheal inflammation as in croup, and must be distinguished from acute supraglottitis. Examination of the larynx reveals erythema, edema, secretions, and occasionally superficial mucosal ulcerations. The presence of exudate or membrane on the pharyngeal or laryngeal mucosa should raise the suspicion of streptococcal infection, mononucleosis, or diphtheria; granulomatous infiltration may be compatible with tuberculosis, sarcoidosis, fungal infection, or syphilis.

The respiratory viruses such as influenza virus, parainfluenza virus, rhinovirus, and adenovirus are most often isolated in cases of laryngitis (90%). *Moraxella catarrhalis* has been isolated from the nasopharynx of 50% to 55% and *H. influenzae* from 8% to 15% of adults with laryngitis. It remains unclear whether these may represent a secondary bacterial invasion. Group A and G streptococci, *Chlamydia pneumoniae*, and *Mycoplasma pneumoniae* have also been associated with acute laryngitis. Laryngeal diphtheria is very

rare and usually results from extension of pharyngeal involvement. It may occur in previously immunized persons.

Fungal infections such as histoplasmosis, coccidioidomycosis, blastomycosis, and cryptococcosis may cause laryngitis. Candidiasis is most often seen in immunosuppressed patients. *T. pallidum,* herpes simplex virus, and herpes zoster virus may also be a cause of acute laryngitis. Laryngeal tuberculosis is very rarely seen in the United States since the advent of effective antimycobacterial therapy. It is associated with a large tuberculous load, and patients often have very active pulmonary involvement. Sarcoidosis, Wegener's granulomatosis, and rhinoscleroma may be considered as a cause of laryngitis.

Therapy

Because most cases of acute laryngitis are viral in etiology and self-limited, treatment usually consists of resting the voice and inhaling moistened air. The role of empiric antibiotic therapy of laryngitis has been examined by prospective double-blinded studies. Penicillin V had no effect on the clinical course. Patients treated with erythromycin (0.5 g twice a day for 5 days) had a marked reduction of *M. catarrhalis* carriage in the nasopharynx and reported a significant improvement of subjective voice disturbances after 1 week and cough after 2 weeks; however, there was no difference in laryngological examination and voice evaluation. Because acute laryngitis in adults is self-limiting and subjective symptoms are spontaneously reduced after 1 week in most cases, empiric antibiotic treatment does not seem warranted as a general policy.

Antimicrobial therapy is indicated only in those patients with a bacterial infection or superinfection; therapy is directed toward the believed causative agent. Usual duration is for 10 to 14 days.

For treatment of laryngeal or pharyngeal diphtheria, see the chapter *Corynebacteria.*

Immunosuppressed patients who present with hoarseness or patients whose hoarseness has persisted longer than 10 to 14 days should have a laryngoscopic examination to exclude other more atypical causes such as herpes simplex virus, bacterial, fungal, mycobacterial, and malignant etiologies of laryngitis.

Suggested Reading

Frantz TD, Rasgon BM, Quesenberry CP: Acute epiglottis in adults. Analysis of 129 cases, *JAMA* 272:1358, 1994.

Klassen TP: Recent advances in the treatment of bronchiolitis and laryngitis in new frontiers in pediatric drug therapy, *Pediatr Clin North Am* 44:249, 1997.

Mayo-Smith MF, et al: Acute epiglottitis: an 18 year experience in Rhode Island, *Chest* 108:1640, 1995.

Rosekrans J: Viral croup: current diagnosis and management, *Mayo Clinic Proc* 73:1102, 1998.

Schalen L, et al: Erythromycin in acute laryngitis in adults, *Ann Otol Rhinol Laryngol* 102(3 pt 1):209, 1993.

ATYPICAL PNEUMONIA

Thomas M. File Jr.
James S. Tan

The term *atypical pneumonia* was first used more than 50 years ago to describe cases of pneumonia caused by an unknown agent(s) that appeared clinically different from pneumococcal pneumonia. It was initially characterized by constitutional symptoms, often with upper and lower respiratory tracts symptoms and signs, a protracted course with gradual resolution, the lack of typical findings of consolidation on chest radiograph, failure to isolate a pathogen on routine bacteriologic methods, and a lack of response to penicillin therapy. In the 1940s, an agent that was believed to be the principal cause was identified as *Mycoplasma pneumoniae*. Subsequently, other pathogens have been linked with atypical pneumonia because of similar clinical presentation, including a variety of respiratory viruses, *Chlamydia psittaci*, *Coxiella burnetti*, and more recently, *Chlamydia pneumoniae*. Less common etiologic agents associated with atypical pneumonia include *Francisella tularensis*, *Yersinia pestis* (plague), and the newly identified sin nombre virus (Hantavirus pulmonary syndrome), although these latter agents are often associated with a more acute clinical syndrome. In addition, although presently exceedingly rare, inhalation anthrax is included in part because of the concern for this pathogen as an agent of bioterrorism. Finally, pneumonia caused by *Legionella* species, albeit often more characteristic of "pyogenic" pneumonia, is also included because it is not isolated using routine microbiologic methods.

Although the original classification of atypical and typical pneumonia arose from the perception that the clinical presentation of patients was different, recent studies have shown there is excessive overlap of clinical manifestations. Thus the designation of "atypical pneumonia" is controversial, and many authorities have suggested that it be discontinued. However, the term remains popular among clinicians and investigators. Moreover, options for appropriate antimicrobial therapy for the most common causes are similar, which is considered justification by some to lump them together.

Mycoplasma pneumoniae, Chlamydia pneumoniae, and *Legionella pneumophila* are the most common causes of atypical pneumonia. The results of recent studies indicate they cause from 15% to as much as 50% (in selected outpatient populations) of cases of community-acquired pneumonia (CAP). Recently published guidelines for management of CAP acknowledge the significance of these three pathogens by suggesting the need for empiric therapy that is active against them. In a recent prospective study from Ohio, of 2776 patients hospitalized with CAP, these three pathogens ranked number 2, 3, and 4 of all etiologic organisms categorized as meeting criteria for "definite" diagnosis. The other causes of atypical pneumonia occur with much less frequency.

■ CLINICAL MANIFESTATIONS

Although the diagnosis of these specific pathogens is difficult to establish on clinical manifestations alone, there are several generalizations that may be helpful. See specific chapters for more detail.

Mycoplasma pneumoniae
M. pneumoniae is a common cause of respiratory infections that range from inapparent infection to upper respiratory infection (URI), tracheobronchitis, and pneumonia. It is estimated that only 3% to 10% of infected persons develop pneumonia.

M. pneumoniae infections are ubiquitous and can affect all age groups. Although previously perceived as a cause of CAP predominantly in young healthy patients, recent data suggest that the incidence of *M. pneumoniae* pneumonia increases with age, highlighting the importance of this pathogen in the elderly as well.

M. pneumoniae pneumonia is considered the classic atypical pneumonia. The onset is usually insidious, over several days to a week. Constitutional symptoms, including headache (usually worse with cough), malaise, myalgias, and sore throat, are commonly present. Cough typically is initially dry, may be paroxysmal and often worse at night, and may become productive of mucopurulent sputum. Sinus and ear pain occasionally are reported. The physical findings often are minimal, seemingly disproportional to the patient's complaints.

The course of *M. pneumoniae* pneumonia is usually mild and self-limiting. However, significant pulmonary complications may occur and include pleural effusion, pneumatocele, lung abscess, pneumothorax, bronchiectasis, chronic interstitial fibrosis, respiratory distress syndrome, and bronchiolitis obliterans. Extrapulmonary manifestations include rash, neurologic involvement (i.e., aseptic meningitis, meningoencephalitis, cerebral ataxia, Guillain-Barré syndrome, and transverse myelitis), hemolytic anemia, myopericarditis, polyarthritis, and pancreatitis.

Chlamydia pneumoniae
Pneumonia caused by *C. pneumoniae* may be sporadic or epidemic. *C. pneumoniae* infections are often acquired early in life. Reinfections or recrudescent processes, both referred to as *recurrent infection,* may occur throughout one's lifetime.

Infections often present initially with sore throat, hoarseness, and headache as important nonclassic pneumonic findings. A subacute course is common, and fever is low grade. Cough is prominent but unproductive and may last if not treated early and effectively for weeks or even months.

Legionella pneumophila
Legionellosis is primarily associated with two clinically distinct syndromes: Legionnaires' disease (LD), a potentially fatal form of pneumonia, and Pontiac fever, a self-limited, nonpneumonic illness. Many of the clinical features of Legionnaires' disease are more typical of pyogenic (bacterial) pneumonias than the previously described atypical pneumonia. However, as LD has become increasingly recognized, less severely ill patients are seen earlier in the course of disease and thus clinical manifestations of unusual severity

once considered distinctive of Legionnaires' disease are now known to be less specific. The onset is often acute, with high fever, myalgias, anorexia, and headache. Temperature often exceeds 104° F (40° C). Diarrhea, hyponatremia, elevated lactate dehydrogenase (LDH), and relative bradycardia may be present.

Other Causes of Atypical Pneumonia (*Coxiella burnetti* [Q Fever], Psittacosis, Tularemia, Hantavirus Pulmonary Syndrome, Plague, Inhalation Anthrax)

Several of the less common causes of the atypical pneumonia syndrome are transmitted from animals to humans. In such cases, epidemiologic clues may be very important; although specific clinical manifestations cannot be considered diagnostic of a particular etiology, there are general findings that are characteristic of these diseases (Table 1).

C. burnetti may be associated with exposure via any mammal, but most commonly cattle, goats, sheep, and pets, including cats and dogs. The mode of transmission is either aerosol or by tick bite; high concentrations of the organism can be found in birth products of infected animals. The acute disease is a self-limiting, flulike illness characterized by high fever, rigor, headache, myalgia, cough, and arthralgia. Pneumonia may be accompanied by granulomatous hepatitis. Radiologic findings include lobar or segmental alveolar opacities, which may be multiple. Other manifestations may include hemolytic anemia, endocarditis, pericarditis, pancreatitis, and epididymoorchitis.

Pneumonia caused by *C. psittaci* usually occurs after exposure to infected birds, which may be asymptomatic. Headache is often prominent. Clinical clues include pharyngeal erythema, splenomegaly, and a specific rash (Horder's spots—pink blanching maculopapular eruption resembling rose spots of typhoid fever), which are seen in a minority of cases.

Primary *Tularemic pneumonia* occurs after direct inhalation of infected aerosols and is most common in persons in high-risk occupations or avocations, such as laboratory workers, farmers, hunters or trappers, or meat handlers. The most important reservoirs and vectors are ticks, hares, and rabbits. The onset is usually abrupt, with high fever, chills, cough (usually nonproductive, occasionally with hemoptysis), pleuritic chest pain, and diaphoresis. Signs and symptoms may be mild and persist for several weeks, especially when occurring as a complication of ulceroglandular disease.

The clinical illness of *Hantavirus pulmonary syndrome (HPS)* typically begins with a prodromal phase, followed by a cardiopulmonary phase in patients with prior exposure to rodent excreta. The prodrome lasts from 3 to 6 days and is characterized by nonspecific manifestations such as fever

Table 1 Common Characteristics and Therapy for the Other Atypical Pneumonias

PATHOGEN	EPIDEMIOLOGIC OR UNDERLYING CONDITION	CLINICAL FEATURES	RECOMMENDED THERAPY
Chlamydia psittaci	Exposure to birds	Headache, myalgia prominent, liver involvement, Horder spots (see text), spleniomegaly	Tetracycline, doxycycline, macrolide
*Coxiella burnetii** (Q fever)	Exposure to farm animals (especially parturient) *and* pets (*especially cats and dogs*)	Headache prominent, liver involvement	Tetracycline, doxycycline, chloramphenicol
*Francisella tularensis** (Tularemia)	Exposure to rabbits	Headache, chest pain prominent; hilar adenopathy	Streptomycin; gentamicin for less serious cases; (alternatives are tetracycline, chloramphenicol, but relapses occur)
*Yersinia pestis** (Pneumonic plague)	Exposure to infected animals (rodents, cats, squirrels, chipmunks, prairie dogs)	For inhalation, acute onset with rapidly severe pneumonia; blood-tinged sputum	Streptomycin (alternatives: gentamicin, tetracycline, chloramphenicol)
*Bacillus anthracis**	Wood mill worker	Biphasic (see text); hallmark radiographic finding is mediastinal widening	Ciprofloxacin (penicillin G or doxycycline if susceptible)
Viruses			
Influenzae	Influenza in community	Influenza pneumonia usually follows tracheobronchitis	Amantadine (influenza A)† Rimantadine (influenza A)† Zanamavir and oseltamivir (influenza A and B)†
Adenovirus		Pharyngitis prominent	
Respiratory syncytial virus (RSV)	Adults: cardiopulmonary disease, chronic obstructive pulmonary disease	Bronchospasm	Ribavirin for selected neonatal/ infants; no recommendation currently available for adults
Hantavirus pulmonary syndrome	Exposure to rodent excreta	Febrile prodrome; followed by noncardiogenic pulmonary edema with shock; thrombocytopenia	Supportive care

*Potential infectious agent for biologic warfare.
†Benefit for primary influenza pneumonia is unknown.

myalgia, headache, nausea, vomiting, and cough. The cardiopulmonary phase starts suddenly with tachypnea and shortness of breath and is followed by respiratory failure and shock. Chest radiography shows noncardiogenic bilateral interstitial edema during this phase. Characteristically, the patient is hemoconcentrated and manifests significant thrombocytopenia.

Pneumonic plague and inhalation anthrax syndrome are of increasing recent interest because of concern as possible agents of bioterrorism. *Plague pneumonia* may occur after hematogenous spread during bacteremia of bubonic or septicemic plague, or after inhalation of bacteria after coming in contact with a person or animal (most often a cat) with plague pneumonia. Inhalation plague pneumonia is rapidly fatal and highly contagious. The disease may have an abrupt onset and usually begins with a painless cough with shortness of breath. Sputum is thin, watery, and blood tinged, and the Gram stain reveals typical *Y. pestis* (bipolar gram-negative bacilli). Untreated pneumonic plague has a 40% to 90% mortality rate. In the natural setting, *inhalation anthrax* is exceedingly uncommon and is classically referred to as *woolsorters disease* because of the association with workers in wool mills who may inhale *B. anthracis* spores. However, the potential use as a biologic weapon has brought increased interest to this pathogen, particularly because of the environmental stability of spores, small amount of inoculum necessary to produce fulminant infection, and high mortality rate.

Several recent reports have suggested respiratory syncytial virus (RSV) to be a more common cause of pneumonia in immunocompetent adults than previously appreciated. Characteristics include seasonal occurrence (winter) and association of bronchospasm.

■ DIAGNOSIS

Laboratory tests used for the diagnosis of the etiologic agents associated with atypical pneumonia are listed in Table 2). In general, there is a lack of rapid, accessible, and accurate diagnostic tests for the most common causes, *C. pneumoniae* and *M. pneumoniae*. Rapid diagnostic tests and accessible culture methods are available for *Legionella* but must be specifically requested from the clinical microbiology laboratory because they are not routinely performed. Hopefully newer tests such as DNA amplification tests (i.e., polymorphic chain reaction [PCR] might be available in the future to provide a cost-effective, rapid means of diagnosis. Serologic tests are less valuable given the requirement for measurement of acute and convalescent specimens (Table 2); however, this remains the most common means of laboratory diagnosis for *C. burnetti* and *C. psittaci*.

■ ANTIMICROBIAL THERAPY

Because most cases of atypical pneumonia are treated empirically, clinicians also need to consider the possibility of other "standard" pathogens (i.e., *S. pneumoniae*, *H. influenzae*) when deciding on antimicrobial therapy. More details of therapy for specific pathogens are provided in the relevant individual chapters.

Mycoplasma and *Chlamydia*

Therapy of *Mycoplasma* and *Chlamydia* has been the subject of some conjecture. A common view is that it really does not matter whether antibiotics are given for most of these infections because the mortality rate is low; however, data indicate that treatment (especially for *M. pneumoniae*) reduces the morbidity.

Erythromycin and tetracyclines have been the old standbys in the treatment of *M. pneumoniae* infections and have been considered effective therapy. The newer macrolides (clarithromycin and azithromycin) and the newer fluoroquinolones (levofloxacin and grepafloxacin) have been shown to be effective in early trials. The duration of doxycycline or erythromycin therapy for adults with *M. pneumoniae* pneumonia is 2 weeks, and 3 weeks if *C. pneumoniae* is suspected or documented. Shorter courses appear to be effective for the newer antimicrobials.

Legionella

There is little debate concerning the need for therapy of *Legionella* pneumonia. Delay in instituting appropriate antimicrobial therapy for *Legionella* pneumonia significantly increases mortality. Therefore empirical anti-*Legionella* therapy should be included in treatment of atypical pneumonia. Fluoroquinolones and the newer macrolides (especially azithromycin) show superior activity compared with erythromycin, which has been the standard of therapy. We prefer the newer fluoroquinolones (i.e., levofloxacin) because of greater activity in vitro against *S. pneumoniae* (including drug-resistant strains) and other common causes of atypical pneumonia that need to be considered for empirical therapy. Doxycycline has also been shown to be effective in limited, well-documented cases. Although LD can undoubtedly cause mild disease amenable to outpatient therapy, in reality, most documented cases are treated in the hospital with parenteral therapy initially.

Therapy for Other Pathogens Associated with Atypical Pneumonia (See Table 1)
C. psittaci

The tetracyclines generally are considered the drugs of choice, with the macrolides as appropriate alternatives. The newer fluoroquinolones are active in vitro and in animal models, but their efficacy for human infection is unknown.

C. burnetti

The tetracyclines and macrolides are both considered effective. Ciprofloxacin and rifampin have been used for Q fever endocarditis.

F. tularensis

The choice of therapy for pneumonic tularemia is streptomycin. Gentamicin can be used, but relapses are known to occur. Alternative agents include doxycycline or chloramphenicol, but experience is limited for pulmonary tularemia.

Hantavirus Pulmonary Syndrome

Treatment options are limited. The use of ribavirin has not been shown to be effective in cases to date; however, its use is still being evaluated. Optimal cardiopulmonary and fluid management is critical for appropriate management.

Table 2   Diagnostic Studies for Pathogens Associated with Atypical Pneumonia

PATHOGEN	RAPID TEST[a]	STANDARD CULTURE OR MICROBIOLOGIC TEST(S)	SEROLOGY, OTHER TESTS
Mycoplasma pneumoniae	PCR[b] [95]	Throat or NP swab [90] (requires 7-10 days for preliminary growth)	ELISA, CF[c] [75-80] (IgM may be present after 1 wk but can persist 2-12 mo) Diagnostic criteria: Definite: four-fold titer rise Possible: IgG ≥1:64 (CF) IgM ≥1:16 (ELISA) Cold agglutinin [50] (less than 50% specificity; takes several weeks to develop)
Chlamydia pneumoniae	PCR[b] [80-90]	Throat or NP swab[d] [50-90]	MIF[c] (IgM may take up to 4-6 wk to appear in primary infection) Diagnostic criteria: Definite: four-fold titer rise Possible: IgG ≥1:512 IgM ≥1:32
Legionella pneumophila	Urine antigen[e] [60] PCR,[b] DFA[f] [25-75]	Sputum, bronchoscopy [75-99] (selective media required, 2-6 days)	IFA[c] [40-75] Diagnostic criteria: Definite: four-fold titer rise Possible: IgG or IgM ≥1:512 (acute titer of 1:256 has positive predictive value of only 15%)
Chlamydia psittaci	PCR[b]	Usually not done (considered laboratory hazard)	CF (Presumptive IgG ≥1:32) MIF for IgM
Coxiella burnetii	PCR[b]	Usually not done (considered laboratory hazard)	ELISA, IFA, CF
Influenza	Antigen detection (EIA), DFA stain, PCR	Virus isolation	CF or HAI
Respiratory syncytial virus (RSV)	Antigen detection (EIA), DFA stain, PCR	Virus isolation	ELISA
Adenovirus	DFA stain, PCR	Virus isolation	ELISA or RIA
Francisella tularensis		Culture (selective media)	ELISA preferred passive hemagglutination
Yersinia pestis	Gram stain, morphology, gram-negative cocco-bacillus exhibiting bipolar staining ["safety pin"]	Culture	
Bacillus anthracis (Inhalation anthrax)		Culture (may be dismissed as Bacillus contaminant)	

PCR, Polymerase chain reaction; *NP,* nasopharyngeal; *ELISA,* enzyme-linked immunosorbent assay; *CF,* complement fixation; *MIF,* microimmunofluorescence; *DFA,* direct fluorescence Ab; *IFA,* indirect fluorescence Ab; *HAI,* hemagglutination inhibition; *RIA,* radioimmunoassay.
[a][] = sensitivity percentage of test.
[b]Available in selected laboratories; reagents are not FDA cleared.
[c]Paired sera generally required.
[d]Rarely done; requires specialized culture techniques.
[e]Only for *L. pneumophila* serogroup 1 (= 60%-70% of cases); can be positive for months.
[f]Primarily for *L. pneumophila* serogroup 1; some false-positive results with other species, technically demanding.

Y. pestis

Untreated plague pneumonia has a mortality up to 90%. Streptomycin is considered the drug of choice; alternatives include gentamicin, tetracycline, and chloramphenicol. Close contacts of patients with pneumonic plague should receive tetracycline (500 mg qid), doxycycline (100 mg bid), or streptomycin (20 mg/kg/day for 7 days for prophylaxis).

Inhalation Anthrax

The mortality rate without treatment is greater than 95%; the mortality rate remains greater than 80% if treatment is not initiated before the development of clinical symptoms. Penicillin intravenously at high dosages has historically been the preferred therapy, but reports of resistance have been published, so some authorities now recommend ciprofloxacin (500 mg bid) as the preferred empiric treatment before susceptibility tests, with doxycycline or penicillin as an alternative.

Influenza

Amantadine or rimantidine appear to reduce symptoms in patients with influenza A uncomplicated respiratory infections; their use for primary influenza A pneumonia is not well established. Zanamivir and oseltamivir are newly released neuraminidase inhibitors, which are active against influenza A and B and have resulted in reduced symptoms if initiated early.

RSV

Ribavirin administered via inhalation has been shown to have some beneficial effect for infants with RSV lower respiratory tract infections. Intravenous administration of immunoglobulin may have some benefit (either alone or in combination with ribavirin). The benefit of ribavirin therapy for healthy or immunocompromised adults has not been established.

Suggested Reading

Bartlett JG, et al: Community-acquired pneumonia in adults: guidelines for management, *Clin Infect Dis* 26:811, 1998.

Cunha BA (Guest Editor): Zoonotic pneumonias, *Semin Resp Infect* 12:1, 1997.

File TM Jr, Tan JS, Plouffe JF Jr: The role of atypical pathogens: *Mycoplasma pneumoniae*, *Chlamydia pneumoniae*, and *Legionella pneumophila* in respiratory infection, *Infect Dis Clin North Am* 12:569, 1998.

Hammerschlag MR: Community-acquired pneumonia due to atypical organisms in adults: diagnosis and treatment, *Infect Dis Clin Pract* 8:232, 1999.

Marston BJ, et al: Incidence of community-acquired pneumonia requiring hospitalization: results of a population-based active surveillance study in Ohio, *Arch Intern Med* 157:1709, 1997.

Tan JS: The other causes of "atypical" pneumonia, *Curr Opin Infect Dis* 12:121, 1999.

COMMUNITY-ACQUIRED PNEUMONIA

Rebecca Edge Martin
Joseph H. Bates

Community-acquired pneumonia is a significant cause of morbidity and mortality in the United States. An estimated 3 million episodes occur annually, and 500,000 require hospitalization. Mortality among those admitted to a hospital averages 14%. Making the diagnosis of pneumonia is usually not difficult; selecting appropriate therapy, however, can be challenging. The purpose of this chapter is to assist the clinician in the selection of antibiotic therapy for community-acquired pneumonia in immunocompetent patients who are not residents of chronic care facilities.

■ DIAGNOSIS AND TREATMENT

The diagnosis of pneumonia is suspected when one or more of the following clinical findings are present: cough, purulent sputum, dyspnea, pleuritic pain, fever, leukocytosis, chest auscultation findings consistent with pneumonia, or a new pulmonary infiltrate. Once the diagnosis is made, the physician must decide whether hospitalization is necessary. A number of risk factors predict a complicated course (Table 1). The PORT (Pneumonia Patient Outcomes Research Team) study provides clinicians a guideline for predicting which patients will have adverse outcomes. The study assigned patients to one of five risk categories. Risk was calculated by giving points to 19 variables based on age and comorbidities similar to those listed in Table 1.

The exact microbial cause of an episode of community-acquired pneumonia is rarely known when antibiotics are started. Accurate historical information, including occupation; travel; exposure to animals, birds, and insects; recent dental work; and history of alcohol or drug abuse, may suggest a cause. Anaerobic infection is suggested by foul-smelling sputum as well as a history of seizure disorder or alcoholism. Hantavirus pulmonary syndrome (HPS), which has now been reported in most areas of the United States, is usually associated with fever, myalgia, and subsequent pulmonary edema, hemoconcentration, thrombocytopenia, and leukocytosis. However, there are no unique clinical features of any pathogen that allow a specific identification by history alone. Human immunodeficiency virus (HIV) disease should be a diagnostic consideration in most patients hospitalized with community-acquired pneumonia, and HIV serology should be obtained (following informed consent) in areas where the rate of newly diagnosed HIV exceeds 1 case per 1000 discharges.

The laboratory studies set out in Table 2 are useful in the diagnosis and management of community-acquired pneumonia. The extent of the evaluation should depend on the degree of illness and response to therapy. Diagnostic studies are usually unnecessary for the patient who is to be treated on an outpatient basis. Many common diagnostic methods are expensive and technically difficult to perform. The value of the Gram stain and culture of expectorated sputum is controversial. The guidelines from the American Thoracic Society (ATS) and the Infectious Diseases Society of America (IDSA) differ on the value of sputum studies for the diagnosis of bacterial etiology of community-acquired pneumonia. The IDSA recommends Gram stain and culture of sputum for all patients hospitalized with community-acquired pneumonia. The sputum specimen should be grossly purulent, obtained by deep cough, and processed in less than 2 hours. Minimum criteria for a specimen suitable for culture are fewer than 10 squamous epithelial cells or more than 25 polymorphonuclear neutrophils (PMNs) per low-power field, and it is claimed that the yield is increased when the stain is examined by an expert. The IDSA guide-

Table 1 Predictors of a Complicated Course in Patients with Community-Acquired Pneumonia

Suspicion of high-risk cause (*Staphylococcus aureus*, gram-negative bacilli, aspiration, or postobstructive process)
Older than 50 years
Prior episode of pneumonia
Consolidation, multilobe involvement, or pleural effusion on chest radiograph
Abnormalities on physical examination:
    Temperature <95° F (35° C) or >104° F (40° C)
    Systolic or diastolic blood pressures <90 mm Hg or 60 mm Hg, respectively
    Respiratory rate ≥30 breaths/min
    Heart rate >125 beats/min
    Extrapulmonary areas of infection
Laboratory factors
    Abnormal renal function (BUN >30 mg/dl or serum creatinine >1.2 mg/dl)
    Sodium ≤130 mg/dl
    Glucose ≥250 mg/dl
    Hematocrit <30%
    WBC count <4000/mm^3 or >30,000/mm^3
    Metabolic acidosis (pH <7.35)
    Pao$_2$ <60 mm Hg breathing room air
Comorbid conditions
    Renal insufficiency
    Congestive heart failure
    Liver disease
    Diabetes mellitus
    Altered mental state
    Neurologic disease
    Alcoholism
    Immunosuppression
    Malignancy
    Splenectomy
No responsible person in the home to assist the patient

BUN, Blood urea nitrogen; *WBC,* white blood cell.

Table 2 Studies Useful in the Diagnosis and Management of Patients Hospitalized with Community-Acquired Pneumonia

Chest radiograph (posterior and lateral)
Arterial blood gas values
Complete blood count with differential
Chemistry panel, including electrolytes, glucose, blood urea nitrogen, and creatinine
Liver function
Blood culture (2 sets drawn 10 minutes or more apart)
Pleural fluid stain, culture, leukocyte count with differential, pH
Sputum studies (for pneumonia unresponsive to usual antibiotics):
    Acid-fast stain and culture
    Fungal stains and culture
    Immunofluorescent antibody, Gomori's methenamine silver, or Giemsa stain for *Pneumocystis carinii*
    Legionella direct fluorescent antibody
    A Gram stain (from an appropriately obtained specimen, examined by an expert within 2 hours of collection before the patient has received antibiotics) may be of value to some patients
Serology
    HIV serology in hospitals with more than 1 newly diagnosed case of HIV per 1000 discharges (after informed consent)
    Legionella species
    Francisella tularensis
    Mycoplasma pneumoniae
    Chlamydia (*pneumoniae* and *psittacosis*) species
    Coxiella burnetii
Urinary antigen for *Legionella*

HIV, Human immunodeficiency virus.

lines state that identifying the causative agent from any appropriately processed sputum allows for the selection of antimicrobials specific for the infecting organism. The ATS guidelines do not recommend sputum studies, claiming that organisms seen on Gram stain do not correlate with organisms grown in sputum culture. Timely and correct processing of sputum is a challenge in most clinical settings. Unfortunately, there are no properly done studies documenting the value or benefit of Gram stain and sputum culture.

Sputum studies can be diagnostic for disease caused by *Legionella* species, mycobacteria, fungi, influenza, respiratory syncytial virus, and *Pneumocystis carinii* (see Table 2). Some 10% to 15% of blood cultures performed on patients hospitalized with community-acquired pneumonia identify a causative organism. Bacteremia is associated with a more complicated course. A parapneumonic pleural effusion is a common complication of pneumonia, and cultures of the fluid will often give a positive result. The incidence of pleural effusion accompanying pneumonia depends on the etiologic agent. Effusions accompany *Streptococcus pyogenes* infections around 95% of the time but accompany only 10% of *S. pneumoniae* infections. Bronchial alveolar lavage may

be useful but should not be relied on to determine a bacterial agent. Protected brush specimens obtained by bronchoscopy are more accurate than expectorated sputum. The gold standards of transthoracic needle aspiration and open lung biopsy are definitive when an organism is found, but they place the patient at added risk. A fourfold rise in serologic titer may aid in diagnosis, but several weeks are usually required for an appropriate serologic response. Cross-reactivity among some organisms lessens the specificity of serology. A definitive microbial cause can be identified in only 50% of patients even after exhaustive investigation using many methods.

■ RECOMMENDATION FOR EMPIRIC SELECTION OF ANTIMICROBIAL AGENTS

Because a definitive pathogen usually will not have been identified when therapy for pneumonia must begin, empiric selection of antimicrobials is necessary, even when treatment will ultimately be based on cultures and sensitivity reports. Selection of appropriate antibiotics may be facilitated by categorizing patients according to age and severity of illness, taking into consideration any comorbidities and epidemiologic factors present. Some microbes cause disease in all ages and types of patients; others are common only in

Table 3   Guidelines for Empiric Antibiotic Therapy for Community-Acquired Pneumonia in Outpatients Younger Than 50 Years with No Comorbid Illness

COMMON PATHOGENS
Streptococcus pneumoniae
Mycoplasma pneumoniae
Chlamydia pneumoniae
Respiratory viruses

ANTIBIOTICS
Erythromycin, 500 mg PO qid, or
    azithromycin, 500 mg PO day 1, then 250 mg daily
    Clarithromycin, 250 mg PO bid
If macrolide intolerant:
    Levofloxacin, 250-500 mg/day PO
    Grepafloxacin, 400-600 mg/day PO
Doxycycline, 100 mg PO bid (only in young adults <40 years
    of age)

Table 4   Guidelines for Empiric Antibiotic Therapy for Community-Acquired Pneumonia in Patients Older Than 50 Years or with Comorbid Illness

COMMON PATHOGENS
Streptococcus pneumoniae
Legionella spp.

LESS COMMON PATHOGENS
Haemophilus influenzae
Moraxella catarrhalis
Other gram-negative bacilli
Respiratory viruses

ANTIBIOTICS
Fluoroquinolone as a single agent
    Levofloxacin, 250-500 mg/day
    Grepafloxacin, 400-600 mg/day
                            or
Macrolide
    Azithromycin, 500 mg PO day 1, then 250 mg daily
    Clarithromycin, 250 mg bid
                            and
Trimethoprim-sulfamethoxazole, 1 DS PO bid, or amoxicillin/
    clavulanate, 875/125 mg PO bid

Table 5   Guidelines for Empiric Antibiotic Therapy for Community-Acquired Pneumonia in Patients Requiring Hospitalization (Not Intensive Care)

COMMON PATHOGENS
Streptococcus pneumoniae
Legionella spp.
*Staphylococcus aureus**
Chlamydia pneumoniae
Other gram-negative bacilli
Respiratory viruses

LESS COMMON PATHOGENS
Haemophilus influenzae
Moraxella catarrhalis

ANTIBIOTICS
Azithromycin, 500 mg/day IV (change to PO when clinically
    improved and normal absorption)
Fluoroquinolone
    Levofloxacin, 250-500 mg/day IV (change to PO dosing
        recommendations when clinically improved and normal
        absorption)
                            with or without
Beta-lactam antibiotic:
    Cefuroxime, 0.75-1.5 g IV q8h
    Ceftriaxone, 1-2 g q24h
    Cefotaxime, 2 g q6h
    Ampicillin/sulbactam, 1.5-3 g IV q6h

*If *S. aureus* is a strong consideration, a beta-lactam with anti-staphyloccocal activity should be included.

patients with certain comorbidities. Tables 3 to 6 list these categories of patients along with common pathogens and appropriate antibiotic therapy.

Among previously healthy patients with mild pneumonia not requiring hospitalization (see Table 3), *Streptococcus pneumoniae* is a common bacterial pathogen, especially during influenza season. The atypical pneumonias (*Mycoplasma pneumoniae* and *Chlamydia pneumoniae*) are more common in this group of patients. Atypical pneumonia generally is benign, with systemic complaints often more prominent than respiratory ones. Fever, headache, and myalgia are common. Leukocytosis is rare, and chest infiltrates consist primarily of segmental lower lobe or hilar infiltrates. Although *M. pneumoniae* is more common among patients younger than 30 years of age, it is recognized with increasing frequency in older persons. *M. pneumoniae* is characterized

by a prominent cough, often occurs in slowly evolving epidemics, and can precipitate reactive airway disease, especially in children. *C. pneumoniae* is a common cause of mild, often biphasic illness. Upper respiratory symptoms and pharyngitis predominate initially with recovery, then pneumonia develops 2 or 3 weeks later. Reinfection is common. Macrolides, fluoroquinolones with enhanced activity against *S. pneumoniae,* and doxycycline are appropriate choices for treatment of outpatient, community-acquired pneumonia in patients younger than 40 years of age. Recent studies have shown increasing pneumococcal resistance to macrolides and fluoroquinolones, so in areas with high pneumococcal resistance, caution should be used.

Patients who are older than 50 years of age or have comorbid illnesses (see Table 4) are more likely to require hospitalization. Some can be managed as outpatients but will require frequent follow-up visits. Gram-negative organisms, such as *Moraxella catarrhalis* and *Haemophilus influenzae,* are more common in this group, particularly in persons who smoke or have chronic obstructive pulmonary disease. About 80% to 90% of *Moraxella* isolates are beta-lactamase producers, as are an increasing number of *H. influenzae* strains. Azithromycin and clarithromycin are effective against these more resistant bacteria, but either of these agents should be given together with another antibiotic active against gram-negative organisms, such as trimethoprim-sulfamethoxazole or amoxicillin/clavulanate. Fluoroquinolones may be useful as single agents; however, there are recent reports of growing resistance, especially in areas of high fluoroquinolone use and high penicillin resistance.

Table 6 Guidelines for Empiric Antibiotic Therapy for Severe Community-Acquired Pneumonia Requiring Admission to the Intensive Care Unit

COMMON PATHOGENS

*Streptococcus pneumoniae**
Legionella spp.
Haemophilus influenzae
Staphylococcus aureus
Chlamydia pneumoniae
Other gram-negative bacilli
Respiratory viruses

ANTIBIOTICS

Azithromycin,† 500 mg/day IV
or
Levofloxacin, 250-500 mg/day IV
and
Beta-lactam antibiotic:
  Cefuroxime, 0.75-1.5 g IV q8h
  Ceftriaxone, 1 g q24h
  Cefotaxime, 2 g q6h

*In areas where highly resistant *Streptococcus pneumoniae* (MIC ≥2 µg/ml) are isolated, fluoroquinolones with enhanced pneumococcal susceptibility (depending on the resistance pattern in the community) or vancomycin may be necessary in the initial regimen.
†If *Legionella* is strongly suspected, rifampin, 600 mg/day PO or IV, should be added.
Additional considerations:
a. Penicillin allergy (anaphylaxis)—a fluoroquinolone may be substituted for the beta-lactam and possibly combined with an aminoglycoside.
b. Structural diseases of the lung—piperacillin/tazobactam or imipenem or meropenem or a fluoroquinolone *and* an aminoglycoside.
c. Suspected aspiration—ampicillin/sulbactam or imipenem or meropenem or clindamycin with a fluoroquinolone.

Patients admitted to the hospital with pneumonia of moderate severity and unknown cause require empiric therapy to cover the organisms listed in Table 5. The incidence of *Legionella* in community-acquired pneumonia is as high as 23% in some studies, particularly those focusing on severe pneumonia. A macrolide or fluoroquinolone may be used as a single agent in cases in which the community resistance patterns do not suggest a high incidence of penicillin-resistant pneumococci and *Staphylococcus aureus* is not a suspected pathogen. A beta-lactam antibiotic may be added for broader coverage when that is desirable. When the etiologic agent and its sensitivity are known, the antibiotic regimen should be as narrow and as cost-effective as possible. Penicillin is the drug of choice for *S. pneumoniae* when the minimum inhibitory concentration (MIC) is less than 0.1 µg/ml.

The importance of subdividing hospital admissions for pneumonia into moderate and severe illness lies in the recognition of increased mortality in patients with severe pneumonia, especially during the first 7 days. Mortality ranges from 50% to 70% in some studies. Severe pneumonia manifests as hypoxia, tachypnea, multilobe involvement or consolidation, and signs of septic shock. These patients should be managed in an intensive care unit. Organisms listed in Table 6 may cause more severe disease, although the severity of the pneumonia and ultimate outcome is more a function of the immune response of the host. Antibiotic coverage should be expanded to include a third-generation cephalosporin, or when there is preexisting structural disease of the lung a carbepenem or piperacillin-tazobactam, in combination with a macrolide, should be used. When a highly resistant pneumococcus is isolated, a fluoroquinolone or vancomycin should be used, based on the susceptibility testing. Antistaphylococcal coverage would be included for severe pneumonia during influenza season or when a chest radiograph suggests *S. aureus* (i.e., pneumatoceles or necrotizing changes). Aminoglycosides are poor choices as single agents for gram-negative pneumonia because of the low concentration of drug found in lung tissue.

A few other organisms deserve special mention. Although rare in most of the United States, tularemic pneumonia should be considered in endemic areas among patients with exposure to wild mammals, especially rabbits, and exposure to ticks. Intravenous gentamicin should be given to a hospitalized patient when tularemic pneumonia is in the differential. *Coxiella burnetii* causes an atypical pneumonia often accompanied by hepatosplenomegaly. It is endemic in many hot, dry areas such as southern Texas. The most common reservoirs are sheep, goats, cattle, and ticks. Tetracycline or doxycycline is the recommended therapy. *Chlamydia psittaci* is another atypical pneumonia that should be considered in patients with exposure to infected birds, especially parrots. Splenomegaly in conjunction with an atypical pneumonia suggests psittacosis. Again, the drug of choice is tetracycline or doxycycline. *Mycobacterium tuberculosis* should be considered early in the differential diagnosis of pneumonia not responding to usual antibiotics. Endemic fungal infections, such as blastomycosis, histoplasmosis, cryptococcosis, and coccidioidomycosis may also present as a community-acquired pneumonia.

■ THERAPY

As a rule, antibiotic choices should not be altered during the first few days of therapy, unless there is marked deterioration or cultures indicate the need for a change. Usually 48 to 72 hours are required for significant clinical improvement. Fever usually lasts 2 to 4 days but may last longer, especially if bacteremia accompanies the pneumonia. The white blood cell count generally returns toward normal after 4 days, and blood cultures become negative 24 to 48 hours after treatment is begun. Duration of therapy should be individualized according to the infecting organism and overall health of the patient. Generally, treatment of bacterial pneumonia requires 7 to 10 days of antibiotics, whereas atypical pneumonia requires a longer period ranging up to 21 days. Because of its long tissue half-life, azithromycin may be given for a shorter duration. Patients with pneumonia caused by *S. pneumonia* should usually receive antibiotic therapy for 72 hours after the resolution of fever. Immunocompromised patients usually require 21 days of treatment. When the patient is hemodynamically stable and improving clinically, oral antimicrobials should be considered, assuming the patient has adequate absorption. It is not necessary that the patient be afebrile, but the fever curve should be trending down.

Resolution of abnormal radiographic findings usually lags behind clinical improvement. It is slower in elderly patients, smokers, and those with comorbidities or multi-lobe involvement. Multiple chest radiographs in the hospital are unnecessary except for intubated patients and those with clinical deterioration. Patients who are older than 40 years of age or are smokers should be followed until complete radiographic resolution of the infiltrate is demonstrated. Follow-up chest radiographs should be obtained between 7 to 12 weeks after completion of therapy. If abnormalities have not resolved or greatly improved, the possibility of an occult neoplasm should be raised.

There are a number of reasons for failure in the treatment of community-acquired pneumonia. The serum level of the chosen antibiotics may not be high enough. Correct dosage and route of administration should be reevaluated when the patient does not respond appropriately. Some antibiotics, such as the aminoglycosides, may not achieve high enough concentrations in the lung tissue. The etiologic agent may be resistant to the antibiotics, or less likely, the organism may develop resistance during therapy. An initial response followed by recurrent fever may be due to thrombophlebitis at the intravenous infusion site, an emerging empyema, or drug fever. In addition, lack of clinical improvement should raise the suspicion of a cause other than routine bacteria, such as viruses, mycobacteria, fungi, or parasites. Clinicians must always keep in mind the possibility of a noninfectious illness that mimics pneumonia, such as pulmonary infarction, carcinoma, pulmonary edema, atelectasis, sarcoidosis, hypersensitivity pneumonitis, and drug-induced pulmonary disease.

Suggested Reading

American Thoracic Society: Guideline for the initial management of adults with community-acquired pneumonia: diagnosis, assessment of severity, and initial antimicrobial therapy, *Am Rev Respir Dis* 148:1418, 1993.

Bartlett JG, Mundy L: Community-acquired pneumonia, *N Engl J Med* 333:1618, 1995.

Bates JH, et al: Microbial etiology of acute pneumonia in hospitalized patients, *Chest* 101:1005, 1992.

Fine MJ, et al: A prediction rule to identify low-risk patients with community-acquired pneumonia, *N Engl J Med* 336:243, 1997.

Infectious Diseases Society of America: Community-acquired pneumonia in adults: guidelines for management, *CID* 26:811, 1998.

Sanyal S, et al: Initial microbiologic studies did not affect outcome in adults hospitalized with community-acquired pneumonia, *Am J Respir Crit Care Med* 160:346, 1999.

NOSOCOMIAL PNEUMONIAS

Burke A. Cunha

Nosocomial pneumonia may be defined as a pneumonia that occurs 1 week or more after hospitalization. This is different from patients admitted with a community-acquired pneumonia, who worsen and are admitted to the intensive care unit within the first week of hospitalization. These patients should properly be regarded as having community-acquired pneumonia. When any patient in the hospital after 1 week develops pneumonia, this is termed *nosocomial pneumonia*. Most of these patients are on ventilators; therefore *nosocomial pneumonia* and *ventilator-associated pneumonia* (VAP) mean essentially the same thing.

The diagnosis of nosocomial pneumonia is more difficult than the therapy. In patients on ventilators, in the ICU/CCU, many develop fevers, leukocytosis with a shift to the left, and pulmonary infiltrates on chest radiographs. The majority of such patients do not have nosocomial pneumonia or VAP. A variety of noninfectious disorders produce a similar picture (i.e., congestive heart failure [CHF], atelectasis, pulmonary emboli/infarction, mucous plugs, adult respiratory distress syndrome [ARDS], pulmonary drug reactions, bronchogenic carcinoma, and connective tissue diseases such as systemic lupus erythematosus pneumonitis). If all patients with fever, leukocytosis, and infiltrates on chest radiograph are treated empirically for nosocomial pneumonia or VAP, then most patients will be treated unnecessarily, resulting in needless expenditure of precious health care resources, subjecting patients to potential adverse drug reactions, drug-drug interactions, bacterial/fungal suprainfections, and may predispose to the emergence of resistant organisms.

When clinically possible, every attempt should be made to arrive at a definitive diagnosis of nosocomial pneumonia, either by definitively diagnosing the condition mimicking nosocomial pneumonia or by using a protected bronchial brushing (PBB) technique. PBB may be carried out by obtaining a sample of respiratory secretion or by bronchoalveolar lavage (BAL). Cultures obtained by either technique are sent to the microbiology laboratory for semiquantitative colony counts. If the specimen obtained by PBB contains 10^3 cfu/ml or more, the patient is likely to have nosocomial pneumonia. Although false-positive results occur with this technique, it is nonetheless a good way to differentiate respiratory tract colonization from infection, if that distinction is not apparent microbiologically.

The respiratory tract is colonized quickly in patients who are intubated, especially in a CCU/ICU environment. The organisms that colonize in the respiratory tract are similar to those in the aquatic environment of the hospital (i.e., *Pseudomonas aeruginosa*, *Enterobacter*, *Citrobacter*, *Flavobacterium*, *Burkholderia cepacia* [*P. cepacia*], *Stenotrophomonas maltophilia* [*P. maltophilia*], and *Serratia*). After a week in the ICU/CCU, the respiratory tracts of all patients have become colonized with one or more of these organisms and less commonly with *Staphylococcus aureus*. Cultures obtained from respiratory secretions of intubated patients are rarely sterile and usually contain one or more of these organisms. It is important to appreciate that pathogens as well as nonpathogens are present in respiratory secretions as colonizers. Fortunately, many of the organisms listed virtually never cause nosocomial pneumonia (i.e., *B. cepacia*, *S. maltophilia, Enterobacter, Citrobacter,* and *Flavobacterium*). The recovery of these organisms from the culture of respiratory secretions may be summarily dismissed as colonization with no clinical relevance. The recovery of other organisms such as *Klebsiella, Acinetobacter, P. aeruginosa,* or *S. aureus,* although they are most often colonizers, cause concern because of their known pathogenic potential.

P. aeruginosa is the most virulent pathogen associated with nosocomial pneumonia/VAP, but it is rarely proved as a cause of nosocomial pneumonia. Most patients do not undergo sufficient diagnostic procedures to determine the etiologic organism responsible for their pneumonia. Statistically, *S. aureus* and *Acinetobacter* are rare causes of nosocomial pneumonia. *Acinetobacter,* although an ICU/CCU colonizer, is basically a cause of nosocomial pneumonia only in outbreak situations and rarely presents as a single case. *S. aureus* and *Pseudomonas* cause fulminant disease with rapid cavitation on the chest radiograph, profound hypoxemia with or without cyanosis, and usually with a fatal outcome. Patients without such a fulminant clinical presentation and appearance on chest radiograph, growing *P. aeruginosa* or *S. aureus* from their respiratory secretion cultures, almost never have pneumonia due to these organisms. Therefore the clinician can almost always dismiss these isolates as colonizers when the clinical presentation is at variance with the known clinical characteristics of the cultured respiratory organism. If *Pseudomonas* or *S. aureus* pneumonia is still strongly suspected despite its clinical unlikeliness, PBB should resolve the issue. Because *S. aureus* nosocomial pneumonia is uncommon, nosocomial pneumonia caused by methicillin-resistant strains (MRSA) is so rare as to be reportable, with no well-documented cases in the literature (Table 1).

■ EMPIRIC THERAPEUTIC APPROACH

The clinician should make every attempt to avoid treating noninfectious infiltrates mimicking nosocomial pneumonias. If noninfectious disorders can be ruled out, as they usually can with a high degree of clinical certainty, then empiric treatment of nosocomial pneumonia is not unreasonable. Coverage should be directed against *P. aeruginosa* whether or not it is the putative organism causing hospital-acquired pneumonia. By directing therapy against *P. aeruginosa,* all other nosocomial pneumonia pathogens (e.g., *Serratia, Klebsiella*) are also covered. As described previously, colonizing organisms should not be treated when recovered from respiratory tract secretions. Antistaphylococcal coverage does not need to be included in the regimen, although many drugs that have anti–*P. aeruginosa* activity have good antistaphylococcal activity. Certainly, coverage against

Table 1 Nosocomial Colonizers and Pathogens

SPUTUM COLONIZERS	RESPIRATORY PATHOGENS IN NOSOCOMIAL PNEUMONIAS
COMMON	**COMMON**
Pseudomonas aeruginosa	*Pseudomonas aeruginosa*
Non–*aeruginosa Pseudomonas**	*Klebsiella*
*Enterobacter**	*Serratia*
Stenotrophomonas maltophilia (*Pseudomonas maltophilia*)	*Escherichia coli*
Burkholderia cepacia (*Pseudomonas cepacia*)	
*Xanthomonas**	
Citrobacter	
Acinetobacter	
*Staphylococcus aureus** (MSSA/MRSA)	
UNCOMMON	**UNCOMMON**
Enterococcus	*Actinobacter**
Flavobacterium	*Legionella*
	Staphylococcus aureus (MSSA/not MRSA)

*Cause of nosocomial pneumonia usually in outbreak, not solitary cases.

MRSA should never be included, even if MRSA is isolated as it commonly is from respiratory secretion specimens.

Because *P. aeruginosa* is the most common pathogen when demonstrated in nosocomial pneumonias, the traditional approach has been to use double-drug therapy. It does not matter which two antipseudomonal drugs are used in combination in terms of outcome. Double-drug combinations with or without synergy have the same outcome in terms of clinical efficacy. Antipseudomonal antibiotics with low minimal inhibitory concentrations (MICs) perform no better than those with higher MICs as long as the isolate is susceptible to both antipseudomonal antibiotics. Antipseudomonal double-drug therapy emerged in the era when the antipseudomonal potency of drugs available (e.g., gentamicin, carbenicillin) was barely adequate. Currently, potent antipseudomonal drugs that permit the monotherapy of nosocomial pneumonia are available.

Monotherapy for nosocomial pneumonia using a well-chosen antibiotic produces the same clinical outcomes as pseudomonal drug combination. Double-drug combinations may have an advantage in leukopenic compromised hosts, but this is not the problem in a patient with hospital-acquired pneumonia. Monotherapy has several advantages over combination therapy. It is less likely to be associated with dosing errors, drug-drug interactions, and drug side effects, and most importantly, it is less expensive. It is a popular misconception that combination therapy will eliminate resistance potential from either antibiotic in the combination. This has been shown to be true only for antibiotic combinations that are no longer clinically used. For example, ceftazidime is known to be associated with the rapid emergence of *Pseudomonas* resistance. Combining ceftazidime with an aminoglycoside, aztreonam, a carbapenem, or

Table 2 Antimicrobial Therapy of Hospital-Acquired/
Nosocomial Pneumonia

MONOTHERAPY
Necessary features
    Antipseudomonal antibiotic
    Least cost to the hospital
    Few/no side effects
    Little/no resistance potential
    Preferred antimicrobials for monotherapy
      regimens
      Cefepime, 2 g IV q12h × 2 wk
      Meropenem, 1 g IV q8h × 2 wk
      Piperacillin/tazobactam, 4.5 g IV q8h
ANTIBIOTICS TO AVOID
Cost
Adverse side effects
Resistance potential
    Ciprofloxacin*
    Imipenem*
    Ceftazidime†
    Trovafloxacin‡

*Associated with seizures, resistance to *P. aeruginosa,* and increased MRSA prevalence.
†Associated with an increased MRSA prevalence.
‡Associated with significant neurologic, hematologic, gastrointestinal, and hepatic side effects.

Table 3 Nosocomial Pneumonia Outbreaks Caused
by Specific Respiratory Pathogens

ACINETOBACTER BAUMANII
Meropenem, 1 g IV q8h × 2 wk
    or
Piperacillin/tazobactam, 4.5 g IV q8h × 2 wk
    or
Cefipime, 2 g IV q12h ×2 wk
LEGIONELLA
Levofloxacin, 500 mg IV q24h × 4 wk
    or
Doxycycline, 200 mg IV q12h × 4 wk
PSEUDOMONAS AERUGINOSA
Meropenem, 1 g IV q8h × 2 wk
    or
Piperacillin/tazobactam, 4.5 g IV q8h ×2 wk
    or
Cefipime, 2 g IV q12h ×2 wk
MULTIRESISTANT *PSEUDOMONAS AERUGINOSA*
Polymyxin B, 5 mg/kg IV q12h × 2 wk

a quinolone does not reduce ceftazidime's resistance potential. Ceftazidime use is also associated with an increase in the prevalence of MRSA in units or institutions using ceftazidime in high volume.

To use monotherapy optimally, the clinician must not only choose a drug with high activity against *P. aeruginosa* but must also choose one that is cost-effective with minimal side effects and little or no resistance potential. Knowing what not to use is as important as knowing what to use, especially in the treatment of hospital-acquired pneumonias. On the basis of their resistance potential, the antibiotics that should be avoided in combination regimens or as monotherapy include ciprofloxacin, imipenem, and ceftazidime. There are no resistance problems with their class counterparts (i.e., meropenem or cefepime). Although staphylococcal activity is not necessary, these preferred antibiotics have good activity against methicillin-sensitive *S. aureus* strains (MSSA) but not against MRSA. As mentioned previously, MRSA coverage only rarely should be included in an antimicrobial regimen against *P. aeruginosa* (Table 2).

On the basis of lowest cost, fewer side effects, and lowest resistance potential, optimal monotherapy for nosocomial pneumonia is best achieved with cefepime or meropenem. Occasionally, nosocomial pneumonia will occur as outbreaks, and these are usually caused by *Acinetobacter, P. aeruginosa,* or *Legionella.* Treatment should be based on susceptibilities (Table 3).

In summary, properly selected monotherapy is the currently accepted standard treatment for hospital-acquired nosocomial/pneumonias. Therapy is usually continued for 2 weeks. Therapy should not be extended for patients with pulmonary infiltrates of undetermined etiology or in patients who are unable to be weaned off respirators. Patients unable to be weaned off respirators and those with persistent pulmonary infiltrates or low-grade fevers, with or without leukocytosis, invariably have a noninfectious or nonbacterial cause for these problems that cannot be corrected by a change in antimicrobial therapy or lengthening the duration of antimicrobial therapy. Causes or such problems should be looked for; for example, herpes simplex virus (HSV) pneumonia is a common cause of inability to wean patients off respirators, patients with low-grade fevers, and pulmonary infiltrates.

Suggested Reading

Collins T, Gerding DA: Aminoglycoside versus β-lactams in gram-negative pneumonia, *Am J Med* 84:1091, 1988.

Cunha BA: Antibiotic pharmacokinetic considerations in pulmonary infections, *Semin Respir Infect* 6:168, 1991.

Cunha BA: Antibiotic resistance, *Crit Care Clin* 14:309, 1998.

LaForce FM: Systemic antimicrobial therapy of nosocomial pneumonia: monotherapy versus combination therapy, *Eur J Clin Microbiol Infect Dis* 8:61, 1989.

Leibovici L, et al: Monotherapy versus β-lactam-aminoglycoside combination treatment for gram-negative bacteremia: a prospective, observational study, *Antimicrob Agents Chemother* 41:1127, 1997.

Lode HM, et al: Nosocomial pneumonia in the critical care unit, *Crit Care Clin* 14:119, 1998.

Rubenstein E, Lode H, Grassi C, Antibiotic Study Group: Ceftazidime monotherapy versus a combination of ceftriaxone and tobramycin in serious hospital-acquired infection, *Clin Infect Dis* 20:1217, 1995.

Schrank JH Jr, McCallister CK: Randomized comparison of cefepime and ceftazidime for treatment of hospitalized patients with gram-negative bacteremia, *Clin Infect Dis* 20:56, 1995.

Spencer RC: The bacterial etiology and resistance patterns in the EPIC study, *Eur J Clin Microbiol Infect Dis* 15:281, 1996.

ASPIRATION PNEUMONIA

C. Hewitt McCuller, Jr.

Aspiration is the introduction of a foreign object or substance into the lower respiratory tract. The objects or substances may be of various sizes and consistency, and this, along with other characteristics, will determine the type and severity of injury. Factors that may influence the effects of aspiration (especially liquid aspirations) include the volume and character of the aspirate (acidic versus inert), frequency of aspiration, presence or absence of solid or particulate matter, and the location of the patient at the time of the event. Several clinical syndromes have been grouped under the term *aspiration pneumonia,* which can lead to some confusion. These syndromes may be distinct, but often there is significant overlap because of aspiration of more than one substance.

■ PREDISPOSING FACTORS

Impairment of the normal swallowing mechanism or lower respiratory tract defenses (cough reflex, mucociliary clearance) can lead to aspiration and its complications. Dysphagia and other abnormalities of the actual swallowing process may result from various disorders. Conditions that lead to an altered level of consciousness increase the risk of aspiration, as can neuromuscular disease, gastrointestinal diseases, and certain mechanical factors (Table 1).

■ NONINFECTIOUS COMPLICATIONS

The severity of injury that occurs after gastric aspiration is directly related to the pH, volume, and particulate nature of the aspirate. An aspirate with a low pH (≤ 2.5) and large volume (≥ 0.4 ml/kg) containing large particles has the worst prognosis, but aspiration of gastric contents at a more alkaline pH (>5) can also cause severe pulmonary inflammation and dysfunction, especially if particulate matter is suspended in the fluid. Clinical indicators of a less favorable prognosis include the occurrence of shock, pulmonary infiltrates that include more than two lobes on a chest radiograph, the onset of adult respiratory distress syndrome (ARDS), or secondary infection.

Aspiration of gastric acid usually results in profound hypoxemia because of ventilation-perfusion mismatching and intrapulmonary shunt. Initially, this may result from closure of small airways and atelectasis resulting from loss of surfactant, which can be destroyed by acid or inactivated by plasma proteins. Pulmonary capillary leak and permeability edema also occur, worsening the shunt. Clinically, a dramatic picture that may include the presence of gastric contents in the oropharynx, wheezing, coughing, cyanosis,

Table 1   Risk Factors for Aspiration

ALTERED LEVEL OF CONSCIOUSNESS
General anesthesia
Narcotic and sedative drugs

ABNORMAL GLOTTIC CLOSURE
Anesthetic induction or postanesthetic recovery
Postextubation
Drug overdose and ethanol toxicity
Structural lesions of the central nervous system (CNS)
    (tumors, cerebrovascular accident, head trauma)
Metabolic encephalopathies (electrolyte imbalances, liver failure,
    uremia, sepsis)
Hypoxia and hypercapnia
CNS infections
Seizures

DECREASED GASTROESOPHAGEAL TONE
Alkaline gastric pH
Gastrointestinal tract dysmotility
Esophagitis (infectious, postradiation)

INCOMPETENT GASTROESOPHAGEAL JUNCTION
Hiatal hernia
Scleroderma
Esophageal motility disorders (achalasia, megaesophagus)
Tracheoesophageal fistula

ELEVATED INTRAGASTRIC PRESSURE OR VOLUME
Ascites
Gastrointestinal bleeding
Malignancy of gastrointestinal tract
Intestinal obstruction or ileus

NEUROMUSCULAR DISEASES
Guillain-Barré syndrome
Botulism
Muscular dystrophy
Parkinson's disease
Polymyositis
Amyotrophic lateral sclerosis
Multiple sclerosis
Myesthenia gravis
Poliomyelitis

MECHANICAL FACTORS
Nasogastric or enteral feeding tubes
Upper endoscopy
Emergency and routine airway manipulation
Surgery to the neck and pharynx
Trauma to the neck and pharynx
Tumors of the upper airway
Tracheostomy
Endotracheal tube

OTHER FACTORS
Diabetes (functional gastric outlet obstruction)
Obesity
Pregnancy
Lack of molar teeth (young children)

fever, hypoxemia, and sometimes shock usually accompanies these changes. Patients may then progress in one of three ways: (1) prompt recovery (usually within 1 week), (2) rapid death from respiratory failure, or (3) initial improvement within 1 week followed by worsening and development of ARDS or secondary bacterial infection.

In addition to the acute effects of gastric and/or oropharyngeal aspiration, chronic long-term effects can occur.

Acute recurrent or chronic pneumonitis may be seen with esophageal disease. Granulomatous interstitial pneumonitis may be related to chronic inhalation of particulate matter. Chronic aspiration can cause interstitial lung disease resembling idiopathic pulmonary fibrosis. Bronchial hyperreactivity can be caused by gastric acid regurgitation, even in the absence of true aspiration. Chronic respiratory symptoms such as cough, dyspnea, or hemoptysis may be associated with aspiration. Chronic bronchitis, with or without chronic air flow obstruction, may be linked to chronic aspiration.

■ INFECTIOUS COMPLICATIONS

Infectious complications of aspiration syndromes may present as either an acute or chronic process. This may include acute pneumonitis, necrotizing pneumonia, lung abscess, bronchiectasis, and empyema.

Acutely, aspiration pneumonia may be a primary event, with clinical manifestations noted within the first 24 to 48 hours. Although primary pneumonia is noted in only 23% to 30% of all cases of aspiration, its occurrence is associated with increased morbidity and mortality rates. The onset of aspiration pneumonia is often heralded by fever, leukocytosis, and development of pulmonary infiltrates; unfortunately, these findings may also arise in noninfectious aspiration pneumonitis. Many patients show initial improvement after aspiration, only to develop pneumonia 2 to 7 days later. These secondary pneumonias result from obstruction or inflammation in the lower respiratory tract that impairs the patient's host defenses. The risk of secondary infection is also increased by mechanical ventilation, hospitalization for more than 5 days, or the use of H_2 blockers.

Aspiration pneumonia can also present as a chronic indolent infection. In this setting, a lung abscess or empyema may have developed. This presentation is more likely to occur in patients with specific risk factors, including swallowing dysfunction, gastroesophageal reflux, poor dentition, alcoholism, and seizure activity. Lung abscess, with or without pleural involvement, may commonly present with fever and nonspecific findings, typically of 3 weeks' duration or more. The chest radiograph often reveals a rounded area of consolidation with or without an air-fluid level, but it may occasionally reveal patchy infiltrates, interstitial changes, or pleural effusion.

Aspiration pneumonia is often polymicrobial, reflecting the variety of pathogens in the oropharynx. The site in which aspiration occurred (community, hospital, nursing home), recent exposure to antibiotics, and the presence of dental caries or gingival disease modify the oropharyngeal flora and the causative pathogens of aspiration pneumonia. In aspiration in the community setting, the most common pathogens are the aerobes *Staphylococcus aureus* and *Streptococcus pneumoniae* and anaerobic organisms such as *Bacteroides* species, *Peptostreptococcus* species, *Fusobacterium nucleatum,* and *Prevotella* species. Although the same spectrum of anaerobic organisms is commonly seen in aspiration pneumonia occurring in the hospital, the spectrum of aerobic pathogens differs, especially if the patient has been hospitalized for more than 4 days, has received prior antibiotics, or is receiving mechanical ventilation. *S. aureus* (which

may be methicillin resistant), enteric gram-negative bacilli (i.e., *Escherichia coli, Klebsiella* species, *Proteus* species), and *Pseudomonas aeruginosa* are commonly isolated in this setting.

Several recent studies have questioned the role of anaerobic organisms as primary pathogens in pneumonia following aspiration. These studies used specific sampling of lower respiratory tract secretions to define the microbial flora of aspiration pneumonia. Their findings indicate that aerobic gram-negative, as well as certain gram-positive organisms, may have greater importance as primary pathogens in this setting. Consequently, anaerobic coverage may not necessarily be required as first-line therapy. The validity of these studies is not established at this time, though, and no broad changes in the therapy of aspiration pneumonia should be based on these findings.

■ TREATMENT

In patients with substantial gastric aspiration, initial therapy involves establishing and maintaining sufficient oxygenation. Patients usually require intubation and mechanical ventilation with the application of positive end-expiratory pressure (PEEP) because of aspiration pneumonitis with resulting noncardiogenic pulmonary edema and intrapulmonary shunt. In severe cases, bronchoscopy may be helpful if there is particulate matter blocking the airway, but large-volume lavage is of little help in minimizing the effects of gastric acid because the acid is dispersed and neutralized very rapidly. Close attention should be given to fluid and electrolyte balance because large amounts of intravascular volume can be lost in the formation of pulmonary edema.

Studies in animals and humans have shown conflicting results regarding the benefit of corticosteroids given either before aspiration or after aspiration has occurred. Corticosteroids predispose patients to infection and can cause fluid and electrolyte imbalance. Considering the unconfirmed benefit and potential risks of corticosteroids in this clinical setting, their use is not recommended either parenterally or via the airway in the treatment of aspiration pneumonia.

The routine use of prophylactic antibiotics following a witnessed aspiration is not recommended because of the possibility of selecting for antibiotic-resistant organisms. Unfortunately, the clinical manifestations of secondary bacterial infection can be confused with those of chemical injury to the lung tissue. After all aspiration events, the patient should be observed closely. If clinical evidence compatible with pneumonia (i.e., new infiltrate, fever, leukocytosis) is noted, empiric antibiotics, based on the most probable spectrum of pathogens, should be initiated for 24 to 48 hours and the patient closely observed. Antibiotics should be discontinued if improvement is noted in less than 24 to 48 hours. Clinical worsening should prompt broadening of antibiotic coverage, with strong consideration given to obtaining respiratory secretions by bronchoscopy or tracheal suctioning for microbiologic evaluation.

Choice of antimicrobial agents is affected by the possible spectrum of pathogens and the probability of antibiotic-resistant organisms (Table 2). With aspiration pneumonia occurring in the community setting, high-dose penicillin

Table 2   Treatment of Aspiration Pneumonia

PRIMARY/STANDARD	COMMENTS
COMMUNITY-ACQUIRED	
Penicillin G	
Clindamycin	Lower failure rates; more rapid reduction of purulent sputum
Metronidazole	Combine with penicillin (PCN) to cover anaerobic and microaeroophilic streptococci
Alternatives	
Imipenem	May afford better coverage if mixed flora (especially anaerobes with aerobic gram-negative organisms) suspected
Chloramphenicol	
Beta-lactam with beta-lactamase inhibitor (ampicillin-sulbactam, ticarcillin-clavulanate, piperacillin-tazobactam)	
HOSPITAL-ACQUIRED	
Imipenem	Base on most common bacterial pathogens and antimicrobial resistance patterns; initial therapy should be aimed at antibiotic-resistant gram-negative bacteria (*P. aeruginosa, Acinetobacter* species) and methicillin-resistant *Staphylococcus aureus*
Meropenem	
Fourth-generation cephalosporins (cefepime)	
Beta-lactam with beta-lactamase inhibitor	
Fluoroquinolone combined with another antibiotic (clindamycin, cephalosporins, beta-lactam with beta-lactamase inhibitor)	
Imipenem plus amikacin plus vancomycin	May be most effective regimen for patients at high risk of developing pneumonia (especially ventilator-associated pneumonia) caused by resistant bacteria

has conventionally been the drug of choice, but the presence of penicillin-resistant organisms, such as *Bacteroides* species and possibly *S. pneumoniae,* has resulted in the increased use of other agents. Clindamycin has been reported to be more effective in resolving fever and sputum production when compared with penicillin, and it may have a lower failure rate. Metranidazole has been used for various anaerobic infections, but because of the relative insensitivity of microaeroophilic streptococci to this drug, it may need to be combined with penicillin. Alternative treatments include imipenem-cilastatin, chloramphenicol, or a beta-lactam antibiotic combined with a beta-lactamase inhibitor. Aspiration in the hospital setting is more likely to involve gram-negative bacilli or *S. aureus,* as well as anaerobic organisms. In the past, empiric antibiotic therapy has often included the use of third-generation cephalosporins. With the growing emergence of resistant organisms, however, other therapies (e.g., imipenem, piperacillin-tazobactam , or fluoroquinolones combined with clindamycin or other agents) are increasingly being used.

Lung abscesses usually require a prolonged course of antibiotics, often for weeks to months. When this is ineffec-tive, as can occur in up to 10% of patients, percutaneous drainage or lobectomy may be needed. Empyemas typically call for either drainage through closed thoracostomy tubes or open surgical drainage, with or without decortication. The availability of video-assisted thoracoscopic surgery (VATS) has now made earlier surgical intervention, with drainage and directed placement of chest tubes, more feasible.

■ PREVENTION

Small-volume liquid aspiration may be prevented by elevation of the head of the bed to 35 to 40 degrees in patients with swallowing disorders or gastroesophageal reflux who are at particularly high risk for aspiration. Correction of reversible risk factors such as treatment of seizures, careful titration of pain medications and sedation, prudent use of nasoenteric tubes, and careful monitoring of gastric volumes with nasoenteric feedings should reduce the risk of aspiration. Small-bore nasoenteric tubes have been considered to be preferable to larger tubes because of the risk of lower esophageal sphincter incompetence with large-bore tubes. However, recent studies have shown that small-caliber nasoenteric tubes may offer no added protection against aspiration, especially in intubated patients. In patients requiring long-term feeding, surgical interventions such as gastrostomy or enterostomy, possibly combined with an antireflux procedure such as a Nissen fundiplication, should be considered; however, many patients may continue to have problems with aspiration after simple gastrostomy. Feeding tubes placed distal to the ligament of Treitz may offer better protection against reflux and aspiration.

Prevention may have its greatest role in massive gastric aspiration, in which case supportive care has not influenced overall outcome. Thought should be given to defining patients at risk because of underlying conditions and attempts made to modify any correctable risk factors. Other factors to be considered are the volume, pH, and the presence of particulate matter in the gastric contents. Patients undergoing surgery are at a significant risk, particularly at the time of anesthetic induction, especially for emergency procedures. Fasting for approximately 8 to 12 hours before surgery may decrease gastric volume and the amount of particulate matter and increase gastric pH. Many fasting patients, however, still have gastric volumes greater than 25 ml as well as a pH of 2.5 or less in gastric secretions. Preoperative therapy with antacids may raise gastric pH, but this advantage may be offset by the increase of gastric volume from the antacids. H_2 antagonists such as cimetidine and ranitidine raise gastric pH and reduce gastric volume. Metaclopramide and cisapride, agents that increase gastric motility and emptying, could be added to further decrease gastric volume and increase gastric pH, although it is still unclear whether this offers any real advantage. At the time of intubation, rapid sequence induction of anesthesia will shorten the period between loss of consciousness and tracheal intubation. The application of cricoid pressure (Sellick's maneuver) during intubation may decrease the risk of aspiration. Premature postoperative extubation should be avoided because of the protracted laryngeal incompetence that occurs after anesthesia. Obtunded patients at risk for large-volume aspiration should be closely observed and placed in the head-down lateral position to reduce the volume of material aspirated in the event that aspiration occurs.

Intractable aspiration that continues despite standard therapy may require surgical intervention to separate the tracheobronchial tree from the alimentary tract. Tracheostomy can cause swallowing problems and may not completely prevent aspiration, but large-volume aspiration will be averted. Other surgical procedures include vocal cord medialization for unilateral vocal cord paralysis or fixation, antiaspiration stents for immediate and short-term relief of reversible causes of aspiration, laryngotracheal separation or diversion techniques for chronic aspirators with potential for recovery, and in rare instances, laryngectomy for permanent and severe aspirators.

Suggested Reading

Bartlett JG: Anaerobic infections of the lung and pleural space, *Clin Infect Dis* 16(suppl 4):S248, 1993.

DePaso WJ: Aspiration pneumonia, *Clin Chest Med* 12:269, 1991.

Lee-Chiong TL Jr: Pulmonary aspiration, *Comp Ther* 23:371, 1997.

Tietjen PA, Kaner RJ, Quinn CE: Aspiration emergencies, *Clin Chest Med* 15:117, 1994.

LUNG ABSCESS

Lisa L. Dever
Waldemar G. Johanson, Jr.

Lung abscess is a chronic or subacute lung infection initiated by the aspiration of contaminated oropharyngeal secretions. The result is an indolent, necrotizing infection in a segmental distribution limited by the pleura. Except for infections with unusual organisms such as *Actinomyces*, the process does not cross interlobar fissures, and pleural effusion is uncommon. The resultant cavity is usually solitary, with a thick, fibrous reaction at its periphery. So defined, lung abscess is almost always associated with anaerobic bacteria, although aerobic bacteria may be present as well.

In contrast, necrotizing pneumonia is an acute, often fulminant, infection characterized by irregular destruction of alveolar walls and therefore multiple cavities. This infection spreads rapidly through lung tissue, frequently crossing interlobar fissures, and is often associated with pleural effusion and empyema. The duration of illness before recognition is usually only a few days. Causative organisms include *Staphylococcus aureus*, *Streptococcus pyogenes*, *Klebsiella pneumoniae*, *Pseudomonas aeruginosa*, and less commonly, other gram-negative bacilli, *Legionella* species, *Nocardia* species, and fungi.

The focus of this discussion will be the diagnosis and therapy of anaerobic lung abscess. Diagnosis can usually be made from the clinical presentation and chest radiograph findings. Many patients have conditions such as seizure disorders, neuromuscular diseases, or alcoholism that predispose them to aspiration of oropharyngeal secretions. Gingival disease and poor dental hygiene, which promote higher concentrations of anaerobic organisms in the mouth, are common. Patients usually give a several-week history of fever and cough; putrid sputum occurs in less than 50% of patients. With chronic infection, patients will often experience weight loss and anemia, mimicking malignancy. Chest radiographs show consolidation in a segmental or lobar distribution with central cavitation. Air-fluid levels may be present. The lung segments most commonly involved are those that are dependent when the person is supine (i.e., posterior segments of the upper lobes and superior segments of the lower lobes). Aspiration and resulting lung abscess are uncommonly found in anterior lung segments because of the up-hill angulation of the trachea when the subject lies prone.

The etiologic diagnosis of lung abscess is hampered by contamination of specimens by the normal anaerobic flora of the mouth. Although the Gram stain of sputum may be helpful in suggesting an etiologic diagnosis, routine sputum cultures are of no value because all contain anaerobic organisms. Techniques used to obtain uncontaminated lower-airway specimens for anaerobic cultures include transtracheal needle aspiration, transthoracic needle aspiration, and open lung biopsy. Using these techniques, early investigators demonstrated anaerobic bacteria in virtually all untreated patients. These invasive techniques are seldom warranted in the clinical management of patients today. More recently, investigators have used quantitative cultures of bronchoalveolar lavage or other bronchoscopically obtained lower-airway specimens, such as those obtained with a protected specimen brush, to recover anaerobic organism. Although these methods may prove useful in the occasional patient suspected of having lung abscess, they are not needed in most. The expanding applications of needle aspiration guided by either ultrasound or computed tomography (CT) into all body organs should be used with caution in the case of lung abscess. Pneumothorax requiring chest tube placement occurs in 10% to 20% of cases; bacterial contamination of the pleural space, although uncommon, is a serious complication that greatly prolongs the recovery period.

Anaerobic organisms most commonly recovered from lung abscesses are listed in Table 1. Multiple anaerobic organisms are commonly present along with aerobic or microaerophilic organisms. One recent report emphasized the role of viridans streptococci, particularly the *S. milleri* group, as potential pathogens causing lung abscess and

Table 1 Anaerobes Most Commonly Isolated in Lung Abscess

ORGANISM
GRAM-NEGATIVE BACILLI
Pigmented *Prevotella* spp.
Pigmented *Porphyromonas* spp.
Nonpigmented *Prevotella* spp.
Bacteroides fragilis group
Fusobacterium nucleatum
Fusobacterium spp.
GRAM-POSITIVE COCCI
Peptostreptoccus spp.
Peptococcus spp.
GRAM-POSITIVE BACILLI
Clostridium perfringens
Clostridium spp.
Propionibacterium acnes
Actinomyces spp.

Table 2 Intravenous Antibiotic Therapy of Anaerobic Lung Abscess

ANTIBIOTIC	INTRAVENOUS DOSAGE*	FREQUENCY
RECOMMENDED REGIMENS		
Penicillin G	2-3 million U	q4h
Clindamycin	900 mg	q8h
Penicillin G plus	2-3 million U	q4h
metronidazole	500 mg	q6h
ALTERNATIVE REGIMENS†		
Chloramphenicol	500 mg	q6h
Cefoxitin	2 g	q6h
Cefotetan	2 g	q12h
Piperacillin	3 g	q6h
Ticarcillin	3 g	q6h
Imipenem	500 mg	q6h
Meropenem	1 g	q8h
Ampicillin/sulbactam	3 g	q6h
Piperacillin/ tazobactam	3.375 g	q6h
Ticarcillin/ clavulanate	3.1 g	q6h

*All dosages are for adults with normal renal function.
†These regimens have not been validated by clinical trials.

empyema. When anaerobic organisms are recovered, in vitro susceptibility testing is seldom warranted.

■ THERAPY

Most lung abscesses are treated empirically. Table 2 provides therapeutic options for intravenous treatment of lung abscess. Traditionally, penicillin has been the antibiotic of choice. Penicillin has good in vitro activity against most anaerobic and microaerophilic bacteria present in the oral cavity. Early studies showed excellent responses when either parenteral or oral penicillin was used as a single agent in the treatment of anaerobic lung infections. Two randomized clinical trials found that clindamycin is superior to penicillin. In both of these studies, the time to resolution of symptoms and the failure rate were significantly lower in clindamycin-treated patients. Failure of penicillin therapy was associated with the isolation of penicillin-resistant *Bacteroides* species in one of these studies. Other evidence suggests that penicillin resistance is increasing among oral gram-negative anaerobes, primarily because of production of beta-lactamases. For these reasons, it is recommended that clindamycin rather than penicillin be used, at least initially, in the treatment of lung abscess.

The combination of metronidazole and penicillin has been used with success for the treatment of anaerobic pulmonary infections. Metronidazole has excellent bactericidal activity against virtually all anaerobes but lacks activity against microaerophilic and aerobic streptococci, as well as *Actinomyces* species, and therefore should not be used as a single agent in the treatment of lung abscess.

A number of other agents have good in vitro activity against anaerobic organisms, including beta-lactamase producers, and may be effective for the treatment of lung abscess. These agents include second-generation cephalosporins, carbapenems, antipseudomonal penicillins, and beta-lactam–beta-lactamase inhibitor combination drugs. In addition, these drugs are attractive because of their activity against many of the aerobes that may be present in

mixed infections. Chloramphenicol has excellent in vitro activity against almost all clinically significant anaerobes, but the potential for hematologic toxicity limits its usefulness. Drugs that have essentially no anaerobic activity should not be used in the treatment of lung abscess; such agents include aminoglycosides, fluoroquinolones other than trovafloxacin, and aztreonam. Although a number of newer antimicrobials have a suitable spectrum of activity in vitro, it is unlikely that any of them will ever prove to be more efficacious than current therapy in prospective clinical trials because of difficulties inherent in conducting trials in this condition. Because no single institution sees large numbers of patients with lung abscess, it is difficult to isolate anaerobic organisms from uncontaminated respiratory specimens for accurate diagnosis and susceptibility testing, and the patients' response to treatment varies widely but is often slow, which can lead to the erroneous conclusion of treatment failure if that decision is made too early.

Duration of Therapy

The duration of therapy for lung abscesses must be individualized, but extended therapy is usually required. Parenteral therapy is recommended initially in seriously ill patients and should be continued until the patient is afebrile and clinically improving. A prolonged course of oral antibiotics follows initial parenteral therapy. Less severely ill patients can be treated effectively with oral antibiotics alone. Options for oral therapy are provided in Table 3. Therapy should be continued until there is complete resolution or at least stabilization of chest radiograph lesions—this may require 8 weeks or more of therapy. Relapses have been reported when therapy has been discontinued before resolution of chest radiograph findings, even when patients are clinically asymptomatic.

Table 3 Oral Antibiotic Therapy of Anaerobic Lung Abscess

ANTIBIOTIC	DOSAGE*	FREQUENCY
Penicillin G	750 mg	qid
Clindamycin	300 mg	qid
Penicillin G plus	750 mg	qid
metronidazole	500 mg	qid
Amoxicillin/clavulanate	875 mg	bid

*All dosages are for adults with normal renal function.

Other Therapy

As with all abscesses, the patient with lung abscess will not improve until drainage has been accomplished. Ideally, drainage is effected via the tracheobronchial tree. Postural drainage may be a useful adjunct. Bronchoscopy should be performed in patients who have unchanged air-fluid levels (or increasing levels) and who remain septic after 3 to 4 days of antibiotic therapy. Bronchoscopy rarely results in direct drainage of the abscess cavity; rather, drainage occurs over hours to days after suctioning of secretions and manipulation of the involved bronchopulmonary segments. The presence of a large abscess cavity (>6 to 8 cm diameter) requires special consideration. Some authorities prefer to drain such abscesses surgically because of the fear of an unplanned and uncontrolled sudden evacuation of the abscess contents into the bronchial tree with resultant asphyxiation. Another approach is to use a rigid bronchoscope to examine and open the involved airways because of the greater capacity for suctioning. A third approach, and the one we favor for most cases, is to perform fiberoptic bronchoscopy through an endotracheal tube with large-bore suction catheters at the ready. It must be remembered that the gross appearance of the bronchial orifice and the results of cytologic examina-tions may falsely suggest the presence of an underlying malignancy because of intense and long-lived inflammation. On the other hand, nearly 50% of lung abscesses in adults older than 50 years of age are associated with carcinoma of the lung, either because of cavitation of the neoplasm or cavitation behind a proximal bronchial obstruction. Patients with lung abscess must be followed to resolution with great care.

In general, the pleura should not be violated unless absolutely necessary. A recent flurry of papers extolling the safety and efficacy of percutaneous catheter drainage in anecdotal series of lung abscesses have appeared in the radiology literature. The safety of this approach depends critically on the degree of synthesis of the two pleural surfaces; in the chronic stages of lung abscess, this has usually been accomplished so that passing a needle through the pleura into the lung does not result in pneumothorax. If the visceral pleura has not been firmly adhered to the chest wall, a pyopneumothorax results, often with bronchopleural fistula—a true disaster. Using CT and ultrasound to guide needle placement can minimize the occurrence of this complication, but it is far better avoided than treated, so our approach is to avoid the temptation to perform percutaneous drainage until attempts to achieve endobronchial drainage have clearly failed.

Suggested Reading

Bartlett JG: Anaerobic bacterial infections of the lung and pleural space, *Clin Infect Dis* 16(suppl 4):S248, 1993.

Davis B, Systrom DM: Lung abscess: pathogenesis, diagnosis and treatment, *Curr Clin Top Infect Dis* 18:252, 1998.

Gudiol F, et al: Clindamycin vs. penicillin for anaerobic lung infections: high rate of penicillin failures associated with penicillin-resistant *Bacteroides melaninogenicus, Arch Intern Med* 150:2525, 1990.

Jerng JS, et al: Empyema thoracis and lung abscess caused by viridans streptococci, *Am J Respir Crit Care Med* 156:1508, 1997.

EMPYEMA AND BRONCHOPLEURAL FISTULA

Dennis J. Shale

Infection of the pleura with the formation of an empyema and the importance of clearing the pus from this space have been recognized since ancient times. The incidence of empyema has decreased markedly since the development of effective antibiotic therapy for pneumonia. However, parapneumonic effusions occur in 30% to 60% of pneumonias, and when empyema occurs, it is associated with significant morbidity and mortality of up to 75%.

Traditionally, parapneumonic effusions have been classified as "uncomplicated," "complicated," and empyema, recognizing the clinical impression of a continuum of disease. Recently, a seven-category classification has been proposed with parallel management options for each category (Table 1). This expansion of the former classification is based on some evidence, although there remains a very limited background of adequate studies on which to base management decisions.

Empyema may be defined broadly as the presence of organisms and numerous neutrophils in pleural fluid, or, more narrowly, as pus apparent to the naked eye. The former definition has the advantage that during its acute phase, with free-flowing fluid, treatment is simpler than in the more chronic fibropurulent state associated with multiple loculations and the need for greater interventional therapy. Bronchopleural fistula (BPF) may be caused by an empyema or may be associated with empyema following surgery, penetrating lung injuries, or lung abscess.

■ ETIOLOGY

Empyema is most commonly associated with bacterial pneumonia. The most common organism associated is *Streptococcus pneumoniae*; although the risk in any one case of pneumococcal pneumonia is low, this remains the major cause because of the common nature of this form of pneumonia. A greater risk of empyema is associated with infections with *Staphylococcus aureus*, *Klebsiella* species, and other gram-negative bacteria, and anaerobic organisms. Other organisms with a tendency to involve the pleura include *Streptococcus milleri*, *Actinomycetes*, and *Nocardia*. Rupture of the esophagus, hepatic or subphrenic abscesses, or penetrating chest injuries may introduce organisms, especially gram-negative or anaerobic organisms, into the pleural space. Amebae may enter the pleural space if an amebic hepatic abscess is involved. Tuberculous empyema is considered a minor problem in western countries but is still seen in reactivation of tuberculosis (TB) in the elderly. In the Third World, with rapid urbanization, continued population in-

creases, and high levels of human immunodeficiency virus (HIV) infection, there is an increasing incidence of tuberculous empyema. All such infections may cause a BPF or be secondary to a BPF. Resectional lung surgery is the major cause of BPF, occurring in 3% to 5% of operations.

■ CLINICAL FEATURES

No specific features differentiate complicated and uncomplicated parapneumonic effusions. The main features are fever, chest pain, sputum production, appropriate clinical signs and peripheral blood leucocytosis. Progression to an empyema is usually indicated by the persistence or recurrence of fever and systemic upset with physical signs of lack of resolution because differentiation of consolidation from a small to medium volume of effusion may not be possible.

Table 1   Classification and Treatment of Parapneumonic Effusions and Empyema

"UNCOMPLICATED" PARAPNEUMONIC EFFUSION	
Class 1 Nonsignificant	Small volume <10 mm thick on decubitus film Thoracentesis not indicated
Class 2 Typical parapneumonic effusion	>10 mm thick, pH >7.2, glucose >40 mg/dl, Gram smear and culture negative Antibiotics alone
"COMPLICATED" PARAPNEUMONIC EFFUSION	
Class 3 Borderline complicated	pH <7.2 but >7.0 and/or glucose >40 mg/dl, LDH >1000 IU/L, Gram smear and culture negative Antibiotics and repeated thoracocentesis
Class 4 Simple complicated	pH <7.0 and/or glucose <40 mg/dl, and/or positive Gram smear or culture, no frank pus or loculation Antibiotics and closed tube drainage
Class 5 Complex complicated	pH <7.0 and/or glucose <40 mg/dl and/or loculated Antibiotics, closed tube drainage, and thrombolytics
EMPYEMA	
Class 6 Simple empyema	Frank free-flowing pus Antibiotics, closed tube drainage, possible decortication
Class 7 Complex empyema	Frank pus with loculation Antibiotics, closed tube drainage, thrombolytics, likely decortication

Other physical features include dyspnea with large effusions, acute finger clubbing, lethargy, and marked weight loss. Purulent sputum may indicate the development of a BPF. However, a more insidious onset may occur with presentation weeks to months after the original pneumonia.

■ INVESTIGATIONS

A chest radiograph usually shows a collection of fluid, although a localized, loculated collection may resemble an intrapulmonary mass. This may be resolved by posteroanterior and lateral chest radiographs. Ultrasonography will help distinguish fluid from solid tissue and can be used to guide a percutaneous diagnostic aspiration if there is pleural thickening or loculation. Occasionally, it is difficult to distinguish between empyema with a BPF and a lung abscess. In this setting, the use of computed tomography (CT) scanning may guide both investigation and management approaches.

Aspirated material should be collected under anaerobic conditions and a portion submitted for anaerobic culture. Routine bacterial and mycobacterial culture should be undertaken with cytologic examination. If appropriate, fungi and parasites should be sought. Other investigations, including pH, glucose concentrations, and lactate dehydrogenase (LDH) activity, may be of use if there is little naked-eye evidence of purulence. A meta-analysis of pleural fluid biochemistry, based on user characteristics, demonstrated that pH, especially less than 7.2, was a guide to the need for tube drainage and that glucose or LDH determinations were of no extra benefit.

Generally, percutaneous pleural biopsy is unhelpful and potentially harmful, although the diagnosis of tuberculosis at times is made only from such material.

■ THERAPY

Small or insignificant effusions (class 1) do not need thoracocentesis. For larger effusions with a pH greater than 7.2 and no evidence of infection in the pleural space (class 2), antibiotic treatment alone should suffice. Classes 1 and 2 equate to the former group of "uncomplicated" parapneumonic effusions. With a pH less than 7.2 but greater than 7.0 and no Gram smear or culture evidence of pleural space infection (class 3), the effusion should be considered borderline complicated and managed with antibiotics and repeated thoracocentesis.

Effusions in classes 4 and 5 represent a spectrum of "complicated" parapneumonic effusions. In class 4 a pH less than 7.0 and evidence of pleural space infection, but free of frank pus or loculation, is managed with antibiotics and closed tube drainage. This is effective if applied early and may stop progression to an empyema. The tube must be placed at the most dependent point possible. The largest-bore tube should be used, and drainage via underwater seal is effective, although negative-pressure suction may be needed if flow is slow and will hasten the obliteration of the empyema space. This approach is contraindicated in patients with a neoplasm causing airway obstruction. Success is usually evident within 48 hours with clinical and radiologic improvement, and drainage should continue until fully resolved. In class 5, with the complication of loculation of the effusion, management requires the addition of a thrombolytic agent such as streptokinase (250,000 IU) or urokinase (100,000 IU). The latter is less likely to produce allergic side effects. Thrombolytics increase the flow of fluid from the chest and are associated with a good outcome. It is unclear whether they reduce the need for surgical intervention by stopping progression to empyema.

The presence of pus defines an empyema (classes 6 and 7), and the free drainage of pus or loculation determines the use of thrombolytics in the latter in addition to the surgical options that might be needed in these groups (Table 1). It requires a balanced decision so that surgery is not contemplated too late, when the patient's condition may reduce the chance of a satisfactory outcome. Decortication aims to remove pus and fibrous tissue lining the pleural cavity but is a major procedure unsuitable for debilitated patients. In general, decortication is not needed for residual pleural thickening from a successful management of classes 3 through 5 unless it persists for more than 6 months, there is extensive pleural thickening, or it causes respiratory symptoms secondary to restrictive effects. Decortication has the benefit of quicker resolution of the empyema over methods of open drainage, which have median healing periods of 6 to 12 months.

This classification has the utility of matching a spectrum of clinical status to a plan of escalating therapeutic options but remains only a guide based on limited evidence. Patients may move in either direction along this spectrum, so careful and repeated reassessment of the patient's status is required, particularly soon after a therapeutic intervention is made, to ensure a continuing appropriate management response.

The aim with BPF is to deal with the air leak and any empyema. The air leak may be dealt with either by surgical or nonsurgical intervention, largely depending on the size and duration of the BPF (Table 2).

Pleural space infections demand major management decisions of physicians. There are various approaches to the patient with empyema and bronchopleural fistula, and the heterogeneity of response means that management of this

Table 2   Management of Bronchopleural Fistula (BPF)
SMALL BPF
Some may close spontaneously:
Without empyema
Transbronchoscopic fibrin glue
Transbronchoscopic tissue glue
Transbronchoscopic vascular occlusion coils
Transbronchoscopic laser/tetracycline/gel foam
Thoracoscopic scaling
With empyema
Antibiotic/tube drainage of empyema and the attempted
closure of BPF
LARGE BPF
Typically associated with an empyema:
Surgical options involve decortication or open drainage for
the empyema and occlusion of the BPF using direct closure,
or well-vascularized muscle or omental flaps

problem should be individualized. There is much literature, but most studies are too small and not designed to demonstrate clear beneficial options.

Suggested Reading

Bouros D, Schiza S, Patsourakis G: Intrapleural streptokinase versus urokinase in the treatment of complicated parapneumonic effusions: a prospective, double-blind study, *Am J Respir Crit Care Med* 155:291, 1997.

Bouros D, et al: Role of streptokinase in the treatment of acute loculated parapneumonic pleural effusions and empyema, *Thorax* 49:852, 1994.

Heffner JE, et al: Pleural fluid chemical analysis in parapneumonic effusions; a meta-analysis, *Am J Respir Crit Care Med* 151:1700, 1995.

Light RW: A new classification of parapneumonic effusions and empyema, *Chest* 108:299, 1995.

ENDOCARDITIS OF NATURAL AND PROSTHETIC VALVES: TREATMENT AND PROPHYLAXIS

Oksana M. Korzeniowski
Mashiul H. Chowdhury

■ DEFINITION AND PATHOGENESIS

The term *infective endocarditis* (IE) denotes an infection of the endothelial surfaces of the heart. This is usually a valvular surface, but extracardiac endothelium can also be infected.

In the past, IE was classified as acute or subacute, depending on the severity of clinical presentation. Since the advent of antibiotics, classification and therefore therapeutic decisions are based on the bacteriology and the valvular tissue involved, that is, native valve versus prosthetic valve.

The animal model of endocarditis has improved the understanding of the in vivo aspects of the pathogenesis of this disease. Any structural abnormalities that cause turbulent blood flow across a high to low pressure gradient denude epithelium from surfaces impacted on by the turbulence. Such damaged areas (most commonly valvular surfaces) are predisposed to platelet and fibrin deposition and eventually to the formation of a sterile vegetation, also known as *nonbacterial thrombotic endocarditis* (NBTE).

When transient bacteremia occurs after injury to mucosal surfaces in the oropharynx, genitourinary tract, or gastrointestinal tract, organisms are deposited onto the NBTE, where they adhere firmly, multiply, and stimulate further deposition of platelets and fibrin. The infected site is sustained by the inaccessibility of the organisms to host defenses. Enlargement of the lesion into a mature vegetation may result in destruction of valves and may cause complications through local bacterial spread or through embolization of fragments of the vegetation. The endovascular location of the lesions causes multiorgan bacterial seeding as well as organ damage through immune complex deposition.

■ NATIVE VALVE ENDOCARDITIS

In most cases of native valve endocarditis, there is an identifiable predisposing cardiac lesion. Mitral valve prolapse is now the most commonly identified underlying cardiac abnormality in patients with IE in the United States. The risk of IE is estimated to be five to eight times greater than that of individuals with a normal mitral valve. Men with mitral valve prolapse are at considerably greater risk than women, although the frequency of mitral valve prolapse is three times greater in women than in men. Rheumatic heart disease accounts for 30% and congenital heart disease for 10% to 20% of the heart lesions in patients with endocarditis. Other recognized predisposing cardiac lesions (Table 1) are ventricular septal defects, subaortic and valvular aortic stenosis, tetralogy of Fallot, coarctation of the aorta, Marfan syndrome, and pulmonary stenosis, but not uncomplicated atrial septal defects. Most cases of native valve endocarditis are caused by the streptococci (50% to 70%), which are normal inhabitants of the oropharynx and elaborate complex polysaccharides that promote their adherence to fibrin platelet matrices. They are highly susceptible to penicillin. Enterococci (10% of cases of native valve IE) present an enhanced risk to elderly men and young women with genitourinary disease. *Staphylococcus aureus* IE (25% of cases) remains the most aggressive form of native valve infection. In recent years, both enterococci and staphylococci have become major pathogens in infections originating from intravascular catheters. Occasionally, almost all species of bacteria can cause infective endocarditis. Fastidious oropharyngeal organisms such as the HACEK group (*Haemophilus parainfluenzae*, *H. aphrophilus*, *H. paraphrophilus*, *Actinobacillus actinomycetem-comitans*, *Cardiobacterium hominis*, *Eikenella corrodens*, and *Kingella kingae*) cause 3% of community-acquired IE. Fungi rarely cause IE on a native valve except in intravenous drug abusers.

■ PROSTHETIC VALVE ENDOCARDITIS

The overall incidence of prosthetic valve endocarditis (PVE) is 1% to 4%. The causative organisms differ in early and late PVE. Infection within 60 days of valve insertion is considered to be early PVE and is usually caused by *Staphylococcus epidermidis* (25% to 30%) or *S. aureus* (15% to 20%). The remaining cases are caused by gram-negative aerobic organisms, diphtheroids, enterococci, and streptococci. Fungal endocarditis may develop in patients with prolonged hospitalization with indwelling central venous catheters and long-

Table 1 Cardiac Conditions Associated with Risk of Endocarditis

HIGH RISK (ENDOCARDITIS PROPHYLAXIS IS NEEDED)	MODERATE RISK (ENDOCARDITIS PROPHYLAXIS IS NEEDED)	LOW RISK (ENDOCARDITIS PROPHYLAXIS IS NOT NEEDED)
Prosthetic heart valves Previous history of endocarditis Cyanotic heart disease Surgically constructed systemic pulmonary shunt or conduit	Patent ductus arteriosus Ventricular septal defect Primum atrial septal defect Coarction of the aorta Bicuspid aortic valve Hypertrophic cardiomyopathy Mitral valve prolapse with regurgitation Acquired valvular dysfunction	Previous coronary artery bypass graft surgery Mitral valve prolapse without regurgitation Physiologic, functional, or innocent heart murmur Previous Kawasaki syndrome without valvular dysfunction Previous rheumatic disease without valvular dysfunction Cardiac pacemakers and implanted defibrillators Surgical repair of atrial septal defect, ventricular septal defect, or patent ductus arteriosus Isolated secundum atrial septal defect

Modified from Dajani AS, et al: Prevention of bacterial endocarditis. Recommendations by the American Heart Association, *Circulation* 96(1):358, 1997.

term antibiotic use. Organisms that cause late PVE closely resemble those of native valve endocarditis, although staphylococci remain predominant.

■ NOSOCOMIAL ENDOCARDITIS

IE can occur as a complication of nosocomial bacteremia. In the last decade, the increased use of intravascular devices and invasive diagnostic procedures, with their consequent complications, have drawn attention to the risk of nosocomial endocarditis. *S. aureus,* including methicillin-resistant *S. aureus* (MRSA); *S. epidermidis;* and enterococcus are the predominant pathogens. A retrospective study in Europe showed a 10-fold increase in the incidence of nosocomial endocarditis from 1978 to 1992, compared with cases from 1960 to 1975. In a recent study of prospectively identified patients with *S. aureus* endocarditis at Duke University Medical Center, 27 of the 59 (45.8%) patients had hospital-acquired *S. aureus* bacteremia. An intravascular device was thought to be the source of the bacteremia in 50.8% of patients. In another large prospective, multicenter, observational study to determine the incidence of PVE resulting from nosocomial bacteremia, 33% had PVE at the time that bacteremia was discovered and 11% developed PVE endocarditis later (a mean of 45 days) regardless of the antibiotic used to treat the bacteremia and the duration of such therapy.

■ INFECTIVE ENDOCARDITIS IN THE INTRAVENOUS DRUG ABUSERS

Endocarditis in intravenous drug abusers (IVDAs) involves mainly normal valves. Only about 20% of the patients have an underlying valvular abnormality when IE is diagnosed. Infection is believed to result from the deposition of bacteria on valves that have sustained microscopic injury through bombardment with drug-associated contaminants injected intravenously. The tricuspid valve is predominantly involved in IVDAs, but the aortic and the mitral valves may also be damaged. Although *S. aureus* is known to be the most common causative organism in patients with IE associated with IVDAs, a variety of microorganisms and fungi, including unusual and fastidious organisms (e.g., the HACEK group), are not uncommon in IVDAs, particularly in patients who are not meticulous in their injection practices. Because of the higher incidence of right-sided lesions and the generally younger age of the affected group, prognosis for recovery in treated IVDA IE is better than in the general population. However, valvular damage sustained in the course of the infection confers an extremely high risk of recurrent IE in those patients who continue to indulge in intravenous drugs.

■ DIAGNOSIS OF INFECTIVE ENDOCARDITIS

Definitive diagnosis of IE requires documentation of sustained bacteremia with a microorganism typical for endocarditis in a patient with an underlying valvular cardiac lesion or by direct demonstration of the pathogen by culture or histopathology of a vegetation or an embolus. The Duke criteria (Table 2) have been in use since 1994 to diagnose IE clinically. The Duke criteria incorporate echocardiographic findings and IVDA as an important epidemiologic risk factor into the previously formulated Von Reyn criteria for IE and expand their sensitivity and specificity.

■ THERAPY

A vegetation consists of microorganisms in high density ($>10^8$ organisms/g of tissue) and in a reduced metabolic

Table 2 Duke Criteria to Diagnose Infective Endocarditis

Definite infective endocarditis
  Pathologic: Microorganism by culture or histology of
    vegetation or emboli
  Histopathologically proven at autopsy or surgery
  Clinical: 2 major or 1 major and 3 minor or 5 minor criteria

MAJOR CRITERIA	MINOR CRITERIA
Positive blood cultures Endocardial involvement by showing vegetation or prosthetic valve dehiscence in echocardiogram or new valvular regurgitation	Predisposing heart condition or intravenous drug use Fever Vascular phenomena Immunologic phenomena Positive blood cultures but short of major criteria or serologic evidence of infection Echo consistent with infective endocarditis but short of major criteria

Table 3 Antibiotic Therapy for Streptococcal Endocarditis

VIRIDANS STREPTOCOCCI OR S. BOVIS MIC ≤0.1 µg/ml	VIRIDANS STREPTOCOCCI OR S. BOVIS MIC >0.1 µg/ml AND <0.5 micg/ml	VIRIDANS STREPTOCOCCI OR S. BOVIS MIC ≥0.5 µg/ml
NATIVE VALVE		
PCN G, 12-18 mU/24 hr IV −4 wk or Ceftriaxone, 2 g/24 hr IV or IM −4 wk PCN G, 12-18 mU/24 hr IV plus Gentamicin, 1 mg/kg q8h IV −2 wk	PCN G, 18 mU/24 hr IV −4 wk plus Gentamicin, 1 mg/kg q8h IV for the first 2 wk PCN G, 18-30 mU/24 hr IV plus	PCN G, 18-30 mU/24 hr IV plus Gentamicin, 1 mg/kg q8h IV −4-6 wk PCN G, 18-30 mU/24 hr IV plus
PROSTHETIC VALVE		
PCN G, 18 mU/24 hr IV −6 wk plus Gentamicin for the first 2 wk	Gentamicin, 1 mg/kg q8h IV −6 wk	Gentamicin, 1 mg/kg q8h IV −6 wk
IF PATIENT IS ALLERGIC TO PCN		
Vancomycin, 1 g q12h 4-6 wk	Vancomycin, 1 g q12h 4-6 wk	Vancomycin, 1 g q12h 4-6 wk

MIC, Minimal inhibitory concentration; *PCN*, penicillin.

state inside an acellular lesion with impaired host defenses. Eradication of IE is thus almost totally dependent on the efficacy of the antimicrobial therapy. To achieve this end, certain principles of therapy are critical:

1. Parenteral antibiotics are usually required to provide a predictably high serum antibiotic level and thus to optimize penetration of the antibiotic into tissue.
2. Bactericidal rather than bacteriostatic antibiotics should be used to compensate for impaired host defenses in the vegetation.
3. Prolonged therapy is required for complete eradication of microorganisms.

In a patient with suspected IE but in whom culture results are not available, empiric antimicrobial therapy should be directed against staphylococci, streptococci, and enterococci unless epidemiologic data point at alternative etiologies. Nafcillin or oxacillin, 2 g IV every 4 hours, and gentamicin, 1 mg/kg IV every 8 hours, may be used as initial therapy. Vancomycin, 15 mg/kg IV every 12 hours, should be used if the patient is allergic to penicillin. Vancomycin should also be the drug of choice in suspected nosocomial endocarditis because of the high incidence of MRSA and coagulase-negative *S. epidermidis* (CoNS) in this subgroup.

Viridans Streptococci and S. Bovis

Antibiotic selection for the therapy of streptococcal endocarditis is based on the minimal inhibitory concentration (MIC) of the isolated organism to penicillin (Table 3). Viridans streptococci or *S. bovis* are generally highly susceptible to penicillin (MIC <0.1 µg/ml) and can be treated with aqueous penicillin G for 4 weeks. The addition of gentamicin can shorten therapy to 2 weeks, but such therapy should be reserved for patients with normal renal function and uncomplicated (i.e., short duration, minimal distal disease) endocarditis. For streptococci with moderate to high resistance to penicillin (MIC >0.1 and >0.5 µg/ml), the addition of gentamicin is always recommended to prevent relapse. This group contains nutritionally variant viri-

dans streptococci and typable streptococci of groups other than A. A duration of therapy of less than 4 weeks of antibiotics is ineffective. The same regimen applies to the therapy of streptococcal prosthetic valve endocarditis, but the duration of treatment is prolonged to 6 weeks. Vancomycin is an option only for the penicillin-allergic patient. In a recent open label, randomized, multicenter trial, ceftriaxone (2 g IV daily) for 2 weeks (with the addition of a single daily dose of gentamicin) or 4 weeks (when used alone) showed full efficacy in treatment of endocarditis caused by viridans streptococci sensitive to penicillin. These data support the revised American Heart Association (AHA) recommendations of 1995 for *S. viridans* endocarditis.

Staphylococci

Most strains of *S. aureus* are resistant to penicillin by virtue of beta-lactamase production. Therapy is based on antistaphylococcal penicillins (i.e., nafcillin, oxacillin) or first-generation cephalosporins (i.e., cefazolin) administered from 4 to 6 weeks (Table 4). The addition of gentamicin to nafcillin enhances the rate of killing of bacteria and the sterilization of blood, but no clinical advantage results from longer than 3- to 5-day use, whereas toxicity increases significantly. Vancomycin should be used only in cases of serious beta-lactam allergy (IgE-mediated hypersensitivity) or if a methicillin-resistant isolate is suspected or documented; otherwise cefazolin can be substituted for nafcillin for a less frequent dosing regimen. In a patient with uncomplicated right-sided *S. aureus* endocarditis (only tricuspid

Table 4 Antibiotic Therapy for Staphylococcal Endocarditis

S. AUREUS OR COAGULASE-NEGATIVE STAPHYLOCOCCI NATIVE VALVES	S. AUREUS OR COAGULASE-NEGATIVE STAPHYLOCOCCI PROSTHETIC VALVES
METHICILLIN SENSITIVE	
Nafcillin, 2 g q4h IV 4-6 wk, plus gentamicin, 1 mg/kg q8h IV 3-5 days or Cefazolin, 2 g q8h IV 4-6 wk, plus gentamicin, 1 mg/kg q8h IV 3-5 days	Nafcillin, 2 g q4h IV, plus rifampin, 300 mg PO q8h 6-8 wk, plus gentamicin, 1 mg/kg q8h IV first 2 wk
METHICILLIN RESISTANT OR PCN ALLERGIC	
Vancomycin, 1 g q12h IV 4-6 wk	Vancomycin, 1 g q12h IV, plus rifampin, 300 mg PO q8h 6-8 wk, plus gentamicin, 1 mg/kg q8h IV first 2 wk

PCN, Penicillin.

Table 5 Antibiotic Therapy for Enterococcal Endocarditis

ENTEROCOCCI AND NUTRITIONALLY VARIANT VIRIDANS STREPTOCOCCI
PCN G, 18-30 mU/24 hr IV, plus gentamicin, 1 mg/kg q8h IV 4-6 wk

or

Ampicillin, 2 g q4h IV, plus gentamicin, 1 mg/kg q8h IV 4-6 wk
IF PATIENT ALLERGIC TO PCN OR PCN-RESISTANT ENTEROCOCCI
Vancomycin, 1 g q12h IV, plus gentamicin, 1 mg/kg q8h IV 4-6 wk

PCN, Penicillin.

valve involved) resulting from IVDA, 2 weeks of intravenous nafcillin with gentamicin for 2 weeks may be adequate therapy. These findings do not extrapolate to treatment with vancomycin.

In prosthetic valve endocarditis, the most common causative agents are S. aureus and coagulase-negative S. epidermidis (see Table 4). Both species are commonly resistant to beta-lactam antibiotics; thus, until sensitivity to methicillin can be confirmed, vancomycin should be used as the primary therapeutic agent. Rifampin and gentamicin are added to improve synergistic killing and to prevent emergence of resistant strains. The duration of therapy is generally longer than that for therapy of native valve endocarditis. Bacteriologic failures are common and surgical valve replacement may be necessary.

Enterococci and Vancomycin-Resistant Enterococcus

The enterococcus is becoming a serious gram-positive nosocomial pathogen. Enterococci are streptococci intrinsically resistant to the bactericidal effect of penicillin or vancomycin. Therefore, for the treatment of endocarditis, the addition of aminoglycoside is needed to promote bactericidal effect. Cephalosporins are always inactive against enterococci and cannot be used interchangeably with penicillin in this setting. Emergence in nosocomial settings of strains of enterococci highly resistant to penicillin, aminoglycosides, and vancomycin has seriously compromised the efficacy of available treatment. To guide the choice of the most effective regimen, all enterococcal isolates in cases of suspected IE should be subjected to in vitro sensitivity testing.

The established course of treatment for a patient with native valve endocarditis caused by a community-acquired enterococcus (i.e., one relatively sensitive to penicillin and susceptible to synergistic killing with aminoglycosides) is 4 to 6 weeks of penicillin (20 to 30 mU $\times$ 10^6 U/day) or vancomycin, 1 g every 12 hours, plus gentamicin, 3 mg/kg/day in divided doses (Table 5). Patients with prosthetic valve infections should have therapy prolonged for 8 weeks. When

penicillin or vancomycin must be used alone because of a high level of resistance to aminoglycosides, 8 to 10 weeks of therapy is recommended. For enterococci highly resistant to ampicillin and highly resistant to aminoglycosides, treatment is based on vancomycin alone. The relapse rate may increase substantially.

Vancomycin-resistant enterococcus (VRE) now accounts for 15% of infections in critical care units. E. faecium is much more commonly vancomycin resistant than E. fecalis. Occasional cases of VRE endocarditis have been reported. In general, VRE isolates are resistant to all currently available antimicrobial agents; thus there is no standard regimen for VRE endocarditis. A number of new antimicrobials with activity against VRE are in development. Clinical success rates for treatment of vancomycin-resistant E. faecium (VREF) infections with quinapristine-dalfopristin (synercid) are as high as 73%, although data are extremely limited with regard to VREF endocarditis. Other agents such as daptomycin and linezolid are active in vitro against a variety of resistant gram-positive organisms, including VRE, but clinical efficacy is as yet undetermined. Studies evaluating such agents are warranted. Figure 1 presents an algorithm that may be helpful in managing enterococcal endocarditis.

Other Treatment Considerations

Gram-negative organisms of the HACEK group grow slowly on standard culture media and may require more than 2 weeks of incubation; susceptibility testing is therefore difficult. Emergence of HACEK resistance to ampicillin has been recognized. Because all strains are susceptible to third-generation cephalosporins, treatment with ceftriaxone sodium, 2 g IV for 4 weeks, has replaced ampicillin (12 g/24 hr) plus gentamicin (10 mg/kg every 8 hours) as the regimen of choice. Alternative regimens based on in vitro data include trimethoprim-sulfamethoxazole, fluoroquinolones, and aztreonam. Most streptococci other than viridans or enterococci (i.e., pneumococcus, group A to G streptococci) remain susceptible to penicillin, but therapy before the availability of their susceptibility profile must take into account the possibility of a resistant isolate. Although pneumococcal endocarditis is rare (<1%), its fulminant course and the increasing incidence of penicillin and cephalosporin resistance have mandated vancomycin with or without ceftriaxone as the empiric regimen. Non–group A strains of streptococci may need gentamicin in addition to penicillin to ensure synergistic killing. Enterobacteriaceae and

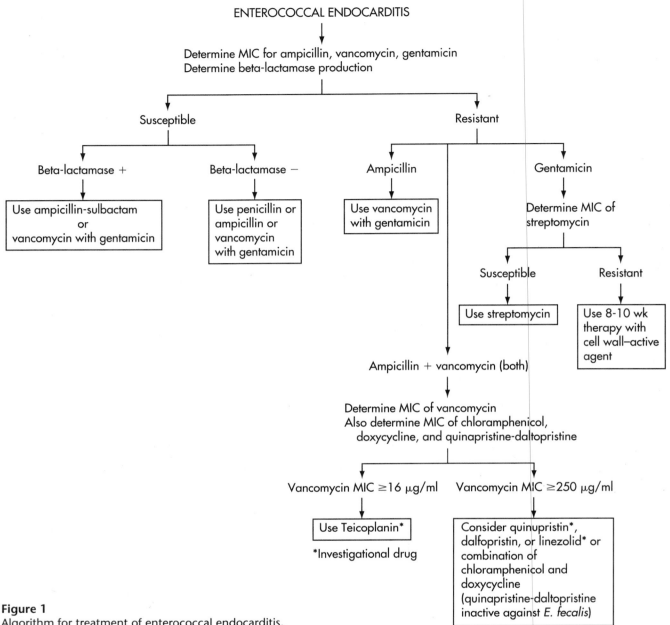

Figure 1
Algorithm for treatment of enterococcal endocarditis.

P. aeruginosa are uncommon causes of endocarditis. Therapy should be determined by in vitro susceptibility testing. Adequacy of the regimen may require monitoring via serum bactericidal activity.

Fungal endocarditis is poorly responsive even to the gold standard of treatment, that is, amphotericin B for 6 to 8 weeks. Surgical valve replacement may be necessary. In patients with hemodynamically stable valves and candidal or aspergillus infections susceptible to imidazoles, long-term suppression with fluconazole *(Candida albicans)* or itraconazole *(Aspergillus* species) may be the preferred therapeutic choice.

Traditionally, oral regimens have not had a role in the treatment of endocarditis because adequate antibiotic serum levels could not be achieved. With newer agents such as the quinolones, the serum concentration after oral administration is equivalent to that seen with parenteral dosing. These agents have been used for the oral treatment of highly susceptible gram-negative pathogens. Also, a 4-week oral regimen of ciprofloxacin plus rifampin has been used to treat uncomplicated right-sided endocarditis in IVDAs. Close monitoring of patients for adequate gastrointestinal function and compliance is mandatory. Clinical outcome data are limited.

Prophylaxis

Despite improvements in diagnostic modalities, in technologies of parenteral therapy and valve replacement, and in

Table 6   Procedures Warranting Endocarditis Prophylaxis

PROPHYLAXIS RECOMMENDED

Dental extractions
Periodontal procedures
Professional teeth cleaning
Tonsillectomy and/or adenoidectomy
Surgery on respiratory mucosa
Sclerotherapy for esophageal varices*
Esophageal stricture dilation*
Endoscopic retrograde cholangiography with biliary
    obstruction*
Biliary tract surgery*
Surgical operations that involve intestinal mucosa
Cystoscopy
Urethral dilation
Prostatic surgery

PROPHYLAXIS NOT RECOMMENDED

Restorative dentistry (filling above the gum line)
Orthodontic appliance adjustment
Injection of local intraoral anesthetic
Endotracheal intubation
Bronchoscopy with a flexible bronchoscope with or without
    biopsy†
Tympanectomy tube insertion
Transesophageal echocardiogram
Endoscopy with or without gastrointestinal biopsy†
Vaginal delivery or vaginal hysterectomy†
Cesarean section
Dilation and curettage

*Prophylaxis recommended for high risk; optional for medium risk.
†Prophylaxis optional for high-risk patients.

Table 7   AHA-Recommended Prophylactic Regimens

PROPHYLACTIC REGIMEN FOR DENTAL, ORAL, RESPIRATORY TRACT, AND ESOPHAGEAL PROCEDURES

Standard
    Amoxicillin, 2 g 1 hr before procedure
Unable to take oral medications
    Ampicillin, 2 g IM or IV 30 min before procedure
Allergic to penicillin
    Clindamycin, 600 mg 1 hr before procedure, or clarithromy-cin, 500 mg, or cephalexin, 2 g 1 hr before procedure
Allergic to penicillin and unable to take oral medications
    Clindamycin, 600 mg IV 30 min before procedure, or cefazo-lin, 1 g IV 30 min before procedure

PROPHYLACTIC REGIMENS FOR GU AND GI (EXCLUDING ESOPHAGEAL) PROCEDURES

High-risk patients
    Ampicillin, 2 g IV or IM plus gentamicin, 1.5 mg/kg within
    30 min before procedure, followed by ampicillin, 1 g IV or IM,
    or amoxicillin, 1 g orally 6 hr later
High-risk but penicillin-allergic patient
    Vancomycin, 1 g IV over 1 hr plus gentamicin, 1.5 mg/kg IV or
    IM, complete infusion within 30 min before procedure
Moderate-risk patients
    Ampicillin, 2 g IV or IM within 30 min of procedure or amox-icillin, 2 g orally 1 hr before procedure
Moderate risk but penicillin-allergic patient
    Vancomycin, 1 g IV over 1 hr, complete infusion within 30
    min before procedure

GU, Genitourinary; *GI*, gastrointestinal.

new antibiotics, IE continues to be a serious problem in the United States. Because the incidence and mortality of IE have both remained steady over the last few decades, prevention remains the goal for individuals at risk for IE. In 1997, the AHA published an updated recommendation for prophylaxis of bacterial endocarditis. Two major factors determine the need for prophylaxis:

1. A cardiac lesion that is in high to moderate risk to predispose to endocarditis (see Table 1)
2. An invasive procedure associated with high incidence of bacteremia (Table 6)

The purpose of prophylaxis is to prevent bacterial attachment and/or multiplication on a susceptible endocardial surface. Based on animal studies, the vulnerable period during surgical procedures is during manipulation of infected tissue. Therefore antibiotics should be delivered just before procedures initiating bacteremia and just long enough to kill any organisms that are adherent to endothelial surfaces and/or multiplying.

In a recent large population-based case control study of IE, the link between dental procedures and the development of IE was not demonstrable even in the presence of high-risk valvular disease. Although these findings have generated a controversial discussion on the merits of prophylaxis, the AHA continues to recommend prophylaxis while awaiting

further review of its recommendation. The regimens recommended by the AHA are aimed at the most likely flora released from the site of the procedure (i.e., viridans streptococci from the oropharynx, enterococcus from the genitourinary and gastrointestinal systems). The regimens are listed in Table 7.

Surgical Indications in the Management of Infective Endocarditis

There are several incontrovertible indications for surgery in IE. Congestive heart failure resulting from acute aortic insufficiency remains the major indication for immediate valve replacement because of the unacceptable high mortality rate in medically treated patients. Nonresponse to antimicrobial therapy may mandate valve removal if no alternative source for the continued bacteremia or fungemia is found. Fungal endocarditis on a prosthetic valve almost always requires valve replacement. With aggressive preoperative and postoperative antibiotic therapy, valve replacement with a mechanical prosthesis during active IE is a safe procedure. The risk of relapse of endocarditis in a newly implanted prosthetic valve is minimal.

Local cardiac complications of IE may require surgical intervention. Transesophageal echocardiography is a powerful tool for detection of valvular dehiscence, rupture, fistula, perforation, perivalvular extension of abscess, a large abscess, or a large vegetation (>10 mm) on an anterior mitral valve leaflet. Because large vegetations tend to embolize, valve replacement or vegetectomy may be indicated in a patient with suspected or documented recurrent CNS or large vessel emboli.

Anticoagulation during IE is a considerable risk for intracerebral hemorrhage. Anticoagulation is not recommended as a therapeutic option; however, maintenance anticoagulation in a patient with a prosthetic valve should be continued regardless of the diagnosis of endocarditis because of the risks of mechanical thrombosis.

Suggested Reading

Bayer AS, et al: Diagnosis and management of infective endocarditis and its complications, *Circulation* 1998:2936, 1998.

Dajani AS, et al: Prevention of bacterial endocarditis. Recommendations by the American Heart Association, *JAMA* 96:358, 1997.

Fang G, et al: Prosthetic valve endocarditis resulting from nosocomial bacteremia: a prospective multicenter study, *Ann Intern Med* 119:560, 1993.

Fernandez-Guerreno ML, et al: Hospital-acquired infectious endocarditis not associated with cardiac surgery: an emerging problem, *Clin Infect Dis* 20:16, 1995.

Fowler VG, et al: Infective endocarditis due to *S. aureus* bacteremia: 59 prospectively identified cases with follow-up, *Clin Infect Dis* 28:106, 1999.

Korzeniowski O, Kaye D: Endocarditis. In Gorbach SL, Bartlett JG, Blacklow NR, eds: *Infectious diseases*, ed 2, Philadelphia, 1998, WB Saunders.

Rybak MJ, et al: Vancomycin-resistant enterococcus: infectious endocarditis treatment, *Curr Infect Dis Rep* 1:2148, 1999.

Sexton DJ, et al: Ceftriaxone once daily for four weeks compared with ceftriaxone plus gentamicin once daily for two weeks for treatment of endocarditis due to penicillin-susceptible streptococci, *Clin Infect Dis* 27:1470, 1998.

Strom BL, et al: Dental and cardiac risk factors for infective endocarditis: a population-based, case-control study, *Ann Intern Med* 129:761, 1998.

PERICARDITIS

A. Martin Lerner

Infections of the heart are common and may be life-threatening. Particularly in immunosuppressed persons, the heart may be affected during bacteremias or fungemias from other sources. The pericardial sac may also be affected by contiguous spread from bacterial pneumonia with empyema involving the left lower lobe. Thoracentesis and pericardiocentesis with specific cultures is definitive evidence of the causative organism. Enteroviruses (e.g., coxsackieviruses, echoviruses), Epstein-Barr virus, cytomegalovirus, pyogenic bacteria including *Borrelia burgdorferi* (Lyme disease), *Mycobacterium tuberculosis,* and fungi are important agents.

The pericardial sac normally contains a fluid volume of 15 to 20 ml. The force of myocardial contraction is diminished by myocarditis or pericarditis. During virus and bacterial infections of the heart the pericardium and myocardium are usually simultaneously involved. However, clinical signs may be predominantly those of myocarditis or pericarditis. During viral myocarditis, myocardial necrosis may occur, but mixed polymorphonuclear leukocytic–mononuclear cell interstitial infiltrates are usual. Acute purulent pericarditis may induce a pericardium 8 to 10 mm deep containing 500 to 2000 ml of viscid fibrinous yellow purulent exudate containing varying quantities of granulation tissue. There may also be a fibrinous granulomatous pericarditis with no free fluid. Bacteremia or fungemia may cause myocardial abscesses. *Staphylococcus aureus* is a common cause of myocardial abscess. Fungemias, especially *Candida* or *Aspergil-*

lus, may accompany the neutropenia of cancer chemotherapy. Abscesses may be present in the heart, kidneys, gastrointestinal tract, lungs, brain, liver, and thyroid. At histologic section stained with periodic acid–Shiff or methenamine silver, the pericardium and myocardium may contain microcolonies of fungi. Depending on the patient's underlying disease and immunologic competence, there may be marked suppuration or no inflammatory response. Myocardial fibers may show coagulative necrosis. Coronary vessels occasionally are invaded by organisms.

■ AGENTS OF DISEASE (Table 1)

At pericardiocentesis or pericardial biopsy, bacteria, fungi, *M. tuberculosis,* and other pathogenic organisms are regularly isolated. Enteroviruses (coxsackieviruses and echoviruses) may also be isolated or identified by antigen capture (enzyme-linked immunosorbent assay [ELISA]) or DNA polymerase studies. *Streptococcus pneumoniae, S. aureus,* and *Streptococcus pyogenes* are the major pathogens causing purulent pericarditis, but gram-negative bacilli are commonly encountered in immunocompromised patients. Cases of tuberculous pericarditis are increasing with the prevalence of isoniazid-resistant strains. Histoplasmosis may also cause a nonconstrictive or chronic constrictive pericarditis. *Candida* and *Aspergillus* pericarditis may be fulminant. Prompt pericardial drainage may be critical. Parasitic infection such as trypanosomiasis (Chagas disease), trichinosis, toxoplasmosis, amebiasis, and echinococcus during systemic disease may produce myopericarditis.

Penicillium citrinum pneumonia and pericarditis in patients with acute leukemia after undergoing induction chemotherapy has been reported. The isolate demonstrated marked in vitro resistance to amphotericin B, itraconazole, fluconazole, and 5-flucytosine with MICs greater than 32 µg/ml and a ketoconazole MIC of 1 µg/ml. In 66 published cases of cardiac tamponade in patients with human immu-

Table 1	Causes of Pericarditis
VIRUSES	**MYCOBACTERIA**
Adenoviruses	*Mycobacterium-avium*
Cytomegalovirus	*intracellulare*
Coxsackieviruses A and B*	*Mycobacterium chelonei*
Epstein-Barr	*Mycobacterium kansasii*
Echoviruses*	*Mycobacterium tuberculosis**
Hepatitis A	**FUNGI AND**
Parvovirus B19	**ACTINOMYCETES**
Polioviruses	*Actinomyces israelii*
Herpes simplex 1 and 2	*Aspergillus* species*
Influenza viruses A and B	*Candida* species*
Lymphocytic choriomeningitis	*Coccidioides immitis*
Mumps	*Cryptococcus neoformans*
Rubella	*Histoplasma capsulatum**
Vaccinia	Agents of mucormycosis
Varicella-zoster	*Nocardia asteroides*
BACTERIA	*Penicillium citrinum*
Borrelia burgdorferi	**PARASITES**
Corynebacterium diphtheriae	*Echinococcus granulosus**
Neisseria gonorrhoeae	*Entamoeba histolytica**
Neisseria meningitidis	*Plasmodium* spp.
Francisella tularensis	*Schistosoma* spp.
Pseudomonas pseudomallei	*Toxoplasma gondii**
Staphylococcus aureus*	*Trichinella spiralis**
Streptococcus milleri	*Trypanosoma cruzi*
Streptococcus pneumoniae*	**RICKETTSIA**
Streptococcus pyogenes	*Coxiella burnetii*
Treponema pallidum	*Rickettsia typhi*
Aerobic gram-negative bacilli*	*Rickettsia rickettsii*
Anaerobic bacteria, includ-	**OTHERS**
ing *Bacteroides* and	*Chlamydia psittaci*
peptostreptococci	*Mycoplasma pneumoniae**

*These infectious agents are most commonly involved in the United States.

nodeficiency virus (HIV) infection, 26% were caused by tuberculosis, 17% were purulent bacterial infections, and 8% were caused by *Mycobacterium-avium intracellulare.* Less common causes were *Cryptococcus neoformans,* cytomegalovirus, and *Mycobacterium kansasii.*

■ CLINICAL MANIFESTATIONS

Patients with pyogenic pericarditis are acutely ill, with anorexia, fever, chills, and precordial chest pain. Physical findings include increased jugular venous pulsations, an adynamic pericardium, impalpable apical pulses, and muffled decreased heart sounds. A paradoxic pulse and varying degrees of cardiac tamponade may occur. Hepatomegaly, pleural effusions, ascites, and pitting edema often follow. The cardinal physical finding of pericarditis, however, is a pericardial friction rub, which is best heard in the fourth intercostal space just to the left of the midsternal border while the patient is sitting up, leaning forward, and not breathing. Pericardial friction rubs are accentuated during inspiration or expiration and may be monophasic, diphasic, or triphasic, corresponding to atrial or ventricular systole or early ventricular diastole. At phonocardiography a systolic

murmur or click may also be detected. At times pericardial or pleuropericardial friction rubs can be palpated.

Abnormal pericardial thickening (>3 mm) confirms the diagnosis of constrictive pericarditis. Nuclear ventriculograms and angiocardiograms show rapid ventricular filling. Tuberculosis, viral pericarditis, histoplasmosis, *Legionella pneumophila,* meningococcal infection, Lassa fever, Whipple's disease, actinomycosis, *Nocardia asteroides,* staphylococcal infection after cardiac surgery, Salmonella, and *Streptococcus milleri* have been reported to cause constrictive pericarditis.

■ LABORATORY FEATURES

A sonolucent space at echocardiography (ultrasonogram) separating the ventricular wall motions from a motionless pericardial sac echo indicates a pericardial effusion. Echocardiography evaluates wall motion, estimates ejection fractions, and validates the presence of significant pericardial effusions, but a negative examination does not exclude a significant pericardial effusion. In fact, pericardiocentesis has occasionally relieved severe cardiac tamponade when echocardiography failed to reveal a diagnostic sonolucent space. The rate of failure to determine the presence of significant pericardial effusion may be as high as 20%, and clinical suspicion should recognize the value of the positive tests only. Sometimes in difficult cases differential diagnosis requires coronary artery catheterization to exclude coronary artery disease.

Intravenous radioisotope (technetium-99m aggregated albumin or sodium pertechnate) outlines the intracardiac blood pool. This scan is compared with the cardiac silhouette chest x-ray film. Electrocardiographs show low voltage and ST segment elevation or depression or both. Leukocytoses, an enlarged cardiac silhouette, increased erythrocyte sedimentation rate, and elevated C-reactive protein are common findings in both pyogenic and viral pericarditis. Analysis of the pericardial fluid is always helpful in reaching a specific diagnosis. Pericardiocentesis carries the risk of a resultant hemopericardium and further cardiac tamponade. The safest procedure is best done by a cardiothoracic surgeon in the operating room with concomitant electrocardiographic monitoring. Specimens must be processed promptly. Special care must be taken by the attending physician that these critical specimens are not mishandled or lost. It is best if the pericardiocentesis is done during the day, when the microbiology and immunology laboratories can participate freely without delay. At pericardiocentesis, contrast material may be injected directly into the pericardial sac. An open pericardial biopsy may be indicated for the diagnosis of chronic pericarditis.

Cultures should also be taken appropriately for the isolation and recognition of viruses. Pyogenic pericarditis is proved by the isolation of a virus, bacterium, or fungus at pericardiocentesis. Tubercle bacilli are isolated in about 40% of the proven cases; when a pericardial biopsy is cultured for tuberculosis, the yield is substantially higher. The pathology of tuberculosis of the pericardium with Langhans giant cells, caseation necrosis, and granulation tissue is characteristic. Special stains may recognize bacteria in these pathogenic materials. Attempts should be made to isolate both aerobic and anaerobic bacteria, fungi, and acid-fast bacilli. Gram, acid-fast, and methenamine silver stain preparations of pericardial exudates should be examined.

Identification of specific bacterial or viral antigens by highly sensitive immunoassays and recognition of pathogenic nucleic acids from these agents by polymerase chain reactions from pericardial biopsies or fluids are diagnostic. Fourfold rises in specific antibodies in paired sera, or high titers that are maintained, are highly suggestive of specific etiologic diagnosis (e.g., *Mycoplasma pneumoniae*).

■ THERAPY (Table 2)

In patients with pyogenic or tuberculous pericarditis, pericardial drainage by pericardiostomy may be insufficient. Adequate relief of constriction may require decortication and resection. For purulent pericarditis, surgical management along with intensive systemic antibacterial therapy for 4 to 6 weeks or longer is often necessary. Antibacterial treatment of tuberculous pericarditis ranges from 6 to 12 months or longer in patients with HIV infections (see

Table 2 Treatment of Pericarditis

AGENT	MEDICAL	SURGICAL*
VIRAL PERICARDITIS		
Enteroviruses (e.g., coxsackievirus, echoviruses; Epstein-Barr virus, cytomegalovirus, human immunodeficiency virus, parvovirus B19)	Acute phase (first 14 days): avoid corticosteroids, alcohol, beta-blockers, anticoagulants, nonsteroidal antiinflammatory agents; give digitalis, diuretics, antiarrhythmic agents; chronic phase: supportive therapy with rest (no exercise) until stable.	Pericardiocentesis Pericardiocentesis or pericardiectomy
PURULENT PERICARDITIS		
Gram-positive cocci *Staphylococcus aureus* *Staphylococcus epidermidis* *Streptococcus pneumoniae* *Streptococcus pyogenes* (See additional agents, Table 1)	For specifically sensitive organisms, penicillin G (20 million-30 million U/day IV for 4-6 wk) or nafcillin 1.5-2 g IV q4h for 4 wk. For oxacillin-resistant *S. aureus* and all strains of *S. epidermidis,* vancomycin IV pharmacokinetic dosing guided by serum levels (C_{max} 25-35 µ/ml, C_{min} 10-15 µ/ml): all antibiotics are continued for 4-6 wk.	Tube drainage, decortication, pericardiectomy as required
Gram-negative bacilli *Escherichia coli, Proteus, Enterobacter, Pseudomonas* spp.	Two appropriate bactericidal antibiotics according to susceptibility studies, usually a penicillin (e.g., timentin) or third-generation cephalosporin (ceftazidime) plus an aminoglycoside (e.g., timentin 3 g IV q6h; ceftazidime 2 g IV q6h; gentamicin, pharmacokinetic dosing, C_{max} 5-8 µ/ml, C_{min} 2 µ/ml). All antibiotics are continued for 4-6 wk. When appropriate ceftriaxone (1.5-2.0 g IV q12h) may be given. All antibiotics are continued for 4-6 wk.	Tube drainage, decortication, pericardiectomy
FUNGI		
Histoplasma, Aspergillus, sporotrichosis, mucormycosis, *Blastomyces, Candida* species	The drug of choice remains amphotericin B 0.4-0.6 mg/kg IV for 10 wk; the following newer agents have potential for efficacy, but they have not been proved useful by clinical trial. Fluconazole and itraconazole have potential for efficacy. Dosages have not been established.	Tube drainage, decortication, pericardiectomy
Mycobacterium tuberculosis	Isoniazid-sensitive strain: A three-drug regimen daily for 12 mo including INH, RIF, and PZA. Isoniazid-resistant strains: A four-drug regimen including INH, RIF, PZA, and SM or EMB; Dosages: INH, 5 mg/kg (max 300 mg); RIF, 10 mg/kg (max 600 mg); PZA, 15-30 mg/kg (max 2 g); EMB, 15-25 mg/kg (max 2.5 g); SM, 15 mg/kg (max 1 g).	Tube drainage, decortication, Isoniazid pericardiectomy

INH, Isoniazid; *RIF,* rifampin; *PZA,* pyrazinamide; *SM,* streptomycin; *EMB,* ethambutol.
*For cardiac tamponade or constrictive pericarditis.

Table 2). When appropriate therapy of acute tuberculous pericarditis is begun promptly, drainage procedures may not be necessary. In areas with isoniazid-resistant strains of *M. tuberculosis,* initial treatment should consider a new infection to be due to a resistant strain until specific susceptibility tests are available. This may require about 6 weeks. When initiating drug treatment for tuberculous pericarditis, prednisone, 80 mg/day, should also be given for 6 to 8 weeks and then tapered off over several weeks. This suppresses inflammation within the pericardium, enhances reabsorption of the effusion, and retards pericardial constriction.

Multiple-drug regimens for multiple-drug–resistant tuberculosis containing older second-line agents, such as paraaminosalicylic acid and cycloserine, and newer drugs, such as amikacin, fluoroquinolones, and beta-lactam–beta-lactamase inhibitor combinations, are in clinical use; prolonged treatment is required, the incidence of serious side effects is high, and only limited data on short- and long-term efficacy are available.

Serum should be collected in the acute phase and at convalescence to test for specific antibodies to viruses and fungi. Continuing fever, chest pain, and elevations in white blood cell counts, creatinine phosphokinase (CPK-MB band), and serum aminotransferases (SGOT) suggest an associated myocardial necrosis.

■ PROGNOSIS

Complete recovery with no residual disease is possible. The outcome depends upon the accuracy of specific diagnosis and therapy.

Suggested Reading

Cameron EWJ: Surgical management of staphylococcal pericarditis, *Thorax* 30:678, 1975.

Estok L, Wallach I: Cardiac tamponade in a patient with AIDS: a review of pericardial disease in patients with HIV infection, *Mount Sinai J Med* 65:33, 1998.

Klacsmann PJ, Bulkley BH, Hutchins GM: The changing spectrum of purulent pericarditis, an 86 year autopsy experience in 200 patients, *Am J Med* 63:666, 1977.

Rooney JJ, Krocco JA, Lyons HA: Tuberclous pericarditis, *Ann Intern Med* 72:73, 1970.

Shuter J, Bellin E: Multidrug-resistant tuberculosis, *Infect Dis Clin Pract* 10:430, 1997.

Turner JA: Parasitic causes of pericarditis, *Western J Med* 122:307, 1975.

MYOCARDITIS

Catherine Diamond
Jeremiah G. Tilles

Myocarditis, inflammation of the myocardium, is an incompletely understood entity. The pathogenesis, diagnostic workup, and treatment of myocarditis remain challenging. Because myocarditis is often undiagnosed and the clinical and histologic definitions of the disease are poorly correlated, the actual incidence of histologic myocarditis is unknown. Myocarditis may be a precursor of dilated cardiomyopathy (DCM), which has an incidence of about 5 to 8 cases per 100,000 population annually.

■ ETIOLOGY

In most cases of clinical myocarditis, the cause is undetermined. Most cases of idiopathic lymphocytic myocarditis in the United States are thought to be viral in origin (Table 1). The most commonly associated viruses are enteroviruses, particularly Coxsackie B viruses. In research studies, enteroviral genomic sequences have been detected in 25% to 45% of endomyocardial biopsies (EMB) from patients with either active myocarditis or dilated cardiomyopathy. Cytomegalovirus (CMV), human immunodeficiency virus (HIV), and influenza viruses have also been implicated; adenovirus may be a common pathogen in children. Autoimmune myocarditis may be the result of a prior viral infection, part of a systemic disorder such as sarcoid, or an isolated finding. Nonviral infectious causes such as *Corynebacterium diphtheriae* (diphtheria), *Borrelia burgdorferi* (Lyme disease), and American trypanosomiasis (Chagas' disease) should be considered in the appropriate epidemiologic setting. Noninfectious causes (Table 2), such as sarcoidosis and peripartum and drug-induced myocarditis, are also in the differential diagnosis of myocarditis.

■ PATHOGENESIS

In a murine model of viral myocarditis, when 2- to 3-week old mice are injected intraperitoneally with Coxsackie B3 virus, the virus can be isolated from the heart and blood during the acute phase of viral replication. Cardiac histology during this phase may show transient inflammatory infiltrates, myocyte necrosis, and dystrophic calcification. Coronary artery microvascular spasm may cause myocardial hypoperfusion. During a following chronic phase, progressive heart failure may develop, characterized by myocardial fibrosis and resulting in a dilated cardiomyopathy. Although viral infection of myocytes appears early, maximal tissue damage occurs later with infiltration of T lymphocytes. In this chronic postviral autoimmune myocarditis, heart-specific autoantibodies against cardiac myosin heavy chain develop, but their role is unclear. On the other hand, cytokines are induced and appear to play an essential role in the pathogenesis of myocarditis.

Table 1   Infectious Causes of Myocarditis

VIRAL	*Neisseria meningitidis* or *Neisseria gonorrhea*
Adenovirus	*Haemophilus influenzae*
Enterovirus	*Streptococcus pneumoniae*
Echovirus	*Actinomyces*
Coxsackie A and B	*Salmonella*
Polio	*Brucella*
Herpesvirus	*Chylamydia psittaci, Chlamydia pneumoniae*
Cytomegalovirus	*Listeria monocytogenes*
Epstein-Barr virus	*Legionella*
Varicella-zoster virus	*Mycoplasma pneumoniae*
Human immunodeficiency virus	*Borrelia burgdorferi* (Lyme disease)
Influenza A and B	Syphilis
Vaccinia	Leptospira
Hepatitis B virus	*Mycobacterium tuberculosis*
Lymphocytic choriomeningitis virus	**RICKETTSIAL**
Mumps	*Coxsiella burnetti* (Q fever)
Rabies	*Rickettsia rickettsii* (Rocky Mountain spotted fever)
Respiratory syncytial virus	*Rickettsia tsutsugamushi* (scrub typhus)
Rubella	**FUNGAL**
Measles	Endemic fungi (histoplasmosis, blastomycosis, cryptococcus,
Variola (smallpox)	coccidioidomycosis)
Arbovirus	*Aspergillus*
Yellow fever	*Candida*
Dengue	**PROTOZOAL**
BACTERIAL	*Entamoeba histolytica*
Corynebacterium diphtheriae (diptheria)	*Trypanosoma cruzi* (Chagas' disease), *Trypanosoma gambiense,*
Clostridium perfringens	*Trypanosoma rhodesiense* (sleeping sickness)
Streptococcus pyogenes	*Trichinella spiralis*
Staphylcoccus aureus	*Toxoplasma gondii*

Table 2   Noninfectious Causes of Myocarditis

IMMUNE	**TOXIC**
Sarcoidosis	Alcohol
Giant cell myocarditis	Cocaine
Systemic lupus	Tetracycline
erythematosus	Sulfonamides
Systemic sclerosis	Penicillins
(scleroderma)	Anthracyclines
Rheumatoid arthritis	Cyclophosphamide
Dermatomyositis/	Methyldopa
polymyositis	Hydrochlorothiazide
Still's disease	Phenylbutazone
Rheumatic fever	Emetine
ENDOCRINE	Catecholamines
Thyrotoxicosis/	Lithium
hypothyroidism	Arsenic
Pheochromocytoma	Carbon monoxide
	Lead
	Radiation
	Scorpion stings
	PERIPARTUM
	KAWASAKI'S DISEASE

CLINICAL PRESENTATION

Most individuals with myocarditis are asymptomatic or suffer a mild, undiagnosed illness and recover without therapy. Some have a subacute presentation with mild ventricular dysfunction and heart failure. A minority of patients present in cardiogenic shock with severe myocarditis. Others present late with chronic dilated cardiomyopathy. Acute myocarditis should be suspected when a patient presents with unexplained congestive heart failure (CHF) or chest pain and creatinine phosphokinase (CPK) elevation without evidence of coronary artery disease. Ventricular tachycardia may be the sole clinical manifestation of myocarditis. Patients with viral myocarditis may give a history of a preceding flulike illness or fever and pharyngitis may still be clinically evident. The physical examination may be normal or there may be tachycardia, a muffled first heart sound, a third heart sound (S_3 gallop), or a mitral regurgitant murmur with ventricular dilation. A pericardial friction rub may be heard with accompanying pericarditis.

DIAGNOSIS

Table 3 includes diagnostic options for infectious myocarditis. There are no laboratory, electrocardiographic (ECG), or echocardiographic features that distinguish between patients with or without histologic evidence of myocarditis. Patients may have an elevated erythrocyte sedimentation rate (ESR) and, less commonly, leukocytosis or leukopenia. The ECG may show low voltage and diffuse ST elevation or T-wave inversion. Holter monitoring may detect arrhythmias. Echocardiography evaluates wall motion, estimates ejection fraction (EF), and detects the presence of pericardial effusion; it generally shows diffuse ventricular dilation with globally reduced contractility. In cases of rapid onset, the left ventricle may be hypokinetic with minimal dilation. Serial echocardiograms obtained a week apart should pro-

Table 3 Diagnostic Clues and Options for Infectious Myocarditis

HISTORY
Chest pain
Palpitations
Shortness of breath/cough
Fever
Arthralgias
Antecedent upper respiratory tract infection

PHYSICAL EXAMINATION
Tachycardia
Muffled first heart sound
Third heart sound (S_3 gallop)
Mitral regurgitant murmur
Pericardial friction rub
Paradoxical pulse
Congestive heart failure (jugular venous distension, hepatomegaly, edema)

CARDIAC TESTING
Electrocardiogram
Chest x-ray study
Echocardiogram
Cardiac catheterization
Radionucleotide scan (indium-111 labeled monoclonal antimyosin antibody or gallium scan)
Magnetic resonance imaging
Endomyocardial biopsy
    Light microscopy
    Polymerase chain reaction
    Immunohistochemistry (viral stains, T cell markers)
    Viral cultures

LABORATORY TESTING
Creatinine phosphokinase
Troponin
Erythrocyte sedimentation rate
White blood cell count
Isolation of virus from throat or rectal swabs, stool, blood, cerebrospinal fluid, or tissue
Serologic testing (four-fold rise in antibody titer or positive IgM)

vide evidence of deterioration or improvement. CPK or troponin may be elevated with myocardial damage. Identification of the specific virus responsible for a recent viral infection may be accomplished serologically either by demonstrating a fourfold increase antibody titer during convalescence or by initial detection of IgM. Alternatively, it may still be possible to isolate an enterovirus by cell culture from a remote site such as from throat or rectal swabs, stool, blood, or cerebrospinal fluid. Secondary causes of myocarditis should be excluded serologically because some causes, such as Chagas' or HIV-related myocarditis, have specific treatments.

Routine chest radiographs may show an enlarged heart or signs of heart failure. Myocyte injury can be studied noninvasively by determining myocardial uptake of indium-111 labeled monoclonal antimyosin antibodies or by gallium scanning. Discrepancies between positive antimyosin and gallium scans and negative histologic findings in the endomyocardial biopsy have been reported, suggesting a high sensitivity but a low specificity of radionucleotide scans for the histologic detection of myocarditis. Radionucleotide scans may be useful in identifying appropriate candidates for endomyocardial biopsy. Recently, magnetic resonance imaging (MRI) has been suggested as a radiographic test for myocarditis.

Of course, the histologic diagnosis of myocarditis during life must be based on the interpretation of endomyocardial biopsy. Given that no specific effective treatments are known for the most common causes of lymphocytic myocarditis and that the clinical manifestations of myocarditis usually resolve with conservative therapy, endomyocardial biopsy is generally not indicated. If there is progressive clinical deterioration, the risks of biopsy may be justified because the long-term prognosis is poor in such cases. In addition, biopsy would be necessary if there were a suspicion of a potentially treatable cause such as giant cell or sarcoid myocarditis. Patients with ventricular tachycardia could be considered for biopsy for prognostic purposes. Because tachyarrhythmias may reverse with recovery, permanent therapies such as an automatic internal cardioverter defibrillator (AICD) or ablation of an arrhythmic focus or lifelong antiarrhythmic therapy may be premature in such cases. Patients with recurrent disease also might be candidates for biopsy. Virus isolation from myocardial tissue, however, is rare unless the patient is immunocompromised.

■ THERAPY

Conventional Therapy
Patients should avoid strenuous exercise (Figure 1, Table 4). Bed rest and oxygen are generally advised. Cardiac monitoring is necessary to detect rhythm disturbances, which may require antiarrhythmics, electrophysiologic evaluation, pacemaker, or an AICD. Patients with CHF with stable hemodynamic status respond to standard measures such as diuretics and salt and fluid restriction; they are particularly sensitive to digoxin. Dobutamine, dopamine, and other inotropic agents may also be used. Angiotensin-converting enzyme (ACE) inhibitors are given to all patients with left ventricular ejection fraction (LVEF) under 40%. If there is a contraindication, hydralazine and isorbide dinitrate are used. In cardiogenic shock, aggressive supportive therapies, including intensive care, intraaortic balloon pumps, extracorporeal membrane oxygenation, or left ventricular assist devices, may be used. Anticoagulation is contraindicated in acute viral myopericarditis because of the danger of inducing cardiac tamponade. Beta-blockers should also be avoided in acute myocarditis, although they have been used successfully in dilated cardiomyopathy. It has been suggested that calcium channel blockers might prevent the coronary microvascular spasm of myocarditis.

Specific Antiviral Therapy
If diagnostic studies or epidemiologic data point to a virus for which specific therapy is available, use of such therapy would be reasonable, although efficacy in human myocarditis has not been demonstrated. Thus, in the initial viral phase, antiviral agents such as ganciclovir for CMV, amantadine for influenza A, or antiretrovirals for HIV could be beneficial.

Immunosuppressants
Studies of immunosuppressive treatment of myocarditis have produced conflicting results. In the murine model,

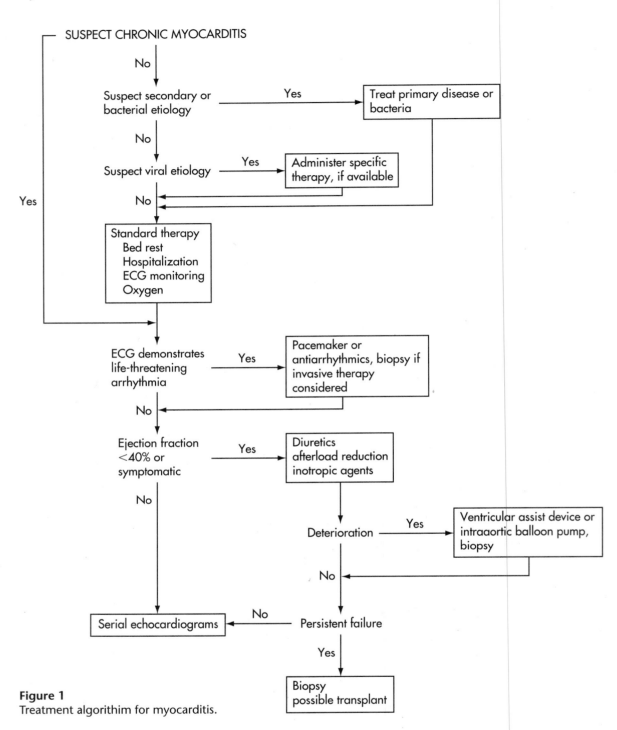

Figure 1
Treatment algorithim for myocarditis.

immunosuppression during the viral replication phases increases myocardial damage and worsens survival. In the best-designed study in humans thus far, the Myocarditis Treatment Trial (MTT), immunosuppressive therapy did not improve left ventricular ejection fraction or survival. However, the study was limited by the small number of biopsies that showed histologic myocarditis by the Dallas criteria and by the lack of agreement in biopsy interpretation between local pathologists and study panel cardiac pathologists. A matched-cohort study demonstrated clini-

cal, hemodynamic, and histologic improvement with prednisone combined with azathioprine or cyclosporin in children with active myocarditis and severe hemodynamic dysfunction. However, the study had methodologic flaws, including lack of blinding, questionable histologic criteria, and a small number of patients. Prednisone alone or combined with azathioprine or cyclosporin has not improved survival or left ventricular function in several other well-designed studies. There appears to be little to support the use of immunosuppressive therapy in acute viral myocardi-

Table 4 Proposed Therapies for Acute, Persistent, or Recurrent, and End-Stage Infectious Myocarditis

THERAPY	ACUTE	PERSISTENT OR RECURRENT	END STAGE
CONVENTIONAL AS INDICATED	+	+	+
Rest			
Reduced salt and fluid intake			
Digoxin			
Diuretics (i.e., furosemide, metolazone)			
Angiotensin-converting enzyme inhibitors (i.e., captopril)			
Hydralazine			
Nitrates			
Dopamine			
Antiarrhythmics			
Anticoagulation	−	±	±
IMMUNOSUPPRESSIVE	−	−	−
Corticosteroids			
Cyclosporin			
Azathioprine			
IMMUNOMODULATING			
Interferon	−	−	−
Intravenous immunoglobulin	+	−	−
TRANSPLANTATION	−	−	±

tis. In addition, because of the conflicting results noted, immunosuppressive therapy cannot be recommended for chronic active forms of myocarditis unless future well-designed studies with sufficient numbers of patients prove its efficacy.

Immunomodulators

In mice, high-dose immunoglobulin markedly improves survival when given at the time of viral infection. When used later in the postviremic phase, intravenous immunoglobulin (IVIG)-treated mice had less necrosis and myocyte inflammation than control animals. In a small, retrospective study of IVIG treatment of presumed acute myocarditis in children, treatment with IVIG was associated with superior recovery of left ventricular function compared with historical controls; there was a trend toward improved survival 1 year after presentation. In a case series of adults with new-onset dilated cardiomyopathy treated with high-dose immunoglobulin (IVIG), left ventricular ejection fraction improved 17 ejection fraction units at 1 year follow-up. Although IVIG treatment of myocarditis has not been evaluated in a prospective, controlled manner, its potential for adverse effects is limited. Thus a single dose of 2 g/kg for patients with decreased left ventricular function might be considered. Experience with other immunomodulating therapies such as interferon, thymus extract, or hyperimmune serum is limited, and they cannot be recommended.

■ PROGNOSIS

Because of the variety in presentation, it is unclear how often myocarditis progresses to dilated cardiomyopathy. Most patients with mild disease seem to recover completely over time. Using conventional therapy, the left ventricular ejection fraction can be expected to improve approximately 10% after 6 months. A proportion of patients will develop residual mild left ventricular dysfunction or dilated cardiomyopathy with concomitant arrhythmias and mural thrombi. Among patients who present in cardiogenic shock, a proportion survive the initial illness, and some will recover completely; however, chronic left ventricular dilation and dysfunction develop in the majority. In the MTT, a multivariate analysis identified a better left ventricular ejection fraction, less intensive conventional therapy, and a shorter duration of disease at baseline as independent predictors of improvement in left ventricular ejection fraction. The overall long-term prognosis was poor, with a rate of death or transplantation that was more than 55% within 5 years despite initial improvement in mean left ventricular ejection fraction. In adults, the 5-year survival in either myocarditis or DCM is about 55%. In a small fraction of patients who recover from myocarditis, the disease recurs. This occasionally has been related to withdrawal of immunosuppressive therapy. After an initial recurrence, subsequent recurrences are likely.

■ THE FUTURE OF MYOCARDITIS THERAPY

The application of immunohistochemical methods such as monoclonal antibodies to identify white blood cell subsets allows more sensitive characterization and localization of infiltrating cells. Polymerase chain reaction (PCR) allows amplification of distinct viral gene regions from endomyocardial biopsies with high sensitivity and specificity but does not allow localization. On the other hand, in situ hybridization using enterovirus probes can localize viral genomes to infected myocardial cells. The European Study of Epidemiology and Treatment of Cardiac Inflammatory Disease

(ESETCID) study is a multicenter, prospective, placebo-controlled, double-blind study that will enroll 250 subjects with biopsy-proven myocarditis and separate them into three subgroups (autoimmune myocarditis, enteroviral myocarditis, and CMV-induced myocarditis). In contrast to the MTT, ESETCID will use new laboratory techniques such as PCR and in situ hybridization as well as conventional histologic methods. Specific therapy will include immunoglobulin with ganciclovir for CMV myocarditis, interferon alpha for enterovirus, and prednisolone with azathioprine for autoimmune myocarditis. Unfortunately, the novel techniques that may allow more exact diagnosis are not widely available outside research settings at this time.

Suggested Reading

Garg A, Shiau J, Guyatt G: The ineffectiveness of immunosuppressive therapy in lymphocytic myocarditis: an overview, *Ann Intern Med* 128:317, 1998.

Maisch B, et al: The European Study of Epidemiology and Treatment of Cardiac Inflammatory Disease (ESETCID), *Eur Heart J* 16(suppl O): 173, 1995.

Mason JW, et al: A clinical trial of immunosuppressive therapy for myocarditis, *N Engl J Med* 333:269, 1995.

MEDIASTINITIS

Lisa S. Tkatch
Nelson M. Gantz

Mediastinitis, an infection involving the structures of the mediastinum, occurs as a result of infection at the surgical site, contiguous infection from the head and neck, extension from proximal infection with rupture into the mediastinum, esophageal perforation, or remote infection with chronic damage (fibrosing mediastinitis) (Table 1). Infection at the surgical site can result from surgery of the heart, neck, or esophagus. Contiguous infection most commonly occurs as a result of descending infection of the head and neck. Proximal infections, such as pneumonia or osteomyelitis of a rib, may rupture into the mediastinal compartments.

Table 1 Causes of Mediastinitis

Surgical site infection
- Cardiac, neck, or esophageal surgery

Contiguous infection from head and neck
- Descending necrotizing mediastinitis

Extension from proximal infection with rupture into mediastinum
- Pneumonia
- Osteomyelitis of rib

Esophageal perforation
- Swallowed foreign bodies
- Trauma
- Complication of endoscopy

Fibrosing mediastinitis
- Histoplasmosis
- Tuberculosis
- Autoimmune processes
- Radiation therapy

Esophageal perforation results from swallowed foreign bodies, esophageal carcinoma, and trauma or as a complication of fibrooptic endoscopy of the upper gastrointestinal tract. Fibrosing mediastinitis, characterized by an excessive fibrotic reaction that occurs in the mediastinum, is most commonly caused by histoplasmosis but may also occur as a result of autoimmune disorders. Of all these disorders, the most common cause of mediastinitis is infection at the surgical site from open-heart surgery, with an incidence of 0.4% to 5.9%.

Risk factors for the development of mediastinitis include the presence of certain underlying medical conditions such as diabetes mellitus, cigarette smoking, obesity, chronic obstructive pulmonary disease, the use of corticosteroids, decreased serum albumin, and prolonged preoperative hospital stay. Intraoperative risk factors, such as removal of chest hair by manual shaving, improper skin preparation, inadequate antibiotic prophylaxis, emergent surgery, prolonged duration of surgery, and/or cardiopulmonary bypass time, increase the risk of mediastinitis. Important postoperative factors that increase the risk of mediastinitis include the need for reoperation, excessive intrathoracic bleeding, prolonged mechanical ventilation, prolonged stay in the intensive care unit, need for tracheotomy, poor left ventricular function, and need for postoperative dialysis.

■ DIAGNOSIS

Characteristic signs and symptoms of mediastinitis depend on the underlying cause. Esophageal perforation initially may present with few symptoms; however, most patients note increased chest pain, respiratory distress, dysphagia, or fever. Infections that originate from a contiguous structure generally have symptoms related to that site. Fever, pain, erythema, or drainage from the surgical site characterizes postcardiothoracic surgical site infections, which usually present weeks to months after surgery. Purulent drainage from the chest wound may be the only physical finding. On the contrary, the incision site may be normal, and the only indication of infection may be a positive blood culture. Other physical findings may include instability of the sternum, bubbling of air from wound, and an audible or palpable mediastinal click or crunching sensation. Laboratory studies usually reveal a moderate leukocytosis with a leftward shift of the white blood cell (WBC) count differential. Computed tomography (CT) of the chest is helpful in diagnosis when mediastinal air, fluid, or both are detected radiographically after the fourteenth postoperative day. However, the most common CT findings are mediastinal soft-tissue swelling and bilateral pleural effusions, which are not specific for mediastinitis and may occur as a routine postoperative finding.

■ THERAPY

Once the diagnosis of mediastinitis is suspected, the entire incision should be reopened and the mediastinum explored. Therapy consists of surgical debridement and the use of antibiotics (Table 2). Aggressive debridement of all necrotic tissue and removal of foreign material is critical. Bone wax, fibrin, hematoma, bone fragments, and sutures must be removed because they can serve as foci for persistent infection. Before the mid 1970s, when the standard of care of mediastinitis was operative debridement followed by antibiotic irrigation or open packing, mortality rates approached 50%. Since then, aggressive surgical debridement and muscle flap or omental transposition for closure of the mediastinum has become more widely used, and morbidity and mortality rates (<10%) have significantly decreased.

Because of the severity and depth of the infection, intravenous antibiotics are preferred over oral antibiotics. The most common bacteria causing sternal wound infections after cardiac surgery are gram-positive cocci. Gram-negative bacilli and yeast play a less important role. Antimicrobial therapy should be guided by the results of susceptibility testing of pathogens recovered from the surgical wound and blood cultures (Table 3). Until these results are available, empiric therapy directed against methicillin-susceptible and methicillin-resistant *Staphylococcus* species using vancomycin is appropriate. The addition of rifampin and gentamicin may shorten time to sterilization with persistently positive blood cultures. Gram-negative coverage, with a third-generation cephalosporin or fluoroquinolone, may be appropriate if the institution has a high rate of gram-negative bacteria causing sternal wound infections. For patients who are allergic to penicillin and fluoroquinolone, aztreonam offers gram-negative coverage. If anaerobic coverage is desired, an extended-spectrum penicillin combined with a beta-lactamase inhibitor (e.g., piperacillin/tazobactam, 3.375 g IV q6h) would be useful because it also has gram-negative (including *Pseudomonas aeruginosa*) and gram-positive activity (including staphylococcus and some entero-

coccus). Empiric antifungal therapy is not warranted; however, if yeast is recovered in the culture, antimicrobial therapy with amphotericin B or fluconazole is indicated. Duration of intravenous antibiotic therapy should be about 6 weeks.

When culture results become available, antibiotic therapy should be guided by susceptibility data (Table 4). If the staphylococci are methicillin susceptible, nafcillin or oxacillin is given at a dosage of 2 g IV every 4 hours. Gentamicin should be given at a dosage of 1 mg/kg every 8 hours in a patient with normal renal function for the first 5 days of therapy. In a patient with an immediate-type allergic reaction to penicillin, vancomycin should be administered for methicillin-susceptible staphylococci. If the patient has a delayed reaction to penicillin, cefazolin, 2 g IV every 8 hours, is appropriate. Cephalosporins should be avoided in patients with methicillin-resistant infections caused by *S. aureus* or *S. epidermidis*. For enterococci, the clinician should administer ampicillin, 2 g IV every 4 hours, plus gentamicin, 1 mg/kg IV every 8 hours. If the patient has a history of a penicillin allergy but has normal renal function, vancomycin, 1 g IV every 12 hours, can be substituted for ampicillin. For strains of enterococci that are resistant to gentamicin, streptomycin may be substituted if the organism is susceptible. Optimal therapy for vancomycin-resistant enterococci is unknown, although chloramphenicol or quinupristin/dalfopristin may be effective in some cases.

P. aeruginosa infections should be treated with two drugs according to the results of susceptibility testing. Possible regimens include piperacillin or ticarcillin plus tobramycin, cefepime plus tobramycin, imipenem-cilastatin plus tobramycin, or aztreonam plus tobramycin. Amikacin, 7.5 mg/kg

---

Table 2 Treatment of Mediastinitis

Surgical treatment
 • Aggressive surgical drainage, debridement, and closure
Medical treatment
 • Intravenous antibiotics for 6 weeks directed against recovered pathogens from culture

---

Table 3 Empiric Antibiotic Therapy of Mediastinitis

SURGICAL SITE INFECTION AFTER OPEN-HEART SURGERY
Vancomycin,* 1 g IV q12h
If gram stain shows gram-negative bacilli or if increased risk of gram-negative infection, cefepime,* 2 g IV q12h, or ciprofloxacin,* 400 mg IV q12h
Amphotericin B, 0.7 mg/kg/day IV, or fluconazole,* 400 mg IV q24h, for documented yeast infection
For penicillin allergic patients with an immediate-type allergic reaction, aztreonam,* 1-2 g IV q6h, may be substituted for cefepime

PROXIMAL INFECTION (ANTIBIOTIC CHOICE DEPENDS ON PRIMARY SITE OF INFECTION)

DESCENDING INFECTION FROM DEEP STRUCTURES OF NECK
Penicillin G, 12-18 million U/day divided q4h, or clindamycin, 600 mg IV q8h

ESOPHAGEAL PERFORATION (NEED TO COVER ANAEROBES, AND AEROBIC GRAM-POSITIVE COCCI AND GRAM-NEGATIVE BACILLI)
Clindamycin, 600 mg IV q8h, plus ceftriaxone, 1 g IV q24h
or
Piperacillin/tazobactam,* 3.375 g IV q6h
or
Ticarcillin/clavulanate,* 3.1 g IV q6h

*Dosage adjustment necessary for renal insufficiency.

Table 4   Suggested Antibiotic Recommendations Against Recovered Pathogens

PATHOGEN	ANTIBIOTIC
Staphylococcus aureus susceptible to methicillin	Nafcillin, 2 g IV q4h, or oxacillin, 2 g IV q4h plus Gentamicin,* 1 mg/kg IV q8h for the first 5 days
• If penicillin allergic—delayed reaction	Cefazolin,* 2 g IV q8h
• If penicillin allergic—immediate reaction	Vancomycin,* 1 g IV q12h
S. aureus resistant to methicillin	Vancomycin,* 1 g IV q12h
Enterococcus species	Ampicillin,* 2 g IV q4h, plus gentamicin,* 1 mg/kg IV q8h
• If penicillin allergic	Vancomycin,* 1 g IV q12h
• If gentamicin resistant by susceptibility testing	Streptomycin,* 7.5 mg/kg IV q12h
Vancomycin-resistant enterococci	Chloramphenicol, 50 mg/kg/day IV divided into q6h doses or Quinupristin/dalfopristin, 7.5 mg/kg IV q8h
Enterobacteriaceae	Ceftriaxone, 1-2 g IV q 24h, plus gentamicin,* 1.5 mg/kg IV q8h or Piperacillin,* 3 g IV q4h, plus gentamicin,* 1.5 mg/kg IV q8h or Imipenem-cilastatin,* 500 mg IV q6h, plus gentamicin,* 1.5 mg/kg IV q8h or Aztreonam,* 1-2 g IV q6h, plus gentamicin,* 1.5 mg/kg IV q8h or Ciprofloxacin,* 400 mg IV q12h, plus gentamicin,* 1.5 mg/kg IV q8h
Pseudomonas aeruginosa	Piperacillin,* 3 g IV q4h, plus tobramycin,* 1.5 mg/kg IV q8h or Cefepime,* 2 g IV q12h, plus tobramycin,* 1.5 mg/kg IV q8h or Imipenem-cilastatin,* 500 mg IV q6h, plus tobramycin,* 1.5 mg/kg IV q8h or Aztreonam,* 1-2 g IV q6h, plus tobramycin,* 1.5 mg/kg IV q8h or Ciprofloxacin,* 400 mg IV q12h, plus tobramycin,* 1.5 mg/kg IV q8h
Candida albicans	Fluconazole,* 400 mg IV q24h or Amphotericin B, 0.7 mg/kg IV q24h
Non–*Candida albicans*	Amphotericin B, 0.7 mg/kg IV q24h

*Dosage adjustment necessary for renal insufficiency.

every 12 hours, should be substituted for tobramycin if the organism is resistant to tobramycin based on the results of susceptibility testing. If organisms are not recovered in culture or identified by pathologic examination and infection is suspected, empiric therapy with vancomycin plus a third-generation cephalosporin such as cefepime may be instituted. Imipenem-cilastatin may be substituted for cefepime. Clinical trials are needed to compare the success rates of the various regimens.

Mediastinitis caused by esophageal perforation and descending infections from the head and neck generally are polymicrobic. Anaerobes play an important role in addition to gram-positive cocci such as viridans streptococci and staphylococcal species. Gram-negative bacilli, including *Enterobacteriaceae* and *Pseudomonas* species, may be seen. Therefore a broad-spectrum antibiotic is appropriate; examples include piperacillin/tazobactam or ticarcillin/clavulanate, which are active against anaerobes, aerobic gram-positive cocci, and gram-negative bacilli. Duration of therapy may range from weeks to months, depending on the clinical response to therapy.

■ FIBROSING MEDIASTINITIS

Fibrosing mediastinitis refers to an excessive fibrotic reaction that occurs in the mediastinum. This reaction may lead to compression and occlusion of mediastinal structures, sometimes with devastating consequences such as superior vena cava syndrome; tracheal, bronchial, or carinal stenosis; esophageal obstruction; or bronchopulmonary fistulas.

Both infectious and noninfectious processes may cause fibrosing mediastinitis. Although it may be a sequela of granulomatous diseases such as tuberculosis or nocardia, the most common infectious cause of fibrosing mediastinitis is exposure to *Histoplasma capsulatum*. Organisms recovered from biopsy specimens are nonviable; therefore this process is not a result of active fungal proliferation but rather a result of a hypersensitivity reaction to healed infection. Noninfectious causes include autoimmune processes, radiation therapy, or association with other fibrosing conditions, such as retroperitoneal fibrosis, orbital pseudotumors, Riedel's sclerosing thyroiditis, and methylsergide therapy.

The most common symptoms of fibrosing mediastinitis

include dyspnea, hemoptysis, postobstructive pneumonia, and superior vena cava obstruction. Chest roentgenograms are almost always abnormal, with the most common finding being a large calcified hilar or subcarinal mass.

■ HISTOPLASMA FIBROSING MEDIASTINITIS

The dense fibrotic reaction invades vital mediastinal structures and obliterates normal tissue planes, making surgical dissection technically difficult and hazardous. Medical therapy is ineffective; steroids do not reverse the fibrosing process, and antifungal agents such as amphotericin B or itraconazole are ineffective because the organisms are nonviable.

Surgical intervention is necessary to manage the complications of mediastinal fibrosis. Biopsies may reveal granulomas with organisms consistent with histoplasmosis seen on silver methenamine stains in approximately one half of the cases.

Amphotericin B should be reserved for patients with active acute infection. However, some authors administer antifungal agents for 3 months to 1 year postoperatively in patients with *H. capsulatum* identified in biopsy material.

Suggested Reading

Jones G, et al: Management of the infected median sternotomy wound with muscle flaps, *Ann Surg* 225:766, 1997.

Mathisen DJ, Grillo HC: Clinical manifestation of mediastinal fibrosis and histoplasmosis, *Ann Thorac Surg* 54:1053, 1992.

McConkey SJ, et al. Results of a comprehensive infection control program for reducing surgical-site infections in coronary artery bypass surgery. *Infect Control Hosp Epidemiol* 20:533, 1999.

Milano CA, et al: Mediastinitis after coronary artery bypass graft surgery, *Circulation* 92:2245, 1995.

Munoz P, et al: Postsurgical mediastinitis: a case-control study, *Clin Infect Dis* 25:1060, 1997.

VASCULAR INFECTION

Susan E. Beekmann
David K. Henderson

Diagnosis and treatment of vascular infections is complex and depends on a variety of factors, including the location of the infected tissue, the microbiology of the infection, and patient-specific factors such as anatomy and immune status. Purulent or suppurative thrombophlebitis is inflammation of a peripheral or central venous wall because of the presence of microorganisms. Endarteritis (or infective arteritis) and mycotic aneurysms are infections of the arterial walls; arterial aneurysms or pseudoaneurysms are usually present because endarteritis may be difficult to diagnose unless an aneurysm is present. The term *mycotic aneurysm* is a misnomer that refers to any arterial aneurysm of infectious cause, fungal or bacterial, and may also include secondary infections of preexisting aneurysms or pseudoaneurysms. Vascular graft infections present an even wider spectrum of disease that depends on the type and location of the graft. Management of infections located on vascular prostheses is further complicated by the fact that prosthesis excision can jeopardize a patient's life and organ function, and alternative grafting techniques, including ex situ bypass and autologous reconstruction, must be considered.

■ PURULENT PHLEBITIS OF PERIPHERAL AND CENTRAL VEINS

Pathogenesis and Diagnosis

Purulent phlebitis is commonly associated with thrombosis, and the thrombus may act as a focus for local entrapment of bacteria that gain access to the site. Superficial suppurative thrombophlebitis is a complication of either dermal infections or indwelling intravenous catheters and is more common with plastic than with steel cannulas. Irritation of the vein wall and subsequent development of purulent thrombophlebitis occurs more often with polyethylene catheters than with Teflon or Silastic catheters and is higher in lower extremity cannulation. Central vein thrombosis is a relatively common complication of central venous catheterization, occurring in as many as one third of patients in some autopsy and clinical series. Central suppurative thrombophlebitis results from the bacterial or fungal contamination (sepsis) of these often asymptomatic thrombi.

Diagnosis of peripheral suppurative thrombophlebitis may be difficult if local findings of inflammation are absent, as often occurs in lower extremity cannulization. Local findings are much more common in suppurative thrombophlebitis of the upper extremities. Bacteremia is present in as many as 90% of patients with peripheral suppurative thrombophlebitis, and gross pus within the vein may be apparent in half of the patients. Suppurative thrombophlebitis of the thoracic central veins should be considered in any septic patient with a central venous catheter when bacteremia (or fungemia) fails to resolve after removal of the catheter and institution of appropriate antimicrobial therapy. Diagnosis can be established by venography with the demonstration of thrombi in a patient with bacteremia or fungemia. Computed tomography (CT) with contrast is also likely to be diagnostic; presence of gas in the venular lumen is typical of this condition. Magnetic resonance imaging (MRI) may be even more sensitive for diagnosis.

Therapy

Treatment of superficial suppurative thrombophlebitis traditionally has consisted of surgical excision plus parenteral antimicrobials. Most of the literature, which is derived primarily from burn center studies, strongly recommends vein excision, indicating that patients treated with antibiotics alone had a much higher death rate than patients who underwent surgical exploration. Other studies suggest that local incision and drainage of the involved site plus appropriate antimicrobial therapy may be sufficient in many nonburn cases. Patients who fail less radical surgery should then be referred for extensive surgical excision with total removal of all involved veins and drainage of contiguous abscesses.

Enterobacteriaceae caused more than half of all cases of suppurative thrombophlebitis in recent reviews, followed by *Pseudomonas aeruginosa, Staphylococcus aureus,* and *Candida albicans.* Initial empiric treatment might include vancomycin and either an aminoglycoside or a third- or fourth-generation cephalosporin with antipseudomonal activity in order to cover the *Enterobacteriaceae, Pseudomonas,* and *S. aureus* (both methicillin resistant and methicillin sensitive) until a culture of the infected material can be performed. Blood cultures should always be drawn before antibiotics are initiated. Empiric antibiotic choices should be tailored for known resistance patterns within hospitals and in geographic areas and may be adjusted based on Gram stain results. For example, a Gram stain of venular material showing gram-negative rods should result in discontinuation of vancomycin. Therapy with an appropriate antibiotic(s) should be continued once culture results are available. Treatment of suppurative thrombophlebitis caused by *C. albicans* is controversial because most of these infections can be cured by vein excision alone. Nonetheless, fluconazole, 400 to 800 mg/day, may be used, and amphotericin B ± 5FC is recommended in the immunosuppressed patient or if metastatic complications occur.

Treatment of central suppurative thrombophlebitis consists of catheter removal and parenteral antibiotics. The addition of full-dose anticoagulation is more controversial. Empiric antibiotic treatment is the same as for peripheral suppurative thrombophlebitis with the potential addition of an antipseudomonal penicillin. The antibiotics appropriate for the organisms identified from cultured material should be continued for at least 2 weeks after catheter removal. A minimum of 4 weeks of antimicrobial treatment is recommended after catheter removal when *S. aureus* is involved. Amphotericin B to a total dosage of at least 22 mg/kg ± 5FC is recommended for suppurative thrombophlebitis of the great central veins caused by *Candida* species; except for the intrinsically resistant species, including *C. glabrata* and *C. krusei;* fluconazole may be an acceptable alternative.

■ ARTERIAL INFECTIONS (MYCOTIC ANEURYSMS AND ARTERITIS)

Pathogenesis and Diagnosis

Mechanisms of arterial infection include (1) embolomycotic aneurysm secondary to septic microemboli (underlying infective endocarditis), (2) extension from a contiguous infected focus, (3) hematogenous seeding during bacteremia originating from a distant site, and (4) trauma to the vessel wall with direct contamination. Normal arterial intima is quite resistant to infection, but congenital or acquired malformation or disease (e.g., atherosclerosis) lowers resistance to infection, and hematogenous seeding of a previously damaged arteriosclerotic vessel currently constitutes the most common mechanism of infection. Mycotic aneurysms complicate infective endocarditis in approximately 5% to 10% of cases, with about half of these aneurysms involving the brain. Gram-positive organisms are the most common pathogens, with *S. aureus* accounting for approximately 30% to 40% of cases. Gram-negative bacteria are the causative organisms in approximately one third of cases, with *Salmonella* species found in about 20% of all cases.

Clinical manifestations depend to a large extent on the site of the aneurysm (Table 1). Although most infected aortic aneurysms occur in elderly atherosclerotic men (4 : 1 ratio, men > women), symptoms are nonspecific and may overlap with those of uninfected aneurysms. Fever and continuing bacteremia despite seemingly appropriate antimicrobial therapy is suggestive of an infected intravascular site.

Therapy

Despite improved prognosis for infected aneurysms of the thoracoabdominal vessels from earlier diagnosis and treatment, the case fatality rate for aortic aneurysms infected with gram-negative organisms may be as high as 75%. Currently accepted management is intravenous antibiotic therapy, excision and debridement of the artery or aneurysm, and extraanatomic vascular reconstruction along an uncontaminated path, where possible. Antibiotic therapy alone usually is insufficient without surgical resection of the infected tissue. Despite this axiom, surgical management of asymptomatic intracranial mycotic aneurysms does depend on their size and location because small lesions may resolve with antibiotic therapy alone. A reasonable approach would be to monitor by MRI every 2 to 3 weeks for 2 months. Surgery is indicated if the infected vessel is accessible or the lesions increase in size and should be considered if the lesions fail to decrease in size.

Basic principles of grafting in this situation include the use of autogenous rather than synthetic grafts and insertion only in clean, noninfected tissue planes. At surgery the aneurysm must be sectioned, Gram stained, and cultured; appropriate antibiotic therapy must be individualized and based on culture and sensitivity results. Bactericidal antibiotics should be continued for 6 to 8 weeks postoperatively.

Table 1 Diagnosis and Management of Mycotic Aneurysms

SITE	FREQUENCY OF DIAGNOSIS (RANGE)	CLINICAL PRESENTATION	IMAGING	MICROBIOLOGY	MANAGEMENT
GENERAL					
All infected aneurysms	100%	Fever common (70%–94%) Malaise, weight loss Pain (100%) Rapidly expanding mass Leukocytosis (65%–85%) Positive blood cultures (50%–75%)	*Findings:* Aneurysm with lack of intimal calcification Perianeurysmal fluid/gas collection *Studies:* CT with contrast MRI Ultrasonography (if accessible) Radionuclide-tagged WBC scans	*Staphylococcus* 30% (19%–34%) *Salmonella* 23% (20%–66%) *Streptococcus* 9% (11%–22%) *Escherichia coli* 6% IVDU: *S. aureus, Pseudomonas* sp. *Enterococcus* sp, *S. viridans*	*Surgical:* Wide debridement, irrigation with antibiotic solution of involved tissues, complete resection of aneurysm if possible *Antibiotic:* Empiric treatment with IV antibiotics for 6–8 wk after surgery based on culture results of resected tissue Follow-up blood cultures Consider chronic suppressive oral antibiotic therapy when extraanatomic bypass is not performed (i.e., for in situ repairs)
SPECIFIC					
Aorta Infrarenal abdominal aorta* Ascending aorta and arch (secondary to endocarditis)	27% (11%–75%)	Abdominal or back pain Palpable abdominal lesions (about 50%–65%) Vertebral osteomyelitis (lumbar/thoracic)	Frontal, lateral abdominal x-ray studies Abdominal ultrasound	*Salmonella* sp. have predilection for aorta	Extraanatomic arterial reconstruction (axillofemoral or aortofemoral)
Visceral artery Superior mesenteric,* splenic, hepatic, celiac, renal	24% (0%–29%)	Colicky abdominal pain Jaundice (hepatic artery) Hemoptysis or hemothorax (celiac artery)	Ultrasound may exclude other causes (e.g., pancreatic masses)	*Bacteroides fragilis* reported from supraceliac aorta and celiac artery	Complete excision may be hazardous; careful drainage and longer-term antibiotic therapy may be necessary
Iliac	4% (0%–25%)	Thigh pain, quadriceps wasting, depressed knee jerk Arterial insufficiency of extremity			Excision and arterial ligation; reconstruction usually can wait until infection has resolved
Arm Radial artery* Brachial artery Subclavian artery	10% (0%–9%)	Pain over site of lesion About 90% palpable May appear as cellulitis, abscess; distal embolic lesions; skin changes common			Proximal ligation of the vessel, resection of the aneurysm and appropriate drainage should be followed by antibiotic therapy

CT, Computed tomography; *MRI*, magnetic resonance imaging; *WBC*, white blood cell; *IV*, intravenous; *IVDU*, intravenous drug user.
*Most common site or manifestation.

Continued

Table 1 Diagnosis and Management of Mycotic Aneurysms—cont'd

SITE	FREQUENCY OF DIAGNOSIS (RANGE)	CLINICAL PRESENTATION	IMAGING	MICROBIOLOGY	MANAGEMENT
Leg Femoral artery*	12% (4%-44%)	Pain over site of lesion About 90% palpable Pulsatile mass, decreased peripheral pulses Possible local suppuration, distal embolic lesions; petechiae, purpura		*S. aureus* incidence as high as 65%	Excision and arterial ligation; reconstruction usually can wait until infection has resolved Autogenous grafting may allow reconstruction through the bed of the resected aneurysm if anastomoses performed in clean tissue planes
Intracranial Peripheral middle cerebral artery*	4%	Usually clinically silent May appear as severe unremitting headache Usually secondary to endocarditis	Four-vessel cerebral arteriography invaluable MRI	*Enterococcus* sp. *S. viridans* *Pseudomonas* sp. *Candida albicans*	

Table 2 Diagnosis and Management of Vascular Graft Infections

SITE	CLINICAL PRESENTATION	MICROBIOLOGY	IMAGING	MANAGEMENT
GENERAL				
Any infected vascular graft	*Early (<4 mo):* Immediate postoperative infections rare; usually associated with wound sepsis Fever, leukocytosis, bacteremia Anastomotic bleeding (most common with gram-negative organisms) Wound healing complication *Late:* Systemic signs few or absent; WBC count often normal Tenderness, erythema of skin over prosthesis Anastomotic false aneurysm Graft-enteric erosion, fistula	*Staphylococcus aureus* Coagulase-negative staphylococci *Streptococcus* *Escherichia coli* *Klebsiella* *Pseudomonas*	*Findings:* Perigraft fluid, gas collection; abnormal appearance of perigraft soft tissues; abscess; pseudoaneurysm formation *Studies: Anatomic imaging study:* 1. CT with contrast, or 2. MRI with contrast and fat saturation; or, for superficial grafts: 3. Ultrasonography *Radioisotope studies that may be useful:* 1. WBC-labeled indium scan, or 2. Tc99-HMPAO-labeled WBC, if available	*Surgical:* Wide debridement, irrigation with antibiotic solution of involved tissues (commonly used but efficacy data not available); graft excision when possible with ex situ bypass reconstruction Consider thorough debridement with myocutaneous flap for patients with a patent graft, intact anastomoses, absence of hemorrhage, and sterile blood cultures *Antibiotic:* Empiric treatment with IV antibiotics for 4 wk after surgery based on culture results of resected tissue Follow-up blood cultures Consider chronic suppressive oral antibiotic therapy if infected graft not removed
SPECIFIC				
Aortoiliac	Higher incidence in months 8-15 First symptoms, fever, slightly increased WBC count Later, abdominal, back pain, false aneurysm formation Finally, hemorrhage	*E. coli* *S. aureus* *Streptococcus* *S. epidermidis* (or coagulase-negative staphylococci)	MRI more sensitive than CT for aortal graft infection	Place axillofemoral or bifemoral graft, then remove entire aortic graft Close arteriotomy sites with monofilament sutures, irrigate with antibiotic solution (no efficacy data)
Aortofemoral	False aneurysm in groin site Wound infection or abscess in inguinal incision Pulsatile mass at groin site	*S. aureus* *S. epidermidis* *Proteus* sp. *E. coli* *Streptococcus* Other gram-negative bacilli	Ultrasonography can be useful in femoral area	May be possible to remove only infected part of graft (one limb), although continued infection likely without removal of entire graft Extraanatomic bypass when possible
Axillofemoral	Same as for aortofemoral	Same as for aortofemoral	Same as for aortofemoral	Remove entire graft Intraabdominal graft may suffice for revascularization; high amputation and death rates
Femoropopliteal	Higher incidence in first 3 mo Small sinus tract, abscess, cellulitis in inguinal incision	*S. aureus* *Streptococcus* *S. epidermidis* Other gram-negative bacilli		Remove entire graft Nonviable limbs must be revascularized or amputated; delay amputation as long as possible to allow maximum development of collaterals

WBC, White blood cell; *MRI*, magnetic resonance imaging; *CT*, computed tomography; *IV*, intravenous.

■ VASCULAR GRAFT INFECTIONS

Pathogenesis and Diagnosis

Reported incidence of vascular graft infections ranges from 0.8% to 6% and varies with the site of graft placement and prosthetic graft material. For example, procedures requiring an inguinal incision have an incidence of infection that is two to three times higher than procedures not requiring an inguinal incision; use of a vascular prosthesis results in significantly higher infection rates than autologous reconstruction. Most contamination likely occurs at the time of implantation, although both hematogenous seeding as well as bacteria harbored in atherosclerotic plaques may account for some late graft infections. Prophylactic systemic antibiotics at time of graft placement have been associated with a decrease in vascular graft infections in recent years. Prophylactic antibiotics should be considered mandatory with placement of vascular grafts.

Staphylococci remain the most prevalent pathogens, with *S. epidermidis* infections often presenting months to years after the operation and *S. aureus* most commonly causing early infections (Table 2). More than 70% of infections involving vascular grafts of the groin and lower extremities develop within 1 to 2 months of surgery, whereas 70% of intraabdominal graft infections do not manifest until months or years after surgery.

Appropriate imaging of the infected area is vital to diagnosis because the extent of local infections may not be recognized if imaging techniques are inadequate. Angiography often is unhelpful in the diagnosis of vascular graft infections, but it is useful for identifying aortoenteric fistulas and guiding the surgical procedure. An anatomic imaging study should be performed. Ultrasound can be used for superficial grafts, including dialysis shunts; a CT with contrast or an MRI with contrast and fat saturation should be performed for deeper grafts. If doubt about infection still exists, radioisotope imaging can be performed using either indium-111-labeled leukocytes or, if available, technetium-99 HMPAO-labeled leukocytes. These studies, although sensitive, are limited by low specificity, particularly in the early postoperative setting (up to 12 weeks after surgery).

Therapy

The greatest likelihood of successful outcome after vascular graft infection requires intensive antibiotic therapy and graft excision with extraanatomic revascularization if distal ischemia is present. Revascularization should be delayed, if possible, to establish potential collateral circulation and to decrease bacterial levels. Although antibiotic treatment and local wound care usually are unsuccessful when used alone, very specific criteria are now defining a subset of patients who may be managed without removal of the entire graft. These criteria include the following (at a minimum): a patent graft, intact and uninvolved anastomoses, absence of hemorrhage, and sterile blood cultures. Diabetic patients and those receiving long-term systemic steroid therapy should be considered at highest risk for continued infection without graft removal and extraanatomic bypass. Likelihood of successful graft preservation appears to be highest with low-grade early staphylococcal infection and lowest with gram-negative infections. The optimal therapy of infected vascular grafts remains removal of the entire graft and revascularization where necessary through uninfected tissue planes.

If a new graft must be placed in the infected field, use of autogenous artery or vein grafts may decrease susceptibility to infection. In the absence of available autologous vessels, polytetrafluoroethylene (PFTE) grafts may constitute the most reasonable alternative. Parenteral antibiotics should be administered for 4 weeks after the infected graft is removed, and some authorities have recommended administering oral antibiotics for an additional 1 to 3 months.

Suggested Reading

Bandyk DF, Esses GE: Prosthetic graft infection, *Surg Clin North Am* 74:571, 1994.

Hannon RJ, Wolfe JHN, Mansfield AO: Aortic prosthetic infection: 50 patients treated by radical or local surgery, *Br J Surg* 654:654, 1996.

Henke PK, et al: Current options in prosthetic vascular graft infection, *Am Surg* 64:39, 1998.

Law NW, Parvin SD, Darke SG: Diagnostic features and management of bacterial arteritis with false aneurysm formation, *Eur J Vasc Surg* 8:199, 1994.

Veith FJ, et al, eds: *Vascular surgery: principles and practice*, ed 2, New York, 1994, McGraw-Hill.

PACEMAKER AND DEFIBRILLATOR INFECTIONS

Stacey R. Vlahakis
James M. Steckelberg

Implantable cardiac pacemakers and defibrillators have greatly decreased the morbidity and mortality rates associated with cardiac arrhythmias. Increasing numbers of people are receiving these devices as the procedures for implantation and device technology improve; as a result, increasing numbers of devices are at risk for infection. The cumulative risk of pacemaker- and defibrillator-related infections after implantation has been estimated to be between 1% and 19% over the lifetime of the device. Infection of these implantable devices is associated with excess morbidity, including prolonged hospital stays and mortality rates as high as 30% in one series.

The first single-chamber permanent pacemakers were introduced for clinical use in the late 1950s. Today, it is estimated that approximately 1 million people in the United States have permanent pacemakers. The pacemaker itself consists of a generator, placed below the pectoral muscle, that serves as the power source. An electrical stimulus from the generator travels through an insulated electrical conductor to the electrodes, which deliver the impulse to the endocardium, or epicardial surface.

Early implantable cardioverter defibrillator devices (ICDs) required surgical placement of epicardial defibrillation patches, which was facilitated by sternotomy, lateral thoracotomy, or subxiphoid approach. Since 1988, transvenous placement of endocardial coils, similar to pacemakers, has become routine practice. In addition, generator packs have become smaller, allowing for pectoral placement as opposed to the traditional abdominal placement of larger, older generators. These technologic advances have reduced the morbidity rates associated with implantation and lowered the incidence of infection. In some cases, however, subcutaneous mesh patch electrodes are necessary for adequate defibrillation thresholds. These patches have been associated with a threefold higher infection rate.

Several risk factors that predispose patients to developing infections of their pacemakers or defibrillators have been identified (Table 1). Infection of pacemakers occurs more

often among patients with diabetes then among nondiabetic patients. However, studies have not adequately determined whether the greater number of device infections in diabetic patients is secondary only to a greater prevalence of implantable antiarrhythmic devices in this population or to an increased incidence of infection among diabetic patients with pacemakers. Other common risk factors include recurrent local surgical procedures after implantation of the device, skin disorders such as a rash or acne, systemic steroid use, and postinsertion hematomas at the generator site.

The microbiology of pacemaker and defibrillator infections is similar to that of other implantable prosthetic devices (Table 2). Early infections, within 4 weeks of implantation of the device, generally are related to device or wound contamination at the time of surgery. *Staphylococcus aureus* is the most common microbial cause. Infections occurring more than 4 weeks after device implantation typically are caused by less virulent organisms, such as coagulase-negative staphylococci. Other gram-positive organisms such as *Enterococcus* species, *Peptostreptococcus* species, or less commonly, gram-negative bacilli such as *Klebsiella* species, *Escherichia coli*, and *Pseudomonas* species, have also been reported. *Aspergillus* species, *Candida* species, and *Mycobacterium avium-intracellulare* infections have also been described but are rare.

Implantable antiarrhythmic device infections are associated with several different clinical syndromes. Infection can involve the generator pocket, the lead wires, native valve endocarditis, or a combination of these. Infections at the generator pocket are most common and may present with localized pain, erythema, and erosion of the skin over the generator or drainage from the pocket. A thick, yellowish, purulent drainage from the pocket with surrounding erythema is more often caused by *S. aureus,* whereas clear drainage without erythema is generally caused by less virulent organisms such as *S. epidermidis.* The fibrous scar tissue surrounding the generator pocket is relatively avascular. This avascular tissue combined with a foreign body has been postulated to predispose the patient to persistent local infection. Patients with electrode or cardiac valve infection may have nonspecific symptoms such as fevers, chills, arthralgias, or wasting.

In patients with local symptoms of infection at the generator pocket, diagnosis is relatively straightforward. Sterilely obtained samples of fluid or drainage from the pocket should be cultured when possible. Blood cultures should also be obtained before beginning antimicrobial treatment to exclude an associated bacteremia. Positive blood cultures strongly suggest lead infection or endocarditis. Endocarditis related to pacemaker or defibrillator lead infections is rare and usually involves the tricuspid valve.

Several series have investigated the ability of echocardiography to identify lead vegetations. Transthoracic echocardiography has a sensitivity of about 30%, and transesophageal echocardiography has a sensitivity of about 95%. Other diagnostic tests that can be used to identify infections on implantable antiarrhythmic devices include computed tomography (CT) and gallium scans. CT scans are most helpful in identifying inflammation at the site of epicardial defibrillator patches, and gallium scans have been used to

Table 1 Patient Risk Factors for Infection of Implantable Pacemakers or Defibrillators
Diabetes mellitus
Multiple surgical procedures
Postinsertion hematoma
Systemic steroids
Skin disorders

Table 2   Most Common Site of Infection and Associated Organism According to Time after Device Implantation

TIME OF ONSET AFTER PLACEMENT		SITE OF INFECTION	SYMPTOMS	MOST COMMON ORGANISM
Early	2-4 wk	Pocket	Local	*Staphylococcus aureus*
Late	>4 wk	Pocket and/or electrodes	Local and/or systemic	Coagulase-negative *Staphylococcus*

Table 3   Recommended Initial Antimicrobial Choice According to the Organism and Its Susceptibilities

ORGANISM	SUSCEPTIBILITY	PRIMARY	ALTERNATIVE
Staphylococcus aureus	Penicillin sensitive	Penicillin G, 2-5 mU q4-6h*	Cefazolin, 1-2 g q8h Ceftriaxone, 1 g q24h
Staphylococcus epidermidis	Penicillin resistant Methicillin sensitive Methicillin resistant	Oxacillin, 1-2 g q4-6h Nafcillin, 1-2 g q4-6h Vancomycin, 15 mg/kg q12h†	Cefazolin, 1-2 g q8h
Enterococcus spp.	Penicillin sensitive Penicillin resistant	Penicillin G, 2-5 mU q4-6h* Ampicillin, 1-2 g q4-6h* Vancomycin, 15 mg/kg q12h†	Vancomycin, 15 mg/kg q12h†
Enterobacteriaceae‡	Empiric treatment Directed treatment (based on cultures)	Cefepime, 1-2 g q12h* Ceftazidime, 1-2 g q8h* Least expensive, least toxic active agent	Quinolone§ Imipenim, 500 mg q6h*
Pseudomonas aeruginosa‡,‖		Cefepime, 1-2 g q12h* Ceftazidime, 1-2 g q12h*	Quinolone§ Imipenem, 500 mg q6h* Aztreonam, 0.5-2 g q8h*

*Dosages adjusted for renal function.
†Monitor and adjust dosage.
‡For some organisms, combination therapy is appropriate.
§For example, ciprofloxacin, 200-400 mg q12h IV/250-750 mg bid PO,* or levofloxacin, 500 mg qd IV or PO.*
‖Based on susceptibilities.

delineate the extent of pacemaker or defibrillator infection; however, gallium scans are more useful when negative.

After appropriate cultures have been obtained, antimicrobial treatment should begin (Table 3). Empiric coverage should include antimicrobials with activity against *S. aureus* and coagulase-negative staphylococci. For methicillin-susceptible staphylococci, a beta-lactamase–resistant penicillin such as oxacillin is appropriate. However, if sensitivities are unknown or the staphylococcus is methicillin resistant, vancomycin should be used. Enterococci are intrinsically resistant to cephalosporins and require penicillin or vancomycin, depending on sensitivities. Treatment for infections caused by gram-negative organisms should be directed by the susceptibilities. Cephalosporins, quinolones, or expanded-spectrum penicillins are often appropriate choices.

Most series report high relapse rates without complete explantation of the pacing or defibrillating system. However, there are a few case reports of salvage of an infected generator, using intravenous antibiotics and 5 days of continuous irrigation to the pocket.

The least invasive surgical procedure possible should be used to explant the device. Removing the leads transvenously with traction through the original site has been shown to be adequate in several series. However, this procedure can be very difficult and result in avulsion of the tricuspid valve, arteriovenous fistulas, or retention of lead tip. Recent advances with laser treatment has improved transvenous lead extraction greatly. A laser sheath is slid over the length of the electrode and used to excise the implanted lead, allowing the entire lead to be withdrawn with little trauma. If complete lead removal is not possible transvenously, if large vegetations are present on the lead, or if epicardial patches need to be removed, an open surgical procedure is required. The risk of untreated infection compared with the risks of thoracotomy must be weighed for each clinical scenario. In one small nonrandomized study, eight patients remained infection free after 4 weeks total of antimicrobial therapy despite retained lead tips after attempted transvenous lead removal.

The new pacing or defibrillating system (when required) should be implanted at a distant site. It is common practice to delay reimplantation and treat with intravenous antibiotics; however, a one-stage procedure was effective in one series of 31 patients. In another small nonrandomized study, 2 weeks of antimicrobial therapy before reimplantation, followed by 10 days of additional antimicrobial treatment, was successful. After the new device is implanted, antimicrobial therapy should be continued for 10 days to 2 weeks for less virulent organisms associated with rapid fever resolution and clinical improvement. A longer course of therapy should be used for more virulent organisms or in patients with prolonged fevers, persistent bacteremia, or endocarditis. Up to 6 weeks of antimicrobial therapy may be appropriate in these latter settings.

Preventing infections of implantable antiarrhythmic devices is fundamental. Because most early infections result from wound contamination at the time of surgery, a good skin preparation before surgery is essential. It remains standard practice to give antistaphylococcal antimicrobial prophylaxis before implantation. Although the evidence for this recommendation remains inconclusive, preoperative antimicrobial prophylaxis has proven successful for other intravascular implantable devices. Regarding endocarditis prophylaxis, the American Heart Association does not recommend antimicrobial prophylaxis for patients with implantable antiarrhythmic devices undergoing dental or other procedures associated with transient bacteremias.

Suggested Reading

Klug D, et al: Systemic infection related to endocarditis on pacemaker leads, *Circulation* 95:2098, 1997.

Molina JE: Undertreatment and overtreatment of patients with infected antiarrhythmic implantable devices, *Ann Thorac Surg* 63:504, 1997.

Smith PN, et al: Infections with nonthoracotomy implantable cardioverter defibrillators: can these be prevented? *PACE* 21:42, 1998.

Victor F, et al: Pacemaker lead infection: echocardiographic features, management, and outcome, *Heart* 81:82, 1999.

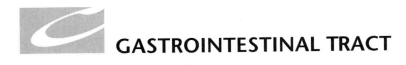

ACUTE VIRAL HEPATITIS

Steven-Huy Han
Paul Martin

Viral hepatitis is a major cause of morbidity and mortality in the United States. Five major hepatotropic viruses (A, B, C, D, and E) cause hepatitis, resulting in necrosis and inflammation of the liver. These viruses differ in their ability to cause acute and chronic hepatitis. Hepatitis A and E viruses cause acute hepatitis only, which is defined as necro-inflammatory activity of the liver of less than 6 months' duration. Hepatitis B, C, and D viruses also cause acute hepatitis but in addition may progress to chronic infection that can ultimately lead to cirrhosis and hepatocellular carcinoma. Hepatitis G virus has also been associated with acute and chronic infection, but its clinical significance remains unclear. Other viruses, such as acute Epstein-Barr virus (EBV) and cytomegalovirus (CMV), can present with prominent hepatic dysfunction, although they are usually multisystem disorders.

■ HEPATITIS A VIRUS

The hepatitis A virus (HAV) is an RNA virus transmitted via the fecal-oral route and is a common cause of acute hepatitis in North America. In the Third World, HAV infection typically occurs in childhood and is subclinical, with most of the population exposed before adulthood. HAV infection, occurring in older children and adults, is more likely to be symptomatic and associated with morbidity and even mortality. The incubation period is 15 to 45 days, with peak fecal viral shedding and infectivity before the onset of clinical symptoms, which can include anorexia, fever, malaise, fatigue, nausea, vomiting, diarrhea, and right upper quadrant discomfort. In acute HAV infection, these symptoms tend to occur 1 to 2 weeks before the onset of jaundice.

The typical serologic course of acute HAV is shown in Figure 1. Recovery is usually uneventful. However, the illness occasionally is bimodal, with apparent recovery followed by return of symptoms before eventual recovery. A prolonged cholestatic phase may also occur, with clinical symptoms characterized by persistent jaundice with prominent pruritis. It is important to recognize the rare fulminant case of HAV infection. Most typically, this occurs in adults. Features that suggest its onset include a prolonged prothrombin time,

hypoglycemia, profound jaundice, or early signs of hepatic encephalopathy. Urgent referral to a liver transplant program is indicated.

The routine diagnosis of HAV infection is made by detection of IgM anti-HAV antibody in serum (Table 1). IgM anti-HAV persists for 3 to 12 months after infection. IgG anti-HAV antibody, present early in infection, persists indefinitely. The presence of IgG anti-HAV alone indicates previous infection with development of immunity to HAV.

Therapy

Acute hepatitis secondary to HAV is self-limited without chronic sequelae. The major goal of therapy in all forms of acute viral hepatitis is supportive. It should include bed rest if the patient is very symptomatic, a high-calorie diet, avoidance of hepatotoxic medications, and abstinence from alcohol (Table 2). Because acute HAV is more likely to lead to hepatocellular failure in adults, the adult with acute HAV needs close follow-up until symptoms resolve.

Prevention of HAV infection consists of proper hygiene and immunization. General measures include careful hand-washing practices, especially with food preparation and handling; proper disposal of waste and sewage; and a clean water supply. Passive prophylaxis before and after exposure with HAV immunoglobulin, 0.02 ml/kg intramuscularly (IM), has been shown to be safe and efficacious. The following high-risk groups should receive prophylaxis: (1) close household and sexual contacts of a patient with documented acute HAV, (2) staff and patients of institutions for the developmentally disabled with outbreaks of HAV, (3) children and staff of day-care centers with an index case of HAV, (4) those exposed to protracted community outbreaks, and (5) travelers and military personnel who plan to visit countries endemic for HAV. A vaccine made with inactivated HAV has been available in the United States since 1995. It is recommended for travelers to endemic areas, nonimmune residents of such areas, others with potential occupational exposures such as caretakers in institutions for the developmentally challenged and any person with underlying chronic liver disease because of reports of severe acute HAV in individuals with underlying liver disease. A dose of 1 ml as an IM injection into the deltoid muscle should be followed by a booster dose 6 to 12 months later. The initial dose should be given at least 1 month before possible exposure.

Earlier studies had suggested that HAV immunoglobulin given passively interferes with the active immune response after vaccination if given simultaneously, resulting in lower antibody titers. However, recent controlled trials comparing antibody responses after concurrent passive immunization and vaccination with passive immunization or vaccination alone have not demonstrated a significant difference in overall protection. In fact, more durable protection was

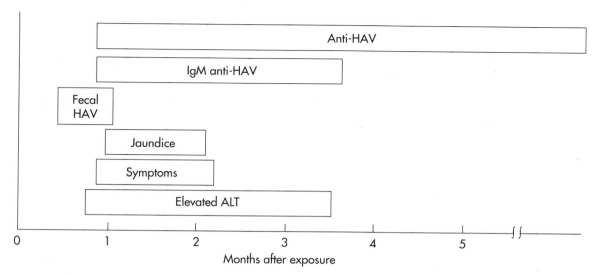

Figure 1
Course of acute hepatitis A. *HAV,* Hepatitis A virus; *ALT,* alanine aminotransferase; *anti-HAV,* antibody to hepatitis A virus. *(Adapted from Martin P, Friedman LS, Dienstag JL: Diagnostic approach to viral hepatitis. In Thomas HC, Zuckerman AJ, eds:* Viral hepatitis, *Edinburgh, 1993, Churchill Livingstone. Used with permission.)*

Table 1   Diagnostic Testing for Viral Hepatitis

TYPE	DIAGNOSTIC TESTS	COMMENTS
Hepatitis A virus (HAV)	IgM anti-HAV	Acute infection
	IgG anti-HAV	Resolved infection
Hepatitis B virus (HBV)	HBsAg	Indicates infection
	IgM anti-HBc	Acute infection
	HBeAg, HBV DNA	Indicates replication
	Anti-HBs	Indicates immunity
	IgG anti-HBc	Current or prior infection
Hepatitis C virus (HCV)	Anti-HCV	Indicates infection
	HCV RNA	Indicates infection/viremia
Hepatits D virus (HDV)	IgM anti-HDV	IgM anti-HBc positive indicates coinfection
		IgG anti-HBc positive indicates superinfection
	Anti-HDV	Indicates infection
	HDV RNA and HDV Antigen	Research tools at present
Hepatitis E virus (HEV)	IgM anti-HEV	Acute infection
	IgG anti-HEV	Resolved infection
Hepatitis G virus (HGV)	Anti-HGV (anti-E2)	Research tool at present
	HGV RNA	Research tool at present
TT virus (TTV)	TTV DNA	Research tool at present

achieved in persons receiving passive immunoglobulin and vaccine than in persons receiving passive immunoglobulin alone. Therefore concurrent administration of HAV immunoglobulin and vaccine is now recommended for preexposure and postexposure prophylaxis in high-risk individuals. Antiviral therapy has no role in the treatment of hepatitis A.

■ HEPATITIS B VIRUS

Hepatitis B virus (HBV) is the most common cause of chronic viral hepatitis worldwide and is a major cause of

acute viral hepatitis. In the Far East and Africa, up to 20% of the population has serologic evidence of current or prior HBV infection. In the United States, HBV infection is less frequent, although 0.5% of the population is chronically infected.

HBV is a DNA virus transmitted predominantly by intimate contact or percutaneous exposure. The incubation period is 45 to 160 days. The typical course of a patient with acute HBV infection is shown in Figure 2. Typically, elevated alanine aminotransferase (ALT) levels and clinical symptoms appear just before the onset of jaundice. However, not all patients with acute HBV infection develop jaundice.

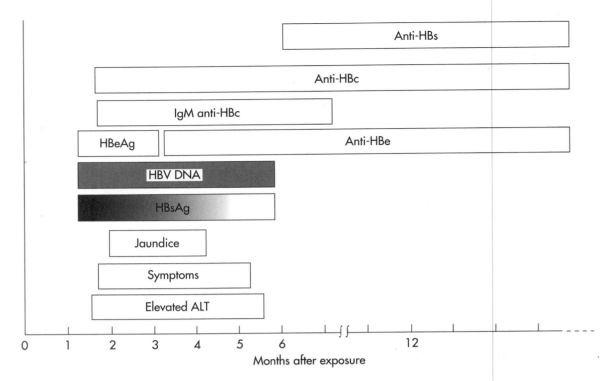

Figure 2
Typical course of acute hepatitis B. *HBsAg,* Hepatitis B surface antigen; *ALT,* alanine aminotransferase; *HBV DNA,* hepatitis B virus DNA; *HBeAg,* hepatitis B e antigen; *Anti-HBc,* antibody to hepatitis B core antigen; *Anti-HBe,* antibody to hepatitis B e antigen; *Anti-HBs,* antibody to hepatitis B surface antigen. *(Adapted from Martin P, Friedman LS, Dienstag JL: Diagnostic approach to viral hepatitis. In Thomas HC, Zuckerman AJ, eds:* Viral hepatitis, *Edinburgh, 1993, Churchill Livingstone. Used with permission.)*

Table 2   Therapy of Acute Viral Hepatitis

TYPE	MAJOR FOCUS	COMMENTS
Hepatitis A	Symptomatic therapy only	Recognition of FHF and referral for orthotopic liver transplantation important
Hepatitis B	Symptomatic therapy for acute disease; (?) lamivudine for therapy of acute infection	Observe for FHF
Hepatitis C	Interferon-alpha for acute infection	Treatment efficacious in acute hepatitis C virus
Hepatitis D	Vaccination against HBV	Liver disease clinically more severe than hepatitis B virus alone
Hepatitis E	Symptomatic therapy only	FHF can be seen in pregnant women
Hepatitis G	No recommended therapy	No information available on role of antiviral agents
TT virus	No recommended therapy	No information available on role of antiviral agents

FHF, Fulminant hepatic failure.

Paradoxically, the patient with anicteric and less clinically severe acute HBV infection is more likely to become chronically infected than the individual with more symptomatic acute infection because a brisk immune response causes more hepatic dysfunction but also a greater chance of clearance of HBV. The symptomatic patient should be reassured that full recovery is likely but should be warned to report back if symptoms such as deepening jaundice, severe

nausea, or somnolence develop because these symptoms may be the first manifestations of possible fulminant hepatic failure.

The diagnosis of acute HBV hepatitis is made by the detection of hepatitis B surface antigen (HBsAg) and IgM anti–hepatitis B core antibody (anti-HBc IgM) in the serum (Table 3). Resolution of HBV infection is characterized by the loss of HbsAg. IgG anti–hepatitis B core antibody (anti-

Table 3 Initial Serologic Workup of Suspected Acute Hepatitis
IgM anti-HAV
HBsAg
(If positive, then IgM anti-HBc)
Anti-HCV

HBc IgG) appears slowly after IgM anti-HBc and persists throughout life. The appearance of anti–hepatitis B surface antibody (anti-HbsAb) indicates immunity to HBV.

In adults, more than 95% of patients with acute HBV infection have successful clearance of HBV; the remainder develop chronic infection. Individuals who are immuno-compromised or have another chronic condition such as renal failure are more likely to develop chronic infection. Children younger than 7 years of age and the elderly also have a greater likelihood of becoming chronically infected. The absence of a brisk immune response during acute HBV infection, manifested by few symptoms, absence of jaundice, and modest ALT elevation, predicts that infection is more likely to become chronic. Chronic HBV infection is diagnosed by documenting HBsAg positivity for longer than 6 months and absence of IgM anti-HBc. The presence of HBeAg and HBV DNA in the serum suggest ongoing active viral replication or "high replicative state" in a patient with chronic infection. The absence of these markers of active replication in a chronically infected patient with no clinical evidence of liver disease is sometimes referred to as the "healthy carrier state," although the preferred term now is *low replicative state.*

Therapy

Interferon-alpha and lamivudine (an oral nucleoside analog) are the only two currently available therapies in the United States for the treatment of chronic HBV infection. Therapy is indicated for patients with HBsAg positivity with increased ALT levels for more than 6 months, active viral replication indicated by serum HBeAg positivity, and compensated liver disease. Therapy for chronic HBV infection is discussed in the chapter *Chronic Hepatitis.*

The highly effective recombinant HBV vaccine is recommended for all newborns, infants, adolescents, health care workers, and emergency services personnel (e.g., paramedics, police). Postexposure prophylaxis should consist of a combination of HBV vaccination and passive protection with hepatitis B immunoglobulin (HBIG).

In the rare case of acute fulminant HBV infection or in the patient with progressive end-stage liver disease, orthotopic liver transplantation (OLT) is an option. HBV tends to recur after transplant with a frequently aggressive course, at times causing failure of the transplanted liver as early as 6 months after the transplant. Transplant centers have had encouraging results with the use of perioperative and postoperative high-dose polyclonal HBIG, which is now usually part of the regimen to prevent reinfection of the transplanted liver. However, indefinite HBIG therapy is both cumbersome and expensive. Accordingly, transplant programs are evaluating the use of alternative schedules of HBIG administration and newer antiviral agents (i.e., lamivudine) to prevent allograft reinfection. Most recently, prophylaxis with combination HBIG and lamivudine has been shown to be effective in preventing HBV reinfection after transplant.

■ HEPATITIS C VIRUS

The hepatitis C virus (HCV) is a single-stranded RNA virus and is the major cause of what was formerly known as posttransfusional non-A, non-B hepatitis. HCV may cause acute hepatitis, with as many as 85% of infected individuals developing chronic infection. Acute HCV is typically subclinical, with less than a third of patients developing jaundice, and thus acute illness usually escapes medical attention. It is usually transmitted parenterally through exposure to blood products, by sharing contaminated needles among intravenous drug abusers, or by other percutaneous or high-risk practices such as tattooing or intranasal cocaine use. Sexual and maternal-neonatal transmission can occur but are generally inefficient routes of transmission.

Figure 3 shows the course of a patient with acute HCV infection progressing to chronicity. The incubation period is 14 to 180 days, after which elevation of ALT levels occurs and symptoms may appear, although, as noted, the acute illness may be subclinical. Routine diagnosis is made by detection of antibodies to HCV (anti-HCV) by enzyme-linked immunosorbent assay (ELISA) testing in the serum. The recombinant immunoblot assay (RIBA) test is used by blood banks to enhance specificity as a supplemental test in ELISA-positive donors. Persistence of abnormal ALT levels for 6 months or longer suggests chronicity. HCV RNA can be detected by the polymerase chain reaction (PCR) technique in serum and liver tissue by a number of experimental techniques. PCR tests can be highly sensitive qualitative tests or less sensitive quantitative tests.

Therapy

At present, indications for therapy in chronic HCV infection include elevation of ALT levels for 6 months or longer and active hepatic inflammation on liver biopsy. Therapy of chronic HCV infection is discussed in more detail in the chapter *Chronic Hepatitis.*

No HCV vaccine is yet available because the virus' heterogeneity makes development of one vaccine problematic. There is no convincing benefit from gamma globulin administration following needlestick exposure to HCV. Universal precautions should be used because the risk of HCV transmission by needlestick to health care workers can be as high as 10%. Routine screening by blood banks for HCV has reduced the risk of transmission by transfusion to a negligible level. In patients with end-stage liver disease secondary to HCV, liver transplantation has been successful. Although recurrent HCV infection of the transplanted liver occurs in many patients, only a subset of patients will have severe recurrence of viral infection after transplantation in the short term. However, the long-term consequences of recurrent HCV are a cause of growing concern because of an accelerated progression to cirrhosis. Transplant centers are currently exploring prophylactic strategies to prevent severe

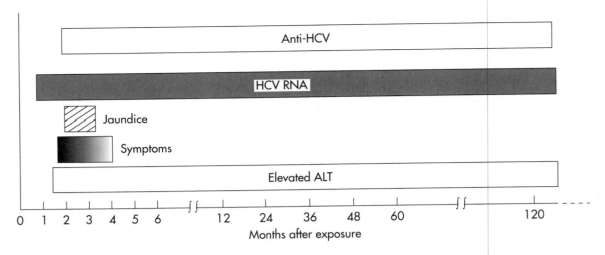

Figure 3
Typical course of acute hepatitis C progressing to chronic hepatitis C. *HCV,* Hepatitis C virus; *anti-HCV,* antibody to the hepatitis C virus. *(Adapted from Martin P, Friedman LS, Dienstag JL: Diagnostic approach to viral hepatitis. In Thomas HC, Zuckerman AJ, ed:* Viral hepatitis, *Edinburgh, 1993, Churchill Livingstone. Used with permission.)*

recurrent HCV, including the use of interferon-alpha in combination with ribavirin after transplant.

Interferon therapy has an important role in the treatment of patients with acute HCV infection, with a high likelihood of cure by decreasing the severity of the acute illness and the risk of chronicity. This is most typically recognized now in a health care worker after a needlestick injury. In a meta-analysis of interferon therapy in acute HCV, a short course of low-dose interferon-alpha (3 million units every 3 weeks) resulted in a significantly lower rate of chronicity. In an additional study, high-dose interferon-alpha (10 million units daily) was also highly efficacious in preventing chronicity.

■ HEPATITIS D VIRUS

The hepatitis delta virus (HDV) is an incomplete RNA virus and requires HBsAg to complete its replicative cycle and thus can occur only in the presence of HBV infection. HDV may be transmitted either simultaneously with HBV (coinfection) or acquired in chronic HBV carriers (superinfection). In the United States, it is spread mainly through intravenous drug abuse, whereas in other areas of high endemicity, such as the Mediterranean, intimate contact is implicated in transmission. Most cases of coinfection of HDV and HBV are self-limited, as in HBV infection, but patients are more likely to develop fulminant hepatitis than with HBV alone. If HDV is acquired by superinfection, progression to cirrhosis is more likely than with HBV alone.

The diagnosis of HDV coinfection is made if IgM anti-HDV, HBsAg, and IgM anti-HBcAb are all present. HDV superinfection is denoted by IgM anti-HDV, HBsAg, and IgG anti-HBcAb with absent IgM anti-HBc. During the acute phase of infection with HDV, serologic detection of antibodies to HDV is often insensitive. The only commercial assay available is a blocking radioimmunoassay for total anti-HDV; however, anti-HDV appears late in the course of acute delta virus infection. If HDV is clinically suspected, repeat testing may be required (see Table 1). Direct serologic tests for delta virus include molecular hybridization techniques for detecting HDV RNA and Western immunoblot techniques for detecting HDV antigen. However, these tests are research tools at present and not widely available.

Therapy

Vaccination against HBV prevents HDV infection. The risk of HDV exposure with intravenous drug use must be stressed to HBsAg-positive patients.

Patients with chronic HDV infection tend to present with progressive and often advanced liver disease, and HDV infection should be considered in a patient with clinically severe disease and HBV infection. Liver transplantation is an option for patients with end-stage disease, and referral to a specialized center should be considered. HDV infection may protect the transplanted liver to some extent from the consequences of HBV recurrence, making recurrence less severe.

■ HEPATITIS E VIRUS

The hepatitis E virus (HEV) is an RNA virus spread by fecal-oral transmission, similar to HAV. HEV disease occurs in developing countries primarily through fecal contamination of water supplies. Several geographic regions, including China, India, Pakistan, and Mexico, have been identified as endemic. HEV infection is self-limited, with no chronic sequelae. The highest attack rate appears to be among individuals between 15 and 40 years of age. A unique feature of this disease is a high mortality rate (20%) among pregnant women in the third trimester. The United States is not an endemic region for the disease, but HEV should be considered in patients with hepatic dysfunction who have traveled to areas endemic for the disease within the last 1 to 2 months. Selected research laboratories can detect HEV RNA and anti-HEV antibodies.

Therapy

As with acute HAV, the disease is self-limited, and therapy is supportive only. Pregnant patients should be discouraged from traveling to endemic areas. During travel to an endemic area, careful handwashing, drinking bottled water only, and abstaining from fresh raw vegetables are common-sense precautions.

■ HEPATITIS G VIRUS

The hepatitis G virus (HGV) is a single-stranded RNA virus with some genomic similarity to HCV. HGV is a bloodborne virus transmitted by transfusion of contaminated blood products or parenteral exposure to blood among intravenous drug abusers or hemodialysis patients. Accordingly, HGV often occurs as a coinfection with other hepatitis viruses because of similar modes of transmission. The worldwide prevalence can reach as high as 10% among volunteer blood donors, compared with 1.7% among volunteer blood donors in the United States. Vertical transmission from mother to infant and sexual transmission are rare.

HGV can establish both acute and chronic infection; however, the role of HGV as a cause of acute or chronic hepatic dysfunction has not been established. Indeed, persistent viremia for many years has been documented in the absence of aminotransferase elevations. HGV prevalence may be as high as 20% to 50% in patients with fulminant hepatitis of unknown etiology and 14% to 36% in patients with cryptogenic cirrhosis, but again, a role has not been defined in the causation of liver disease.

■ TT VIRUS

TT virus (TTV) is a single-stranded, nonenveloped DNA virus first isolated in Japan in 1997 from the serum of a patient (initials, T.T.) with posttransfusion, non–A-to-G hepatitis. Subsequent studies in a cohort of patients in the United States demonstrated a high prevalence among patients with cryptogenic cirrhosis and idiopathic fulminant hepatitis and those with prior exposure to blood products. This high prevalence in patients with prior transfusion exposure subsequently resulted in the term *transfusion transmitted virus* for TTV.

Since its initial discovery, TTV has been increasingly reported to be highly prevalent worldwide, with a strong predilection for areas in South America, Central Africa, and Papua New Guinea. High prevalence rates found among healthy volunteer blood donors underline the ubiquitous nature of TTV and its worldwide prevalence. Viremia has been documented in patients in the absence of elevated aminotransferases. Coinfection with other chronic viral hepatitis viruses commonly occurs and most likely reflects similar modes of transmission. However, TTV does not significantly worsen liver disease in coinfected patients. Therefore, despite early interest in TTV as a possible etiologic agent in cryptogenic cirrhosis and/or idiopathic fulminant liver failure, current data suggest that TTV does not play a significant role in the genesis of acute or chronic liver disease.

Suggested Reading

Camma C, Almasio P, Craxi A: Interferon as treatment for acute hepatitis C. A meta-analysis, *Dig Dis Sci* 41:1248, 1996.

Charlton M, et al: TT-virus infection in North American blood donors, patients with fulminant hepatic failure, and cryptogenic cirrhosis, *Hepatology* 28:839, 1998.

Kanda T, et al: The role of TT virus infection in acute viral hepatitis, *Hepatology* 29:1905, 1999.

Karaylannis P, et al: Natural history and molecular biology of hepatitis G virus/GB virus C, *Clin Diagn Virol* 10:103, 1998.

Markowitz JS, et al: Prophylaxis against hepatitis B recurrence following liver transplantation using combination lamivudine and hepatitis B immune globulin, *Hepatology* 28:585, 1998.

Seeff LB: Acute viral hepatitis. In Kaplowitz N, ed: *Liver and biliary diseases*, Baltimore, 1996, Williams & Wilkins.

Sjogren M: Serologic diagnosis of viral hepatitis, *Med Clin North Am* 80:929, 1996.

Vogel W, et al: High-dose interferon-alpha 2b prevents chronicity in acute hepatitis C: a pilot study, *Dig Dis Sci* 41(12 suppl):81S, 1996.

CHRONIC HEPATITIS

William N. Katkov
Gary Gitnick

The term *chronic hepatitis* encompasses a number of infectious and noninfectious diagnoses. The long-term consequences of chronic hepatitis include cirrhosis, hepatocellular carcinoma, and end-stage liver disease, for which orthotopic liver transplantation remains the intervention of last resort. During the past decade, antiviral therapy has become established as a treatment for chronic viral hepatitis B (HBV) and C (HCV). Refined interferon regimens, along with the arrival of new therapeutic agents, provide significantly greater efficacy in treating these common chronic viral infections.

■ INTERFERONS

Interferons are endogenous, naturally occurring glycoproteins whose antiviral and immunomodulatory effects make them ideal candidates for the treatment of chronic viral hepatitis. Initial clinical trials with small doses of relatively unstable interferon showed benefits in patients with viral hepatitis. Recombinant DNA technology can produce stable pure interferon, which has now been used in numerous multicenter trials. Several forms of recombinant interferon are now licensed in the United States for the treatment of chronic HBV and HCV. Of the three types of interferon (alpha, beta, and gamma), interferon alpha, of which more than 20 subtypes exist, has been studied and used most widely. It is derived from monocytes, in contrast to interferon beta, which is made from activated fibroblasts, and interferon gamma, which derives from stimulated T cells. Interferons alpha and beta are similar in molecular structure, suggesting that they exert comparable antiviral and immunomodulatory effects. Interferon gamma tends to have fewer antiviral effects.

■ CHRONIC HEPATITIS B

Interferon

A large, randomized U.S. multicenter trial of interferon alfa-2b enrolled 169 patients and 43 untreated controls, permitting a comparison of the natural history of chronic hepatitis B with interferon treatment. When treated with 5 million units of interferon alfa-2b daily by subcutaneous injection for 16 weeks, 37% of patients lost hepatitis B e antigen (HbeAg) and HBV DNA. A number of clinical trials from various countries replicated these findings.

Interferon therapy that eradicates HBV DNA usually also results in normal aminotransferase levels. Follow-up suggests that most responses to treatment are sustained. Reacti-

vation occurs in a small number of patients, who often can be re-treated successfully. Loss of hepatitis B surface antigen (HbsAg) either during treatment or after 1 year of follow-up is uncommon, occurring in only 10% to 15% of responders. Korenman and colleagues at the National Institutes of Health (NIH) reported on 5 to 7 years of follow-up and found a strikingly high frequency of HbsAg loss, with 13 of 20 (65%) interferon responders having lost HbsAg during a mean follow-up period of 4 years. In many of the HbsAg-negative patients, HBV DNA became undetectable in serum by polymerase chain reaction.

Perrillo and associates have presented evidence that histologic improvement in the liver follows successful interferon therapy and may be most apparent 4 or more years after treatment.

A U.S. multicenter trial identified variables that influence the likelihood of response to interferon. In general, patients with high pretreatment alanine aminotransferase (ALT) values and low HBV DNA levels (<200 pg/ml) were more likely to respond. Among patients with HBV DNA levels of less than 100 pg/ml, approximately 50% responded to 5 million units of interferon compared with approximately 7% of those with HBV DNA levels greater than 200 pg/ml ($p < .0001$). Thus a favorable pretreatment profile consisted of an active immune response to HBV (higher ALT) and a relatively low level of viral replication as measured by HBV DNA.

An important event that occurs for most responders during interferon therapy for chronic HBV is a flare, or transient rise, of ALT. This elevation, most commonly seen during the second or third months of therapy, is associated with a decrease in HBV DNA levels. It can mimic acute hepatitis clinically and precipitate hepatic failure in a marginally compensated liver. Consequently, interferon is not recommended for patients with decompensated chronic HBV (prolonged prothrombin time, elevated serum bilirubin level, or hypoalbuminemia). All patients require close monitoring during and after interferon therapy.

Lamivudine

In early HBV trials, nucleoside analogs, including acyclovir, adenine arabinoside, and ribavirin, were either ineffective or associated with unacceptable toxicities. Among these, fialuridine (FIAU) was a potent inhibitor of HBV replication but led to an often fatal syndrome of lactic acidosis and liver failure.

New-generation nucleoside analogs developed for the treatment of human immunodeficiency virus (HIV) have shown promise for HBV treatment as well. These drugs interfere with the reverse transcriptase that the HIV virus uses for replication. The hepatitis B virus also replicates via an intermediate, HBV DNA polymerase. In vitro and in vivo evidence shows that new nucleoside analogs such as lamivudine, famciclovir, adefovir dipivoxil, and lobucavir all inhibit HBV replication.

Lamivudine is the only nucleoside analog that the U.S. Food and Drug Administration (FDA) has licensed for the treatment of HBV, following several large, randomized, clinical trials. In a multicenter study carried out in the United States, lamivudine, 100 mg/day, for 1 year led to HbeAg seroconversion (i.e., development of antibody to

Hbe) in 17% of patients and HbeAg clearance in 32%. In most patients, this response was durable.

Other trials of lamivudine suggest that the drug is also efficacious in the liver transplant population. In combination with hepatitis B immunoglobulin, lamivudine may be particularly effective as prophylaxis against recurrent hepatitis B virus infection in these patients.

Lamivudine is associated with remarkably few side effects. Malaise, headache, nausea, and abdominal discomfort have been noted in both treated and control groups. Emergence of resistant HBV often occurs during and after therapy. Breakthrough can occur during treatment, although ALT and HBV DNA levels rarely reach or exceed pretreatment levels. Therefore therapy should continue in the face of breakthrough unless ALT levels exceed pretreatment values.

In summary, lamivudine is now considered first-line therapy for patients with chronic HBV and evidence of ongoing replication (HbeAg positive with detectable HBV DNA). The recommended dosage is 100 mg/day orally continued until there is evidence of HbeAg seroconversion. Close monitoring is required, especially after treatment. Studies of combination therapy with interferon and lamivudine have not shown an advantage over therapy with lamivudine alone. Combination therapy with several nucleoside analogs may be capable of preventing or delaying the emergence of resistant viral strains, but such regimens await clinical trials.

■ HEPATITIS D (Delta) VIRUS

Hepatitis D virus (HDV) is a defective RNA virus that infects the liver in the presence of HBV infection. HDV can infect a person either concomitantly with acute HBV infection or as a superinfection after chronic HBV infection is established. The experience with antiviral therapy for HDV is limited. Interferon often leads to a decrease in aminotransferase levels; however, elimination of the infection is uncommon. Effective treatment of HDV with interferon may require higher dosages and longer duration of therapy than that required to treat chronic HBV infection. Once HbsAg is cleared, HDV infection does not recur. Recurrence of HBV infection after liver transplantation appears to be unlikely when a patient is coinfected with HDV.

■ CHRONIC HEPATITIS C

The epidemiology of chronic hepatitis C virus infection is a difficult topic to study because the disease is often asymptomatic, serious complications of chronic hepatitis C may occur in only a minority of cases, and chronic hepatitis C usually progresses slowly over many years, necessitating long follow-up periods.

Despite these challenges, several conclusions can be drawn about the natural history of hepatitis C virus infection. After having an acute infection, as many as 70% to 80% of patients will become chronically infected. More than 30% of these chronically infected patients will develop cirrhosis. The rate of progression to cirrhosis is directly related to the degree of fibrosis seen on liver biopsy. Additional factors that may influence progression to cirrhosis include age of onset, duration of infection, gender, excessive alcohol use, route of infection, and immune status. Thus far, virologic factors such as genotype and viral titer do not appear to influence the course of the disease.

In addition to decompensated cirrhosis, progression to hepatocellular carcinoma remains the most serious consequence of chronic hepatitis C virus infection. The likelihood of developing hepatocellular carcinoma (HCC) is strongly linked to the presence of fibrosis and/or cirrhosis on liver biopsy. In one study in the United States of 112 patients, the annual rate of decompensation was 4.4%, HCC development was 2.4%, and mortality was 3%. It can be concluded that chronic hepatitis C virus infection is a slowly progressive disease with potentially life-threatening consequences that occur in a substantial minority of infected individuals.

Numerous clinical trials established the role of interferon as a single agent (monotherapy) for the treatment of chronic HCV. In a U.S. multicenter trial that used interferon alfa-2b three times weekly by subcutaneous injection for 6 months, ALT levels normalized in 38% of the patients. The encouraging response rate after 6 months of treatment stands in contrast to the frequency of relapse once interferon is discontinued; ALT elevations recur in as many as 80% of responders to interferon monotherapy.

Combination Therapy (Interferon and Ribavirin)

Large, multicenter trials of both relapsed and previously untreated chronic HCV patients have demonstrated that a combination of interferon and ribavirin, a nucleoside analog taken orally, is far more likely to result in sustained virologic, histologic, and biochemical benefit than is interferon alone. Sustained virologic responses are increased twofold to threefold in patients treated with combination versus monotherapy. Thus interferon-ribavirin combination therapy has become the standard initial treatment for chronic hepatitis C virus infection in most patients and for those who have relapsed following interferon monotherapy. Combination therapy with interferon and ribavirin has led to response rates as high as 80% with up to half of the patients maintaining a virologic response 6 months after treatment ends.

The recommended dose of interferon remains 3 million IU three times per week subcutaneously. The dosage of ribavirin is determined by weight: 1000 mg (weight <75 kg) or 1200 mg (weight ≥75 kg) taken orally in a divided daily dose. Data from controlled trials indicate that several factors lead to enhanced treatment efficacy, including infection with a hepatitis C viral genotype other than type 1, an absence of cirrhosis, and a low pretreatment viral titer. Furthermore, patients with this favorable clinical profile may achieve a sustained response to antiviral therapy with 6 months of treatment.

Although factors such as genotype, histology, and viral titer may affect the likelihood of response, it is the loss of detectable HCV RNA measured by polymerase chain reaction during treatment that remains the most reliable predictor of end-of-treatment response. With monotherapy (interferon alone), the absence of HCV RNA at 12 weeks of treatment is the strongest predictor of response at 24 or

48 weeks. In combination therapy with interferon and ribavirin, detectable HCV RNA at 24 weeks of treatment is a more reliable indicator of ultimate treatment efficacy. Follow-up of patients treated for hepatitis C has shown that those individuals who remain HCV RNA negative 6 months after the end of treatment are likely to maintain a response for a number of years. Histologic improvement has consistently been demonstrated among responders. There may be histologic improvement even among nonresponders compared with untreated controls. Patients who received combination therapy have demonstrated a greater degree of histologic improvement compared with patients who received monotherapy.

Side Effects of Interferon

Interferon is often associated with side effects. Although most of these effects are identifiable and manageable, they necessitate regular and close monitoring during therapy. Initially, myalgias, fever, malaise, and nausea can accompany subcutaneously injected interferon. These flulike effects are most pronounced at the initiation of treatment and become milder and more tolerable after 1 to 2 weeks. Acetaminophen and bedtime dosing are usually sufficient management.

Bone marrow suppression with associated cytopenias is a more serious potential effect of interferon therapy. Leukopenia and thrombocytopenia occasionally warrant a reduction in dosage or even cessation of therapy.

Interferon commonly affects a patient's mood and emotional life, leading to some degree of malaise and moodiness, effects that may become dominant issues during treatment. Less commonly, interferon exacerbates depression; it has been associated rarely with psychosis. In patients with a history of psychiatric illness, interferon therapy should be instituted with great care, if at all.

Interferon is an immunomodulating agent and, in theory, can enhance autoimmune activity. Some patients treated with interferon develop hypothyroidism caused by an autoimmune process and require hormone replacement therapy. This hypothyroidism is reversible in many cases. Ribavirin can be associated with a reversible normocytic, normochromic hemolytic anemia. In clinical trials, the mean fall in hemoglobin seen with ribavirin therapy was 2 to 3 g/dl, with fewer than 10% of patients experiencing a decrease in hemoglobin below 10 g/dl. Reducing the dosage often arrests treatment-associated hemolytic anemia. Coronary artery disease, or any condition that could be exacerbated by anemia, must be considered a relative contraindication to treatment with ribavirin. Ribavirin has been shown to be teratogenic and embryocidal. Therefore it is mandatory that both male and female patients taking ribavirin practice effective contraception during therapy and for 6 months after therapy.

■ LIVER TRANSPLANTATION

Chronic viral hepatitis is a common cause of advanced liver disease necessitating liver transplantation. The short-term prognosis of patients with chronic viral hepatitis after liver transplantation is no different from that of liver transplant patients with other diagnoses.

HBV infection often recurs after liver transplantation. Posttransplantation immunosuppression allows viral replication to thrive, and HBV DNA levels may reach very high levels. When liver transplantation patients have fulminant HBV and/or coexistent HDV infection, the likelihood of posttransplantation HBV recurrence is much lower. For patients with chronic HBV facing liver transplantation, the most important variable predicting posttransplantation recurrence is the pretransplant viral replicative status. The likelihood of recurrence is significantly lower in patients negative for HbeAg and HBV DNA than in patients positive for these measures of viral replicative activity.

Strategies to prevent HBV recurrence after transplantation have included pretransplant antiviral therapy with interferon. Interferon in decompensated HBV must be administered with caution, if at all. The ALT flare often seen with therapy can precipitate further decompensation and hepatic failure. Administration of hepatitis B surface antibody immunoglobulin in the perioperative and postoperative periods, combined with the nucleoside analog lamivudine, is emerging as the treatment of choice for patients with HBV undergoing liver transplantation.

Like hepatitis B, hepatitis C often recurs in patients undergoing liver transplantation for chronic hepatitis. The clinical course after transplantation varies from mild aminotransferase elevations to an aggressive hepatitis rapidly leading to liver failure. The efficacy of interferon therapy in posttransplantation patients remains unclear. Virtually all patients treated with interferon alone have recurrent HCV viremia when treatment ends. Combination therapy with interferon and ribavirin has shown more promise in the transplant population and requires further study.

Suggested Reading

Davis GL, et al: Interferon alfa-2b alone or in combination with ribavirin for the treatment of relapse of chronic hepatitis C, *N Engl J Med* 339:1493, 1998.

DiBisceglie A, ed: Treatment advances in chronic hepatitis C, *Semin Liver Dis* 19:1S, 1999.

Dienstag JL, et al: A preliminary trial of lamivudine for chronic hepatitis B infection, *N Engl J Med* 333:1657, 1995.

McHutchinson JG, et al: Interferon alfa-2b alone or in combination with ribavirin as initial therapy for chronic hepatitis C, *N Engl J Med* 338:1485, 1998.

Rosenberg PM, Dienstag JL: Therapy with nucleoside analogues for hepatitis B virus infection, *Clin Liver Dis* 349, 1999.

Seef LB: Natural history of hepatitis C, *Hepatology* 26:21S, 1997.

BILIARY INFECTION: CHOLECYSTITIS AND CHOLANGITIS

D. Rohan Jeyarajah
Robert V. Rege

*C*holecystitis and *cholangitis* refer to infections and inflammatory processes of the bile ducts and gallbladder. The causes of these conditions are variable but often involve gallstone disease as an important pathologic entity. This chapter outlines the pathogenesis of acute cholecystitis and cholangitis and discusses the available treatment options.

■ ACUTE CHOLECYSTITIS

Acute cholecystitis refers to acute inflammation of the gallbladder. In the United States, the most common cause of this condition is gallstone disease. Obstruction of the cystic duct by a gallstone leads to stasis of bile and inflammation. As a consequence, the patient may experience pain in the right upper quadrant of the abdomen and systemic signs of infections, including fever and leukocytosis. Gallstones can also migrate into the common bile duct and lead to choledocholithiasis or biliary pancreatitis. Rarely, acute cholecystitis can be present without gallstones, which is termed *acalculous cholecystitis*. This entity often presents in debilitated patients who have not emptied their gallbladder in a long period (usually related to not having anything by mouth [NPO] for extended periods). It is thought that stasis of bile leads to superinfection in this case.

Diagnosis

Patients with acute cholecystitis often have systemic signs of inflammation and tenderness in the right upper quadrant of the abdomen for more than 12 hours. The history of back pain should heighten one's suspicion of biliary pancreatitis. On physical examination, tenderness in the right upper quadrant, especially with inspiration (Murphy's sign) suggests gallbladder pathology. This tenderness is usually well localized to an area directly over the gallbladder. More diffuse right upper quadrant pain suggests a liver problem, gallbladder perforation, or another upper abdominal cause of pain. The presence of dark urine, acholic stool, and jaundice should raise the question of choledocholithiasis. Laboratory testing should include complete blood count (CBC) with differential, liver function tests, and lipase assay. The white blood cell count is usually elevated, reflecting inflammation. Ultrasound of the right upper quadrant should then be obtained to look for gallstones. The presence of gallstones with a suggestive history and examination suffices for the diagnosis of acute cholecystitis if the findings

are typical and gallstones are present. If the patient does not have gallstones on ultrasound or if further confirmation of the diagnosis is necessary, a technetium radionucleotide cholescintigraphy (HIDA) scan would be helpful. Nonvisualization of the gallbladder on HIDA scan indicates cystic duct obstruction and is highly suggestive of acute cholecystitis; 98% of patients with nonvisualization of the gallbladder have acute cholecystitis.

Bacteriology

Bacteria are not always isolated from bile early during the course of acute cholecystitis, but the incidence of bactibilia increases with time. The most common organisms are gram-positive organisms, especially *Enterococcus* (Table 1). The gram-negative bacteria *Klebsiella, Proteus,* and *Pseudomonas* are also frequently cultured. Anaerobic bacteria are isolated in only approximately 10% of cases but may represent the difficulty in culturing these organisms using standard techniques. *Bacteroides* and *Clostridium* species may be evident in as many as 50% of cases of biliary disease. *Candida* species are often isolated from immunosuppressed patients and patients with malignancy. Considering the possible bacteria involved, patients with acute cholecystitis require broad-spectrum antibiotic coverage.

Treatment

Initial therapy for the patient with acute cholecystitis includes fluid resuscitation, intravenous fluid replacement, bowel rest, and antibiotics. Most patients will be well covered by a second-generation cephalosporin. Alternatively, ampicillin-sulbactam (Unasyn) can be used. Surgical removal of the gallbladder is necessary. The timing of cholecystectomy is debatable. It is our preference to perform early cholecystectomy. The patient is admitted to the hospital, medical therapy is instituted, and operation is performed within 24 to 72 hours. Early operation is safe in the hands of an experienced biliary surgeon and prevents recurrent cholecystitis and other complications of biliary disease, which occur in as many as 30% of patients. Some groups emphasize a delay of 6 weeks from the time of presentation to surgical resection. This approach is certainly indicated in seriously ill patients who have contraindications to surgery. Percutaneous drainage of the gallbladder with cholecystos-

---

Table 1 Bacteriology of Patients Who Develop Acute Cholecystitis or Acute Cholangitis
GRAM-NEGATIVE ORGANISMS
Klebsiella species
Proteus species
Pseudomonas species
GRAM-POSITIVE ORGANISMS
Enterococcus
Streptococcus species
ANAEROBES
Bacteroides species
OTHER
Fungus
Cytomegalovirus
Cryptosporidium

tomy tube is also an option for critically ill patients who fail medical therapy and are at high risk for immediate surgical therapy.

Minimally invasive procedures (laparoscopic cholecystectomy) have become the standard of care, but open operation or conversion to open operation may be required in patients with marked inflammation or fibrosis. The rate of conversion from laparoscopic to open operation increases markedly 96 hours after the onset of symptoms. Patients with choledocholithiasis and biliary pancreatitis should be considered for endoscopic retrograde cholangiopancreatography (ERCP) if the laboratory tests do not show improvement. This modality should be considered both diagnostic and therapeutic as stones can be extracted.

■ ACUTE CHOLANGITIS

Acute cholangitis refers to infection and inflammation of the biliary tree itself. It is most often caused by bacteria but can be caused by parasites and chemical irritants. Terms such as *suppurative cholangitis* and *ascending cholangitis* are traditional, but we favor the term *toxic cholangitis* in those patients who are critically ill as a result of pus in their biliary ducts. The pathogenesis of acute cholangitis involves two abnormalities: obstruction of the biliary tree and bacteria in bile. Partial obstruction is more commonly associated with acute cholangitis than complete obstruction, possibly a result of the ability of bacteria to ascend the biliary tree more easily in this circumstance. Causes of obstruction are shown in Table 2. The treatment of acute cholangitis requires addressing both the infection and the cause of biliary obstruction.

Gallstones are the most common cause of cholangitis in the United States. Malignant obstruction of the bile duct is also a common cause of cholangitis, although most patients with malignant obstruction present with painless jaundice and sterile bile. Iatrogenic cholangitis after manipulation of the biliary tract is increasing because of a growing use of endocoscopic and radiologic procedures on the bile duct.

Diagnosis

The classic presentation of patients with acute cholangitis includes abdominal pain, fever, and jaundice—Charcot's triad. However, only approximately 50% of patients present with the complete triad. Fever and chills are present in 90% of patients. Physical examination most often reveals jaundice and tenderness in the right upper quadrant of the abdomen. However, about 20% of patients with acute cholangitis have a serum bilirubin level of less than 2.0 mg/dl, so lack of jaundice does not exclude a diagnosis of acute cholangitis. Physical findings are usually accompanied by leukocytosis and abnormal liver function tests. Some patients present with sepsis and require management in an intensive care unit. Patients with Charcot's triad, hypotension, and altered sensorium are said to have Reynold's pentad, which is indicative of toxic cholangitis. Ultrasound should be performed urgently to distinguish "medical" from "surgical" jaundice: the presence of dilated bile ducts is indicative of obstruction and "surgical" jaundice. If there is no intrahepatic biliary dilation, medical causes of jaundice

should be considered. Endoscopic retrograde cholangiography (ERC; see the following) is usually diagnostic but can also be therapeutic. Percutaneous transhepatic cholangiography is helpful when ERC is unsuccessful.

Bacteriology

As with acute cholecystitis, gram-negative organisms are the most common bacteria cultured from patients with acute cholangitis. Table 3 outlines the organisms found and the differences in malignant versus benign causes of acute cholangitis in a large series.

Treatment

Patients with acute cholangitis should be placed in the intensive care unit and aggressively monitored. Intravenous hydration should be started and urine output followed closely. Coagulation parameters should be repleted with fresh frozen plasma (FFP) and platelets because these patients often have profound coagulopathy related to liver dysfunction, poor nutrition, and sequestration of both clotting factors and platelets. Antibiotic therapy is essential. Initially, broad-spectrum coverage should be started, and once organisms have been isolated and sensitivities ascertained, the antibiotic coverage can be narrowed. Ampicillin and an aminoglycoside provide excellent coverage for the major culprits, specifically covering well for *Enterococcus* species, but they may cause nephrotoxicity. First- and second-generation cephalosporins provide good prophylaxis for elective biliary surgery but do not provide good gram-negative coverage for patients with acute cholangitis. Third-generation cephalosporins provide excellent gram-negative coverage but are not good agents to treat *Staphylococcus* and *Enterococcus* species. The latter organism is present in 34% of patients with acute cholangitis, and ampicillin is often added to provide coverage for these bacteria. To cover anaerobic bacteria, which can be cultured often if strict conditions are used, metronidazole may be added. Hence, the combination of ceftazadime, ampicillin, and metronidazole has been used for many years. It has been shown, however, that single-drug therapy with ciprofloxacin is as efficacious as triple-drug therapy (Table 4). This drug regimen is particularly helpful in patients with recurrent

Table 2   Causes of Biliary Obstruction
Gallstones
Strictures of the biliary tree
Benign
Primary sclerosing cholangitis (PSC)
Iatrogenic (e.g., postcholecystectomy)
Ischemic (e.g., anastomotic)
Congenital anomalies (e.g., choledochocyst)
Malignant
Cholangiocarcinoma
Pancreatic or ampullary neoplasm
Extrinsic compression (e.g., metastatic node)
Hematobilia
Parasites
Clonorchis sinensis
Ascaris lumbricoides

Table 3 Organisms Isolated from the Bile in Malignant and Benign Causes of Cholangitis

	TOTAL (N = 96% OF PATIENTS)	BENIGN CAUSES (N = 42% OF PATIENTS)	MALIGNANT CAUSES (N = 54% OF PATIENTS)
GRAM NEGATIVE			
Klebsiella species	54	31	72
Escherichia coli	39	43	35
Enterobacter species	34	17	48
Pseudomonas species	24	12	33
Citrobacter species	21	17	24
Proteus species	13	12	13
Aeromonas species	5	2	7
Serratia species	3	0	6
GRAM POSITIVE			
Enterococcus	34	36	33
Streptococcal species	38	24	48
ANAEROBES			
Bacteroides species	15	17	13
Clostridium species	5	2	7
FUNGI			
Candida species	18	5	28
OTHERS	14	19	9

Adapted from Thompson JE Jr, et al: Broad spectrum penicillin as adequate therapy for acute cholangitis, *Surg Gynecol Obstet* 171:279, 1990.

Table 4 Summary of Antibiotic Regimens for Acute Cholecystitis and Acute Cholangitis

ACUTE CHOLECYSTITIS
Cefoxitin, 1 g IV q8h or 2 g IV q4h
Ampicillin-sulbactam (Unasyn), 3 g IV q6h
ACUTE CHOLANGITIS
Single agents
    Ciprofloxacin, 400-800 mg IV q12h
    Piperacillin-tazobactam (Zosyn), 3.375 IV q6h
    Imipenem, 500 mg IV q6h
Multidrug therapy
    Ceftazadime, 1-2 g IV q8-12h
    Ampicillin, 2 g IV q6h
    Metronidazole, 500 mg IV q6h, up to q12h

cholangitis because it can be administered long term as an outpatient. Piperacillin should also be considered as a single agent because it appears as efficacious as ampicillin and tobramycin but is less nephrotoxic. Newer combinations, such as piperacillin-tazobactam (Zosyn) may also be considered. In patients with biliary obstruction secondary to *Ascaris* or *Clonorchis* infection, specific antiparasitic therapy is indicated (see specific chapters).

After resuscitation and antibiotics have been started, the main aim should be drainage of the biliary tree. This can be obtained in two ways: (1) percutaneous transhepatic cholangiography (PTC) or (2) ERCP. The risk of ERCP is less than that with PTC in these sick patients, and this should be the intervention of choice. ERCP can also provide other information. For example, cancers of the biliary tree can be visualized and a biopsy performed and stones can be extracted, providing therapy as well as diagnosis. If ERCP fails to provide adequate drainage, PTC should be undertaken. If the patient has a high cholangiocarcinoma, PTC may actually be safer than ERCP. Rarely, decompression of the biliary tree is impossible by these methods; in this case, the patient will require laparotomy and open drainage of the common bile duct with a T-tube.

Once the acute obstruction has been managed by drainage, the patient should improve. The patient should then undergo a definitive procedure to treat the cause of biliary obstruction. Common bile duct stones may be removed, and benign and malignant strictures stented endoscopically. Cholecystectomy should be performed if choledocholithiasis was the inciting event. Curable malignancies should be resected. Benign strictures require balloon dilation or choledochointestinal bypass, and unresectable tumors are either bypassed or palliated with internal or external stents.

Suggested Reading

Lipsett P, Pitt H: Acute cholangitis, *Surg Clin North Am* 170:1297, 1990.
Rege R: Cholecystitis and cholelithiasis. In Rakel RE, ed: *Conn's current surgical therapy*, Philadelphia, 1999, WB Saunders.
Sinanan MN: Acute cholangitis, *Infect Dis Clin North Am* 6:571, 1992.
Thompson J Jr, et al: Doty, MD, FACS, Broad spectrum penicillin as an adequate therapy for acute cholangitis, *Surg Gynecol Obstet* 171:275, 1990.

PYOGENIC LIVER ABSCESS

H. Franklin Herlong

Although the liver is exposed to bacteria through its dual systemic and portal circulations, bacterial infections of the liver are relatively rare. This is largely because of the abundant network of Kupffer cells that line the hepatic sinusoids, resulting in efficient bacterial clearance. Pyogenic liver abscesses represent the most common serious bacterial infections of the liver, with mortality rates approaching 80% in the preantibiotic era. However, the availability of sensitive imaging techniques, effective antimicrobial agents, and better drainage procedures have reduced the mortality to 10% to 20%.

■ ETIOLOGY AND CLINICAL CHARACTERISTICS

Bacteria causing pyogenic liver abscesses reach the liver via the bile ducts, the portal vein or artery, or extension of contiguous infections. Formerly, most abscesses resulted from portal pylephlebitis caused by diverticular disease, intraabdominal abscess, appendicitis, or inflammatory bowel disease. In more recent series, cholangitis, caused by calculi or strictures of the bile duct, accounts for up to 40% of cases. Extension of contiguous infection from subhepatic abscesses, cholecystitis, or pancreatitis can cause liver abscesses. No associated conditions are found in approximately one quarter of cases, with most of these occurring in individuals with some form of immunosuppression, including old age, diabetes, sickle cell disease, or chemotherapy.

Cultures from liver abscesses usually show a polymicrobial flora with a mixture of aerobic and anaerobic bacteria (Table 1). Organisms most commonly isolated include aerobic gram-negative bacilli, streptococci (aerobic and anaerobic), and anaerobic gram-negative bacilli. *Staphylococcus aureus* is a common cause of liver abscesses in childhood and trauma patients. Microbiologic profiles can help determine the source of the liver abscesses, with facultative gram-negative bacilli originating commonly from the biliary tract, whereas anaerobic organisms come from portal bacteremias. An unusual pathogen, *Yersinia enterocolitica,* causes abscesses in patients with diabetes or underlying liver disease, particularly hemochromatosis.

Most patients with pyogenic liver abscesses appear acutely ill with fever, chills, and right upper quadrant pain. However, in elderly, debilitated patients, clinical signs may be minimal, delaying diagnosis. Most patients have tender hepatomegaly, occasionally with focal tenderness over the intercostal spaces of the right upper quadrant. However, in patients with liver transplants, denervation may prevent the pain of hepatic enlargement. Jaundice is unusual unless the abscess compresses the biliary tract. An associated pleural effusion may obliterate breath sounds at the right base.

Table 1 Bacteriology of Pyogenic Liver Abscess

ORGANISM	INCIDENCE (%)
AEROBES (GRAM-NEGATIVE BACILLI)	50-70
Escherichia coli	
Enterobacter	
Klebsiella	
Pseudomonas	
AEROBES (GRAM-POSITIVE COCCI)	30
Streptococci	
Group A	
Group B	
Enterococcus	
Staphylococci	
OTHER	1
Yersinia	
Listeria monocytogenes	
Salmonella	
Actinobacter	
ANAEROBES	50
Bacteroides	
Fusobacterium	
Peptostreptococci	
Clostridium	
Actinomyces	

Table 2 Clinical Findings in Pyogenic Liver Abscess

	INCIDENCE (%)
SIGN OF SYMPTOM	
Chills	60
Abdominal pain	60
Weight loss	30
Fever	75
Hepatomegaly	50
Right upper quadrant tenderness	40
Jaundice	25
LABORATORY VALUES	
Leukocytosis	70
Elevated bilirubin (2 mg/dl)	40
Elevated alkaline phosphatase	50
Elevated aminotransferases	60

Laboratory abnormalities include the typical findings seen in systemic infection or other liver diseases. Modest elevations of the alkaline phosphatase, aminotransferases, and bilirubin values are common. A leukocytosis with a left shift is present in most patients, and half will have positive blood cultures (Table 2).

■ DIAGNOSIS AND TREATMENT

The availability of accurate imaging techniques is probably the most significant factor in the reduction in mortality rates from pyogenic liver abscesses in most recent series. Ultrasonographic examination of the abdomen shows variable patterns of echogenicity. Typically, the abscesses are cystic, round lesions with irregular walls. They may be septated and multiloculated and contain internal echoes caused by debris. Although the sensitivity is usually about 75%, small abscesses may go undetected. Computed tomography (CT) is the most widely used modality to confirm the presence of pyogenic liver abscesses. When performed with contrast, sensitivities approach 95%. CT can detect smaller lesions than ultrasonography and may also help identify other sites of intraabdominal infection. Technitium-99m sulfacolloid and gallium citrate scans are rarely used because they cannot reliably detect small lesions or distinguish abscesses from neoplasm. At present, there is no evidence that magnetic resonance imaging is superior to CT.

When pyogenic liver abscess is suspected, prompt introduction of antibiotic therapy is essential. Empiric regimens are similar to those used in other causes of intraabdominal sepsis. Many combinations are appropriate (e.g., metronidazole, ampicillin, and an aminoglycoside or a third-generation cephalosporin combined with metronidazole or clindamycin). The regimen can be altered appropriately based on the results of culture data obtained at aspiration.

Although there are anecdotal reports of successful treatment of pyogenic liver abscesses with antibiotics alone, some form of drainage procedure is advocated in most patients. Percutaneous aspiration and drainage, under ultrasonographic or CT guidance, has largely replaced surgical drainage, the former mainstay of treatment. Although there are no randomized trials comparing nonoperative approaches with surgery, published experience suggests that mortality and morbidity rates from percutaneous drainage are equal to or better than those achieved with surgery. As a result,

surgery should be reserved for those patients who fail to respond to percutaneous drainage. Surgery may be necessary in patients with multiple loculated abscesses or when an appropriate site for safe placement of the catheter cannot be ascertained. Two surgical approaches have been used: extraserous drainage and transperitoneal drainage. The former was previously selected because of the potential to eliminate peritoneal contamination. However, because of reduced capacity to explore the liver for accessory abscesses and the inability to identify other intraabdominal sources of infection, this approach is rarely used. Most surgeons prefer the transperitoneal approach using appropriate antibiotic coverage.

Multiple small abscesses are not amenable to surgical or catheter drainage and must be treated with intravenous antibiotic administration alone. Not surprisingly, this group has the highest mortality. (Amoebic liver abscess is discussed in the chapter *Extraintestinal Amoebic Infection.*)

Suggested Reading

Bartlett JG: Pyogenic liver abscess. In Gorbach SL, Bartlett JG, Blacklow NR, eds: *Infectious diseases,* ed 2, Philadelphia, 1998, WB Saunders.

Bertel CK, van Heerden JA, Sheedy PF: Treatment of pyogenic hepatic abscesses. Surgical vs. percutaneous drainage, *Arch Surg* 121:554, 1986.

McDonald MI, et al: Single and multiple pyogenic liver abscesses: natural history, diagnosis and treatment, with emphasis on percutaneous drainage, *Medicine* (Baltimore) 63:291, 1984.

Pitt HA: Surgical management of hepatic abscesses, *World J Surg* 14:498, 1990.

Wong KP: Percutaneous drainage of pyogenic liver abscesses, *World J Surg* 14:492, 1990.

INFECTIOUS COMPLICATIONS IN ACUTE PANCREATITIS

Jamie S. Barkin
Jeffrey A. Goldstein

Acute pancreatitis (AP) is an acute inflammatory process of the pancreas with a variable involvement of peripancreatic tissue, remote organ systems, or both. The proposed etiology of AP is loss of compartmentalization, obstruction of secretory transport, and intracellular activation of pancreatic enzymes. The clinical consequence of these events varies from a mild attack with edematous pancreatitis to a life-threatening situation with pancreatic necrosis and multiple organ failure. Approximately 80% of cases of AP are edematous and self-limited, undergoing rapid resolution with supportive care. However, 20% are complicated with necrosis and possibly multiorgan system failure (MOSF). It is this select population with pancreatic necrosis that is most at risk for infectious complications, with the necrotic focus serving as the nidus for infection. Pancreatic infection is the leading cause of death in patients with AP, unfortunately, accounting for up to 70% to 80% mortality.

Overall, AP is complicated by infection in 10% of patients. The greater the amount of necrotic reaction, the greater the risk for subsequent infection of the gland. In addition, infection has also been linked to the time course of the pancreatic necrosis, with the highest yield detected in the first 4 weeks after onset of the disease. Thus patients with severe pancreatitis have pancreatic necrosis with or without secondary bacterial infections and with increased morbidity and/or mortality. There is a growing awareness of the importance of a superimposed or primary pancreatic infectious process. The warm, wet, dark, and proteinaceous dead pancreatic and peripancreatic tissue is an ideal medium for pathogens. The cause of pancreatitis does not appear to influence the frequency of these infections.

■ DEFINITIONS AND PROGNOSTIC INDICATORS

The presence of pancreatic necrosis and fluid collections is a sine qua non for the development of a variety of infectious complications seen in AP. *Pancreatic necrosis* is one or more diffuse or focal areas of nonviable pancreatic parenchyma typically associated with peripancreatic fat necrosis and found in patients with severe AP. Acute fluid collections, which occur early in the course of AP, are in or near the pancreas and may be sterile or infected. Infectious processes are classified as those that occur within 2 weeks, in which there is infection or necrosis causing a cellulitis of the pancreas, and those that occur later, usually after 2 weeks, in which there is a localized infected fluid collection. Other terms and definitions include *pseudocyst,* which is a collection of pancreatic juice enclosed by a nonepithelized wall that arises as a consequence of AP and may remain sterile or become infected, and *pancreatic abscess,* which is a circumscribed intraabdominal collection of pus, usually near the pancreas, arising as a consequence of AP or pancreatic trauma.

The prognosis and severity of a pancreatitis attack may be accurately assessed on clinical grounds alone, including the presence of peritonitis, respiratory decompensation, and shock. Several scoring systems, including Ranson's Criteria and APACHE II scores, all with inherent limitations, have been developed in an attempt to predict the outcome of an attack of acute pancreatitis. These systems are based on (1) single biochemical factors, (2) multiple prognostic criteria, and/or (3) results of peritoneal lavage. Abdominal computed tomography (CT) allows the physician to determine the severity as well as to confirm the presence of pancreatic necrosis.

Single Biochemical Factors

A variety of laboratory tests have been suggested as markers of severe pancreatitis. A urea-to-glucose ratio over 0.67 mmol/L and presence of serum trypsinogen–activated peptides appear promising in selecting patients with severe disease. Severe AP also has been correlated with a C-reactive protein (CRP) level greater than 120 mg/L and a lactate dehydrogenase (LDH) level greater than 270 mg/L. The level of interleukin-6, which rises 24 to 36 hours before that of CRP, has been an accurate marker of AP. These are not sufficiently sensitive or specific to be adopted and used widely for detecting patients with severe pancreatitis.

Multiple Prognostic Criteria

The Multiple Organ System Failure (MOSF) scoring system may be more accurate than the other criteria (Table 1). The combination of the APACHE II score with the MOSF score and the patient's age is very useful to identify the patients who are at risk for increased morbidity and mortality.

Peritoneal Lavage

Analysis of peritoneal lavage has been used to predict outcomes in patients with AP. Criteria predicting severe pancreatitis include one or more of the following: (1) more than 20 ml of ascitic fluid, (2) the presence of dark ascitic fluid, and (3) return of peritoneal lavage fluid that is darker than a pale straw color obtained after peritoneal lavage with 1 L of normal saline. Its major advantages are (1) rapid diagnosis of severe pancreatitis, (2) ability to detect other causes of an acute abdomen, and (3) possible therapeutic benefit of peritoneal lavage.

Computed Tomography

Rapid bolus CT scanning using intravenous (IV) contrast effectively and accurately (>95%) detects pancreatic necrosis. CT scanning should be restricted to patients who have severe acute pancreatitis, who do not show signs of clinical improvement despite supportive care over several days, and whose infection is suspected (i.e., temperature >101° F [38.3° C] or positive blood cultures) (Figure 1).

The severity of AP can be estimated by the findings on abdominal CT. The presence of pancreatic enlargement, peripancreatic inflammatory changes, and the number and locations of fluid collections increasingly show disease severity. Although these criteria are useful, it is important to determine whether pancreatic necrosis is present and, if so, to what extent. Necrosis is characterized by lack of pancreatic vascular perfusion, which on CT is seen as nonenhancement of pancreatic tissue (see Figure 1).

CT or ultrasound-guided fine-needle aspiration (FNA) of pancreatic necrosis and/or fluid collections is the most accurate, expedient, and reliable method to detect infected

Table 1	Criteria for Organ System Failure
ORGAN SYSTEM	**CRITERIA**
Cardiovascular	Mean arterial pressure ≤50 mm Hg; need for volume loading and/or vasoactive drugs to maintain systolic arterial pressure >100 mm Hg; heart rate ≤50 beats/min; ventricular tachycardia or fibrillation; cardiac arrest; acute myocardial infarction
Pulmonary	Respiratory rate ≤5 breaths/min or ≥50 breaths/min; mechanical ventilation for ≥3 days or Fio_2 >0.4 and/or PEEP >5 cm H_2O
Renal	Serum creatinine ≥280 µmol/L (3.5 mg/dl); dialysis/ultrafiltration
Neurologic	Glasgow Coma Scale score ≤6 in the absence of sedation
Hematologic	Hct ≤20%; leukocyte count ≤0.3 × 10⁹ L; thrombocyte count ≤50 × 10⁹ L; disseminated intravascular coagulation
Hepatic	Clinical jaundice or total bilirubin level ≥51 µmol/L (3 mg/dl) in the absence of hemolysis; serum glutamic-pyruvic transaminase >2× normal; hepatic encephalopathy
Gastrointestinal	Stress ulcer necessitating transfusion of >2 U of blood/24 hr; hemorrhagic pancreatitis; acalculous cholecystitis; necrotizing enterocolitis; bowel perforation

From Larvin M, McMahon M: *Lancet* 22:201, 1989.
PEEP, Positive end-expiratory pressure; *Hct,* hematocrit.

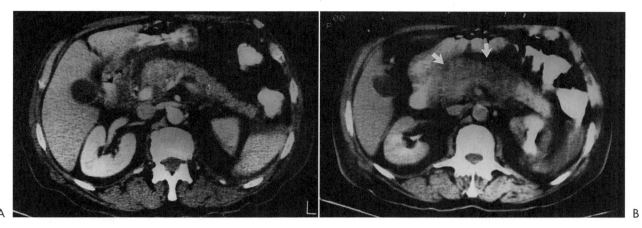

Figure 1
A, Dynamic computed tomography (CT) scan of an 80-year-old man with acute pancreatitis showing homogeneous contrast enhancement of the pancreas. **B,** Same patient 7 days later. CT shows 80% necrosis of the pancreatic gland with a well-demonstrated parenchymal area of unenhancement *(closed arrows).*

pancreatic necrosis or fluid. The fluid and/or tissue is then sent for Gram stain and culture analysis. The most common enteric pathogens cultured in decreasing order of frequency are *Escherichia coli, Klebsiella pneumoniae, Enterococcus, Staphylococcus* species, *Pseudomonas* species, *Proteus,* aerobic streptococcus, *Enterobacter,* and *Bacteroides.* Fungi, anaerobes, and viral pathogen are less commonly found. The mode of secondary infection of pancreatic necrosis is unclear but is speculated to arise from bacterial translocation from the small bowel or colon and/or biliary tract reflux into the pancreatic duct.

Antibiotic Prophylaxis

Antibiotic prophylaxis has been used to decrease mortality in patients with necrotizing pancreatitis. However, its use in patients with AP is not standardized throughout the world, as Dr. Paul Lankisch emphasizes. The American Society of Gastrointestinal Endoscopy guidelines suggest that it is reasonable to initiate antibiotics in the setting of marked pancreatitis. Conversely, the practice guidelines in the United Kingdom are uncertain whether antibiotic prophylaxis is helpful. Interestingly, in Great Britain it is the practice that prophylactic antibiotics are indicated in patients with severe AP. The preferred antibiotic is cefuroxime, and treatment is extended for a minimum of 7 to 10 days. The German Society of Gastroenterology recommends prophylactic antibiotics in patients with severe AP, especially in those with necrosis. Individual studies have had conflicting results; however, most of the recent studies have found prophylactic antibiotics to be beneficial. This was confirmed in a meta-analysis of eight randomized prospective clinical trials conducted by Golub and colleagues, which was published in the *Journal of Gastrointestinal Surgery.* They found that the use of broad-spectrum antibiotics for prophylaxis in severe AP significantly reduced mortality. In particular, Sainio and others noted that a 14-day prophylaxis with a 1.5 g/day cefuroxime was helpful in decreasing the number of infections as well as mortality in patients with AP.

Antibiotic Selection

The antibiotic chosen for prophylaxis requires a broad spectrum of activity against gram-positive, gram-negative, and anaerobic bacteria with good penetration into the pancreatic tissue. The two antibiotics that are first-line therapies are imipenem and the quinolones. Quinolones (ciprofloxacin) have good gram-positive and gram-negative antibacterial activity and good penetration into the pancreatic tissue. However, some believe the quinolones should be used in combination with clindamycin or metronidazole for better anaerobic coverage. Second-line therapies include piperacillin, cefotaxime, or ceftazidine in combination with clindamycin or metronidazole. A recent multicenter study compared imipenem with pefloxacin (a quinolone) in 60 patients with severe AP with necrosis and found that imipenem was the preferred prophylactic antibiotic choice.

■ INFECTIOUS COMPLICATIONS

Infected Necrotizing Pancreatitis

Pancreatic necrosis as a consequence of AP is seen in up to 20% of patients. Infection or contamination of necrosis occurs early in the course of necrotizing pancreatitis, usually within the initial 14 days. The usual contaminant is a single bacterium with 75% of the pathogens cultured being gram-negative, 10% gram-positive, and 10% anaerobes. *Candida* species may be a primary pathogen, although it is found in fewer than 10% of patients. It may have an indolent course but also requires surgical debridement, as well as antifungal medication, and it has high mortality. The nature of isolated pathogens suggests an enteric source, but the exact mechanism of contamination of the necrotic tissue is obscure. A variety of routes, including hematogenous, lymphogenous, bilious routes and translocation of bacteria from the bowel, have been suggested. In addition, a transient immunosuppressive state during AP has been implicated as a predisposing condition for bacterial contamination.

To decrease the infectious complications and the associated high morbidity and mortality in AP, several studies have used prophylactic antibiotics with high pancreatic penetration. Further studies are necessary to evaluate the potential benefit and side effects (resistance and fungal superinfection) of antibiotics in this situation. However, some antibiotics are known to penetrate pancreatic tissue and have been found in clinical studies to be beneficial; these include ciprofloxacin, cefotaxime, and imipenem.

Clinically, it is difficult, if not impossible, to differentiate between sterile and infected pancreatic necrosis because multiorgan failure, fever, and leukocytosis may occur in both instances. Similar CT findings are found in patients with infected and sterile necrosis, but the presence of air in the fluid collection is almost pathognomic of the presence of gas-producing organisms. However, rupture of the fluid collection into the bowel can also result in the presence of air in the fluid collection. Therefore a CT-guided aspiration of any necrotic area is indicated for patients with suspected infection (Figure 2). Gram stain of the aspirate reveals organisms in approximately 90% of infected patients, and positive cultures are found in 10% of patients with negative Gram stain. The true-false negative rate is unknown. The management of patients with bacteria or fungi on Gram stain or culture is surgical drainage, debridement, and antibiotics or antifungal agents. Peritoneal lavage or any other percutaneous drainage procedure that does not address the retroperitoneum and remove all the necrotic tissue is doomed to failure.

The management of patients with sterile pancreatic necrosis is supportive and includes nutritional support and prophylactic antibiotics. If there is no clinical improvement

after 3 to 4 weeks of supportive measures, surgical debridement should be considered to remove the necrotic focus that is fueling the inflammatory process that produces chemokines and cytokines.

The surgical treatment of infected pancreatic necrosis has evolved to include necrosectomy with open and/or closed drainage and with reexplorations (Figure 3). The surgical technique that we prefer is to debride and then pack the surgical wound and leave it open to allow for subsequent planned reexplorations every 2 to 3 days. Some surgeons prefer to close the wound and leave large-bore lavage cath-

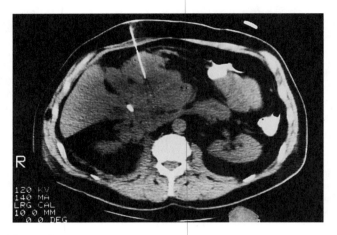

Figure 2
CT-guided aspiration of a peripancreatic collection with early gas formation.

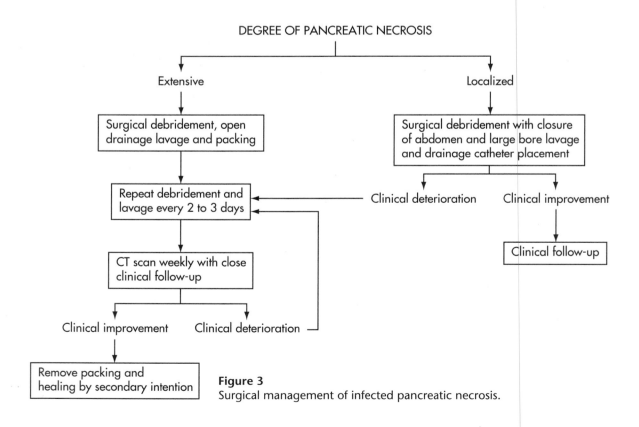

Figure 3
Surgical management of infected pancreatic necrosis.

eters in the retroperitoneum, to be removed once the patient improves. A literature review of this topic suggests better results with open management plus lavage of 1 L/hr of sterile saline than with a single necrosectomy and drainage. Despite these aggressive surgical treatments, high surgical morbidity results from abscess formation, pancreatic fistula, colonic fistula and necrosis, incisional hernia, and intraperitoneal bleeding. An approach to patients with necrotizing pancreatitis is depicted in Figure 4.

Pancreatic Abscess

In contrast to infected necrotizing pancreatitis, a pancreatic abscess is a localized collection of pus in a capsule. It occurs in 4% of patients and usually develops 3 to 6 weeks after the onset of severe pancreatitis. Unfortunately, it is fatal if not treated. Patients present with fever, abdominal pain, an-

orexia, weight loss, and possibly a palpable mass after an episode of acute pancreatitis. However, in some instances, an indolent presentation is seen with absence of toxic manifestation. Most patients have an elevated white blood cell count and positive blood cultures. The presence of retroperitoneal air on a plain abdominal x-ray film or air in a fluid collection usually indicates an abscess but can result from a fistula to a hollow viscus (Figure 5). Ultrasound- or CT-directed fine-needle aspiration of any suspicious collection will confirm the diagnosis. The flora recovered from these collections is usually polymicrobial; most of the organisms are gram-negative Enterobacteriaceae and anaerobes. Gram-positive organisms and yeast are seen in fewer than 15% of cases. In contrast to infected pancreatic necrosis, which may require several debridements, this localized collection of pus can be drained by a variety of nonsurgical techniques,

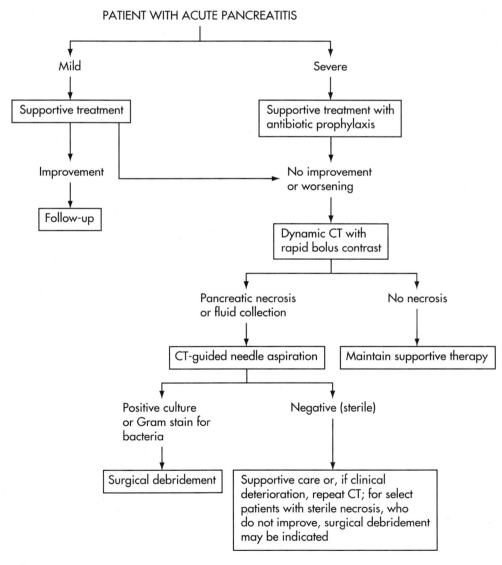

Figure 4
Approach to the patient with necrotizing pancreatitis. Acute pancreatitis classified clinically or by evaluation system (Ranson, APACHE score, MOSF) with laboraotry criteria.

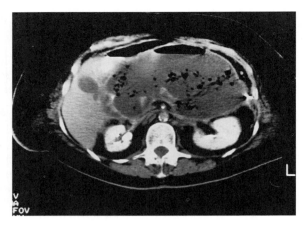

Figure 5
Large abscess 4 weeks after acute necrotizing pancreatitis.

including percutaneous-guided aspiration with catheter placement and endoscopic-guided drainage. Over the past 10 years, percutaneous drainage has replaced the traditional surgical approach for drainage of pancreatic abscess and other pancreatic collections. Unfortunately, throughout the literature, there is confusion and inconsistency regarding the description of the infected complications of AP, with mislabeling of pancreatic abscess, infected pseudocyst, and infected fluid collections. If one uses the definition of pancreatic abscess as a localized collection of infected fluid in or around the pancreas in these single, well-loculated, relatively small collections without thick necrotic debris in patients without MOSF, current evidence supports the use of percutaneous or endoscopic drainage for their management. In addition, percutaneous drainage can be used as an adjuvant measure for drainage of infected fluid collection in the postoperative drainage stage. Percutaneous drainage can also be used as a temporizing measure in the critically ill patient who is not a surgical candidate but who is an ideal candidate for percutaneous aspiration. Patients who are toxic with MOSF probably should undergo surgical debridement.

■ INFECTED PANCREATIC COLLECTIONS AND PSEUDOCYSTS

Up to 40% of patients with AP have acute fluid collections (AFCs) that consist of enzyme-rich pancreatic secretions, which occur during the first 2 weeks of the episode. An AFC is usually peripancreatic, without a capsule, and confined to the anatomic space within which it arises. Extrapancreatic fluid collections can also occur in the lesser sac, perirenal and peripancreatic space, spleen, and liver. These collections, which can be single or multiple, result from pancreatic and gastrointestinal fistulas that usually close spontaneously. If these collections do not resolve spontaneously, they evolve into a pseudocyst, which can become infected and, according to the bacterial load, form an abscess. Most AFC and pseudocysts resolve spontaneously, especially if they are smaller than 6 mm, so they do not need to be drained unless they become infected. If infected, percutaneous or endoscopic drainage of an infected pseudocyst or fluid collection is successful in most selected cases. The catheter should be carefully removed when drainage ceases, communication closes, the infection is controlled, and the collection is resolved.

Suggested Reading

Aloia T, Solomkin J, Fink AS: Candida in pancreatic infection: a clinical experience, *Am Surg* 60:703, 1994.

Bassi C, et al: Controlled clinical trial of pefloxacin versus imipenem in severe acute pancreatitis, *Gastroenterology* 115:1513, 1998.

Bjornson HS: Pancreatic "abscess": diagnosis and management, *Pancreas* 6(suppl):31, 1991.

Bradley EL III: A clinical based classification system for acute pancreatitis, *Arch Surg* 128:586, 1993.

Buchler P, Reber HA: Surgical approach in patients with acute pancreatitis: is infected or sterile necrosis an indication: in whom should this be done, when and why? *Gastroenterol Clin North Am* (in press).

Golub R, Siddiqi F, Pohl D: Role of antibiotics in acute pancreatitis: a meta-analysis, *J Gastrointest Surg* 2:496, 1998.

Johnson CD, Stephens DH, Sarr MG: CT of acute pancreatitis: correlation between lack of contrast enhancement and pancreatic necrosis, *Am J Roentgenol* 156:93, 1991.

Lang EK, Paolini RM, Pottmeyer A: The efficacy of palliative and definitive percutaneous versus surgical drainage of pancreatic abscess and pseudocysts: a prospective study of 85 patients, *South Med J* 84:55, 1991.

Neustater BR, Barkin JS: Acute pancreatitis. In McNally PR, ed: *GI/liver secrets*, Philadelphia, 1996, Hanley & Belfus.

Ratschko M, Fenner T, Lankisch PG: The role of antibiotic prophylaxis in the treatment of acute pancreatitis, *Gastroenterol Clin North Am* 38:641, 1999.

Widdison AL, Karanja ND, Alvarez C: Sources of pancreatic pathogens in acute necrotizing pancreatitis, *Gastroenterology* 100:A:304, 1991.

Witt MD, Edwards JE: Pancreatic abscess and infected pancreatic pseudocyst: diagnosis and treatment, *Curr Clin Top Infect Dis* 12:111, 1992.

ESOPHAGEAL INFECTIONS

Qian Yun Xie
Jean-Pierre Raufman

Fungal, viral, or bacterial infection of the esophagus (Table 1) results in mucosal inflammation that, in addition to painful swallowing, may cause erosions, ulcers, or fistulae. Infectious esophagitis commonly complicates predisposing conditions, such as diabetes mellitus, corticosteroid or antibiotic use, hematologic cancers, or immunosuppression (e.g., organ transplant recipients and those infected with human immunodeficiency virus [HIV]), and contributes to their morbidity and mortality. Some pathogens, such as herpes simplex virus type 1, may cause infectious esophagitis in otherwise healthy people. It is important to identify and treat promptly the infecting organism because, in contrast to underlying diseases that predispose patients to their occurrence, esophageal infections generally respond rapidly to appropriate treatment. In recent years, the acquired immunodeficiency syndrome (AIDS) epidemic and the increasing use of organ transplantation with its attendant immunosuppressive therapy have precipitated an increased incidence of esophageal infections.

■ FUNGAL INFECTIONS OF THE ESOPHAGUS

Candida Species
Candida albicans is the most common fungal organism causing esophageal infection, but other *Candida* species (*C. tropicalis, C. parapsilosis,* and *Torulopsis glabrata*) must also be considered. Candida organisms are normal components of the oral flora that may become pathogenic if their numbers increase (e.g., antibiotic use) or the host becomes immunosuppressed (e.g., steroid or cyclosporin therapy, hematologic malignancies, or AIDS). It is common, but not necessarily correct, to view mucosal infection with *Candida* species as a two-stage process. The first stage, colonization, is one of mucosal adherence and proliferation. The second stage, invasion of the epithelium, commonly requires defective cellular immunity. In practice, differentiating between these two stages relies on the gross endoscopic appearance and the microscopic appearance of material obtained by brushing or biopsy. Because fungal hyphae and masses of budding yeast are rarely seen with colonization alone, their presence indicates invasive infection. Moreover, *C. albicans* infection results in adherent plaques that reveal a denuded, friable surface when removed. The spectrum of esophageal involvement with *Candida* species ranges from scattered white plaques to a dense pseudomembrane consisting of fungi, sloughed mucosal cells, and fibrin overlying severely damaged mucosa. Ultimately, this process may result in

Table 1   Organisms Associated with Infectious Esophagitis

Fungi
    Candida species (especially *C. albicans*)
    Aspergillus species
    Histoplasma capsulatum
    Blastomyces dermatitides
Viruses
    Herpes simplex virus type 1
    Cytomegalovirus
    Varicella-zoster virus
Bacteria
    Mycobacterium tuberculosis and *M. avium*
    Actinomyces israelii
    Staphylococcus aureus
    Streptococcus viridans
    Lactobacillus acidophilus
    Treponema pallidum
Idiopathic ulcerative esophagitis in AIDS

luminal narrowing and the development of pseudodiverticulae and fistulae.

Clinical Presentation and Complications
Candida esophagitis may not cause symptoms, particularly in those who are immunocompetent with few adherent esophageal plaques. However, when symptomatic, the most common complaint is odynophagia (painful swallowing). This symptom may result in minimal difficulty swallowing, or the pain may be so intense that the patient avoids eating or swallowing his or her saliva. In severe cases, retrosternal chest pain or burning may be present without swallowing. In granulocytopenic patients, fungal infection may be disseminated, thereby resulting in fever, sepsis, and signs and symptoms related to hepatic, splenic, or renal fungal abscesses.

In AIDS, esophageal candidiasis is commonly associated with oropharyngeal thrush. In this setting, the presence of esophageal symptoms (odynophagia or dysphagia) plus oral candidiasis predicts the presence of Candida esophagitis in 71% to 100% of cases. Nevertheless, Candida esophagitis may occur independently of thrush up to 25% of the time.

Severe complications of esophageal candidiasis include esophageal bleeding from ulceration; luminal obstruction from a fungal ball; mucosal scarring and stricture; fistulization into the trachea, bronchi, or mediastinum; and esophageal mucosal sloughing with replacement by pseudomembrane. Although life-threatening hemorrhage has been reported, bleeding from esophageal candidiasis is usually mild, not requiring transfusion.

Diagnosis
Candida esophagitis should be suspected when persons at risk complain of odynophagia or dysphagia. In this setting, many authorities recommend empiric therapy, with further workup reserved for those who do not respond within a reasonable time (7 to 10 days). If necessary, the most accurate method for diagnosing fungal esophagitis is endoscopy with brushing and biopsy of lesions (Figure 1). Endoscopic appearance alone may be suggestive but is insufficient

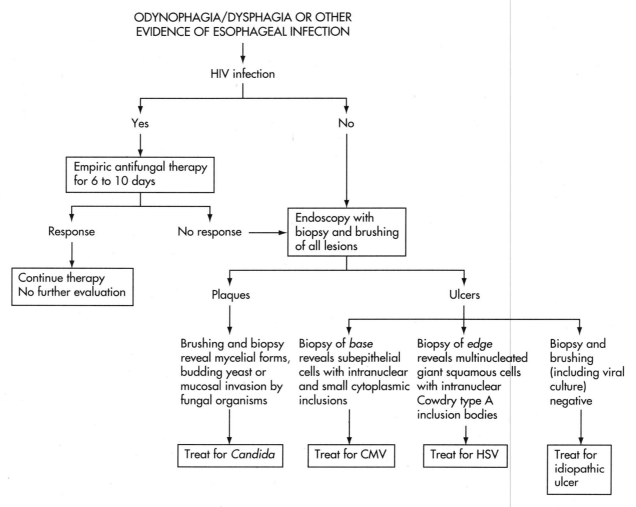

Figure 1
Suggested diagnostic approaches to common esophageal infections. *HIV,* Human immuno-deficiency virus; *CMV,* cytomegalovirus; *HSV,* herpes simplex virus type 1.

to diagnose Candida esophagitis. Typical candidal plaques are creamy white or pale yellow. At endoscopy, the gross appearance is graded: grade 1—a few raised white plaques up to 2 mm wide, without ulceration; grade 2—multiple raised white plaques more than 2 mm wide, without ulceration (Figure 2, *A*); grade 3—confluent, linear, and nodular elevated plaques with superficial ulceration; and, grade 4—finding of grade 3 plus narrowing of the esophageal lumen.

Brushings from involved surfaces and ulcers can be obtained with a sheathed cytology brush spread onto slides and stained by the PAS, silver, or Gram methods. Mycelial forms and masses of budding yeast are consistent with *Candida* infection (Figure 2, *B*). Fungal cultures are generally not helpful unless an unusual pathogen (e.g., a resistant *Candida* species, such as *Torulopsis glabrata*) is suspected.

Because findings are often nonspecific and concurrent infections (e.g., *C. albicans* plus a virus) will be missed, radiographic studies of the esophagus are not helpful in establishing an accurate diagnosis of esophageal infection.

Barium esophagrams may reveal a "shaggy" esophagus, plaques, pseudomembranes, cobblestoning, nodules, strictures, fistulae, or mucosal bridges. Radiographic examination is useful when endoscopy is not available, when endoscopic biopsies are precluded because of coagulopathy, or when dysphagia or coughing associated with eating are prominent symptoms, thereby suggesting the presence of perforation, stricture, or fistula.

Treatment

Three classes of agents are used to treat esophageal fungal infections: (1) imidazoles (e.g., fluconazole, ketoconazole, itraconazole, clotrimazole) alter fungal cell membrane permeability by inhibiting the synthesis of ergosterols. (2) Polyene antibiotics (nystatin and amphotericin) irreversibly bind to fungal membrane sterols, thereby altering membrane permeability. (3) Flucytosine, a fluorinated pyrimidine, interferes with fungal translation of RNA. Fungi rapidly develop resistance to this agent, so it should be used only in combination with amphotericin.

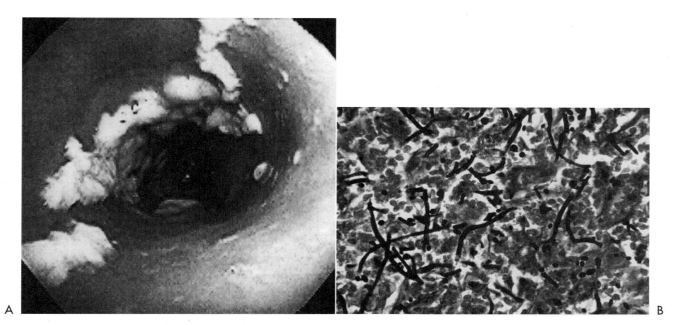

Figure 2
A, Endoscopic appearance of grade 3 Candida esophagitis with multiple raised white plaques greater than 2 mm. **B,** Biopsy revealing budding yeast cells, hyphae, pseudohyphae, and mucosal invasion by the organisms.

The aggressiveness of treatment for Candida and other forms of infectious esophagitis should be tailored to the immunocompetence of the host and the severity of infection (Table 2). Topical antifungal agents will suffice for most immunocompetent patients with fungal esophagitis (see Table 2). Advantages of these nonabsorbable agents include fewer side effects and drug interactions. Clotrimazole (10-mg troches dissolved in the mouth five times daily for at least 1 week) is a nonabsorbable imidazole that is well tolerated. Nystatin (1 to 3 million units orally four times daily for at least 1 week) is an effective nonabsorbable agent that is generally less palatable than clotrimazole. Miconazole and amphotericin are rarely used orally and demonstrate no obvious advantage when compared with clotrimazole or nystatin.

Moderately or severely impaired host defenses result in more extensive infection and require more aggressive treatment. Based on the severity of immunocompromise and infection, one can initiate oral therapy with fluconazole, itraconazole, or ketoconazole (Table 2). Fluconazole has a longer half-life, has more reliable gastrointestinal absorption regardless of gastric acidity, has fewer drug interactions, and perhaps most importantly, is associated with fewer treatment failures than ketoconazole. However, fluconazole is more costly. In immunocompromised patients with esophageal candidiasis, particularly those with AIDS, fluconazole (100 to 200 mg/day orally for 10 to 14 days) is the preferred treatment.

In granulocytopenic patients, Candida esophagitis must be treated with intravenous amphotericin to prevent potential systemic dissemination of Candida infection. Patients who are febrile or have disseminated infection should be treated with amphotericin, 0.5 mg/kg/day intravenously,

with the duration of therapy dictated by the degree and duration of granulocytopenia. In a persistently granulocytopenic patient, successful treatment of disseminated Candida infection generally requires a cumulative amphotericin dose of 1.5 to 2.0 g infused over 6 to 12 weeks. In patients without evidence of infection beyond epithelial tissues, less aggressive treatment with amphotericin (0.3 mg/kg/day intravenously for 7 to 10 days) may be effective. With recovery of granulocytes, resolution of fever, and symptomatic improvement, therapy may be changed from amphotericin to a 10- to 14-day course of fluconazole. Combination therapy with fluconazole plus amphotericin should be avoided because of theoretic concerns regarding competing modes of action for these agents. However, for life-threatening fungal infections, amphotericin may be combined with flucytosine (every 6 hours to 50 to 150 mg/kg/day). Adjunctive therapy with colony-stimulating factors may help restore granulocyte counts in some leukopenic patients.

Other Fungal Infections of the Esophagus

Esophageal aspergillosis, histoplasmosis, and blastomycosis, acquired from the environment rather than from endogenous flora, are much less common than infection with *Candida* species. Blastomycosis and histoplasmosis commonly invade the esophagus from paraesophageal lymph nodes. *Aspergillus* infection results in large, deep ulcers, whereas esophageal histoplasmosis and blastomycosis are characterized by focal lesions and abscesses. With involvement of muscle layers, severe odynophagia results. Complications of these noncandidal fungal infections include esophageal stricture and tracheoesophageal fistula. *Aspergillus* species have a distinctive microscopic appearance. *Histoplasma* organisms usually do not invade the esophageal

Table 2   Recommended Treatment of Common Esophageal Infections

ORGANISM	HOST IMMUNE STATUS	TREATMENT
Candida albicans	Normal	Nystatin suspension, 1-3 million units PO 4 times daily for 7 days or Clotrimazole troche, 10 mg dissolved in the mouth 5 times daily for 7 days
	Impaired	Fluconazole, 100 mg PO once daily for 14 days or Ketoconazole, 200 mg PO once daily for 14 days or Clotrimazole troche, 100 mg dissolved in the mouth 3 times daily for 14 days or Fluconazole, 100-200 mg IV once daily
	Impaired/granulocytopenic	Amphotericin, 0.5 mg/kg/day IV to a cumulative dose of 1.5 to 2.0 g over 6 to 12 wk
Herpes simplex virus		Acyclovir, 250 mg/m² IV q8h for 7-10 days or Foscarnet, 90 mg/kg IV q12h for 14-21 days or Famciclovir, 500 mg PO twice daily for 14 days
Cytomegalovirus		Ganciclovir, 5 mg/kg IV q12h for 14 days, followed by maintenance therapy until immunosuppression resolves or Foscarnet, 90 mg/kg IV q12h for 14-21 days, followed by maintenance therapy with 90-120 mg/kg/day
Varicella-zoster virus		Acyclovir, 250 mg/m² IV q8h for 7-10 days or Foscarnet, 90 mg/kg IV q12h for 14-21 days or Famciclovir, 500 mg PO twice daily for 14 days

mucosa. Hence, endoscopic brushing and biopsy specimens may be nondiagnostic, and bronchoscopy, mediastinoscopy, or surgery may be needed to diagnose this infection. Intravenous amphotericin is the preferred treatment for *Aspergillus* infections and is also used for complicated histoplasmosis and blastomycosis or for ketoconazole-resistant organisms.

■ VIRAL INFECTIONS OF THE ESOPHAGUS

Herpes Simplex Virus Type 1

Herpes simplex virus type 1 (HSV) is the most common of the three herpes viruses that may infect the esophagus; the others are cytomegalovirus (CMV) and varicella-zoster virus (VZV). In contrast to CMV, VZV, and *Candida* species, HSV can infect the esophagus in otherwise healthy people without a risk factor.

HSV, a large, enveloped, double-stranded DNA virus, causes an acute infection of squamous epithelium with the formation of characteristic painful herpetic vesicles with erythematous bases. Latency in the root ganglia of nerves supplying the affected regions may follow resolution of acute HSV infection. Thus, although primary HSV esophagitis occurs, it is most often a result of reactivation of latent virus in the distribution of the laryngeal, superior cervical, or vagus nerves.

The abrupt onset of severe odynophagia is a common presenting symptom of HSV esophagitis. Other symptoms include persistent retrosternal pain, nausea, and vomiting. Bone marrow transplant recipients may have continuous nausea and vomiting as the sole manifestation of HSV esophagitis. Herpes labialis (i.e., cold sores) or skin involvement may precede or occur concurrent with esophageal infection. In untreated immunocompetent persons, HSV esophagitis resolves 1 to 2 weeks after the onset of symptoms, although early initiation of antiviral therapy may hasten recovery. In immunodeficient patients, esophageal infection with HSV can cause hemorrhage and perforation with tracheoesophageal fistulae or can disseminate to involve the liver, lungs, and central nervous system.

Diagnosis of HSV esophagitis is usually established by endoscopy (see Figure 1). Early, vesicular herpetic lesions (round 1- to 3-mm vesicles in the mid to distal esophagus) are rarely seen. More commonly, by the time the clinician has performed endoscopy, the centers of the vesicles have sloughed to reveal discrete, circumscribed ulcers with raised edges (Figure 3, *A*). These "volcano" lesions result in the classic appearance of HSV esophagitis on double-contrast barium studies of the esophagus, although similar radiographic findings may rarely be seen in Candida esophagitis. Discrete HSV ulcers seen at early stages can coalesce into large lesions or, in severe cases, to near-total denudation of the esophageal epithelium. Hence, diffuse herpetic esophagitis results in cobblestoning or a "shaggy" mucosa that, because of the similar appearance to Candida esophagitis, further confuses the diagnosis. Endoscopic brushings and

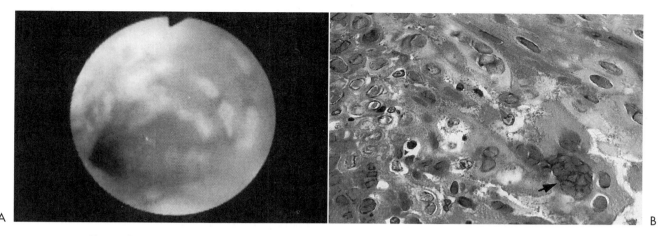

Figure 3
A, Endoscopic photograph revealing multiple aphthous ulcers in distal third of esophagus.
B, Biopsy demonstrating multinucleated giant cells *(arrow).*

biopsies for cytologic or histologic examination, respectively, should be taken from ulcer edges because HSV preferentially infects squamous epithelial cells. Additional biopsy samples should be submitted in transport media for HSV culture. Multinucleated giant cells, ballooning degeneration, "ground-glass" intranuclear Cowdry type A inclusions, and margination of chromatin are among the features that may be observed with histologic staining of HSV-infected epithelial cells (Figure 3, *B*).

Treatment of HSV esophagitis is with intravenous acyclovir, 250 mg/m^2 every 8 hours for 7 to 14 days (Table 2). In trials comprising immunocompromised patients with HSV-1 and HSV-2 oral and genital infections, this nucleoside analog shortened periods of viral shedding, lessened pain, and hastened healing. Adverse effects of acyclovir therapy include rash and irritation of veins used for drug infusion. Because it is safe and effective, acyclovir is usually given to all patients with HSV esophagitis regardless of immune status. Foscarnet is used to treat those infected with acyclovir-resistant HSV. Prophylaxis with oral acyclovir may be indicated for immunocompromised persons at high risk for reactivation of HSV (e.g., HSV-seropositive transplant recipients and AIDS patients with recurrent herpetic infections). Famciclovir is an acyclovir analog with a similar spectrum of activity and better bioavailability that may eventually replace acyclovir for oral prophylaxis and treatment.

Cytomegalovirus

CMV, a ubiquitous herpesvirus, infects most of the world's adults. In healthy people with latent infection, CMV viral DNA can be detected in many tissues, including circulating leukocytes. Latent infection is responsible for the high transmission rate of the virus from CMV-seropositive donors to CMV-seronegative recipients after blood transfusion or organ transplant. In contrast to HSV, esophageal infection with CMV, either primary or reactivation of latent virus, occurs only in immunodeficiency states (AIDS and others). Other differences between these herpesviruses is that, in

CMV esophagitis, the virus infects subepithelial fibroblasts and endothelial cells of the esophagus, not squamous epithelial cells, and the onset of symptoms with CMV is typically more gradual than with HSV or Candida esophagitis. Because CMV disease is systemic and involves multiple organs, nausea, vomiting, fever, epigastric pain, diarrhea, and weight loss are prominent symptoms, whereas dysphagia and odynophagia are less commonly observed than in HSV infection.

In CMV esophagitis, barium studies may reveal focal ulcerations in the distal third of the esophagus that are indistinguishable from those seen with HSV. In some cases, radiographs may show flat elongate, tear-drop, or stellate giant ulcers that can be confused with those observed with HIV-associated idiopathic esophageal ulcers (see the following). Hence, because neither clinical assessment, radiographs, nor endoscopic appearance are sufficiently accurate, the diagnosis of CMV esophagitis commonly depends on endoscopic biopsies (see Figure 1). Endoscopic findings suggestive of CMV esophagitis include superficial erosions or deep ulcers with geographic, serpiginous, flat borders in the mid to distal esophagus. Deep ulcers may extend longitudinally for several centimeters and may reach the muscularis, occasionally resulting in stricture formation. Numerous biopsy samples should be taken from ulcer bases, where CMV-infected subepithelial fibroblasts and endothelial cells are most likely to be present. Specimens containing only squamous epithelium are not helpful, and superficial brushings for cytologic examination do not increase the diagnostic yield. Because CMV may infect gastric and intestinal epithelial and lamina propria cells, biopsy of abnormal mucosa in these areas should also be obtained for histology and viral culture. Biopsy specimens are important for confirmation of CMV infection and to exclude concurrent fungal, viral (HSV), or bacterial pathogens.

Histologic features indicative of CMV infection are large cells in the subepithelial layer with amphophilic intranuclear inclusions, a "halo" surrounding the nucleus, and, in contrast to HSV and VZV, multiple, small cytoplasmic inclu-

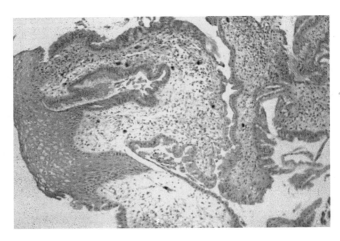

Figure 4
Biopsy at gastroesophageal junction revealing subepithelial CMV by immunohistochemical staining *(Courtesy L.W. Lamps, M.D., Little Rock, AR.)*

sions. Although immunohistochemical staining and in situ hybridization can confirm CMV infection (Figure 4), viral cultures are more sensitive.

Effective treatment for CMV esophagitis is ganciclovir and foscarnet, alone or in combination (see Table 2). Ganciclovir (5 mg/kg IV every 12 hours for 2 weeks) is very effective in eliminating CMV from esophageal ulcers. However, without restoration of the normal immune system, recurrence after short courses of therapy is common. Therefore it is recommended that full-dose antiviral therapy for 2 weeks be followed by maintenance therapy until immunosuppression resolves (see Table 2). Persons with AIDS and recurrent CMV infection often require indefinite maintenance therapy with ganciclovir. Bone marrow suppression is the major adverse effect of ganciclovir. An additional concern is the emergence of ganciclovir-resistant CMV with long-term therapy. Ganciclovir-resistant CMV is usually responsive to foscarnet (90 mg/kg IV every 12 hours for 2 to 3 weeks) followed by maintenance therapy (90 to 120 mg/kg/day).

Varicella-Zoster Virus

The frequency of VZV esophagitis during the course of chickenpox or herpes zoster infections is unknown. Symptomatic VZV esophagitis is extremely rare. However, VZV esophagitis may be severe in profoundly immunocompromised individuals but is relatively minor compared with other manifestations of disseminated infection such as varicella encephalitis, pneumonitis, and fulminant hepatitis. The clinical presentations and esophageal lesions with VZV mimic HSV esophagitis. Finding concurrent dermatologic VZV lesions (shingles) is often crucial for diagnosing VZV esophagitis. VZV esophagitis may be treated with acyclovir or famciclovir. Foscarnet is an alternative for acyclovir-resistant VZV (see Table 2).

Idiopathic Ulcerative Esophagitis in AIDS

HIV infection is often associated with esophageal ulcers that lack identifiable pathogens. These lesions, called *HIV-associated* or *idiopathic esophageal ulcers,* appear as multiple, small aphthoid ulcers during seroconversion in early HIV infection and, later, as giant, deep ulcers extending up to several centimeters. The latter are associated with severe, incapacitating odynophagia. Radiologic and endoscopic studies reveal ulcers that mimic those caused by CMV. Clinical and endoscopic improvement has been reported following systemic prednisone (40 mg/day for 4 weeks) or intralesional corticosteroid therapy. A thorough search for infectious pathogens, including endoscopic brushing and biopsy, must be undertaken before corticosteroid therapy is initiated. Thalidomide, a sedative with immunomodulatory properties related to inhibition of tumor necrosis factor-alpha has also been used successfully to treat these ulcers.

Bacterial, Mycobacterial, and Treponemal Infections

Esophageal infection with normal oropharyngeal flora rarely occurs, although invasive bacteria may account for 11% to 16% of infectious esophagitis in immunodeficient patients, especially those with granulocytopenia. As with other organisms, symptoms of bacterial esophagitis include dysphagia and odynophagia. Fever is an uncommon finding, probably because of agranulocytosis. Endoscopic findings are nonspecific, including mucosal friability, plaques, pseudomembranes, and ulcerations. Diagnostic biopsies reveal sheets of confluent bacteria invading subepithelial tissues. Bacterial culture of biopsy material is often contaminated by multiple organisms and consequently of little utility. Bacterial esophagitis is treated with a broad-spectrum, beta-lactam antibiotic combined with an aminoglycoside.

Formerly, esophageal infection with *Mycobacterium tuberculosis* or *M. avium* was considered a rare finding that occurred in fewer than 0.15% of autopsies. However, with the advent of the AIDS epidemic, the prevalence of tuberculosis has increased. Esophageal involvement with tuberculosis almost always results from direct extension of infection from adjacent mediastinal structures, with few cases of primary esophageal tuberculosis. Symptoms of esophageal mycobacterial infection include odynophagia, dysphagia, weight loss, cough, chest pain, and fever, depending on the extent of involvement. Fistulae within the wall of the esophagus (so-called double-barrelled esophagus) and connecting to the mediastinum, trachea, or bronchi are not infrequent. Contrast radiology findings, including ulcers, fistulae, and strictures, are not specific. Gross endoscopic findings include shallow ulcers, heaped-up lesions mimicking cancer, and extrinsic compression of esophagus from adenopathy (the latter can also be evaluated by computed tomography of the chest). Mycobacterial infection of the esophagus can be diagnosed when endoscopic biopsies reveal granulomas or acid-fast bacilli. Biopsy specimens can be cultured for confirmation of infection and determination of sensitivity to antimycobacterial agents. Esophageal infection with mycobacteria is treated with standard multidrug therapy, guided in part by the sensitivity profile in the community. In addition to pharmacologic therapy, endoscopic stenting or surgery are sometimes required to treat fistulas and perforations.

In the current era, esophageal syphilis is very rare. Tertiary syphilis may be associated with gummas, diffuse ulceration, fistulas, and stricture of the upper third of the esophagus. Syphilitic esophagitis may be considered in a patient with tertiary syphilis and an inflammatory esophageal stricture. The diagnosis may be suspected if syphilitic periarteritis is present on endoscopic biopsy specimens; however, specific immunostaining for *Treponema pallidum* should be performed for definitive diagnosis.

Suggested Reading

Baehr PH, McDonald GB: Esophageal infections: risk factors, presentation, diagnosis, and treatment, *Gastroenterology* 106:509, 1994.

Baehr PH, McDonald GB: Esophageal disorders caused by infections. In Sleisenger M, ed: *Sleisenger & Fordtran's gastrointestinal and liver disease,* ed 6, Philadelphia, 1998, Saunders.

Raufman JP: Infectious esophagitis. In Hurst JW, ed: *Medicine for the practicing physician,* ed 4, Norwalk, CT, 1996, Appleton & Lange.

Wilcox CM: Esophageal infections. In Yamada T, ed: *Textbook of gastroenterology,* ed 3, Philadelphia, 1999, Lippincott.

Wilcox CM, Schwartz DA, Clark WS: Esophageal ulceration in HIV infection: causes, response to therapy, and long-term outcome, *Ann Intern Med* 123:143, 1995.

GASTROENTERITIS

Douglas R. Morgan
Robert L. Owen

■ GASTROENTERITIS

The term *gastroenteritis,* rigorously defined, refers to any inflammatory process of the stomach or intestinal mucosal surface. However, the term usually refers to acute infectious diarrhea, a diarrheal syndrome of less than 2 weeks' duration that may be accompanied by fever, nausea, vomiting, abdominal pain, dehydration, and weight loss. This chapter provides an overview of the infectious enteritides. Other chapters consider food poisoning, traveler's diarrhea, antibiotic-associated diarrhea, sexually transmitted enteric infections, and *Helicobacter pylori* disease.

In developed countries, gastroenteritis, like the common cold, is common and annoying, but it usually does not require a physician visit, laboratory evaluation, or antibiotic treatment. On a global scale, it is second only to cardiovascular disease as a cause of death. It remains the leading worldwide cause of childhood death and of years of productive life lost, with approximately 12,600 deaths per day. Annual per-person attack rates range from 1 to 5 in the United States and Europe and up to 5 to 20 in the developing world. There are approximately 100 million cases per year among adults in the United States, nearly 50% of which require patients to limit their activities for more than 24 hours, while 8% require consultation with a physician and fewer than 0.3% result in hospitalization.

■ PATHOPHYSIOLOGY

The normal gastrointestinal (GI) tract is remarkably efficient at fluid reabsorption. Normally, of the 1 to 2 L of fluid ingested orally and the 7 L that enter the upper tract from saliva, gastric, pancreatic, and biliary sources, less than 200 ml of fluid are excreted daily in the feces. Thus small increases in secretory rate or decreases in the absorptive rate can easily overwhelm the colonic absorptive capacity of about 4 L/day—leading to diarrhea, defined as increased frequency (more than three bowel movements) or increased volume (>200 ml/day).

Intestinal infection with bacteria, viruses, and parasites that produce gastroenteritis usually follows fecal-oral transmission. Host defenses, which protect the human intestine, are reviewed in Table 1. The principal defenses include the physical barrier of the mucosa itself and gastric acidity. A gastric pH below 4 will rapidly kill more than 99% of ingested organisms, although rotavirus and protozoal cysts can survive. Patients with achlorhydria from gastric surgery, human immunodeficiency virus (HIV) infection, chronic atrophic gastritis, or use of proton pump inhibitors (PPIs) are at increased risk of developing infectious diarrhea. Destruction of the mucosal barrier, as is the case with mucositis associated with chemotherapy or irradiation, predisposes patients to gram-negative sepsis. In gastroenteritis there is an increase in peristalsis, which propels organisms along the GI tract, analogous to the cough clearing the lungs. The intestinal flora forms a critical element of the host defense, both in terms of quantity and composition. The small intestine and colon contain approximately 10^4 and 10^{11} organisms per gram, respectively. More than 99% of the colonic bacteria are anaerobes. Their production of fatty acids with an acidic pH and their competition for mucosal attachment sites prevent colonization by invading organisms. At the extremes of age, in children and the elderly, and after recent antibiotic use, the flora is altered and the risk for gastroenteritis increased. Impairment of intestinal immunity is also a risk factor for intestinal infections.

Virulence factors play a complementary role in acute infectious diarrhea. Whether an individual ingests an inoculum sufficient to establish clinical gastroenteritis is directly related to community sanitation and personal hygiene. Most organisms require an inoculum of 10^5 to 10^8 to establish infection. Exceptions include *Shigella* and protozoa such as *Giardia, Cryptosporidium,* and *Entamoeba,* which may cause diarrhea when only 10 to 100 organisms are ingested. Bacteria produce several types of toxins, which lead to different

Table 1 Host Defenses

HOST DEFENSE FACTOR	EXAMPLE DISEASE STATE
Barrier	
Gastric acid	Achlorhydria (PPI, HIV, gastric surgery)
Mucosal integrity	Mucositis (chemotherapy)
Intestinal motility	
Peristalsis	Blind loop, antimotility drugs, hypomotility states (diabetes, scleroderma)
Commensal microflora	Antibiotics, age extremes
Sanitation	Contaminated water
Intestinal immunity	
Phagocytic	Neutropenia
Cellular	HIV
Humoral	IgA deficiency

PPI, Proton pump inhibitor; HIV, human immunodeficiency virus.

Table 2 Virulence Factors

VIRULENCE FACTORS	EXAMPLES
Inoculum size	*Shigella, Entamoeba, Giardia*
Adherence	Cholera, EPEC
Invasion	*Shigella, Salmonella typhi, Yersinia,* EIEC
Toxins	
Enterotoxin	Cholera, *Salmonella,* ETEC
Cytotoxin	*Shigella, Clostridium difficile,* EHEC
Neurotoxin	*Clostridium botulinum, Staphylococcus aureus, Bacillus cereus*

EPEC, Enteropathogenic *Escherichia coli*; EIEC, enteroinvasive *E. coli*; ETEC, enterotoxigenic *E. coli*; EHEC, enterohemorrhagic *E. coli*.

clinical syndromes, including enterotoxin (watery diarrhea), cytotoxin (dysentery), and neurotoxin. Botulinum toxin is the classic example of a preformed neurotoxin, but interestingly, both *Staphylococcus aureus* and *Bacillus cereus* also produce neurotoxins, which act on the central nervous system to produce emesis. Adherence and invasion factors facilitate colonization and contribute to virulence. Various forms of *Escherichia coli* express the gamut of virulence factors (Table 2).

■ CLINICAL SYNDROMES

The acute infectious diarrheas can be divided into noninflammatory, inflammatory, and invasive (Table 3). Most attacks are caused by organisms from the noninflammatory, or secretory, category. The bacteria in this group, such as *Vibrio cholerae* and enterotoxigenic *E. coli* (ETEC), typically secrete an enterotoxin, which affects the small intestine, producing a large volume of watery diarrhea without fecal leukocytes. Most forms of viral gastroenteritis (e.g., *Rotavirus* and *Calicivirus* [Norwalk agent]) also fall into this group.

The inflammatory diarrheas typically infect the colon, causing frequent small-volume stools, often with fecal white cells and either gross or occult blood. Fever, tenesmus, and bloody diarrhea are characteristic of dysentery. Some bacteria that cause inflammatory diarrhea produce cytotoxins. The invasive diarrheas may be considered a subset of the inflammatory diarrheas because there is invasion of the intestinal wall, but with a propensity to cause bacteremia and metastatic disease. *Salmonella typhi* is the prototype. Typhoid bacteria invade the Peyer's patches of the distal ileum, then disseminate and multiply in the reticuloendothelial system to produce systemic disease.

Certain subpopulations of patients with gastroenteritis merit close surveillance because of the organisms involved, the potential for severe disease, and the possible need for intervention. These are listed in Table 4. Foodborne disease should be considered in outbreaks of acute GI symptoms affecting two or more persons. The most common causes include *Salmonella* species, *S. aureus, Shigella* species, *B. cereus,* and *C. perfringens.* Patients with the acquired immunodeficiency syndrome (AIDS) are predisposed to a number of unique infections (microsporidia, cytomegalovirus) or more severe manifestations of otherwise common infections (*Salmonella, Campylobacter, Cryptosporidium*). The microbial pathogens responsible for traveler's diarrhea are dependent upon the region visited. Enterotoxigenic *E. coli* is the most commonly isolated organism, ranging between 20% and 60% of isolates in areas of Asia and Latin America, respectively. Acute infectious proctitis, which is often sexually transmitted, leads to tenesmus, hematochezia, and rectal pain. Syphilis, gonorrhea, and chlamydia are additional organisms to consider. The incidence of sexually transmitted proctitis is decreasing in the AIDS era with safer sex practices. Other important subpopulations include patients with antibiotic-associated diarrhea, especially those from hospitals or chronic care facilities.

Gastroenteritis is a major cause of worldwide mortality and morbidity among infants and children. In developed countries, acute diarrheal illnesses account for 7% of pediatric ambulatory visits as well as hospitalizations. Peak attack rates involve young schoolchildren and their younger siblings. Most cases are caused by viral agents: rotaviruses (10% to 50%), calcivirus (Norwalk agent, 10% to 30%), and the enteric adenoviruses (2% to 5%). Bacterial agents cause less than 15% of disease but may cause severe disease in patients with *Campylobacter* species, *E. coli* species, *Salmonella* species, or *Yersinia* species. EHEC O157:H7 is an important cause of hemolytic-uremic syndrome in children. *Yersinia* causes a watery diarrhea in children ages 1 to 5, but it may mimic appendicitis in older children and adolescents. Important pathogens in day-care and institutional settings are the above-mentioned bacterial species, as well as *Giardia lamblia, Cryptosporidium parvum,* and *Clostridium difficile.*

H. pylori infection is a form of GI infection localized to the stomach. This gram-negative spiral bacterium is now known to be a cause of acute gastritis, chronic atrophic gastritis, and peptic ulcer disease. Based on epidemiologic data, it is also a major causative factor in the development of gastric adenocarcinoma and low-grade, mucosa-associated lymphoid tissue (MALT) lymphoma. It is likely acquired in

Table 3 Clinical Syndromes

		NONINFLAMMATORY	INFLAMMATORY	INVASIVE
Syndrome		Watery diarrhea, emesis	Dysentery	Enteric fever
Site		Small intestine	Colon	Ileum, colon
Stool				
	Volume	Large	Small	Small
	Fecal WBCs	Absent	Present	Present
Common organisms				
	Bacteria	*Vibrio cholerae* ETEC	Shigella spp. *Salmonella* spp. *Campylobacter jejuni*	*Salmonella typhi* *Yersinia* spp. *Brucella*
	Viruses	Rotavirus Calicivirus* Adenovirus Astrovirus	—	—
	Parasites	*Giardia* *Cryptosporidium*	*Entamoeba*	*Entamoeba*

WBC, White blood cells; *ETEC*, enterotoxigenic *E. coli*; *EIEC*, enteroinvasive *E. coli*.
*Formerly known as the Norwalk agent.

Table 4 Etiologic Agents by Clinical Presentation

POPULATION	BACTERIA	VIRUSES	PARASITES	OTHER
Food poisoning	*Salmonella* *Staphylococcus aureus* *Shigella* *Clostridium perfringens* *Bacillus cereus* *Listeria*	Norwalk Hepatitis A	*Trichinella* *Giardia* *Cryptosporidium*	Ciguatera Histamine fish
AIDS	*Salmonella* *Campylobacter* *Shigella* MAC	CMV	*Cryptosporidium* *Isospora belli* *Microsporidia*	AIDS enteropathy
Traveler's diarrhea	*Escherichia coli* ETEC *Shigella* *Aeromonas* *E. coli*, other	Rotavirus	*Giardia*	No pathogen (40%)
Acute proctitis	*Gonorrhea* *Chlamydia* *Treponema pallidum* *Shigella* *Salmonella*	HSV Condyloma, HPV CMV	*Entamoeba* *Cryptosporidium*	
Day-care centers	*Shigella* *Campylobacter jejuni*	Rotavirus	*Giardia* *Cryptosporidium*	
Antibiotic associated	*Clostridium difficile*			*Candida albicans*
Seafood ingestion	*Vibrio* spp.		Anisakidae	

AIDS, Acquired immunodeficiency virus; *CMV*, cytomegalovirus; *MAC*, *Mycobacterium avium* complex; *ETEC*, enterotoxigenic *E. coli*; *HSV*, herpes simplex virus; *HPV*, human papilloma virus.

childhood via oral-oral or fecal-oral transmission, and the prevalence within a population is directly related to the socioeconomic status of the cohort in childhood. Approximately 60% of the world's population is chronically infected; in the United States, 30% to 40% of adults and 5% to 10% of adolescents are infected. More than 50% of peptic ulcers are caused by *H. pylori*, and there is substantial prospective evidence that eradication of the organism prevents their recurrence. Studies to date fail to demonstrate an association between *H. pylori* and nonulcer dyspepsia or that its eradication in this setting relieves symptoms. Documen-

tation of infection is done with serology, the urea breath test, and gastric biopsy (rapid urease tests, histology). (See the chapter on *Helicobacter pylori* for further details).

■ PATIENT EVALUATION

Most cases of acute gastroenteritis are self-limited and do not require medical attention. Physician consultation generally is advised for patients with a fever (>38.5° C [101.3° F]), dysentery (bloody stools), significant abdominal pain, dehydration, and risk factors for disease requiring intervention. Initial evaluation consists of the history, physical examination, and screening stool examination. Laboratory testing and antimicrobial therapy are recommended in a limited subset of patients based on this initial evaluation.

The history should focus on the severity of disease and the risk factors for specific types of infectious diarrhea. The patient should be questioned regarding symptom duration, fever, abdominal pain, tenesmus, and dehydration. The description of the diarrhea is important: frequency, volume, and any blood, pus, or mucus. Diarrhea persisting longer than 2 to 4 weeks qualifies as chronic, has an alternate differential, and should be fully investigated. Inquiry should also be made into factors that may place the patient in a specific subpopulation at increased risk for significant infection. Examples include age over 70, recent international travel or camping, antibiotic use within the last 2 months, HIV disease or risk factors, other immunosuppression (including prednisone therapy), anal eroticism, seafood consumption, household contacts of day-care workers or children, and the potential for a common source outbreak (e.g., friends or relatives with similar symptoms). Short incubation periods of less than 6 hours, or 6 to 12 hours, suggest ingestion of an enterotoxin produced by *S. aureus* and *B. cereus*, or *C. perfringens*, respectively. A viral infection or food poisoning is suggested when vomiting is the dominant complaint.

A broad differential diagnosis is considered initially because acute diarrhea may be the initial presentation of noninfectious and also potentially life-threatening diseases. Important diagnoses to consider include inflammatory bowel disease, mesenteric vascular disease, bowel obstruction, and GI hemorrhage. Patients should be questioned regarding medications that may cause diarrhea, such as metformin, colchicine, diuretics, angiotensin-converting enzyme (ACE) inhibitors, PPIs, and magnesium-containing antacids.

The physical examination is important to gauge the severity of the disease. Orthostasis, tachycardia, decreased skin turgor, and dry mucous membranes are signs of significant dehydration. The presence of fever, abdominal tenderness, and any skin rashes should be documented. All patients should undergo a rectal examination when rectal bleeding is present.

All patients who merit medical evaluation should have a screening stool examination. A fresh-cup specimen is preferred because there is evidence that swab and diaper specimens have decreased sensitivity. The stool should be evaluated for fecal leukocytes and fecal occult blood. Fecal leukocytes are detected in the clinical laboratory either with staining techniques or lactoferrin (a leukocyte product) testing. In the office or at the bedside, microscopic examination of the stool is facilitated by the methylene blue stain. A wet mount is prepared with two drops of methylene blue mixed with fecal mucus; 2 minutes should be allowed for adequate staining of the leukocyte nuclei before high-power microscopy of the cover-slipped slide. The presence of three or more fecal leukocytes per high-powered field in at least four fields is considered a positive examination. Table 5 lists the degree of association of the usual enteric pathogens with

Table 5 Fecal Leukocytes		
PRESENT	**VARIABLE**	**ABSENT**
Campylobacter	Salmonella	Toxigenic bacteria
Shigella	Yersinia	ETEC, EPEC
EIEC, EHEC	Clostridium difficile	Viruses
	Vibrio parahemolyticus	Parasites
	Noninfectious causes	
	Ischemic colitis	
	IBD	

EIEC, Enteroinvasive *E. coli*; *EHEC*, enterohemorrhagic *E. coli*; *IBD*, inflammatory bowel disease; *ETEC*, enterotoxigenic *E. coli*; *EPEC*, enteropathogenic *E. coli*.

fecal leukocytes. With fecal leukocytes, there is some overlap between the inflammatory and noninflammatory diarrheas. The finding on screening stool examination of either fecal leukocytes, lactoferrin, or occult blood have equal predictive values for diffuse colonic disease, positive stool cultures, and disease requiring antimicrobial therapy. The organisms most commonly associated with a positive screening test include *Salmonella, Shigella, Campylobacter, Yersinia, Aeromonas, Vibrio,* and *C. difficile*.

The history, physical examination, and office stool evaluation serve as screening steps before further laboratory evaluation and possible need for treatment. Most patients with self-limited noninflammatory infectious diarrhea require only symptomatic therapy. Laboratory evaluation is indicated in three situations: patients with severe or persistent disease (fever greater than 38.5° C [101.3° F], dehydration, grossly bloody stools, duration of more than 1 week), patients from the aforementioned subpopulations, and patients with positive stool screening examinations (fecal leukocytes or occult blood). The initial laboratory evaluation should include a complete blood count, serum electrolytes, and stool processed for bacterial culture (*Salmonella, Shigella, Campylobacter*). Many stool cultures are ordered inappropriately. The probability of a positive culture is less than 2% to 5% for patients without fever, occult blood, or fecal leukocytes. The yield increases to approximately 20% and 50%, respectively, when one or two of the three findings are present. Formed stools should not be sent for testing. Patients hospitalized for more than 3 days who subsequently develop diarrhea are unlikely to have a bacterial or parasitic pathogen, and stool cultures are inappropriate.

Additional laboratory or diagnostic evaluation depends on the clinical situation. Routine stool examination for ova and parasites are not recommended. Studies for parasites are indicated in the setting of persistent diarrhea, international or wilderness travel, AIDS, and infants attending a day-care center (or persons exposed to such infants). In addition, fecal leukocyte-negative, bloody diarrhea is associated with *Entamoeba histolytica, Schistosoma, Dientamoeba fragilis,* and *Balantidium coli*. The sensitivity of three ova and parasite examinations on three separate days is 95% to 98%. Stool testing for *C. difficile* cytotoxin is appropriate in patients who have been taking antibiotics or who have been hospitalized within the past 2 months. Differentiation of

Table 6   Symptomatic Therapy for Diarrhea

GENERAL	INTRALUMINAL	ANTIMOTILITY	ANTISECRETORY
Rehydration	Bulking agents	Opiates	BSS
ORS	Psyllium	Loperamide	Octreotide
IV	Adsorbents	Diphenoxylate	
Diet therapy	Kaolin-pectin	Codeine	
	Attapulgite	Tincture of opium	
	Cholestyramine	Anticholinergics	
	Bacterial agents	Atropine	
	Lactobacilli	Scopolamine	
	Saccaromyces		

ORS, Oral rehydration solution; *IV*, intravenous; *BSS*, bismuth subsalicylate.

pathogenic and nonpathogenic strains of *E. coli* requires serotyping in specialized laboratories and is not generally indicated, except in an outbreak situation in which *E. coli* O157:H7 may be involved. Commercial EIA kits are available for detection of rotavirus and enteric adenovirus and may be useful in the pediatric population. Routine stool cultures identify most *Yersinia* species strains but may require special culture techniques if indicated. Sigmoidoscopy with biopsy should be considered for cases of acute proctitis, dysentery, and persistent infectious diarrhea. Colonoscopy or abdominal imaging (computed tomography [CT] scan, small-bowel-follow-through) may be helpful in complex presentations to help differentiate infectious and noninfectious causes of acute diarrhea.

The initial evaluation of AIDS-associated diarrhea should include stool examination for culture, ova and parasites, and acid-fast and *Cyclospora* smear (*Cryptosporidium*). Specialized stool studies are required for the detection of *Cyclospora*, microsporidiosis, and *Isospora belli*. Mucosal biopsies are required for the diagnosis of cytomegalovirus and *Mycobacterium avium-intracellulare* complex (MAC). Sigmoidoscopy may be considered for persistent or severe cases in patients with CD4 counts of less than 100 or those who have experienced weight loss. Colonoscopy and upper endoscopy generally are reserved for refractory cases.

■ MANAGEMENT

Rehydration is the goal of initial management. This can usually be accomplished with oral fluids. Oral rehydration solutions (ORS) have decreased worldwide cholera mortality rates from 50% to 1%. The World Health Organization (WHO) ORS is made up of 3.5 g sodium chloride, 2.5 g sodium bicarbonate, 1.5 g potassium chloride, and 20 g glucose per liter of water. Rice-based ORS also may be used. Prepared forms are available in solution (e.g., Pedialyte, Rehydrolyte) and packets (e.g., Orlyte). Various homemade recipes exist. One example includes alternating a glass of fruit juice (8 oz) with honey (½ tsp) and salt (¼ tsp), with a second glass of water (8 oz) with baking soda (¼ tsp). Sport drinks such as Gatorade are reasonable in nondehydrated adults. The goal is the passage of relatively dilute urine every 2 to 4 hours. Patients are advised to eat judiciously until

Table 7   Antidiarrheal Therapy

AGENT	DOSING	COMMENTS
Loperamide* (Imodium)	2 mg PO q3h	Initial dose, 4 mg Maximum, 16 mg/day
Diphenoxylate (Lomotil)	2 tablets or 10 ml PO qid	Maximum, 8 tablets/day
BSS† (Pepto-Bismol)	2 tablets or 30 ml PO qid	Maximum, 8 tablets/day
Tincture of opium	0.5-1.0 ml PO q4-6h	
Octreotide	100-500 µg SC tid	

BSS, Bismuth subsalicylate.
*Loperamide is the drug of choice. BSS may be used in presentations with significant vomiting.
†BSS should not be used in patients with human immunodeficiency virus because of the risk of bismuth encephalopathy.

stools are again formed. Cereals (rice, pasta), boiled foods (potatoes, vegetables), bananas, and crackers are recommended initial foods. Alcohol (cathartic effect), caffeine (increases intestinal motility), and carbonated drinks (gastric distension with reflex colonic contraction) should be avoided. Recommendations vary regarding dairy products, but transient lactose intolerance may occur.

In addition to rehydration, symptomatic therapy includes administering agents to control the diarrhea. These agents include bulking agents, antimotility drugs, and antisecretory medications. They are outlined in Tables 6 and 7. Antimotility agents should not be used if there is a possibility of a severe inflammatory bacterial diarrhea, particularly a febrile dysentery syndrome. Loperamide (Imodium) is the drug of choice in most situations because of its efficacy and safety. Bismuth subsalicylate (BSS) has antisecretory and antibacterial properties and is the drug of choice when vomiting is a significant part of the patient's presentation. It should not be used in the immunosuppressed patient, particularly the HIV population, because bismuth encephalopathy may occur. Diphenoxylate-atropine (Lomotil), which has both antimotility and antisecretory activity, may cause central nervous system depression, especially in children. Despite their popularity, kaopectate, cholestyramine, lactobacilli, and the anticholinergics have not been shown to be

Table 8   Antibiotic Therapy by Etiologic Agent

ETIOLOGIC AGENT	THERAPY	DURATION	COMMENTS
BACTERIA			
Empiric therapy*	Quinolone†	5-7 days	Indications:
			Fever and positive stool screen‡
			Dysentery syndrome
			Traveler's diarrhea, severe
Campylobacter	Erythromycin, 500 mg PO qid	5 days	See text for treatment indication
	Quinolone†		
	Azithromycin, 500 mg PO qd		
*Clostridium difficile**	Metronidazole, 250 mg PO qid	7-10 days	Metronidazole is the drug of choice
			given VRE risk.
	Vancomycin, 125 mg PO qid		
EIEC, ETEC*	Quinolone†	5 days	Treatment is not indicated for EHEC,
			including O157:H7.
	TMP-SMX-DS PO bid		
EPEC	Quinolone†	5 days	
Salmonella	Quinolone†	3-7 days	See text for treatment indication.
	TMP-SMX-DS PO bid		
	Chloramphenicol, 500 mg PO qid		
*Shigella**	Quinolone†	3-5 days	
	TMP-SMX-DS PO bid		
	Azithromycin, 250-500 mg PO qd		
*Vibrio cholerae**	Doxycycline, 300 mg PO	1 dose	
	Ciprofloxacin, 1 g PO		
Yersinia	Ceftriaxone, 2 g IV qd	5 days	For severe infection.
	Quinolone†		
PARASITES			
Cyclospora	TMP-SMX-DS PO bid	7 days	
*Entamoeba**	Metronidazole, 750 mg PO tid	10 days	Follow with cyst eradication regimen.
*Giardia**	Metronidazole, 250 mg PO tid	5 days	
Isospora	TMP-SMX-DS PO bid	7 days	

VRE, Vancomycin-resistant enterococcus; *EIEC*, enteroinvasive *E. coli*; *ETEC*, enterotoxigenic *E. coli*; *TMP-SMX-DS*, trimethoprim-sulfamethoxazole, 160-800 mg double-strength tablet; *EHEC*, enterohemorrhagic *E. coli*; *EPEC*, enteropathogenic *Escherichia coli*.
*Treatment clearly indicated. Treatment for the other listed microbes will depend on the clincal situation.
†Quinolone oral therapy options include: ciprofloxacin 500 mg bid, ofloxacin 300 mg bid, levofloxacin 250 mg qd.
‡Positive stool screen: fecal leukocytes or hemoccult positive.

consistently effective. With the exception of octreotide for prolonged secretory diarrhea, no new antidiarrheals have been released in several decades, but several agents are currently in clinical trials.

Severe AIDS diarrhea should be treated in stepwise fashion with Imodium (2 to 4 mg PO four times daily), lomotil (1 to 2 tablets PO four times daily), morphine (MS Contin 30 mg twice daily) or tincture of opium (DTO 0.5 to 1 ml PO four times daily), and octreotide (100 to 500 µg SC three times daily, increasing the dosage 200 µg every 3 days until response is seen).

Antibiotic therapy is indicated in a limited subset of patients with acute infectious diarrhea, as outlined in Table 8. Empiric therapy with a quinolone pending stool study is recommended for severe traveler's diarrhea and for patients with a fever and a positive stool screening study (leukocytes or blood). Patients with a positive stool culture or parasite examination should be treated in specified situations. Standard indications include symptomatic infections with certain bacteria (*Shigella*, enteroinvasive *E. coli*, *C. difficile*, *V. cholerae*), the sexually transmitted pathogens,

and the parasites. Therapy is reserved for specific situations for *Salmonella*, *Campylobacter*, *Yersinia*, *Aeromonas*, noncholera *Vibrio*, and other strains of *E. coli* (EPEC, EAEC). Treatment of *Salmonella* and *Campylobacter* is indicated for patients with dysentery; systemic illness, including bacteremia; or significant comorbidity (immunosuppression, malignancy, sickle cell anemia, prosthetic device, age extremes). Although controversial because of the possible association with the hemolytic-uremic syndrome, antimicrobial therapy is not recommended for enterohemorrhagic *E. coli*, including *E. coli* O157:H7. Metronidazole is the drug of choice for *C. difficile* colitis, given the risk of vancomycin-resistant enterococcus. Evolving eradication regimens for *H. pylori* are outlined in the chapter on *Helicobacter pylori*.

In summary, acute gastroenteritis, although common, is usually a self-limited disease. Oral rehydration and symptomatic therapy are appropriate for most patients. Medical evaluation is advised for patients with significant fever, dysentery, abdominal pain, dehydration, or risk factors for disease requiring intervention. Laboratory evaluation and antibiotic treatment should be limited to specific situations.

Suggested Reading

DuPont HL: Practice guidelines on acute infectious diarrhea, *Am J Gastro* 92:1962, 1997.

Fekety R: Practice guidelines for the diagnosis and management of *Clostridium difficile*-associated diarrhea and colitis, *Am J Gastro* 92:739, 1997.

Hamer DH, Gorbach SL: Infectious diarrhea and food poisoning. In Feldman M, Scharschmidt BF, eds: *Gastrointestinal and liver disease,* ed 6, Philadelphia, 1998, WB Saunders.

Heyman HB, Johnson AO, Synder JD: Diarrhea in infants and children. In Surawicz C, Owen RL, eds: *Gastrointestinal and hepatic infections,* Philadelphia, 1995, WB Saunders.

Hines J, Nachamkin I: Effective use of the clinical microbiology laboratory for diagnosing diarrheal diseases, *Clin Infect Dis* 23:1292, 1996.

Powell DW, Szauter KE: Nonantibiotic therapy and pharmacotherapy of acute infectious diarrhea, *Gastro Clin North Am* 22:683, 1993.

FOOD POISONING

Andrew T. Pavia

Foodborne illnesses are caused by ingestion of foods containing microbial and chemical toxins or pathogenic microorganisms. This chapter concentrates on toxin-mediated syndromes, usually called *food poisoning,* rather than on syndromes reflecting enteric infection, such as salmonellosis, shigellosis, vibriosis, and *Escherichia coli* O157:H7 infection. Treatment of these infections is covered in the chapter on gastroenteritis and in chapters on the specific organisms.

■ CLINICAL PRESENTATION AND DIAGNOSIS

Initially, the diagnosis of specific food poisoning syndromes is suggested by the clinical presentation, the incubation period from exposure to onset of symptoms, and the food consumed. The incubation periods, symptoms, and commonly associated foods for specific syndromes are shown in Table 1. Incubation periods range from a few hours or less in the case of preformed chemical and bacterial toxins such as histamine poisoning (scombroid), staphylococcal food poisoning, and *Bacillus cereus,* to several days for bacterial infections (e.g., *Campylobacter jejuni, Salmonella, Yersinia enterocolitica,* and *E. coli* O157:H7 or other enterohemorrhagic *E. coli*) and some types of mushroom poisoning. Therefore it is essential to obtain a diet history covering 3 to 4 days before the onset of symptoms. A careful history of illness in meal companions may help point to the responsible food. It is clinically useful to consider syndromes grouped by incubation period and symptoms.

Nausea and Vomiting Within 1 Hour

Symptoms developing within 5 to 15 minutes of exposure that resolve over 1 to 2 hours are typical of contamination of food or drink with heavy metals or other nonspecific chemical irritants.

Nausea, Vomiting, or Diarrhea Within 1 to 16 Hours

When gastrointestinal symptoms develop 1 to 16 hours after exposure, the likely agents include *Staphylococcus aureus, B. cereus,* and *Clostridium perfringens.* Vomiting is the dominant feature of *S. aureus* and short-incubation, or emetic, *B. cereus* food poisoning. These syndromes result from preformed centrally acting toxins elaborated by the organisms in food when the food is mishandled. In contrast, abdominal cramps and diarrhea are most prominent in long-incubation, or diarrheal, *B. cereus* poisoning and *C. perfringens* food poisoning. In these syndromes, toxins are also elaborated in the small intestine. The duration of illness is usually less than 24 hours. Diagnosis of these syndromes is usually made on epidemiologic and clinical grounds. Laboratory confirmation of *S. aureus* food poisoning is based on isolation of *S. aureus* from food handlers and demonstration of more than 10^5 colonies per gram of the same strain in food or enterotoxin production. Laboratory confirmation of *B. cereus* and *C. perfringens* can be performed in epidemiologic investigations; it requires collection of food and stool for quantitative cultures.

Watery Diarrhea and Cramps Within 16 to 48 Hours

Diarrhea following a slightly longer incubation period is typical of viral foodborne illness, particularly Norwalk virus, and enterotoxin-producing bacteria, including enterotoxigenic *E. coli* (ETEC), *Vibrio cholerae* O1 and non-O1, and other *Vibrio* species. Most microbiology laboratories can diagnose *Vibrio* infections from stool culture provided the laboratory is aware that *Vibrio* is being considered. Diagnosis of ETEC infection requires detection of enterotoxin production by *E. coli* isolates and is limited to reference laboratories. Antigen detection–based enzyme immunoassays using recombinant antigens have been developed for the diagnosis of Norwalk and other gastroenteritis-causing viruses; these are limited to research laboratories but may soon become commercially available.

Fever, Diarrhea, and Abdominal Cramps Within 16 to 96 Hours

Bacterial infections of the gastrointestinal tract and gut-associated lymphatics with *Salmonella, Shigella, C. jejuni, Y. enterocolitica,* and enterohemorrhagic *E. coli* (EHEC) typically follow a longer incubation period and are marked

Table 1 Incubation Period, Symptoms, and Common Vehicles for Microbial Causes of Food Poisoning

ORGANISM	INCUBATION PERIOD (HR) MEDIAN (RANGE)	VOMITING	DIARRHEA	FEVER	COMMON VEHICLES
Staphylococcus aureus	3 (1-6)	+++	++	0	Ham, poultry, cream-filled pastries, potato and egg salad
Bacillus cereus (emetic syndrome)	2 (1-6)	+++	++	0	Fried rice
Bacillus cereus (diarrheal syndrome)	9 (6-16)	+	+++	0	Beef, pork, chicken, vanilla sauce
Clostridium perfringens	12 (6-24)	+	+++	0	Beef, poultry, gravy
Vibrio parahemolyticus	15 (4-96)	++	+++	++	Fish, shellfish
Vibrio cholerae O1 and non-O1	24 (12-120)	++	+++	+	Shellfish
Norwalk virus	24 (12-48)	+++	++	++	Shellfish, salads, ice
Shigella	24 (7-168)	+	+++	+++	Egg salads, lettuce, sandwiches
Clostridium botulinum	24 (12-168)	++	+	0	Canned vegetables, fruits, sauces and fish; salted fish; bottled garlic, baked potatoes
Salmonella	36 (12-72)	+	+++	++	Beef, poultry, pork, eggs, dairy products, fruit and vegetables, sprouts
Campylobacter jejuni	48 (24-168)	+	+++	+++	Poultry, raw milk
Entereohemorrhagic *Escherichia coli* (e.g., O157:H7)	96 (48-120)	++	+++	+	Beef (especially hamburger), raw milk, salad dressings, lettuce, sprouts, apple cider
Yersinia enterocolitica	96 (48-240)	+	+++	+++	Pork, chitterlings, tofu, milk
Cyclospora cayatensis	168 (24-336)	+	+++	++	Raspberries, basil, lettuce

0, Rare (<10%); +, infrequent (11%-33%); ++, frequent (33%-66%); +++, classic (>67%).

by more prominent signs of colonic inflammation or systemic illness. Diarrhea that becomes bloody after 12 to 36 hours is typical of *E. coli* O157:H7 and other EHEC. These organisms are now among the most common causes of bacterial gastroenteritis in North America (see the chapter on gastroenteritis).

Diarrhea, Fatigue, and Weight Loss Within 1 to 14 Days

Cyclospora infection should be suspected in a patient with diarrhea of several days' duration associated with loss of appetite and weight and prominent fatigue. The incubation period is highly variable, ranging from 1 to 14 days, with a median of 7 days. Recent outbreaks have definitively shown that *Cyclospora* infections in developed countries can result from consumption of contaminated foods, notably fresh raspberries, mesclun lettuce, and basil.

Paresthesias Within 6 Hours

Chemical food poisoning caused by niacin, Chinese restaurant syndrome (monosodium glutamate), histamine fish poisoning, ciguatera poisoning, and neurotoxic and paralytic shellfish poisoning present with paresthesias and other symptoms after a brief incubation period. Chinese restaurant syndrome is characterized by a burning sensation in

the neck, chest, and abdomen with chest tightness and occasionally facial flushing, headache, nausea, and abdominal cramps.

The features of fish and shellfish poisoning are summarized in Table 2. Histamine fish poisoning (scombroid) is caused by bacterial decarboxylation of histidine in fish that are inadequately refrigerated, resulting in production of large amounts of histamine. Signs and symptoms are facial flushing, headache, nausea, and less commonly, urticaria or diarrhea. The fish is often reported to have a peppery or bitter taste. Demonstration of high levels of histamine in the implicated fish confirms the diagnosis.

Ciguatera fish poisoning results from ingestion of fish containing toxins produced by the dinoflagellate *Gambierdiscus toxicus*. Predatory fish such as grouper, amberjack, snapper, and barracuda are usually implicated. The symptoms, which are quite distinctive, usually involve the combination of gastrointestinal and neurologic symptoms, most commonly perioral and distal extremity paresthesias, and reversal of hot and cold sensation. Other symptoms include sensation of loose teeth, arthralgias, headaches, muscle weakness, pruritus, lancinating pains, and hallucinations. Bradycardia, hypotension, and respiratory paralysis may occur. The symptoms may last from a few days to 6 months. The diagnosis is based on the clinical picture; detection of

Table 2   Clinical Features of Fish and Shellfish Poisoning

SYNDROME	INCUBATION PERIOD	SYMPTOMS	VEHICLES	DURATION
Histamine (scombroid)	5 min–1 hr	Facial flushing, headache, nausea, cramps, diarrhea, urticaria	Tuna, mackerel, bonito, mahi-mahi, bluefish	Hours
Ciguatera	1–6 hr	Diarrhea, nausea, vomiting, myalgia, arthralgia, shooting pains, perioral and extremity paresthesias, hot-cold reversal, fatigue	Barracuda, snapper, grouper, amberjack	Days to months
Neurotoxic shellfish poisoning	5 min–4 hr	Paresthesias, nausea, vomiting, ataxia	Shellfish	Hours to days
Paralytic shellfish poisoning	5 min–4 hr	Paresthesias, cranial nerve weakness, ataxia, muscle weakness, respiratory paralysis	Shellfish	Hours to days
Domoic acid	15 min–38 hr	Vomiting, cramps, diarrhea, confusion, amnesia, cardiac irritability	Mussels	Indefinite
Haff disease		Muscle pain, stiffness, brown urine	Buffalo fish	2–3 days

ciguatoxin in the fish by high-performance lipid chromatography (HPLC), radioimmunoassay (RIA) or enzyme-linked immunoassay (EIA), or bioassay is confirmatory.

Paralytic shellfish poisoning (PSP) and neurotoxic shellfish poisoning (NSP) are closely related syndromes caused by heat-stable neurotoxins produced by dinoflagellates (*Gonyaulax catonella* and *Gonyaulax tamarensis* cause PSP; *Gymnodinium breve* causes NSP). During periodic blooms of the dinoflagellates, which may cause red tides, shellfish concentrate the heat-stable toxins. PSP is more severe and occurs in colder waters. Patients develop symptoms a median of 30 minutes after exposure. Symptoms consist of paresthesias and dysesthesias, beginning with the lips, mouth, and face and progressing to the extremities; then dysphonia, dysphagia, ataxia, muscle weakness, and in severe cases, respiratory paralysis occur. NSP occurs primarily near warmer waters and is characterized by similar paresthesias, reversal of hot and cold sensation, nausea, vomiting, and ataxia. Toxin can be detected in samples of the shellfish by bioassay. Anamnestic shellfish poisoning is a recently described syndrome associated with mussels contaminated with domoic acid elaborated by *Nitzchia pungens*. In some patients, gastrointestinal symptoms are followed by memory loss, coma, cardiac arrhythmias, and death. Haff disease is a syndrome of acute rhabdomyolysis that is caused by an unidentified toxin in certain bottom-feeding fish, notably buffalo fish and burbot. Patients present 6 to 21 hours after ingestion with vomiting, severe myalgia, and stiffness. Elevated creatine phosphokinase (CPK) and other muscle enzyme levels confirm the diagnosis.

Nausea, Vomiting, Diarrhea, and Paralysis Within 18 to 36 Hours

Foodborne botulism results from exposure to one of three distinct botulinum toxins, A, B, and E, produced when *Clostridium botulinum* spores germinate in food in an anaerobic environment. Gastrointestinal symptoms occur before the onset of neurologic symptoms in about 50% of patients

with acute foodborne botulism. Descending paralysis begins with cranial nerve weakness manifested as dysphonia, dysphagia, diplopia, and blurred vision, followed by muscle weakness and respiratory insufficiency. Larger doses of toxin result in shorter incubation periods and more severe symptoms. Botulism can be differentiated from acute myasthenia gravis and Guillain-Barré syndrome (which may follow *C. jejuni* infection) by botulism's normal cerebrospinal fluid protein, the descending nature of the paralysis, absence of sensory symptoms, normal nerve conduction studies, and typical electromyographic findings of increase in the action potential with rapid repetitive stimulation. Confirmation is based on detection of toxin in food or in serum or stool of patients by mouse toxicity assay or of *C. botulinum* spores in the stool by selective culture.

Mushroom Poisoning Syndromes

Syndromes of food poisoning from mushrooms fall into eight major categories, outlined in Table 3. Parasympathetic syndromes, delirium, disulfiram (Antabuse)-like symptoms, hallucinations, or gastroenteritis may occur after a short incubation period. The more serious syndromes of monomethylhydrazine poisoning, hepatorenal failure from amatoxin-containing mushrooms, and tubulointerstitial nephritis develop after longer incubation periods and may not be suspected initially. If available, specimens of the mushrooms should be examined promptly by a mycologist or poison control expert to confirm the diagnosis. Toxins can be detected in gastric contents, blood, or urine by thin-layer chromatography.

■ THERAPY

Nonspecific Therapy

Most food poisoning syndromes are self-limited, and for the majority of episodes, nonspecific supportive therapy is all that is required. Exceptions include botulism, listeriosis,

Table 3   Clinical Syndromes of Mushroom Poisoning

SYNDROME (TOXINS)	INCUBATION PERIOD	SYMPTOMS	MUSHROOMS
Parasympathetic (Muscarine)	30 min-2 hr	Sweating, salivation, lacrimation, blurred vision, diarrhea, bradycardia, hypotension	*Inocybe* spp *Clitocybe* spp.
Delirium (Ibotenic acid, muscimol)	30 min-2 hr	Dizziness, incoordination, ataxia, hyperactivity, visual disturbance, stupor	*Amanita muscaria, Amanita pantherina*
Disulfuram-like (Coprine)	30 min after alcohol	Flushing, metallic taste, nausea, vomiting, sweating, hypotension	*Coprinus atramentarius, Clitocybe clavipes*
Hallucinations (Psilocybin)	30-60 min	Mood elevation, anxiety, muscle weakness, hallucination	*Psilocybe cubensis,* Panaleolus spp.
Gastroenteritis	30 min-2 hr	Nausea, vomiting, abdominal cramps, diarrhea	Various
Methemoglobin poisoning (Monomethylhydrazine gyromitrin)	6-12 hr	Nausea, vomiting, bloody diarrhea, abdominal pain, convulsion, coma, liver failure, hemolysis	*Gyromitra* spp.
Hepatorenal failure (Amatoxins, phallotoxins)	6-24 hr	Nausea, vomiting, abdominal pain, diarrhea; then jaundice, liver and kidney failure, coma, death	*Amanita phalloides, A. verna, A. virosa, Galerina autumnalis, G. marginata*
Tubulointerstitial nephritis (Orellanine)	36 hr-14 days	Thirst, nausea, vomiting, flank pain, chills, oliguria	*Cortinarius orellanus, C. speciosissimus*

some enteric infections in infants and compromised hosts, and some types of mushroom poisoning.

The mainstay of treatment is fluid and electrolyte replacement to prevent and treat dehydration. The first step is to assess the degree of volume depletion by examining the skin turgor, mucous membranes, vital signs, and mental status. Measuring postural changes in pulse and blood pressure is also helpful in quantifying the volume loss. Slightly dry mucous membranes and thirst indicate mild dehydration (5% to 6% deficit, or 50 to 60 ml/kg); loss of skin turgor, very dry mucous membranes, postural pulse increases, and sunken eyes indicate moderate dehydration (7% to 9%); and the additional presence of weak pulse, postural hypotension, cold extremities, or depressed consciousness indicates severe volume depletion, above 10%.

Most children and adults with diarrhea can be treated successfully with oral rehydration. This therapy is possible because of the coupled transport of glucose with water and sodium even in severely damaged small bowel. Diarrheal stool contains significant concentrations of sodium, potassium, and bicarbonate, and fluid therapy should replace these losses.

One liter of the World Health Organization's recommended replacement solution contains 90 mmol of sodium, 20 g of glucose, 20 mmol of potassium, 80 mmol of chloride, and 30 mmol of citrate (as a bicarbonate source); this is close to an ideal solution. Commercial solutions such as Rehydralyte, Ricelyte, and Pedialyte have a slightly lower sodium concentration, but they are convenient and readily available, if expensive. A homemade approximation of the oral solution can be made by adding a pinch of salt, a pinch of baking soda, and a spoonful of sugar or honey to an 8-oz glass of fruit juice. For patients with altered consciousness or uncontrolled vomiting, intravenous rehydration with Ringer's lactate should be used initially. The estimated volume deficit should be replaced over 4 hours; after that, ongoing losses should be replaced. Gatorade and commer-

cial soft drinks are poor choices because the low sodium content can lead to hyponatremia and the high osmolarity can exacerbate diarrhea.

Water intake should be allowed ad lib, and solid food can be introduced as soon as it is tolerated. Some patients will develop lactose intolerance after severe or protracted diarrhea, and dairy products should be avoided if they appear to exacerbate symptoms.

Phenothiazine antiemetics may be useful for severe or prolonged vomiting. Promethazine (Pheneragan), 12.5 to 25 mg, and prochlorperazine (Compazine), 5 to 10 mg orally or intramuscularly (IM), 25 mg rectally, can be given orally, as suppositories, or intramuscularly. Alternatively, droperidol (Inapsine), 1 to 2 ml, can be used intravenously. Antidiarrheals should be used cautiously, especially in children. Pepto-Bismol 30 ml orally every 4 to 6 hours, may be reasonable if an antidiarrheal is used because it has been shown to bind some enterotoxins. Care must be taken because of the salicylate content.

Specific Therapy

Specific therapies for food poisoning are outlined in Table 4. Gastric emptying and administration of active charcoal and cathartics are important for virtually all cases of mushroom poisoning. If vomiting has not occurred spontaneously in patients with botulism or ciguatera, the remaining food should be removed from the gut. In botulism, paralytic shellfish poisoning, and ciguatera, death from respiratory failure is the major risk, and monitoring the vital capacity can be lifesaving.

Polyvalent equine antitoxin, which binds botulinum toxins A, B, and E, is available in the United States through state health departments and the Centers for Disease Control and Prevention (404-639-2206, 8:00 to 4:30 Eastern Time workdays; 404-639-2888 nights, weekends, and holidays). It may prevent further paralysis but does not reverse established symptoms. To be effective, it should be administered early.

Table 4 Specific Treatment for Food Poisoning Syndromes

SYNDROME	FIRST-LINE TREATMENT	COMMENT
Staphylococcus aureus, Bacillus cereus, Clostridium perfringens, Norwalk virus	Fluid replacement, antiemetics (e.g., promethazine [Pheneragan], prochlorperazine [Compazine], droperidol [Inapsine])	Oral rehydration is usually adequate if vomiting can be controlled
Bacterial gastroenteritis	Fluid replacement; antimicrobials helpful for some syndromes	See chapters on specific organisms and the chapter Gastroenteritis for specific antimicrobial therapy
Clostridium botulinum	Gastric empying, cathartics if food still in gastrointestinal tract; respiratory support, polyvalent antitoxin*	Antitoxin should be given as soon as possible
Cyclospora	Trimethoprim-sulfamethoxazole (160 mg trimethoprim component bid for 7 days)	If not treated, symptoms may be protracted and relapsing
Histamine (scombroid)	Antihistamine (e.g., diphenhydramine 25-50 mg IM or IV)	H2 receptor antagonists (cimetidine) have been helpful for refractory symptoms
Ciguatera	Empty stomach if vomiting has not occurred; analgesia, antiemetics, supportive measures; atropine for symptomatic bradycardia	Amitryptiline (25-50 mg/day) or tocainide may help paresthesias; mannitol infusion, calcium gluconate infusion have been used
Neurotoxic shellfish poisoning	Supportive therapy	
Paralytic shellfish poisoning	Supportive therapy, monitor vital capacity	
Haff disease	Intravenous hydration	Mannitol and bicarbonate have also been used to protect renal tubules
Muscarine-containing mushrooms	Gastric emptying, activated charcoal, cathartics; atropine 0.01 mg/kg IV up to 1 mg	Titrate atropine to drying of secretions
Muscimol- and ibotenic acid–containing mushrooms	Gastric emptying, activated charcoal, cathartics; supportive measures	Physostigmine may be used if anticholinergic symptoms are severe
Hallucinogen-containing mushrooms	Reassurance, quiet room; diazepam for severe agitation	
Monomethylhydrazine-containing mushrooms (*Gyromitra* spp.)	Gastric emptying, activated charcoal, cathartics; for delirium, pyridoxine, 25 mg/kg IV	For methemoglobinemia, methylene blue 1% solution 0.1-0.2 ml/kg over 5 min
Amatoxin-containing mushrooms	Gastric emptying, activated charcoal, cathartics; correction of fluid and electrolytes; monitoring glucose, liver, and renal function	Thioctic acid†, silibinin, high dosages of steroids, and intravenous penicillin have been advocated, but controlled data are lacking; hemodialysis, charcoal hemoperfusion, and liver transplantation may be necessary
Orellanine-containing mushrooms	Gastric emptying, activated charcoal, cathartics; cautious correction of fluid and electrolyte problems	Hemodialysis is often necessary

*Available through State Health Department, or Foodborne and Diarrheal Diseases Branch, Centers for Disease Control and Prevention 404-639-2206 8:00 to 4:30 EST workdays; 404-639-2888 nights, weekends, and holidays.
†Assistance in obtaining thioctic acid can be sought through regional Poison Control Centers.

Dosage and a protocol for desensitization in the case of a positive skin test are listed in the package insert.

In ciguatera poisoning, analgesia and avoidance of unpleasant stimuli such as warm baths are usually adequate. Anecdotal reports in the literature suggest that amitriptyline, 25 to 50 mg/day orally, and tocainide may be useful for dysesthesias. Intravenous mannitol has also been reported to be effective for severe neurologic manifestations. For histamine fish poisoning, conventional antihistamines, such as diphenhydramine, 25 to 50 mg IM or intravenously (IV), are helpful. Epinephrine or albuterol should be given for bronchospasm. Intravenous cimetidine can be tried for refractory symptoms.

Atropine is a specific antidote for poisoning from muscarine-containing mushrooms, but the dosage (0.01 mg/kg up to a maximum of 1 mg) should be titrated to control excess respiratory secretions and bradycardia rather than other symptoms.

Specific treatment is usually not necessary for poisoning caused by acid–containing ibotenic or muscimol-containing mushrooms. If severe anticholinergic symptoms such as hyperpyrexia, hypertension, or severe agitation are present, physostigmine, 0.01 mg/kg IV, should be used. Cardiac and blood pressure monitoring are necessary because hypotension and bradycardia can result.

For poisoning caused by monomethylhydrazine-containing mushrooms, pyridoxine, 25 mg/kg IV, should be given; the dose can be repeated every 5 to 10 minutes. The methemoglobin level should be measured if possible. If there is symptomatic methemoglobinemia with central cyanosis, methylene blue, 0.1 to 0.2 ml/kg of a 1% solution, should be given over 5 minutes.

The high fatality rate associated with poisoning by *Amanita phalloides* and related amatoxin-containing mushrooms makes it a special concern. Toxin removal should be attempted with activated charcoal and cathartics even after several days because of the extensive enterohepatic cycling. During the initial phase, gastrointestinal symptoms may cause hypotension. This first stage often is followed by a stage of apparent improvement, but hepatic transaminases usually are elevated by 24 to 48 hours. Fulminant hepatic necrosis and acute renal failure begin after 48 to 96 hours. Supportive treatment consists of careful fluid replacement and monitoring of serum glucose and liver function tests. Thioctic acid may be partially effective at 300 mg/kg/day IV with glucose infusion in divided doses every 6 hours; contact the regional poison control center for help in obtaining it. The roles of intravenous penicillin, silibinin, and high-dose steroids are unclear. Charcoal hemoperfusion is theoretically attractive if it can be begun within the first 10 to 16 hours. Liver transplant has been successful in some cases.

Reporting

Reporting of suspected foodborne outbreaks to local or state health departments is an important part of management because epidemiologic investigation can clearly establish the responsible food and may prevent many additional cases.

Suggested Reading

Avery ME, Snyder JD: Oral therapy for acute diarrhea: the underused simple solution, N Engl J Med 323:891, 1990.

Hall AH, Spoerke DG, Rumack BH: Mushroom poisoning: identification, diagnosis and treatment, Pediatr Rev 8:291, 1987.

Pavia AT: Foodborne and waterborne disease. In Long S, Pickering L, and Prober C, eds: Principles and practices of pediatric infectious diseases, New York, 1977, Churchill Livingstone.

Slutsker L, Altekruse SF, Swerdlow DL: Foodborne diseases. Emerging pathogens and trends, Infect Dis Clin North Am 12:199, 1998.

TRAVELERS' DIARRHEA

Harumi Gomi
Herbert L. DuPont

Travelers' diarrhea (TD) is a syndrome that is acquired when a person travels from industrialized countries to tropical developing countries. TD can be defined as the passage of three or more unformed stools in a 24-hour period in association with at least one of the following symptoms or signs of enteric infection: nausea, vomiting, abdominal pain or cramps, fever, fecal urgency, tenesmus, or the passage of bloody/mucoid (dysenteric) stools. This definition should also consist of illness occurring during the first 7 to 10 days after travelers return to their home countries. Acute TD lasts for less than 2 weeks. Illness lasting more than 2 weeks is considered "persistent," and diarrhea lasting longer than a month is considered "chronic." Cases of TD can be categorized by severity as being mild (no disturbance in normal activities), moderate (modified travel activities required), or severe (illness requires confinement to bed). Previous prospective studies have demonstrated that approximately 40% of the more than 20 million people crossing international borders each year from the industrialized to the developing countries suffer from this illness. Fewer than 1% are admitted to a hospital, 20% to 30% are confined to bed, and 40% are required to change their travel schedule.

■ ETIOLOGY

Bacterial enteropathogens cause at least 80% of TD cases. Geographically different areas have different predominant organisms. However, Escherichia coli, particularly enterotoxigenic E. coli (ETEC), is the major etiologic organism in TD in most areas of the developing world. Other causes are Shigella species, Campylobacter jejuni, Aeromonas species, Plesiomonas shigelloides, Salmonella species, and non-cholera Vibrio. Enteroaggregative E. coli also represents an important cause of TD. The causes of TD in some areas of the world are also affected by the regional climate. ETEC was shown to be the major pathogen in the rainy, summer season in Mexico and Morocco, whereas C. jejuni was found to be the most important pathogen in the dry winter season.

Other than bacterial pathogens, parasites and viruses are also noted to cause TD. Giardia is an important pathogen in mountainous areas of North America and Russia. Cryptosporidium species has been noted to be an important cause of diarrhea in travelers to St. Petersburg, Russia. Entamoeba histolytica is rarely a cause of TD in short-term travelers living in hotels. It is seen in those living close to the local poor residents in those areas. Cyclospora cayetanensis has been found to be an important causative organism of TD occurring in Nepal. Rotavirus and Norwalk virus cause approximately 10% of TD cases.

■ TREATMENT

Hydration and Dietary Recommendations

TD can cause dehydration in infants, the elderly, or persons who have underlying medical illness such as human immunodeficiency virus (HIV) infection, diabetes, or malnutrition. Fluids combined with electrolytes is the most important form of therapy. In the nondehydrated person with no underlying medical illness, commercially available sports drinks, diluted fruit juices, and other flavored soft drinks taken with saltine crackers and/or soups are usually enough to meet the fluid and salt needs during TD. Oral rehydration powders or solutions are also commercially available.

During the early hours of diarrheal illness, it may be

helpful and prudent to temporarily withhold solid food as a stimulant of intestinal motility. In most cases of diarrhea carbohydrates (noodles, rice, potatoes, oat, wheat, banana) and white meats (fish and chicken) can be taken. As illness improves, fruits, vegetables, and red meats may be ingested. In general, dairy products should be avoided in adults for the first day or two. It is important to feed patients with diarrhea to facilitate enterocyte renewal.

Nonantimicrobial Therapy

Symptomatic therapy can be used in cases of mild TD. Bismuth subsalicylate (BSS) is a commonly used antidiarrheal drug. This agent has a direct antibacterial, antiinflammatory, and antisecretory activity. BSS can decrease the number of unformed stools passed in cases of TD by approximately 50%. BSS can rarely cause tinnitus, and it commonly produces harmless blackening of the tongue and stools. If a person is taking doxycycline as a malaria prophylaxis, BSS should not be used concomitantly because it may prevent absorption of the antibiotic.

Attapulgite and kaolin are hydrated aluminum silicate clays that lead to the passage of more formed stools without important effect on water and electrolytes loss.

Antimotility agents such as loperamide (Imodium) and diphenoxylate with atropine (Lomotil) are synthetic opioids that have selective effects on the intestine. These agents can improve diarrhea by slowing intestinal transit, leading to greater absorption of fluids and electrolytes. Loperamide is a drug of choice for symptomatic treatment in the most cases of diarrhea because it is safe and effective. This agent will reduce the number of stools passed during a diarrhea episode by approximately 80%. The antimotility agents should not be used in patients with febrile dysentery because they may rarely prolong or worsen illness.

Zaldaride is an antisecretory agent that reduces diarrhea by inhibiting intestinal calmodulin. In a previous clinical study in U.S. students who traveled to Mexico, zaldaride reduced the duration of diarrhea from 42 hours in untreated persons to 20 hours in those treated.

Antimicrobial Therapy

Antimicrobial therapy in patients with TD shortens the duration of diarrhea from approximately 3 days to 1 day. Antibiotic therapy is indicated in patients with moderate to severe diseases. We also recommend that antibiotic therapy be initiated after passage of the third unformed stool within 24 hours.

Presently, the most active antibiotic agents to use in the treatment of TD are fluoroquinolones such as norfloxacin, ciprofloxacin, and levofloxacin. The dosage and duration of fluoroquinolones to use are given in Tables 1 and 2. The drug is ordinarily given for 1 day in patients without fever or dysentery. It should be taken again on day 2 and 3 if symptoms continue. All patients with fever and dysentery should receive 3 days of fluoroquinolone treatment. Fluoroquinolones should not be used in children and pregnant women because they have been shown to damage articular cartilage in growing animals. These agents may interfere with xanthine metabolism, so patients taking theophylline may need to adjust their dosage of the drug.

Table 1 Dosage of Pharmacologic Agents for Treatment of Travelers' Diarrhea in Adults

AGENT	DOSAGES	COMMENTS
Loperamide	4 mg initially, then 2 mg after each stool, not to exceed 16 mg/day*	Should not use in patients with fever and dysentery
Bismuth subsalicyte	30 ml or 2 tablets (262 mg/tablet) PO q30min up to 8 doses/day*	Should not use with doxycycline; malaria prophylaxis
Fluoroquinolones		
Ciprofloxacin	500 mg PO bid	Fluoroquinolones are equivalent in therapy of TD
Norfloxacin	400 mg PO bid	
Levofloxacin	500 mg PO qd	

*To be used for no more than 48 hours.

Table 2 Treatment of Travelers' Diarrhea in Adults Based on Clinical Severity of Illness

CLINICAL SEVERITY	PHARMACOLOGIC THERAPY
Mild (no disturbance in activities)	No therapy or symptomatic therapy: loperamide or BSS (preferred if vomiting is predominant)
Moderate to severe (modified activities to confinement to bed)	
Without fever and dysentery	Combination therapy with loperamide and a fluoroquinolone for 1 to 3 days
With fever and dysentery	Fluoroquinolones alone for 3 days

Because of the emerging trimethoprim-sulfamethoxazole (TMP-SMX) resistance among ETEC and other bacterial enteropathogens commonly causing TD worldwide, this agent should not be used as a first choice for treatment.

Azithromycin is an azalide antibiotic related to macrolides and is more active than erythromycin against ETEC, *Salmonella* species, *Shigella* species, *Vibrio cholerae,* and *C. jejuni.* In a clinical trial in Thailand, where *Campylobacter* has become resistant to ciprofloxacin, azithromycin was more effective than ciprofloxacin against *Campylobacter.*

Nonabsorbable agents, such as rifaximin are currently under evaluation.

Combination Therapy

The combination of loperamide with a 1- to 5-day course of a fluoroquinolone was shown to significantly reduce the duration of diarrhea when compared with either agent alone. Combination therapy represents the treatment of choice for afebrile, nondysenteric TD.

■ PREVENTION AND CHEMOPROPHYLAXIS

Prevention measures consist of travelers education (behavioral modification), chemoprophylaxis, and vaccination. Travelers should be instructed to avoid potentially contaminated food and water (including ice cubes). Food served steaming hot, dry foods (e.g., bread), fruits that can be peeled, and foods with high sugar content (e.g., syrup or jelly) generally are safe.

Chemoprophylaxis generally is not recommended for most travelers who do not have an underlying medical illness. Prophylaxis may be used for short-term travel in patients with achlorhydria (from prior gastric surgery or regular use of proton pump inhibitors) and in patients with inflammatory bowel diseases or HIV infection or in persons who are otherwise immunosuppressed. Chemoprophylaxis may be considered in patients with critical trips or missions where an illness rendered short-term by appropriate therapy could destroy the purpose of the trip. All travelers considering this approach should be fully informed of the risks and benefits of use of antibiotic chemoprophylaxis. They should be given an option of self-treatment rather than prophylaxis and should be encouraged to pursue this course.

BSS is modestly effective in the prevention of TD with protection rates of approximately 65%. The dosage recommended for prophylaxis is two tablets (262 mg/tablet) orally with meals and at bedtime (8 tablets/day). Antimicrobial agents show protection rates of 90%. A fluoroquinolone can be taken one tablet per day (see Table 1). The prophylactic agent should be initiated on the day of travel and continued daily and for 2 days after leaving the region of risks.

Immunologic protection against ETEC diarrhea is feasible. A new vaccine consisting of cholera toxin B subunit and inactivated whole cell ETEC strains has become available in some parts of the world. This vaccine protects against ETEC diarrhea and probably cholera. Vaccination for TD with an anti-ETEC preparation can never be completely protective because TD is a syndrome caused by multiple organisms.

Suggested Reading

DuPont HL: Guidelines on acute infectious diarrhea in adults, *Am J Gastroenterol* 92:1963, 1997.

DuPont HL, Ericsson CD: Prevention and treatment of traveler's diarrhea, *N Engl J Med* 328:1821, 1993.

Ericsson CD: Travelers' diarrhea: epidemiology, prevention, and self-treatment, *Infect Dis Clin North Am* 12:285, 1998.

Ericsson CD, DuPont HL: Travelers' diarrhea: approaches to prevention and treatment, *Clin Infect Dis* 16:616, 1993.

Petrucelli BP, Kollaritsh H, Taylor DN: Treatment of travelers' diarrhea. In DuPont HL, Steffen R, eds: *Textbook of travel medicine and health*, Hamilton, Canada, 1997, BC Decker.

ANTIBIOTIC-ASSOCIATED DIARRHEA

John G. Bartlett

Diarrhea is a relatively common complication of antibiotic use. Nearly all agents with an antibiotic spectrum of activity have been implicated. The great majority of cases are either enigmatic or caused by *Clostridium difficile*.

■ DIAGNOSTIC STUDIES

C. difficile–associated disease should be suspected in any patient who has diarrhea in association with antibiotic exposure. The most common inducing agents are clindamycin, ampicillin or amoxicillin, and cephalosporins. Nevertheless, nearly any antimicrobial agent with an antibacterial spectrum of activity can cause this complication.

The usual method for identifying cases of diarrhea caused by *C. difficile* is the toxin assay. The standard technique is with a tissue culture assay for detection of cytotoxin or toxin B; more recently most laboratories have used alternative detection methods, most commonly the enzyme immunoassay (EIA) for detection of toxin A or toxin A plus B. Some authorities consider the culture using selective media to be the most sensitive, and some use culture in combination with the toxin assay. Studies of the EIA compared with the tissue culture assay indicate that it is relatively sensitive and specific and has the advantage of providing results within 2 to 3 hours.

Other diagnostic tests include fecal leukocyte examination, preferably using lactoferrin. Anatomic studies, usually sigmoidoscopy or colonoscopy, were far more common before the general availability of *C. difficile* toxin assays in the late 1970s. This also was when pseudomembranous colitis (PMC) was a relatively common complication because of the lack of treatment to interrupt the natural history of the disease. Endoscopy is still indicated in some patients who have negative toxin assays or pose other problems in diagnosis. Computed tomography (CT) and x-ray studies with contrast are sometimes done for other conditions and will occasionally show changes that are highly suggestive of antibiotic-associated colitis caused by *C. difficile*; nevertheless, these are substantially less sensitive than endoscopy.

■ *CLOSTRIDIUM DIFFICILE*

The first principle of treatment is discontinuation of the implicated antimicrobial agent. Supportive measures include fluid and electrolyte restoration and avoidance of antiperistaltic agents such as loperamide. Many patients respond to simple withdrawal of the implicated antimicrobial agent and appropriate supportive care.

If the condition being treated requires continued antibiotic treatment, the recommendation is to change to an agent that is infrequently associated with this complication, such as sulfonamide, tetracycline, aminoglycoside, vancomycin, or fluoroquinolone.

Antibiotic treatment directed against *C. difficile* is readily available and highly effective. The usual agent is vancomycin or metronidazole (Table 1). Response is impressive; generally, fever resolves within 24 hours and diarrhea over an average of 4 to 5 days. Overall response rates are usually reported at 95% to 100%. Vancomycin has ideal pharmacokinetic properties and is active against all strains of *C. difficile* in vitro. Vancomycin is poorly absorbed with oral administration, so mean levels in the colon lumen are several hundredfold higher than the minimum inhibitory concentration. This is a disease whose putative agent is entirely restricted to the colon lumen, so tissue levels are irrelevant to therapy. The disadvantages of vancomycin treatment are relatively high rates of relapse, relatively high costs, occasional poor tolerance to the drug, and implication of its use in promotion of vancomycin-resistant *Enterococcus faecium*. This last problem has resulted in the admonition to avoid oral administration of vancomycin to hospitalized patients.

Metronidazole is active against virtually all strains of *C. difficile* and has a track record of efficacy comparable with that of vancomycin in comparative trials. Theoretic disadvantages are the low levels of the drug in the colon lumen because of almost complete absorption. This drug is substantially less expensive than vancomycin. Most authorities recommend it as initial therapy for most patients with *C. difficile*–associated disease. Vancomycin is reserved for patients who fail to respond to metronidazole. The rate of relapse for metronidazole is comparable with that for vancomycin.

Relapses of *C. difficile* diarrhea are seen only with antibiotic therapy. The typical clinical presentation is recurrence of the initial symptoms 3 to 10 days after discontinuation of metronidazole or vancomycin. Patients generally respond to readministration of either agent, but occasional patients have multiple relapses that can be a major therapeutic problem; several therapeutic options are summarized in Table 2. The problem of relapses has prompted many to scrutinize the necessity of treating all patients, because most cases resolve after simple discontinuation of the implicated agent. For this reason, a common recommendation is to restrict antibiotic therapy to patients with any of the following indications: (1) persistent disease despite discontinuation of the implicated agent, (2) the necessity to continue antibiotic therapy for the infection being treated, (3) severe disease as indicated by devastating diarrhea or diarrhea associated with systemic complaints such as fever and systemic toxicity, or (4) the endoscopic demonstration of PMC or advanced colitis.

C. difficile–associated enteric disease is now largely a nosocomial problem. Recommendations to control spread include (1) isolating patients, especially those with incontinence; (2) enforcing handwashing with soap or detergent; and (3) replacement of electronic thermometers. With outbreaks, it may be necessary to restrict use of selected antimicrobials, especially clindamycin.

■ OTHER CAUSES

Most patients with antibiotic-associated diarrhea or colitis have negative diagnostic studies for *C. difficile* toxin and

---

Table 1   Treatment of *C. difficile* Diarrhea and Colitis

NONSPECIFIC MEASURES

Discontinue the implicated antibiotic; if continued antibiotic treatment is necessary, change to an alternative agent that is unlikely to cause or promote *C. difficile*–associated enteric disease.

Change to another agent infrequently associated with this complication.

Provide supportive measures.

Avoid antiperistaltic agents.

Use enteric precautions for hospitalized patients.

SPECIFIC TREATMENT

Antimicrobial agents if symptoms are severe or persist

    Oral agent (preferred)

        Vancomycin, 125 mg PO qid, 7-14 days*

        Metronidazole, 250 mg PO tid, 7-14 days*

    Parenteral agents (only until oral agents are tolerated):

        Metronidazole, 500 mg IV q12h

Alternative treatments

    Anion exchange resins

        Cholestyramine, 4 g packet PO tid, 7-14 days*

        Cholestipol, 5 g packet PO tid, 7-14 days

    Alter fecal flora

        Lactinex or alternative lactobacillus preparation, 1 g packet PO qid, 7-14 days

*Established efficacy.

Table 2   Methods to Manage Multiple Relapses of *C. difficile* Diarrhea or Colitis

Metronidazole or vancomycin PO ×10-14 days followed by cholestyramine (4 g tid) with or without lactobacilli (as Lactinex, 1 g PO qid) × ≥4 wk.

Vancomycin, 125 mg PO qid ×10-14 days, followed by vancomycin, 125 mg PO qid × ≥4 wk.

Vancomycin, 125 mg PO qid ×4-6 wk, then taper over 4-8 wk.

Vancomycin, 125 mg PO qid, plus rifampin, 600 mg PO qd ×10-14 days.

Vancomycin, 125 mg PO qid, plus *Saccharomyces boulardii* (investigational drug) ×10-14 days, then *Saccharomyces boulardii* for 4 wk.

Intravenous gamma globulin, 400 mg/kg q3wk (reported in pediatric patients only).

Lactobacillus G-G (1 g PO qid) (investigational drug) or Lactinex, 1 g PO qid (available over the counter) ×3 wk.

have no established agent or mechanism. Some believe the best explanation is dysbiosis of the colonic flora, which simply means a disruption in the concentrations and types of bacteria that are presumably critical for maintaining homeostasis in the colonic lumen. The antimicrobial agents implicated are the same that cause *C. difficile* disease. However, some of the clinical differences include the facts that this form of diarrhea is usually dose related, symptoms usually resolve when the implicated agent is discontinued or reduced in dose, systemic symptoms are unusual, it is rarely serious or life threatening, and colitis (fecal leukocytes, fever, or evidence of colitis by endoscopy or CT scan) is unusual. This form of diarrhea also tends to be sporadic, whereas *C. difficile* may be endemic or epidemic within hospitals or nursing homes.

The usual treatment for antibiotic-associated diarrhea with a negative toxin assay is to discontinue the implicated agent; most patients respond. Patients with serious disease, evidence of colitis, or persistent symptoms after discontinuation of antibiotics should have repeat toxin assays for *C. difficile*. The tissue culture assay rarely shows false-negative results, but this degree of confidence does not apply to any of the alternative tests now used by most laboratories. Patients with persistent or serious symptoms in the face of negative assays should undergo anatomic studies using endoscopy and exploration of alternative causes, for example idiopathic inflammatory bowel disease, diarrhea enteric pathogens, and diarrhea caused by other medications.

Suggested Reading

Bartlett JG: *Clostridium difficile:* clinical considerations, *Rev Infect Dis* 12:S243, 1990.

Fekety R, Shah AB: Diagnosis and treatment of *Clostridium difficile* colitis, *JAMA* 269:71, 1993.

Gerding DN, et al: *Clostridium difficile*–associated diarrhea and colitis, *Infect Control Hosp Epid* 16:495, 1995.

Johnson S, et al: Epidemics of diarrhea caused by a clindamycin-resistant strain of *Clostridium difficile* in four hospitals, *N Engl J Med* 341:1645, 1999.

Merz CS, et al: Comparison of four commercially available rapid enzyme immunoassays with cytotoxin assay for detection of *Clostridium difficile* toxin(s) from stool specimens, *J Clin Microbiol* 32:1142, 1994.

Tsutaoka B, et al: Antibiotic-associated pseudomembranous enteritis due to *Clostridium difficile*, *Clin Infect Dis* 18:982, 1994.

SEXUALLY TRANSMITTED ENTERIC INFECTIONS

Thomas C. Quinn

A wide variety of microbial pathogens may be transmitted sexually by the oral-anal or genital-anal routes. Sexually transmitted enteric infections may involve multiple sites of the gastrointestinal tract, resulting in proctitis, proctocolitis, and enteritis. These infections occur primarily in homosexual men and heterosexual women who engage in anal-rectal intercourse or in sexual practices that allow for fecal-oral transmission. Anorectal infections with syphilis, gonorrhea, condyloma acuminata, lymphogranuloma venereum (LGV), and granuloma inguinale (donovanosis) have been recognized for many years. Over the past two decades, other sexually transmitted pathogens such as herpes simplex virus (HSV) and *Chlamydia trachomatis* have also been recognized as causing anorectal infection. Enteric pathogens traditionally associated with food or waterborne acquisition but that also may be transmitted sexually include *Giardia lamblia, Entamoeba histolytica, Campylobacter, Shigella,* and *Salmonella*. In patients with acquired immunodeficiency syndrome (AIDS), other opportunistic infections, including *Candida, Microsporida, Cryptosporidia, Isospora, Cyclo-* *spora, Mycobacterium avium* complex, and cytomegalovirus (CMV), may also cause intestinal disorders.

Depending on the pathogen and the location of the infection, symptoms and clinical manifestations vary widely. Perianal lesions are usually caused by syphilis, HSV, granuloma inguinale, chancroid, and condyloma acuminata. Rectal infections cause inflammation of the rectal mucosa, commonly referred to as *proctitis*. Symptoms include constipation, tenesmus, rectal discomfort or pain, hematochezia, and a mucopurulent rectal discharge. Proctitis can be caused by gonorrhea, chlamydia, syphilis, and HSV. Proctocolitis involves inflammation extending from the rectum to the colon, and in addition to the organisms causing proctitis, other enteric pathogens such as *Shigella, Salmonella, Campylobacter, E. histolytica,* and CMV may be involved. Enteritis is an inflammatory illness of the duodenum, jejunum, and/or ileum. Sigmoidoscopy results are often normal, and symptoms consist of diarrhea, abdominal pain, bloating, cramps, and nausea. Additional symptoms may include fever, weight loss, myalgias, flatulence, urgency, and in severe cases, melena. Sexually transmitted pathogens usually associated with enteritis include *Shigella, Salmonella, Campylobacter, Giardia,* CMV, and potentially, *Cryptosporidia, Isospora,* and *Microsporida*.

The large number of infectious agents that cause enteric and anorectal infections necessitate a systematic approach to the management of these conditions. While obtaining the medical history, the clinician should attempt to differentiate between proctitis, proctocolitis, and enteritis and should assess the constellation of symptoms that suggest one or another likely infectious cause. The history should be used to investigate types of sexual practices and possible exposure to the pathogens known to cause intestinal infections. Examination should include inspection of the anus, digital rectal examination, and anoscopy to identify general mucosal abnormalities. Initial laboratory tests should include a Gram stain of any rectal exudate obtained with the use of an anuscope. The demonstration of leukocytes provides objective evidence of the presence of an infectious or inflammatory disorder. Cultures for gonorrhea should be obtained from the rectum, urethra, and pharynx, and if possible, rectal culture for chlamydia should be performed. Serologic tests for syphilis should be performed in all cases. Darkfield examination of any ulcerations and a rapid plasma reagin test should be performed. Cultures for HSV should be performed if ulcerative lesions are present. If proctocolitis is present, additional stool cultures for *Campylobacter,* *Salmonella,* and *Shigella* should be obtained, and stool examination for *E. histolytica* is indicated. For human immunodeficiency virus (HIV)-positive patients, other pathogens, including *Microsporida,* CMV, atypical *Mycobacteria, Cryptosporidia,* and *Isospora,* should be screened for by stool examination and cultured. Specific information on clinical presentation, diagnosis, and therapy is provided in other chapters on gastroenteritis, intestinal protozoa, and individual enteric pathogens.

■ GONOCOCCAL PROCTITIS

Rectal infection with *Neisseria gonorrhoeae* occurs predominantly among homosexual men and women engaging in anal-rectal intercourse. In many cases of women, the patient has no history of rectal intercourse and the infection is thought to have resulted from contiguous spread of infected secretions from the vagina. Symptoms, when present, develop approximately 5 to 7 days after exposure. Symptoms are usually mild and include constipation, anorectal discomfort, tenesmus, and a mucopurulent rectal discharge that may cause secondary skin irritation, resulting in rectal itching and perirectal erythema. Although asymptomatic or mild local disease is common, complications such as fistulas, abscesses, strictures, and disseminated gonococcal infection may occur.

Findings of rectal gonorrhea during anoscopy are nonspecific and limited to the distal rectum. The most common finding is the presence of mucopus in the rectum. The rectal mucosa may appear completely normal or demonstrate generalized erythema with local areas of easily induced bleeding, primarily near the anal-rectal junction. Diagnosis is usually made by Gram stain and culture of material obtained by swabbing the mucosa of the rectal area. The sensitivity of Gram stain of rectal exudate for identification of gram-negative intracellular diplococci is approximately 80% when obtained through an anoscope versus 53% for blindly inserted swabs. Cultures inoculated on selective media provide the definitive diagnosis; however, the precise sensitivity of a single rectal culture for gonorrhea may be no greater than 80%.

Therapy for *N. gonorrhoeae* has focused on a single-dose therapy effective against beta-lactamase–inducing strains. A single dose of ceftriaxone, 250 mg intramuscularly (IM); cefixime; 400 mg orally; ciprofloxacin, 500 mg orally; or ofloxacin, 400 mg orally, are recommended regimens for uncomplicated anal infection. These regimens are effective in treating more than 95% of rectal infections. Alternative regimens include spectinomycin, 2 g, intramuscularly in a single dose, but it should be noted that this regimen is relatively ineffective against pharyngeal infection. Ciprofloxaxin and ofloxacin should be avoided in pregnant women and children younger than 17 years of age. Because of the established efficacy of these regimens, routine repeat testing for cures generally is not recommended unless therapeutic compliance is questionable or symptoms persist after treatment. If there is continued evidence of proctitis, further evaluation for other agents such as chlamydia, syphilis, enteric bacterial pathogens, and HSV should be considered.

■ CHLAMYDIA PROCTITIS

Rectal infection with LGV and non-LGV immunotypes of *C. trachomatis* have been well documented. LGV infections are endemic in tropical countries, but they have also been seen in the United States and Europe and more often in homosexual men than in heterosexual men and women. LGV infections usually cause a severe proctocolitis characterized by severe anorectal pain, bloody mucopurulent discharge, and tenesmus. Inguinal adenopathy, which is characteristic of genital LGV, is often present. Sigmoidoscopy typically reveals diffuse friability with discrete ulcerations in the rectum that occasionally extend to the descending colon. Strictures and fistulas may become prominent and can be easily misdiagnosed clinically as Crohn's disease or carcinoma. Histologically, rectal LGV may be confused with Crohn's disease because giant cells, crypt abscesses, and granulomas may be present.

The non-LGV immunotypes of *C. trachomatis* are less invasive than LGV and cause a mild proctitis characterized by rectal discharge, tenesmus, and anorectal pain. Many infected individuals may be asymptomatic and can be diagnosed only by routine cultures. However, even in asymptomatic cases, abnormal numbers of fecal leukocytes are usually present. Sigmoidoscopy results may be normal or may reveal mild inflammatory changes with small erosions or follicles in the lower 10 cm of the rectum.

Diagnosis of chlamydia proctitis is best made by isolation of *C. trachomatis* from the rectum, together with an appropriate response to therapy. Serology is useful for the diagnosis of LGV, particularly with the microimmunofluorescence (micro-IF) technique. Direct fluorescent antibody staining with monoclonal antibody of rectal secretions can also be used to establish the diagnosis. Azithromycin, tetracycline, and doxycycline are the drugs of choice for infection with *C. trachomatis.* Azithromycin, 1 g as a single dose, is effective for urethritis and cervicitis and has been recommended for uncomplicated rectal infections. Doxycyline, 100 mg twice a day for 7 to 10 days, is effective, except for treating LGV infection, which should be treated for 3 weeks with doxycycline. Patients should be followed carefully with repeat sigmoidoscopy, particularly when there is any question about the differential diagnosis of LGV versus inflammatory bowel disease.

■ ANORECTAL SYPHILIS

Treponema pallidum can be seen in its early infectious stages, with a primary anorectal lesion appearing 2 to 6 weeks after exposure to rectal intercourse. However, clinicians often fail to recognize anorectal chancres, and consequently, syphilis in homosexual men is diagnosed in a secondary or early latent stage much more often than in the primary stage. Careful perianal examination can reveal unsuspected perianal chancres, but digital rectal examination and anoscopy may be required to detect asymptomatic chancres higher in the anal canal or rectum. When anorectal syphilis causes symptoms, it is often misdiagnosed as a traumatic lesion, fissure, or hemorrhoiditis. When symptoms are present, they include mild anal pain or discomfort, constipation, rectal bleeding, and occasionally a rectal discharge. Primary anorectal syphilis may appear as a single or multiple, mirror-image perianal ulcers ("kissing chancres"). It can also present as an ulcerated mass typically located on the anterior wall of the rectum. Inguinal adenopathy with rubbery, nonsuppurative, painless nodes may be associated with anorectal syphilis; it helps distinguish it from fissures. Secondary syphilis may cause discrete polyps, smooth lobulated masses, mucosal alterations, and nonspecific mucosal erythema or bleeding. In secondary syphilis, condyloma lata may be found near or within the anal canal. These are smooth, warty masses and should be differentiated from the more highly keratinized condyloma acuminata.

Diagnosis of anorectal syphilis is based on serology, perirectal and digital rectal examination, and anoscopy. Detection of motile treponemes by darkfield examination is useful for evaluation of perianal and anal lesions but may be less specific for rectal lesions because pathogenic treponemes can be found in the intestine. Biopsies of rectal lesions or masses should be processed for silver staining if syphilis is suspected. Serologic diagnosis of syphilis is based on the presence of antibodies to nontreponemal and treponemal antigens. A positive VDRL or RPR test must be confirmed by a positive specific test such as the fluorescent treponemal antibody absorption test (FTA-ABS) or the microhemagglutination assay (MHA). Concomitant HIV infection may alter serologic manifestations of syphilis. There has been delayed or absent RPR reactivity in some patients infected with HIV and proved secondary syphilis.

Treatment for anorectal syphilis is standard treatment for early syphilis and consists of benzathine penicillin, 2.4 million U IM. Penicillin-allergic patients may be treated with a 15-day course of doxycycline, 100 mg twice daily, or tetracycline, 500 mg four times a day.

■ *SHIGELLA, SALMONELLA,* AND *CAMPYLOBACTER* INFECTIONS

Shigellosis presents with an abrupt onset of diarrhea, fever, nausea, and cramps. Diarrhea is usually watery but may contain mucus or blood. Sigmoidoscopy usually reveals an inflamed mucosa with friability not limited to the distal rectum, and histologic examination shows diffuse inflammation with bacteria scattered throughout the submucosa. *Shigella sonnei* and *S. flexneri* account for most of the *Shigella* infections in the United States. Diagnosis is made by culturing the organism from the stool on selective media. Treatment is usually supportive with fluid replacement, and antimotility agents should be avoided. Antibiotics are useful in the management of shigellosis because use of appropriate therapy has reportedly shortened the period of fecal excretion and limited the clinical course. However, some authorities believe that antibiotic therapy should be reserved for the severely ill only or the immunocompromised patient because the infection is typically self-limited and resistance has been common. HIV-infected patients who develop *Shigella* infections may require prolonged treatment or suppressive therapy similar to those infected with salmonella. Antibiotic therapy should be chosen according to the sensitivity pattern of the *Shigella* species isolated. Ciprofloxacin, 500 mg twice a day for 7 days, is usually effective unless resistance is evident.

Campylobacter jejuni and *Campylobacter*-like organisms such as *Helicobacter cinaedi* and *Helicobacter fennelliae* have also been associated with proctocolitis in homosexual men. Clinical manifestations of infections resulting from all *Campylobacter* species appear nearly identical. There is often a prodrome with fever, headache, myalgia, and malaise 12 to 24 hours before the onset of intestinal symptoms. The most common symptoms are diarrhea, malaise, fever, and abdominal pain. Abdominal pain is usually cramping and may be associated with 10 or more bowel movements per day. *C. enteritis* is often self-limiting with gradual improvement in symptoms over several days. Illnesses lasting longer than 1 week occur in approximately 10% to 20% of patients seeking medical attention, and relapses are often seen in HIV-infected patients. Fecal leukocytes are uniformly present, and diagnosis is confirmed by isolation of the organisms on selective media in a microaerophilic atmosphere. Therapy consists of fluid and electrolyte replacement and antibiotic treatment. Erythromycin remains the treatment of choice at a dosage of 500 mg four times daily for 1 week, although resistance has been increasing. Treatment with azithromycin, 500 mg once daily for 3 days, or ciprofloxacin, 500 mg twice a day for 7 days, have also been used successfully, but resistance to these antibiotics has also been increasing within recent years.

Salmonella infections of the intestinal tract are primarily caused by *S. typhimurium* and *S. enteritidis*. Salmonella has been reported among homosexual male partners, suggesting sexual transmission and salmonella bacteremia in an HIV-infected individual are now diagnostic of AIDS. Clinical presentation often depends on the host-immune status. In an immunocompetent person, salmonellosis is usually self-limited and causes gastroenteritis. No antibiotic therapy is recommended because symptoms fade within days, and antibiotics have been associated with prolonged salmonella intestinal carriage. In HIV-infected individuals, salmonella infections may cause severe invasive disease and often result in bacteremia with widespread infection. The fluoroquinolones are effective drugs of choice for *Salmonella* infections in immunocompromised individuals. Despite adequate therapy for bacteremia, virtually all HIV-infected patients may suffer recurrent salmonella septicemia. Ciprofloxacin, 500 to 750 mg twice daily, has been effective in suppressing recurrences in such patients.

■ PARASITIC INFECTIONS

Homosexual men engaging in sexual activities involving fecal contamination such as oral-anal sex are at increased risk for a number of parasitic infections, including *Giardia lamblia, Iodamoeba butschlii, Dientamoeba fragilis, Enterobius vermicularis, Cryptosporidia, Isospora,* and *Microsporidia.* Of these infections, *Giardia* and *E. histolytica* appear to be the most common sexually transmitted parasitic infections. *G. lamblia* is associated with symptoms of enteritis, and *E. histolytica* may cause proctocolitis. Most *E. histolytica* infections are asymptomatic and fewer than 10% of those infected develop invasive disease with amoebic dysentery or liver abscess. Most *E. histolytica* strains isolated from homosexual men are the nonpathogenic strains that are not usually associated with gastrointestinal symptoms. However, when symptoms are present, they may vary from mild diarrhea to fulminant bloody dysentery. These symptoms may wax and wane for weeks to months.

Diagnosis is based on demonstration of *E. histolytica* in the stool in a wet mount of a swab or in biopsy of rectal mucosal lesions. Occasionally, multiple fresh stool examinations are necessary to demonstrate the cysts or trophozoites or *E. histolytica.* Invasive intestinal disease should be treated with metronidazole.

G. lamblia also appears to be sexually transmitted through oral-anal contact. Giardiasis is typically an infection of the small intestine, and symptoms vary from mild abdominal discomfort to diarrhea, abdominal cramps, bloating, and nausea. Multiple stool examinations may be necessary to document infection with *G. lamblia.* When stool examination is negative, sampling of the jejunal mucus by the Enterotest or small-bowel biopsy may be necessary to confirm the diagnosis. (See the chapter on intestinal protozoa for details of treatment of amebiasis and giardiasis.)

Although sexual transmission of *Cryptosporidia, Isospora belli,* and *Microsporida* are commonly seen in HIV-infected homosexual men, evidence for sexual transmission is limited. These protozoa primarily infect the small bowel and cause nonspecific watery diarrhea, abdominal cramping, and bloating. Diagnosis is established by a modified acid-fast stain or fluoramine stain of the stool or by concentration and identification of the organism by the sugar-flotation method. A commercially available fluorescein monoclonal antibody assay increases the sensitivity for detection of cryptosporidia. Treatment of cryptosporidia or *Isospora* infections in immunocompetent patients with self-limited diarrhea is rarely required. Among HIV-infected individuals, treatment should be directed toward symptomatic treatment of the diarrhea with dehydration and repletion of electrolyte losses by either oral or intravenous route. Although several antibiotics have been used, including paromomycin and azithromycin, chronic infection and relapses are common. The most effective therapy currently is a reversal of immunosuppression with the use of highly active antiretroviral therapy. It is common for patients with severe diarrhea from *Cryptosporidia* and *Microsporida* to clear their infections by taking combination antiretroviral agents with reduction in the viral load below detectable limits. Successful treatment of the infection presumably results from a subsequent rise in CD4 count and restoration of immune competence sufficient to clear the intestinal infection.

Suggested Reading

Centers for Disease Control and Prevention: 1998 guidelines for treatment of sexually transmitted diseases, *MMWR* 47:104, 1998.

Quinn TC, et al: The polymicrobial origin of intestinal infections in homosexual men, *N Engl J Med* 309:576, 1983.

Rompalo AR, Quinn TC: Enteric bacterial diseases. In Dolin R, Masur H, Saag MS, eds: *AIDS Therapy,* New York, 1999, Churchill Livingstone.

Verley JR, Quinn TC: Sexually transmitted intestinal syndromes. In Holmes KK, et al, eds: *Sexually transmitted diseases,* ed 3, New York, 1999, McGraw-Hill.

ACUTE APPENDICITIS

S. Frank Redo

Acute appendicitis may occur in all age groups but is most common in older children and young adults. It is rare in infants, probably because of the conical nature of the appendix, which permits easier entry and exit of stool. In children up to 4 to 6 years of age and in the elderly, diagnosis is difficult and often not made until perforation has occurred. The incidence is equal in males and females but increases in males during early adulthood, after which the sex ratio again becomes equal.

■ PATHOGENESIS

Acute appendicitis is initiated by obstruction of the lumen by stool (fecalith), fibrous band, lymphoid hyperplasia, or a foreign body. The normal mucosal secretion of the appendix collects distal to the site of the obstruction, which leads to an increase in intraluminal pressure. This causes first interference with venous outflow and subsequently, as pressure increases, with arterial blood inflow. Ulceration of the mucosa occurs with infiltration of the wall of the appendix by bacteria. The resultant infection may lead to gangrene, necrosis, and perforation.

■ DIAGNOSIS

Symptoms and Signs

In a classical case of acute appendicitis, the patient gives a history of periumbilical pain associated with nausea and vomiting that migrates and localizes in the right lower quadrant. This may occur within 1 to 2 or 12 to 18 hours. Vomiting usually consists of only one or two episodes and begins after the onset of pain. If vomiting precedes the pain, the patient probably does not have appendicitis. Anorexia is common.

Unfortunately, this classical history does not exist in all cases. If the appendix is retrocecal, the pain may be described as being in the right flank or right back. When the appendix lies in the pelvis, the pain may be in the testicle or suprapubic (bladder) region. Diarrhea, in such instances, may be a presenting associated problem.

On physical examination, the abdomen usually is tense with spasm and guarding in the right lower quadrant. If the pain has had moderately long duration, the entire abdomen may be rigid, suggesting peritonitis and probable perforated appendix. Discrete tenderness at McBurney's point is diagnostic for acute appendicitis. Rebound, shake, and toe-heel tenderness are indicative of peritoneal irritation. When the appendix is retrocecal, rebound tenderness may not be evident. In such instances, however, there usually is a positive psoas sign.

The abdomen should be palpated for a mass in the right lower quadrant and auscultated for bowel sounds. Bowel sounds may be normal in the early phase of infection but become less active or quiet as the process progresses.

Percussion over the flank and back may cause pain when the appendix is retrocecal. Temperature rarely exceeds 38.5° C (101.3° F) unless there has been perforation and peritonitis has developed.

On rectal examination, a mass may be palpable in the right lower quadrant. Pain may be elicited in this region by pressure of the examining finger on the anterior aspect of the right rectal wall.

Laboratory

Laboratory workup should begin with a complete blood count, urinalysis, serum electrolyte determinations, and supine and upright radiographs of the abdomen. The hemoglobin and hematocrit levels are helpful in assessing dehydration and hemoconcentration. The white blood cell (WBC) count is usually elevated to 15,000 or more with a differential high in polymorphonuclear cells and bands.

The urinalysis provides another clue with respect to degree of hydration. In addition, results of microscopic examination reveal WBC count, red blood cell (RBC) count, and bacteria content. A small number of WBCs or RBCs may be seen in the urine, especially when the appendix lies on or near the ureter. Large numbers of bacteria or pus in urine, not found in appendicitis, indicate probable urinary tract infection.

Abdominal radiographs confirm or rule out small-bowel obstruction, right lower quadrant mass, or fecalith. If the presentation and clinical and laboratory findings are not diagnostic, sonography, computed tomography (CT), or barium enema may be required for the diagnosis.

Differential Diagnosis

Many conditions may present with symptoms and signs that mimic acute appendicitis. These conditions include gastroenteritis (particularly that caused by *Yersinia enterocolitica*, *Salmonella enteriditis*, and *Campylobacter jejuni*); mesenteric adenitis (in younger patients), usually associated with enterecolitis; *Yersinia pseudotuberculosis*; and occasionally streptococcal infection, urinary tract infections, constipation, intussusception, primary peritonitis, duodenal ulcer, measles, Crohn's disease, sickle cell disease, hemophilia, leukemia, Meckel's diverticulum, or pneumonia and pelvic inflammatory disease, ovarian pathology, or mittelschmerz in females. In most instances, history and physical and laboratory findings may differentiate these problems from acute appendicitis, although the gastroenteritis and mesenteric adenitis syndromes just referred to may be particularly misleading, and their mimicry is often termed *pseudoappendicitis*. In patients with acquired immunodeficiency syndrome (AIDS), pseudoappendicitis also may be caused by bacterial typhlitis, cecal cytomegalovirus (CMV) infection, or tuberculosis.

Types of Appendicitis

Appendicitis is seen in five forms: simple acute, suppurative, gangrenous, perforated, and abscess (Table 1).

Table 1 Types of Appendicitis

TYPE	CHARACTERISTICS
Simple acute	Mild hyperemia, edema, no serosal exudate
Suppurative	Edematous, congested vessels, fibrinopurulent exudate; peritoneal fluid increased, clear or turbid; may be early walling off by omentum and adjacent bowel or mesentery
Gangrenous	As above plus areas of gangrene, microperforations, increased and purulent peritoneal fluid
Perforated	Obvious defect in wall of appendix; peritoneal fluid thick and purulent; ileal obstruction possible
Abscess	Appendix may be sloughed; abscess at site of perforation: right iliac fossa, retrocecal, subcecal, or pelvic; may present rectally; thick, malodorous pus

■ THERAPY

The treatment of appendicitis is surgical removal of the affected organ. Surgery should be performed as soon as possible after diagnosis. Patients with signs of peritonitis with dehydration and electrolyte abnormalities should have fluid and electrolyte resuscitation for a few hours before surgery. This should be started promptly, but complete restoration of normality before the operation is not necessary. Ringer's lactate solution and normal saline may be infused to correct fluid and electrolyte abnormalities. If there is evidence to suggest a ruptured appendix with peritonitis, a nasogastric tube should be inserted and placed on suction.

The operation is performed using a McBurney or Rocky-Davis incision, except in those instances in which the diagnosis is in doubt, especially in females. In those cases, a lower midline or right paramedian approach is preferred.

If there is an associated abscess, the appendix should be removed, unless extensive dissection is required to locate the appendix. The peritoneal cavity is irrigated copiously with saline. There is some question about the efficacy of antibiotics in the irrigant.

The abscess cavity should be drained and the drains brought out through a separate stab wound, not the incision. Usually three soft rubber (Penrose) drains are placed, one up to the subhepatic region on the right, a second into the pelvis, and a third down to the right gutter near the base of the cecum. The drains are left in place for 7 days, after which they are gradually removed over the next 2 to 3 days, by which time a definite tract should have developed. The tract should be allowed to close from the deeper to the superficial portion. The skin edges must not be allowed to seal until the tract has closed.

If the patient is not seen early in the course of the disease and when seen is improving and there is a palpable, nonobstructing right lower quadrant mass, nonoperative treatment is used by some. In such cases, an interval appendectomy is usually done 2 to 3 months after the patient has recovered and is free of abdominal complaints. Similarly, in patients in whom surgery reveals a well-walled-off periappendiceal abscess, many surgeons simply drain the abscess to avoid general peritoneal contamination and perform an elective appendectomy 2 to 3 months later. This can be done laparoscopically.

Given the minimal morbidity of the procedure, some investigators believe that interval appendectomy done laparoscopically should be considered for most patients. Laparoscopic appendectomy may replace conventional appendectomy. In the pediatric surgery literature, it is suggested that laparoscopic appendectomy be avoided in children who have complicated appendicitis because of the increased risk for postoperative intraabdominal abscesses. Laparoscopic appendectomy is currently widely used and has been reported as a safe alternative to open appendectomy in uncomplicated cases of acute appendicitis, but because of an increased rate of postlaparoscopic complications, it may be contraindicated in patients with gangrenous appendicitis, peritonitis, or abscess. The advocates of laparoscopic appendectomy stress that it can be done safely with minimal morbidity. The procedure takes more time and costs more. However, postdischarge recovery is shortened, and there is a better cosmetic result. There is no significant difference in length of hospital stay, oral feedings, or wound complications between open and laparoscopic appendectomy.

Antibiotic Regimens

The use of antibiotic prophylaxis for appendicitis is controversial. Many surgeons think antibiotics are not needed for a patient suspected of having acute appendicitis without evidence of peritonitis to suggest perforation or abscess. However, the efficacy of preoperative antibiotics in decreasing the infectious complications of appendicitis has been demonstrated. Also, the possibility of perforation at the time of initial evaluation of a patient has led to widespread use of preoperative antibiotics.

Triple-drug coverage consisting of ampicillin, gentamicin, and clindamycin in appropriate dosages for age and weight should be given within 4 hours of surgery (usually 1 hour before). Some surgeons use only a single antibiotic, cefoxitin, cefotetan, or ampicillin-sulbactam. Further treatment depends on findings at surgery.

For acute, nonperforated appendicitis, antibiotics may not be necessary for more than 24 hours. In most instances, the single preoperative dose is all that is given. If an acute perforated appendix is found, antibiotics are given for 10 days. If a definite abscess is encountered, in addition to adequate drainage, antibiotic therapy should be continued for as long as 21 days. This is a conservative regimen. The patient may be discharged when there are no longer signs of active disease and continue the remainder of the course of antibiotics on a home intravenous program (Tables 2 and 3).

There is no universal regimen for antibiotic use. In many institutions, a single drug, cefoxitan, cefotetan, or ampicillin-sulbactam, is used rather than triple-drug management. Ampicillin and cefoxitan have been used in combination. Metronidazole (Flagyl) has been used as an oral medication for 7 to 10 days after completion of 14 days of intravenous antibiotics in patients who have had abscess and drainage.

Basically, the choice of antibiotics depends on the results of culture and sensitivity determinations of specimens obtained at the time of surgery. Because the disease is polymi-

Table 2   Antibiotic Regimens in Appendicitis

TYPE OF APPENDICITIS	ANTIBIOTIC REGIMEN*
Simple acute	Triple drug, cefoxitin, or ampicillin-sulbactam alone preoperatively and for 12-24 hr postoperatively
Acute with perforation	Triple drug preoperatively and for 10 days postoperatively
Acute with abscess	Triple drug preoperatively and for as long as 21 days postoperatively

*See Table 3 for dosages.

Table 3   Recommended Dosages for Antibiotics in Appendicitis

DRUG	CHILD	ADULT
Triple drug		
Ampicillin	100-200 mg/kg/day q6h	1-2 g q4-q6h
Gentamycin	3-5 mg/kg/day q8h	1-1.7 mg/kg q8h
Clindamicin	2.5-10 mg/kg q6h	15-900 mg q6h
Single drug*		
Cefoxitin	20-25 mg/kg q4-q6h	1-2 g q6h
Ampicillin-sulbactam	25-50 mg/kg q6h	1.5-3 g q6h

*Single-drug therapy is less often recommended in cases of perforation or abscess.

crobial, with aerobic and anaerobic organisms, antibiotics must be effective against both aerobic and anaerobic bacteria.

Suggested Reading

Bauer T, et al: Antibiotic prophylaxis in acute nonoperative appendicitis: the Danish multicenter study group III, *Ann Surg* 209:307, 1989.

Bonanni F, et al: Laparoscopic versus conventional appendectomy, *J Am Coll Surg* 179:273, 1994.

Brown JJ: Acute appendicitis: the radiologist's role, *Radiology* 180:13, 1991.

Gilbert SR, Emmens RW, Putnam TC: Appendicitis in children, *Surg Gynecol Obstet* 161:261, 1985.

Horattas MC, Guyton DP, Wu D: A reappraisal of appendicitis in the elderly, *Am J Surg* 160:291, 1990.

Lund D, Murphy EU: Perforated appendicitis in children: a decade of aggressive treatment, *J Pediatr Surg* 29:1130, 1994.

Paul RH, et al: Pediatric appendectomy, *J Pediatr Surg* 30:173, 1995.

Sherlock DJ: Acute appendicitis in the over 60 age group, *Br J Surg* 72:245, 1985.

DIVERTICULITIS

Ronald Lee Nichols
James Wm. C. Holmes

Diverticulosis coli is an anatomic abnormality of the large bowel wall that manifests itself in various ways. Its occurrence varies greatly with such factors as geographic location, dietary habits, race, and age. In the United States, a third of the population over age 50 is affected.

The diagnosis of diverticulosis coli is often made incidentally in otherwise asymptomatic patients at the time of routine surveillance endoscopy or barium enema x-ray examination. However, unless a stricture is present, most of these patients require only counseling about possible infectious or hemorrhagic complications of the disease and the need for prophylactic measures such as a fiber-rich diet, adequate fluid consumption, and the prevention of constipation.

When clinical manifestations of diverticulosis occur, surgical intervention is necessary in only a minority of patients. These patients may have massive, or recurrent, gastrointestinal bleeding, but more commonly have localized intraabdominal abscess or generalized peritonitis that has developed after diverticular perforation.

Clinically significant diverticular disease and its complications continue to tax the diagnostic and therapeutic skills of physicians. Physical findings range from diffuse slight abdominal tenderness to shock secondary to either massive hemorrhage or overwhelming sepsis. During such life-threatening emergencies, the physician must be prepared to resuscitate the patient quickly and proceed to surgical intervention without benefit of a definite diagnosis.

■ DIAGNOSIS OF INFECTION

The most common clinically significant manifestations of diverticulosis are hemorrhage and infection (diverticulitis). In patients with signs of abdominal infection, including fever and abdominal pain and tenderness, usually in the left lower quadrant, it is often possible to make a presumptive diagnosis of acute diverticulitis on the basis of history, physical examination, and initial laboratory tests. This allows for the initiation of resuscitative measures, including empiric antibiotic therapy. Although further diagnostic endoscopic and radiographic procedures can be delayed for up to 2 days, if the patient continues to show signs of improvement, it is best to perform them as soon as possible to confirm the presumptive diagnosis.

Few if any patients with acute diverticulitis will tolerate proctoscopy above 15 to 20 cm. Sigmoidoscopy is better tolerated, but force must be avoided. In addition, the examiner must be careful to avoid insufflating large amounts of air during the examination and be ready to discontinue the procedure immediately if the patient complains of abdominal pain.

Although ultrasonography is an effective and relatively inexpensive method of evaluating the abdomen and pelvis, particularly for imaging abscesses and their relationship to adnexal structures, most consider computed tomography (CT) to be superior, notably in the evaluation of right colon lesions, and safer than contrast enema studies. Others prefer the contrast enema as the most effective method of colonic imaging. We prefer water-soluble contrast materials to barium to avoid barium peritonitis in case of perforation or leakage.

Once diverticulitis has been documented radiographically, further clinical decisions depend on the resolution of signs and symptoms of infection. If they resolve completely and the patient is stable, examine the entire large bowel endoscopically for neoplastic disease. Colonoscopy is best performed 4 to 6 weeks after symptoms of diverticulitis have subsided so that enough time passes for resolution of any partial obstruction secondary to inflammatory changes in the bowel wall. We routinely perform flexible sigmoidoscopy at 4 to 6 weeks to determine whether sigmoid compliance and patency have returned to normal before preparing the patient for total colonoscopy.

■ MANAGEMENT OF COMPLICATIONS

The greatest number of complications in colonic diverticular disease result from infection. They range from localized short segments of diverticulitis to abscesses and/or fistulas, to free perforation with generalized peritonitis and overwhelming intraabdominal sepsis (Figure 1). The cause of the diverticular perforation is not clear. Some authorities postulate that a surge in intraluminal pressure is often the cause, and others suggest ulceration, ischemia, and foreign-body perforation.

Peridiverticulitis

When ulceration or ischemia is not accompanied by free communication with the peritoneal cavity, penetration of mixed bacterial flora into the wall initiates peridiverticular infection.

Patients with localized peridiverticular disease usually complain of abdominal pain localized to the left lower quadrant. In some cases, however, a redundant sigmoid colon may have sufficient mobility to produce local symptoms in the right lower or right upper abdominal quadrant as well as in the midepigastrium. These patients are often febrile and have mild leukocytosis. However, they respond well to bowel rest, parenteral fluids, and antibiotic therapy. Nasogastric tube insertion is usually unnecessary unless obstructive signs and symptoms are present.

It is important that patients take nothing by mouth to abolish the gastrocolic reflex. Morphine sulfate should not be administered because it can increase intracolonic pressure. Most patients require a 3- to 5-day course of appropriate parenteral antimicrobials (Table 1). If they continue to improve, with normalization of the white blood cell (WBC) count, temperature, and abdominal examination, we discontinue their parenteral antibiotics and advance them to a regular diet that is devoid of poorly digestible foods (e.g., whole corn).

Patients must be followed carefully after resolution of abdominal symptoms. If no disease other than diverticulosis is found on follow-up endoscopy, each patient should follow a fiber-supplemented diet with a generous consumption of fluids.

We do not recommend surgery after a single, uncomplicated episode of diverticulitis in otherwise healthy patients. Rather, we recommend medical therapy when the first episode is mild and uncomplicated and advise patients younger than 40 years of age that a more aggressive form of the disease may develop.

Although the medical approach rarely fails to control the signs and symptoms of peridiverticulitis, surgical resection may become necessary if the infection does not resolve with prolonged parenteral antibiotic therapy. Occasionally, a major complication such as liver abscess or bacteremia develops and requires colonic resection. However, patients with very limited symptoms and no signs of systemic sepsis may respond to oral regimens of antibiotics aimed at covering these colonic aerobes and anaerobes (Table 2).

Pericolic Disease

If the peridiverticular process fails to respond to antibiotic therapy or the patient presents in a late stage of the infectious process, an abscess may be present. Such a pericolic abscess can often be demonstrated by ultrasound, CT, or contrast-enhanced radiography. If any of these studies reveals a small cavity communicating freely with the colon and the patient is improving dramatically, continuation of medical therapy and antibiotics may be warranted. In selected patients, percutaneous drainage of the abscess may be a useful adjunct to surgery. Decompressing the purulent contents of an abscess via CT-guided percutaneous catheter placement gains time to improve the patient's status with volume replacement, parenteral hyperalimentation, and appropriate antibiotic therapy. Once the abscess cavity has been resolved by catheter drainage, it is possible to prepare the bowel for elective resection of the diseased colon, often with primary anastomosis (Table 3).

Smaller symptomatic pericolic abscesses confined to the mesocolon and larger collections associated with peritonitis are best treated surgically. There are two essential operative goals. The first is to resect the inflamed colon and control the associated septic complications; we believe surgical resection of the infectious source is superior to simple

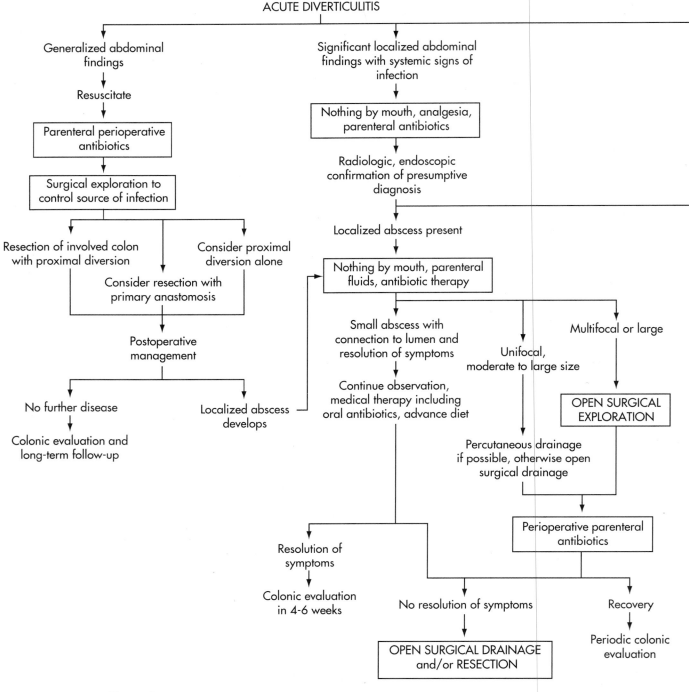

Figure 1
Algorithm for the workup and treatment of acute diverticulitis.

diversion of colonic contents (colostomy) and drainage. The second goal is to restore intestinal continuity. Although this may require a second procedure in some cases, we believe it can be accomplished safely during the same operation (single-stage procedure) in most patients. This is particularly true in individuals who are not hemodynamically compromised, who have localized diverticulitis or who have diverticulitis with an associated mesocolonic abscess amena-

ble to en bloc resection and with no intraabdominal spillage of purulent material. Some surgeons perform an abdominal colectomy with ileorectostomy in patients who have not had preoperative mechanical bowel preparation.

Another somewhat controversial technique is resection of the involved colon, usually the sigmoid, intraoperative lavage, and primary anastomosis. This procedure requires a team effort to keep control of either the proximal or distal

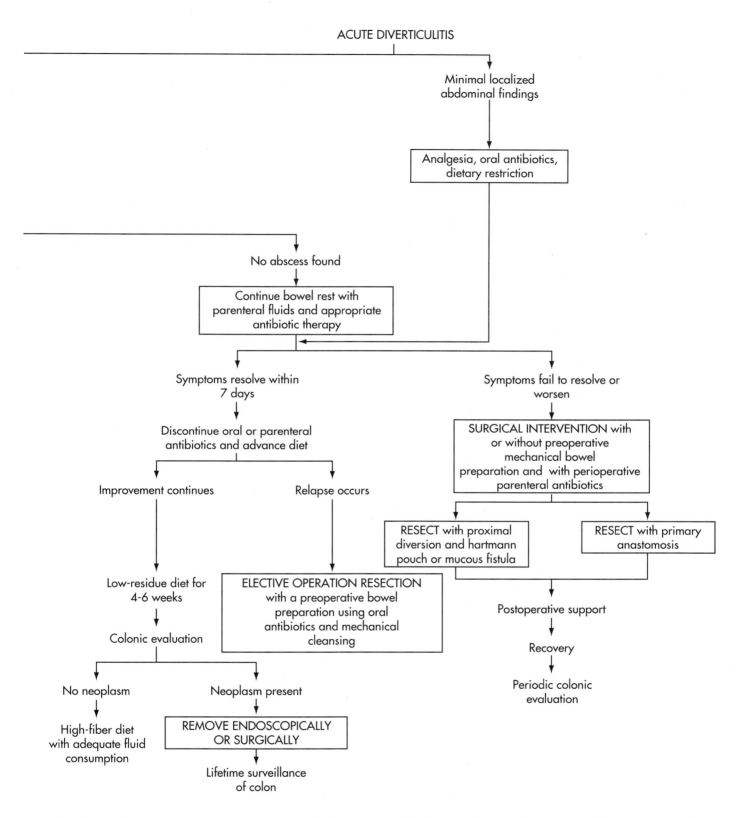

colon during lavage, preventing gross peritoneal fecal contamination with its accompanying disastrous effects.

In summary, if emergency surgery is necessary for localized diverticulitis, we try to remove the inflamed colon, most often performing a primary anastomosis. If this is inadvis-

able because of hemodynamic instability or gross evidence of peritoneal contamination, we do an end colostomy with a distal pouch, usually using the Hartmann procedure or distal mucous fistula. In modern surgery, diversion alone is rarely done.

Table 1 Intravenous Antibiotics for Aerobic and Anaerobic Human Colonic Microflora

DRUG	DOSAGE	FREQUENCY
COMBINATION THERAPY		
Aerobic coverage*		
Amikacin	15 mg/kg/day	bid-tid
Aztreonam	1-2 g	q8-12h
Ceftriaxone	1-2 g	qd
Cefotaxime	1-2 g	q8-12h
Ciprofloxacin	200-400 mg	q12h
Gentamicin	3 mg/kg/day	q8h
Tobramycin	3 mg/kg/day	q8h
Anaerobic coverage†		
Clindamycin	600-900 mg	q8h
Metronidazole	7.5 mg/kg	q6h
SINGLE-DRUG THERAPY		
Aerobic-anaerobic coverage		
Ampicillin-sulbactam	1.5-3 g	q6h
Cefotetan	1-2 g	q8-12h
Cefoxitin	1-2 g	q6-8h
Ceftizoxime	1-2 g	q8-12h
Imipenem-cilastatin	500 mg	q6h
Meropenem	1 g	q8h
Piperacillin-tazobactam	3.375-4.5 g	q6h
Ticarcillin-clavulanic acid	3.1 g	q6h

*To be combined with a drug exhibiting anaerobic activity.
†To be combined with a drug exhibiting aerobic activity.

Table 2 Oral Antibiotic Regimens for Treatment of a Mild Episode of Acute Diverticulitis

ANTIBIOTIC	DOSAGE (mg)	FREQUENCY-DURATION
Ciprofloxacin	500	bid
	500	bid
Ciprofloxacin and metronidazole	500	bid
TMP-SMX DS and metronidazole	800	bid
	500	bid
Amoxicillin-clavulanic acid	250-500	tid
Doxycycline	100	q24h

TMP-SMX DS, Trimethoprim-sulfamethoxazole (Bactrim) double strength.

Generalized Intraabdominal Sepsis

The cause of generalized abdominal findings suggesting intraabdominal sepsis is often unknown before exploratory laporatomy. These patients require prompt fluid resuscitation and empiric antibiotic coverage with an agent or combination of agents that will control both aerobic and anaerobic enteric organisms (see Table 1). If there is evidence of

Table 3 Suggested Approach to Preoperative Preparation for Elective Colon Resection

TWO DAYS BEFORE SURGERY (AT HOME)
1. Low-residue or liquid diet *plus*
   sodium phosphate (Phosphosoda), 1½ oz PO at 6 PM
   or
2. Nothing additional until next day

ONE DAY BEFORE SURGERY (AT HOME OR IN HOSPITAL IF NECESSARY)
Admit in morning (if necessary and allowed)
1. Continue clear liquid diet, IV fluids as needed *plus*
   Sodium phosphate (Phosphosoda), 1½ oz PO at 6 AM
   or
2. Start clear liquid diet *plus*
   Whole-gut lavage with polyethylene glycol, 1 L/hr PO starting at 8 AM until diarrhea is clear (no longer than 3-4 hr)
No enemas
All patients receive 1 g neomycin PO and 1 g erythromycin base PO at 1 PM, 2 PM, and 11 PM

DAY OF SURGERY
Operation at 8 AM
A single dose of antibiotic with broad-spectrum aerobic/anaerobic activity given IV by anesthesia personnel in the operating room just before incision; repeat dosage if operation lasts more than 2 hr

perforation or if the patient is in shock, laparotomy as soon as the patient is stable is often necessary. Laparotomy often reveals fibrinous exudate, free pus, or abscesses throughout the abdominal cavity. If we find diverticulitis, we resect the involved segment and perform a proximal colostomy. Under these conditions, we do not consider performing a primary anastomosis. We prefer to leave a closed distal pouch, but only if a preoperative endoscopic examination has ensured that there is no other obstructing or significant neoplastic lesion present. Such a lesion could produce a blind-loop syndrome and leakage of the distal pouch, or could require another operation for its removal.

After resection, we copiously irrigate the abdominal cavity with normal saline. If a localized abscess is identified, a closed drainage system is used; however, drains are not placed if diffuse peritonitis is present. We strongly believe that if gross peritonitis is present, the skin wound should not be closed tightly if at all. Patients who have undergone such surgery usually require careful monitoring in an intensive care unit and appropriate antibiotic coverage.

Many of these patients develop secondary intraabdominal or pelvic abscesses, which are detectable with CT or ultrasound. If surgical drainage is required, we use an extraperitoneal approach (ribs, transvaginal, transanal) when possible because we believe it lowers postoperative morbidity when percutaneous drainage is not feasible. Many of these patients will also have prolonged ileus and therefore require parenteral hyperalimentation to meet the extraordinary metabolic demands of controlling intraabdominal sepsis. Of course, enteral nutrition should be resumed as soon as possible.

See also the chapter *Abdominal Abscess.*

Suggested Reading

Lambert ME, et al: Management of the septic complications of diverticular disease, *Br J Surg* 73:576, 1986.

Mueller PR, et al: Sigmoid diverticular abscesses: percutaneous drainage as an adjunct to surgical resection in 24 cases, *Radiology* 164:321, 1987.

Nichols RL: Bowel preparation. In Wilmore DW, et al, eds: *Care of the surgical patient*, New York, 1995, Scientific American.

Nichols RL, et al, eds: *Decision making in surgical sepsis*, Philadelphia, 1991, BC Decker.

Nichols RL, et al: Current practices of preoperative bowel preparation among North American colorectal surgeons, *Clin Infect Dis* 24:609, 1997.

Schecter S, Mulvey J, Eisenstat TE: Management of uncomplicated acute diverticulitis: results of a survey, *Dis Colon Rectum* 42:470, 1999.

ABDOMINAL ABSCESS

Donald D. Trunkey

Abdominal abscess can follow primary intraabdominal disease such as diverticulitis, appendicitis, biliary tract disease, pancreatitis, or perforated viscus; abdominal surgery; penetrating and blunt abdominal trauma; and bacteremic spread of infection from a distant source to an intraabdominal site, particularly in the immunocompromised patient. The mortality rate is reported as high as 40%; however, recent studies suggest a mortality rate of 20%, with the reduction most likely the result of earlier diagnosis. The three distinct anatomic locations of abdominal abscesses are intraperitoneal, retroperitoneal, and visceral, the last developing in liver, gallbladder, spleen, pancreas, and kidney. Liver abscesses are covered in the chapter *Liver Abscess,* and pancreatic abscesses in the chapter *Infectious Complications in Acute Pancreatitis.*

Bacteria in the peritoneal cavity are subject to the normal influences of gravity and pressure gradients. If the patient is upright, peritoneal fluid will collect within the dependent portion of the pelvis. Patients who are sick with an intraperitoneal process such as peritonitis typically are supine, and their dependent positions are the subphrenic space and the pericolic gutters. Pressure gradients within the peritoneal cavity are due to motion of the diaphragm. With expiration, relative negative pressure beneath the diaphragm sets up a current of movement that favors fluid moving from the pericolic space to the subhepatic and subphrenic space. These currents allow the bacteria to come into contact with the diaphragmatic surface, which has lymphatic fenestrations and is an important means of clearing bacteria from the celomic cavity. Equally important is the clearance of bacteria by macrophages and neutrophils.

Initially, macrophages are the primary white cells in peritonitis; they are followed in a few hours by neutrophils. The exudate typically associated with peritonitis may approach 300 to 500 ml of fluid per hour. This contributes not only to hypovolemia and shock but perhaps also to impaired clearance of bacteria when fibrin blocks the fenestrations in the diaphragm.

Other factors contributing to abscess formation are adjuvants, which include hemoglobin, hematoma, dead tissue, and foreign bodies. Hypovolemia and hemorrhagic shock also enhance the frequency and severity of infection. Blood transfusion has been indicted as a potential contributor to intraperitoneal sepsis because it is immunosuppressive. The diabetic patient may be at increased risk because some host defense mechanisms are impaired. Protein-calorie malnutrition and antecedent steroid therapy also may contribute to formation of intraabdominal abscess.

Finally, abdominal abscess should be viewed as a continuum in the systemic inflammatory response syndrome. On one hand, formation of an abdominal abscess may represent a success from the host defense viewpoint because the infection is now localized and walled off. On the other hand, many abdominal abscesses progress to severe sepsis and septic shock, particularly when left untreated.

■ CLINICAL FEATURES

The clinical presentation of an abdominal abscess is greatly influenced by the immunocompetence of the host. The nonimmunocompromised patient typically has a spiking fever, abdominal pain, and tenderness. There is a leukocytosis of 15,000 to 25,000/mm^3. Pleural fluid is present in about 80% of patients with subphrenic abscess. Occasionally, there is intrathoracic spread of an abdominal abscess, which presents as empyema, cough, and even formation of a bronchopleural fistula with resultant thick, foul-smelling sputum. Less often, the patient may develop a chronic intraabdominal abscess that smolders for many weeks or even months. These patients have a fever of unknown origin and as time progresses often become cachectic.

In contrast, the immunocompromised patient has blunting of the clinical symptoms. Fever may be absent, rebound tenderness and guarding are markedly diminished or absent, and leukocytosis is not a reliable indicator of sepsis. Unfortunately, intraabdominal abscess is increasing in the immunocompromised patient, and mortality is significantly higher than in the nonimmunocompromised patient.

■ DIAGNOSIS

At present, computed tomography (CT) is the gold standard for diagnosis of abdominal abscess. CT has a sensitivity of 78% to 100%, and ultrasound has a sensitivity of 75% to

82%. Magnetic resonance imaging (MRI) is no better than CT. CT is superior to ultrasound for all anatomic sites with the possible exception of the pelvis. CT scan can be done in almost all patients, including those with wounds, dressings, ostomies, and drains. In an era of managed care, it is imprudent from a cost standpoint to do plain films, which help with fewer than 50% of patients. Similarly, scintigraphy, arteriograms, and radio contrast studies lack sensitivity and specificity. Sequential testing is more costly than CT scanning, and with spiral CT, time is no longer a major consideration. The interventional radiologist should be aware when the CT is done that abdominal abscess is being considered. If an abscess is found, the patient can often have percutaneous drainage immediately upon diagnosis.

■ THERAPY

There are three major considerations for optimal management of the patient with abdominal abscess. First and foremost is drainage of the abscess. Second is appropriate antibiotic therapy, and third is physiologic support for the patient.

Since 1980, there has been a shift from open abdominal to percutaneous drainage. The results of percutaneous drainage appear to be equal clinically and more cost effective in the nonimmunocompromised patient. Although there have been no randomized trials, the only advantage of abdominal drainage is that the length of stay in the hospital is shorter than with percutaneous drainage. However, percutaneous drainage has been more problematic in the immunocompromised host. This may be because of a higher incidence of fungal infections which are associated with tissue invasion.

Percutaneous drainage is done with CT or ultrasound guidance. If the patient's symptoms have not improved within 48 to 72 hours, open abdominal drainage should be strongly considered. In certain high-risk immunocompromised patients, open abdominal drainage may be the procedure of choice. This depends on the infecting organism and the extent of the abscess. Percutaneous drainage can also be used for splenic and renal abscess. A contraindication to percutaneous drainage is lack of a safe access route. A safe drainage route is identified in 85% to 90% of patients. Pelvic abscess may be best drained by transrectal technique.

In complex abscesses and immunocompromised patients, open drainage allows debridement of the abscess wall. A modification of open abdominal drainage is planned relaparotomy (etappenlavage). One study suggests a diminishing point of return after three laparotomies or when the bacterial count falls below 10^5 organisms per milliliter.

Antimicrobial Treatment

In the nonimmunocompromised patient, anaerobic bacteria are isolated in up to 60% to 70% of abdominal abscesses. Commonly isolated bacteria include *Bacteroides fragilis*, peptostreptococci and peptococci, *Clostridium* species, *Escherichia coli*, *Enterobacter* and *Klebsiella* organisms, and enterococci. *Staphylococcus aureus* is uncommon in intraabdominal abscess and suggests bacteremic seeding, an immunocompromised patient, or vertebral osteomyelitis. *Candida* also suggests an immunocompromised host or

previous antimicrobial therapy. *Pseudomonas* species, *Serratia* species, cytomegalovirus, *Coccidioides immitis*, *Cryptococcus neoformans*, and *Mycobacterium avium* are also found in the immunocompromised patient.

Antimicrobial therapy for abdominal abscesses should be based on specific cultures when possible. If the organism is not known, therapy should be directed by Gram stain. Broad-spectrum coverage should be avoided when possible, and when it does become necessary, cyclic administration of antibiotics within the institution may avoid resistance problems and opportunistic infections. Until definitive cultures are available, broad-spectrum antibiotics including anaerobic coverage are indicated. An aminoglycoside plus metronidazole is a good choice for the patient who is only mildly to moderately ill. *B. fragilis* has an increasing prevalence of resistance to clindamycin, making clindamycin less dependable as a first-line agent. If the patient is at risk for aminoglycoside toxicity (antecedent renal failure, hypovolemic shock, severe trauma), an alternative therapeutic regimen is the substitution of a quinolone or a third-generation cephalosporin for the aminoglycoside. The monobactam aztreonam is also a good choice when *Pseudomonas* is strongly suspected; however, anaerobic coverage must be added to this drug. Additional useful agents are the combinations piperacillin-tazobactam or imipenem-cilastatin or ampicillin-sulbactam. If the patient is immunocompromised or has recent isolation of *Candida* from the urine or tracheobronchial tree, amphotericin B or fluconazole should accompany the initial treatment. A Gram stain and fungal preparations should always be obtained from the abscess cavity. If the Gram stain shows a predominance of grampositive cocci in chains, ampicillin may be added for activity against *Enterococcus* species.

■ COMPLICATIONS

Open drainage of the abdominal abscess has been associated with enteric fistula formation. Percutaneous drainage has a small but predictable failure rate; failure requires open drainage. All abdominal abscesses may progress to septicemia, septic shock, and sequential organ failure. Abdominal abscess is a major cause of adult respiratory distress syndrome, renal failure, and liver failure. In addition to the appropriate individual organ support measures carried out in an intensive care setting, attention must be directed to adequate nutrition. Studies show that enteral nutrition is superior to parenteral nutrition.

Suggested Reading

Bone RC: Sepsis, the sepsis syndrome, multi-organ failure: a plea for comparable definition, *Ann Intern Med* 114:332, 1991.

Fry DE, Clevenger FW: Reoperation for intraabdominal abscess, *Surg Clin North Am* 71:159, 1991.

McClean KL, Sheehan AG, Harding GKM: Intraabdominal infection: a review, *Clin Infect Dis* 19:100, 1994.

Rangel-Frausto MS, et al: The natural history of the systemic inflammatory response syndrome (SIRS), *JAMA* 273:117, 1995.

Swartz MN, Simon HB: Peritonitis and intraabdominal abscesses, *Sci Am* 23:1, 1995.

SPLENIC ABSCESS

Thomas R. Howdieshell
Thomas R. Gadacz

The diagnosis of splenic abscess is often overlooked because of its rarity and misleading clinical features, as well as the presence of predisposing conditions that obscure its clinical presentation. Hence, it is not surprising that splenic abscess is often diagnosed during postmortem examinations, even in the era of antibiotics.

■ INCIDENCE AND PREDISPOSING FACTORS

Splenic abscesses occur more commonly in males (55% to 60% in several series), with the average age ranging from 37 to 54 years. Nelken and colleagues describe a bimodal distribution: patients younger than 40 years of age; generally immunosuppressed or drug addicts, who usually present with a multilocular abscess; and patients older than 70 years of age who are suffering from diabetes and/or a nonendocarditic septic focus and develop a unilocular abscess.

The primary predisposing causes of splenic abscess include metastatic hematogenous infection, contiguous disease processes extending to the spleen, splenic trauma, hematologic disorders (collagen-vascular diseases, hemoglobinopathies), and immunodeficiency states (acquired, congenital). The incidence of these predisposing causes or risk factors is shown in Table 1.

Table 1 Primary Predisposing Causes or Risk Factors for Splenic Abscess

FACTORS	PERCENTAGE
INFECTIOUS ETIOLOGY	**68.8**
Endocarditis	15.3
Urinary infection	7.1
Otitis	3.3
Appendicitis	2.8
Pneumonia	2.8
Brucellosis	2.3
Lung abscess	2.3
Malaria	1.9
Diverticulitis	1.9
Urologic surgery	0.95
Amebiasis	0.95
Miscellany	11.9
Septic syndrome	11.9
NONINFECTIOUS ETIOLOGY	**31.2**
Trauma	16.7
Hemoglobinopathies	11.9
Contiguous diseases	23.0

■ METASTATIC HEMATOGENOUS INFECTIONS

Infective endocarditis is the most common condition predisposing a patient to splenic abscess (Figure 1). Although the exact incidence is difficult to determine, several studies demonstrated the occurrence of splenic embolization in 31% to 44% of the patients with endocarditis. Histologic examination disclosed splenitis in at least 20% of patients. Splenic infarction occurred in 30% to 67% of patients with endocarditis during the preantibiotic era and in 33% to 44% of these patients during the antibiotic era. In 1977, Pelletier and Petersdorf reported the incidence of splenic abscess in patients with subacute bacterial endocarditis to be approximately 2.4%. Mycotic aneurysms are seen angiographically within abscesses, but whether these predispose a patient to, or result from, splenic abscess remains uncertain.

In addition to endocarditis, a multitude of other infections have been reported as primary causes of splenic abscess (see Table 1). Miscellaneous infections include dental abscess, bacteremia after dental extraction, tonsillectomy, hemodialysis, peritonsillar abscess, acute parotitis, bronchiectasis, perinephric abscess, decubitus ulcer, complicated infectious mononucleosis, tuberculosis, yellow fever, diphtheria, and anthrax.

■ CONTIGUOUS INFECTION

On occasion, splenic abscesses result from the direct extension of diseases having their primary foci in adjacent organs. Contiguous extension from diverticulitis, pancreatic infection or carcinoma, gastric ulcer, perihepatic abscess, carcinoma of the stomach, perinephric and subphrenic abscess, and carcinoma of the descending colon have been reported.

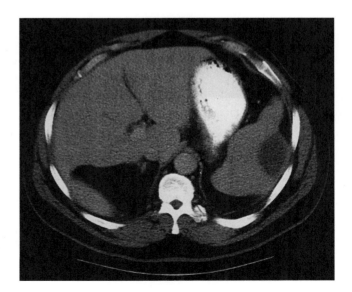

Figure 1
Unilocular splenic abscess in a patient with bacterial endocarditis.

■ TRAUMATIC ABSCESS

Traumatic abscess results from secondary infection and suppuration of contused parenchyma or of a hematoma arising from injury to splenic tissue. In a report by Inlow, the initial traumatic injury was not easily recognized or reported, and most patients developed signs and symptoms of splenic infection after a latent period of 2 weeks to 4 months after sustaining injuries to the left upper quadrant. Splenic abscess has been reported after splenorrhaphy, and nonoperative management of blunt splenic injuries diagnosed by computed tomography (CT) scan. On rare occasions, radiologic procedures such as splenic artery embolization for thrombocytopenia or splenoportography for portocaval shunt evaluation have been implicated as a cause of splenic abscess.

■ HEMATOLOGIC DISORDERS

Hemoglobinopathies accounted for approximately 12% of splenic abscesses reported by Alsono-Cohen. Patients with sickle cell disease have an increased risk of acquiring systemic bacterial infections as a result of hyposplenism and a variety of functional defects in opsonization, phagocytic function, and cell-mediated immunity.

One of the main organs to be affected in sickle cell disease is the spleen. Sometimes, splenomegaly persists beyond the first decade of life, and these patients are susceptible to splenic abscess.

The spleen may also be a site of infection in patients with collagen-vascular diseases. Splenic abscesses have been reported in patients with rheumatoid arthritis, systemic lupus erythematosus, and polyarteritis nodosa. Pathologic features of the spleen in these illnesses include capsulitis and small infarcts.

■ IMMUNODEFICIENCY STATES

Splenic abscess has been reported complicating acquired immunodeficiency syndrome (AIDS), chemotherapy, cancer (leukemia, lymphoma), and long-term steroid use, as well as conditions such as diabetes mellitus and alcoholism.

■ DIAGNOSIS

History and Physical Examination

The signs and symptoms of a splenic abscess are often insidious, nonspecific, and related to the underlying disease. Table 2 characterizes the clinical findings in 227 patients. Fever is the most common symptom, but pain in the left hypochondrium appears in a minority of cases, with vague abdominal pain being more common. Pain is probably caused by splenitis with capsular involvement. Abscesses located in the upper pole of the spleen tend to irritate the diaphragm causing radiation of pain toward the left shoulder and an elevated, immobile left hemidiaphragm. Splenic rupture also commonly manifests as left shoulder pain. An abscess located in the lower pole of the spleen more often

Table 2 Clinical Findings in Splenic Abscess

CLINICAL FEATURE	PERCENTAGE
Fever	92.5
Abdominal pain	57.5
Left upper quadrant pain	39.2
Pleuritic pain	15.8
Toxic syndrome	15.4
Vomiting	14.0
Abdominal tenderness	60.1
Splenomegaly	56.0

irritates the peritoneal surface, resulting predominantly in signs and symptoms of peritonitis. A deep-seated abscess that does not involve the splenic capsule may be accompanied only by general symptoms of infection without pain or other localizing signs.

Laboratory Findings

Leukocytosis is present in 70% to 80% of patients but is a variable finding. In one large series, the white cell count varied between 2400 and 41,000 cells/mm^3. In general, other serum laboratory studies were not helpful. Blood cultures were positive in 59.7% of patients. Of these positive blood cultures, 74% grew the same organisms as those subsequently isolated from the splenic abscess.

The infecting organisms and their incidence from a review of 189 patients of Nelken and others are reported in Table 3. The increasing number of splenic abscesses resulting from gram-negative organisms appears to be related to the widespread use of broad-spectrum antibiotics, the improved survival of critically ill patients colonized with these bacteria, and prolonged hospitalization, which increases the risk of nosocomial infection. *Candida* abscesses of the spleen are seen almost exclusively in neutropenic patients with the exception of disseminated candidiasis as a complication of abdominal surgery. Fungal abscesses due to *Candida* are more likely to complicate the use of broad-spectrum antibiotics, indwelling intravenous cannulas, hyperalimentation fluids, systemic steroids, cytotoxic chemotherapy, or immunosuppression after organ transplantation. Organisms responsible for AIDS-related splenic abscesses include *Salmonella*, *Mycobacterium avium-intracellulare*, fungi, and *Pneumocystis carinii*. In several series, approximately one fourth of patients with a splenic abscess did not have an organism cultured from the abscess cavity or from blood.

Radiographic Findings

The most common finding on chest radiography is an elevated left hemidiaphragm (31%), pleural effusion (28%), and left basilar pulmonary consolidation (18%). Plain abdominal films reveal abnormalities in 69% of patients. CT scanning, with a sensitivity of 96% and an associated specificity between 90% and 95%, is currently the best diagnostic test for splenic abscess. CT scan may show a homogeneous low-density area, with or without rim enhancement; lucent areas within the spleen containing fluid levels of different densities; and intrasplenic gas formation. This gas may be dispersed diffusely through the abscess as fine low attenua-

Table 3 Infecting Organisms and Their Incidence in Splenic Abscess

ORGANISM	PERCENTAGE
ANAEROBIC BACTERIA (n = 28)	**18**
Mixed	30
Bacteroides	23
Propionobacterium species	20
Clostridium	13
Streptococcus	10
Fusobacterium	4
Actinomyces	0
AEROBIC BACTERIA (n = 90)	**56**
All staphylococcus	20
All *Salmonella*	15
Escherichia coli	15
Enterococcus	8
Salmonella typhi	7
Unspecified *Streptococcus*	6
Unspecified coliforms	6
Staphylococcus epidermidis	4
α-*Streptococcus*	4
Klebsiella	3
Enterobacter	2
Proteus	2
Pseudomonas aeruginosa	2
Shigella	2
Diphtheroids	2
Beta-hemolytic *Streptococcus*	1
Nonhemolytic *Streptococcus*	1
Pneumococcus	0
Nocardia	0
Brucella	0
Pseudomonas pseudomallei	0
FUNGI (n = 41)	**26**
Candida albicans	42
Candida tropicalis	21
Aspergillus	10
Blastomycosis	5
Aureobassidium pullulans	2

tion bubbles or may coalesce into one or more larger collections.

Ultrasonography has a sensitivity of 76% in the detection of splenic abscess. The ultrasound appearance of splenic abscess generally is characterized as a hypoechoic or nearly anechoic, ovoid-, or round-shaped area in the spleen, with varying internal echogenicity, irregular wall, and mild to moderate distal acoustic enhancement. Differential diagnoses of splenic abscess in CT and ultrasound images should include splenic infarct, hematoma, neoplasm, and complicated cysts.

Differential Diagnosis

The differential diagnosis should include subphrenic abscess, pulmonary empyema, splenic infarction, perinephric abscess, neoplasm, and leukemic infiltration. In a review of 3372 subphrenic abscesses, Ochsner and Graves found a primary lesion in the spleen in approximately 4% of the cases. Therefore the possibility of coexistent splenic abscess should be considered in the presence of a subphrenic abscess. Pulmonary empyema as a complication of splenic

abscess (4%) may also divert the clinician's attention from the primary lesion.

■ TREATMENT

There is no place for long-term medical management of a clinically overt splenic abscess. The mainstay of treatment consists of splenectomy and appropriate antibiotics, with a success rate of 86% to 94%. Recent evidence has shown that percutaneous drainage plus effective antibiotics is a safe and efficacious therapy. Percutaneous drainage may be used if the patient has a unilocular abscess, is in unstable condition from a recent operation, has had multiple previous operations, or has significant risks for general anesthesia or standard surgical drainage. The catheter can be removed when the drainage is minimal and the cavity has decreased in size as evidenced by sinogram, ultrasound, or CT scan. If the patient does not improve clinically, splenectomy is advised. Percutaneous drainage is most likely to succeed when the abscess collection is unilocular, has a discrete wall, and has no internal septation. Abscesses containing thick, tenacious, necrotic debris are less likely to be successfully drained percutaneously, as are phlegmons, poorly defined cavities, microabscesses, multiple abscesses, and abscesses originating from a contiguous process. Percutaneous drainage of a multiloculated abscess is almost uniformly unsuccessful. However, for a single loculation, percutaneous drainage has been reported to be effective in 68% to 75% of cases.

Broad-spectrum antibiotics should be initiated when a splenic abscess is diagnosed. This therapy should include agents effective against staphylococci, streptococci, and gram-negative bacteria. A semisynthetic penicillin or cephalosporin plus an aminoglycoside are recommended. If a contiguous abdominal process is suspected, anaerobic agents such as clindamycin or metronidazole should be added. In immunosuppressed patients, antifungal coverage such as fluconazole should be initiated early in the disease process. Some authors recommend continuing antibiotics for 2 weeks after splenectomy or discontinuation of percutaneous drainage.

The optimal management of fungal splenic abscess remains to be defined. Some authors have suggested prolonged courses of amphotericin B with a total dose ranging from 530 mg to 2 g. Others have suggested splenectomy in conjunction with amphotericin B for the treatment for fungal splenic abscess. The argument in support of splenectomy for fungal abscess is based primarily on reports of bacterial abscesses of the spleen in which case nonoperative therapy was associated with high mortality. However, because most cases of splenic candidiasis represent disseminated infection, splenectomy does not address the problem of *Candida* present in other tissues, most notably the liver. There are many reports of confirmed splenic fungal abscesses resolving with antifungal drugs alone. Several case reports and a recent multicenter randomized trial in patients without neutropenia or major immune deficiency indicate that fluconazole may be as efficacious as amphotericin B. Patients suspected of having a fungal abscess should have a specific diagnosis made by percutaneous aspiration of the liver or spleen or open biopsy of the lesions. This is important because the differential diagnosis includes leukemic infiltrates, metastatic tumor, and fungal and bacterial abscesses.

Splenic abscess may rupture into the peritoneal cavity, thus causing acute peritonitis. A mortality rate of 50% has been reported in cases of splenic rupture. A splenic abscess may also drain into the stomach, colon, or pleura. However, splenic abscesses most commonly produce repeated bacteremia, which ends in septic shock if not treated. Two thirds of all splenic abscesses in adults are solitary, and one third are multiple. In children, however, the opposite is true. Solitary abscesses generally are easier to diagnose and treat and usually are caused by streptococci, staphylococci, hemoglobinopathies, or *Salmonella.* Multiple abscesses tend to be caused by *Candida.* The prognosis is clearly related to multisystem organ failure, age, and associated diseases.

With early diagnosis and treatment of splenic abscess, the mortality rate can be as low as 7%. Medical therapy appears appropriate for patients with mycobacterial, *Pneumocystis carinii,* and fungal disease. Percutaneous drainage appears reasonable for patients with a singular, unilocular abscess without associated intraabdominal disease. In patients in whom there is any question as to the accessibility, locularity, or singularity of the abscess, or if there is a question of intraabdominal pathology, splenectomy remains the treatment of choice.

Suggested Reading

Alonso-Cohen MA, et al: Splenic abscess, *World J Surg* 14:513, 1990.

Al-Salem AH, et al: Splenectomy in patients with sickle-cell disease, *Am J Surg* 172:254, 1996.

Chou YH, et al: Splenic abscess: sonographic diagnosis and percutaneous drainage or aspiration, *Gastrointest Radiol* 17:262, 1992.

Johnson JD, et al: Splenic abscess complicating infectious endocarditis, *Arch Int Med* 143:906, 1983.

Nelken N, et al: Changing clinical spectrum of splenic abscess: a multicenter study and review of the literature, *Am J Surg* 154:27, 1987.

Rex JH, et al: A randomized trial comparing fluconazole with amphotericin B for the treatment of candidemia in patients without neutropenia, *N Engl J Med* 331:1325, 1994.

Tikkakoski T, et al: Splenic abscess: imaging and intervention, *Acta Radiologica* 33:561, 1992.

PERITONITIS

Linda A. Slavoski
Matthew E. Levison

Peritonitis is inflammation of the serous lining of the peritoneal cavity. This inflammation may result from a response to microorganisms or chemical irritants, such as blood, bile, pancreatic secretions, or antimicrobial agents. The peritoneal cavity is lubricated with 20 to 50 ml of clear yellow transudative fluid, normally with fewer than 300 cells/mm³, a specific gravity below 1.016, and protein below 3 g/dl.

Infectious causes of peritonitis are considered in this chapter. Two major types of infective peritonitis exist: (1) primary (spontaneous or idiopathic) and (2) secondary. When signs of peritonitis and sepsis persist after treatment for secondary peritonitis and no pathogens or only low-grade pathogens are isolated, the clinical entity has been termed *tertiary peritonitis.* Intraperitoneal abscesses can result from localization of the initially diffuse peritoneal inflammatory response to one or more dependent sites or at the site of the underlying condition (e.g., periappendiceal, pericholecystic, or peridiverticular abscess). Peritonitis may also result from the use of a peritoneal catheter for dialysis or central nervous system ventriculoperitoneal shunting. For management of peritoneal catheter–related peritonitis, see the chapter *Dialysis-Related Infections.*

■ PRIMARY PERITONITIS

Primary peritonitis is best defined as infection of the peritoneal cavity without an evident source in the abdominal cavity. Primary peritonitis occurs at all ages. In children it particularly occurs in association with postnecrotic cirrhosis and with nephrotic syndrome. Primary peritonitis, also called *spontaneous bacterial peritonitis,* in the adult is seen most commonly in association with alcoholic cirrhosis, especially in its end stage. It has been seen also with ascites caused by postnecrotic cirrhosis, chronic active hepatitis, acute viral hepatitis, congestive heart failure, malignancy, systemic lupus erythematosus, and nephrotic syndrome. Rarely, primary peritonitis occurs with no apparent underlying disease.

The organisms reported to cause primary peritonitis in children were *Streptococcus pneumoniae* and group A streptococci. These organisms are much less important now and have been replaced by gram-negative bacilli and to a lesser extent staphylococci. In adults gram-negative bacilli also dominate, followed by streptococci and other gram-positive cocci. *Escherichia coli* is the most frequently isolated pathogen, followed by *Klebsiella* species, *S. pneumoniae,* and other streptococcal species, including enterococci. *Staphylococcus aureus* is rare in primary peritonitis. Anaerobes and microaerophilic organisms are also infrequently isolated. Recovery of anaerobes from ascitic fluid, particularly in polymicrobial cases, should raise the possibility of secondary peritonitis.

Cases with positive ascitic fluid culture but with low leukocyte counts and no clinical findings of peritonitis have been designated as bacterascites. This may represent early colonization of the peritoneal cavity. Conversely, some patients have clinical evidence of peritonitis, elevated leukocyte counts in the ascitic fluid, but negative cultures. These have been called *culture-negative neutrocytic ascites.*

The route of infection in primary peritonitis may be hematogenous, lymphogenous, via transmural migration through the intact bowel wall or, in women, from the vagina via the fallopian tubes. Seeding of ascitic fluid during bacteremia is probably the most common route. A major pathogenetic mechanism is likely to be impaired clearance of bacteria from blood. Patients with cirrhosis exhibit decreased phagocytic activity within the reticuloendothelial system, impaired intracellular killing by neutrophils and monocytes, impaired opsinization, and low serum and ascific complement levels.

The clinical features of primary peritonitis are variable. In children it is often confused with acute appendicitis. Common signs and symptoms include fever (often low grade), abdominal pain, nausea, vomiting, diarrhea, diffuse abdominal tenderness, rebound tenderness, and hypoactive to absent bowel sounds. Atypical signs such as hypothermia, hypotension, and unexplained decline in renal function may be present, as well as unexplained encephalopathy, hepatorenal syndrome, and variceal bleeding in cirrhotic patients. Because peritonitis may be clinically inapparent in a patient with ascites and decompensated liver disease, routine paracentesis may be necessary to disclose its presence in these patients.

The diagnosis of primary peritonitis requires that the possibility of an intraabdominal source of infection be excluded. Examination of the ascitic fluid is required. The ascitic fluid leukocyte count is generally greater than 300 polymorphonuclear leukocyte/mm^3. Gram stain of the fluid is commonly negative. The diagnostic yield of ascitic fluid culture can be enhanced by culturing a relatively large volume (e.g., 10 ml). Blood cultures should also be obtained.

Because the Gram stain is often negative in primary peritonitis, the initial choice of antimicrobial agents is often empiric and is modified once results of cultures and susceptibility testing are available. Initial therapy should be directed against enteric gram-negative bacilli and grampositive cocci. Acceptable regimens include the thirdgeneration cephalosporins ceftriaxone and cefotaxime, the fourth-generation cephalosporin cefepime, or one of the newer fluoroquinolones (e.g., levofloxacin, gatifloxacin, or moxifloxacin) that have improved activity against *S. pneumoniae,* including those strains that are relatively penicillin resistant, carbapenems (e.g., imipenem or meropenem), and beta-lactam antibiotic–beta-lactamase inhibitor combinations (e.g., ampicillin-sulbactam, ticarcillin-clavulanate, or piperacillin-tazobactam), with or without an aminoglycoside. If peritonitis develops during hospitalization, antimicrobial therapy should have activity against *Pseudomonas aeruginosa.*

S. pneumoniae and group A streptococci are best treated with high-dose penicillin G, ceftriaxone, or cefotaxime. Methicillin-sensitive *S. aureus* is best treated with a penicillinase-resistant penicillin (nafcillin) or with a firstgeneration cephalosporin (cefazolin). If the strain is methicillin-resistant or the patient is allergic to penicillin, vancomycin is used. If *Pseudomonas aeruginosa* is isolated, an aminoglycoside is given in combination with an antipseudomonal penicillin or cephalosporin, aztreonam, or imipenem or meropenem; or ciprofloxacin combined with

another antipseudomonal agent should be used. Antimicrobial therapy should be continued for 10 to 14 days if improvement is noted; however, shorter-course (5 day) therapy has been shown to be efficacious. Intraperitoneal antimicrobial administration has not been shown to be of benefit. A clinical response should be evident by 48 hours in patients receiving appropriate antimicrobial therapy. Failure to respond in this manner should prompt an examination for an alternative or additional diagnoses.

Recurrence of primary peritonitis is relatively common in patients with advanced liver disease; 70% of patients will have a recurrence in the first year after their initial episode. Prophylactic maintenance therapy with norfloxacin (400 mg daily), ciprofloxacin (750 mg once a week), or trimethoprim-sulfamethoxazole (one double-strength tablet once daily for 5 days each week) can reduce the frequency of recurrent episodes, perhaps by selective decontamination of the bowel, and may be an option in patients awaiting liver transplantation but may not otherwise prolong survival. Occasionally, peritonitis may be caused by *Mycobacterium tuberculosis,* usually from hematogenous dissemination from remote foci of tuberculous infection or extension of infection in mesenteric lymph nodes. The diagnosis of tuberculous peritonitis can usually be confirmed by histologic examination and culture of a peritoneal biopsy specimen and fluid. Diagnosis of *Coccidioides immitis* peritonitis can be made by wet mount of ascitic fluid, histology, and culture of the peritoneal biopsy specimen and fluid.

■ SECONDARY PERITONITIS

By definition, secondary peritonitis is associated with a predisposing intraabdominal lesion, and it usually involves components of the gastrointestinal flora. Any of numerous intraabdominal processes may give rise to secondary peritonitis; a partial list includes perforation of a peptic ulcer; traumatic perforation of the uterus, urinary bladder, stomach, or small or large bowel; appendicitis; pancreatitis; diverticulitis; bowel infarction; cholecystitis; biliary obstruction; rupture of an intraabdominal abscess; operative contamination of the peritoneum; and disease of the female genital tract such as septic abortion, postoperative uterine infection, endometritis, or salpingitis.

Although any type of microorganism may be responsible, secondary peritonitis is usually an endogenously acquired polymicrobial infection. On average, about five bacterial species are isolated and they include both obligate and facultative anaerobes. *Candida* species and gram-positive bacteria may be isolated, especially following gastric perforation, whereas components of the colonic flora with particular pathogenic potential predominate when the intraabdominal pathology involves the distal small or large bowel. In descending order of frequency they include *E. coli, Bacteroides fragilis,* enterococci, other *Bacteroides* species, *Fusobacterium, Clostridium perfringens,* other clostridia, *Peptostreptococcus,* and *Eubacterium.* Concomitant bacteremia has been reported in 20% to 30% of patients. Organisms most frequently recovered from the blood are *E. coli* and *B. fragilis.* In patients who acquire their infection after admission to a hospital, antibiotic-resistant organisms such as *Enterobacter, Serratia, Acinetobacter,* vancomycin-resistant enterococci, and *P. aeruginosa* are more frequently isolated.

The presenting symptoms are similar to those of primary peritonitis. Pain is the predominant symptom and can often localize to the site of the initiating process (e.g., cholecystitis, appendicitis, diverticulitis). Other findings include fever, nausea, vomiting, and abdominal distension. Blood pressure is usually normal early but may fall with onset of septic shock, and there may be an increase in respiratory rate and tachycardia. Direct and rebound abdominal tenderness and abdominal wall rigidity are often present. Bowel sounds are absent. Rectal and vaginal examinations, and in women in whom an ectopic pregnancy is suspected, a urinary β-HCG determination, are necessary.

Often, the diagnostic evaluation must be brief but thorough because of the patient's critical condition. Laboratory studies include a complete blood count, serum chemistry profile, liver profile, and amylase and lipase determinations. Appropriate cultures (blood, urine, and peritoneal) should be done promptly. The peritoneal fluid is evaluated for cell count, bacteria, blood, bile, and feces. In patients without free peritoneal fluid, peritoneal lavage may be indicated, with lactated Ringer's solution infused into the peritoneum and then drained to gravity and evaluated. Chest radiographs should be obtained to exclude chest conditions that might simulate clinically an intraabdominal process. Plain radiographs of the abdomen may also be helpful, sometimes revealing free air or fluid, bowel distention, ileus, or bowel wall edema. Computed tomography (CT) of the abdomen and pelvis with contrast is most helpful to localize the infection and indicate its probable source.

Antimicrobial therapy is initiated early to control bacteremia and to minimize the local spread of infection. Patients with hemodynamic, respiratory, renal, and other critical organ system dysfunction require immediate appropriate supportive therapy. Surgery is often necessary to drain purulent material, debride devitalized tissue, and control continued peritoneal contamination by removing the initiating process (e.g., cholecystitis, appendicitis, diverticulitis).

Antibiotic therapy should be begun as soon as blood cultures are obtained but often before peritoneal fluid can be obtained for culture. Peritoneal fluid cultures should be obtained at the time of paracentesis, percutaneous drainage of an intraperitoneal abscess, or laparotomy. Recent data suggest that survival of patients is diminished if initial therapy is inadequate, regardless of the adequacy of subsequent therapy. Initial therapy is consequently empirical and must have broad-spectrum activity against both beta-lactamase–producing anaerobes, such as *Bacteroides fragilis,* and facultative enteric gram-negative bacilli, such as *E. coli.*

Because these infections are commonly polymicrobial, a broad-spectrum agent or combination of agents should be used. Traditional therapy has been a combination of clindamycin plus an aminoglycoside or an alternative agent, such as aztreonam, third- or fourth-generation cephalosporin, or fluoroquinolone. Aztreonam and the fluroquinolones should be combined with an agent that covers anaerobes and gram-positive cocci (clindamycin). Third- or fourth-generation cephalosporins should be combined with an agent that covers colonic anaerobes (clindamycin or metronidazole). All these regimens fail to cover enterococci, which may be a significant component of the polymicrobial flora. Drugs such as the beta-lactam–beta-lactamase inhibitor combinations, ampicillin-sulbactam and piperacillin-tazobactam or the carbapenems, imipenem and meropenem, which usually cover most components of the polymicrobial flora, including enterococci, have made single-agent therapy possible. Single-agent therapy is most useful in community-acquired infection, which usually involves antibiotic-sensitive organisms. In hospitalized patients or patients who have recently received antibiotics, resistant organisms may be present and require more specific antibiotic therapy. The duration of antimicrobial therapy after adequate surgery is usually 5 to 10 days but depends on severity of infection, clinical response to therapy, and normalization of the white blood cell count. Only a short course of antimicrobial therapy (about 24 hours) is required for sterile peritonitis that occurs around an infected but resected intraabdominal organ, such as an appendix or gallbladder. Once the patient can tolerate oral therapy, antimicrobial agents can be given orally rather than intravenously, if oral agents are available that have antimicrobial activity equivalent to that of the intravenous regimen.

Peritoneal catheter–related peritonitis usually results from contamination of the catheter by skin flora. The most common pathogens include *Staphylococcus epidermidis, S. aureus, Streptococcus* species, and diphtheroids. Other less frequently isolated pathogens include *E. coli, Klebsiella, Enterobacter, Proteus,* and fungi. Symptoms include abdominal pain and tenderness, nausea, and vomiting.

Suggested Reading

Bohnen JMA, et al: Guidelines for clinical care: anti-infective agents for intra-abdominal infection, *Arch Surg,* 127:83, 1992.

Burnett RJ, et al: Definition of the role of enterococcus in intraabdominal infection: analysis of a prospective randomized trial, *Surgery* 188:716, 1995.

Christou NV, et al: Intra-abdominal infection study, *Arch Surg* 128:193, 1993.

Levison ME, Bush LM: Peritonitis and other intra-abdominal infections. In Mandell GL, Bennett JE, Dolin R, eds: *Principles and practice of infectious diseases,* ed 4, New York, 1995, Churchill Livingstone.

Pacelli F, et al: Prognosis in intraabdominal infections, Multivariate analysis on 604 patients, *Arch Surg* 131:641, 1996.

Schein M, Hirshberg A, Hashmonai M: Current surgical management of severe intraabdominal infection, *Surgery* 112:489, 1992.

Solomkin JS, et al: Results of a randomized trial comparing sequential intravenous/oral treatment with ciprofloxacin plus metronidazole to imipenem/cilastatin for intra-abdominal infections, *Ann Surg* 223:303, 1996.

Wilcox CM, Dismukes WE: Spontaneous bacterial peritonitis: a review of pathogenesis, diagnosis and treatment, *Medicine* 66:447, 1987.

Wittman DH, Schein M, Condon RE: Management of secondary peritonitis, *Ann Surg* 224:10, 1996.

WHIPPLE'S DISEASE AND SPRUE

Phillip B. Amidon
John G. Banwell

◼ WHIPPLE'S DISEASE

Whipple's disease is a rare multisystem disease with only 664 known cases before 1985 and 20 new cases being reported per year worldwide. Before antibiotic therapy, the disease was uniformly fatal. Symptoms are often present for 5 to 10 years before treatment, and because of the manifold clinical findings, merely considering this diagnosis is one of the most important steps regarding therapy. Beginning insidiously with complaints of arthralgia, myalgia, fever, and weight loss and progressing to malabsorbion and diarrhea, it is usually diagnosed only when chronic diarrhea occurs. Steatorrhea is present as well as malabsorption of proteins, carbohydrates, vitamins, and minerals. Joint pain and swelling are usual, but the most feared manifestation, central nervous system (CNS) Whipple's disease, is associated with headache, ataxia, personality change, ophthalmoplegia, seizures, and dementia. Cardiac involvement includes endocarditis of all valves, pericarditis, and myocarditis. The eye is less commonly involved, with uveitis, chorioretinitis, or keratosis.

The etiologic agent, *Tropheryma whippelii*, is a gram-positive, PAS-positive, non–acid-fast, rod-shaped bacillus with typical electron microscopy morphology. Only within the past year has it been possible to grow the organism in cell culture, using peripheral blood monocytes. Host interaction is probably involved in the pathogenesis of Whipple's disease. In autopsy series, the frequency is less than 0.1%; 40- to 50-year-old men predominate, and 97% are Caucasian. HLA-B27 is found in 28% to 44% of patients, compared with an HLA-B27 incidence of 8% in the general population. In 1992, investigators using polymerase chain reaction (PCR) technology identified the unique gene segment that encodes the 16S ribosomal RNA of the bacillus. PCR testing has a very high sensitivity (96.6%) and specificity (100%) and has shown *T. whippelii* in tissues that demonstrate no evidence of disease.

Biopsy is necessary to make the diagnosis. The intestine is nearly always involved, with endoscopic biopsy of the distal duodenum or proximal jejunum being sufficient. Classic lesions are yellow-white granulated mucosa found between Kerckring folds. Histologic findings are flattened villi, cuboid deformation of the epithelium, large extracellular fat accumulation, and PAS-positive macrophages in the lamina propria, adjacent to the lumen. PAS-positive macrophages are detectable in the joint, bone marrow, spleen, adrenal, kidney, heart, and brain tissue.

The disease can often be identified on the basis of infected mesenteric lymph nodes. Because the CNS is considered the most serious site of involvement in Whipple's disease, treatment should include PCR analysis of cerebrospinal fluid (CSF). This test is potentially useful for diagnosis and for monitoring response to therapy, even in patients without neurologic symptoms.

Before antibiotic therapy, the disease was invariably fatal. Because of the rarity of the disease, no large-scale controlled studies have been done to determine optimal therapy. In the past, the inability to culture *T. whippelii* precluded the determination of antibiotic sensitivity and resistance. Treatment is therefore based on clinical experience and retrospective studies involving small numbers of patients. The first cure was reported with chloramphenicol in 1952. Later, tetracycline was commonly used. However, the problem of relapse and CNS involvement has led to reevaluation of therapy. The now-recognized high prevalence of CNS disease requires drugs that cross the blood-brain barrier. A look-back study of 88 patients by Keinath found a 35% relapse occurring on average 4 years after stopping antibiotic treatment. Of those, 43% of the relapsers had been treated only with tetracycline and 68% of that group had a CNS relapse. No CNS relapses were noted in the group treated initially with parenteral penicillin and streptomycin followed by oral trimethoprim-sulfamethaxone (TMP-SMX). In other reports, some patients had developed symptomatic Whipple's disease of the CNS while undergoing treatment with TMP-SMX alone. Two such patients were found to be CSF PCR positive and were treated with ceftriaxone and chloramphenicol with conversion to PCR-negative status. There is a case report of a patient presenting with neurologic symptoms and a magnetic resonance imaging (MRI) scan suggesting Whipple's disease in whom a relapse occurred 7 years after the onset of symptoms. The CSF PCR was negative, but the symptoms and MRI findings improved with antibiotic therapy.

Based on the clinical findings published to date, recommended treatment is parenteral streptomycin, 1 g, and penicillin G, 1.2 million U daily for 14 days, followed by TMP-SMX DS twice daily for 1 year (Table 1). Alternative therapies that have been used are parenteral ampicillin, 2 g three times daily, and ceftriaxone, 2 g daily for 14 days, followed by twice-daily TMP-SMX DS for 1 year. Also, parenteral ceftriaxone, 2 g twice daily, and streptomycin, 1 g daily for 14 days, followed by TMP-SMX DS twice daily or cefixime, 400 mg orally for 1 year.

With treatment, the steatorrhea may persist up to 7 months. The bacteria may be visible by electron microscope for up to 4 months. The mucosal changes seen by light microscopy take an average of 14 months to normalize, and PAS-laden macrophages can still be found up to 2 years after therapy. Currently, the optimal length of treatment is unknown, and proof of cure does not exist. Follow up should continue for at least 20 years. Relapses occur on average after 4 years (20 months to 20 years). Therapy for relapse is outlined in Table 2. CNS relapses typically occur late and are not associated with intestinal symptoms. It is not yet clear that CSF PCR is an accepted criterion, but recent experience suggests a potential value of monitoring the CSF PCR as a

Table 1 Recommended Regimens of Antibiotic Therapy for Whipple's Disease: Initial Presentation

A. Penicillin G plus	1.2 million U/day	IM	×14 days
Streptomycin (followed by)	1 g daily	IM	×14 days
TMP-SMX or	1 DS tab bid	PO	×1 yr
B. Ampicillin plus	2 g tid	PO	×14 days
Ceftriaxone (followed by)	2 g daily	IV	×14 days
TMP-SMX or	1 DS tab bid	PO	×1 yr
C. Ceftriaxone plus	2 g bid	IV	×14 days
Streptomycin (followed by)	1 g daily	IM	×14 days
TMP-SMX	1 DS tab bid	PO	×1 yr

Table 2 Recommended Regimens of Antibiotic Therapy for Whipple's Disease: Relapse

A. Chloramphenicol	1 g qid	IV	×2-4 wk
B. Penicillin G	1.2 million U/day	IM	×14 days
C. Streptomycin	1 g qid	IM	×2-4 wk
D. Ceftriaxone (followed by)	2 g qid	IV	×2-4 wk
TMP-SMX or	1 DS tab bid	PO	×1-2 yr
Cefixime	400 mg bid	PO	×1-2 yr

Table 3 Recommended Therapy for Tropical Sprue

Tetracycline	250 mg qid	PO	×3-6 mo
Folic acid	5 mg	PO	×3-6 mo
Vitamin B$_{12}$	1000 µg weekly	IM	×2 mo

parameter of the therapeutic response; a positive result often turns negative with successful therapy.

■ SPRUE

Sprue is a general term applied to disorders of intestinal malabsorption. Only two of these disorders, tropical sprue and small intestinal bacterial overgrowth syndrome, have infectious causes.

Tropical Sprue

Tropical sprue affects the entire length of the small intestine and causes diarrhea and malabsorption with multiple and severe nutritional deficiencies. The diagnosis requires demonstration of intestinal malabsorption of at least two nutrients, exclusion of other diseases that cause malabsorption, a compatible jejunal biopsy, and response to therapy. Tropical sprue occurs between the tropics of Capricorn and Cancer. Visitors to these areas can develop disease within weeks, but it is more likely to occur in those who have lived there for more than a year. An illness resembling tropical sprue appears in the Indian medical literature between 1600 and 1300 BC. Tropical sprue occurred in British troops in Singapore during the 1700s and in American soldiers and service personnel in the Philippines, Puerto Rico, and Viet-

nam. Patients have malabsorption of fat with steatorrhea and abnormal D-xylose absorption, with deficiencies of folate, B$_{12}$, vitamins A and D, protein, magnesium, and calcium. Jejunal biopsies normally demonstrate finger-shaped villi with a paucity of intraepithelial lymphocytes, delicate subendothelial basement membrane, and sparse mononuclear cell population of the villous core. In tropical sprue the jejunal biopsy reveals thick, leaf-shaped villi, infiltration of the epithelium with lymphocytes, thickened and collagenous basement membrane, and infiltration of the villous core by chronic inflammatory cells. The mucosal lesion coincides with the onset of tissue folate deficiency. Persistent contamination of the small bowel by enterotoxigenic *Escherichia coli*, which are unusually adherent to the mucosa, may be the precipitating cause. Tropical sprue should be considered in anyone returning from the tropics with persistent diarrhea. Demonstrating malabsorption of fat, B$_{12}$, and D-xylose, along with a compatible jejunal biopsy, should result in a response to therapy. Treatment with tetracycline, 250 mg orally four times daily, and folic acid, 5 mg daily for 3 to 6 months, is usually effective (Table 3). Vitamin B$_{12}$, 1000 µg, is recommended weekly for several weeks to replenish tissue stores. Treatment typically results in subjective and objective improvement within weeks, although up to 2 years of therapy may be required for complete resolution of tropical sprue.

■ SMALL BOWEL BACTERIAL OVERGROWTH SYNDROME

Small bowel bacterial overgrowth syndrome condition occurs when the normal flora of the small intestine is repopulated in numbers and species by the flora of the colon. The colonic flora compete with the human host for ingested nutrients, and the toxic byproducts of colonic fermentation in the small bowel cause a wide spectrum of symptoms. These symptoms include diarrhea, malabsorption, and malnutrition. Conditions associated with small bowel bacterial overgrowth syndrome are as follows:

1. Profound gastric hypocholorhydria
2. Structural changes in the small bowel such as jejunal diverticulae, afferent loop, blind loop, and gastrocolic and jejunocolic fistula
3. Disordered intestinal motility from idiopathic intestinal pseudoobstruction and scleroderma
4. Immunodeficiency syndromes and occasionally in cirrhosis and chronic pancreatitis with narcotic overuse

Therapy of symptomatic disease requires reduction the bacterial overgrowth in the small bowel. Surgical correction of an underlying structural abnormality responsible for the intestinal stasis is seldom possible. Patient management is

Table 4 Recommended Therapy for Small Bowel Overgrowth Syndrome

Amoxicillin-clavulanate or	875 mg bid	PO	×7-10 days
Cephalexin or	250 mg qid	PO	×7-10 days
Metronidazole	250 mg tid	PO	×7-10 days

For recurrent disease, cycle antibiotics, 1 week out of every 4 weeks.

therefore medical, with broad-spectrum antibiotic therapy, often for the patient's lifetime. Traditional therapy has been tetracycline, but the high incidence of bacterial resistance limits its effectiveness. Aerobic and anaerobic flora can be suppressed with amoxicillin-clavulanate, 875 mg twice daily; cephalexin, 250 mg four times daily; or metronidazole, 250 mg three times daily (Table 4). Antibiotics are given for 7 to 10 days. If symptoms are recurrent, cyclic therapy of 1 week out of every 4 with rotating coverage to avoid bacterial resistance is often necessary. Currently available prokinetics have not been found useful. Attention to the nutritional status is important. Vitamin B_{12}, 1000 μg intravenously (IM), calcium, and vitamin K are very often necessary to correct secondary deficiency states.

Suggested Reading

Haghighi P, Wolf PL: Tropical sprue and subclinical enteropathy: a vision for the nineties, *Crit Rev Clin Lab Sci* 34:313, 1997.

Herbay AV, et al: Whipple's disease: staging and monitoring by cytology and polymerase chain reaction analysis of cerebrospinal fluid, *Gastroenterology* 113:434, 1997.

Lange U, et al: Whipple's disease—current status of diagnostics and therapy, *Euro J Med Res* 20:331, 1998.

Pereira SP, Gainsborough H, Dowling RH: Drug induced hypochlorhydria causes high duodenal bacterial counts in the elderly, *Ailment Pharmacol Ther* 12:99, 1998.

URETHRITIS AND DYSURIA

William R. Bowie

Dysuria, or burning on urination, strongly suggests the presence of urethritis or cystitis, but can also be associated with other infectious and noninfectious diseases. Management differs between genders, but most individuals with acute or recent onset of dysuria can be managed appropriately at the time they are first seen.

■ DYSURIA IN FEMALES

Management of dysuria in women is complicated because of the overlap in symptoms of urinary tract infection (UTI) and sexually transmitted diseases (STDs). Acute dysuria may indicate cystitis, urethritis, or vulvitis (Table 1). Furthermore, sexual activity, use of diaphragms, and use of spermicides all contribute to increased risk of UTIs and the possibility of concurrent infections. Management of a woman with acute onset of dysuria requires consideration of the overlap, and investigations performed will vary depending on clinical features suggesting UTI, such as the previous occurrence of similar symptoms in conjunction with a proven UTI, and the woman's risk of having an STD, which will primarily be estimated by the age, sexual history obtained (e.g., new sexual partner, or STD in a partner) and where care is being provided (e.g., an adolescent clinic versus a family practice clinic).

Internal Dysuria

The clinical distinction between presentations is helped by differentiating internal dysuria, where discomfort is perceived as urine passes through the urethra, from external dysuria where the discomfort is felt as urine passes over the meatal or introital region. Internal dysuria strongly suggests urethritis or cystitis caused by classical urinary tract pathogens or, less commonly, STDs such as *Chlamydia trachomatis*, *Neisseria gonorrhoeae*, or herpes simplex virus. UTI is further suggested by acute onset of frequency, hematuria, nocturia, urgency, incontinence, suprapubic or pelvic discomfort, and possibly fever and flank pain. Nevertheless, in one third of these, a UTI is not present, with about one half of this subset having an STD, especially if pyuria is detected by microscopy or a leukocyte esterase test (LET).

For women with internal dysuria, a test to detect pyuria should be performed. Routine urine cultures for an acute previously untreated episode of typical cystitis are not required. Availability of highly sensitive urine-based testing for *C. trachomatis* and *N. gonorrhoeae* may aid in the investigation of some women where the diagnosis seems less clear.

Urinary Tract Infection

When a UTI is considered, initial treatment decisions depend on making the distinction between uncomplicated and complicated UTI. Management of UTIs in women is discussed in more detail in the chapter *Urinary Tract Infection*. Uncomplicated UTI mainly occurs in otherwise healthy women with structurally normal urinary tracts and normal voiding mechanisms. There is usually only a single organism isolated, and infection responds readily to short courses of antimicrobials to which the pathogen is susceptible. Three-day fluoroquinolone regimens, but not trimethoprim-sulfamethoxazole (TMP-SMX) or trimethoprim alone, would typically also cure *N. gonorrhoeae*, but none would predictably cure *C. trachomatis*. Although not usually recommended as a first-line treatment for acute cystitis, doxycycline, 100 mg orally twice daily for 7 days, directed against *C. trachomatis* would cure many UTIs caused by *Escherichia coli* and *Staphylococcus saprophyticus*.

With complicated UTI, there is usually a structural or functional abnormality or underlying disease. It is typically associated with more resistant organisms and several pathogens and responds less well to treatment.

The most useful guide to the presence of upper tract infection is clinical: fever, flank and/or low back pain, systemic symptoms, pyuria and bacteriuria, in conjunction with dysuria and related symptoms.

Table 1	Acute Dysuria in Women	
SITE OF INFECTION	**TYPE OF DYSURIA**	**MAIN INFECTIOUS CAUSES**
Cystitis	Internal	Usually coliforms or *Staphylococcus saprophyticus*
Urethritis	Internal	Often coliforms or *Staphylococcus saprophyticus*
		Often *Chlamydia trachomatis*
		Occasionally *Neisseria gonorrhoeae* or herpes simplex virus
Vulvitis	External	Usually herpes simplex virus or yeasts
		Occasionally *Trichomonas vaginalis*

External Dysuria and Evaluation for Sexually Transmitted Disease

External dysuria is strongly suggestive of vulvitis or vulvovaginitis most often caused by infection with herpes simplex virus, yeasts or *Trichomonas vaginalis*. Vaginitis or vulvovaginitis is further suggested by a new or changed vaginal discharge, vaginal odor, itch, and genital edema, erythema or lesions, particularly when these symptoms arise after unprotected intercourse with a new sexual partner.

If the possibility of an STD is considered, genital examination and laboratory testing are indicated. Management of STD in women is discussed in the chapters *Vaginitis and Cervicitis, Genital Ulcer Adenopathy Syndrome,* and *Pelvic Inflammatory Disease.*

◼ DYSURIA IN MALES

Acute onset of dysuria in males strongly suggests urethritis and is usually associated with urethral discharge, which is the classic symptom and sign of urethritis in men. An itch in the meatus or distal urethra is also commonly present. Urethral discharge may be present spontaneously or may be hard to detect. Urethral secretions show increased numbers of polymorphonuclear leukocytes (PMNs). The most important causes of urethritis in males are *C. trachomatis* and *N. gonorrhoeae*. Diagnosis of urethritis and microbiologic detection of *C. trachomatis* and *N. gonorrhoeae* are not synonymous. Infection can often be present without evident urethral inflammation or symptoms. There are also other additional causes of urethritis.

Etiology and Changing Epidemiology

Gonorrhea or gonococcal urethritis is diagnosed when *N. gonorrhoeae* is detected (usually by Gram stain or culture). Approximately 20% to 30% of those with gonococcal urethritis have concurrent infection with *C. trachomatis*. Nongonococcal urethritis (NGU) is diagnosed in men with increased numbers of PMNs in urethral secretions, but where *N. gonorrhoeae* is not detected. In developed countries, NGU is many times more common than gonococcal urethritis. *C. trachomatis* is the most important cause of NGU, but whereas in the 1970s it was recovered from 30% to 50% of cases, it is now identified in 15% to 30% of cases, with the lower rates most likely in areas with well-established *C. trachomatis* control programs. Less important but common causes of NGU are *Ureaplasma urealyticum* and probably *Mycoplasma genitalium*. However, many men have none of these detected. In most of these cases, the cause is not apparent, but occasionally *T. vaginalis* and herpes simplex virus are detected.

◼ CLINICAL AND LABORATORY DIAGNOSIS

Figure 1 shows an algorithm outlining an approach to the initial diagnosis and management of urethritis.

Detection of urethritis is usually straightforward. When examined under optimal conditions, most men with the onset of new symptoms of dysuria or urethral discharge will have objective evidence of urethritis (increased numbers of PMNs in urethral secretions detected by a Gram stain or in first voided urine, or alternatively by a positive LET). Of those with symptoms, most but not all will also have a detectable urethral discharge. The more pronounced the discharge and the more acute the symptoms, the greater the likelihood of gonorrhea. Nevertheless, for a specific patient, distinguishing between gonorrhea and NGU requires laboratory evaluation.

Strictly speaking, to detect urethritis, all that is required is documentation of increased numbers of PMNs. How-

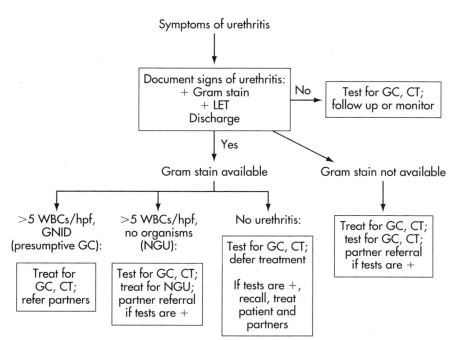

Figure 1

Algorithm for initial diagnosis and management of urethritis in males. CT, *Chlamydia trachomatis* infection; *GC,* gonococcal infection; *GNID,* gram-negative intracellular diplococci; *hpf,* high-powered field; *LET,* leukocyte esterase test; *NGU,* nongonococcal urethritis; +, positive. *(Used with permission from Burstein GR, Zenilman JM: Nongonococcal urethritis—a new paradigm, Clin Infect Dis 28[suppl 1]:S66, 1999.)*

ever, specimens should usually be taken for detection of *N. gonorrhoeae*, preferably by culture, and for detection of *C. trachomatis*. The results of these tests are particularly important for contact tracing efforts. Routine initial evaluation for *U. urealyticum* and other less usual causes is not indicated. Symptomatic men who do not have urethritis documented at an initial visit should be reevaluated. However, if urethritis is strongly suspected and reevaluation is not possible, treatment should usually be offered.

This discussion focuses on men with dysuria, but it is important to again stress that absence of symptoms does not exclude the presence of urethral infection, so detection of infection in such men requires similar testing.

■ TREATMENT

Treatment of the Initial Presentation

Urethritis is readily managed on a syndromic basis. This allows a rational choice of therapy, treatment at the time the man is seen, and initiation of efforts to ensure diagnosis and treatment of sexual partners. The key determinants for choice of the specific therapy are whether urethritis is documented and whether infection with *N. gonorrhoeae* has been excluded.

Regimens for *Neisseria gonorrhoeae*

Treatment for presumptive (smear showing gram-negative intracellular diplococci), proven (by culture or other diagnostic method), or suspected (test results not available) gonorrhea requires a regimen active against both *N. gonorrhoeae* and *C. trachomatis*, currently necessitating use of two drugs. Recommended for *N. gonorrhoeae* are a single oral dose of cefixime, 400 mg; ciprofloxacin, 500 mg; or ofloxacin, 400 mg; or a single injection of ceftriaxone 125 mg intramuscularly (IM). All are followed by a regimen active against *C. trachomatis*, using azithromycin, 1 g orally as a single dose, or doxycycline, 100 mg orally twice daily for 7 days. Quinolones are not recommended for patients younger than 17 years of age and are not recommended when gonorrhea may have been acquired directly or indirectly from Southeast Asia.

Regimens for Chlamydia trachomatis and Nonchlamydial Nongonococcal Urethritis

Either a single oral dose of azithromycin, 1 g, or 7 days of doxycycline, 100 mg orally twice daily, is recommended. When treatment is taken as recommended, outcomes are similar with either. Azithromycin has the benefit of single-dose therapy, but it has the disadvantage of added cost.

Alternative recommended regimens are erythromycin in doses comparable to 500 mg of base orally four times daily for 7 days, or ofloxacin, 300 mg orally twice daily for 7 days. The latter is no more effective than doxycycline or azithromycin and is much more expensive. For children younger than 8 years, erythromycins in appropriate doses are recommended for those under 45 kg, and azithromycin, 1 g, if the child weighs 45 kg or above.

Expected Microbiologic Outcomes

When recommended regimens are used as prescribed and men are not reexposed to new or untreated partners, persis-

tence of *N. gonorrhoeae* and *C. trachomatis* is so unusual that routine diagnostic test of cure evaluations are not recommended. Positive tests after treatment usually indicate reinfection from an inadequately treated or new sexual partner, poor compliance, or false-positive results. This situation may change with the increasing detection of isolates of *N. gonorrhoeae* demonstrating in vitro resistance to fluoroquinolones.

Treatment When Symptoms Continue

Almost all men with gonorrhea will improve and remain clinically cured. In contrast, although more than 95% of men with NGU will initially improve, up to one-third will have symptoms recur or fail to entirely resolve. In the small group who show no initial improvement, infection with *T. vaginalis,* herpes simplex virus, or tetracycline-resistant isolates of *U. urealyticum* account for approximately half of infections. In the larger group who show initial improvement, a cause is usually not apparent. Use of newer detection methods for *T. vaginalis* may increase its rate of detection in this setting.

Management is complicated by the persistence of symptoms in some men without objective evidence of urethritis, and increased numbers of PMNs in others without symptoms. Clear or mucoid urethral discharge at follow-up is not necessarily abnormal. This type of discharge, or symptoms of dysuria or an itch, in the absence of a PMN response does not constitute failure. For men who have documented persistent or recurrent urethritis, no history of reexposure or failure to take the initial course of treatment, and in whom no apparent cause is detected, my recommended treatment is 2 weeks of erythromycin, 500 mg orally four times daily, if a tetracycline was used initially. Alternatively, doxycycline, 100 mg orally twice daily for 2 weeks, would seem reasonable, particularly if azithromycin or erythromycin had been used initially. However, no studies have conclusively shown that such an approach expedites recovery. The Centers for Disease Control and Prevention (CDC) has proposed a regimen of metronidazole, 2 g orally in a single dose, plus 1 week of an erythromycin regimen equivalent to erythromycin base 500 mg four times daily.

With use of a second course of treatment, most men will again improve, but approximately one-third will have symptoms recur or incompletely resolve. Thus approximately 10% of men treated twice will be in this state. Most of these men will ultimately improve spontaneously, and further antimicrobial therapy does not appear warranted. There is also little benefit from conducting urologic investigations unless there are other indications to do so. Because many of these men have additional concerns, a careful explanation of the frequency of residual minimal urethritis, and the apparent absence of long-term physical consequences to the patient and partner(s) is often beneficial in allaying concerns.

Treatment of Partners

Recommendations for detection and initial treatment of urethritis are aggressive, mainly to decrease consequences for women. Men can have infection with *N. gonorrhoeae* or *C. trachomatis* for long periods with little risk of significant sequelae. Fewer than 1% will develop epididymitis, and even this is unlikely to result in sterility. In contrast, a high proportion of women who are infected with *C. trachomatis* or *N. gonorrhoeae* are at significant risk of spread of infection to the endometrium or above, with the associated risk of sterility, ectopic pregnancy, or chronic pelvic pain. These sequelae can arise without any evident symptoms or signs in the woman.

Thus detection of urethritis in men, and especially if testing in the male shows one or both of *N. gonorrhoeae* or *C. trachomatis,* should result in urgent evaluation and treatment of the sexual partner(s) with a regimen similar to that used for the male. Although evaluation is strongly recommended, if this will impede treatment or cannot be arranged in a timely manner, medication is sometimes prescribed to contacts even without evaluation. Unprotected intercourse should be avoided until the index case and the partner(s) have been treated.

■ OTHER PRESENTATIONS WITH DYSURIA

In men with urethritis, symptoms other than dysuria, urethral discharge, and itch in the urethra are unusual. When associated with symptoms of fever, abdominal or flank pain, hematuria, irritative symptoms such as frequency or nocturia, or problems with the flow of urine, including difficulty initiating the urinary stream or with postvoid dribbling, diseases such as prostatitis or pyelonephritis are much more likely and are discussed in the chapter *Prostatitis and Urinary Tract Infection.* The small proportion of patients who develop epididymitis are more likely to present with findings of epididymitis (see the chapter *Epididymoorchitis*), and the urethritis is recognized subsequently.

Suggested Reading

Burstein GR, Zenilman JM: Nongonococcal urethritis—a new paradigm, *Clin Infect Dis* 28(suppl 1):S66, 1999.

Centers for Disease Control and Prevention: 1998 Sexually transmitted diseases treatment guidelines, *MMWR* 47(RR-1):1, 1998.

Holmes KK, Stamm WE: Lower genital tract infection syndromes in women. In Holmes KK, et al, eds: *Sexually transmitted diseases,* ed 3, New York, 1999, McGraw-Hill, p. 761.

Martin DH, Bowie WR: Urethritis in males. In Holmes KK, et al, eds: *Sexually transmitted diseases,* ed 3, New York, 1999, McGraw-Hill, p. 833.

VAGINITIS AND CERVICITIS

Sebastian Faro

■ VAGINAL ECOSYSTEM

The vaginal ecosystem is complex, made up of several interacting components, such as host metabolites, immunoglobulins, cytokines, microorganisms, hormones, and so on. A healthy vaginal ecosystem is characterized by several factors (Table 1).

Lactobacillus acidophilus, as well as other species that produce lactic acid, hydrogen peroxide, and bacterocin, is able to suppress the growth of other bacteria. The bacteriology of the vaginal ecosystem is made-up of a variety of gram-positive and gram-negative bacteria (Table 2).

In a healthy vaginal ecosystem, the difference in concentration of lactobacilli and other bacteria is, in large part, controlled by the pH or acidity of the environment. At a pH of 4.5 or less, nonlactobacilli grow either not at all or very poorly. Although the lactobacilli grow best at a pH of 5 or more, in vitro, they are able to grow at a pH of 5 or less. Suppression of bacterial growth is further enhanced by the production of bacterocin, a protein that inhibits growth of gram-positive and gram-negative facultative as well as obligate anaerobic bacteria. In addition, some strains of lactobacilli produce hydrogen peroxide, which is toxic to obligate anaerobic bacteria.

Table 1	Vaginal Exudate Characteristics				
	HEALTHY	**BACTERIAL VAGINOSIS**	**TRICHOMONIASIS**	**CANDIDIASIS**	**OTHER**
Discharge	White to slate-gray	Dirty-gray	Dirty-gray	White	White to purulent
pH	3.8-4.2	>5	>5	<4.5	>5
Whiff test	(−)	(+)	(±)*	(−)	(−)
Clue cells	(−)	(+)	(±)*	(−)	(−)
White blood cells	<5/hpf	<5/hpf	>5/hpf	>5/hpf	>5/hpf
Lactobacillus	Dominant	No	No	Present	No

*If bacterial vaginosis also present, whiff test will be positive and clue cells will be present.

Table 2 Bacteria Endogenous to the Lower Genital Tract	
GRAM POSITIVE	**GRAM NEGATIVE**
FACULTATIVE ANAEROBES	**FACULTATIVE ANAEROBES**
Lactobacillus acidophilus	*Escherichia coli*
Corynebacterium	*Enterobacter cloacae*
Diphtheroids	*Gardnerella vaginalis*
Staphylococcus epidermidis	*Klebsiella*
Streptococcus*	*Morganella*
Enterococcus faecalis	*Proteus*
OBLIGATE ANAEROBES	**OBLIGATE ANAEROBES**
Peptococcus	*Bacteroides*
Peptostreptococcus	*Fusobacterium*
	Prevotella

*There are a variety of species (e.g., agalactine, viridous).

■ BACTERIAL VAGINOSIS

Bacterial vaginosis (BV) is not an infection but an alteration or disruption in the vaginal ecosystem. BV is characterized by a pH of 5 or more, the presence of an odor described as "fishlike" or "foul," the absence of white blood cells (WBCs), and the presence of clue cells, squamous epithelial cells that are densely covered with adherent bacteria. In addition, there is a noticeable absence of lactobacilli and the presence of a variety of morphotypes of bacteria. These clinical criteria can easily be recognized by determining the pH, performing a whiff test (mix a drop of KOH with a drop of vaginal discharge to detect a fishlike odor), and examining the discharge microscopically for presence of clue cells and various bacteria and absence of lactobacilli and WBCs.

This examination should be performed on every woman who complains of vaginal discharge, odor, discomfort, itching, or soreness, and asymptomatic women whose discharge is a color other than white or slate-gray or who has a vaginal odor.

The patient with BV and WBCs should be evaluated for additional vaginal and cervical infections (see the following). Treatment of BV is directed at reducing the numbers of obligate anaerobic bacteria below a critical number ($\leq 10^3$ bacteria/ml of vaginal fluid). This, in turn, will eliminate the competition between bacteria, thus allowing lactobacilli to grow. Active growth of lactobacillus is accompanied by the secretion of lactic acid, which will reduce the pH to less than 4.5, suppressing the growth of BV bacteria (e.g., *Gardnerella vaginalis, Prevotella, Mobiluncus*). Treatment regimens are listed in Table 3.

Although BV is not considered sexually transmitted, there does appear to be a correlation between the number of sexual partners and recurrences. Condoms should be worn with each episode of intercourse until the patient can be reevaluated. There are three outcomes that can be expected:

1. Resolution of BV and restoration of a healthy vaginal ecosystem
2. Resolution of BV but failure to restore the vaginal ecosystem to a healthy state
3. Failure to resolve BV

Patients who have resolution of BV but fail to achieve restoration of a healthy vaginal ecosystem can be identified

Table 3 Treatment Regimens for Bacterial Vaginosis
Metronidazole, 500 mg orally twice a day for 7 days
Metronidazole, 2 g orally in a single dose
Clindamycin, 300 mg twice a day for 7 days
Clindamycin cream 2%, one full applicator intravaginally at bedtime for 7 days
Metronidazole gel 0.75%, one full applicator intravaginally twice a day for 5 days

by a pH of 5 or more and microscopic analysis of the vaginal fluid demonstrating an absence of lactobacilli. There may be a dominant bacterium, but usually there is a scant number of bacteria, giving the discharge a sterile appearance. The patient should insert one applicator full of Aci-Jel gel nightly for 4 weeks. The vaginal ecosystem should be reevaluated 1 week after completion of therapy. Failure to restore the pH to 4.5 or less will likely result in recurrent BV or replacement of BV with another bacterium (e.g., *Escherichia coli* or *Streptococcus agalactiae*), which should then be treated with appropriate systemic antimicrobials.

■ CANDIDIASIS

Vulvovaginal candidiasis (VVC) is a common infection that is experienced by 75% of women at least once in a lifetime. Approximately 5% of these women will experience a recurrent episode, with a smaller percentage going on to develop chronic or persistent disease. Because *Candida* can be found as a member of the endogenous vaginal microflora in 30% to 40% of women, a cure should be confined to the elimination of signs and symptoms.

The most common cause of VVC is *Candida albicans*, which is responsible for 75% of the cases, followed by *C. glabrata (Torulopsis glabrata)*, which causes 15% to 20%. The remainder are caused by less common species. Differentiating *C. albicans* from *C. glabrata* can be easily accomplished with microscopic examination of vaginal fluid. *C. albicans* will form hyphae, whereas *C. glabrata* develops only budding yeast cells. *C. albicans* cannot be differentiated from other species that produce hyphae on microscopic evaluation because the hyphal forms appear similar.

The distinction between *C. glabrata* and other species is important because it tends to be resistant to the antifungal agents that are commonly used. The other non-*albicans* species also tend to be resistant to the commonly used antifungal agents, but less so than *C. glabrata*.

The clinical presentation of VVC is highlighted by erythema, itching, and burning. Typically, especially in severe cases, the erythema involves the external genitalia as well as the vagina and cervix. There may be excoriations that resemble fissures, and the patient may report bleeding. The vaginal discharge is typically white, and the consistency may vary from a paste (cottage cheese) to a liquid. The external genitalia are often covered by thin white exudates.

The diagnosis can easily be established by examining discharge microscopically for the presence of yeast cells, either hyphal forms or budding. Culturing specimens from the external genitalia and vagina should be performed when

Table 4 Antifungal Agents Commonly Used in the Treatment of Vulvovaginal Candidiasis

GENERIC NAME	BRAND NAME
Miconazole	Monistat
Butoconazole	Femstat
Clotrimazole	Lotrimin
Tioconazole	Monistat-1, Vagistat-1
Terconazole	Terazol
Ketoconazole	Nizoral
Fluconazole	Diflucan

Table 5 Metronidazole Treatment Regimens for Vulvovaginal Trichomoniasis

The following are all administered orally.
1. 2 g as a single dose
2. 250 mg three times a day for 7 days
3. 500 mg twice a day for 7 days
4. Flagyl ER, 750 mg tablet once a day for 7 days

the clinical signs and symptoms suggest yeast but no fungal elements can be identified microscopically and when a correct diagnosis has been established but there has been an unsatisfactory response to therapy. Therapeutic choices are listed in Table 4.

Patients with acute VVC who have tried all the over-the-counter antifungals can be treated with fluconazole, 100 mg orally twice a day on the first day followed by 100 mg a day on days 2, 3, 4, 5, and 6. In my experience, fluconazole, 150 mg given as a single oral treatment, has not been satisfactory.

Patients who fail to respond to therapy listed in Table 4 should be treated with boric acid (600 mg) suppositories twice daily for 10 days or topical application of gentian violet.

Once the patient's acute episode has been resolved, she should be monitored for recurrent episodes. Individuals who experience four or more episodes within a year should be classified as having recurrent VVC and should be started on suppressive therapy. One effective regimen is fluconazole, 150 mg orally once a month for 6 months. The medication should be administered with the onset, or shortly before the start, of the menses. An alternative regimen is fluconazole, 150 mg orally once a week for 6 to 8 weeks. Patients who do not want to take the oral medication or who are allergic to fluconazole can be treated with weekly applications of clotrimazole, 500 mg vaginal suppository.

The presence of recurrent or persistent VVC may be an indicator of diabetes or of an immunosuppressive disorder. All medications should be reviewed to determine whether the patient is taking antibiotics or receiving immunosuppressive therapy. The patient's sexual partner may also be infected or serving as a carrier. A common complaint of the male sexual partner is penile burning shortly after sexual intercourse. The male may also report penile itching and areas of erythema.

For patients with persistent VVC who do not respond to one of the treatment regimens outlined here, I use a regimen as follows:

1. Perform antifungal sensitivities in vitro and administer an antifungal agent that the organism is sensitive to.
2. Administer oral nystatin, 200,000 to 400,000 units/ml three times a day for 10 days, to reduce the fecal carriage of yeast.
3. Treat the sexual partner with nystatin plus triamcilocone cream applied to the penis two to three times a day for 10 days.

■ TRICHOMONIASIS

Trichomoniasis is caused by the protozoan *Trichomonas vaginalis,* a sexually transmitted organism. Nonsexual transmission (e.g., from fomites) is rare, and physicians should always consider that the infection was acquired through sexual intercourse. Therefore the patient with trichomoniasis should be evaluated for the presence of other STDs (e.g., *Neisseria gonorrhoeae, Chlamydia trachomatis, Treponem pallidum,* herpes simplex, human papillomavirus, hepatitis B, and human immunodeficiency virus (HIV).

Trichomoniasis is not restricted to the vagina, and therefore does not cause solely vaginitis but may simultaneously infect Bartholin's and Skene's glands, the urethra, the bladder, and the upper genital tract. Thus, to treat this infection, medication that achieves systemic levels of the antiprotozoan drug must be administered.

The patient with vulvovaginal trichomoniasis (VVT) usually presents with a copious discharge, edema of the labia, petechial hemorrhages on the surface of the vaginal epithelium, vaginal soreness, and a foul odor.

The vaginal discharge ranges in color from dirty gray to green and is noted spilling from the vagina and covering the labia minora, the posterior fourchette, and perineum; it often appears frothy. WBCs and elliptical motile cells that represent *Trichomonas vaginalis* are seen microscopically. Adjusting the fine focus will allow the examiner to see the characteristic flagella of *T. vaginalis.*

In those cases in which the patient has clinical signs and symptoms of vaginitis (i.e., numerous WBCs, erythema of the vaginal epithelium, and green or dirty gray and frothy discharge) but no specific pathogen can be identified, a culture for the isolation of *T. vaginalis* may be performed by inoculating Diamond's medium.

Currently, there is only one antiprotozoan agent available in the United States for the treatment of trichomoniasis—metronidazole (Table 5). During treatment and until a follow-up evaluation can be completed the patient should refrain from sexual intercourse or use condoms.

Treatment should be administered to both the patient and her partner within the same time period. In addition, they should both refrain from consuming any alcoholic beverages while taking metronidazole because of the disulfiram-type reaction that can occur.

Treatment of patients with persistent trichomoniasis can require higher dosages of metronidazole. The organism can also be isolated and tested for resistance to metronidazole. One approach is to combine delivery of metronidazole (e.g., oral and by vaginal or rectal suppository [Metro gel]). Metronidazole can be administered orally, 500 mg twice daily, and the suppositories once or twice daily for 7 days.

This should provide sustained blood and tissue levels with a high concentration in the vaginal environment. If the daily dose exceeds 2 g a day, the patient is at risk for suffering the usual side effects of metronidazole, as well as peripheral neuropathy and seizures.

Patients who are truly allergic to metronidazole should undergo desensitization. Before instituting desensitization, the patient's allergy should be documented. If the patient has developed a rash and experienced difficulty breathing and this has been documented and attributed to metronidazole exposure, no further investigation is necessary. If the allergy is questionable, a small amount of metronidazole gel can be placed on the lateral vaginal wall and within 30 minutes an area of erythema will appear. I have desensitized patients by modifying the Pearlman protocol (see Suggested Reading) and administering metronidazole intravenously until a total dose of 2 g has been administered. This is followed by treatment with oral metronidazole, 500 mg twice a day for 7 days.

If the patient has a strain of *T. vaginalis* that is resistant to metronidazole, treatment may require increased dosage of metronidazole or use of an agent (e.g., tinidazole, not approved for use in the United States).

■ CERVICITIS

Cervicitis is an inflammatory condition often caused by infection. It is unique because it is typically asymptomatic.

Any sexually transmitted disease can infect the cervix (Table 6). In fact, any microorganism that can either gain entrance to the columnar epithelium or invade the squamous epithelium can cause cervicitis. The most common presentation of cervicitis is a Pap smear that is reported as inflammatory.

The clinical clues that a patient may have cervicitis are often overlooked, but they can be distinctive and should encourage evaluation. For example, the patient may relate the sudden onset of postcoital bleeding or dyspareunia or when obtaining a Pap smear, there may be brisk cervical bleeding. Examination of the cervix may reveal hypertrophy of the endocervical columnar epithelium or the presence of petechial hemorrhages. Thus, if any of these clinical features are present or cervical cytologic examination reveals inflammation, the patient's history should be reviewed to determine whether she is at risk for STD. During the pelvic examination, the cervix can be evaluated by gently cleansing the surface to remove vaginal discharge and mucus. A

cotton- or dacron-tipped swab can be inserted into the endocervical canal and rotated 360 degrees several times and withdrawn. The top of the swab should be inspected for the presence of mucopus and inserted into 2 ml of saline. The swab should be agitated in the saline, and one to two drops of saline should be examined microscopically. The presence of WBCs suggests inflammation. Specimens should be sent for detection of *N. gonorrhoeae*, *C. trachomatis*, *H. simplex*, and human papillomavirus (Table 7).

Once a specific diagnosis has been established, treatment should be directed against the documented infection. If the patient is found to have gonorrhea and/or chlamydia, I prefer a 7-day regimen (Table 8) because upper genital tract infection may be present. Because of the high incidence of coinfection, identification of gonnococcal infection mandates empirical treatment for chlamydia also. In addition, therapy for chlamydia need not await laboratory confirmation, especially if no other pathogen is identified or suspected as the cause of cervicitis. All patients with STDs should have serologic testing for syphilis and HIV, and their partners treated and investigated similarly. Organism-specific regimens are provided in more detail in the chapters *Gonnococcus*, *Herpes Simplex*, *Papillomavirus*, and *Syphilis and Other Treponematoses*.

Table 7 Diagnostic Tests Used in Evaluating the Vaginal Microflora

VAGINA	CERVIX
Trichomoniasis—culture	*Neisseria gonorrhoeae*—culture, nucleic acid detection (PCR)
Candidiasis—culture	*Chlamydia trachomatis*—culture, nucleic acid detection
HPV—PCR	Trichomoniasis—culture
Herpes—culture	*Mycoplasma* and *ureaplasma*—culture

PCR, Polymerase chain reaction; *HPV*, human papillomavirus.

Table 8 CDC Recommendations for Treatment of STD

CHLAMYDIA CERVICITIS
Azithromycin, 1 g orally in a single dose
Doxycycline, 100 mg orally bid × 7 days*
Ofloxacin, 300 mg orally bid × 7 days
GONOCOCCAL CERVICITIS
Cefixime, 400 mg orally in a single dose
Ceftriaxone, 125 mg orally in a single dose
Ciprofloxacin, 500 mg orally in a single dose
Ofloxacin, 400 mg orally in a single dose
Azithromycin, 1 g orally in a single dose
Doxycycline, 100 mg orally bid × 7 days*
Spectinomycin, 2 g IM in a single dose

From Centers for Disease Control and Prevention: 1998 Guidelines for treatment of sexually transmitted diseases, *MMWR* 47:1-11, 1998.
*My preference.

Table 6 Microorganisms That Can Cause Cervicitis

Neisseria gonorrhoeae
Chlamydia trachomatis
Trichomonas vaginalis
Herpes simplex
Human papillomavirus
Treponema pallidum
Candida
Streptococcus agalactiae

Suggested Reading

Centers for Disease Control and Prevention: 1998 Guidelines for the treatment of sexually transmitted diseases, *MMWR* 47:70, 1998.

Faro S: Systemic vs topical therapy for the treatment of vulvovaginal candidiasis, *Infect Dis Obstet Gynecol* 1:202, 1994.

Lin L, et al: The role of bacterial vaginosis in infection after major gynecologic surgery, *Infect Dis Obstet Gynecol* 7:169, 1999.

Pearlman MD, et al: An incremental dosing protocol for women with severe vaginal trichomoniasis and adverse reactions to metronidazole, *Am J Obstet Gynecol* 174:934, 1996.

Reynolds M, Wilson J: Is *Trichomonas vaginalis* still a marker for other sexually transmitted infections in women? *Int J STD AIDS* 7:131, 1996.

Sobel JD: Candidal vulvovaginitis, *Clin Obstet Gynecol* 36:153, 1993.

Sobel JD: Treatment of recurrent vulvovaginal candidiasis with maintenance fluconazole, *Int J Obstet Gynecol* 37:17, 1992.

White DJ, Johnson EM, Warnock DW: Management of persistent vulvovaginal candidosis due to azole-resistant *Candida glabrata, Genitourinary Med* 69:112, 1993.

EPIDIDYMO-ORCHITIS

Andrew J. Deck
Robert H. Shapiro
Richard E. Berger

■ PRESENTATION AND EVALUATION

Acute epididymitis, or epididymo-orchitis, is a clinical entity involving inflammation with swelling and pain of the epididymis and testicle. Many patients give a history of symptoms of either urethritis (urethral discharge, dysuria, and penile pain or burning) or urinary tract infection (frequency, urgency, dysuria). However, many young men with epididymitis secondary to sexually transmitted urethritis will deny urethral symptoms or discharge and may not have had sexual exposure for months before presentation. Examination reveals an indurated, swollen epididymis that, often along with the testicle, is exquisitely tender. There can be diffuse scrotal swelling, erythema, and edema, and in the later stages of the infection, a reactive hydrocele may be present. The inflammation often involves tenderness and swelling in the ipsilateral spermatic cord with associated groin pain.

Appropriate laboratory evaluation of epididymitis is important to determine the organism responsible for the infection. In men for whom sexually transmitted urethritis is a risk, a swab of the urethra should be Gram-stained and cultured for *Chlamydia trachomatis* and *Neisseria gonorrhoeae.* This must be performed *before* having the patient void because urination may wash away urethral organisms or white blood cells, giving a false-negative result. Gram-negative intracellular diplococci on the Gram stain are diagnostic of *N. gonorrhoeae.* If no gram-negative diplococci are present but more than 5 white blood cells per high-powered field are seen, the diagnosis is nongonococcal

urethritis. Nucleic acid amplification tests (ligase chain reaction) for gonococcus and chlamydia that can be performed on voided urine, obviating the need for a urethral swab, are also becoming available. Midstream urine should be sent for Gram stain and culture to rule out bacterial cystitis. If the patient appears systemically ill or is febrile, serum white blood count with differential and blood cultures should also be sent.

■ DIFFERENTIAL DIAGNOSIS

Before diagnosing and treating epididymitis in a man who presents with an acute scrotum, it is imperative to rule out testicular torsion. Figure 1 presents an algorithm for managing a patient with acute scrotum. In men younger than age 35, both epididymitis (usually related to sexually transmitted organisms) and torsion are common. Physical examination can be quite equivocal. Of patients with early torsion, 15% will have swelling of the epididymis. Patients with advanced epididymo-orchitis may have diffuse scrotal swelling and tenderness, making adequate examination of the testis impossible. Children may have torsion of an appendix, testis, or epididymis, resulting in a reactive epididymitis.

Imaging studies are often helpful in confirming a diagnosis of epididymitis. This can be accomplished with either a radionuclide scan or a scrotal ultrasound with Doppler to evaluate venous and arterial testicular blood flow.

Torsion is a surgical emergency requiring prompt intervention; delay in its diagnosis can result in loss of a testicle. The presence of urethritis or bacteriuria, with *enhanced* arterial flow to the testis and epididymis on imaging, suggests that the patient has epididymitis. Any uncertainty or question of the diagnosis, however, should lead to consultation with a urologist. In these cases, scrotal exploration may be necessary to rule out torsion.

■ ETIOLOGY

Epididymitis is an ascending infection from the genitourinary tract. It results from spread of organisms from the bladder or urethra in a retrograde fashion into the vas

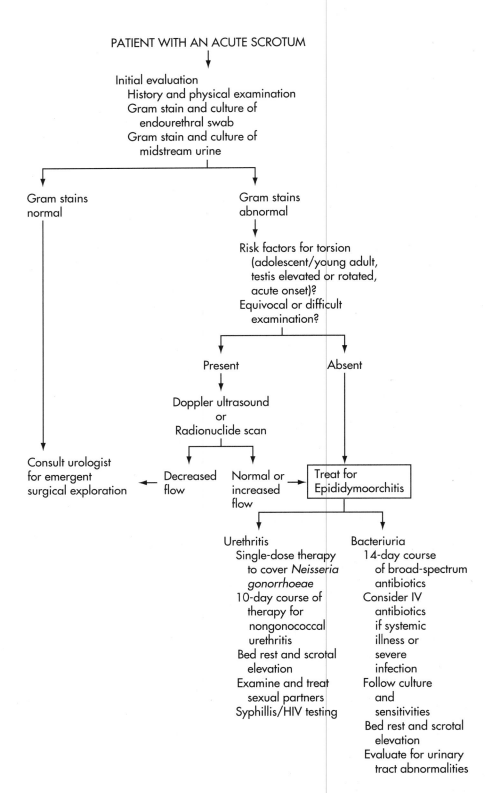

Figure 1
Algorithm for management of the acute scrotum.

deferens. The most likely causative organism corresponds to the most common cause of genitourinary infection in that age group.

In sexually active men who are younger than 35 years of age, sexually transmitted urethritis is common, whereas bacteriuria is uncommon. The most likely causative organisms of epididymitis in this group are *N. gonorrhoeae* and *C. trachomatis*. In men who practice anal intercourse, infection resulting from coliforms may be the most common cause of epididymitis. *Haemophilus influenzae* may also be found in these patients.

Most cases of epididymitis in children who are not yet sexually active and in older men result from bacteriuria from the common urinary pathogens. In men older than 35, sexually transmitted urethritis is uncommon, whereas acquired urinary tract obstruction or recent urologic instrumentation causing bacterial cystitis is more likely. The organism causing epididymitis in these populations is usually *Escherichia coli*.

In a small number of cases, epididymitis in any age group may be caused by a systemic infection such as tuberculosis, brucellosis, or other bloodborne organisms. In the immunocompromised man, *Cryptococcus* and *Candida albicans* have been documented as causative pathogens of epididymo-orchitis. Finally, the antiarrhythmic drug amiodarone has been shown to produce an inflammatory epididymitis. This swelling occurs in the head of the epididymis and results from a selective concentration of the drug in the epididymis. Symptoms respond to a decrease in dosage.

■ TREATMENT

The treatment for acute epididymo-orchitis involves two aspects: antibiotic therapy and scrotal rest. Antimicrobial therapy should be directed at the causative organism. For the severely ill, febrile, or noncompliant patient, consideration should be given to hospitalization and treatment with intravenous (IV) broad-spectrum antibiotics. Immunocompromised patients do not automatically require inpatient or longer outpatient therapy, but close follow-up and consideration of unusual organisms is important.

Deciding on the antibiotic depends on the suspected source of infection. For epididymo-orchitis secondary to bacteriuria, a combination of ampicillin and an aminoglycoside is appropriate for inpatient IV treatment and trimethoprim-sulfamethoxazole or a fluoroquinolone for oral outpatient therapy. Treatment should extend for 14 days of antibiotics. For epididymitis secondary to urethritis, the patient should be given single-dose therapy to cover *N. gonorrhoeae* (Table 1) and a 10-day course of treatment for nongonococcal urethritis, primarily to cover chlamydia, because two thirds of nongonococcal urethritis is caused by *C. trachomatis*. In addition, 30% to 50% of patients with gonococcal urethritis will have a concomitant *C. trachomatis* infection. Single-dose azithromycin commonly is used to treat nongonococcal urethritis instead of a 10-day course of doxycycline. However, the efficacy of this regimen for the treatment of epididymitis secondary to urethritis has not been studied. In addition, patients with sexually transmitted urethritis should be tested for syphilis and offered human immunodeficiency virus (HIV) counseling. Because *N. gonorrhea* and *C. trachomatis* are reportable infections, all sexual partners within 60 days should be notified and treated. Patients should not engage in sexual activity until treatment is complete.

The second but equally important, aspect of treatment of epididymitis is strict bedrest with elevation of the scrotum. Until the swelling and induration begins to resolve, the

Table 1   Antibiotic Choices for Epididymo-Orchitis Secondary to Urethritis
SINGLE-DOSE REGIMENS TO COVER *N. GONORRHOEAE*:
1. Ceftriaxone, 250 mg IM
2. Cefixime, 400 mg PO
3. Ciprofloxacin, 500 mg PO
4. Ofloxacin, 400 mg PO
10-DAY COURSE TO COVER *C. TRACHOMATIS*:
1. Doxycycline, 100 mg PO bid
2. Erythromycin base, 500 mg PO qid
3. Erythromycin ethylsuccinate, 800 mg PO qid
4. Ofloxacin, 400 mg PO bid
5. Ciprofloxacin, 500 mg PO bid

patient is unlikely to experience symptom relief. The patient should lie supine with the scrotum elevated as much as possible until the pain and swelling have subsided. Nonsteroidal antiinflammatory medications are also often helpful. Corticosteroid treatment has been found to be of no significant benefit in the treatment of epididymo-orchitis.

■ FOLLOW-UP

After initiating therapy, the patient should be seen in 3 to 5 days to be sure that he is responding to treatment. Culture results should be examined, and antibiotic regimens should be adjusted if necessary. Failure of antibiotic therapy may be the result of patient noncompliance with rest and scrotal elevation, contributing to persistent swelling and induration. In patients who fail to improve with treatment, consideration should also be given to other diagnoses, including abscess, tumor, infarction, fungal infection, or tuberculosis. An abscess can be diagnosed by scrotal ultrasound and requires urgent surgical exploration and drainage. Complications of inadequately treated epididymo-orchitis include sepsis, abscess formation, testicular infarction, chronic pain, and infertility.

Young men who are found to have uncomplicated urethritis as a cause for epididymitis and who respond well to therapy are unlikely to have a structural urinary tract abnormality. In contrast, young boys or older men with bacteriuria often will have anatomic pathology (usually obstructive) and should be referred to a urologist for complete evaluation.

Suggested Reading

Ball TP Jr: Epididymitis and orchitis. In Seidmon EJ, Hanno PM, eds: *Current urologic therapy*, Philadelphia, 1994, WB Saunders.

Berger RE: Sexually transmitted diseases: the classic diseases. In Walsh, et al, eds: *Campbell's urology*, Philadelphia, 1998, WB Saunders.

Centers for Disease Control and Prevention: 1998 Guidelines for treatment of sexually transmitted diseases, *MMWR* 47:1, Jan 23, 1998.

GENITAL ULCER ADENOPATHY SYNDROME

Allan Ronald
Shurjeel Choudhri

Control of genital ulcer disease (GUD) is an important public health priority because most sexually transmitted etiologic agents of GUD enhance the risk of human immunodeficiency virus (HIV) acquisition and transmission in both heterosexual and homosexual populations. Table 1 lists the infectious and noninfectious etiologies that may produce genital ulcerations with or without adenopathy. The most common sexually transmitted etiologies of GUD include syphilis, which is caused by *Treponema pallidum;* genital herpes caused by herpes simplex viruses 1 and 2 (HSV); chancroid, caused by *Hemophilus ducreyi;* lymphogranuloma venereum (LGV), caused by the L1, L2, and L3 serovars of *Chlamydia trachomatis;* and granuloma inguinale (donovanosis), caused by *Calymmatobacterium granulomatis.* Trauma, erosive balanitis, and fixed-drug eruptions are the most common noninfectious causes of GUD, and neoplasia and fungal and mycobacterial disease should be considered if a genital ulcer persists. Because of the limita-

tions of current diagnostic tests, a specific diagnosis is obtained in about 80% of patients.

Remarkable geographic variation exists in the etiology and prevalence of GUD (Table 2). In Europe and North America, fewer than 5% of patients present to sexually transmitted disease (STD) clinics with a genital ulcer compared with 20% to 70% of patients presenting to such clinics in Africa and Asia. HSV is the most common cause of genital ulcerations in Europe and North America, whereas chancroid has been the most common cause of genital ulcerations in Africa and Asia. However, genital herpes is becoming much more common in patients coinfected with HIV. LGV is endemic in some areas of the tropics. Donovanosis is endemic in Papua New Guinea, India, and Southern Africa. Syphilis continues to be a global pandemic, but transmission has been largely interrupted in regions of North America and Europe.

■ CLINICAL PRESENTATIONS

Clinical features of GUD are listed in Table 3. The incubation period is short for genital herpes and chancroid, intermediate for LGV, and intermediate to long for syphilis and donovanosis. Depending on the etiology, the initial lesion can be a papule, pustule, or vesicle, but this quickly erodes to form an ulcer. In men the ulcers are often located on the coronal sulcus but may also be found on the glans, prepuce, and shaft of the penis. Herpes and chancroid have a predilection for involving the frenulum. In women the ulcers may occur on the labia, in the vagina, on the cervix, or on the fourchette and perianal area. Perianal ulcers are also seen in homosexual men. Occasionally, ulcers may be seen on the scrotum and extragenitally on the lips or orpharynx. Unfortunately, a correct clinical etiologic diagnosis is possible in only 50% of patients with GUD.

Genital Herpes

Genital herpes are classically multiple, small vesicles that rapidly become superficial ulcers with erythematous margins. Dysuria, urethritis, and gynecologic symptoms may predominate. Systemic symptoms of fever, myalgias, and headache can occur with a primary infection. A prodome of paresthesias 12 to 48 hours before the appearance of vesicles is often reported with recurrences. Painful lymphadenopa-

Table 1   Etiologies of Genital Ulcer Disease
INFECTIOUS
Bacterial
Haemophilus ducreyi (chancroid)
Treponema pallidum (syphilis)
Chlamydia trachomatis (lymphogranuloma venereum)
Calymmatobacterium granulomatis (donovanosis)
Balanitis (often polymicrobial but *C. albicans* is often present)
Viral
Herpes simplex
Varicella zoster*
Epstein-Barr virus*
Cytomegalovirus*
Parasitic
*Sarcoptes scabiei**
*Phthirus pubis**
*Entamoeba histolytica**
*Trichomonas vaginalis**
NONINFECTIOUS
Trauma
Fixed drug eruptions
Pyoderma gangrenosum*
Behçet's disease*
Reiter's syndrome*
Wegener's granulomatosis*
Neoplasms*
Unknown

*Unusual.

Table 2 Geographic Variation in the Prevalence of Genital Ulcer Diseases	SOUTH EAST ASIA INDIA	AFRICA	NORTH AMERICA EUROPE
Chancroid	+++	++++	±
Syphilis	+++	+++	++
Genital herpes	++	+++	++++
Lymphogranuloma venereum	++	+	±
Donovanosis	++	+	±

±, Sporadic or imported cases only.

thy can be present with a primary infection. Systemic dissemination may occur in the presence of immunodeficiency.

Syphilis

The ulcer seen with syphilis is classically solitary, painless, and minimally tender and has elevated, well-demarcated margins with an indurated nonpurulent base. Multiple ulcers are present in about half of patients. Lymphadenopathy, if present, is usually bilateral with firm, nontender nodes.

Chancroid

Chancroid typically produces painful, excavated ulcers with irregular, undermined margins and a purulent base. The ulcers can be superficial and may resemble herpetic ulcers. Approximately 50% of the patients will develop painful inguinal lymphadenopathy, which is often unilateral. Lymph nodes may become fluctuant and rupture. Untreated ulcers may persist for up to 8 to 24 weeks and heal with scarring. Late complications include cicatrization with phimosis, which may require circumcision. Systemic dissemination has not been described.

Lymphogranuloma Venereum

The ulcer of LGV is a small, transient, usually superficial, painless lesion that precedes the development of inguinal lymphadenopathy by 7 to 30 days; fewer than a third of the patients remember having had an ulcer. The lymph nodes are tender and may become fluctuant with eventual rupture and formation of draining sinuses. A "groove" sign may be present if nodes above and below Poupart's ligament are involved. Women and homosexual men may have involvement of perianal and perirectal tissues. Complications of

untreated infection include genital elephantiasis, rectal strictures, and perianal fistulas. Other manifestations include meningoencephalitis, hepatitis, erythema nodosum, and erythema multiforme.

Donovanosis

The patient presents with slowly progressive disease of the genital area characterized by heaped up granulomatous tissue and painless genital ulceration. Local extension, healing, and fibrosis may occur simultaneously. Lymphadenopathy is unusual, but "pseudobuboes" caused by subcutaneous extension of the granulomatous process into the inguinal area are common. Systemic spread with involvement of liver, thorax, and bones has been reported but is rare.

Laboratory Diagnosis of GUD

Clinical diagnosis of GUD is imprecise because of overlap between the clinical syndromes, presence of mixed infections, and atypical presentations. Because of these limitations, the diagnosis must be confirmed using the relevant laboratory tests (Table 4). Specimens should be collected for *H. ducreyi, C. trachomatis,* and *H. simplex* cultures and DNA identification with polymerase chain reaction (PCR). If possible, a darkfield examination should be performed in all patients presenting with GUD. The lesion is washed with saline, dried with a cotton gauze, and squeezed between the thumb and forefinger until an exudate appears. This can be collected directly onto a coverslip for darkfield microscopy. Vesicles and pustules should be aspirated with a fine-gauge needle or deroofed and swabbed for viral culture. Fluctuant lymph nodes should be aspirated for *H. ducreyi* and *C. trachomatis* culture. Both treponemal (FTA-ABS, MHA-TP) and nontreponemal (RPR, VDRL) serologic tests

Table 3   Clinical Characteristics of Genital Ulcer Adenopathy Syndromes

	SYPHILIS	HERPES SIMPLEX VIRUS	CHANCROID	LYMPHO-GRANULOMA VENEREUM	DONOVANOSIS
Incubation period	9-90 days	2-7 days	1-14 days	7-21 days	8-80 days
Primary lesion	Papule	Vesicle	Papule or pustule	Papule, pustule, or vesicle	Papule
Number of lesions	Usually solitary	Multiple	Multiple	Usually solitary	Variable
CLASSICAL ULCER CHARACTERISTICS					
Size (mm)	5-15	1-10	2-20	2-10	Variable
Margins	Well demarcated Elevated Round or oval	Erythematous	Ragged, irregular Undermined	Elevated Round or oval	Variable Elevated, irregular
Depth	Superficial or deep	Superficial	Excavated	Superficial or deep	Elevated
Base	Red, smooth, nonpurulent	Red, smooth, serous discharge	Purulent exudate	Variable	"Beefy" red, rough
Induration	++	—	—	—	++
Pain	—	++	++	±	—
Lymphadenopathy	++[B]	++[B]	++[U]	++[U]	—[P]
CHARACTERISTICS OF LYMPHADENOPATHY					
Consistency	Firm	Firm	Fluctuant	Fluctuant	—
Tenderness	—	++	++	++	—

[B]Bilateral; [U]unilateral; [P]pseudolymphadenopathy.

Table 4   Recommended Tests for Diagnosing Genital Ulcer Diseases

	RECOMMENDED TESTS	OTHER TESTS
Chancroid	Culture	Gram stain/PCR
Syphilis	Darkfield examination	PCR
	Direct fluorescent antibody test	
	Serology (e.g., RPR/VDRL, FTA-ABS, MHA-TP)	
Genital herpes	Viral culture	Antigen detection (ELISA), PCR
		Serology
Lymphogranuloma venereum	Serology (complement fixation, microimmunofluorescence)	Chlamydia culture, PCR
Donovanosis	Giemsa or Wright stains of tissue smears	
	Histopathology	

PCR, Polymerase chain reaction.

should be obtained in all patients with GUD to exclude syphilis. The diagnosis of LGV is confirmed if antibody titers are 1:64 or greater by complement fixation or 1:512 or greater by microimmunofluorescence.

Approach to the Patient with GUD

An algorithm for approaching a patient with genital ulceration is given in Figure 1. The history is crucial. Information should be collected about the sexual risk factors, demographics, medication, and travel. Risk factors such as sex work or recent prostitute contact are associated with syphilis and chancroid. Travel may suggest the diagnosis of an otherwise uncommon cause such as donovanosis. Finally, the occurrence of a lesion at the same location as previous ulcers or a history of recent self-medication may be caused by a fixed drug eruption. Self-medication with topical or systemic antibiotics can limit the utility of diagnostic testing by producing a false-negative darkfield examination or *H. ducreyi* culture.

Treatment

No single antibiotic is effective against all causes of GUD. The drug regimens currently recommended for treating GUD are given in Table 5. Treatment traditionally has been initiated only once a definitive diagnosis has been established; however, the delay inherent in obtaining laboratory results makes it necessary to initiate empiric therapy at the time of the initial visit. Such therapy should always treat syphilis and include chancroid if it is known to be endemic in the community. Fluctuant bubos should be incised or aspirated with a large-gauge needle because of the viscous nature of bubo fluid. Repeated aspirations may be required. All patients with GUD should be tested for HIV infection after appropriate pretest counseling.

Patients should be reassessed at 7 days to assess response to therapy. Most patients with chancroid and donovanosis will show improvement; failure of the lesions to respond should prompt a search for an alternative diagnosis. The RPR or VDRL as well as a treponemal test should be repeated in all patients who had a negative test on initial evaluation because the test may give a false-negative result when the patient first presents with primary syphilis. Specific treatment recommendations for the common causes of GUD are given in the following sections.

Syphilis

A single intramuscular (IM) injection of benzathine penicillin G, 2.4 million U, is the treatment of choice for both HIV-infected and uninfected patients with primary syphilis. Doxycycline or tetracycline can be used in patients with a documented penicillin allergy. HIV-seronegative patients should be followed with a quantitative RPR or VDRL at 3, 6, 12, and 24 months after treatment. Treatment failure is diagnosed if clinical signs persist or recur, a sustained fourfold rise in titer occurs, or an initially high titer fails to decline by at least fourfold at 6 months. In HIV-infected patients, the RPR or VDRL should be followed at 1, 2, 3, 6, 9, and 12 months. Patients who fail treatment as determined by the criteria outlined should undergo a lumbar puncture and be treated with benzathine penicillin G, 2.4 million U IM weekly for 3 weeks, if the cerebrospinal fluid (CSF) is normal. Because doxycycline and tetracycline are contraindicated in pregnancy, pregnant patients with a true penicillin allergy must be desensitized and then treated with penicillin. Persons who had sexual contact with the infected individual in the preceding 90 days should be treated even if they are asymptomatic.

Chancroid

Trimethoprim-sulfamethoxazole (TMP-SMX) is no longer recommended for the treatment of chancroid because *H. ducreyi* has become resistant to this regimen in most areas of the world. Erythromycin, 500 mg PO four times daily for 7 days, is recommended as the treatment of choice. However, a prospective study in Kenya found that erythromycin, 250 mg three times daily for 7 days, is as effective in both HIV-infected and uninfected patients. A single dose of azithromycin is an alternative to erythromycin. Single-dose regimens with ciprofloxacin, 500 mg, are also effective, although ceftriaxone prescribed as a single-dose regimen is less effective in patients coinfected with HIV. HIV-infected patients may also take longer to heal despite adequate therapy, and treatment failure should be diagnosed only if there has been no response to treatment at 14 days. All chancroid patients with initially negative serologies for HIV and syphilis should have these tests repeated at 3 months. All persons who had sexual contact with the patient in the preceding 3 weeks should be treated regardless of symptoms. Erythromycin can be used in pregnant patients.

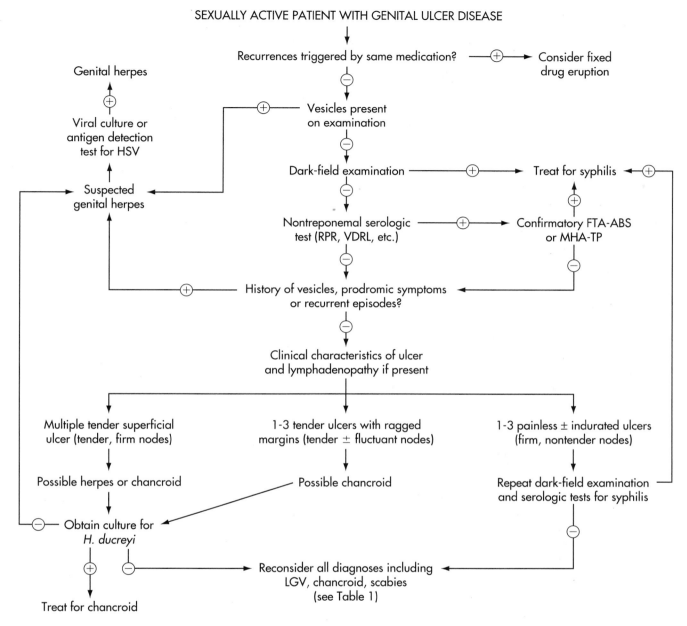

Figure 1
Diagnostic algorithm for patients with genital ulcer disease.

Lymphogranuloma Venereum
Doxycycline is the treatment of choice for LGV, but treatment failures may occur, especially in the presence of proctocolitis, and repeated courses should be prescribed. Pregnant patients should be treated with erythromcin. All sexual contacts within the last 30 days should be investigated for urethral or cervical chlamydial infection and treated accordingly.

Donovanosis
Doxycycline remains the treatment of choice for donovanosis, although treatment failures occur. When therapy fails,

patients should be treated with TMP-SMX or ciprofloxacin. TMP-SMX should be used during pregnancy.

Genital Herpes
Acyclovir, valacyclovir, or famciclovir should be used to treat the initial clinical episode of genital herpes, and for severe cases, intravenous acyclovir therapy may be required. Most immunocompetent patients with recurrent disease do not require treatment. However, preventive treatment is indicated for patients with frequent recurrences. Acyclovir, 400 mg twice daily; famciclovir, 250 three times daily; or valacyclovir, 1 g once daily, will each prevent 90% or more of

Table 5 Treatment Regimens for Infectious Causes of the Genital Ulcer Adenopathy Syndrome

DISEASE	RECOMMENDED REGIMEN	ALTERNATIVE REGIMENS	COMMENTS
Primary syphilis	Benzathine penicillin G (2.4 million U IM)	Doxycycline (100 mg PO bid × 14 days) or Tetracycline (500 mg PO qid × 14 days)	The Jarisch-Herxheimer (J-H) reaction (acute onset of fever accompanied by headache, myalgia, malaise, nausea, and tachycardia) may occur 2-24 hr after initiating therapy for syphilis. Although the J-H reaction may produce fetal distress or premature labour in a pregnant woman, this is not an indication to delay therapy.
Chancroid	Erythromycin (250 mg PO qid × 7 days) Erythromycin (500 mg PO qid × 7 days)	Azithromycin (1 g PO × 1 dose) or Ciprofloxacin (500 mg PO × 1 dose) or Amoxicillin-clavulanic acid (500/125 mg PO tid × 7 days)	Single-dose regimens are contraindicated in HIV-seropositive patients because of unexpectedly high failure rates.
Lymphogranuloma venereum	Doxycycline (100 mg PO bid × 21 days)	Erythromycin (500 mg PO qid × 21 days) or Sulfisoxazole (500 mg PO qid × 21 days)	Contacts may require treatment.
Donovanosis	Doxycycline (100 mg PO bid)	Cotrimoxazole (TMP-SMX 160/800 PO bid) Ciprofloxacin (500 mg PO bid) Tetracycline (500 mg PO qid)	Treat until all lesions are healed (may take up to 4 wk).
Genital herpes (primary)	Acyclovir (200 mg PO 5× daily × 10 days) Famciclovir (250 mg PO tid × 5-10 days) Valacyclovir (1 g PO bid × 5-10 days)		Recurrences require treatment only if severe.

HIV, Human immunodeficiency virus.

recurrences. See the chapter *Herpes Simplex Viruses* for more details of treatment.

Suggested Reading

Ballard R: Genital ulcer adenopathy syndrome. In Holmes KK et al, eds: *Sexually transmitted diseases*, New York, 1999, McGraw-Hill.

Centers for Disease Control and Prevention: 1998 Sexually transmitted diseases treatment guidelines, *Clin Infect Dis* 28(suppl 1):S14, 1999.

Dickerson MC, et al: The causal role for genital ulcer disease as a risk factor for transmission of human immunodeficiency virus, *Sex Transm Dis* 23:429, 1996.

Gourevitch MN, et al: Effect of HIV infection on the serologic manifestations and response to treatment of syphilis in intravenous drug users, *Ann Intern Med* 121:94, 1993.

Hart G: Donovanosis in Australia, *Venerology* 8:15, 1995.

Jessamine PG, et al: Human immunodeficiency virus, genital ulcers and the male foreskin: synergism in HIV-1 transmission, *Scand J Infect Dis*, 69(suppl):181, 1990.

Morse SA, et al: Comparison of clinical diagnosis and standard laboratory and molecular methods for the diagnosis of genital ulcer disease in Lesotho: association with human immunodeficiency virus infection, *J Infect Dis* 175:583, 1997.

Ronald AR, Albritton W: Chancroid and *Haemophilus ducreyi*. In Holmes KK et al, eds: *Sexually transmitted diseases*, New York, 1999, McGraw-Hill.

PROSTATITIS

Jonathan M. Zenilman

Prostatitis is a common clinical problem and can result from infectious or noninfectious causes. Data from the U.S. National Center for Health Statistics suggest that more than 2 million people seek medical attention annually for prostatitis, most of whom are seen by internists and family practitioners.

Prostatitis is the clinical expression of inflammatory exudate within the ducts and prostate gland tissue. In acute prostatitis, the inflammatory cells are polymorphonuclear leukocytes (PMNs). In chronic prostatitis, a lymphocytic and mononuclear inflammatory process is present. Chronic prostatitis is often focal. Furthermore, noninfectious events may contribute to the chronic prostatitis syndrome. For example, prostatic concretions may serve as a nidus for the development of chronic bacterial prostatitis. Focal prostatic necrosis (as part of benign prostatic hyperplasia) may cause prostatic inflammation, even without infection.

Most cases of bacterial prostatitis occur as a result of reflux of infected urine into the prostatic ducts and canaliculi. Although large-scale, formal epidemiologic studies have not been done, prostatitis not surprisingly is seen most commonly in older men. Bacterial prostatitis is more common in patients with previous prostate disease, diabetes mellitus, and a history of urethral instrumentation (e.g., catheterization).

Infectious prostatitis is rarely caused by sexually transmitted organisms. Because urethritis is the initial symptom of gonococcal and chlamydial infection, patients seek care early, and with the widespread availability of effective treatments, the infection is eradicated. Prostatitis caused by hematogenously disseminated organisms is usually seen as part of those disease syndromes. Organisms implicated have been *Mycobacterium tuberculosis, Cryptococcus neoformans, Coccidioides immitis, Histoplasma capsulatum, Aspergillus* species, and *Candida.* With the exception of *Candida,* these infections present as granulomatous disease and are often confused with malignancy.

The long-term sequelae of bacterial prostatitis are not well described. Some authorities believe that prostatitis may be a contributing factor in male infertility.

■ CLINICAL SYNDROMES

Except for acute prostatitis, the accurate clinical diagnosis of prostatitis is difficult. Clinical symptoms are typically nonspecific, and the differential diagnosis often includes a host of noninfectious urologic problems. Many patients seek urologic or infectious disease consultation for prostatitis evaluation after previous diagnoses of lower urinary tract infection or sexually transmitted disease (STD) syndromes; therefore they have often been treated with antibiotics previously. Because of the gland's location, definitive histopathologic diagnosis by biopsy is rarely an option, unless malignancy is strongly suspected.

Acute prostatitis is characterized by an abrupt, febrile illness with symptoms referable to the lower genitourinary tract. Chills, leukocytosis, urinary frequency, and occasional bladder outlet obstruction are present. A rectal examination typically shows an enlarged, boggy, exquisitely tender prostate.

Chronic prostatitis actually is divided by etiology into those resulting from bacterial etiologies and those in which inflammation is present but no bacteria can be identified. There is a large variety of presenting symptoms, including urinary urgency, frequency, nocturia, dysuria. Lower back pain or pain in the inguinal, suprapubic, or scrotal areas may be present. Hematospermia or hematuria is seen in approximately 10% of patients. Systemic symptoms are unusual. Rectal examination of the prostate is typically unremarkable. In practice, most men come for evaluation after being treated initially with antibiotics for community-acquired urinary tract infection.

The differential diagnosis also includes urinary tract infection caused by cystitis, prostatic hyperplasia caused by either benign prostatic hypertrophy or tumor, and urethral stricture caused by previous undertreated urethritis. Carcinoma of the bladder should be considered, especially in patients with hematuria. Urine cytologic examination is useful in ruling out this diagnosis. Neuromuscular urologic disorders may also be involved and should be considered in consultation with the urologist if laboratory investigations fail to reveal a cause for the symptoms.

■ LABORATORY EVALUATION

The only way chronic bacterial prostatitis can be diagnosed with certainty is by evaluating the expressed prostatic secretions for inflammatory cells and bacterial pathogens. Stamey and Meares' technique of segmental urinary tract culture is widely accepted.

Procedure

The patient should have a full bladder and should not have taken antibiotics for 48 hours. The penis is washed with sterile water (no antibacterials are used because they may reduce culture yield). In uncircumcised men, the foreskin is retracted. The patient is then asked to void. The first 10 ml are collected (VB_1), and a midstream sample is collected (VB_2). After voiding 200 ml, the patient is instructed to kneel. The physician vigorously massages the prostate, and the expressed prostatic secretions (EPS) are collected in a sterile container as they drip from the urethral meatus. The patient is then asked to empty his bladder, and the first 10 ml of this final void (VB_3) are collected. Gram stain smear is prepared from the EPS specimens. The midstream urine and prostatic secretions are sent to the laboratory (chilled) for culture. The laboratory should be asked to perform low colony count cultures.

Table 1   Differential Diagnosis of Prostatitis

	MIDSTREAM URINE		EPS	
	WBC	CULTURE	WBC	CULTURE
Acute bacterial prostatitis	++	+	++	+
Chronic bacterial prostatitis	+	+	+	+
Chronic nonbacterial prostatitis	−	−	+	−
Prostadynia	−	−	−	−

Adapted from Meares, Stamey.

Evaluation of Results

Differential diagnosis of prostatitis is achieved by using the data from the expressed prostatic secretions and the midstream urine (VB_2) and are summarized in Table 1. The number of white blood cells (WBCs) in prostatic secretions necessary to make the diagnosis varies in the literature. However, nearly all have more than 12 WBC/hpf (high-powered field). Acute bacterial prostatitis has a large number of organisms and PMNs; the diagnosis is seldom subtle. Chronic prostatitis is diagnosed by presence of PMNs in the expressed prostatic secretions. Culture results from the EPS differentiate bacterial and nonbacterial causes. Patients with nonbacterial chronic prostatitis should be referred to the urologist for further evaluation. Sexually transmitted organisms such as *Chlamydia* or *Trichomonas* are rarely implicated. *Prostadynia* is diagnosed in settings in which the prostatic secretions demonstrate no inflammation and cultures are negative. In some studies, as many as 40% of patients have prostadynia. Delineation of this syndrome is important because antimicrobials would have no effect and should not be prescribed.

■ BACTERIAL ETIOLOGIES

Determination of bacterial etiology is desirable because antimicrobial therapy for prostatitis is usually required for at least 4 weeks. If the patient has taken antibiotics before the evaluation, false-negative culture results will occur. Except in cases of acute prostatitis, the clinician may want to consider discontinuing antibiotic therapy, waiting for 48 to 72 hours, and then obtaining the prostatic fluid and urine cultures.

The organisms typically isolated are those associated with lower urinary tract infection (Table 2). Enteric gram-negative rods are most common, followed by *Enterococcus, S. saprophyticus,* and *Pseudomonas*. Streptococci and anaerobes are rarely involved. If the patient has been recently instrumented or catheterized in a hospital setting, especially if he has been treated with antibiotics, *Pseudomonas* and *Enterococcus* would be the major concerns. In some studies, *Mycoplasma hominis* and *Ureaplasma urealyticum* have been cultured in up to 25% of cases. Routine culture for these organisms is not recommended as special media, and bacteriologic techniques are required. Furthermore, both these organisms are found frequently as commensals in normal hosts and their role as pathogens is controversial.

In sexually active patients, especially those with multiple partners, *Chlamydia* and *Trichomonas* are rarely found.

Table 2   Organisms Implicated in Bacterial Prostatitis

GRAM-NEGATIVE
  Escherichia coli
  Proteus mirabilis
  Klebsiella
  Pseudomonas aeruginosa
GRAM-POSITIVE
  Enterococcus
  Staphylococcus saprophyticus

These organisms are difficult to culture. New nucleic acid amplification tests (LCR and PCR) have been recently approved for use in urine and may be helpful in ascertaining chlamydial infection. Fungal and mycobacterial causes can be usually diagnosed only by prostatic biopsy.

■ TREATMENT

Evaluating treatment efficacy of prostatitis is complicated by the following:

1. Making an accurate clinical diagnosis is difficult, especially in the substantial fraction of patients with prior antibiotic therapy for lower urinary tract infections.
2. No standardized definition of cure exists. Most studies of treatment, even those that evaluate prostatic secretions for bacteriology, do not repeat the procedure at post-therapy evaluation.
3. The optimal duration of therapy is not definitively known.
4. There are few longitudinal, randomized controlled trials that have evaluated prostatitis treatment efficacy.

Acknowledging these difficulties, most authorities believe that treatment regimens for bacterial prostatitis should include the following:

1. Use an antimicrobial effective against the most likely organisms.
2. Use an antimicrobial that is well absorbed into prostate tissue and that has an acid dissociation coefficient (pK_a) that is favorable to trap the drug in prostate tissue (compared with the acidic urinary tract environment).
3. The treatment duration should be 1 month. Therefore drugs that require less frequent dosing would be preferred to facilitate compliance.

Table 3 Therapy Recommendations for Prostatitis

Trimethoprim-sulfamethoxazole DS (160/800 mg) bid
Ciprofloxacin, 500 mg bid, or ofloxacin, 300 mg bid
Oral therapy duration is 4 weeks

The quinolones and sulfamethoxazole-trimethoprim (Table 3) meet these criteria. I prefer to use the quinolones because they are associated with fewer side effects, especially in older patients, and are more active against the grampositive organisms. However, they are two to five times more costly than trimethoprim-sulfamethoxazole (TMP-SMX). Quinolones are also poorly absorbed if the gastric pH is greater than 5, a consideration in patients who are taking antacids or H_2 blockers.

Because many patients are referred for evaluation after being given a course of antibiotic therapy, accurate bacteriologic evaluation may be impossible. The trap here is that antibiotic treatment of nonbacterial chronic prostatitis is ineffective. One option is to discontinue antibiotics and evaluate 72 hours after discontinuation.

Recurrent disease is common and is reported in as many as 40% of patients. In patients with well-documented disease, antimicrobials should be resumed for a minimum of 3 months. If a second recurrence occurs, chronic prophylaxis should be considered. Recurrence after cessation of antibiotics in patients with poorly documented disease should be viewed as an opportunity to fully evaluate the syndrome.

Suggested Reading

del la Rosette JJMC, et al: Diagnosis and treatment of 409 patients with prostatitis syndromes, *Urology* 41:301, 1993.

Domingue GJ, Hellstrom WJG: Prostatitis, *Clin Microbiol Rev* 11:604, 1998.

Johansen TEB, et al: The role of antibiotics in the treatment of chronic prostatitis: a consensus statement, *Euro Urol* 34:457, 1998.

Meares EM, Stamey EA: Bacteriologic localization patterns in bacterial prostatitis and urethritis, *Invest Urol* 5:492, 1968.

Roberts RO, et al: A review of clinical and pathological prostatitis syndromes, *Urology* 49:809, 1997.

PELVIC INFLAMMATORY DISEASE

William J. Ledger

Our biologic scientific heritage of classification serves us poorly when we evaluate pelvic infection in the sexually active, nonpregnant female. *Pelvic inflammatory disease* (PID) is a single term that attempts to encompass too wide a range of clinical syndromes. Women with this diagnosis include those seriously ill with a tuboovarian abscess who require hospitalization and for whom intravenous antibiotics and, in some cases operative intervention, either drainage or removal of pelvic organs, is needed for a cure. In contrast, most women with pelvic infection (PID) either are asymptomatic or have such mild symptoms that they never seek medical care. A frustration for any policy of intervention is the knowledge that these patients with "silent" infections can have irreversible tubal damage.

■ MICROBIOLOGY

There are diverse multitudes of bacteria involved in PID, and most of these infections are polymicrobial; that is, more than one species is involved. The bacteria causing infection can be placed into one of three categories. One group of infected women has *Neisseria gonorrhoeae* as one of the involved pathogens. These women have symptomatic infections with diffuse lower abdominal and pelvic pain, as well as an elevated temperature. In contrast, the second group of women, infected with *Chlamydia trachomatis,* has a much more subtle clinical presentation. They have minimal or no symptoms, are usually afebrile, and often have no abnormal blood studies. Although they do not appear ill, these women can have widespread tissue damage, and it is likely that the process of tissue damage with this intracellular organism is an autoimmune phenomenon. The third microbiologic category is the catch-all term, *other*. These patients are infected with neither *N. gonorrhoeae* nor *Chlamydia trachomatis*. Organisms recovered from these patients include grampositive and gram-negative aerobes and anaerobes. Gram-negative anaerobes are particularly important in patients with more severe infections, that is, those with pelvic abscess formation.

■ CLINICAL DIAGNOSIS

Clinical diagnosis is a difficult undertaking because of the tremendous variation in patient response to infection. In some women the diagnosis of PID is obvious. This is particularly true in patients visiting urban emergency rooms. When *N. gonorrhoeae* is one of the involved pathogens, these women have severe lower abdominal discomfort, pelvic pain on examination, and an elevated temperature. Another group, patients with pelvic abscesses, is also obviously sick. The patients are febrile and have tender pelvic masses detected by pelvic examination using an imaging technique. In contrast, most women with PID are infected with *C. trachomatis* and have minimal or no symptoms.

Because so many women have few signs or symptoms, I remain unconvinced of the validity of the minimal criteria set forth by the Centers for Disease Control and Prevention (CDC) for the diagnosis of PID, that is, lower abdominal tenderness, adnexal tenderness, and cervical motion tenderness. This is a carryover from a formulation published by four obstetrician/gynecologists in 1983. Unfortunately, these physical examination screens have never been subjected to a clinical evaluation to test their specificity. In fact, a large published study of laparoscopy in women with PID showed these minimal criteria did not distinguish between women who had a pelvic infection and those who did not. What are clinicians to do? They must heighten their level of awareness. Suspect a pelvic infection in any sexually active woman who has either a new sexual partner or a promiscuous male partner who does not use condoms. Consider this diagnosis when the woman complains of urgency and frequency on urination, has irregular vaginal bleeding with no obvious pathologic condition present on pelvic examination, or most commonly, has a new vaginal discharge.

The most sensitive office test to detect PID in this population is a vaginal smear examined microscopically that is loaded with white cells. This microscopic examination should be part of the initial workup by any physician who suspects PID.

This heightened physician awareness is only one portion of the strategy to ensure that women with a pelvic infection will be diagnosed and treated. The current reality in the United States is that women with few or no symptoms do not avail themselves of medical care so that a diagnosis can be made. Women need to be educated about the risks of exposure to a new male partner who does not use a condom and to the subtle signs of pelvic infection. One possible future strategy will be that these women will self-test themselves for the presence of *C. trachomatis*. At least one study has shown this to be a sensitive method of testing.

■ LABORATORY DIAGNOSIS

The traditional tests for a bacterial infection (i.e., an elevated white blood cell count and an increase in the number of immature cells) are neither sensitive nor specific markers for a pelvic infection. The most feared current pathogen is *C. trachomatis* because of its frequency of involvement and the paucity of symptoms. Physicians should use the polymerase chain reaction (PCR) test. It is more sensitive than either the DNA probe or the cell culture technique.

■ TREATMENT

The CDC has recommended a variety of parenteral (Table 1) and outpatient (Table 2) regimens. The criteria for admission and the effectiveness of intravenous antibiotic treatment versus oral antibiotic treatment have never been subjected to a prospective clinical comparison. Patients who fail to respond to the systemic antibiotic treatment should be evaluated to determine whether pelvic abscess formation has occurred. In women in whom an abscess is discovered, aspiration can be done by laparoscopy or transabdominal

Table 1   Suggested Parenteral Regimens for Pelvic Inflammatory Disease

A. Cefotetan, 2 g q12h
                    or
   Cefoxitin, 2 g q6h
                    plus
   Doxycycline, 100 mg IV or orally q12h
B. Clindamycin, 900 mg IV q8h
                    plus
   Gentamicin—loading dose IV or IM (2 mg/kg body weight) followed by a maintenance dosage of 1.5 mg/kg q8h
C. Alternative parenteral regimens
   1. Ofloxacin, 400 mg IV q12h
                    plus
      Metronidazole, 500 mg IV q8h
   2. Ampicillin-sulbactum, 3.0 g IV q6h
                    plus
      Doxycycline, 100 mg IV or orally q12h
   3. Ciprofloxacin, 200 mg IV q12h
                    plus
      Doxycycline, 100 mg IV or orally q12h
                    plus
      Metronidazole, 500 mg IV q8h

Table 2   Suggested Outpatient Regimens for Pelvic Inflammatory Disease

A. Ofloxacin, 400 mg PO twice a day for 14 days
                    plus
   Metronidazole, 500 mg PO twice a day for 14 days
B. Ceftriaxone, 250 mg IM single dose
                    or
   Cefoxitin, 2 g IM plus probenecid 1 g PO single dose
                    or
   Other parenteral third-generation cephalosporin (ceftizoxime or cefotaxime)
                    plus
   Doxycycline, 100 mg PO twice a day for 14 days

needle aspiration. Patients who fail to respond to this treatment are few in number. These few are the ones who could need operative removal of the infected tissue to finally achieve a cure.

Suggested Reading

Centers for Disease Control and Prevention: 1998 Guidelines for treatment of sexually transmitted diseases, *MMWR* 47:1, 1998.

Curran JW, et al: Female gonorrhea. Its relation to abnormal uterine bleeding, urinary tract symptoms and cervicitis, *Obstet Gynecol* 45:195, 1975.

Hager WD, et al: Criteria for diagnosis and grading of salpingitis, *Obstet Gynecol* 61:113, 1983.

Holland SN, et al: Demonstration of chlamydia RNA and DNA during a culture negative state, *Infect Immunol* 60:2040, 1992.

Jacobson I, Westrom L: Objectivized diagnosis of acute pelvic inflammatory disease. Diagnostic and prognostic value of routine laparoscopy, *Am J Obstet Gynecol* 105:1088, 1969.

Landers DV, Sweet RL: Tubo-ovarian abscess: contemporary approach to management, *Rev Infect Dis* 5:876, 1983.

Ledger WJ, Sweet RL, Headington JT: *Bacteroides* species as a cause of severe infection in obstetric and gynecologic patients, *Surg Gynecol Obstet* 133:837, 1971.

Montgomery RS, Wilson SE: Intra-abdominal abscesses: image-guided diagnosis and therapy, *Clin Infect Dis* 23:28, 1996.

Peipert JF, et al: Laboratory evaluation of acute upper genital tract infection, *Obstet Gynecol* 87:730, 1996.

Polaneczky M, et al: The use of self-collected vaginal introital specimens for the detection of *Chlamydia trachomatis* infections in women, *Obstet Gynecol* 91:375, 1998.

Reich H, McGlynn F: Laparoscopic treatment of tubo-ovarian and pelvic abscess, *J Reprod Med* 32:747, 1987.

Soper DE, Brockwell NJ, Dalton HP: Microbial etiology of urban emergency department acute salpingitis, *Am J Obstet Gynecol* 167:648, 1992.

Witkin SS, et al: Cell mediated immune response to the recombinant 57Kda heat shock protein of *Chlamydia trachomatis* in women with salpingitis, *J Infect Dis* 167:1379, 1993.

Witkin SS, et al: Detection of *Chlamydia trachomatis* by the polymerase chain reaction in the cervices of women with acute salpingitis, *Am J Obstet Gynecol* 168:1438, 1993.

URINARY TRACT INFECTION

Judith A. O'Donnell
Elias Abrutyn

Urinary tract infections (UTIs) are exceedingly common in both the outpatient and inpatient settings. They occur in patients of all ages, affecting females throughout life and males at each end of the age spectrum. It is estimated that more than 6 million visits are made annually to physicians' offices for evaluation of symptoms such as dysuria, urinary frequency, or urgency. In addition, UTIs are the leading cause of gram-negative bacillary sepsis in hospitalized patients. The phrase *urinary tract infection* encompasses a broad array of diagnoses, including cystitis, pyelonephritis, asymptomatic bacteriuria, complicated infections associated with nephrolithiasis or bladder catheters, and recurrent infections. The appropriate management of a patient with infection of the urinary tract entails the consideration of a number of factors, including the patient's age and sex, the presence of underlying diseases or pregnancy, the history and timing of prior UTIs, the differentiation between cystitis and pyelonephritis, and the expected microbial pathogen involved.

The delineation of upper versus lower tract infection is essential to understanding the approach to therapy. *Lower urinary tract infection* is infection involving the bladder (cystitis) and describes the syndrome of dysuria, pyuria, increased urinary frequency, or urgency. *Upper urinary tract infection*, or *pyelonephritis*, is infection involving the bladder and kidney and clinically presents with fever, flank pain, or tenderness, along with the signs and symptoms of lower tract infection. The pathogenesis of most cases of upper and lower urinary tract infection is related to the ability of microorganisms to establish colonization in the periurethral area, and subsequently *ascend* into the urinary tract, thus causing infection. The hematogenous route is a less common mechanism for establishing UTIs.

The majority of both upper and lower tract infections are monomicrobial. *Escherichia coli* is the single most common pathogen; however, other members of the *Enterobacteriaceae* family such as *Proteus* species, *Enterobacter* species, and *Klebsiella* species are also uropathogens. *Staphylococcus saprophyticus* and *Enterococcus* species are the most common gram-positive pathogens; however, they are isolated much less often than enteric gram-negative rods. Many other bacteria can also serve as the infecting organism, especially when an indwelling bladder catheter is present. A polymicrobial infection in the absence of a bladder catheter may suggest an enterovesical fistula. Fungi can also be pathogens, usually when a bladder catheter is chronic. *Candida albicans* and other *Candida* species are the most common isolates when funguria is identified.

The distinction between uncomplicated and complicated UTI is of paramount importance. An uncomplicated infection of the urinary tract is a lower tract infection in an individual who has no functional or structural abnormalities of the kidneys, ureters, bladder, or urethra. Most women with UTIs fall into this category. Complicated infections of the urinary tract are those infections occurring in the setting of functional or anatomic abnormalities of the upper or lower tract, are associated with nephrolithiasis, occur in the presence of an indwelling bladder catheter, or are seen in patients with underlying conditions such as pregnancy, diabetes mellitus, renal transplantation, or sickle cell anemia. These conditions are recognized as factors influencing response to therapy.

It is necessary to determine whether each patient diagnosed with a UTI has an uncomplicated or complicated infection. This differentiation will determine the management and duration of therapy. Uncomplicated lower UTIs respond well to therapy of short duration (3 days) and are not associated with sequelae. Complicated infections are thought to require longer courses of therapy (10 days or more) and are more likely to be associated with bacteremia or recurrence. It is important to recognize that the definition of complicated UTI as used by different authors is variable and that few studies have been performed to evaluate the implications for treatment.

■ CYSTITIS

Women are much more likely to develop cystitis than men, in part because bacteria are able to ascend into the bladder of women with greater efficiency. Diagnosis can be made through microscopic examination of the sediment from a midstream, "clean-voided" urine specimen. The presence of pyuria, defined as 10 white blood cells per high-powered field or more, and significant bacteriuria ($>10^5$ organisms per milliliter of urine) are indicative of UTI. In recent studies, however, lower colony counts of bacteria in the urine (10^2 to 10^4 per milliliter of urine) in association with signs and symptoms of cystitis in young women, has been accepted as significant and diagnostic for infection. Similar studies have not been performed in men or older adults, and as such the 10^5 colony count number should probably still be used in these patient populations.

Bacteria can be readily seen by examining a wet mount preparation or by Gram stain of unspun urine. The gram-stained preparations are particularly useful in differentiating vaginal flora from gram-negative rods and for determining whether the likely uropathogen is a gram-positive organism. Quantitative culture of the specimen can provide a specific microbiologic diagnosis, and susceptibility testing can offer the most effective means for determining adequate therapy. However, in most young women with uncomplicated UTI, the diagnosis can be made by the presence of pyuria and bacteriuria. A urine culture need not be performed in this particular setting because presumptive therapy for the expected uropathogens (*E. coli, S. saprophyticus*) is usually successful.

Therapy of uncomplicated cystitis is directed at eradicating pathogenic bacteria from the bladder as well as the periurethral area, and this can be accomplished with a short course of an effective antimicrobial agent. In well-designed clinical studies, 3-day regimens have been shown to be significantly more effective than 1-day regimens. Short-course therapy can be recommended only for women with acute uncomplicated cystitis because there have not yet been clinical studies in men with UTI. Regimens composed of either a fluoroquinolone (ciprofloxacin, ofloxacin, norfloxacin, enoxacin, lomefloxacin, levofloxacin, sparfloxacin) or trimethoprim-sulfamethoxazole (TMP-SMX) are more effective than those containing a beta-lactam or tetracycline in eradication of infection and periurethral colonization. TMP-SMX given as one double-strength tablet every 12 hours; trimethoprim alone, 100 mg every 12 hours or 200 mg daily; ciprofloxacin, 100, 250, or 500 mg every 12 hours; norfloxacin, 400 mg every 12 hours; ofloxacin, 200, 300 or 400 mg every 12 hours; enoxacin, 200 mg twice daily; levofloxacin, 250 mg daily; lomefloxacin, 400 mg daily; and sparfloxacin in a 400 mg loading dose with 200 mg daily thereafter are all equally effective when prescribed for a 3-day course of therapy (Table 1).

Recently, a meta-analysis of the treatment of cystitis and pyelonephritis was performed by a panel established by the Infectious Diseases Society of America (IDSA). The results were used to develop guidelines for treatment. They recommended TMP-SMX for 3 days as standard initial therapy with trimethoprim and ofloxacin as equally effective alternatives. Other quinolones such as norfloxacin, ciprofloxacin, and fleroxacin were considered similarly effective, but quinolones were not recommended as initial therapy because of high expense unless resistance to TMP-SMX or TMP exceeded 10% to 20%. Beta-lactam therapy for 3 days was found to be less effective.

Although there are a number of new fluoroquinolones on the market and more are being developed, the choice of a particular agent from this class need not be confusing. In general, these agents are all equally efficacious and usually well tolerated. It should be noted that these agents cannot be taken orally in conjunction with preparations containing divalent or trivalent cations (e.g., iron salts or antacids containing magnesium or aluminum) or sucralfate. Fluoroquinolones should be taken 2 hours after sucralfate, or 4 hours before or after these other compounds, to ensure adequate absorption. There are cost differences and some disparities in side effect profiles with which prescribing clinicians should be familiar. Specifically, photosensitivity is more common with sparfloxacin and lomefloxacin.

Fosfomycin tromethamine has recently been marketed in the United States for treatment of uncomplicated UTI in women. This agent and a related compound have been used extensively in Europe. The drug is recommended as a single 3-g dose, provided in granule form, and dissolved in one-half cup of water before taken. In the currently recommended dose above, fosfomycin was less effective than ciprofloxacin or TMP-SMX in eradicating bacteriuria immediately after treatment and at 6-week follow-up. Thus it should not be considered a first-line agent in the UTI treatment armamentarium.

Ampicillin and amoxicillin, which were mainstays of therapy, for uncomplicated lower UTIs in the past, should no longer be considered first-line agents. Thirty to forty percent of community-acquired *E. coli* strains produce beta-lactamase and are resistant to these beta-lactam drugs, and recent studies have shown that these agents are inferior in their ability to eradicate uropathogens from perirectal and periurethral colonization sites when compared with the fluoroquinolones or TMP-SMX. Moreover, TMP-SMX and the fluoroquinolones, when given for 3 days, will eliminate *E. coli* and other pathogens from the vaginal reservoir without disturbing the normal vaginal and fecal flora. The beta-lactam drugs, including newer cephalosporins, cannot achieve this desired endpoint.

Cystitis that is less likely to respond adequately to short-course therapy is seen in women with more than 1 week of symptoms at the time of presentation, women with a history of recurrent infections, pregnant women, or patients with infection from resistant bacteria. In addition, because men with lower UTI have not been adequately studied, they should be considered as having complicated UTI and should not be prescribed short-course therapy. The management of such patients with complicated lower UTIs must include performing a urine culture and susceptibility testing, the results of which should be used to guide the clinician's choice of an antimicrobial regimen. Fluoroquinolones and TMP-SMX are again the appropriate empiric choices in this setting because of their superior tissue levels and enhanced ability to eradicate uropathogens from the perineal colonization sites. Successful therapy of complicated lower UTI hinges upon the duration of treatment. Regimens given for a 7- to 10-day course are preferred.

■ PYELONEPHRITIS

The diagnosis of pyelonephritis remains a clinical one that includes fever, flank pain or tenderness, pyuria, and bacteri-

Table 1   Summary of Treatment Recommendations for Lower Urinary Tract Infections

INFECTION	FIRST-LINE THERAPY	MISCELLANEOUS
Uncomplicated lower tract infection in women (duration of therapy is 3 days)	TMP-SMX one double-strength tab q12h TMP, 100 mg q12h, 200 mg daily Ciprofloxacin, 100, 250, 500 mg q12h Ofloxacin, 200, 300, 400 mg q12h Norfloxacin, 400 mg q12h Enoxacin, 200 mg twice daily Lomefloxacin, 400 mg daily Levofloxacin, 250 mg daily Sparfloxacin, 400 then 200 mg daily Gatifloxacin, 200 mg PO daily	Best anti-*Pseudomonas* activity (avoid divalent and trivalent cations with all fluoroquinolones) High rate of photosensitivity Well tolerated High rate of photosensitivity
Complicated lower tract infections (duration of therapy is 7-10 days)	Same as uncomplicated	Therapy guided by C/S

C/S, Culture and sensitivity.

Table 2   Summary of Treatment Recommendations for Pyelonephritis

DESCRIPTION	THERAPY*	OTHER MANAGEMENT RECOMMENDATIONS
Outpatient	TMP-SMX one double-strength tab q12h Ciprofloxacin, 500 mg twice daily Levofloxacin, 250 mg daily Lomefloxacin, 400 mg daily Gatifloxacin, 400 mg PO daily	Therapy directed by urine Gram stain; must follow-up in 72 hours to determine response
Hospitalized	TMP-SMX, 10 mg/kg/day, 2-4 divided doses Ciprofloxacin, 400 mg IV q12h Levofloxacin, 250-400 mg IV daily Gatifloxacin, 400 mg IV daily Ceftriaxone, 1 g q24h Cefotaxime, 1 g q8h Aztreonam, 1 g q8h Piperacillin, 4 g q6h Gentamicin or tobramycin, 2 mg/kg load, then 1.8 mg/kg q8h *or* 5 mg/kg (7 mg/kg critically ill) q24h Amikacin or kanamycin, 7.5 mg/kg q12h *or* 15 mg/kg q24h	Streamline therapy based on C/S data; can switch to orals once patient responds

*Duration of therapy is 14 days with all regimens.
C/S, Culture and sensitivity.

uria. The decision to hospitalize a patient with pyelonephritis should be based on the likelihood of bacteremia associated with the infection (presence of hypotension, rigors, or septic shock), as well as the patient's ability to tolerate and be compliant with an oral antimicrobial regimen.

If the patient is deemed an appropriate candidate for outpatient oral therapy, any of a number of antimicrobials can be prescribed after a urine Gram stain is performed and culture is obtained (Table 2). Again, either TMP-SMX at the usual dosage or a fluoroquinolone (some in the larger doses mentioned previously), would be appropriate empiric choices when the gram-stained urine reveals gram-negative bacilli. When gram-positive cocci in chains and pairs are identified, suggesting an enterococcal infection, amoxicillin, 500 mg three times daily, is reasonable empiric therapy as long as vancomycin-resistant enterococci are not likely; amoxicillin-clavulanic acid is an alternative. The IDSA guidelines indicate that a 14-day course is generally appropriate, but courses as short as 7 days may be appropriate in mild to moderate cases when highly active agents are used.

Patients should have follow-up within 48 to 72 hours after beginning antimicrobial therapy to ensure clinical response and confirm bacteriologic diagnosis. If patients are not improving clinically (i.e., presence of persistent fever, pyuria, flank pain), then further diagnostic evaluation of the kidneys and urinary tract is warranted to establish the presence of abscess or obstruction. Hospitalization and intravenous therapy should be considered as well.

Patients who require hospitalization for management and initial treatment of pyelonephritis can be given parenteral therapy with any of several antiinfective agents. According to the IDSA guidelines, therapy with a parenteral quinolone, an aminoglycoside with or without ampicillin, or an extended-spectrum cephalosporin with or without aminoglycoside should be considered. If gram-positive cocci were found, therapy with ampicillin-sulbactam with or without an aminoglycoside can be used. After clinical improvement, oral therapy with a fluoroquinolone or TMP-SMX should be administered; amoxicillin or amoxicillin-clavulanate should be given for gram-positive infection. Dosages for antimicrobials that can be used to treat pyelonephritis can be found in Table 2. It is important to remember that empiric therapy should be reevaluated once the microbiologic diagnosis and susceptibilities are known. Therapy should be tailored to the specific pathogen with cost-effectiveness in mind. Patients can be switched to oral therapy once clinical response has been documented. A 14-day course of therapy is necessary to ensure cure. In the event that no response to therapy is seen within the first 72 hours, renal ultrasound to evaluate for obstruction, abscess, or other infectious complication is suggested.

■ CATHETER-ASSOCIATED UTI

Catheter-associated UTI can be extremely difficult to manage. Virtually all individuals with an indwelling catheter in place for 1 to 2 weeks or more will have asymptomatic bacteriuria. A low number of white blood cells and red blood cells (10 to 20 cells per high-powered field) may also be seen on microscopic examination of such urine specimens. As such, the diagnosis of a catheter-associated UTI can be challenging. Clinical signs and symptoms may be most helpful in association with very large numbers of white blood cells in the urine. Urine cultures should always be obtained in this setting because these UTI are often polymicrobial. When possible, the catheter should be removed as part of the management.

Antimicrobial therapy should be broader in coverage for the catheter-associated UTI in the hospitalized or nursing home patient. Empiric oral therapy with a fluoroquinolone with *Pseudomonas aeruginosa* activity, such as ciprofloxacin or levofloxacin, is recommended. If intravenous therapy is necessary, again ciprofloxacin or levofloxacin are reasonable empiric choices. Other possible choices include piperacillin, ceftazidime, aztreonam, cefotaxime, ticarcillin clavulanate, or piperacillin tazobactam. Therapy should be tailored once susceptibilities are known.

Fungal pathogens can be a problem in this setting, as can vancomycin-resistant enterococci (VRE). Funguria alone should never be treated. Fungal UTI is identified by pyuria and a positive urine culture with 10^5 organisms per milliliter. When fungal UTI is caused by *Candida albicans,* oral fluconazole, 100 mg daily for 3 to 5 days, may be prescribed. Because of its excessive cost, intravenous fluconazole should be used only when the patient cannot tolerate oral medications. When other *Candida* species or *Torulopsis glabrata* are the fungal pathogens identified in urine culture, amphotericin B either in low-dose intravenous form (1 mg/kg/day) or as a continuous bladder irrigation (50 mg/L of sterile water) is effective when given for 2 to 5 days.

VRE are even more problematic than fungi as catheter-associated UTI pathogens. Many of these VRE are susceptible to nitrofurantoin, and if this is so, nitrofurantoin should be prescribed for the UTI. If the organism is a vancomycin-resistant *Enterococcus faecalis,* ampicillin susceptibility is often present and may be used. If the organism is a vancomycin-resistant *Enterococcus faecium,* susceptibilities are often variable and extremely limited. Doxycycline, tetracycline, ciprofloxacin, rifampin (in combination only), novobiocin, and chloramphenicol have all been used alone or in combination to treat these VRE UTI with limited success. Treatment of these infections should be guided in consultation with an infectious diseases specialist.

Prevention of catheter-associated UTI is greatly desired but still imperfect. Obviously, patients who do not absolutely require indwelling catheters should have them removed. Antibiotic prophylaxis for patients with chronic catheters is not recommended and only serves to allow for colonization with more resistant bacteria and fungi. Silver alloy–coated urinary catheters, although more expensive, are significantly more effective at preventing UTI than silver oxide catheters; the cost-effective use of these catheters needs to be defined.

■ ASYMPTOMATIC BACTERIURIA

Asymptomatic bacteriuria is the presence of significant bacteria in the urine ($>10^5$ cfu/ml) in the absence of signs or symptoms of UTI. The diagnosis of asymptomatic bacteriuria is made in women after two separate urine specimens demonstrate the same organism. Only one sample is required to make the diagnosis in males. The appropriate management of this entity depends on the patient's age, the presence or absence of pregnancy, or a planned genitourinary procedure for the patient. Significant bacteriuria will occur in 1% of neonates, 1% to 3% of nonpregnant women ages 15 to 24, 4% to 10% of pregnant women, and up to 20% of ambulatory women in the sixth and seventh decades of life. Moreover, the prevalence rate of asymptomatic bacteriuria is even greater among nonambulatory elderly persons, and 100% in the chronically catheterized nursing home population. Asymptomatic bacteriuria in the elderly should neither be sought nor treated. Pyuria in the elderly is often present and in and of itself is not a reliable predictor of infection. In addition, incontinence or a perceived change in the pattern of incontinence is also not an indication for therapy in the presence of asymptomatic bacteriuria.

Children who are found to have asymptomatic bacteriuria should be treated as though they have a complicated UTI. Pregnant women and candidates for urologic surgery are the only two subsets of the adult population who have been shown to benefit from treatment of asymptomatic bacteriuria. Patients undergoing urologic procedures should be screened and, if culture positive, treated to lower their risk of postprocedure infection. As many as 60% of pregnant women with asymptomatic bacteriuria develop symptomatic lower or upper UTI during their pregnancy. Moreover, acute pyelonephritis in this setting has been associated with premature birth. For these reasons, pregnant women with asymptomatic bacteriuria should be treated with antimicrobials that are safe for use in pregnancy. Thus fluoroquinolones and tetracyclines should be avoided throughout gestation and sulfonamide-containing preparations avoided in the third trimester. Empiric choices include amoxicillin, 500 mg orally three times daily, or cephalexin, 500 mg orally four times daily. TMP-SMX twice daily may also be used if the woman is not in her third trimester. Duration of therapy should be 7 days, with follow-up urine cultures obtained at the completion of therapy to document sterilization of

Table 3 Summary of Treatment Recommendations for Recurrent Urinary Tract Infections

PROPHYLAXIS TYPE	ANTIMICROBIAL AGENT	DOSE	MISCELLANEOUS
Postcoital	TMP-SMX	40 mg/200 mg	Eliminates vaginal reservoir without disturbing other flora
	Nitrofurantoin	50 mg	Can be used in pregnancy
	Cephalexin	125-250 mg	Disrupts vaginal flora
	Cinoxacin	250 mg	Not available in the United States
Continuous*	TMP-SMX	40 mg/200 mg	As above; safe with years of use
	TMP alone	100 mg	As above
	Nitrofurantoin	50-100 mg	As above, safe with years of use
	Norfloxacin	200 mg	Eliminates vaginal reservoir without disturbing other flora
	Cephalexin	125-250 mg	As above
	Cefaclor	250 mg	Disrupts vaginal flora
	Sulfa	500 mg	

*Continuous therapy can be given either daily or three times weekly at bedtime.

urine. If bacteriuria persists or recurs, prolonged therapy may be necessary (4 to 6 weeks' duration).

■ RECURRENT UTI

Recurrent UTIs are three or more infections per year. There are two distinct types: (1) *reinfection* with different bacterial pathogens or (2) *relapse* of infection with the same pathogen. Reinfection accounts for 80% of recurrent infections and can be seen weeks to months after initial infection. Relapse accounts for 20% of recurrent infections and usually occurs within 2 weeks of initial therapy. Relapsing UTIs usually result from inadequate length of therapy, structural abnormalities, or chronic bacterial prostatitis.

Treatment of relapse is as follows: failure of short-course therapy should receive a 2-week regimen; failure of 2-week therapy should receive a 6-week regimen; failure of 6-week therapy should be considered for a 6-month regimen. When structural abnormalities or prostatitis are suspected, further investigation of the genitourinary tract is also warranted in patients with relapse.

For women with frequent reinfection, three management strategies are possible. First, in the educated patient with two or fewer UTIs per year, patient-initiated self-treatment may be used with either TMP-SMX or a fluoroquinolone. Second, in patients with three or more UTIs per year who can temporally associate their UTI recurrences with sexual activity, postcoital prophylaxis can be offered. In the remainder of women with three or more UTIs per year, continuous low-dose antimicrobial prophylaxis is recommended and has been shown to be highly effective. Continuous prophylaxis may be given for 6 to 12 months, prescribed either nightly or three times weekly, and a variety of agents may be used (Table 3). Postcoital regimens that have been studied include TMP-SMX, cephalexin, nitrofurantoin, and cinoxacin (see Table 3). Continuous antimicrobial prophylaxis choices include TMP-SMX, cephalexin, nitrofurantoin, tri-

methoprim alone, norfloxacin, nitrofurantoin, sulfa, or cefaclor. As noted earlier, only TMP-SMX and the fluoroquinolones have a positive effect on the vaginal flora. In general, when prophylaxis is discontinued, women with recurrent UTI usually revert back to their baseline pattern of recurrent infection. If this occurs, prophylaxis can be reinitiated. Both TMP-SMX and nitrofurantoin have been shown to be safe over years of use.

In postmenopausal women with recurrent UTI, one additional measure may be used: estrogen replacement therapy. Loss of estrogen with menopause leads to an elevated vaginal pH, a loss of lactobacilli in the vagina, and a more uropathogen-dominant vaginal flora. Use of topical estriol has been shown to decrease the incidence of UTI in one large-study population. Because the outcomes of this single study have not been reproduced, routine use of hormonal therapy as an adjunct to the management of recurrent UTI cannot yet be recommended for all patients. Oral estrogen replacement is thought to have similar effects but has not been formerly evaluated as yet.

Suggested Reading

Hooton TM, et al: Randomized comparative trial and cost analysis of 3-day antimicrobial regimens for treatment of acute cystitis in women, *JAMA* 273:41, 1995.

Kunin CM: Urinary tract infections in females, *Clin Infect Dis* 18:1, 1994.

Lipsky BA: Urinary tract infections in men: epidemiology, pathophysiology, diagnosis, and treatment, *Ann Intern Med* 110:138, 1989.

Ronald AR, Harding GKM: Complicated urinary tract infections, *Infect Dis Clin North Am* 11:583, 1997.

Stamm WE, Hooton TM: Management of urinary tract infections in adults, *N Engl J Med* 329:1328, 1993.

Stapleton A, Stamm WE: Prevention of urinary tract infections, *Infect Dis Clin Am* 11:719, 1997.

Warren JA, et al: Guidelines for antimicrobial therapy of uncomplicated acute bacterial cystitis and acute pyelonephritis, *Clin Infect Dis* 29:745, 1999.

Wood CA, Abrutyn E: Urinary tract infection in older adults, *Clin Geriatr Med* 14:267, 1998.

CANDIDURIA

Jack D. Sobel

The prevalence of candiduria in hospitals has increased by 200% to 300% in the last decade such that in a community hospital, 5% of urine cultures may yield *Candida,* and in tertiary care centers, *Candida* accounts for almost 10% of urinary isolates, including a quarter of Foley catheter–associated infections. Most positive *Candida* urine cultures are isolated or transient findings of little significance and represent colonization rather than true infection. Although fewer than 10% of candidemias are the consequence of candiduria, *Candida* urinary tract infections (UTIs) have emerged as important nosocomial infections.

Candida albicans is the most common species isolated from the urine, whereas non-*albicans Candida* species account for almost half the *Candida* urine isolates. *Candida glabrata* is responsible for 25% to 35% of infections.

■ PREDISPOSING FACTORS

Candiduria is rare in the absence of predisposing factors. Most infections are associated with use of Foley catheters, internal stents, and percutaneous nephrostomy tubes. Diabetic patients, especially when their diabetes is poorly controlled, are particularly at risk primarily because of increased instrumentation, urinary stasis, and obstruction secondary to autonomic neuropathy. Concomitant bacteriuria is common. Antimicrobials similarly play a critical role in that candiduria almost always emerges during or immediately after antibiotic therapy. Antibiotics, especially broad-spectrum agents, act by suppressing protective indigenous bacterial flora in the gastrointestinal (GI) tract and lower genital tract, facilitating *Candida* colonization of these sites with ready access to the urinary tract. The pool of critically ill, immunosuppressed medical and surgical patients has increased, and this increase, together with improved technology, provides an expanded population at risk of developing *Candida* infection.

Most lower UTIs are caused by retrograde infection from an indwelling catheter or genital or perineal colonization. The upper urinary tract is uncommonly involved during ascending infection and then only in the presence of urinary obstruction, reflux, or diabetes. Renal candidiasis is usually the consequence of secondary hematogenous seeding of the renal parenchyma; *Candida* species have a unique tropism for the kidney.

■ CLINICAL ASPECTS

Most patients with candiduria are asymptomatic, especially those with indwelling bladder catheters. Clinical manifestations depend on the site of infection. *Candida* cystitis may present with frequency, dysuria, urgency, hematuria, and pyuria. Ascending infection resulting in *Candida* pyelonephritis is characterized by fever, leukocytosis, and rigors and is indistinguishable from bacterial pyelonephritis. Excretory urography may reveal ureteropelvic fungus balls or papillary narcosis. Renal candidiasis is difficult to diagnose when secondary to hematogenous spread and presents with fever and other signs of sepsis. By the time renal candidiasis is considered, blood cultures are usually no longer positive; however, unexplained deteriorating renal function is often evident.

Because isolation of *Candida* from a urine specimen may represent contamination, colonization, or superficial or deep infection of the lower or upper urinary tract, diagnosis is difficult and management depends on the site of infection. Contamination of the sample is particularly common in women with vulvovaginal colonization and may be excluded by repeating urine culture with special attention to proper collection techniques. Differentiating infection from colonization may be extremely difficult if not impossible in some patients, especially if they are catheterized. Accordingly, I often rely on accompanying clinical features to determine the significance of candiduria; unfortunately these are often nonspecific in critically ill patients, and fever and leukocytosis may have several other sources.

Quantitative urine colony counts have some value in separating infection from colonization but only in the absence of a Foley catheter. The latter negates any diagnostic value of quantitative cultures. In noncatheterized patients, counts greater than 10^4 CFU/ml are usually associated with infection. It is rare for patients with invasive disease of the kidney, pelvis, or bladder to have 10^3 CFU/ml or less. Most patients with urinary tract *Candida* infection have pyuria, but the value of this finding is similarly diminished in the presence of a catheter or concomitant bacteriuria and in neutropenic subjects. Serologic tests of *Candida* tissue invasion are not available. Treatment is preceded by attempts to localize the source or anatomic level of infection. Unfortunately, no reliable tests to differentiate renal candidiasis from the more frequent lower tract infections exist. The extremely rare finding of *Candida* microorganisms and pseudohyphae enmeshed in renal tubular casts is useful when present. Ultrasonography and computed tomography (CT) scans have a useful but limited role in localization. A 5-day bladder irrigation with amphotericin B may be of value in localizing the source of candiduria in catheterized subjects in that postirrigation persistent candiduria originates from above the bladder, thus identifying patients with need for further studies. Unfortunately, the lengthy nature of this diagnostic test excludes its utility in most febrile, critically ill subjects.

■ PROGNOSIS

Prognosis depends on the anatomic site of *Candida* infection and the presence of urinary drainage tubes, obstruction, and concomitant renal failure. A high mortality rate of 20% is found in candiduria patients, which is more a reflection of the multiple serious illnesses found in these patients than the consequence of candiduria per se.

■ MANAGEMENT

More important than the knowledge of antifungal agents for treating candiduria is understanding the indications and rational basis for initiating treatment. Regrettably, despite the availability of a variety of potent antifungal agents, data from controlled studies are scant.

■ ASYMPTOMATIC CANDIDURIA

No antifungal therapy is required for asymptomatic candiduria, a common condition, because candiduria often is transient only and even if persistent rarely results in serious morbidity. Moreover, relapse of candiduria is common if the patient remains catheterized: An exception to observation only is the presence of asymptomatic candiduria after renal transplantation. In catheterized patients, removal of the catheter and discontinuation of antibiotics often results in cessation of candiduria (40%). Change of catheter results in elimination of candiduria in only approximately 20% of patients. However, persistent candiduria in noncatheterized patients should be investigated because the likelihood of obstruction and stasis is high. Patients with asymptomatic candiduria in whom urologic instrumentation or surgery is planned should have candiduria eliminated or suppressed before and during the procedure to prevent precipitating invasive candidiasis and candidemia. Successful elimination can be achieved by amphotericin B irrigation using a concentration of 50 μg/dl of sterile water for 7 days or with systemic therapy using amphotericin B, flucytosine, or fluconazole. Fluconazole, 200 mg/day, oral therapy should continue for at least 14 days to maximize cure rates.

■ *CANDIDA* CYSTITIS

Symptomatic cystitis requires treatment with either amphotericin B bladder irrigation (50 μg/dl) or systemic therapy, once more using intravenous (IV) amphotericin B, flucytosine, or oral azole agents. Of the oral azole agents, both ketoconazole and itraconazole are poorly excreted in the urine and there is limited and suboptimal clinical experience only. In contrast, fluconazole is water soluble, well absorbed orally with more than 80% excreted unchanged in the urine, and despite limited experience, appears highly effective. The optimal dose and duration of fluconazole therapy has yet to be determined, but usually 200 mg/day is prescribed for 7 to 10 days. Similarly, the duration of therapeutic bladder irrigation with amphotericin B is arbitrary, lasting 5 to 7 days. This amphotericin B therapy is extremely labor intensive. Flucytosine is also excreted unchanged in high concentrations in the urine and is highly active against most *Candida* species, including *C. glabrata;* nevertheless, because resistance develops rapidly to flucytosine when used alone, this agent is rarely used.

Single-dose IV amphotericin B, 0.3 mg/kg, has also been shown to be highly efficacious in the treatment of lower urinary tract candidiasis, achieving therapeutic urine concentrations for considerable time after the single administration. More prolonged systemic IV amphotericin B (7 to 10 days) and at conventional dosage of 0.5 to 0.7 mg/kg/day is preferable for resistant fungal species.

■ ASCENDING PYELONEPHRITIS AND *CANDIDA* UROSEPSIS

Invasive upper UTI requires systemic antifungal therapy as well as immediate investigation and visualization of the urinary drainage system to exclude obstruction, papillary necrosis, and fungus ball formation. Appropriate therapy includes IV amphotericin B, 0.5 to 0.7 mg/kg/day, for a variable duration depending on severity of infection, presence of candidemia, and response to therapy, in general 1 to 2 g total dose. Systemic therapy with fluconazole, 5 to 10 mg/kg/day (IV or oral) for at least 2 weeks offers an effective and less-toxic alternative regimen. Infection refractory to medical management should be treated surgically with drainage, or in cases of a nonviable kidney, nephrectomy may be indicated. An obstructed kidney with hydronephrosis requires a percutaneous nephrostomy. In some cases, nephrostomy drainage must be combined with local amphotericin B irrigation (50 μg/dl), particularly with end-stage renal disease and low urinary levels of antifungal agents.

■ RENAL AND DISSEMINATED CANDIDIASIS

Management of renal candidiasis secondary to hematogenous spread is that of systemic candidiasis, including IV amphotericin B, 0.6 to 1.0 mg/kg/day, or IV fluconazole, 5 to 10 mg/kg/day. Dosage modifications of fluconazole are necessary in the presence of moderate to severe azotemia. Prognosis depends on correction of underlying factors, that is, resolution of neutropenia, removal of responsible intravascular catheters, and susceptibility of the *Candida* species, but most importantly the nature and prognosis of the underlying disease per se. Systemic candidiasis involving metastatic sites of infection requires prolonged therapy for approximately 4 to 6 weeks.

Suggested Reading

Ang BSP, et al: Candidemia from a urinary tract source: microbiological aspects and clinical significance, *Clin Infect Dis* 17:622, 1993.

Conzo JA, Dismukes WE: Oral azole drugs as systemic antifungal therapy, *N Engl J Med* 330:263, 1994.

Fisher JF, et al: Urinary tract infections due to *Candida albicans, Rev Infect Dis* 4:1107, 1982.

Kauffman CA, et al: A prospective multicenter surveillance study of funguria in hospitalized patients, *Clin Infect Dis* 30:14, 2000.

Rivett AG, Perry JA, Cohen J: Urinary candidiasis: a prospective study in hospitalized patients, *Urol Res* 14:153, 1986.

Sobel JD, et al: Candiduria—a randomized double blind study of treatment with fluconazole and placebo, *Clin Infect Dis* 30:19, 2000.

Wise GJ, Silver DA: Fungal infections of the genitourinary system, *J Urol* 149:1377, 1993.

FOCAL RENAL INFECTIONS AND PAPILLARY NECROSIS

L.M. Dembry
V.T. Andriole

Focal infections of the kidney can be divided into intrarenal and perirenal pathology (Table 1). The classification of intrarenal abscess encompasses renal cortical abscess and renal corticomedullary abscess; the latter includes acute focal bacterial nephritis, acute multifocal bacterial nephritis, and xanthogranulomatous pyelonephritis. Perirenal abscesses are found in the perinephric fascia external to the capsule of the kidney, generally occurring as a result of extension of an intrarenal abscess. Papillary necrosis is a clinicopathologic syndrome that develops during the course of a variety of syndromes, including pyelonephritis, affecting the renal medullary vasculature, which in turn leads to ischemic necrosis of the renal medulla.

■ RENAL CORTICAL ABSCESS

A renal cortical abscess results from hematogenous spread of bacteria from a primary focus of infection outside the kidney, often the skin. The most common causative agent is *Staphylococcus aureus* (90%). Predisposing conditions include entities associated with an increased risk for staphylococcal bacteremia, such as hemodialysis, diabetes mellitus, and injection drug use. The primary focus of infection may not be apparent in up to one third of cases. Ascending infection is an uncommon cause of renal cortical abscess formation. Ten percent of renal cortical abscesses rupture through the renal capsule, forming a perinephric abscess.

Patients present with chills, fever, and back or abdominal pain, with few or no localizing signs (Table 2). Most patients do not have urinary symptoms because the process is circumscribed in the cortex and does not generally communicate with the excretory passages. Costovertebral angle tenderness and involuntary guarding in the upper lumbar and abdominal musculature are often present on physical examination. A flank mass or bulge in the lumbar region with loss of lumbar lordosis may be present.

Table 1   Focal Renal Infections
Intrarenal abscesses
Renal cortical abscesses
Renal corticomedullary abscesses
Acute focal bacterial nephritis
Acute multifocal bacterial nephritis
Xanthogranulomatous pyelonephritis
Perinephric Abscesses

Radiologic techniques are useful in characterizing the renal mass and making the diagnosis. Ultrasonography is useful in the diagnosis of this entity and may be used to drain the abscess percutaneously and follow its response to therapy. Computed tomography (CT) is the most precise noninvasive technique for diagnosis because it yields the most accurate anatomic information. It may also be used as a guide to percutaneous aspiration.

Renal cortical abscesses often respond to antistaphylococcal antibiotics alone, and surgical intervention usually is not required. If the diagnosis of renal cortical abscess is suspected and bacteriologic evaluation of the urine reveals large, gram-positive cocci or no bacteria, antistaphylococcal therapy should be started promptly. A semisynthetic penicillin (oxacillin or nafcillin), 1 to 2 g every 4 to 6 hours, is appropriate empiric therapy. For penicillin-allergic patients, a first-generation cephalosporin, such as cefazolin, 2 g every 8 hours, may be used. Vancomycin, 15 mg/kg every 12 hours, should be used for patients with a severe immediate beta-lactam allergy. Parenteral antibiotics are administered for 10 days to 2 weeks, followed by oral antistaphylococcal therapy for at least an additional 2 to 4 weeks. Fever generally resolves after 5 to 6 days of antimicrobial therapy. If no response to therapy is seen in 48 hours, percutaneous aspiration should be considered, and if unsuccessful, open drainage should be undertaken. The prognosis is good if the diagnosis is made promptly and effective therapy is instituted immediately.

■ RENAL CORTICOMEDULLARY ABSCESS

Renal corticomedullary abscesses occur most commonly as a complication of bacteriuria and ascending infection accompanied by an underlying urinary tract abnormality. The most common abnormalities include obstructive processes, genitourinary abnormalities associated with diabetes mellitus or primary hyperparathyroidism, and vesicoureteral reflux. Enteric aerobic gram-negative bacilli, including *Escherichia coli*, *Klebsiella* species, and *Proteus* species, are commonly responsible for this infection. Acute focal bacterial nephritis, a severe form of acute bacterial interstitial nephritis involving a single renal lobe, represents focal inflammation of the kidney without frank abscess formation and may be an early phase of acute multifocal bacterial nephritis. Xanthogranulomatous pyelonephritis is an uncommon but severe chronic infection of the renal parenchyma. It may be related to a combination of renal obstruction and chronic urinary tract infection. Predisposing factors include renal calculi, urinary obstruction, lymphatic obstruction, partially treated chronic urosepsis, renal ischemia and secondary metabolic alterations in lipid metabolism, abnormal host immune response, diabetes mellitus, and primary hyperparathyroidism.

Patients typically present with fever, chills, and flank or abdominal pain. Two thirds of patients have nausea and vomiting, and dysuria may not be present. Patients may have a history of recurrent urinary tract infections, renal calculi, or prior genitourinary instrumentation. On examination, 60% of patients will have a flank mass and 30% will have hepatomegaly. Patients with acute focal or multifocal bacte-

Table 2 Clinical and Laboratory Findings of Renal and Perirenal Abscesses

	RENAL CORTICAL ABSCESS	RENAL CORTICOMEDULLARY ABSCESS	PERINEPHRIC ABSCESS
Epidemiology	Males 3× > females, second through fourth decades, hematogenous seeding of the kidneys	Males = females (females > males in xanthogranuloma-tous pyelonephritis), incidence increases with age, associated with an underlying abnormality of the urinary tract	Males = females, 25% of patients are diabetic, rupture of an intra-renal suppurative focus into the perinephric space
Clinical presentation	Chills, fever, localized back or abdominal pain	Chills, fever, flank or abdominal pain, nausea and vomiting (65%)	Insidious onset over 2-3 wk; fever (early), flank pain (late)
Urinary symptoms	None*	Dysuria or other urinary tract symptoms variably present	Dysuria 40%
Physical examination	Flank mass	Flank mass in 60%, hepatomegaly in 30%	Flank or abdominal mass in <50%, 60% have abdominal tenderness
Organisms	*Staphylococcus aureus*	Enteric aerobic gram-negative rods (*Escherichia coli, Klebsiella* species, *Proteus mirabilis*)	Enteric aerobic gram-negative rods and *S. aureus;* occasionally *Pseudomonas* species, gram-positive bacteria, obligate anaerobic bacteria, fungi, mycobacteria; 25% polymicrobial
Urinalysis	Normal*	Abnormal in 70% of patients	Abnormal in 70% of patients
Urine cultures	Negative*	Generally positive	Positive in 60%
Blood cultures	Often negative	Often positive	Positive in 40%

*If there is no communication between the abscess and the collecting system.

rial nephritis are often bacteremic. Many patients (75%) are anemic, and up to 50% of patients with xanthogranuloma-tous pyelonephritis have hyperuricemia.

The nonspecific clinical presentation is associated with a variety of renal processes, including renal cortical abscess, perinephric abscess, renal cysts, and tumors. Radiographic techniques are necessary to differentiate these various processes. Ultrasonography and CT scanning are both used for diagnosing renal corticomedullary abscesses except for xanthogranulomatous pyelonephritis, in which ultrasound findings are less specific than CT findings.

Most patients with acute focal and multifocal bacterial nephritis manifest a clinical response to antibiotic treatment alone within 1 week of starting therapy. Patients generally have no sequelae after treatment. Radiologic techniques should be used to ensure resolution of the parenchymal abnormalities after clinical resolution. A large, well-established abscess may be more difficult to treat successfully with antimicrobial agents alone than an abscess identified early. An intensive trial of appropriate antibiotic therapy can be attempted before considering surgical drainage for lesions localized to the renal parenchyma. Parenteral antimicrobial agents and intravenous hydration should be administered promptly when the diagnosis is considered. Empiric antimicrobial therapy is directed against the common bacterial organisms in this setting, including *E. coli, Klebsiella,* and *Proteus* species (Table 3). An extended-spectrum penicillin (mezlocillin or piperacillin), an extended-spectrum cephalosporin (ceftriaxone or cefotaxime), or ciprofloxacin are all appropriate choices. Alternatively, an intravenous beta-lactam antibiotic, such as ampicillin or cefazolin, along with an aminoglycoside, can be administered until culture and sensitivity results are known. Antimicrobial therapy should be modified based on the results of culture and

sensitivity testing. Duration of therapy should be determined on a case-by-case basis. Current recommendations are to continue parenteral antimicrobial therapy for at least 24 to 48 hours after clinical improvement of symptoms and resolution of fever. Oral antibiotic therapy, based on antimicrobial susceptibility results, can then be administered for an additional 2 weeks.

Acute focal bacterial nephritis typically responds to antimicrobial therapy alone, with follow-up radiographic studies showing complete resolution of the intrarenal lesion. Most patients with acute multifocal bacterial nephritis improve with antibiotics alone, albeit slowly, and only occasionally is a drainage procedure necessary. Factors associated with failure to respond to antimicrobial therapy alone include large abscesses, obstructive uropathy, advanced age, and urosepsis. Percutaneous aspiration of the abscess combined with parenteral antibiotics has been successful in those requiring drainage. If obstructive uropathy is present, prompt drainage by percutaneous nephrostomy until the patient is stable and afebrile is appropriate, at which time the lesion should then be corrected. If open drainage is required, incision and drainage are done when possible. Nephrectomy is reserved for patients with diffusely damaged renal parenchyma or patients requiring urgent intervention for survival.

Patients with xanthogranulomatous pyelonephritis generally require surgical excision of the xanthogranulomatous process for cure of the disease, although there have been several case reports of successful treatment without surgical intervention. Once the tissue is removed, the xanthogranulomatous process ceases and does not recur; however, bacteriuria may recur and require treatment. After excision, the prognosis in those without other urinary pathologic conditions is excellent.

Table 3 Therapy of Renal and Perirenal Abscesses

	EMPIRIC THERAPY	DURATION	DRAINAGE	SURGERY
RENAL CORTICAL ABSCESS	Semisynthetic penicillin: oxacillin or nafcillin (1-2 g IV q4-6h) *Penicillin allergy:* First-generation cephalosporin (cefazolin, 2 g IV q8h; cephalothin 2 g IV q4h) or vancomycin (15 mg/kg IV q12h) if severe immediate beta-lactam allergy	Intravenous antibiotics for 10 days to 2 wk followed by 2-4 wk of an oral antistaphylococcal antibiotic (dicloxacillin, 500 mg q6h, or cephalexin, 500 mg q6h)	If no response to treatment after 48 hr, then percutaneous drainage followed by open drainage if no response	
RENAL CORTICOMEDULLARY ABSCESS				
Acute focal bacterial nephritis	Extended-spectrum penicillin (mezlocillin, 3 g IV q4h, or piperacillin 3-4 g IV q4-6h), extended-spectrum cephalosporin (ceftriaxone 1 g IV q24h, or cefotaxime, 1 g q8h), fluoroquinolone (ciprofloxacin, 200-400 mg IV q12h), ampicillin (1 g IV q4-6h) with gentamicin, or cefazolin (1 g q8h) with gentamicin	Intravenous for 24-48 hr after resolution of symptoms and fever followed by 2 wk of oral antibiotics based on results of susceptibility testing (cefpodoxime, 200 mg q12h, or ciprofloxacin, 500 mg q12h)	Generally not necessary	
Acute multifocal bacterial nephritis	Same as acute focal bacterial nephritis	Intravenous for 24-48 hr after resolution of symptoms and fever followed by 2 wk of oral antibiotics	If slow response to antibiotics or large abscess, presence of obstructive uropathy, urosepsis, or advanced age	
Xanthogranulomatous pyelonephritis	Same as acute focal bacteria nephritis	Intravenous for 24-48 hr after resolution of symptoms and fever followed by 2 wk of oral antibiotics		Surgical excision usually necessary for cure (partial nephrectomy or total nephrectomy)
PERINEPHRIC ABSCESS	Antistaphylococcal agent with an aminoglycoside or an extended-spectrum beta-lactam agent. If *Pseudomonas aeruginosa* is isolated, an antipseudomonal beta-lactam (mezlocillin, piperacillin, cefoperazone, 2 g IV q12h; ceftazidime, 2 g IV q8h) should be added to the aminoglycoside Alternatively, ciprofloxacin, 200-400 mg IV q12h, can be added and the aminoglycoside discontinued; for enterococcus, the treatment of choice is ampicillin, 2 g IV q4-6h (or vancomycin, 15 mg/kg IV q12h for penicillin-allergic patients) plus gentamicin	Initial parenteral therapy until clinical improvement, change to appropriate oral therapy until radiographic studies indicate resolution of process	Requires percutaneous drainage followed by open surgical drainage if no resolution	Nephrectomy in cases that do not resolve with antibiotics and drainage

■ PERINEPHRIC ABSCESS

The common etiologic agents of intrarenal abscesses, *E. coli, Proteus* species, and *S. aureus,* are also the common organisms associated with perinephric abscesses. Other gram-negative bacilli associated with this entity are *Klebsiella* species, *Enterobacter* species, *Pseudomonas* species, *Serratia* species, and *Citrobacter* species. Occasionally, enterococci are implicated, and anaerobic bacteria may account for culture-negative abscesses. Fungi, particularly *Candida* species, are also important, as is *Mycobacterium tuberculosis.* Perinephric abscesses may be polymicrobial in up to 25% of cases.

A perinephric abscess is a collection of suppurative material in the perinephric space between the renal capsule and Gerota's fascia. Most perirenal abscesses result from the rupture of an intrarenal abscess into the perinephric space, chronic or recurrent pyelonephritis (particularly in the presence of obstruction), or xanthogranulomatous pyelonephritis. Predisposing conditions for perinephric abscesses are similar to those for intrarenal abscesses. Most patients have underlying urinary tract abnormalities, usually obstruction. Patients with chronic or recurrent urinary tract infections, with or without calculi, may also be at increased risk. Up to 25% of patients are diabetic.

The symptoms develop insidiously over 2 to 3 weeks. Fever is the most common presenting symptom and is present in virtually all patients. Unilateral flank pain is common (70% to 80%), and chills and dysuria are less common (40%). Flank and costovertebral angle tenderness is often present on examination, and 60% of patients may have abdominal tenderness. Half the patients have a flank or abdominal mass, and referred pain is not uncommon.

The key to making this diagnosis is considering this entity in the differential and doing the appropriate radiographic studies. CT scanning is the study of choice because it identifies the abscess and defines its extent beyond the renal capsule and the surrounding anatomy, including extension into the psoas muscle. The diagnosis should be strongly considered in any patient with a febrile illness and unilateral flank pain that does not respond to therapy for acute pyelonephritis.

Early recognition, prompt drainage, and antimicrobial therapy have all contributed to a decrease in the mortality associated with this entity. However, antimicrobial therapy alone is not adequate and should be used in conjunction with percutaneous drainage performed under CT or ultrasound guidance. Surgical drainage is considered when percutaneous drainage fails or is contraindicated. Acute nephrectomy is occasionally indicated. Empiric antimicrobial therapy should be directed against the most common gram-negative pathogens and *S. aureus.* An aminoglycoside (gentamicin or tobramycin) and an antistaphylococcal beta-lactam (oxacillin, nafcillin, or cefazolin) are appropriate initial antibiotics. An extended-spectrum beta-lactam may be used in place of an aminoglycoside for gram-negative coverage in patients with abnormal renal function. Once culture results are obtained, therapy should be modified accordingly. When *Pseudomonas aeruginosa* is cultured, an antipseudomonal beta-lactam (mezlocillin, piperacillin, cefoperazone, or ceftazidime) should be added to the ami-

Table 4 Conditions Associated with Development of Papillary Necrosis
Diabetes mellitus
Pyelonephritis
Obstruction
Analgesic abuse
Sickle cell disease
Renal transplantation

noglycoside; alternatively, the aminoglycoside may be discontinued and ciprofloxacin given. If enterococcus is isolated, ampicillin plus gentamicin is the treatment of choice. Isoniazid plus rifampin are indicated for *Mycobacterium tuberculosis* infections; ethambutol and streptomycin may also be used in combination with these. (Refer to the chapter *Tuberculosis* for more detail.) Amphotericin B is necessary for treatment of fungal abscesses. Perirenal abscesses may cause ureteral compression, giving rise to hydronephrosis. Even after drainage, ureteral stenosis from periureteritis may evolve during the healing process, which is a late complication of this disease.

■ RENAL PAPILLARY NECROSIS

Renal papillary necrosis is an uncommon severe complication of pyelonephritis (2% to 5% of patients) that occurs most often in patients with underlying structural renal abnormalities or host immunocompromise (more than half of patients are diabetic) (Table 4). When papillary necrosis is caused by infection, both kidneys are often affected, with one or more pyramids involved. As the lesion progresses, a portion of the necrotic papilla may break off, producing a calyceal deformity that results in a recognizable radiologic filling defect. The sloughed portion may be voided and in some instances can be recovered from the urine.

Patients present with worsening symptoms of preexisting pyelonephritis. They may have lumbar pain, hematuria, and fever. The diagnosis should be considered in diabetic patients with active pyelonephritis who experience a rapid clinical deterioration and/or worsening renal function.

Therapy is directed toward control of infection generally caused by the common uropathogens, including *E. coli, Proteus* species, and *Klebsiella* species (see recommendations for treatment of renal corticomedullary abscesses, Table 3). If the patient does not respond promptly to appropriate antimicrobial therapy and infection is not controlled, nephrectomy may need to be considered.

Suggested Reading

Brown BS, Dodson M, Weintraub PS: Xanthogranulomatous pyelonephritis: report of nonsurgical management of a case and review of the literature, *Clin Infect Dis* 22:308, 1996.

Dembry LM, Andriole VT: Renal and perirenal abscesses, *Infect Dis Clin North Am* 11:663, 1997.

Eknoyan G, Qunibi WY, Grissom RT: Renal papillary necrosis: an update, *Medicine* 61:55, 1982.

Kaplan DM, Rosenfield AT, Smith RC: Advances in the imaging of renal infection, *Infect Dis Clin North Am* 11:681, 1997.

C MUSCULOSKELETAL SYSTEM

INFECTION OF NATIVE AND PROSTHETIC JOINTS

Shahbaz Hasan
James W. Smith

■ NATIVE JOINT INFECTIONS

Infections of native joints generally occur in patients with predisposing factors such as trauma, underlying arthritis, immunosuppressive therapy, diabetes mellitus, malignancies, intravenous drug abuse, and other infections (e.g., endocarditis, skin infections, urinary tract infections). Hematogenous spread of the organism through the highly vascular synovial space leads to an influx of polymorphonuclear leukocytes (PMLs) into the synovium, then to a release of enzymes that destroy the articular surface.

Diagnosis

Patients present with pain and limited motion of the joint. Fever may be mild, with only a few patients having a temperature higher than 39° C (102.2° F). Joint tenderness can be minimal to severe, but most patients have swelling as a result of joint effusions in response to the infection. Involvement of multiple joints is seen in 10% to 20% of cases, especially in viral arthritis and rheumatoid arthritis. Laboratory findings suggestive of septic arthritis include an elevated erythrocyte sedimentation rate and synovial fluid cell counts exceeding 50,000/ml, with more than 75% PMLs. In no individual case do any of these findings distinguish infected from inflammatory arthritis, such as rheumatoid or crystalline arthropathy, so the diagnosis is based on cultures of synovial fluid. On occasion, blood cultures may be positive. In patients with a chronic monarticular process caused by mycobacterial or fungal organisms, synovial tissue cultures provide a better yield than synovial fluid cultures. Serum antibody tests provide the diagnosis of Lyme or viral arthritis. Polymerase chain reaction (PCR) assay of the joint fluid may yield the diagnosis in partially treated patients or in patients infections caused by fastidious organisms such as *Mycoplasma, Chlamydia,* or *Borrelia burgdorferi* (Lyme disease). Plain radiographs are seldom of use diagnostically.

Computed tomography (CT) and magnetic resonance imaging (MRI) provide more detail of the surrounding soft tissue and may reveal adjacent osteomyelitis. Radionuclear scans may be needed to visualize the sacroiliac joint; however, they are unable to distinguish septic arthritis from other inflammatory arthritis.

Staphylococcus aureus is the most common organism isolated in native bacterial arthritis. However, a variety of other gram-positive and gram-negative organisms have been reported as agents in monarticular bacterial arthritis. *Neisseria gonorrhoeae* is the main cause of bacterial arthritis in sexually active individuals with no underlying joint disease. It presents with a syndrome of fever, skin lesions, and polyarticular involvement, often with associated tenosynovitis. Any of a number of mycobacterial and fungal organisms can cause a chronic, slowly progressive infection of a single joint with tenosynovitis. Viral agents commonly associated with arthritis include rubella and parvovirus B19 (erythema infectiosum, or fifth disease) in women and mumps in men. Hepatitis B infection may manifest as a prodromal syndrome consisting of arthritis and urticaria that disappear with the onset of jaundice.

Therapy

Empiric antimicrobial therapy for suspected bacterial arthritis is started after obtaining appropriate fluid specimens for analysis and culture. The choice of antibiotics depends on the patient's age, risk factors, and results of the synovial fluid Gram stain (Figure 1). The antibiotics are modified after obtaining the culture results. The usual course of antibiotics is 2 weeks. Infections from staphylococci and gram-negative bacilli require 3 weeks of treatment. Mycobacterial and fungal infections are treated for up to a year. Initial therapy by causative organism is given in Table 1.

Infected joint effusions require repeated needle aspirations of recurrent joint effusions during the first 5 to 7 days of antimicrobial therapy. Most patients respond to needle aspiration. If the volume of fluid and number and percentage of PMLs decrease with each aspiration, no drainage is required. However, if the effusion persists for more than 7 days or the cell count does not decrease, surgical drainage is indicated. Surgical drainage is also indicated when effective decompression with needle aspiration is unlikely (hip joint) or when the joint is not accessible for aspiration (sternoclavicular and sacroiliac joints); if the joint space has become loculated as a result of formation of adhesions; or if thick, purulent material resisting aspiration is encountered. Arthroscopic drainage is an alternative to open drainage for the knee, shoulder, and ankle joints.

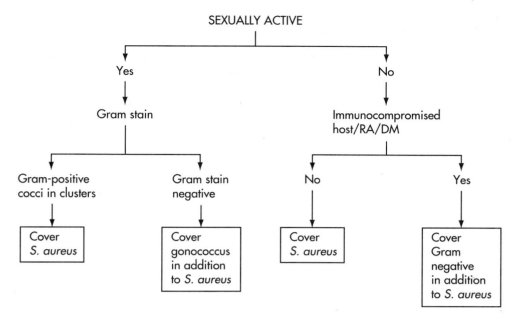

Figure 1
Empiric antibiotic coverage for nontraumatic, acute monoarticular arthritis.

Table 1   Therapy for Bacterial Arthritis of Native Joints

MICROORGANISM/INFECTION	TREATMENT	DURATION
Staphylococcus aureus	Penicillinase-resistant penicillins,* first-generation cephalosporin,† or cefuroxime, 1.5 g q8h	3 wk
Methicillin-resistant *S. aureus* or patient allergic to penicillin	Vancomycin, 1 g q12h	3 wk
Streptococci	Penicillin G, 4 million units q6h, or first-generation cephalosporin† or clindamycin, 300 mg q8h	2 wk
Gram-negative bacilli	Antipseudomonal cephalosporins,‡ carbapenem,§ quinolone‖	3 wk
Disseminated gonococcal infection	Ceftriaxone, 1 g q24h until response, then cefixime, 400 mg PO bid	7-10 days
Septic gonococcal arthritis	Ceftriaxone, 1 g q24h, or quinolone	3 wk
Lyme arthritis	Doxycycline, 100 mg PO bid, or ceftriaxone, 2 g q24h IV	4 wk, 2 wk
Mycobacterium tuberculosis	Isoniazid, 300 mg/day, plus rifampin, 600 mg/day, with ethambutol, 15 mg/kg/day, and pyrazinamide, 1500 mg/day for the first 2 mo	1 yr
Fungal arthritis	Amphotericin B, 0.5-0.7 mg/kg/day for a total of 2 g, then itraconazole, 200-400 mg/day PO, or fluconazole, 200-400 mg/day PO	1 yr

*Nafcillin, 2 g q6h IV.
†Cefazolin, 1 g q8h IV, or cephalothin, 1-2 g q6h IV.
‡Ceftazidime, 2 g q8h IV, or cefepime, 1 g q12h IV.
§Imipenem-cilastatin, 500 mg q6h IV, or meropenem, 500 mg q8h IV.
‖Ciprofloxacin, 400 mg q12h IV, or levofloxacin, 500 mg q24h IV.

Prognosis

Bacterial arthritis is associated with a mortality of 10% to 15%. Up to 25% to 50% of surviving patients are left with residual loss of joint function. Poor outcomes are commonly seen in the elderly and those with severe underlying joint disease, hip infections, or infections caused by mycobacterial or fungal agents.

■ PROSTHETIC JOINT INFECTIONS

Prosthetic joint surgery has been used with increasing frequency over the past three decades. About 400,000 arthroplasties are performed in the United States each year. Although most procedures involve the hip and knee joints, arthroplasties of the elbow, shoulder, and wrist are also

Table 2   Microbiology of Prosthetic Joint Infections

ORGANISM	PERCENTAGE
Staphylococcus aureus	25
Coagulase-negative staphylococci	25
Streptococci	5-10
Enterococci	3-5
Gram-negative bacilli	8-10
Anaerobes	5-10
Mixed	10-15
Others (fungi, mycobacteria, actinomyces, brucella)	1-2

being performed. Primary indications for surgery generally include rheumatoid arthritis, degenerative joint disease, fractures, and septic arthritis.

Ten-year implant survival rates of 70% to 90% are being achieved at most centers as a result of recent technical advances. Most failures result from aseptic loosening of the prosthesis, with infectious complications accounting for fewer than 1% of implant failures. These prosthesis infections necessitate extensive surgical procedures and prolonged use of antibiotics, all of which result in increased cost, morbidity, and rarely, mortality. Risk factors for the development of prosthesis infection include rheumatoid arthritis, previous surgeries at the joint, postoperative wound infection, hematoma, and unhealed or draining wounds at hospital discharge. Other risk factors reported by some authors include skin ulcers, obesity, age, use of steroids, diabetes mellitus, and distant site infections, especially urinary tract and skin infections. Varying frequency of infection is noted with different joints: incidence of infections for hip arthroplasties is less than 1%; for knees, 1% to 2%; and for elbows, 4% to 9%.

Direct inoculation of the joint at the time of surgery and intraoperative airborne contamination probably account for most infections. Evidence of the importance of this is demonstrated by the preponderance of infections caused by skin commensals (Table 2) and by reduction in frequency of infection that accompanies the use of prophylactic antibiotics. Hematogenous seeding of the implants is implicated in infections occurring more than 2 years postoperatively.

Diagnosis

The diagnosis of acute prosthetic joint infection is suspected in those who develop pain and fever within 6 months of the procedure. These findings are similar to those of acute septic arthritis in a native joint. However, most infections tend to be indolent and manifest with local pain and mechanical loosening of the prosthesis. Clinical features, laboratory tests, and imaging techniques may be insufficient to differentiate between aseptic and septic complications (Table 3). Infection must be suspected because aseptic loosening would be managed with a one-stage revision, whereas infections require extensive debridement, prolonged antibiotics, and often delayed reimplantation. Hence, the diagnosis of an infection often has to be confirmed on the basis of the intraoperative appearance of the tissues and the presence or absence of acute inflammatory reaction on the intraoperative histopathology specimens. Given the heterogeneity of

organisms (see Table 2), the joint fluid and tissues must be submitted for aerobic and anaerobic bacterial, fungal, and mycobacterial cultures.

Therapy

The object of successful management of prosthetic joint infections is twofold: eradication of infection and maintenance of functional integrity of the joint. Two-stage reimplantations offer the best possible outcome. However, not all patients may be suitable candidates for this extreme surgical undertaking because of poor bone stock, inability to withstand prolonged immobilization, or inability to eradicate the infectious agent. Such cases may call for other salvage techniques that usually sacrifice joint function for microbiologic cure (Table 4). Antibiotic selection is based on the susceptibility pattern of the organisms isolated through joint aspiration or intraoperative joint tissue and fluid cultures. The antibiotics of choice for the isolated organisms are similar to those used in native joint infections (see Table 1). Unlike native joint infections, the most common organisms isolated in prosthetic joint infections are coagulase-negative staphylococci (see Table 2). Therefore this organism should not be considered a contaminant but should be treated with vancomycin, 1 g intravenously (IV) twice daily, to which some would add rifampin. If the prosthesis is removed, parentral antibiotics are administered for 6 weeks; however, if management includes retention of the prosthesis, a prolonged course of oral antibiotics (6 months to 1 year) should be given after the completion of the course of parenteral antibiotics. With regard to staphylococci, oral agents may include quinolones, if susceptible, such as ciprofloxacin, 750 mg twice daily, or levofloxacin, 500 mg once daily, combined with rifampin, 600 mg once daily. Other alternatives include minocycline or doxycycline, 100 mg twice daily.

Prevention

Prophylactic antibiotic coverage generally includes agents directed against the most common causative agents, that is, gram-positive cocci. A penicillinase-resistant penicillin or a first-generation cephalosporin may achieve this. The antimicrobial agents are administered within 30 to 60 minutes of surgery and are continued for up to 24 postoperatively. Antibiotic-impregnated beads and cement have also been used extensively because they have the advantage of delivering high local levels of antibiotics with minimal systemic toxicity. Laminar air-flow devices and body exhaust suits have been recommended to prevent intraoperative contamination; however, it is unclear whether these considerably expensive techniques are cost-effective.

There is no convincing evidence of benefit of routine prophylaxis with antibiotics for patients with prosthetic joints undergoing uncomplicated dental, urinary, or gastrointestinal procedures. The risk of infection is similar to that of endocarditis developing in the general population. In a joint advisory statement, however, the American Dental Association and the American Academy of Orthopedic Surgeons have suggested prophylaxis regimens similar to those set out by the American Heart Association for endocarditis in certain high-risk patients undergoing high-risk dental procedures. See the chapter *Nonsurgical Antimicrobial Prophylaxis.*

Table 3   Diagnostic Features of Prosthetic Joint Infections

	SUGGESTIVE FINDINGS	COMMENTS
History	Rest pain; lack of postoperative pain-free interval; difficult wound healing; fever	These findings are not specific; they may also be found in aseptic loosening of the prosthesis. Infected prosthesis may be asymptomatic.
Physical findings	Swelling; tenderness; limitation of motion; fever	As above.
Laboratory tests	Leukocytosis; ESR >30 mm; raised CRP	Elevations in these parameters noted in most acute infections but may be normal in chronic, indolent infections.
Radiology	Periostitis; endosteal scalloping; focal or diffuse osteolysis	Radiologic findings may be normal. Cannot distinguish mechanical loosening from septic arthritis.
Nuclear imaging	Enhanced uptake in the region of the prosthesis	Subjective and reader dependent. Sequential bone and tagged white cell scans provide greater sensitivity and specificity than if done alone. Provides no information about organisms.
Joint aspiration	Positive cultures	Sensitivity 60%-80%; specificity 85%-95%; dry taps 10%-15%. More useful in symptomatic cases; provides specific information about organisms and sensitivities; detection of previously undetected infections.

ESR, Erythrocyte sedimentation rate; *CRP,* C-reactive protein.

Table 4   Treatment Options for Prosthetic Joint Infections

TECHNIQUE	METHOD	COMMENTS
Reimplantation (exchange arthroplasty)	Removal of prosthesis and cement, immediate reimplantation (one stage) or delayed reimplantation (two stages)	Technique of choice. Excellent functional results and good microbiologic cure. Patient must be physically able to undergo major surgery and prolonged immobilization. Adequate bone stock necessary for reimplantation.
Resection arthroplasty	Removal of prosthesis and cement, extensive debridement of adjacent bone	Used if reimplantation not possible because of major bone loss, recurrent infections, poorly responsive organisms (e.g., fungi) and patient mobility not essential. Provides good microbiologic cure at the expense of joint function.
Arthrodesis	Removal of prosthesis and cement and fusion of joint	If mobility is needed but patient cannot undergo reimplantation. May require prolonged immobilization.
Amputation		Radical treatment may be necessary following multiple revision attempts, intractable pain, or life-threatening infection.
Implant salvage	Chronic antibiotic suppression, alone or with local debridement and retention of prosthesis	Indicated if patient is unable or refuses to undergo major surgery. May be successful in <20% provided duration of symptoms <2 wk, no sinus drainage, no radiologic evidence of loosening, and the microorganism is highly susceptible to antibiotics.

Suggested Reading

Donatto KC: Orthopedic management of septic arthritis, *Rheum Clin North Am* 24:275, 1998.

Garvin KL, Hanssen AD: Infection after total hip arthroplasty: past, present and future, *J Bone Joint Surg* 77-A:1576, 1995.

Kaandorp CJE, et al: Risk factors for septic arthritis in patients with joint disease: a prospective study, *Arthritis Rheum* 38:1819, 1995.

Karchmer AW: Editorial response: salvage of infected orthopedic devices, *Clin Infect Dis* 27:714, 1998.

Smith JW, Piercy E: Infectious arthritis, *Clin Infect Dis* 20:225, 1995.

BURSITIS

Richard H. Parker

Inflammation of bursal sacs, or bursitis, is a common condition that may involve any one of the more than 150 bursal sacs in the human body. However, most cases of bursitis involve the olecranon or the prepatellar bursa. Approximately one third of cases may be septic, with the majority being related to trauma and a few secondary to rheumatologic disorders. It is important to recognize that trauma can cause both septic and nonseptic bursitis. Septic bursitis can occur as a complication of bacteremia without a history of trauma to the involved area. A common cause of septic bursitis is the injection of medication, often corticosteroids, into a bursa as treatment for nonseptic bursitis.

Clinical features often help differentiate septic from nonseptic bursitis when superficial bursa such as the olecranon and prepatellar bursa are inflamed, but both may be inflamed and tender. Bursitis of deeper bursa is more often nonseptic, but tuberculous bursitis of the greater trochanter and other sites have occurred. *Staphylococcus aureus* is the most common microorganism isolated from infected bursa, but any microorganism can infect these spaces if introduced. As with other infectious diseases, the immunocompromised host may be infected with unusual opportunistic microorganisms.

Diagnosis of septic bursitis requires aspiration of fluid for microscopy, culture, cell counts, and glucose (Table 1).

■ THERAPY

Following a decision as to whether the inflammation is infectious or noninfectious, therapy is started (Figure 1). Noninfectious bursitis is treated with immobilization, heat, and antiinflammatory agents and referred to orthopedics depending on the severity or response to therapy. Septic

Figure 1
Algorithm for the management of musculo-skeletal pain in area of a bursa.

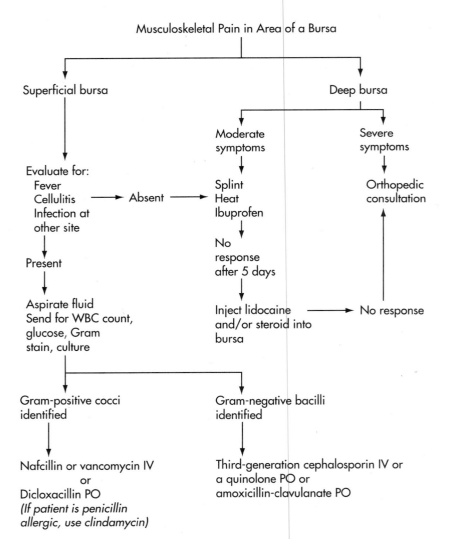

Musculoskeletal Pain in Area of a Bursa

Table 1   Findings in Bursal Fluid Related to Causes of Bursitis

FINDING	NORMAL	TRAUMA	SEPSIS	RHEUMATOID INFLAMMATION	MICROCRYSTALLINE INFLAMMATION
Color	Clear yellow	Bloody xanthochromic	Yellow, cloudy	Yellow, cloudy	Yellow, cloudy
WBC	0-200	<5000	1000-200,000	1000-20,000	1000-20,000
RBC	0	Many	Few	Few	Few
Glucose	Normal*	Normal*	Decreased	Decreased (slight)	Variable
Gram stain, culture	Negative	Negative	Positive	Negative	Negative

WBC, White blood cell; *RBC,* red blood cell.
*Fluid glucose/blood glucose = 0.6-1.

bursitis might require hospitalization for surgical drainage and intravenous antimicrobial therapy. However, if the patient is not septic or toxic, is not immunocompromised, and is considered compliant, therapy can be initiated with oral antimicrobial agents and the patient followed closely as an outpatient. Home intravenous infusion therapy is an option but must be restricted to therapy of methicillin-resistant *S. aureus* (MRSA) and similar other pathogens that require use of an intravenous drug such as vancomycin or patients who cannot tolerate oral medications.

Initial therapy must use a good antistaphylococcal agent. In areas where MRSA are common, intravenous vancomycin should be initiated. Therapy to cover an infection caused by gram-negative bacilli and/or anaerobes should be started if the septic bursitis occurs in the lower extremity or in an immunocompromised patient. Oral antimicrobial agents, if not started initially, can be used within 48 to 72 hours. Depending on Gram stain and culture results, the oral drug

could be dicloxacillin, amoxicillin-clavulanate, advanced-generation quinolone, or a cephalosporin. Well-tolerated, once-a-day therapy is considered preferable for compliance. Total duration of therapy is usually 3 to 4 weeks. The recurrence of fluid after initial aspiration requires re-aspiration and consideration for surgical drainage or bursectomy.

Suggested Reading

Garcia-Porrua C, et al: The clinical spectrum of severe septic bursitis in northwestern Spain: a 10 year study, *J Rheumatol* 26:663, 1999.

Ho G, Tice AD: Comparison of nonseptic and septic bursitis, *Arch Intern Med* 139:1269, 1979.

Jaovisidha S, et al: Tuberculous tenosynovitis and bursitis: imaging findings in 21 cases, *Radiology* 201:507, 1996.

Stell IM: Septic and non-septic olecranon bursitis in the accident and emergency department—an approach to management, *J Accid Emerg Med* 13:351, 1996.

ACUTE AND CHRONIC OSTEOMYELITIS

Daniel P. Lew
Francis A. Waldvogel

Osteomyelitis is a progressive infectious process involving the various components of bone, namely periosteum, medullary cavity, and cortical bone. The disease is characterized by progressive, inflammatory destruction of bone; by necrosis; and by new bone apposition.

Acute osteomyelitis evolves over several days to weeks: the term *acute* is used in opposition to *chronic* osteomyelitis,

a disease characterized by clinical symptoms that persist for several weeks followed by long-standing infection that evolves over months or even years, by the persistence of microorganisms, by low-grade inflammation, by the presence of necrotic bone (sequestra) and foreign material, and by fistulous tracts. The terms *acute* and *chronic* do not have a sharp demarcation and are often used somewhat loosely. Nevertheless, they are useful clinical concepts in infectious diseases because they describe two different patterns of the same disease, caused by the same microorganisms, but with different evolutions.

■ CLINICAL MANIFESTATIONS AND CHARACTERISTICS OF THE PATHOGEN

From a practical point of view, it is useful to distinguish three types of osteomyelitis, which are described separately. Hematogenous osteomyelitis follows bacteremic spread, is seen mostly in prepubertal children and in elderly patients, and is characterized by local multiplication of bacteria within bone during septicemia. In most cases, infection is located in the metaphyseal area of long bones or in the spine. Osteomyelitis secondary to a contiguous focus of infection without vascular insufficiency follows trauma, organ perforation, or an orthopedic procedure. It implies a first infection, which by continuity gains access to bone. By definition, it can occur at any age and can involve any bone. It is useful to distinguish in this group patients with a foreign body implant because of its high susceptibility and necessity to remove the prosthesis to achieve cure.

Diabetic foot osteomyelitis has several important contributing factors leading to bone destruction: diabetes and its metabolic consequences, bone ischemia resulting from poor vascularisation, neuropathy, and infection.

■ TREATMENT

Basic Principles

The many pathogenic factors, modes of contamination, clinical presentations, and types of orthopedic procedures related to osteomyelitis have precluded a very scientific approach to therapy, with well-controlled, statistically valid studies; however, experimental models have helped clinicians understand some basic principles of antibiotic therapy. Thus, except for the fluoroquinolones, which penetrate unusually well into bone, bone antibiotic levels 3 to 4 hours after administration are usually low compared with serum levels; antibiotic treatment given parenterally has to be given for several weeks to achieve an acceptable cure rate; and early antibiotic treatment, given before extensive bone destruction has occurred, produces the best results. Finally, a combined antimicrobial and surgical approach should at least be discussed in all cases: whereas at one end of the spectrum (e.g., hematogenous osteomyelitis) surgery usually is unnecessary, at the other end (a consolidated infected fracture) cure may be achieved with minimal antibiotic treatment provided the foreign material is removed.

Microbiologic and Pathologic Criteria

If there is one area in which adequate sampling for bacteriology is important, this is the case of osteomyelitis because treatment will be given for many weeks, most often by a parenteral route following the results of the initial culture. Adequate sampling of deep infected tissue is thus extremely useful (in contrast to specimens obtained superficially from ulcers or from fistula, which are often misleading).

Results of Gram stain and culture, obtained ideally before therapy, should be analyzed carefully. The importance of histology (and intraoperative frozen section histology searching for neutrophil infiltrates) has also been shown in the setting of prosthetic joint infection.

Antimicrobial Therapy

Single-agent chemotherapy is usually adequate for the treatment of osteomyelitis of any type. A conventional choice of antimicrobial agents for the most commonly encountered microorganisms is given in Table 1. As a general principle, these antibiotics should be given parenterally for 4 to 6 weeks, as substantiated by experimental models.

In recent years, new approaches to antimicrobial therapy have been developed experimentally and validated clinically. Thus, in hematogenous osteomyelitis of childhood, initial parenteral administration of antibiotics may be followed with an equal success rate by completion of treatment with oral therapy for several weeks, provided that the organism is known, clinical signs abate rapidly, patient compliance is good, and serum antibiotic levels can be monitored. This approach has now also been validated in small series of adult patients. Another approach that is gaining acceptance because of its reduced cost is parenteral administration of antibiotics, first in hospital, then on an outpatient basis: effective as it is for hematogenous osteomyelitis, the question remains open whether this mode can be used for postsurgical osteomyelitis. Long-term oral therapy extending over months and more rarely years is aimed at palliation of acute flare-ups of chronic, refractory osteomyelitis. Recently, the combination of rifampin-quinolone orally has been used with success in small groups of patients for the therapy of staphylococcal osteomyelitis and particularly prosthetic infections. Local administration of antibiotics, either by instillation or by gentamicin-laden beads, has its advocates both in the United States and in Europe, but it has not been submitted to critical, controlled studies; antibiotic diffusion is limited in time and space but may be of some additional benefit in osteomyelitis secondary to a contiguous focus of infection. The fluoroquinolones have been one of the most interesting developments in this domain and have been shown to be quite efficient in experimental infections and in several randomized and nonrandomized studies in adults. Whereas their efficacy in the treatment of osteomyelitis caused by most *Enterobacteriaceae* seems undisputed, their advantage over conventional therapy in osteomyelitis caused by *Pseudomonas* or *Serratia* species as well as gram-positive organisms (in particular *Staphylococcus aureus*) remains to be demonstrated.

Finally, considerable progress has been achieved in the development of novel surgical approaches (bone graft, revascularization procedure, muscle flaps) that allow more rapid formation of new bone.

■ CLINICAL RESPONSE

Because of the protracted characteristics of osteomyelitis, *cure* is defined as the resolution of all signs and symptoms of active disease at the end of therapy and after a minimal posttreatment observation period of 1 year. By contrast, *failure* is defined as a lack of apparent response to therapy, as evidenced by one or more of the following: (1) persistence of drainage, (2) recurrence of a sinus tract or failure of a sinus tract to close, (3) persistence of systemic signs of infection (chills, fever, weight loss, bone pain), and (4) progression of bone infection shown by imaging methods (e.g., radiography, computed tomography [CT], or magnetic resonance imaging [MRI]).

■ HEMATOGENOUS OSTEOMYELITIS

Historically, hematogenous osteomyelitis has been described in children. It involves mostly the metaphysis of long bones

Table 1   Antibiotic Treatment of Osteomyelitis in Adults

MICROORGANISMS ISOLATED	TREATMENT OF CHOICE	ALTERNATIVES
Staphylococcus aureus		
Penicillin sensitive	Penicillin G (5 million units q6h)	A cephalosporin II[a] clindamycin (600 mg q6h), or vancomycin
Penicillin resistant	Nafcillin[b] (2 g q6h)	A cephalosporin II, clindamycin (600 mg q6h), or vancomycin Ciprofloxacin (750 mg q12h) and rifampicine (600 mg q24h oral)
Methicillin resistant	Vancomycin (1 g q12h)	Teicoplanin[c] (400 mg q12-24h, first day q12h)
Various streptococci (group A or B beta-hemolytic; *Streptococcus pneumoniae*)	Penicillin G (3 million units q4-6h)	Clindamycin (600 mg q6h), erythromycin (500 mg q6h), or vancomycin
Enteric gram-negative rods	Quinolone (ciprofloxacine, 500-750 mg q12h IV or PO)	A cephalosporin III[d]
Serratia sp. Pseudomonas aeruginosa*	Piperacillin[e] (2-4 g q4h) and gentamycin (1.5 mg/kg/day)	A cephalosporin III[e] or a quinolone (with aminoglycosides)
Anaerobes	Clindamycin (600 mg q6h)	Amoxicillin-clavulanic acid (2.2 q8h) or metronidazole for gram-negative anaerobes (500 mg q8h)
Mixed infection (aerobic and anaerobic microorganisms)	Amoxicillin-clavulanic acid (2.2 g q8h)	Imipenem[f] (500 mg q6h)

[a]*II*, Second generation.
[b]Flucloxacillin in Europe.
[c]Teicoplanin is presently available only in Europe.
[d]*III*, Third or fourth generation (ceftazidime or cefepime).
[e]Depends on sensitivities: piperacillin/tazobactam and imipenem are useful alternatives.
[f]In cases of aerobic gram-negative microorganisms resistant to amoxicillin-clavulanic acid.

(particularly tibia and femur), usually as a single focus. Although rare in adults, it most commonly involves the vertebral bodies.

The clinical features of hematogenous osteomyelitis in long bones are quite typical: chills, fever, and malaise reflect the bacteremic spread of microorganisms; pain and local swelling are the hallmarks of the local infectious process.

Bacteria responsible for hematogenous osteomyelitis reflect essentially their bacteremic incidence as a function of age, so the organisms most commonly encountered in neonates include *S. aureus* and group B streptococci; in infants, most infections are caused by *S. aureus,* coagulase-negative staphylococci, and various streptococci. Later in life, *S. aureus* predominates; in elderly persons, who are often subject to gram-negative bacteremias, an increased incidence of vertebral osteomyelitis caused by gram-negative rods is found.

Fungal osteomyelitis is a complication of intravenous device infections, neutropenia, or profound immune deficiency; *Pseudomonas aeruginosa* hematogenous osteomyelitis is often seen in drug addicts and has a predilection for the cervical vertebrae.

Treatment of Acute Hematogenous Osteomyelitis

Hematogenous osteomyelitis of the long bones rarely occurs in adults. When it develops, debridement and/or incision and drainage of soft-tissue abscesses are usually required. Appropriate deep-tissue samples should be obtained, a parenteral administration of an antimicrobial regimen may be begun as empirical therapy aimed at the clinically suspected pathogen(s). Once one or more organisms are isolated, in vitro susceptibility testing can be done as a guide to treatment. The current standard of care is parenteral antimicrobial treatment for 4 to 6 weeks, with the start of this interval dating from the first day of treatment judged to be appropriate in light of in vitro susceptibility results.

■ VERTEBRAL OSTEOMYELITIS

The management of vertebral osteomyelitis requires effective antimicrobial therapy and may necessitate early surgery and stabilization of the spine. The choice of an antimicrobial drug is guided by the results of cultures of specimens obtained by biopsy or debridement. Needle biopsy obtained through CT guidance currently is the process of choice to obtain samples, which are submitted in parallel to bacteriologic and pathologic evaluation. Pathology is particularly useful in patients with previous antibiotic therapy and suspected mycobacterial disease. If the first biopsy is culture negative, a second biopsy guided by CT scan should be obtained. In case of a second failure to establish diagnosis the physician faces the choice to propose empirical therapy or to request a surgical biopsy for diagnosis.

Depending on the pharmacologic characteristics of a specific drug, the drug may be administered by the oral or the parenteral route. The antimicrobial agent should be given for 4 to 6 weeks. The duration of treatment is usually dated either from the initial use of an effective antimicrobial agent or from the last major debridement. The indications for surgery in vertebral osteomyelitis are similar to those in hematogenous infections of bone: failure of medical management, formation of soft-tissue abscesses, impending instability, or neurologic signs indicating spinal cord compression. In the last case, surgery becomes an emergency procedure. Therefore the neurologic status of the patient must be monitored frequently. Eventual fusion of adjacent infected vertebral bodies is a major goal of therapy.

■ OSTEOMYELITIS SECONDARY TO A CONTIGUOUS INFECTION WITHOUT VASCULAR DISEASE

The situation and the clinical picture are more complex in cases of osteomyelitis associated with a contiguous focus of infection, for example, as a complication of the insertion of a total hip prosthesis. After a few days' pain following usual surgery, the situation improves and the patient is progressively mobilized. During that period, the pain reappears, mostly on weight bearing. The patient is mildly febrile, and the wound is slightly erythematous with a slight discharge. No other clinical signs point toward the diagnosis of osteomyelitis, and no radiographic examination or other imaging procedure is fully diagnostic. Similar clinical reasoning has to be used to diagnose osteomyelitis secondary to a contiguous infection such as a comminuted fracture, which can become contaminated by wound infection. Any other prosthetic material can become contaminated during surgery and produce signs of infection during the ensuing weeks.

Acute purulent frontal sinusitis can lead to bone involvement, with a characteristic edema of the forehead (Pott's puffy tumor).

Dental root infection can lead to local bone destruction. Deep-seated pressure sores can lead to local bone destruction, usually of the sacrum. Under all these conditions, the inflammatory reaction may be mild, and the bone destruction difficult to assess.

In the past, *S. aureus* and coagulase-negative staphylococci were the most frequently reported microorganisms. In recent years, various types of streptococci, *Propionibacterium acnei*, anaerobic microorganisms, *Enterobacteriaceae*, and *Pseudomonas aeruginosa* (the last mostly in the setting of chronic osteomyelitis, comminuted fractures, and puncture wounds to the heel) are being encountered. Finally, osteomyelitis of the mandible and secondary to pressure sores often also contains anaerobic flora, as do human and animal bites.

Practical Approach and Therapy

Adequate drainage, thorough debridement, obliteration of dead space, wound protection, and specific antimicrobial therapy are the mainstays of management. After clinical evaluation, a bone biopsy should be performed, and the sample obtained should be submitted for aerobic and anaerobic cultures and histopathologic evaluation. Often, the patient receives antimicrobial agents only after the results of cultures and susceptibility tests become available. However, if immediate debridement is required, the patient may receive empirical antimicrobial therapy before the bacteriologic data are reported. This antimicrobial regimen can be modified, if necessary, on the basis of culture and susceptibility results.

Almost always, surgical debridement is an important adjunctive therapy. Ideally, specific antimicrobial therapy is initiated before debridement is undertaken. Debridement includes removal of all orthopedic appliances except those deemed absolutely necessary for stability. Often, debridement must be repeated at least once for the removal of all nonviable tissue.

Posttraumatic infected fractures are especially difficult to treat. A variety of techniques have evolved for management of the exposed bone and/or the dead space(s) created by the trauma and debridement (i.e., use of local tissue flaps and of vascularized tissue transferred from a distant site). Other experimental modalities that are occasionally used include cancellous bone grafting and implantation of acrylic beads impregnated with one or more antibacterial agents. Finally, in patients with osteomyelitis, the Ilizarov fixation device allows major segmental resections, in combination with new bone growth, to fill in the defect.

Antimicrobial agents are used to treat viable infected bone and to protect bone that is undergoing revascularization. Because revascularization of bone after debridement takes 3 to 4 weeks, the patient should be treated with parenteral antimicrobial agents for 4 to 6 weeks. The start of this therapy is usually dated from the last major debridement.

■ DIABETIC FOOT OSTEOMYELITIS

Diabetic foot osteomyelitis is a special entity observed in patients with diabetes and is located almost exclusively on the lower extremities. The disease starts insidiously in a patient who has complained of intermittent claudication in an area of previously traumatized skin. Cellulitis may be kept at a minimum, and infection progressively burrows its way to the underlying bone (e.g., toe, metatarsal head, tarsal bone). Physical examination elicits either no pain (with advanced neuropathy) or excruciating pain if bone destruction has been acute; an area of cellulitis may or may not be present; crepitus can be felt occasionally, which points toward the presence of either anaerobes or *Enterobacteriaceae*. Physical examination includes a careful examination of the vascular supply to the affected limb and the evaluation of a concomitant neuropathy.

Here again, the whole gamut of human pathogenic bacteria can be isolated, often in multiple combinations. *S. aureus* still predominates, but any other gram-positive or gram-negative, aerobic or anaerobic bacteria may be involved, particularly in more severe infection. To distinguish between superficial colonization/infection and bone infection, several experts propose bone biopsy for histopathology and culture. This procedure is supposed to firmly establish diagnosis and optimize therapy.

The ability to reach bone by gently advancing a sterile surgical probe combined with plain radiography is the best initial approach to the diagnosis of diabetic foot osteomyelitis. If bone is detected on probing, treatment for osteomyelitis is recommended. If bone cannot be detected by probing and the plain radiography does not suggest osteomyelitis, the recommended treatment is a course of antibiotics directed at soft-tissue infection. Because occult osteomyelitis may be present, radiography should be repeated in 2 weeks. Further studies, such as MRI are recommended in doubtful cases.

Practical Approach and Therapy

The prognosis for cure of diabetic foot osteomyelitis is poor because of the impaired ability of the host to assist in the eradication of the infectious agent. The vascular insufficiency may be the result of trauma, atherosclerotic peripheral vascular disease, secondary manifestations of diabetes mellitus, or some combination of these processes.

It is important to determine the amount of vascular compromise. This assessment can be made by measurement of transcutaneous oximetry (once inflammation has been controlled) and of pulse pressures with Doppler ultrasonography. If serious ischemia is suspected, arteriography of the lower extremity, including the foot vessels, should be performed.

Because of impaired vascular perfusion, a case may be managed by antimicrobial therapy, debridement surgery, or ablative surgery. The type of treatment offered depends on the oxygen tensions of tissue at the infected site, the extent of osteomyelitis and time damage, the potential for revascularization, and the preference of the patient.

Revascularization often proves to be useful before amputation is considered. There is no convincing evidence that hyperbaric oxygen is useful for the treatment of diabetic osteomyelitis. Poor prognostic factors on admission include fever, increased serum creatinine levels, prior hospitalization for diabetic foot lesions, and gangrenous lesions.

Suggested Reading

Caputo GM, et al: Assessment and management of foot disease in patients with diabetes, *N Engl J Med* 331:854, 1994.

Jauregui LE, Senour CL: Chronic osteomyelitis. In Jauregui LE, ed: *Diagnosis and management of bone infections*, New York, 1995, Marcel Dekker.

Lew DP, Waldvogel FA: Osteomyelitis, *N Engl J Med* 336:999, 1997.

Lew DP, Waldvogel FA: Use of quinolones in osteomyelitis and infected orthopedic prosthesis, *Drugs* 58(suppl 2):85, 1999.

Lipsky BA: Osteomyelitis of the foot in diabetic patients, *Clin Infect Dis* 25:1318, 1997.

Pillet D, et al: Outcome of diabetic foot infections treated conservatively, *Arch Intern Med* 159:851, 1999.

Mader JT, et al: Evaluation of new anti-infective drugs for the treatment of osteomyelitis in adults. Infectious Diseases Society of America and the Food and Drug Administration, *Clin Infect Dis* 15(Suppl 1):S155, 1992.

POLYARTHRITIS AND FEVER

Robert S. Pinals
Alexander Ackley, Jr.

Polyarthritis and fever may be manifestations of a wide variety of infectious and noninfectious diseases (Table 1). Prompt identification of treatable infectious diseases is important; even the diagnosis of nontreatable infections may have important consequences for the individual or for public health. In all cases, treatment is based on specifics that apply to the known or presumptive pathogen.

■ BACTERIAL INFECTIONS

Suppurative bacterial arthritis caused by *Staphylococcus aureus,* group A streptococci, and gram-negative bacteria usually is monoarticular, but 10% of patients have polyarticular involvement, occurring simultaneously or within 1 to 2 days. Risk factors for bacterial polyarthritis are listed in Table 2. Septic joints in such persons are not always red, hot, or exquisitely painful. The mortality rate is higher with polyarticular infection (>30%) than with monoarticular infection (<10%) and has not changed in recent years.

Therefore, just as for a monoarticular arthritis, prompt arthrocentesis of a polyarthritis is essential because delay in the diagnosis and treatment is the best predictor of an unfavorable outcome. Broad-spectrum antibiotic treatment should be started immediately.

The bacteria listed in Table 2 are more likely than others to produce polyarthritis. Neisserial arthritis, which is most often polyarticular, presents as migratory arthritis with chills, fever, and tenosynovitis in the wrist and ankle extensor tendon sheaths. Characteristic pustular or vesicular skin lesions often aid in diagnosis. Disseminated gonococcal infections occur more often in women, especially during menses and the second and third trimesters of pregnancy. Therapy should be started immediately after cultures are obtained. Dramatic improvement in fever and joint symptoms within 24 hours supports a presumptive diagnosis of gonococcal arthritis even when cultures are negative. Chronic or episodic "benign" meningococcemia can present in a similar fashion.

In bacterial endocarditis, musculoskeletal symptoms may be the initial manifestation of infection. Low back pain and arthralgias are most common, but polyarthritis with effusions may occur. The synovial fluid cell count generally is lower than with septic arthritis, and the fluid usually is sterile. In suspect cases, blood cultures should be held 2 weeks to increase the yield of fastidious organisms. Rheumatoid factor is present in about one third of patients.

Brucellosis is an acute, chronic, or undulant febrile illness. Joint involvement occurs in 20% to 80% of patients. The frequency and type of articular involvement depends on the patient's age and the particular species causing infection.

Table 1   Causes of Polyarthritis and Fever

Bacterial infections	Systemic rheumatic illnesses
Septic arthritis	Systemic vasculitis
Bacterial endocarditis	Systemic lupus
Brucella species	erythematosus
Lyme disease	Crystal-induced arthritis
Syphilis	Gout and pseudogout
Whipple's disease	Mucocutaneous disorders
Mycobacteria	Dermatomyositis
M. tuberculosis	Behçet's disease
Atypical organisms	Henoch-Schönlein purpura
Leprosy	Kawasaki disease (muco-
Mycoplasma infections	cutaneous lymph node
Viral infections	syndrome)
Fungal infections	Erythema nodosum
Parasitic infections	Erythema multiforme
Postinfectious or reactive	Pyoderma gangrenosum
arthritis	Pustular psoriasis
Enteric infection	Other diseases
Chlamydia	Familial Mediterranean
Rheumatic fever	fever
Inflammatory bowel disease	Angioimmunoblastic
Serum sickness	lymphadenopathy
Antibiotics and other drugs	Cancers and lymphomas
Rheumatoid arthritis	Sarcoidosis
Still's disease	

Table 2   Risk Factors for Polyarticular Infection

PATHOGENS	HOST FACTORS
Neisseria gonorrhoeae	Intravenous drug abuse
Neisseria meningitidis	Immunosuppression
Streptocobacillus moniliformis	Rheumatoid arthritis
Streptococcus pneumoniae	Gout
Haemophilus influenzae	Other polyarthropathies
Group G streptococcus	
Bacteroides fragilis	

Sacroiliitis and a peripheral monoarthritis are most common. A nondestructive polyarthritis similar to a reactive arthritis occurs in about 1% of the arthritis cases.

In early Lyme disease, disseminated infection with *Borrelia burgdorferi* can cause fever and polyarthralgias. Frank arthritis is uncommon, but when it is present, pain and restriction of movement in the temporomandibular joints are highly suggestive. IgM antibodies may be detected 4 to 6 weeks after the tick bite. If the patient lives in or has traveled to an endemic area, presumptive treatment should be given even when there is no diagnostic erythema chronicum migrans (ECM) lesion and the serology is negative. Late Lyme arthritis, occurring weeks to months after the tick bite, usually is monoarticular and most often involves a knee. Less often, it is episodic and polyarticular, involving both small and large joints. Serology usually is strongly positive.

Rarely, another spirochetal infection, secondary syphilis, presents with a febrile symmetric polyarthritis that can mimic rheumatoid arthritis. Most patients have a maculopapular rash on the palms and soles, and the serology is always positive.

Whipple's disease is caused by an intracellular bacillus that has never been grown in culture but was recently characterized by amplification of an RNA sequence obtained from involved tissue. The clinical picture resembles that of inflammatory bowel disease, but arthritis is a common early complication, with several patterns, including migratory and persistent oligoarticular synovitis. The diagnosis is made by biopsy of the intestinal mucosa or lymph nodes. Long-term treatment with tetracycline and/or other antibiotics is required for cure.

■ MYCOBACTERIA

Tuberculosis causes indolent monoarthritis (85%) or oligoarthritis (15%). Rarely, a patient with pulmonary or visceral tuberculosis will manifest an acute polyarthritis without evidence of joint infection (Poncet's disease). The symptoms resolve within weeks of starting conventional treatment.

Atypical mycobacteria can also infect joints, tendons, and bursae. Only occasionally is the infection polyarticular and then usually in patients who have underlying joint problems from trauma, surgery, steroid injections, acquired immunodeficiency syndrome (AIDS), or systemic arthritis. Diagnosis is by culture, and treatment includes multiple drugs. Synovectomy may be necessary.

Lepromatous leprosy can cause acute polyarthritis with fever, and all forms (lepromatous, tuberculoid, borderline) can be associated with an indolent polyarthritis. Therefore this diagnosis must always be considered in evaluating polyarthritis in residents of endemic areas.

■ MYCOPLASMAS

Arthralgias are common with *Mycoplasma pneumoniae* infection, and rarely a true migratory polyarthritis occurs. Most reported cases with a prominent rheumatic syndrome have been in children with obvious respiratory infection, and the arthritis has lasted for weeks or even months.

A distinctly different syndrome of septic arthritis is caused by *Mycoplasma hominis, Ureaplasma urealyticum,* and other members of the family in variously immunocompromised persons. This septic arthritis usually is monoarticular, although a few patients with hypogammaglobulinemia have a polyarthritis resembling rheumatoid arthritis. If mycoplasmal joint infection is suspected, both blood and joint fluid should be cultured using commercial enriched media. Joint irrigation and prolonged therapy with tetracycline or erythromycin are required.

■ VIRAL ARTHRITIS

Arthritis can occur with infection caused by any of several viral agents (Table 3). Viral invasion per se, joint damage from normal immune responses, and alteration of the host immune system by the virus have all been identified or proposed as mechanisms of injury. Symmetric and asymmetric polyarthritis and polyarthralgia are the most com-

Table 3 Viral Infections Associated with Arthritis	
OFTEN	**OCCASIONALLY**
Parvovirus B19	Hepatitis C virus
Hepatitis B virus	Adenoviruses
Rubella virus and vaccine	Herpesviruses
Alphaviruses	Enteroviruses
Mumps	Lymphocytic choriomeningitis virus

mon patterns of joint involvement. Diagnosis is usually made by serology, but polymerase chain reaction on joint fluid is occasionally available.

In hepatitis B infection, polyarthritis with or without a rash may precede any symptoms of hepatitis. At the time of arthritic symptoms, transaminases usually are elevated and hepatitis B surface antigen (HbsAg) is present in serum in very high titer. Such patients may be highly contagious. Hepatitis B infection should be considered in any sexually active person or suspected drug user with an acute polyarthritis.

Occasionally, hepatitis C can cause polyarthritis without fever. Painful small joint nondestructive synovitis and tenosynovitis are the typical presentation. Patients with obscure cases of polyarthritis should be tested for hepatitis C, and a few have been reported to have had improvement in the arthritis when their hepatitis was treated with interferon.

Rubella and parvovirus B19 can cause a similar clinical syndrome, especially in young women. Because rubella is now uncommon and rubella vaccine has been modified to reduce arthritogenic strains, parvovirus arthropathy, which can occur in epidemics, is probably more common. An acute-onset, symmetric polyarthritis involving the hands and feet is typical. Rash is more common in children, but the arthritis is more prominent in adults. The presence of serum IgM antibody to parvovirus B19 is diagnostic.

Several causes of polyarthritis are recognized with human immunodeficiency virus (HIV) infection (Table 4). Many are secondary processes, but an HIV–related arthritis has been described. Whatever the cause, arthritis can be a presenting feature of HIV disease, and patients with an obscure polyarthritis of new onset should be asked about risk factors for HIV exposure and testing with consent advised as necessary.

■ FUNGAL INFECTIONS

A migratory polyarthralgia or polyarthritis sometimes accompanies acute histoplasmosis. Similarly, polyarticular "desert rheumatism" with or without erythema nodosum may occur at the onset of symptomatic coccidioidomycosis. Both resolve without sequelae. Chronic pathogenic fungal infections occasionally lead to arthritis, but they are almost always monoarticular or pauciarticular.

Among opportunistic fungi only *Candida* species are reported to cause arthritis with any frequency. Disseminated candidiasis of immunocompromised neonates, infants, and adults can produce polyarthritis as well as monoarthritis

Table 4 Polyarthritis Associated with HIV Infection	
TYPE	**CHARACTERISTIC FEATURES**
Nonspecific synovitis (HIV-associated arthritis)	Lower extremity oligoarthritis often with noninflammatory synovial fluid despite severe pain and signs of inflammation; persistent symmetric polyarthritis
Seronegative spondyloarthropathy Reiter's syndrome Psoriatic arthritis Reactive arthritis	Frequent heel pain and other enthesopathy; strong association with HLA-B27; more severe than in patients without HIV
Septic arthritis	Infection may be opportunistic, related to intravenous drug abuse, or sexually transmitted; axial joints likely to be affected

HIV, Human immunodeficiency virus.

Table 5 Parasites and Arthritis*	
ORGANISM	**FEATURES**
Giardia lamblia	Oligoarthritis or polyarthritis
Cryptosporidium	Reactive polyarthritis
Toxoplasma gondii	Symmetric polyarthritis
Strongyloides	Reactive arthritis; oligoarticular or polyarticular
Taenia saginata	Muscle pain and stiffness
Toxocara canis	Elevated ESR
Schistosoma species	Acute febrile symmetric polyarthritis with morning stiffness
	Chronic low back pain, thigh, knee, and heel pain
Filaria species	Acute or chronic monoarthritis; occasional oligoarticular or polyarticular involvement

ESR, Erythrocyte sedimentation rate.
*These syndromes are all uncommon or rare.

or oligoarthritis. Diagnosis is by culture of joint fluid, synovium, adjacent bone, or other extraarticular sites.

■ PARASITIC INFECTIONS

Joint inflammation is relatively rare in these diseases, but because hundreds of millions of people are afflicted by them, they occasionally must be considered in the differential diagnosis of polyarthritis occurring in migrants, travelers, and immunocompromised persons from endemic regions. The parasites most likely to be associated with polyarthritis are listed in Table 5. Identification of the parasite and improvement after antiparasitic treatment support the diagnosis. Antiinflammatory drugs usually are not effective.

■ POSTINFECTIOUS OR REACTIVE ARTHRITIS

Rheumatic fever is the prototype for postinfectious polyarthritis. Adults with arthritis and fever after group A streptococcal pharyngitis seldom have carditis and often do not demonstrate the classical migratory pattern, high fever, and dramatic response to salicylates. This poststreptococcal reactive arthritis may be additive and asymmetric, primarily affecting the lower extremities. A similar reactive arthritis pattern is also seen after various genitourinary and enteric infections (Table 6). Fever may accompany the primary infection but is mild or absent during the subsequent polyarthritis except in a few patients with intense joint inflammation. A genetic predisposition is an important determinant for the rheumatic syndrome. Except in rheumatic fever, human leukocyte antigen (HLA)-B27 is found with high frequency, especially in patients with the triad of urethritis, conjunctivitis, and arthritis (Reiter's syndrome). In some infections, bacterial antigen may be identified in the synovial fluid or membrane, but there are no viable organisms. This suggests that dissemination has resulted in an immune reaction in synovial and other tissues. Treatment with tetracyclines may shorten the course and diminish the likelihood of recurrence in chlamydial arthritis. With enteric arthritis, the value of antibiotic treatment is controversial, but some reports suggest that sulfasalazine may be effective.

■ NONINFECTIOUS CAUSES

Polyarthritis and fever may be presenting features of many noninfectious systemic illnesses (see Table 1). This discussion focuses on those that most closely simulate infections, namely Still's disease and crystal-induced synovitis.

Still's disease is the systemic form of juvenile rheumatoid arthritis, which occasionally occurs in adults. High spiking fever, chills, and marked polymorphonuclear leukocytosis, often preceded by a nonstreptococcal sore throat, are highly suggestive of a bacterial infection. Arthralgia and myalgia are early features; joint swelling appears days or weeks after the onset of fever. There are no diagnostic laboratory tests, but a typical evanescent pink macular rash that accompanies fever spikes is a useful finding. Its recognition may obviate unnecessary imaging and the invasive diagnostic procedures and multiple courses of antibiotics to which patients with persistent high fever are often subjected. The diagnosis of Still's disease is confirmed by the course, in which chronic polyarthritis is the dominant feature. Most patients have elevations of serum ferritin levels well in excess of those seen with infectious and inflammatory reactions. This finding is nonspecific but may be a useful diagnostic clue.

Adult rheumatoid arthritis rarely has a febrile presentation. When fever accompanies exacerbations of synovitis, a superimposed septic arthritis must be ruled out by joint

Table 6	Causes of Reactive Arthritis
Chlamydia trachomatis	
Ureaplasma urealyticum	
Yersinia enterocolitica, Yersinia pseudotuberculosis	
Campylobacter species	
Salmonella species	
Shigella species	
Clostridium difficile	

aspiration. Some patients have episodes of severe monoarticular or oligoarticular sterile inflammation accompanied by fever and synovial fluid white blood cell counts greater than 50,000/mm³. This "pseudosepsis" improves either spontaneously or with antiinflammatory medication.

Systemic lupus erythematosus may feature high fever and polyarthritis, but the latter usually includes more small than large joints, in contrast to the pattern in septic arthritis. In lupus induced by procainamide and other drugs, this presentation is particularly common.

In *crystal-induced arthritis* (gout and pseudogout), acute monoarticular or polyarticular synovitis resembling septic arthritis may occasionally be accompanied by high fever. A few of these patients may indeed have bacterial superinfection, but most have sterile synovial fluids in which polarizing microscopy will identify the causative crystals. Patients with polyarticular gout are often normouricemic at the time of the acute episode. Therefore serum uric acid is not a useful diagnostic test.

Inflammatory bowel disease may present with fever and/or with an oligoarticular arthritis in large joints, but the two features are usually not simultaneous. The synovitis is low grade with prominent effusion and little pain.

Polymyalgia rheumatica may present with low-grade and occasionally high fever. Proximal myalgia and arthralgia is seldom accompanied by joint swelling, and morning stiffness is generally a prominent symptom. Joint effusions are most commonly observed in the knee; these are seldom confused with septic arthritis because pain is much less severe and cell counts fall in the low inflammatory range.

Familial Mediterranean fever presents in childhood with brief episodes that may include fever, arthritis, serositis, and an erysipelas-like rash. An infectious etiology may be suspected initially, but a history of prior episodes and familial occurrence point away from this.

Suggested Reading

Dubost JJ, et al: Polyarticular septic arthritis, *Medicine* 72:296, 1993.

Espinoza L, ed: Infectious arthritis, *Rheum Dis Clin North Am* 19:2279, 1993.

Goldenberg DL: Septic arthritis, *Lancet* 351:197, 1998.

Koopman WJ, ed: *Arthritis and allied conditions: a textbook of rheumatology,* ed 13, Baltimore, 1997, Williams & Wilkins.

Pinals R: Polyarthritis and fever, *N Engl J Med* 330:769, 1994.

INFECTIOUS POLYMYOSITIS

Upinder Singh

Infectious polymyositis is an entity in which there is generalized muscle damage (rhabdomyolysis) caused by an infectious agent. The syndrome of rhabdomyolysis is characterized by elevated serum creatinine phosphokinase (CPK) concentrations and myoglobinuria leading to renal dysfunction. The muscle injury in rhabdomyolysis occurs in a generalized pattern and lacks a specific focus of abscess or infection as is seen in pyomyositis. The entity of pyomyositis is discussed in a separate chapter, *Deep Soft-Tissue Infection: Fasciitis and Myositis.*

A variety of precipitating factors can lead to rhabdomyolysis. These include crush and compression injuries, drug and alcohol ingestion, metabolic and electrolyte disturbances, hypothermia and hyperthermia, and a variety of miscellaneous infections. This review focuses on infectious causes. It is important to distinguish rhabdomyolysis caused by a pathogen from that caused by sepsis, hypotension, or electrolyte imbalances that accompany a severe systemic infection.

■ VIRAL INFECTIONS

The wide spectrum of viral infections that have been reported to cause rhabdomyolysis are listed in Table 1. Influenza is the most common viral etiology reported to precipitate rhabdomyolysis, followed by human immunodeficiency virus (HIV) and enteroviral infection. The presenting symptoms in these patients include myalgias, weakness, muscle tenderness, and edema. Whether the association with influenza results primarily from a special predilection of the virus for the muscle tissue or frequent reporting of the association because of physician awareness and relative ease of diagnosis is unclear. Severe renal dysfunction in rhabdomyolysis secondary to influenza infection is common and apparently not related solely to the level of CPK elevation. The precise mechanism predisposing to renal damage from influenza-induced rhabdomyolysis is unclear; however, the association is intriguing and clinically significant, and aggressive measures should be taken to preserve renal function in these individuals.

Rhabdomyolysis caused by HIV infection adds to the spectrum of clinical presentations of HIV infection. Many musculoskeletal syndromes associated with HIV infection have been documented, ranging from myopathy to rhabdomyolysis. Muscle damage can occur in a variety of clinical scenarios in association with HIV infection, including acute seroconversion and antigenemia, end-stage disease with myopathy, and myositis resulting from medication side effects (specifically zidovudine and stavudine). Muscle biopsies of patients with HIV-induced rhabdomyolysis reveal a nonspecific inflammatory myopathy with focal necrotic areas and regenerating fibers.

The precise pathophysiology underlying viral-induced myoglobinuria is unknown; however, two mechanisms have been postulated: direct viral invasion and toxin generation. Some authors have suggested that direct viral invasion of muscle fibers causes muscle necrosis. Data to support this hypothesis include the identification of viral inclusions, viral DNA, and the isolation of viruses in tissue culture from the muscles of infected patients. In addition, electron microscopy has identified viral particles, and biopsies reveal a lymphocytic infiltrate in the infected muscles. This evidence strongly suggests that direct viral invasion may have a causative role in precipitating rhabdomyolysis. However, various reports documenting normal muscle biopsies or hyaline degeneration and myonecrosis but no viral particles by immunofluorescence and electron microscopy are used to refute this theory. Biopsies of clinically affected musculature that are essentially normal raise the possibility of a circulating "toxin" or cytokine causing rhabdomyolysis. However, to date no putative toxins have been isolated from cases of viral induced rhabdomyolysis.

■ BACTERIAL INFECTIONS

Many bacterial agents have been reported to cause rhabdomyolysis (Table 2). The most common associations are with *Legionella* species, followed by *Streptococcus* species, *Francisella tularensis,* and *Salmonella* infections. An ever-increasing number of bacterial agents are being associated with this entity, probably because of many factors, including better diagnostic techniques, increasing population of immunocompromised individuals susceptible to infection, and increasing physician awareness. Individuals with bacterial infections resulting in rhabdomyolysis have significant morbidity (57% with renal failure in one study) and mortality (38% in one series).

Many other infections have been reported to result in muscle damage and include fungal, rickettsial, spirochetal, and protozoal infections (Tables 3 to 6). In these cases, the clinician will most likely identify the infectious agent

Table 1 Viral Causes of Rhabdomyolysis

Influenza virus A and B
Influenza A H5N1 (avian)
Human immunodeficiency virus
Coxsackie virus
Epstein-Barr virus
Echovirus
Cytomegalovirus
Adenovirus
Herpes simplex virus
Parainfluenza virus
Varicella-zoster virus
Picornavirus, including coxsackie and echovirus
Measles virus
Hepatitis C

Table 2 Bacterial Causes of Rhabdomyolysis

GRAM-POSITIVE BACTERIA	GRAM-NEGATIVE BACTERIA
Streptococcus pneumoniae	Legionella spp.
Staphylococcus aureus	Francesella tularensis
Group B streptococcus	Salmonella spp.
Streptococcus pyogenes	Vibrio spp.
Listeria spp.	Brucella spp.
Staphylococcus epidermidis	Escherichia coli
Bacillus spp.	Herbicola lathyri
Clostridium spp.	Klebsiella spp.
Viridans streptococci	Aeromonas
Streptococcus suis	Haemophilus influenzae
Beta-hemolytic streptococci	Neisseria spp.
Streptococcus pyogenes	

Table 3 Fungal Causes of Rhabdomyolysis

Candida spp.
Aspergillus spp.
Mucor spp.

Table 4 Protozoal and Helminthic Causes of Rhabdomyolysis

Plasmodium spp.
Toxoplasma gondii
Trichinosis

Table 5 Miscellaneous Causes of Rhabdomyolysis

SPIROCHETES	RICKETTSIAL	MYCOPLASMA
Leptospira spp.	Rickettsia conorii	Mycoplasma pneumoniae
Borrelia burgdorferi	Ehrlichia equi	
	Ehrlichia chaffeensis	
	Coxiella burnetti	

Table 6 Other Infections and Related Causes of Rhabdomyolysis

Intravesical instillation of BCG
Tuberculosis

Table 7 Envenomations Reported to Cause Rhabdomyolysis

SNAKES	OTHER
South American rattlesnake	Hornets
Tiger snake	Wasps
Mojave rattlesnake	Bees
Russel viper	Desert centipede
	Redback spider
	Taipan

through obtaining epidemiologic, environmental, and exposure histories. However, once the infectious agent is identified, a high index of suspicion must be maintained for concomitant muscle injury, and therapies (e.g., antibiotics, antifungals, contrast agents) that may exacerbate renal dysfunction must be carefully considered.

Two proposed mechanisms of muscle injury by bacteria include toxin generation and direct bacterial invasion. Legionella is believed to release an endotoxin or exotoxin that causes rhabdomyolysis. Biopsies that are negative for the organism by immunofluorescence (IF) support this hypothesis. Organisms such as Streptococcus and Salmonella cause muscle damage by direct bacterial invasion as well as by decreasing the oxidative and glycolytic enzyme activity of skeletal muscle and activating lysosomal enzymes. A number of bacterial pathogens, including Staphylococcus aureus, Streptococcus pyogenes, Vibrio species, and Bacillus species, have been demonstrated in muscle biopsy specimens, lending credence to the hypothesis of direct bacterial invasion. Rickettsial illnesses such as Q fever and Rocky Mountain spotted fever can cause muscle injury through a vasculitis, as well as direct muscle invasion. A variety of cytokines, such as tumor necrosis factor alpha and interleukin-1, released during systemic infections from a broad range of infections, can result in skeletal muscle proteolysis.

ENVENOMATIONS

Envenomations reported to cause rhabdomyolysis are listed in Table 7. Snake bites are commonly reported to cause muscle injury and include bites inflicted by the Mojave rattlesnake, Russel viper, Croatus durissus terrificus (South American rattlesnake), Australian snake, tiger snake, and seasnake. These patients present with obviously swollen, tender muscles and high CPK levels. In contrast to viral and bacterial causes of rhabdomyolysis, envenomations generally cause a larger myotoxic insult. A large proportion of these patients also subsequently develop acute renal failure, presumably directly related to the increased renal toxicity from myoglobin. The mechanism of muscle damage in these cases appears to be a direct myotoxic activity of the various venoms. Muscle biopsies from patients reveal myonecrosis, loss of cross striations, contraction band formation, and mitochondrial swelling.

RENAL FAILURE IN RHABDOMYOLYSIS

The renal dysfunction associated with rhabdomyolysis arises from a variety of interrelated factors. In muscle injury, both myoglobin and heme proteins are released, although neither is directly toxic to the glomerulus. Heme protein can result in renal tubular injury through a variety of mechanisms: (1) renal vasoconstriction, (2) direct renal tubular cell cytotoxicity, or (3) intraluminal cast formation and tubular obstruction. Therapeutic measures that increase renal blood flow and decrease tubular obstruction are useful in preventing renal injury in these patients.

In a variety of case series, an interesting association of rhabdomyolysis from influenza infection resulting in renal failure has been noted. This association is not the result of higher levels of muscle injury as measured by CPK levels and may point to another mechanism of renal injury in influenza infection. In *Legionella* infection, a variety of renal pathologies have been observed, including acute tubulointerstitial nephritis, acute pyelonephritis, mesangioglomerulonephritis, and rapidly progressive glomerulonephritis. The organism has also been demonstrated in renal tissue by electron microscopy and indirect immunofluorescence. Thus renal injury in rhabdomyolysis may be caused by a combination of heme-induced injury and direct effect of the infectious agent.

■ THERAPY AND MANAGEMENT

General issues in the management of rhabdomyolysis include supportive care and treatment of the underlying predisposing condition or infection. These measures would apply to the infectious etiologies just discussed. For detailed information on the management of renal failure from rhabdomyolysis, see the review by Visweswaran and other critical care manuals. The general approach is as follows: (1) maintenance of a high degree of suspicion for rhabdomyolysis in the appropriate clinical setting; (2) appropriate diagnostic workup, including CPK levels, urinalysis, and urine myoglobin levels; (3) rapid institution of organism-specific drug therapy; and (4) supportive renal care. The renal function can be protected by maneuvers such as volume expansion and urine alkalinization. Other metabolic disturbances resulting from muscle injury, such as hyperkalemia and metabolic acidosis, also may need specific therapy.

Suggested Reading

Falasca GF, Reginato AJ: The spectrum of myositis and rhabdomyolysis associated with bacterial infection, *J Rheumatol* 10:1932, 1994.

Gabow PA, Kaehny WD, Kelleher SP: The spectrum of rhabdomyolysis, *Medicine* 61:141, 1982.

Knochel JP: Mechanisms of rhabdomyolysis, *Curr Opin Rheumatol* 5:725, 1993.

Singh U, Scheld WM: Infectious etiologies of rhabdomyolysis: three case reports and review, *Clin Infect Dis* 22:642, 1996.

Visweswaran P, Guntupalli J: Rhabdomyolysis, *Crit Care Clin* 15:415, 1999.

PSOAS ABSCESS

Pamela A. Lipsett

Iliopsoas abscess is an uncommon but important and potentially life-threatening infection that can be difficult to recognize. Most of the literature on psoas abscess includes case reports and small case series, with few institutions seeing more than one case of iliopsoas abscess in a year and with slightly more than 500 cases reported in the world's literature. The causes of this infection vary internationally and have changed over time. Early in the twentieth century and even in some countries today, *Mycobacterium tuberculosis* has been responsible for most iliopsoas abscesses seen by physicians. Following the control of *M. tuberculosis* in some countries, iliopsoas abscess was then most commonly associated with gastrointestinal and genitourinary tract abnormalities. These iliopsoas abscesses, when arising from another local source, have been termed a *secondary iliopsoas abscess,* and those without an identified or suspected local direct extension are termed *primary* in origin. Primary iliopsoas abscesses reflect different pathogens, most typically *Staphylococcus aureus,* and can be similar to tropical myositis in clinical appearance. Today in some centers, especially those with a large population of patients with intravenous drug abuse, primary iliopsoas abscesses are the single most common type of iliopsoas abscesses seen.

The most common abnormalities involving the iliopsoas compartment are neoplasms, abscesses, and hematomas. The fascia that envelops the iliopsoas compartment covers the iliacus, psoas major, and psoas minor and courses through the retroperitoneum from the lower part of the thorax to the lower lumbar vertebrae and defines the iliopsoas compartment. The psoas muscle is susceptible to both hematogenous spread and local direct extension of infectious processes. An endofascia envelops the psoas muscle, and an infectious process that involves the psoas muscles via direct extension lies outside this fascial envelope, while a hematogenously spread infection lies within this fascia. The psoas muscle is extremely rich in vascular supply, with venous supply from the lumbar spine and lymphatic channels from overlying muscle. Thus venous drainage from an infected spine, as in Potts' disease, or from lymphatic spread, such as can occur with *Salmonella* species, are seen with an iliopsoas abscess.

■ ETIOLOGY AND CLINICAL PRESENTATION

The anatomy of the psoas muscle just described appears to predispose the area to infection both via the local direct extension route and via hematogenous and lymphatic dissemination. Although the etiology and predisposing factors associated with this disease have changed over the last 50 years, today "primary" or hematogenous dissemination and infection of the psoas compartment accounts for about 40% of all cases. In such "primary" cases, patients may use intravenous drugs as a means of contaminating the blood and retroperitoneum, or they may have chronic debilitating diseases, such as severe malnutrition and immunosuppression. Secondary iliopsoas abscesses occur as related to the gastrointestinal or genitourinary tract, or from contamination of the musculoskeletal tree via injury or operation. Gastrointestinal diseases known to be associated with psoas abscess include Crohn's disease, enteric fistula from any cause, perforating cancer, and *Salmonella* enteritis. Local extension from a genitourinary source such as from a prostatic or renal abscess is the origin of a few cases, whereas back or hip osteomyelitis can explain a small number of additional case reports of iliopsoas abscess.

The clinical presentation of a patient with an iliopsoas abscess is protean. The age of presentation in reported series ranges from neonates to those older than 80 years of age, depending on associated risk factors. However, the median age at presentation is 45 years. Clinical presenting signs and symptoms are shown in Table 1. Most patients present with a somewhat vague history of fever, flank, hip, back, or abdominal pain. Symptoms of associated gastrointestinal or genitourinary involvement, recent injury, or surgery should be specifically sought. In addition to fever, night sweats and weight loss may also be seen. On physical examination, the patient classically presents with a unilateral flexion deformity of the lower extremity on the side of the psoas abscess. As many as 24% of patients have swelling in the flank with local erythema. A mass may be seen in the back, flank, hip, groin, or abdomen. Pain is almost uniformly present on attempted hip extension (psoas sign). Because the symptoms are nonspecific and nonlocalizing, patients often present for examination 2 weeks after the onset of symptoms, and the diagnosis may not be obvious for 5 to 7 days after presentation until alternative, more common, diagnoses are excluded.

Laboratory abnormalities are typically present and include an elevated white blood cell count in the range of $16,000/mm^3$, an elevated erythrocyte sedimentation rate, and an elevated blood urea nitrogen and creatinine, usually reflecting the chronicity of the presentation and dehydration. When obtained, blood cultures are positive in almost 70% of all patients. Blood cultures should be obtained in a patient with the symptom complex of fever and back, flank, or abdominal pain. The type of microorganism isolated from the blood may well provide additional insight as to the underlying etiology of the iliopsoas abscess because etiologies are linked to specific microbial pathogens.

■ DIAGNOSIS AND CLINICAL MANAGEMENT

The diagnosis of an iliopsoas abscess is relatively easy to confirm once it is considered. As mentioned, however, the diagnosis is often delayed in prehospital presentation and in considering an iliopsoas abscess as the underlying condition responsible for fever and flank, back, abdominal, or hip pain. Diagnosis and localization of disorders of the psoas muscle are most efficiently and accurately made using computed tomographic (CT) scans. The CT scan ensures a reliable distinction of iliopsoas disorders but is less reliable in differentiating neoplasms, abscesses, and hematomas. In a recent study, an iliopsoas neoplasm was more likely (67%) if irregular margins were seen on CT scan, whereas diffuse involvement of the compartment was more common in hematomas (88%) along with a hyperdense appearance. Destruction of tissue planes was equally common among the three disease categories, while a low attenuation reading seen with a lesion was most typical for an abscess (Figure 1),

Table 1 Clinical Signs and Symptoms of Patients with an Iliopsoas Abscess	
CLINICAL SIGN OR SYMPTOM	PERCENTAGE OF PATIENTS WITH SIGN OR SYMPTOMS
Fever	82-90
Pain	64-100
Abdominal	35-100
Flank/back	30-35
Hip	29
Psoas sign	100
Unilateral flexion deformity	29
Mass	18-80
Swelling or erythema	24
Nausea and vomiting	30
Chills and night sweats	6
Elevated white blood cell count	90-100
Positive blood cultures	70

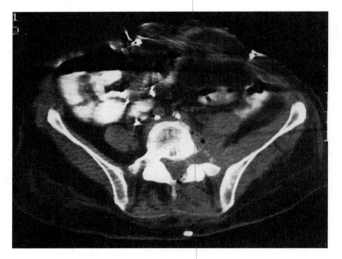

Figure 1
Computed tomography scan of a 78-year-old woman with recent (1 month ago) lumbar surgery and a left psoas abscess. Note the air bubbles located in the lumbar space in continuity with the beginning of a low attenuation area in the left psoas and iliacus muscles. The patient was treated successfully with operative drainage.

although there was low specificity. Although classically gas seen on a CT scan is associated with an abscess, this finding was actually more common in neoplasms (20%) than in abscesses (10%). This study attempted to differentiate whether an iliopsoas process was secondary to infection, neoplasms, or hematoma. These CT scans were interpreted by a radiologist who was blinded to any clinical information. The sensitivity for any single CT finding was reported to be between 67% and 100%, depending on characteristic (Table 2), with specificity ranging between 57% and 80%. Thus, without aspiration and/or biopsy, the exact etiology of an iliopsoas abnormality is difficult to determine. In another study, even when the radiologist knew the clinical history, CT could not be used to characterize the lesion in about 20% of cases. Thus the CT scan can point to the iliopsoas compartment as an etiology for symptoms and signs, but subsequent diagnostic aspiration, biopsy, or drainage should be considered. The CT scan may also identify additional intraabdominal or retroperitoneal structures that are involved and contributing to the formation of the abscess. Both intravenous and oral contrast are indicated to help distinguish additional concurrent pathology. Magnetic resonance imaging (MRI) may offer better anatomic definition of the retroperitoneum, but MRI cannot delineate air bubbles in an abscess, and concurrent gastrointestinal pathology when present may be difficult to determine using MRI. In patients who have a lumbar process such as an epidural abscess or osteomyelitis causing the abscess, the MRI may be preferable to the CT scan. Additional radiographic imaging studies may point to an iliopsoas abscess as a potential source, such as an abdominal roentgenogram that shows the absence of the iliopsoas shadow.

An abdominal ultrasound may be helpful, depending on the patient's body habitus, but usually is not sensitive enough to be diagnostic of an iliopsoas abscess. However, the ultrasound has been used effectively in some institutions as a screening examination in patients with fever, flank, hip, back, or abdominal pain. Thus, in institutions where ultrasonography is commonly used as a screening modality in the emergency department, psoas abscesses may be identified more quickly. If ultrasonography is not available, CT scan should be considered early on in the patient's presentation. The gallium-67 uptake scan is occasionally used in patients with fever of unknown origin and may indicate a gallium-67 avid lesion oriented in the direction of the psoas muscle.

However, this study contributed to the diagnosis or management of patients with an iliopsoas abscess only 54% of the time and therefore cannot be routinely recommended. Gastrointestinal studies with barium or contrast studies through sinus tracts may provide some additional information if it is a suspected source of the abscess, especially when the patient has a history of inflammatory bowel disease or recent surgery.

Immediately upon diagnosis of an iliopsoas abscess, prompt treatment is necessary. Blood cultures should have been obtained and, because they are often positive, should assist in directing antimicrobial therapy. Determining the ultimate appropriate antimicrobial therapy of course depends on the results of systemic and direct cultures. The organisms likely to be causative are determined principally by the pathogenesis of the infection. Thus identifying risk factors for primary infections (intravenous drug abuse, chronic disease, immunosuppression) and for secondary disease (gastrointestinal or pancreatic illness, urinary symptoms, recent hip or back surgery) will help determine likely pathogens (Table 3). In our study population, 75% of patients with a primary iliopsoas abscess had a *Staphylococcus aureus* infection, and thus empiric therapy for this disease should include adequate staphylococcal coverage. In patients with a secondary abscess, enteric organisms were present in 78% of all patients; therefore empiric antimicrobial therapy should include enteric organisms when a secondary abscess is suspected. Once the etiology of the abscess is known and pathogens identified by blood culture and direct aspiration, antibiotics can be tailored. Because most of these patients are ill and bacteremic at the time of presentation, initial antimicrobial therapy should be given intravenously. Later, appropriate oral therapy can be used when indicated by the patient's clinical course. For a primary abscess, staphylococcal coverage can be instituted by a variety of appropriate agents, including oxacillin and nafcillin, the cephalosporins, or clindamycin. In institutions where methicillin-resistant staphylococci are prominent, whether *S. aureus* or coagulase-negative staphylococci, vancomycin therapy may be required. Vancomycin therapy should be considered empirically when the patient is thought to have a primary abscess, especially if a large proportion of staphylococci (either community or nosocomially acquired) are known to be methicillin resistant *and* the patient is critically ill. Patients with an iliopsoas abscess following hip or back

Table 2 Comparison of Different CT Features in Distinguishing Abscesses from Neoplasms and Hematomas of the Iliopsoas Compartment

CT FEATURE	SENSITIVITY %	SPECIFICITY %	ACCURACY %
Enlargement of both psoas and muscle	29	52	41
Low attenuation of the lesion	100	43	70
Diffuse involvement of the entire muscle by lesion	19	52	36
Irregular lesion margins	52	43	48
Fat infiltration	62	48	55
Fascial disruption	57	57	57

Modified from Lenchik L, Dogvan DJ, Kier R: CT of the iliopsoas compartment: value in differentiating tumor, abscess, and hematoma, *AJR Am J Roentgenol* 162:83, 1994. www.arrs.org.
CT, Computed tomography.

Table 3 Pathogens Found in Iliopsoas Abscesses

ILIOPSOAS ETIOLOGY	PATHOGEN
PRIMARY	
Intravenous drug abuse	*Staphylococcus aureus*, coagulase-negative staphylococcus
Immunocompromised	*S. aureus*, *Mycobacterium tuberculosis* Occasional gram-negative organism
SECONDARY	
Gastrointestinal (i.e., Crohn's, fistula, cancer, pancreatic, recent operation)	*Escherichia coli*, *Klebsiella*, *Enterococcus* species, *Proteus* species, *Bacteroides* species, *Peptostreptococcus*, *Clostridium*, *Salmonella enteriditis*
Genitourinary	*E. coli*, *M. tuberculosis*, *Enterococcus* species
Lumbar/back	*M. tuberculosis*, *S. aureus*, coagulase-negative staphylococcus
Trauma	Enteric and *staphylococcal* organisms

Table 4 Treatment Options for Iliopsoas Abscesses

ILIOPSOAS ETIOLOGY	TREATMENT OPTION
PRIMARY	
Intravenous drug abuse	Initial coverage should include specific coverage for *Staphylococcus aureus* but should also include gram-negative coverage until the final organism(s) are known
Immunocompromised	*Options:* Oxacillin (or nafcillin) and aminoglycoside, cephalosporins, especially cefipime, fluoroquinolones, clindamycin, and aminoglycoside
SECONDARY	
Gastrointestinal (i.e., Crohn's, fistula, cancer, pancreatic, recent operation)	Initial coverage for all secondary abscesses should be broad-spectrum and should include gram-negative aerobes and anaerobes
Genitourinary	*Options:* monotherapy: moderate illness: Cefotetan (cefoxitin), piperacillin-tazobactam
Lumbar/back	
Trauma	*Severe illness:* Piperacillin-tazobactam, imipenem, meropenem, alatrofloxacin (except urinary source)
	Combination therapy: clindamycin and aminoglycoside, clindamycin and third-generation cephalosporin (cefotaxime, ceftriaxone), clindamycin, and aztreonam

surgery or those with lumbar osteomyelitis are also likely to have infection with a gram-positive organism, although infection with *Mycobacterium tuberculosis* or *Brucella* species must be suspected when spinal pathology is present. Specific stains and cultures must be obtained. The presence of concurrent hepatosplenomegaly may indicate that spinal brucellosis is present. In children, an iliopsoas abscess is more often related to the hip, and gram-positive organisms predominate.

For patients with a secondary abscess, enteric organisms, most commonly *Escherichia coli*, *Klebsiella*, and *Enterococcus* species are present. Occasionally, *Pseudomonas* species have been isolated. However, much like intraabdominal abscesses, the microbiology of a secondary iliopsoas abscess when an enteric or pancreatic source is likely usually is polymicrobial. Anaerobes are commonly present. When a gastrointestinal source is suspected or identified, broad-spectrum coverage, including the facultative gram-negative aerobes and anaerobes, should be initiated. Thus either monomicrobial therapy or combination therapy can be used as long as the agent covers both aerobes and anaerobes (Table 4). Total duration of antimicrobial therapy should be determined by clinical course, but signs and symptoms of infection may take 5 to 10 days to completely resolve. Antibiotics probably should be continued for 48 to 72 hours beyond the resolution of fever, leukocytosis, and any local signs of erythema.

Antibiotics are not necessary for the entire duration of the drainage catheter, only while clinical signs are present; usually this is at least 7 days and most typically 10 days to 18 days total. Oral antibiotics may be used if the patient has a susceptible organism(s) and the gastrointestinal tract is functional.

Patients with an iliopsoas abscess must undergo some sort of drainage procedure, either operative or percutaneous, usually with radiologic guidance. The decision regarding which of the two approaches should be used is individualized and is based in part on the presence of concurrent disease that would require treatment such as with an enteric source. Other factors that might favor operative drainage include multiple loculations within the abscess and the need for debridement of local tissue. Percutaneous drainage can temporize and stabilize a critically ill patient. In some cases, percutaneous drainage of the abscess cavity may be curative. If the patient is treated with percutaneous drainage, the cavity must be completely obliterated before the catheter is removed. Failure to obliterate the abscess cavity before removing the catheter often results in a recurrent abscess. A sinogram, or dye study through the catheter, along with a CT confirming complete resolution of the collection should be obtained before removal of the catheter. Percutaneous drainage is a useful treatment modality, but recurrence is higher than when operative drainage is used.

■ OUTCOME

The outcome from an iliopsoas abscess depends on the underlying cause, associated diseases, a prompt diagnosis, and timely treatment. Survival is certainly complicated by the presence of underlying cancer and also by the presence of immunosuppression.

The method of treatment, operative versus percutaneous drainage, has not been linked to survival. In fact, treatment options have never been subjected to a clinical trial. In our retrospective review, patients with either concurrent surgical abdominal disease or those who failed percutaneous drainage were treated with operative drainage. Surprisingly, patients with operative drainage had statistically shorter length of hospital stay and a lower recurrence rate when compared with the patients who were treated with percutaneous drainage. This finding has not been reported or examined in any other reports of patients with an iliopsoas abscess and thus may be subject to selection and institutional bias.

Suggested Reading

Chern CH, et al: Psoas abscess: making an early diagnosis in the ED, *Am J Emerg Med* 15:83, 1997.

Kang M, et al: Ilio-psoas abscess in the paediatric population: treatment by US-guided percutaneous drainage, *Pediatr Radiol* 28:478, 1998.

Lenchik L, Dogvan DJ, Kier R: CT of the iliopsoas compartment: value in differentiating tumor, abscess, and hematoma, *AJR Am J Roentgenol* 162:83, 1994.

Macgillvray DC, Valentine RJ, Johnson JA: Strategies in the management of pyogenic psoas abscesses, *Am Surg* 57:701, 1991.

Santaella RO, Fishman EK, Lipsett PA: Primary vs secondary iliopsoas abscess presentation, *Arch Surg* 130:1309, 1995.

Walsh TR, et al: Changing etiology of iliopsoas abscess, *Am J Surg* 163:413, 1992.

BACTERIAL MENINGITIS

Allan R. Tunkel

■ CLINICAL PRESENTATION

The classic clinical presentation in patients with bacterial meningitis is that of fever, headache, meningismus, and signs of cerebral dysfunction (confusion, delirium, or a declining level of consciousness). In a review of 493 cases of acute bacterial meningitis in adults, the classic triad (i.e., fever, nuchal rigidity, and change in mental status) was found in only two thirds of patients, but all had at least one of these findings. The meningismus may be subtle, marked, or accompanied by Kernig's and/or Brudzinski's signs; however, these signs are elicited in only about 50% of adult patients with bacterial meningitis, so their absence never rules out the diagnosis. Cranial nerve palsies and focal cerebral signs are seen in 10% to 20% of cases. Seizures occur in about 30% of patients. Papilledema is observed in less than 1% of cases early in infection, and its presence should suggest an alternative diagnosis. As meningitis progresses, patients may develop signs of increased intracranial pressure (e.g., coma, hypertension, bradycardia, and palsy of cranial nerve III).

Certain symptoms or signs may suggest an etiologic diagnosis in patients with bacterial meningitis. About half of the patients with meningococcemia, with or without meningitis, present with a prominent rash that is localized principally to the extremities. The rash typically is macular and erythematous early in the course of illness, but it quickly evolves into a petechial phase with further coalescence into a purpuric form; the rash may evolve rapidly, with new petechiae appearing during the physical examination. Patients with *Listeria monocytogenes* meningitis have an increased tendency toward focal deficits and seizures early in the course of infection; some patients may present with ataxia, cranial nerve palsies, or nystagmus as a result of rhombencephalitis.

Furthermore, some patients may not present with many of the classic symptoms or signs of bacterial meningitis. Elderly patients, particularly those with underlying medical conditions (e.g., diabetes mellitus, cardiopulmonary disease) may present insidiously with lethargy or obtundation, no fever, and variable signs of meningeal inflammation. Neutropenic patients may also present in a subtle manner because of the impaired ability of the patient to mount a subarachnoid space inflammatory response.

■ DIAGNOSIS

Bacterial meningitis is diagnosed by examination of cerebrospinal fluid (CSF) obtained via lumbar puncture. In virtually all patients with bacterial meningitis, the opening pressure is elevated (>180 mm H_2O), with values greater than 600 mm H_2O suggesting the presence of cerebral edema, intracranial suppurative foci, or communicating hydrocephalus. The CSF white blood cell count is elevated (usually 1000 to 5000 cells/mm^3, with a range of <100 to >10,000/mm^3); patients with low CSF white blood cell counts (from 0 to 20/mm^3), despite high CSF bacterial concentrations, tend to have a poor prognosis. There is usually a neutrophilic predominance (≥80%), although approximately 10% of patients with acute bacterial meningitis will present with a lymphocytic predominance in CSF (more common in neonates with gram-negative bacillary meningitis and patients with *L. monocytogenes* meningitis). A decreased CSF glucose concentration (<40 mg/dl) is found in about 60% of patients; a CSF-to-serum glucose ratio of less than 0.31 is observed in about 70% of patients. The CSF protein is elevated in virtually all cases (usually 100 to 500 mg/dl). Gram stain examination of CSF permits a rapid, accurate identification of the causative microorganism in about 60% to 90% of patients with bacterial meningitis; the specificity is nearly 100%, and the likelihood of detecting the organism is greater with higher CSF bacterial densities. CSF cultures are positive in 70% to 85% of patients with bacterial meningitis. The yield of culture is decreased in patients who have received prior antimicrobial therapy.

In patients with bacterial meningitis and a negative CSF Gram stain, several rapid diagnostic tests for detection of specific bacterial antigens in CSF have been developed to aid in the etiologic diagnosis. Currently available latex agglutination techniques have a sensitivity ranging from 50% to 100% (although these tests are highly specific) and detect the antigens of *Haemophilus influenzae* type b, *Streptococcus pneumoniae*, *Neisseria meningitidis*, *Escherichia coli* K1, and *Streptococcus agalactiae*. Performance of one of these tests may be considered on CSF samples from all patients with presumed bacterial meningitis and a negative CSF Gram stain, although it must be emphasized that a negative test never rules out the diagnosis of meningitis caused by a specific bacterial pathogen. Polymerase chain reaction (PCR) has been used to amplify DNA from patients with meningitis caused by several meningeal pathogens. In one study of patients with meningococcal meningitis, the sensitivity and specificity of PCR were both 91%. However, there are problems with false-positive results when using PCR, and further refinements are needed before this technique can be used in patients with presumed bacterial meningitis when CSF Gram stain, bacterial antigen tests, and cultures are negative.

■ THERAPY

Initial Approach to Management

In patients with the clinical presentation of acute bacterial meningitis, the initial management includes performance of a lumbar puncture. If the CSF formula is consistent with the diagnosis of bacterial meningitis, empiric antimicrobial therapy should be initiated based on results of Gram stain or rapid bacterial antigen tests (Table 1). However, if no etiologic agent can be identified on initial CSF analysis, empiric antimicrobial therapy should be initiated rapidly based on the patient's age (Table 2). In patients with a clinical presentation of bacterial meningitis who have focal neurologic

deficits or papilledema on funduscopic examination, a computed tomography (CT) scan of the head should be performed before lumbar puncture to obviate the potential risk of herniation if an intracranial mass lesion is present. However, because the time involved in obtaining a CT scan can significantly delay the performance of lumbar puncture, empiric antimicrobial therapy, after obtaining blood cultures, should be initiated before sending the patient to the CT scanner to potentially reduce the increased morbidity and mortality associated with bacterial meningitis when initiation of antimicrobial therapy is delayed. Although there are no prospective data on the timing of administration of antimicrobial therapy in patients with bacterial meningitis, a retrospective cohort study in patients with community-acquired bacterial meningitis demonstrated that a delay in initiation of antimicrobial therapy after patient arrival in the emergency room was associated with an adverse clinical outcome when the patient's condition advanced to a high stage of prognostic severity, supporting the assumption that treatment of bacterial meningitis before it advances to a high level of clinical severity improves clinical outcome. Although the yield of positive CSF cultures may decrease with initiation of antimicrobial therapy prior to obtaining CSF for analysis, the pretreatment blood cultures, CSF formula, Gram stain, and/or bacterial antigen tests will likely provide evidence for or against a diagnosis of bacterial meningitis.

Antimicrobial Therapy

Once the infecting meningeal pathogen is isolated and susceptibility testing known, antimicrobial therapy can be modified for optimal treatment (Table 3). Recommended antimicrobial dosages for meningitis in adults with normal renal and hepatic function are shown in Table 4. The following sections review recommendations for use of antimicrobial therapy in patients with bacterial meningitis based on the isolated meningeal pathogen.

Streptococcus pneumoniae

The recommended therapy of pneumococcal meningitis has recently been changed based on recent pneumococcal sus-

---

Table 1 Recommended Antimicrobial Therapy for Acute Bacterial Meningitis Based on Presumptive Identification of the Pathogen*

MICROORGANISM	THERAPY
Streptococcus pneumoniae	Vancomycin plus a third-generation cephalosporin†‡
Neisseria meningitidis	Penicillin G or ampicillin§
Listeria monocytogenes	Ampicillin or penicillin G¶
Haemophilus influenzae type b	Third-generation cephalosporin†
Streptococcus agalactiae	Ampicillin or penicillin G¶
Escherichia coli	Third-generation cephalosporin†

*Positive Gram stain or bacterial antigen test.
†Cefotaxime or ceftriaxone.
‡Addition of rifampin may be considered.
§Some authorities would use a third-generation cephalosporin (cefotaxime or ceftriaxone) as empiric therapy.
¶Addition of an aminoglycoside should be considered.

Table 2 Common Bacterial Pathogens and Empiric Therapeutic Recommendations Based on Age in Patients with Meningitis*

AGE	COMMON BACTERIAL PATHOGENS	EMPIRIC ANTIMICROBIAL THERAPY
0-4 wk	*Streptococcus agalactiae, Escherichia coli, Listeria monocytogenes, Klebsiella pneumoniae, Enterococcus* species, *Salmonella* species	Ampicillin plus cefotaxime, or ampicillin plus an aminoglycoside
4-12 wk	*S. agalactiae, E. coli, L. monocytogenes, Haemophilus influenzae, Streptococcus pneumoniae, Neisseria meningitidis*	Ampicillin plus a third-generation cephalosporin†
3 mon-18 yr	*H. influenzae, N. meningitidis, S. pneumoniae*	Third generation cephalosporin,† or ampicillin plus chloramphenicol
18-50 yr	*S. pneumoniae, N. meningitidis*	Third-generation cephalosporin†‡
>50 yr	*S. pneumoniae, N. meningitidis, L. monocytogenes,* aerobic gram-negative bacilli	Ampicillin plus a third-generation cephalosporin†

*Vancomycin should be added to empiric therapeutic regimens when highly penicillin- or cephalosporin-resistant pneumococcal meningitis is suspected; see text for details.
†Cefotaxime or ceftriaxone.
‡Add ampicillin if meningitis caused by *Listeria monocytogenes* is suspected.

Table 3   Specific Antimicrobial Therapy for Acute Bacterial Meningitis

MICROORGANISM	STANDARD THERAPY	DURATION OF THERAPY
Streptococcus pneumoniae		10-14 days
Penicillin MIC <0.1 µg/ml	Penicillin G or ampicillin	
Penicillin MIC 0.1-1.0 µg/ml	Third-generation cephalosporin*	
Penicillin MIC ≥2.0 µg/ml	Vancomycin plus a third-generation cephalosporin*†	
Neisseria meningitidis		7 days
Penicillin MIC <0.1 µg/ml	Penicillin G or ampicillin	
Penicillin MIC 0.1-1.0 µg/ml	Third-generation cephalosporin*	
Listeria monocytogenes	Ampicillin or penicillin G‡	14-21 days
Streptococcus agalactiae	Ampicillin or penicillin G‡	14-21 days
Haemophilus influenzae		7 days
Beta-lactamase–negative	Ampicillin	
Beta-lactamase–positive	Third-generation cephalosporin*	
Enterobacteriaceae	Third-generation cephalosporin*	21 days
Pseudomonas aeruginosa	Ceftazidime‡	21 days
Staphylococcus aureus		10-14 days
Methicillin-sensitive	Nafcillin or oxacillin	
Methicillin-resistant	Vancomycin	
Staphylococcus epidermidis	Vancomycin†	10-14 days

*Cefotaxime or ceftriaxone.
†Addition of rifampin should be considered.
‡Addition of an aminoglycoside should be considered.

ceptibility patterns. Pneumococcal strains with minimal inhibitory concentrations (MICs) less than 0.1 µg/ml are considered susceptible to penicillin, those with MICs ranging from 0.1 to 1.0 µg/ml are relatively resistant, and those with MICs 2.0 µg/ml or greater are highly resistant. Resistant strains have been reported from many countries throughout the world, including the United States. Because initial CSF concentrations of penicillin are only approximately 1 µg/ml after parenteral administration of standard high dosages, penicillin can no longer be recommended as empiric antimicrobial therapy when *S. pneumoniae* is considered a likely infecting pathogen in patients with purulent meningitis. Of additional concern is that pneumococcal strains resistant to the third-generation cephalosporins have also been described in patients with meningitis; in one study of three such patients in the United States, two responded to initial therapy with vancomycin plus chloramphenicol followed by chloramphenicol alone. However, clinical failures with chloramphenicol have been reported in patients with penicillin-resistant isolates. Furthermore, one report has suggested that vancomycin may also be suboptimal for therapy of pneumococcal meningitis.

Based on these data, it is recommended that for empiric therapy of suspected pneumococcal meningitis, the combination of vancomycin and a third-generation cephalosporin (either cefotaxime or ceftriaxone) should be used pending susceptibility results. This combination was synergistic in a rabbit model of penicillin-resistant pneumococcal meningitis and was synergistic, or at least additive, in the CSF of children with meningitis. If the organism is sensitive to penicillin (MIC <0.1 µg/ml), penicillin is the drug of choice. For relatively resistant strains (MIC 0.1 to 1.0 µg/ml), a third-generation cephalosporin is used. However, if highly resistant strains are documented by susceptibility

testing, vancomycin plus the third-generation cephalosporin are continued for the entire treatment period. Some investigators have also recommended the addition of rifampin, although no clinical data support this recommendation; rifampin should be added only if the organism is susceptible and there is a delay in the expected clinical or bacteriologic response.

Several other antimicrobial agents appear promising for the therapy of penicillin-resistant pneumococcal meningitis. Meropenem, a new carbapenem with less proconvulsant activity than imipenem, is currently under study in patients with pneumococcal meningitis and was used successfully in one patient with a multiply drug-resistant organism. However, further studies are needed to determine the efficacy of meropenem in pneumococcal meningitis caused by penicillin- and cephalosporin-resistant strains. Newer fluoroquinolones (trovafloxacin, moxifloxacin) have also been shown to have efficacy in experimental animal models of penicillin-resistant pneumococcal meningitis, although clinical trials are necessary to determine the usefulness of these agents in patients with bacterial meningitis.

Neisseria meningitidis

The antimicrobial agent of choice for therapy of *N. meningitidis* meningitis is penicillin G or ampicillin. These recommendations may change in the future as a result of the emergence of meningococcal strains that are resistant to penicillin G, with an MIC range of 0.1 to 1.0 µg/ml. In a population-based surveillance study for invasive meningococcal disease in selected areas of the United States, 3 of 100 isolates had penicillin MICs of 0.125 µg/ml. However, the clinical significance of these isolates is unclear because patients with meningitis caused by these organisms have recovered with standard penicillin therapy. Some authorities

Table 4 Recommended Dosages of Antimicrobial Agents for Meningitis in Adults with Normal Renal and Hepatic Function

ANTIMICROBIAL AGENT	TOTAL DAILY DOSE	DOSING INTERVAL (HR)
Amikacin*	15 mg/kg	8
Ampicillin	12 g	4
Cefepime	6 g	8
Cefotaxime	8-12 g	4-6
Ceftazidime	6 g	8
Ceftriaxone	4 g	12-24
Chloramphenicol†	4-6 g	6
Ciprofloxacin	800-1200 mg	8-12
Gentamicin*‡	3-5 mg/kg	8
Meropenem	6 g	8
Nafcillin	9-12 g	4
Oxacillin	9-12 g	4
Penicillin G	24 million U	4
Rifampin§	600 mg	24
Tobramycin*	3-5 mg/kg	8
Trimethoprim-sulfamethoxazole¶	10-20 mg/kg	6-12
Vancomycin‖	2-3 g	8-12

*Need to monitor peak and trough serum concentrations.
†Higher dosage recommended for pneumococcal meningitis.
‡Intrathecal dosage is 4-8 mg; intrathecal dosing should always be used in combination with a parenteral agent.
§Oral administration.
¶Dosage based on trimethoprim component.
‖May need to monitor cerebrospinal fluid concentrations in severely ill patients.

would treat patients with meningococcal meningitis with a third-generation cephalosporin (either cefotaxime or ceftriaxone) pending susceptibility testing of the isolate.

Listeria monocytogenes

Despite their broad range of in vitro activity, the third-generation cephalosporins are inactive against *L. monocytogenes*. Therapy for *Listeria* meningitis should consist of ampicillin or penicillin G, with addition of an aminoglycoside considered in proven infection because of documented in vitro synergy. In the penicillin-allergic patient, trimethoprim-sulfamethoxazole, which is bactericidal against *Listeria* in vitro, should be used. Despite favorable in vitro susceptibility results, chloramphenicol and vancomycin are associated with unacceptable high failure rates, although intraventricular vancomycin was efficacious in one case of recurrent *L. monocytogenes* meningitis. Meropenem, which is active in vitro and in experimental animal models of *Listeria* meningitis, may be a useful alternative in the future.

Haemophilus influenzae

The therapy of bacterial meningitis caused by *H. influenzae* type b depends on whether the strain produces beta-lactamase; these strains accounted for approximately 24% of isolates in the United States in a surveillance study of 27 states from 1978 through 1981, and 32% of isolates in a

subsequent surveillance study of five states and Los Angeles county in 1986. For beta-lactamase–negative strains, ampicillin is recommended, and for strains that produce beta-lactamase, a third-generation cephalosporin (either cefotaxime or ceftriaxone) should be used. In addition, a third-generation cephalosporin should be used as empiric therapy in all patients in whom *H. influenzae* type b is a possible pathogen. Chloramphenicol is not recommended because chloramphenicol-resistant isolates have been reported throughout the world, and even in patients with chloramphenicol-sensitive isolates, a prospective study found chloramphenicol to be bacteriologically and clinically inferior to ampicillin, ceftriaxone, or cefotaxime in the therapy of childhood bacterial meningitis caused predominantly by *H. influenzae* type b. Although cefuroxime, a second-generation cephalosporin, initially appeared to be efficacious in the therapy of *H. influenzae* type b meningitis, a recent study comparing cefuroxime with ceftriaxone for childhood bacterial meningitis documented delayed CSF sterilization and a higher incidence of hearing impairment in the patients receiving cefuroxime; other studies have reported the development of *H. influenzae* meningitis in patients receiving cefuroxime for nonmeningeal *H. influenzae* disease. Recently, cefepime has been compared with cefotaxime in a prospective randomized trial for treatment of meningitis in infants and children; cefepime was found to be safe and therapeutically equivalent to cefotaxime and can be considered a suitable therapeutic alternative for treatment of patients with this disease.

Aerobic Gram-Negative Bacilli

Outcome from meningitis caused by enteric gram-negative bacilli has been greatly improved with the availability of the third-generation cephalosporins (cure rates of 78% to 94%). Ceftazidime, a third-generation cephalosporin with enhanced in vitro activity against *Pseudomonas aeruginosa*, led to cure in 19 of 24 patients with *P. aeruginosa* meningitis in one study when used alone or in combination with an aminoglycoside. Similar results were observed in a study of pediatric patients in which seven patients were cured clinically and nine were cured bacteriologically when receiving ceftazidime-containing regimens. In patients with enteric gram-negative bacillary meningitis not responding to conventional parenteral antimicrobial therapy, concomitant intraventricular or intrathecal aminoglycoside therapy should be considered, although this mode of therapy was associated with a higher mortality rate than systemic therapy alone in infants with gram-negative meningitis and ventriculitis.

Other antimicrobial agents have also been used in patients with aerobic gram-negative meningitis. Imipenem has been efficacious in some isolated cases and larger series, although a high rate of seizure activity (33% in one study) limits its usefulness in patients with bacterial meningitis. The new carbapenem meropenem has been useful in some cases, although further study with this agent as well as newer cephalosporins (e.g., cefepime, cefpirome) are needed before definitive recommendations can be made for the use of these agents in patients with aerobic gram-negative bacillary meningitis. The fluoroquinolones (ciprofloxacin, pefloxacin) have also been used in some patients with bacterial meningitis, although their primary usefulness is for therapy of meningitis caused by multidrug-resistant gram-negative organisms or when the response to conventional therapy is inadequate; these agents should never be used as first-line empiric therapy in patients with meningitis of unknown etiology because of their poor in vitro activity against *S. pneumoniae* and *L. monocytogenes*.

Staphylococci and Streptococci

Meningitis caused by *Staphylococcus aureus* should be treated with nafcillin or oxacillin; vancomycin is used for patients who are allergic to penicillin or when the organism is methicillin resistant. For meningitis caused by coagulase-negative staphylococci (e.g., *S. epidermidis*), vancomycin is recommended; rifampin should be added if the patient fails to improve. In patients with meningitis caused by *S. agalactiae,* ampicillin plus an aminoglycoside is recommended based on documented in vitro synergy and because of the emergence of penicillin-tolerant strains; alternatives include the third-generation cephalosporins and vancomycin.

Adjunctive Therapy

Because of the unacceptable morbidity and mortality rates in patients with bacterial meningitis, even in the antibiotic era, investigators have been studying the pathogenic and pathophysiologic mechanisms operable in bacterial meningitis in the hopes of improving outcome from this disorder. Initial experimental studies focused on the subarachnoid space inflammatory response that occurs during bacterial meningitis to determine whether attenuation of this response would improve outcome. Through the use of experimental animal models of infection, it was determined that one corticosteroid agent, dexamethasone, was effective in reducing the CSF white blood cell response and CSF tumor necrosis factor concentrations, with a trend toward earlier improvement in CSF concentrations of glucose, protein, and lactate; these parameters improved without any apparent decrease in the rate of CSF bacterial killing.

Based on these and other studies in experimental animal models, numerous clinical trials were undertaken to determine the effects of adjunctive dexamethasone on the outcome in patients with bacterial meningitis. A recently published meta-analysis of these clinical studies confirms the benefit of adjunctive dexamethasone (0.15 mg/kg every 6 hours for 2 to 4 days) for *H. influenzae* type b meningitis and, if commenced with or before parenteral antimicrobial therapy, suggests benefit for pneumococcal meningitis in childhood. Evidence of clinical benefit was strongest for hearing outcomes. In adults or in patients with meningitis caused by other bacteria, the routine use of adjunctive dexamethasone is controversial, although some authors recommend their use in all cases of meningitis with a likely bacterial etiology (i.e., demonstrable bacteria on Gram stain, which may predict the patients at high risk of subarachnoid space inflammation after bacterial lysis); however, no clinical data support this recommendation. When adjunctive dexamethasone is used, the timing of administration is crucial; administration before or concomitant with the first dose of the antimicrobial agent is optimal for maximal attenuation of the subarachnoid space inflammatory response.

The use of adjunctive dexamethasone is of particular concern in patients with pneumococcal meningitis caused by highly penicillin- and cephalosporin-resistant strains, in which patients may require antimicrobial therapy with vancomycin. In this instance, a diminished CSF inflammatory response after dexamethasone administration might significantly reduce vancomycin penetration into CSF and delay CSF sterilization. For any patient receiving adjunctive dexamethasone who is not improving as expected or who has a pneumococcal isolate for which the cefotaxime or ceftriaxone MIC is 2.0 µg/ml or greater, a repeat lumbar puncture 36 to 48 hours after initiation of antimicrobial therapy is recommended to document sterility of CSF.

■ PREVENTION

It has become clear in recent years that the spread of several types of bacterial meningitis can be prevented by chemoprophylaxis of contacts of patients with meningitis. The rationale is for eradication of nasopharyngeal colonization, thereby preventing transmission to susceptible contacts and the development of invasive disease in those already colonized. For *H. influenzae*, chemoprophylaxis is recommended for all individuals, including adults, in households with at least one child younger than 4 years of age; the index case should also receive prophylaxis if the antimicrobial agent given for the invasive infection does not eliminate nasopharyngeal colonization. Chemoprophylaxis is not currently recommended for day-care contacts 2 years of age or older unless two or more cases occur in the center within a 60-day period. For children younger than 2 years of age, the question of whether to administer prophylaxis needs to be individualized and should be more strongly considered in centers that resemble households where children have prolonged contact. To prevent transmission of *H. influenzae* type b, the recommended chemoprophylactic agent of choice is rifampin (20 mg/kg/day for 4 days).

Chemoprophylaxis is also recommended for contacts of a case of meningococcal meningitis. Therapy is recommended for close contacts of the index case, defined as household contacts, day-care center members, and anyone directly exposed to the patient's oral secretions (e.g., through kissing, mouth-to-mouth resuscitation, endotracheal intubation, or endotracheal tube management); the index case may also need to receive prophylaxis if he or she is treated with an antimicrobial agent (e.g., penicillin or chloramphenicol) that does not reliably eradicate meningococci from the nasopharynx of colonized patients. The optimal regimen to prevent invasive meningococcal disease is controversial. At present, the Centers for Disease Control and Prevention recommend rifampin (600 mg in adults, 10 mg/kg in children beyond the neonatal period, and 5 mg/kg in infants younger than 1 month of age) given at 12-hour intervals for 2 days. However, eradication rates are only 80% with rifampin, and adverse events, need for multiple dosing, and emergence of resistant organisms have made it less than an ideal agent. Alternatively, ceftriaxone (250 mg intramuscularly in adults and 125 mg intramuscularly in children) or a single dose of oral ciprofloxacin (500 or 750 mg) has been found to be efficacious. Ceftriaxone is probably the safest alternative in the pregnant patient.

Suggested Reading

Aronin SI, Peduzzi P, Quagliarello VJ: Community-acquired bacterial meningitis: risk stratification for adverse clinical outcome and effect of antibiotic timing, *Ann Intern Med* 129:862, 1998.

Kaplan SL, Mason EO Jr: Management of infections due to antibiotic-resistant *Streptococcus pneumoniae, Clin Microbiol Rev* 11:628, 1998.

McIntyre PB, et al: Dexamethasone as adjunctive therapy in bacterial meningitis. A meta-analysis of randomized clinical trials since 1988, *JAMA* 278:925, 1997.

Roos KL, Tunkel AR, Scheld WM: Acute bacterial meningitis in children and adults. In Scheld WM, Whitley RJ, Durack DT, eds: *Infections of the central nervous system,* ed 2, Philadelphia, 1997, Lippincott-Raven.

Tunkel AR, Scheld WM: Acute bacterial meningitis, *Lancet* 346:1675, 1995.

Tunkel AR, Scheld WM: Acute meningitis. In Mandell GL, Bennett JE, Dolin R, eds: *Principles and practice of infectious diseases,* ed 5, Philadelphia, 1999, Churchill Livingstone.

ASEPTIC MENINGITIS SYNDROME

Burt R. Meyers

Fernando Borrego

Alejandra Gurtman

Aseptic meningitis syndrome is associated with symptoms, signs, and laboratory evidence of meningeal inflammation. Clinically, patients usually appear nontoxic but may have changes in mental status, including irritability. Classically, some or all of the following are noted: headache, nausea, vomiting, meningismus, and photophobia. A stiff neck with or without a Brudzinski or Kernig sign may be observed. Other signs of viral infection may include pharyngitis, adenopathy, morbilliform rash, and evidence of systemic viral infection, including myalgia, fatigue, and anorexia. There are usually no signs of vascular instability.

Aseptic meningitis is a syndrome of multiple etiologies (Table 1), including infections from bacteria and higher-order organisms such as mycobacteria, fungi, rickettsia, viruses, and parasites. Noninfectious causes include collagen-vascular diseases (i.e., lupus erythematosus), granulomatous arteritis, sarcoidosis, cerebral vascular lesions, epidermal cysts, meningeal carcinomatosis, serum sickness, drug reactions, and nonfocal lesions of the central nervous system (CNS). Specific syndromes (i.e., Mollaret's meningitis, Still's disease) may produce a similar clinical picture.

■ PATHOPHYSIOLOGY

Viral Meningitis

The most common causes of viral meningitis are the enteroviruses, herpes viruses, and human immunodeficiency virus (HIV). Some viruses passively enter through the skin or respiratory, gastrointestinal, or urogenital tract and may cause initial infection at the entrance site. Growth in extraneural tissue relates to the ability to infect susceptible cells with receptors for the virus and then to replicate viral particles intracellularly. Viruses spread through nerve endings by retrograde transmission via neuronal axons (i.e., poliovirus, rabies virus, herpes virus). Viruses may multiply within an axon as well as within interstitial and lymphatic tissue between nerve fibers. Enteroviruses, lymphocytic choriomeningitis (LCM) virus, mumps, and arthropodborne viruses replicate initially in muscle cells or mesodermal cells. Other viruses enter via the nose, cause infection of the submucosa, and then enter the subarachnoid space. In experimental models, herpes simplex virus (HSV) has been shown to enter by this route. Most viruses probably enter the CNS following viremia with primary replication at the site of entry and dissemination into the systemic circulation to either anchor and grow in the choroid plexus or pass directly through it into the CNS. Enteroviruses and HIV are carried by way of this route.

Nonviral Etiologies

Nonviral causes of meningitis have often a more complicated course than viral meningitis and must be recognized because they may have specific therapy. Agents such as bacteria, mycobacteria, and fungi enter the body through the respiratory tract, including the pharynx, sinuses, skin, or lung, and travel to the CNS via the bloodstream. Pneumonitis may be followed by fungemia or bacteremia. *Treponema pallidum* and *Borrelia burgdorferi* enter the CNS after bloodstream invasion.

Noninfectious Etiologies of Aseptic Meningitis

Entities that should be considered include neurosarcoidosis, connective-tissue disorders, meningeal carcinomatosis or lymphomatosis, CNS vasculitis, migraine-associated pleocytosis, and postviral/postvaccination syndromes. Mechanisms whereby meningeal carcinomatosis, collagen-vascular disease, brain tumors, and epidural or subdural abscess cause changes in the cerebrospinal fluid (CSF) have not been described. Antineoplastic agents, immunosuppressants, including orthoclone (OKT-3), trimethoprim-sulfamethoxazole, and nonsteroidal antiinflammatory drugs (NSAIDs) may produce aseptic meningitis syndrome; the pathophysiology is unknown.

Table 1 Differential Diagnosis of Aseptic Meningitis

NONVIRAL		VIRAL—cont'd	
Bacteria	Partially treated bacterial meningitis	Flavivirus	Japanese encephalitis virus
	Listeria monocytogenes		Murray Valley encephalitis virus
	Brucella species		St. Louis encephalitis virus
	Nocardia		West Nile virus
	Streptococcus pneumoniae (uncommon)	Bunyavirus	California encephalitis virus
	Neisseria meningitidis (uncommon)		LaCrosse encephalitis virus
	Haemophilus influenzae (uncommon)	Reovirus	Colorado tick fever virus
Fungi	*Histoplasma capsulatum*	Arenavirus	Lymphocytic choriomeningitis virus
	Cryptococcus neoformans	Rhabdovirus	Rabies virus
	Coccidiodes immitis	Retrovirus	Human immunodeficiency virus
	Candida spp.	**NONINFECTIOUS**	
	Aspergillus	Drug reactions	Nonsteroidal antiinflammatory agents
	Phycomycetes		Antineoplastic agents
Mycobacteria	Mycobacterium tuberculosis		Antibiotics (trimethoprim-
Rickettsia	Rickettsia rickettsii		sulfamethoxazole)
	Ehrlichia spp.		Immunosuppressants (orthoclone,
Mycoplasma	*Mycoplasma pneumoniae*		azathioprime
Spirochetes	*Treponema pallidum*		Isoniazid
	Borrelia burgdorferi		Immunoglobulin
	Leptospira spp.	Chemicals	Contrast agents
Parasites	Angiostrongylus		Disinfectants, glove powder
	Cysticercosis	Neurologic	Cerebral vascular lesions
	Amoebae	disorders	Epidermal cysts
VIRAL			Brain tumors
Enterovirus	Poliovirus	Systemic	Epidural, subdural abscess
	Echovirus	disorders	Sarcoidosis
	Coxsackie virus		Vasculitis
	New enteroviruses		Behçet's
Herpesvirus	Herpesvirus (HSV) 1 and 2	Miscellaneous	Adult-onset Still's disease
	Varicella-zoster virus		Serum sickness
	Epstein-Barr virus		Mollaret's meningitis
	Cytomegalovirus		Subacute bacterial endocarditis
	HSV-6		Meningeal carcinomatosis
Paramyxovirus	Mumps virus		Vaccination
	Measles virus		Postinfectious viral syndromes
Togavirus	Rubivirus, rubella virus		Post-transplantation lymphoprolifera-
Alphavirus	Eastern equine encephalitis virus		tive disorder
	Western equine encephalitis virus		
	Venezuelan encephalitis virus		

■ DIAGNOSTIC WORKUP

The approach to patients with this syndrome should be careful elucidation of the history and then complete physical and CSF examination (Table 2).

Time of the year may be an important clue because many viral infections are seasonal, occurring during late summer and early fall. Examples of this are the enteroviruses, including echovirus and coxsackievirus. Furthermore, a history of exposure to patients with known viral illness often suggests infection. Enteroviral infection should be considered in patients with aseptic meningitis. These viruses are responsible for up to 90% of cases of aseptic meningitis. Included in this group are the three polioviruses, group A coxsackievirus (24 types), group B coxsackievirus (6 types), echovirus (33 or 34 types), and enterovirus types 68 through 71. Enteroviruses are most commonly isolated in summer and fall, and they decrease through December. Enteroviruses, although most commonly causing aseptic meningitis, may also cause encephalitis, ataxia, peripheral neuritis, and even paralysis. The incubation period is 1 to 5 days. Meningeal

involvement usually occurs within 7 to 10 days. Most cases occur in children 5 years of age or younger, with a male predominance of 1.5:1. Children most commonly have fever, rash, and/or other signs of viral infection of the respiratory or gastrointestinal tract accompanied by irritability and lethargy. In adults, headache is a more prominent finding.

Exposure to mice and rodents suggests infection with LCM, less commonly *Leptospira* species, or the recently described hantavirus, which may cause a severe pulmonary syndrome; history of sexual contacts should be elicited because HSV and, in appropriate risk groups, HIV may present initially with this syndrome. All patients, including the elderly, should be questioned about risk factors for HIV infection, including sexual promiscuity, intravenous drug use, sexual preference, and history of transfusions with blood or blood products.

Syphilitic meningitis has become a more common diagnostic consideration for the aseptic meningitis syndrome in the AIDS era. Syphilitic meningitis may coexist with the primary infection or follow it by as much as 2 years.

Table 2 Diagnostic Workup for Aseptic
Meningitis Syndrome

CLINICAL EVALUATION

History

    Season (summer, enteroviruses, Rocky Mountain spotted
       fever)

    Geographic area (Colorado tick fever, babesia, Lyme disease)

    Exposure to other patients (mumps, varicella)

    Tick, mosquito bites (malaria, Lyme disease)

    Exposure to animals (rabies, hantavirus)

    Sexual history (HIV, HSV, syphilis)

    IVDU (endocarditis)

    Drug reactions (immunoglobulin, OKT-3, NSAIDs,
       antibiotics)

Physical examination

SPINAL FLUID

Opening pressure low

Leukocyte count predominance

    Neutrophils (initial echo [especially 9], polio, TB)

    Lymphocytes (Coxsackie, enterovirus)

    Eosinophils (cysticercosis, angiostrongylus)

    Abnormal cells (Mollaret's, lymphoma)

Protein <40 mg/dl

Glucose <40 mg/dl or <50% serum

Gram stain, AFB smear

Cryptococcal antigen, India ink

Immunoelectrophoresis

VDRL

Latex agglutination for *Haemophilus influenzae* type b,
    Streptococcus pneumoniae, Neisseria meningitidis

Wet mount (toxoplasmosis, amoebae)

Bacterial, viral, mycobacterial, fungal cultures

Lactate, C-reactive protein, adenosine deaminase

PCR for HSV, VZV (in immunocompromised patients), CMV,
    EBV, Mycobacteria

Antibodies to *Borrelia burgdorferi, Brucella, Histoplasma,*
    Coccidioides (chronic or recurrent presentation)

SEROLOGIC TESTING

Cryptococcal antigen

Histoplasma capsulatum, Coccidioides immitis antibody titer

Mycoplasma complement fixation

Lyme disease, ELISA, Western blot

Rocky Mountain spotted fever complement fixation

ANA

HIV-I, HIV-2

VDRL (if positive, FTA-ABS or MHATP)

OTHER

PPD

Chest x-ray film

Computed tomography, magnetic resonance imaging

Echocardiogram

HIV, Human immunodeficiency virus; *HSV,* herpes simplex virus;
IVDU, intravenous drug use; *OKT3,* orthoclone; *NSAIDs,* nonsteroidal antiinflammatory drugs; *AFB,* acid-fast bacilli; *VDRL,* Venereal Drug Research Laboratory; *ELISA,* enzyme-linked immunoab-
sorbent assay; *ANA,* antinuclear antibody.

Geographic location, in terms of domicile and travel
history, should be evaluated. *Histoplasma capsulatum, Coccidioides immitis,* and *B. burgdorferi* occur mainly in certain
sections of the United States. Those who have recently been
in contact with a pet or been camping may risk infection
with *Rickettsia* or *Borrelia* related to a tick bite. Rabies,
although rare, should be considered if there was contact
with or a bite from a sick animal, including skunk, raccoon,
dog, fox, and bat (even, in the bat's case, if there is no
recollection by the patient of been bitten). Drinking local
water on backpacking trips may be associated with *Leptospira;* ingestion of unpasteurized milk and cheeses suggests
brucellosis; and processed meats (i.e., frankfurters) suggest
Listeria. Fungal meningitis is a consideration primarily in
the acquired immunodeficiency syndrome (AIDS) population and in those who have organ transplantation, immunosuppressive chemotherapy, or chronic corticosteroid
therapy. However, the most common fungal meningitis
pathogen, *Cryptococcus neoformans,* can occur in immunocompetent hosts.

Vasculitides found in patients of Mediterranean origin
include Behçet's syndrome and familial Mediterranean fever. Certain drugs, including NSAIDs and immunosuppressants, the latter especially in the transplant patient, have
been associated with aseptic meningitis syndrome. Intracranial infections may present with headache and fever. Brain
abscess and epidural or subdural abscesses should be considered in patients with a history of upper respiratory tract
infection (i.e., otitis media, sinusitis) or infection of the
teeth or gums. Computed tomography (CT) scan or magnetic resonance imaging (MRI) may aid in this diagnosis.
Subacute bacterial endocarditis has been associated with
aseptic meningitis syndrome; physical stigmata, including
conjunctival petechiae, cardiac murmurs, retinal lesions,
and evidence of embolic phenomenon, may be found. Infection with either mycobacteria or fungi or a history of
malignancy must be considered.

Equine-associated meningoencephalitis outbreaks occur
from late summer to early fall; there is usually an association
with infections reported in horses. Avian or equine sources
with spread via mosquitoes is the presumed route of infection to humans.

Partially treated bacterial meningitis should be suspected
if the patient that has received prior oral antimicrobial
therapy and has persistently low CSF glucose or polymorphonuclear pleocytosis, with a negative Gram stain. Recurrent bouts of meningitis with a benign clinical picture and
unknown cause suggest Mollaret's meningitis.

■ PHYSICAL EXAMINATION

The patient is usually febrile and nontoxic appearing, with
or without evidence of meningismus. Low-grade fever may
be present, and the pulse and respiration are usually within
normal limits. Examination of the skin may reveal a morbilliform or vesicular rash or evidence of a tick bite. The scalp
should be examined carefully along with the area behind the
ears. Petechial lesions of the hands and feet usually suggest
rickettsial infection. Examination of the eyes for conjunctival petechiae and funduscopic examination are important
because they may reveal typical lesions of infectious endocarditis. Other lesions usually diagnosed by funduscopic
examination include cytomegalovirus (CMV) retinitis or
toxoplasmosis, especially if there is suspicion of HIV. Examination of the oral cavity may show a mild pharyngitis or
even vesiculopapular lesions on the buccal mucosa gum
margin with or without cervical adenopathy. The chest

examination is usually normal, but a murmur in this setting suggests endocarditis; a pericardial rub suggests a collagen or vascular syndrome. Hepatomegaly, splenomegaly, or adenopathy suggests a systemic disease, including disseminated viral or fungal infection. Examination of the genital area may reveal vesicular or ulcerative lesions. Ulcerative lesions in the vagina have been noted in vascular syndromes such as lupus erythematosus. Joint inflammation, particularly monoarthritis, suggests mycobacterial infection. Examination of the neck may reveal evidence of stiffness on flexion and a positive Brudzinski and/or Kernig sign. Focal or multiple cranial nerve involvement suggests central lesions such as a brain, subdural, or epidural abscess; embolic phenomena may also produce these lesions. Physical examination may reveal a typical malar rash or other stigmata of collagen-vascular disease.

■ LABORATORY DATA

The CSF should be examined and opening pressure recorded. Microscopic examination usually reveals a predominance of lymphocytes. Initially echovirus, polio, mumps, and HSV may have a predominance of polymorphonuclear leukocytes. The cell count is usually less than 100 lymphocytes/ml. Pleocytosis has been reported in 25% of patients with enteroviral infection. Meningeal carcinomatosis is suggested when abnormal cells are seen; large endothelial cells with indistinct cytoplasm suggest Mollaret's meningitis. Fat droplets have been seen following epidermoid cyst rupture. A wet prep of CSF should be examined on suspicion of *Toxoplasma gondii* or *amoebae*. Gram stain and culture should be performed because partially treated bacterial infection or infection with *Listeria monocytogenes* may cause a predominance of lymphocytes. Acid-fast smears to rule out mycobacterial infections and India ink stain for cryptococcal infection should be performed. CSF should be sent for routine fungal, viral, and mycobacterial cultures. If indicated, simultaneous viral cultures should be obtained from throat washings and stool specimens. Eosinophils in the CSF suggest parasitic disease such as angiostrongylus or cysticercosis.

Spinal fluid glucose may be compared with simultaneously drawn blood glucose. Normal levels of CSF glucose (40 mg/dl or more than 50% to 66% of the blood levels) suggest viral meningitis. However, viruses like herpes, mumps, LCM, and polio can cause hypoglycorrhachia (Table 3). The protein is usually elevated in this syndrome; levels greater than 800 mg suggest CSF block with infection or tumor, although it has been described in chemical meningitis.

Latex agglutination for *Haemophilus influenzae* type b (Hib), *Streptococcus pneumoniae*, *Neisseria meningitidis*, done regularly, despite the lack of sensitivity shown in the adult population, providing an accurate and fast diagnosis of potentially treatable entities mainly in the pediatric population.

When aseptic meningitis is suspected, a sample of CSF should be sent for polymerase chain reaction (PCR), which is available for the detection of a range of pathogens, particularly viruses. This technique is highly sensitive and

Table 3 Differential Diagnosis of Cerebrospinal Fluid (CSF) Lymphocytic Pleocytosis

NORMAL CSF GLUCOSE CONCENTRATION	DECREASED CSF GLUCOSE CONCENTRATION
Enteroviruses	Partially treated bacterial meningitis
Mumps virus	*Listeria monocytogenes*
Arthropodborne viruses	
Herpes simplex virus-1 and -2	*Mycobacterium tuberculosis*
Human immunodeficiency virus	
Influenza virus types A and B	*Cryptococcus neoformans*
Measles, SSPE	*Coccidioides immitis*
Varicella-zoster virus	*Histoplasma capsulatum*
Cytomegalovirus	*Candida*
	Blastomyces dermatitidis
Treponema pallidum	
Borrelia burgdorferi	Herpes simplex virus-1
Leptospirosis	Mumps virus
	Lymphocytic choriomeningitis virus
Rickettsia rickettsii	Polio
Human monocytic ehrlichiosis	
Human granulocytic ehrlichiosis	Sarcoidosis
	Leptomeningeal carcinomatosis
Behçet's disease	
Migraine	
Vasculitis	
Postinfectious encephalomyelitis	
Nonsteroidal antiinflammatory agents	
Orthoclone	
Azathioprine	
Trimethoprim-sulfamethoxazole	
Isoniazid	
Intravenous immunoglobulin	

specific, with results available within 24 hours, requiring only small volumes of CSF. Recent studies have devised simple and robust PCR strategies to detect a wide range of viruses, bacteria, and parasites, suggesting that this technique will soon become the "gold standard" test for infections of the CNS. The use of polymerase chain reaction for the diagnosis of aseptic meningitis has resulted in increased identification of the enterovirus, for example, which allows the discontinuation of antimicrobial therapy, decreases hospital length of stay and costs, and enables patients to return to their usual environments. Multiple studies are also exploring the changes in neurochemical (i.e., amino acids, nitrites, concentration of neurotransmitters) and immunologic markers (i.e., IL-1B, IL-6, TNF-a) in the CSF as a tool for the diagnosis and differentiation of the diverse mechanisms and etiologies. For instance, patients with tuberculous meningitis are particularly prone to have vitamin B_{12} deficiency and increased homocysteine levels in the CSF.

Examination of the peripheral blood reveals a white count that is usually normal or may be less than 5000/mm³.

The differential is also normal, although occasionally a left shift of polymorphonuclear leukocytes has been observed. Eosinophilia has been described with drug and serum sickness reactions. Sedimentation rate may be normal or elevated. Blood cultures should be always performed because *L. monocytogenes, Brucella,* and rarely some typical pathogens, such as *Streptococcus pneumoniae, Neisseria meningitidis,* and *H. influenzae,* may present with a predominance of lymphocytes in the CSF. Infectious endocarditis from either bacteria or fungi can be considered in the appropriate clinical setting when a patient has positive blood cultures.

If fungal disease is suspected, serologic studies should be performed for cryptococcal antigen, *H. capsulatum,* and *C. immitis.* Complement fixation for *Mycoplasma pneumoniae* is also warranted. Venereal Disease Research Laboratory (VDRL) test should be performed on CSF. When rickettsial diseases are suspected (i.e., Rocky Mountain spotted fever or Lyme disease), appropriate serologic tests should be performed. If rabies is suspected, an immunofluorescence test on conjunctival scrapings or subcutaneous neck fascial biopsy are the best method for establishing the diagnosis. Other serologic tests include antinuclear antibody (ANA) to rule out systemic lupus erythematosus. Given the appropriate clinical setting, HIV testing may be warranted. Patients with genital HSV-2 infection and meningitis should have serologic tests performed over 3 to 4 weeks, looking for fourfold rise of antibody titer. The virus may be isolated from CSF as well or detected through PCR examination.

If vesicular lesions are present, immunofluorescent staining for HSV-1, HSV-2, and varicella-zoster virus (VZV) should be performed, as should viral culture. If lesions other than vesicular lesions are found, careful examination by darkfield may reveal evidence of *T. pallidum.* Petechial lesions should be stained and cultured for bacteria and stained with immunofluorescence antibody for *R. rickettsii.* Throat and stool cultures should be obtained for confirmation of enteroviral infection.

A roentgenogram film specifically looking for diffuse infiltrates, cavitation, and pleural or pericardial involvement may suggest mycoplasmal, mycobacterial, or fungal infection in that order. Evidence of a mass lesion in this setting suggests carcinoma and possibly meningeal carcinomatosis. With physical findings of focal involvement, a CT scan should be performed to look for evidence of an intracranial infection or malignancy.

■ THERAPY

The diagnosis and treatment of the aseptic meningitis syndrome is a challenge; differentiating between infectious and noninfectious aseptic meningitis can be difficult (see Table 1). Although there is no specific treatment for most patients with aseptic meningitis, the management of those with a syndrome of viral origin includes supportive care in most cases, although therapy exists for specific viral pathogens. Acyclovir, ganciclovir, and zidovudine (AZT) may be used to treat meningitis caused by HSV and VZV, CMV, and meningitis secondary to HIV infection, respectively. Specifi-

cally, acyclovir, 10 to 12 mg/kg every 8 hours, is used for HSV and VZV; ganciclovir, 5 mg/kg twice a day, for CMV, and AZT, 1200 mg/day, for the treatment of HIV. Ribavirin for treatment of hantavirus infection is still experimental.

Although no specific antiviral therapy is indicated for enteroviral and rhinoviral infection, the administration of gamma globulin has led to improvement in patients with agammaglobulinemia who have chronic enteroviral meningitis as well as in neonates with enteroviral sepsis and meningitis. Pleconaril is a novel inhibitor of enteroviruses and rhinoviruses that has been developed for the treatment of diseases associated with the aforementioned virus infections. The drug is in late-stage clinical trials for the treatment of viral meningitis, showing very promising results (good tolerance at prophylactic and therapeutic dosing; dramatic decrease in virus load; increased survival).

Most viral meningitides are benign and require no therapy. For bacterial, fungal, and spirochetal disease antimicrobial therapy directed against the offending agent is required (see specific chapters) and should not be delayed while awaiting the results of CSF assay. Treatment with doxycycline or chloramphenicol may be indicated for patients suspected of having *Brucella* or Rocky Mountain spotted fever. Specific therapy with ampicillin plus gentamicin is suggested when *L. monocytogenes* is the suspected agent, especially in immunocompromised hosts.

Because the differential diagnosis of aseptic meningitis syndrome is so broad, the initial evaluation of the patient in conjunction with the results of CSF studies will determine whether the patient needs to continue empiric antimicrobial therapy to treat bacterial meningitis, pending culture results from blood and CSF. Patients who are toxic appearing, in the extremes of life, or with serious underlying disease should be admitted to the hospital and treated empirically until a clear diagnosis is made. Isolation precautions for contagious diseases should be instituted.

Suggested Reading

Conolly KJ, Hammer SM: The acute aseptic meningitis syndrome, *Infect Dis Clin Am* 4:599, 1990.

Fishman RA: *Cerebrospinal fluid in diseases of the central nervous system,* ed 2, Philadelphia, 1992, WB Saunders.

Greenlee JE: Cerebrospinal fluid in central nervous system infections. In Scheld WM, Whitley RI, Durack DT, eds: *Infections of the central nervous system,* New York, 1991, Raven Press.

Hosoya M, et al: Application of PCR for various neurotropic viruses on the diagnosis of viral meningitis, *J Clin Virol* 11:1174, 1998.

Johnson RT: The pathogenesis of acute viral encephalitis and postinfectious encephalomyelitis, *J Infect Dis* 155:359, 1987.

Melnick JL: Enteroviruses: polioviruses, coxsackieviruses, echoviruses and newer enteroviruses. In Fields BM, Knipe DM, eds: *Virology,* New York, 1990, Raven Press.

Moris G, et al: The challenge of drug-induced aseptic meningitis, *Arch Intern Med* 159:1185, 1999.

Pevear DC, et al: Activity of pleconaril against enteroviruses, *Antimicrob Agents Chemother* 43:2109, 1999.

Qureshi GA, et al: The neurochemical markers in cerebrospinal fluid to differentiate between aseptic meningitis and tuberculous meningitis, *Neurochem Int* 32:197, 1997.

Townsend GC, et al: Infections of the central nervous system, *Adv Intern Med* 43:403, 1998.

ACUTE VIRAL ENCEPHALITIS

Diane Griffin

Roger T. Inouye

Encephalitis is inflammation of the brain parenchyma. In contrast, meningitis is an inflammatory process limited to the leptomeninges and the subarachnoid space, but it can often coincide with encephalitis; hence the overlap term *meningoencephalitis*. Encephalitis or meningoencephalitis is suggested by signs and symptoms of brain parenchymal invasion such as mental status and behavioral changes, seizures, and focal neurologic findings.

■ ETIOLOGY

Viral encephalitis can be subdivided into several clinical and pathogenic categories. These include acute viral encephalitis, slow virus infections, postinfectious encephalitis, and cryptogenic central nervous system (CNS) processes with probable direct or indirect viral associations such as Reye's syndrome. Several viral families are associated with acute encephalitis, the most common of which are *Herpesviridae*, *Picornaviridae*, *Retroviridae*, *Paramyxoviridae*, assorted respiratory and zoonotic viruses, and the group of RNA viruses formerly called *arboviruses*, now designated as the families *Togaviridae*, *Flaviviridae*, *Bunyaviridae*, and *Reoviridae* (Table 1). The acquired immunodeficiency syndrome (AIDS) epidemic and therapeutic immunosuppression in transplant recipients and oncologic chemotherapy patients have redefined the differential of infectious disease processes that can cause symptoms and signs consistent with encephalitis. These changes have made the clinician's diagnostic task when confronted with an encephalitic patient all the more complex and challenging and require the discrimination between an extensive list of potential viral and nonviral causes of encephalitis (Table 2).

■ EPIDEMIOLOGY

The many virus types that can cause encephalitis vary significantly in their epidemiologic profiles. Therefore the identification of a particular virus can be aided by clues derived from a careful review of the patient's epidemiologic background, including sexual behavior, intravenous drug use, travel, occupation, arthropod or animal contacts, vaccine history, and exposures to ill persons. A summary of representative associations with specific viral and nonviral entities is outlined in Table 3.

■ PATHOGENESIS

Depending on the specific pathogen, viruses gain entry into the CNS mainly through hematogenous or neural spread

Table 1 Significant Causes of Viral Encephalitis in the United States

HERPESVIRIDAE	***REOVIRIDAE***
Herpes simplex virus	Colorado tick fever virus
Varicella-zoster	***PICORNAVIRIDAE***
Cytomegalovirus	Echovirus
Epstein-Barr virus	Coxsackievirus
Human herpes virus 6	Poliovirus
B virus	Enterovirus
BUNYAVIRIDAE	***RETROVIRIDAE***
California encephalitis serogroup	Human immunodeficiency virus type 1
LaCrosse virus	***PAPOVAVIRIDAE***
Jamestown virus	JC virus
Snowshoe hare virus	***ORTHOMYXOVIRIDAE***
TOGAVIRIDAE	Influenza virus
Alphavirus	***PARAMYXOVIRIDAE***
Eastern equine encephalitis virus	Measles virus
Western equine encephalitis virus	Mumps virus
	MISCELLANEOUS VIRUSES
Venezuelan equine encephalitis virus	Adenovirus
FLAVIVIRIDAE	Rubella virus (non–arthropod-borne member of *Togaviridae*)
St. Louis encephalitis virus	Lymphocytic choriomeningitis virus
West Nile virus	Rabies virus
Dengue viruses	
Powassan virus	

and cause either direct cytopathic effects or indirect pathology via immune-mediated processes. *Bunyaviridae*, *Flaviviridae*, and *Togaviridae* hematogenously seed the CNS following replication in local tissues after subcutaneous inoculation by the insect vector. In addition to the integument, the initial portal of entry by neurotropic viruses can be the respiratory tract (e.g., adenovirus, measles, influenza), the gastrointestinal tract (e.g., enteroviruses), or the placenta (e.g., cytomegalovirus [CMV]). Rabies virus is a neurotropic virus that reaches the CNS via intraaxonal transport. In the case of adult herpes simplex virus (HSV) encephalitis, either primary or reactivated, the pathogenesis remains unfully characterized, but virus passage along the olfactory and trigeminal tracts, respectively, would explain the classic temporal lobe localization.

Once the CNS parenchyma has been seeded, predominantly mononuclear cell perivascular infiltrates, glial nodules, and neuronophagia characterize histopathologic changes commonly seen in acute viral encephalitis. Inclusion bodies, such as Negri and Cowdry bodies caused by rabies and herpes viruses, respectively, can reflect infections with specific viruses. The type of CNS parechymal cell predominantly affected during encephalitis can vary among neurotropic viruses.

Further clarification of the effect of cytokines in the pathogenesis of encephalitis continues. Interferons (alpha, beta, and gamma) and their regulatory transacting proteins as well as various interleukins (IL-2, IL-4, IL-8, and IL-10) appear to play an important and necessary role in the pathogenesis of and protection against HSV and other encephalitides such as the Venezuelan equine encephalitis.

Nitric oxide (NO) may also be involved in encephalitis pathogenesis. High levels of NO observed in various brain

Table 2 Nonviral Causes of Encephalitis-Like Presentations

INFECTIOUS	NONINFECTIOUS
Bacterial	Parainfectious
Parameningeal infections	Reye's syndrome
Central nervous system	Viral postinfectious
infections	syndromes
Subdural empyema	Postvaccination syndromes
Venous sinus	Primary central nervous
thrombophlebitis	system or metastatic
Neisseria meningitidis	neoplastic disease
Streptococcus pneumoniae	Cerebrovascular disease
Haemophilus spp.	Subdural hematoma
Listeria monocytogenes	Endocrine disorders
Mycoplasma spp.	Toxic metabolic
Rickettsia spp.	encephalopathy
Ehrlichia spp.	Connective tissue disease (e.g.,
Borrelia burgdorferi	systemic lupus erythemato-
Treponema pallidum	sus, Behçet's disease)
Legionella spp.	Paraneoplastic syndromes
Mycobacterium spp.	Seizures/postictal state
Brucella spp.	
Leptospira spp.	
Actinomyces spp.	
Nocardia spp.	
Bartonella henselae	
Trophyrema whippelii	
Bacterial toxin–mediated	
processes	
Fungal	
Zygomycetes	
Aspergillus spp.	
Cryptococcus neoformans	
Coccidioides immitis	
Histoplasma capsulatum	
Parasitic	
Toxoplasma gondii	
Plasmodium spp.	
Trypanosoma spp.	
Naegleria fowleri	
Acanthamoeba spp.	
Strongyloides stercoralis	

regions that coincide with those of viral propagation appear to be a pathogenic factor in models of HSV-1 encephalitis. An NO synthase inhibitor significantly ameliorates clinical symptoms such as paralysis and seizures and mortality in the same models. NO-mediated pathogenesis needs to be further studied and could potentially reveal new therapeutic approaches for encephalitis.

In postinfectious encephalitis, pathogenesis occurs via immune-mediated mechanisms rather than through direct cytopathic effects and manifests as multifocal perivascular demyelination. Viruses implicated in this type of encephalitis include measles, mumps, rubella, varicella-zoster virus (VZV), and Epstein-Barr virus (EBV). This form of encephalitis may manifest either acutely or many years after infection.

Host factors clearly play a role in the susceptibility to and severity of viral encephalitis. For example, chronic enteroviral meningoencephalitis is seen most commonly in patients with agammaglobulinemia; acute measles, CMV, and VZV encephalitis usually occur in immunosuppressed patients.

■ CLINICAL MANIFESTATIONS

Usually, the clinical features of a particular neurotropic virus alone are not pathognomonic. The clinical presentation of viral encephalitis can vary from no symptoms to a fulminantly fatal disease. Although the literature is replete with case reports of unique neurologic manifestations of viral encephalitis, the clinical presentation of acute viral encephalitis is generally characterized by a rapidly progressive constellation of symptoms. These typically include fever, altered mental status, headache, nausea, and vomiting. Nuchal rigidity and seizures, either partial or generalized, can also be prominent. Cranial nerve abnormalities and hyperreflexia are commonly seen in certain encephalitic processes such as HIV-related CMV ventriculoencephalitis.

Certain viral pathogens are associated with focal CNS predilections and can cause corresponding deficits. Archetypal of such viruses are HSV with the temporal and frontoorbital lobes, CMV with the periventricular areas, rabies with the limbic system, and VZV with the cerebellum. Respiratory syncytial virus (RSV) may also give a cerebellitis picture. Decerebration or decortication, flaccid paralysis, focal neurologic signs as well as movement disorders are common with Japanese encephalitis (JE) virus infections.

Extraneural manifestations of a particular neurotropic virus may be helpful when present, such as parotitis with mumps, pharyngitis and lymphadenopathy with EBV, pharyngitis and myalgia with Venzuelan equine encephalitis, and a dermatomal rash with VZV. Nonspecific associated extraneural complications of viral encephalitis may include inappropriate antidiuretic hormone (ADH) secretion and diabetes insipidus.

■ DIAGNOSIS

General chemistries and cell counts have relatively limited value. A peripheral blood examination showing atypical lymphocytes or a positive Monospot may suggest EBV infection; hyperamylasemia may suggest mumps virus. Rectal and throat swabs may provide evidence of neurotropic viruses such as enteroviruses. Immunocytochemical analysis of corneal smears occasionally aids in the diagnosis of rabies. However, the absence of such findings does not exclude a particular virus.

Examination of the cerebrospinal fluid (CSF) can show nonspecifically abnormal cell counts and chemistries. For example, with HSV encephalitis, except in the initial stages, most patients have a mononuclear pleocytosis typically less than 1000 cells/mm^3 with a median of approximately 130 cells/mm^3. Significant numbers of polymorphonuclear cells (at least 40%) can be seen in as many as 10% to 15% of patients if the lumbar puncture is done early; red blood cells (RBCs) are usually present. Although in half of the patients with HSV encephalitis the total protein may be normal in the first week, CSF protein levels are usually elevated, with a range of 7 to 755 and a mean value of 80 mg/dl. In HSV encephalitis, hypoglycorrhachia is relatively uncommon.

The yield, and consequently the utility, of CSF viral culture in adults with encephalitis is low. Because cytologic and chemical CSF results are relatively nonspecific and may

Table 3   Clinical and Epidemiologic Characteristics of Major Causes of Viral Encephalitis in the United States

VIRUS	MOST AFFECTED HOST	PEAK SEASON	GEOGRAPHIC DISTRIBUTION	CLUES IN PRESENTATION	EPIDEMIOLOGIC CLUES
HERPESVIRIDAE					
Herpes simplex type 1	All ages	Year-round	Ubiquitous	Focal neurologic findings such as hemiparesis, ataxia, visual field loss, dysphasia, seizures	
Varicella–zoster	Healthy and immunocompromised adults; infants	Year-round	Ubiquitous	Cerebellar ataxia	Primary varicella rash or herpes zoster dermatomal rash possible; onset usually within 2 wk of rash
Cytomegalovirus	Immunocompromised (e.g., person with AIDS; transplant recipients; neonates)	Year-round	Ubiquitous	Cranial nerve palsies; radiographic findings of ventriculomegaly or periventricular enhancement	In known HIV+ individuals, CD4 <100, prior CMV disease; posttransplant individuals: donor and recipient CMV serologic status, most cases occur 3 wk to 4 mo after transplant; in patients with unknown immune status must elicit HIV risk factors
RETROVIRIDAE					
Human immunodeficiency virus	All ages	Year-round	Ubiquitous	Subacute onset of cognitive, motor deficits in an HIV+ individual; focal findings rare	HIV risk factor history: sexual practices, intravenous drug use, transfusions
PAPOVAVIRIDAE					
JC virus	Immunocompromised (e.g., person with AIDS; transplant recipients)	Year-round	Ubiquitous	Cognitive or focal neurologic deficits with MRI findings of multifocal white matter disease	History of immunodeficiency (e.g., HIV+ individuals, CD4 <100; posttransplant individuals)
TOGAVIRIDAE					
Eastern equine	Young and elderly	Summer, fall	East, Gulf Coast	High morbidity and mortality, especially in the elderly and young	Contact with *Culiseta* mosquito; outdoor occupation or activities
Western equine	Young and elderly	Summer, fall	Western North America, Central and South America	Nonfocal presentation common	Contact with *Culex* mosquito; outdoor occupation or activities; travel or habitation in rural areas
Venezuelan equine	Adults	Summer, fall	South	Nonfocal presentation common	Contact with *Culex* or *Aedes* mosquito; outdoor occupation or activities
St. Louis encephalitis	Elderly	Summer, fall	Nationwide	Nonfocal presentation common	Contact with *Culex* mosquito; in the West endemic in rural areas; in the East, sporadic urban outbreaks
Powassan	Young	Summer, fall	Nationwide	Nonfocal presentation common	Contact with ticks; possible transmission through unpasteurized dairy products
BUNYAVIRIDAE					
LaCrosse	Young	Summer, fall	Midwest, East	Usually asymptomatic	Contact with *Aedes* mosquito; outdoor activities
PICORNAVIRIDAE					
Echo Coxsackie Polio Enterovirus	Young, especially agammaglobulinemic children	Summer, fall	Nationwide	Accompanying viral exanthem, conjunctivitis, myopericarditis, herpangina, hand-foot-and-mouth disease	Known community epidemic of picornavirus
RHABDOVIRIDAE					
Rabies	All ages		Nationwide except Hawaii	Animal bite or scratch	Animal contact

AIDS, Acquired immunodeficiency syndrome; *HIV*, human immunodeficiency virus; *CMV*, cytomegalovirus; *MRI*, magnetic resonance imaging.

even be normal in early disease, several other diagnostic modalities have been used.

Radiologic and Electroencephalographic Evidence

The electroencephalogram (EEG) may assist in the diagnosis of acute focal encephalitis such as HSV. Periodic lateralized epileptiform discharges in the temporal lobe can be seen within the first days after onset. Although having low specificity, the EEG is reported to have a sensitivity of about 81% versus 59% for computed tomography (CT) and 50% for nuclear scans. Encephalitis-induced EEG abnormalities can precede CT changes, which may not be seen until 4 to 5 days after the onset of symptoms. Epileptic seizures early during the course of the disease correlate significantly with outcome. The presence of diffuse slowing of background activity or irritative features acutely is not as important as previously thought. In contrast, the emergence of diffuse slow background activity at follow-up is associated with a less favorable outcome.

Radiographic imaging, namely CT or magnetic resonance imaging (MRI), may aid in the workup of encephalitis. CT abnormalities in HSV, for example, are typically characterized by low-density lesions in one or both of the inferomedial temporal lobes. MRI, however, allows for earlier radiographic evidence of HSV encephalitis and more precise imaging of the inferomedial temporal lobes. Thus MRI is the radiographic imaging study of choice in patients with suspected encephalitis.

MRI has been used extensively in the diagnosis and follow-up of other encephalitides. Basal ganglia lesions are seen with EBV. A wide range of abnormalities, with white matter lesions initially and gray matter involvement later as well as brainstem and cervical cord lesions, are described with VZV. Characteristic bilateral thalamic hyperintense lesions in T_2-weighted images are seen in JE. Diffuse involvement of the cerebral cortex with brain edema and symmetric thalamic lesions as well as focal encephalitis have been reported in influenza encephalitis. Focal lesions in the basal ganglia have been associated with Eastern equine virus (EEE).

In cases of a negative MRI, newer imaging modalities such as brain perfusion single photon emission tomography (SPECT) examination may be useful in identifying areas of marked hyperperfusion. In a study of patients with acute encephalitis, unilateral hyperperfusion with SPECT was an independent predictor of poor prognosis, whereas clinical outcome variables, such as seizures, state of consciousness, and focal neurologic findings, or CSF and EEG findings were not. Applications of this technique require further exploration.

Pathogen-Specific CSF and Serologic Assays

Serum and CSF immunoglobulin assays are available for most neurotropic viruses, including the *Herpesviridae, Bunyaviridae, Togaviridae, Picornaviridae,* and *Rhabdoviridae.* Unfortunately, viral-specific antibodies are difficult to detect early in the disease process. CSF antibodies may be elevated because of nonencephalitic processes such as viremia without CNS involvement; therefore serum-to-CSF antibody ratios may be used to help distinguish between CNS and non-CNS viral processes. Acute and convalescent serum titers alone can retrospectively suggest acute infection, but again, they are of limited utility when initial therapeutic decisions are made.

PCR has been used to detect a number of neurotropic viruses in CSF, biopsy, and autopsy specimens, including HSV, VZV, CMV, EBV, human herpesvirus type 6 (HHV-6), HHV-7, HHV-8, HIV, measles virus, JC virus, enteroviruses, and certain arthropodborne viruses. The sensitivity and specificity of PCR of CSF-extracted DNA from patients with presumed HSV encephalitis is 95% to 100%. Positive results are reported as early as a day after onset of symptoms. In comparison, HSV antigen detection had a sensitivity of 33%, and HSV-specific intrathecal antibody assay by indirect enzyme-linked immunosorbent assay (ELISA) had a sensitivity of 23%. HSV PCR can be negative early in disease, and some authors advocate sequential testing of CSF if the clinical suspicion is high despite an initial negative assay.

Brain Biopsy

The utility of a diagnostic brain biopsy in the management of encephalitis remains controversial, especially in light of the ability to institute effective empiric antiviral drugs for viruses such as HSV and the rivaling sensitivity and specificity of relatively noninvasive PCR-based assays. However, when a diagnosis remains elusive or there is lack of response to initial therapy, brain biopsy continues to play an important role.

■ THERAPY

General Supportive Care

No effective treatment is yet available for many neurotropic viruses such as the *Bunyaviridae, Togaviridae,* and *Picornaviridae.* Therefore particular attention is required in preventing and treating complications that can arise in any patient with a depressed sensorium who may require an extended intensive care unit stay with ventilatory support. These include nosocomial infectious diseases such as pneumonias with potentially resistant bacterial organisms; device-related infections such as those involving intracranial pressure monitoring bolts, central lines, and indwelling urinary catheters; and antibiotic-related colitis. CNS complications of encephalitis, such as seizures and intracranial hypertension, may necessitate anticonvulsants and intracranial pressure-lowering techniques such as hyperventilation, osmotic agents, and barbiturates. The possibility of noninfectious complications, such as deep vein thrombosis, pulmonary embolism, gastrointestinal stress ulcers, decubitus ulcers, musculoskeletal contractures, and malnutrition, requires appropriate attention as well.

Antiviral Therapy

Although numerous viruses are associated with encephalitis, there remain relatively few effective regimens. Nevertheless, several drugs have demonstrated activity against some of the more commonly encountered viral pathogens (Table 4).

Herpesviridae

In the United States, HSV-1 is the most common cause of sporadic encephalitis. Acyclovir is the mainstay of therapy

Table 4 Treatment Regimens for Herpes Viral Encephalitis

VIRUS	DRUG OF CHOICE	MAJOR TOXICITIES	ALTERNATIVE REGIMENS	MAJOR TOXICITIES
Herpes simplex virus	Acyclovir, 10 mg/kg IV q8h for 10-14 days	Nephrotoxicity, vomiting, diarrhea, mental status changes	Foscarnet, 60 mg/kg IV q8h or 90 mg/kg IV q12h for 10-14 days	Nephrotoxicity, electrolyte disturbances, Nausea, fever
Cytomegalovirus	Foscarnet induction, 60 mg/kg IV q8h or 90 mg/kg IV q12h for 21 days; consider maintenance therapy in HIV+ patients	Nephrotoxicity, electrolyte disturbances, Nausea, fever	Foscarnet can be combined with ganciclovir	As above
	Ganciclovir induction, 5 mg/kg IV q12h for 21 days; consider maintenance therapy in HIV+ patients	Bone marrow suppression, rash, fevers	Cidofovir, 5 mg/kg IV qwk with probenecid (2 g PO 3 hr before cidofovir dose, 1 g 2 hr immediately after dose, and 1 g 8 hr after dose) and 1 L of normal saline IV 1 hr before cidofovir infusion	Nephrotoxicity, rash cardiomyopathy
Varicella-zoster virus	Acyclovir, 10 mg/kg IV q8h for 10-14 days	As above		
Epstein-Barr virus	Acyclovir, 10 mg/kg IV q8h for 10-14 days	As above		

HIV, Human immunodeficiency virus.

for this clinical entity. The age of the patient (older than 30 years), level of consciousness at presentation (Glasgow Coma Scale score greater than 10), and duration of disease (less than 4 days) before acyclovir therapy are significant determinants of improved survival. In contrast to adults, trials comparing acyclovir with vidarabine in neonatal HSV encephalitis failed to show significant differences in outcome.

Relapses have occurred after the administration of standard regimens of both acyclovir and vidarabine and are thought to occur in up to 5% of cases. Treatment failures have been attributed to postinfectious encephalomyelitis, reactivation of latent virus, failure of the standard 10-day regimen to eradicate the virus, and possibly drug resistance.

Although no surgical therapy of HSV encephalitis exists, anterior temporal lobe resection and decompressive craniotomy may be of benefit in selected cases complicated by massive brain edema and tentorial herniation.

In the era of the AIDS epidemic, CMV infections, including encephalitis, have become more common. Ganciclovir, one of the mainstays in the treatment of CMV retinitis, has yielded inconsistent results in the treatment of CMV encephalitis and ventriculitis. Its use is also limited by its significant myelosuppressive effects. Foscarnet, in general, readily crosses the blood-brain barrier, attaining virustatic concentrations in CSF, and therefore is a reasonable alternative to ganciclovir. However, this agent's significant renal and electrolyte adverse effects require careful monitoring. Recently, combinations of ganciclovir and foscarnet have been reported to yield successful results (see *AIDS: Treatment of Opportunistic Infections,* and *Cytomegalovirus*).

High-dose parenteral acyclovir has been used in the treatment of VZV encephalitis, although the use of antiviral drugs in this disease has yet to be proved to have clinical benefit. Encephalitis is a rare complication of EBV. The therapeutic effects of acyclovir in EBV encephalitis remain unproved as well, but should be strongly considered, given the lack of alternative regimens and the relatively low toxicity of acyclovir. Vaccination for VZV is recommended for healthy children, patients with leukemia, and patients with chronic diseases receiving immunosuppressive therapy.

Successful treatment of human herpesvirus 6 encephalitis with ganciclovir or foscarnet has been described in immunocompromised patients.

Drug-resistant herpesvirus is most commonly associated with HSV thymidine kinase alternation or deficiency (TK-). Resistant strains have been described as causing acyclovir-refractory HSV meningoencephalitis in HIV-infected individuals and should be considered in the setting of worsening clinical picture and isolation of HSV from persisting lesions despite appropriate doses and blood levels of acyclovir. Cross-resistance between acyclovir and other drugs (i.e., valacyclovir, famciclovir, ganciclovir) may be expected with TK-deficient mutants. Intravenous foscarnet is recommended for most cases of acyclovir-resistant isolates. Lobucavir, a ganciclovir analog that is partially dependent on viral TK, is now under evaluation. Nucleotide analogs (e.g., cidofovir) may also be effective for TK-deficient mutants.

Paramyxoviridae

Invasion of the CNS by measles virus is associated with several distinct syndromes, including two forms of acute

Patient with FEVERS,
HEADACHE, MENTAL STATUS
OR BEHAVIORAL CHANGES, and
SEIZURES

Consider viral and
nonviral infectious and noninfectious
causes

INITIAL DIAGNOSTIC WORKUP:
Cranial MRI or CT; EEG; lumbar
puncture (if no contraindications); blood and CSF for microbiologic, serologic, and special
studies (e.g., PCR)

Consider brain biopsy if
diagnosis remains elusive and
patient is not improving

OBTAIN DETAILED EPIDEMIOLOGIC HISTORY INCLUDING
Season of onset
Travel
Sexual behavior
Intravenous drug use
Transfusion
Occupation
Insect bites
Hobbies and outdoor activities
Exposure to animals or pets
Dietary habits
Ill contacts
Tuberculosis history or exposure
Vaccine history

PHYSICAL EXAMINATION
Focal neurologic findings, e.g., hemiparesis,
    cranial nerve deficits, dysphasia, focal seizures,
    ataxia, visual field deficit
Associated findings, e.g., papilledema, retinal
    lesions, zosteriform rashes, mucocutaneous
    herpetic lesions, insect or animal bites

DIAGNOSTIC WORKUP AND EMPIRIC THERAPY
In immunocompetent host, acyclovir should be
    emergently initiated, particularly if temporal
    lobe localization is suggested by the initial
    assessment.
In suspected or documented immunosuppressed
    host, empiric therapy for herpesviruses
    (HSV, CMV, VZV) and toxoplasmosis should be
    considered. Drug resistance may be an issue.
CSF should be sent for Gram stain, routine culture,
    acid-fast stain and culture, fungal stain and
    culture, viral culture, PCR for specific likely
    pathogens if available, CSF antigen studies
    such as cryptococcal antigen if clinically
    appropriate.
Blood tests for routine laboratories and specific
    serologies should be based on the above
    epidemiologic and clinical data.
Repeat MRI, CT, EEG, or CSF studies may be
    useful. If no response to appropriate therapy,
    drug resistance may be considered and
    alternative therapy administered.

Figure 1
Diagnostic and therapeutic considerations in acute encephalitis.

encephalitis. One is characterized by direct cytopathic effects, the other by immunologically mediated mechanisms. The former usually occurs in immunocompromised hosts. Early ribavirin administration in PCR-diagnosed measles encephalitis of this variety has been reported effective in young immunocompromised hosts. The role of steroids in postinfectious immune-mediated measles and other parainfectious encephalitides related to other viruses has yet to be clearly established. Interferon-alpha or intraventricular interferon-alpha plus ribavirin as well as newer compounds such as isoprinosine continue to be evaluated for subacute sclerosing panencephalitis.

Rhabdoviridae
Because of the lack of effective therapies, the approach to rabies must concentrate on preexposure vaccination of

high-risk individuals such as veterinarians and postexposure prophylaxis because there are only extremely rare survivors with symptomatic disease (see the chapter *Rabies*).

Retroviridae

Human Immunodeficiency Virus. With the advent of more potent antiretroviral therapy, the prevalence of HIV-related encephalopathy has diminished. Early in the natural course of HIV, an encephalitic picture may occur. As the infection progresses to clinically advanced disease, development of HIV encephalopathy and dementia may also appear. A number of antiretroviral agents have been reported to have an effect on primary HIV-related encephalopathy (see the chapter *AIDS: Antiretroviral Therapy*). The most-studied and best-proved of these agents are the reverse transcriptase inhibitors, most notably zidovudine.

Papovaviridae

Several compounds have been employed for the treatment of JC virus, the etiologic agent of progressive multifocal leukoencephalopathy (PML). Reconstitution of immune function with potent antiretroviral therapy in these patients may be an indirect means of treating PML (see the chapter *Progressive Multifocal Leukoencephalopathy*).

Picornaviridae

The mainstay of picornaviral encephalitis treatment is supportive care. Several experimental agents that interfere with the picornaviral capsid hold promise for treatment. The intraventricular administration of gamma globulin may be beneficial in the treatment of picornaviral encephalitis in agammaglobulinemic children. Pleconaril inhibits enterovirus and rhinovirus replication and has shown promise in recent studies.

Bunyaviridae, Flaviviridae, Togaviridae, and Reoviridae

Because of a general lack of effective antiviral therapy for arthropod-transmitted encephalitis, treatment is also generally supportive. As a consequence, interventions for these diseases involve immunization and control of insect vectors.

For example, inactivated JE has been shown to induce significant neutralizing antibody titers and should be strongly considered for individuals who plan on traveling to endemic areas, especially for extended periods or during the peak summer months. Immunization is available for tick-borne encephalitides in Europe.

■ CLINICAL APPROACH

Several factors should be taken into account when approaching a patient with an encephalitic presentation (Figure 1). Host factors such as immune status and age should be noted and combined with a full review of epidemiologic clues. Next, associated physical examination findings and general laboratory values should be assessed. Given the significant morbidity and mortality associated with untreated HSV encephalitis, for which effective therapies now exist, combined with the relatively common prevalence of this entity, empiric anti-HSV therapy should be initiated on an urgent basis in the appropriate clinical setting. Concurrently, alternative viral, nonviral, and noninfectious causes should be diagnostically and therapeutically addressed. When typically effective antiviral therapy fails, the possibility of emergent drug resistance should be entertained. Non–cross-resistant alternative regimens should be initiated when available.

Suggested Reading

Arribas JR, et al: Cytomegalovirus encephalitis, *Ann Intern Med* 125:577, 1996.

Deresiewicz RL, et al: Clinical and neuroradiographic manifestations of eastern equine encephalitis, *N Engl J Med* 336:1867, 1997.

Fishbein DB, Robinson LE: Rabies, *N Engl J Med* 329:1632, 1993.

Koskiniemi M, Vaheri A, Taskinen E: Cerebrospinal fluid alterations in herpes simplex virus encephalitis, *Rev Infect Dis* 6:608, 1984.

Tsai TP: Arboviral infections in the United States, *Infect Dis Clin North Am* 5:73, 1994.

Whitley RJ, Lakeman F: Herpes simplex virus infections of the central nervous system: therapeutic and diagnostic considerations, *Clin Infect Dis* 20:414, 1995.

INTRACRANIAL SUPPURATION

Brian Wispelwey
Carole A. Sable

■ BRAIN ABSCESS

Brain abscess is a focal suppuration within the brain parenchyma. The incidence is estimated to be 1 in 10,000 hospital admissions, and in large autopsy series, brain abscess occurs in 0.18% to 1.3% of all patients. Brain abscesses occur most commonly in men ages 30 to 45 years. The age distribution varies with cause; abscesses secondary to otitis media have a bimodal distribution, with peaks in childhood and after age 40, and paranasal sinusitis occurs most commonly in patients ages 10 to 30 years.

Pathogenesis

Four clinical settings are associated with brain abscess (Table 1). Brain abscesses are located most commonly in the frontal or temporal area, followed in frequency by frontoparietal, parietal, cerebellar, and occipital areas. The location of a brain abscess may provide important information about the underlying predisposing factor. Brainstem abscesses and multiple abscesses most commonly indicate hematogenous dissemination from a distant site. Frontal and temporal abscesses are more commonly related to infection in the associated contiguous space.

It is postulated that brain abscess develops from a contiguous site by either direct extension through adjacent osteitis or osteomyelitis or via retrograde thrombophlebitis of the diploic or emissary vein. In otogenic infections spread may also occur through an existing channel such as the internal auditory canal or the vestibular or cochlear aqueduct. However, these proposed mechanisms do not entirely explain the pathogenesis of brain abscess, including the mechanism by which organisms cross an intact dura.

Brain abscesses secondary to hematogenous dissemination have several characteristics in common: (1) distant focus of infection, often in the chest; (2) middle cerebral artery distribution; (3) location at gray-white junction; (4) poor encapsulation; and (5) association with high mortality.

Brain abscesses rarely accompany bacteremia if the blood-brain barrier is intact. For example, brain abscess rarely complicates infective endocarditis (9 brain abscesses in 218 cases), although infective endocarditis is defined by sustained bacteremia.

Causes

The organisms isolated from brain abscesses are outlined in Table 2. Some 30% to 60% of pyogenic abscesses are mixed infections caused by a combination of streptococci, anaerobes, and *Enterobacteriaceae*. Conversely, *Staphylococcus aureus* is commonly isolated in pure culture.

Yeasts and dimorphic fungi have been implicated as causes of a minority of brain abscesses, typically in immunocompromised patients. Protozoa and helminths should also be considered in the appropriate epidemiologic setting.

Immunocompromised patients are susceptible to a wider array of pathogens. Patients with defects in cell-mediated immunity may develop brain abscesses with *Toxoplasma gondii, Nocardia asteroides, Cryptococcus neoformans,* mycobacteria, and *Listeria monocytogenes.* Neutrophil defects are associated with an increased incidence of infections caused

---

Table 1 Clinical Settings Associated with Brain Abscess

SPREAD FROM A CONTIGUOUS FOCUS
Otitis media, mastoiditis; 40% of all brain abscesses
Sinusitis, frontal
Dental infections (<10%), typically with molar infections; abscesses usually frontal but may be temporal
Meningitis; rarely complicated by brain abscess (must be considered in neonates with *Citrobacter diversus* meningitis, of whom 70% develop brain abscess)

HEMATOGENOUS SPREAD FROM A DISTANT FOCUS OF INFECTION
Empyema, lung abscess, bronchiectasis, cystic fibrosis, wound infections, pelvic infections, intraabdominal sepsis

TRAUMA
After penetrating head trauma, brain abscess develops in about 3%, more commonly after gunshot wounds
Neurosurgical procedures; complicated by brain abscess in only 6 to 17 per 10,000 clean neurosurgical procedures

CRYPTOGENIC
Asymptomatic pulmonary arteriovenous malformation (AVM), a consideration in cases of cryptogenic brain abscess
Cyanotic congenital heart disease is present in 5% to 10% of brain abscesses and is the most common predisposing factor in some pediatric series

---

Table 2 Pathogens in Brain Abscess

AGENT	FREQUENCY (%)
Streptococci (*S. intermedius,* including *S. anginosis*)	60-70
Bacteroides and *Prevotella* spp.	20-40
Enterobacteriaceae	23-33
Staphylococcus aureus	10-15
Fungi*	10-15
Streptococcus pneumoniae	<1
Haemophilus influenzae	<1
Protozoa, helminths† (vary geographically)	<1

*Yeasts, fungi
  Aspergillus
  Agents of mucor
  Candida
  Cryptococci
  Coccidiodoides
  Cladosporium trichoides
  Pseudallescheria boydii

†Protozoa, helminths
  Entamoeba histolytica
  Schistosomes
  Paragonimus
  Cysticerci

Table 3   Causes of Parenchymal Central Nervous System Lesions in Patients with AIDS

TOXOPLASMA GONDII
Most common focal lesion
Occurs in about 10% of all AIDS patients
>1 lesion seen on MRI with surrounding edema, mass effect, and ring enhancement
Most common location is the basal ganglia; most Toxo IgG positive

PRIMARY LYMPHOMA
Occurs in about 2% of AIDS patients
Lymphoma is B cell in origin
Lesions and hyperdense or isodense on CT with edema, mass effect, and variable enhancement CNS caused by Epstein-Barr virus

PROGRESSIVE MULTIFOCAL LEUKOENCEPHALOPATHY
Occurs in 2%-5% of AIDS patients
Lesions occur at gray-white junction and adjacent white matter —caused by JC virus (Papovavirus)
On imaging lesions are hypodense without mass effect

LESS COMMON
*Cryptococcus neoformans**
*Histoplasma capsulatum**
*Coccidioides immitis**
Other fungi—*Aspergillus, Candida*, agents of mucor
*Mycobacterium tuberculosis**
Mycobacterium avium complex
Cytomegalovirus†
Metastatic malignancy, notably KS
Acanthamoeba
Bacterial brain abscess of *Listeria, Nocardia, Salmonella*
Syphilis*

AIDS, Acquired immunodeficiency syndrome; *MRI*, magnetic resonance imaging; *CT*, computed tomography; *KS*, Kaposi's sarcoma.
*More commonly meningitis.
†More commonly encephalitis.

Table 4   Clinical Manifestations of Brain Abscess*

Headache	70%	Nuchal rigidity	≈25%
Fever	50%	Papilledema	≈25%
Altered mental status	>50%	Focal neurologic findings	≈50%
Seizures	25-35%		

*Fewer than half have classic triad of fever, headache, and neurologic deficits.

Table 5   Laboratory Tests and Imaging Studies

LABORATORY TESTS*
WBC: moderate leukocytosis present in about 50% (only 10% WBC >20,000) and normal WBC in 40%
Moderate increase in ESR
Chest x-ray film is useful in detecting the origin of hematogenous brain abscess
EEG abnormal in most patients, lateralizes to side of lesion

IMAGING STUDIES
CT scan: useful in evaluating the brain, sinuses, mastoids, and middle ear
MRI: appears more sensitive early in illness and in detecting cerebral edema
^{99m}Tc very sensitive; useful where CT or MRI not available

WBC, White blood cell count; *ESR*, erythrocyte sedimentation rate; *EEG*, electroencephalograph; *CT*, computed tomography; *MRI*, magnetic resonance imaging.
*Lumbar puncture is contraindicated in patients with known or suspected brain abscess.

by *Enterobacteriaceae, Pseudomonas,* and fungi. Patients with acquired immunodeficiency syndrome (AIDS) may develop focal central nervous system (CNS) lesions as a result of a variety of pathogens (Table 3).

Clinical Manifestations

The clinical courses of patients with brain abscess vary dramatically. In approximately 75% of patients, symptoms are present for fewer than 2 weeks. The prominent symptoms are secondary to mass effect, not infection (Table 4). Headache, the most common symptom, may be hemicranial or generalized. Varying degrees of altered mental status are present in most patients.

Brain abscesses in certain locations may cause additional symptoms. For example, cerebellar abscesses are often associated with nystagmus, ataxia, vomiting, and dysmetria. Frontal lobe abscesses induce headaches, drowsiness, inattention, and decline in mental function. Temporal lobe abscesses are associated with early ipsilateral headaches and, if in the dominant hemisphere, aphasia. Intrasellar abscesses simulate pituitary tumors. Brainstem abscesses often cause facial weakness, headache, fever, hemiparesis, dysphagia, and vomiting.

Laboratory Findings

Most laboratory tests are not diagnostic for brain abscess (Table 5). Lumbar puncture is contraindicated in patients with known or suspected brain abscess. Not only are cerebrospinal fluid (CSF) findings nonspecific, but patients may herniate after the procedure. In one series, 41 of 140 patients deteriorated within 48 hours after lumbar puncture, and 25 died. Similar results have been reported in other studies.

Imaging studies are most useful in making a diagnosis of brain abscess. Computed tomography (CT) can be used to evaluate all cranial structures. It can detect edema, hydrocephalus, shift, or imminent ventricular rupture. A brain abscess appears as a hypodense center with an outlying uniform ring of enhancement surrounded by a variable hypodense region of brain edema. Contrast enhancement is essential. Although CT is very sensitive for detecting brain abscess, the findings are not specific, particularly early in disease. Magnetic resonance imaging (MRI) is rapidly becoming the diagnostic procedure of choice. It appears more sensitive than CT for detecting cerebral edema and early changes associated with brain abscess and is more accurate in differentiating the central necrosis of brain abscess from other fluid accumulations. Gadolinium enhancement provides additional information about brain abscess structure. Magnetic resonance spectroscopy and positron emission tomography (PET) may have better sensitivity and specificity for the diagnosis of brain abscess but are not currently available in most clinical settings.

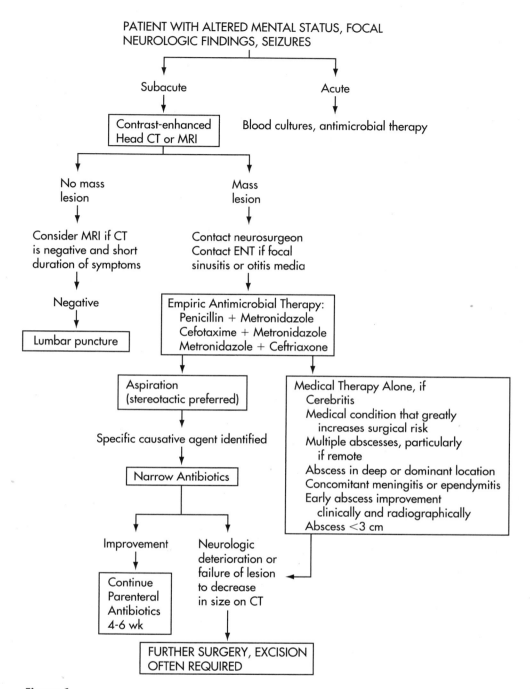

Figure 1
Algorithm for the treatment of suspected brain abscess. If neurologic deterioration, signs of cerebral edema, or increased intracranial pressure is present, the clinician should treat with corticosteroids, mannitol, and hyperventilation.

Therapy

The major distinction in treating focal CNS lesions is whether the patient has cerebritis or a brain abscess (Figure 1). Cerebritis is an area of low density on imaging studies surrounded by ring enhancement that does not decay on contrasted scans 60 minutes later. An encapsulated abscess shows a faint ring on unenhanced scans that is more pronounced on enhanced images and decays on delayed CT. It represents the early stages of a focal CNS infection. The difference is important because cerebritis can be cured with antibiotics alone.

There were 67 cases of brain abscesses reportedly cured by medical therapy alone from 1975 to 1985. (1) The initial diagnosis and resolution of the abscess were documented by

CT. (2) Patients were treated with parenteral antibiotics for more than 8 weeks. (3) There was no surgical or histopathologic evidence of encapsulation. It is possible that these results actually signify successful treatment of cerebritis and not abscess. In addition, several patients underwent diagnostic aspirations, which may bias the results toward a more favorable outcome because diagnostic aspiration is often therapeutic.

Approach to the Patient with Suspected Brain Abscess

Patients who present with altered consciousness, focal CNS signs, or seizures usually are candidates for contrast-enhanced CT or MRI. In hospitals where these imaging techniques are not available, ^{99m}Tc brain scan can be used. Lumbar puncture usually is postponed until a space-occupying CNS lesion is excluded. If rapid clinical progression is occurring, blood cultures for bacteria and fungi may be done and empiric antimicrobial therapy begun before neuroimaging. In every case, management should be done in conjunction with a neurosurgeon. A probable focus in the paranasal sinus or middle ear should prompt consultation also with an otolaryngologist. Empiric treatment depends on the presence or absence of immunosuppression, particularly AIDS, as follows.

Patients with a lesion on CT or MRI consistent with bacterial brain abscess are begun on empiric antibiotic therapy even if urgent neurosurgical intervention is indicated. The most commonly recommended regimen for adults is to begin with penicillin G, 4 million units IV every 4 hours, plus metronidazole, 7.5 mg/kg (often rounded out to 500 mg) every 6 hours. Chloramphenicol is used less often. Cefotaxime, 2 g IV every 4 to 6 hours, is an acceptable and perhaps favored replacement for penicillin in this regimen, according to recent preliminary information. Antibiotic therapy should not preclude efforts to isolate the organism by aerobic and anaerobic culture of surgical material obtained later; additional antibiotics may be necessary (Table 6).

Most patients require surgery. If the patient remains stable and the abscess is accessible, aspiration (CT guided, if possible) is desirable to make a specific bacteriologic diagnosis and narrow the antimicrobial regimen. Although delay may render cultures negative, aspiration during the cerebritis stage may be dangerous, causing hemorrhage. Certain poor prognostic parameters, clinical or radiographic, may necessitate earlier aspiration. If the lesion appears encapsulated by CT scan criteria, antibiotic treatment can be started and aspiration for diagnosis and drainage performed without delay. Subsequent management depends on clinical and radiographic (CT) parameters. Later neurologic deterioration or failure of the abscess to decrease in size as detected by biweekly CT scan or MRI are indications for further surgery, often excision, if feasible. The duration of microbial therapy remains unsettled. Many authorities treat parenterally for approximately 4 to 6 weeks. Duration cannot be determined by resolution of all CT or MRI abnormalities. A cured brain abscess may continue to appear as nodular contrast enhancement on CT scans for 4 weeks to 6 months after completion of successful therapy. No empiric regimen consisting solely of oral agents is recommended, even in the

Table 6 Antimicrobial Therapy for Brain Abscess

ANTIMICROBIAL AGENT	TOTAL DAILY DOSE
Cefotaxime	8-12 g
Ceftazidime	6-12 g
Ceftriaxone	4 g
Chloramphenicol	4-6 g
Metronidazole	30 mg/kg
Nafcillin	9-12 g
Penicillin G	24 million U
Vancomycin	2 g

later stages of therapy. Administration of an anticonvulsant is recommended for at least 1 year because of the high incidence of seizures among brain abscess patients.

AIDS Patients and Other Immunocompromised Patients

Patients with advanced HIV infection or AIDS and who have CNS lesions on MRI or contrast-enhanced CT consistent with toxoplasmosis are usually begun on empiric therapy with pyrimethamine and sulfadiazine. Pyrimethamine is given to adults as a single loading dose of 75 to 100 mg followed by 25 to 50 mg daily. Folinic acid is given as 10 mg daily to decrease bone marrow suppression from pyrimethamine. Sulfadiazine is given as 1 g orally every 6 hours. If sulfadiazine is not available, clindamycin is an acceptable substitute at 600 mg IV every 6 hours. Low-grade fever and a gradual onset also prompt this approach. The limitation of empiric therapy is that radiologic distinction between toxoplasmosis and other lesions is not accurate. Progressive deterioration, an atypical CT or MRI, or failure to show clinical and imaging improvement during 2 weeks of therapy generally prompts biopsy or aspiration. Some physicians also use a negative *Toxoplasma* serology to prompt early neurosurgical intervention. Patients taking trimethoprim-sulfamethoxazole (TMP-SMX) prophylaxis for pneumocystosis may be at a lower risk of toxoplasmosis and are therefore more likely to have another diagnosis (see the Chapter *AIDS: Therapy for Opportunistic Infections*). Newer diagnostic modalities, such as single photon emission computed tomography (SPECT), may allow immediate differentiation between *toxoplasma* and other pathologic processes.

The range of pathogens for brain abscess is so broad in other immunocompromised patients that empiric therapy has limited value. Early neurosurgical intervention is usually indicated.

Corticosteroids

Corticosteroids may be lifesaving in certain settings, including when rapid neurologic deterioration is associated with an increase in intracranial pressure. The role of corticosteroids in the treatment of brain abscess remains controversial. Concerns include the possibility of delayed antibiotic entry into CNS, delayed healing, and alteration in CT scan appearance as inflammation decreases.

Prognosis

Several factors are associated with a poor prognosis (Table 7). In addition, characteristics such as patient's age,

Table 7   Adverse Prognostic Factors in Brain Abscess
Delayed or missed diagnosis
Poor localization, especially in the posterior fossa (before CT)
Multiple, deep, or multiloculated abscesses
Ventricular rupture (80%-100% mortality)
Fungal cause
Inappropriate antibiotics

CT, Computed tomography.

Table 8 Pathogens in Subdural Empyema	
Aerobic streptococci	32%
Anaerobic streptococci	16%
Staphylococcus aureus	11%
CNS	5%
Aerobic gram-negative bacilli	8%
Anaerobes	5%
No organism isolated	34%

CNS, Coagulase-negative staphylococci.

Table 9 Clinical Presentation of Subdural Empyema	
Headache	
Altered mental staus	≈50%
Fever (>39° C [102.2° F])	Majority
Focal neurologic findings	In all, eventually
Hemiparesis, ocular palsies, dysphagia, cerebellar signs	
Seizures	>50%
Meningismus	≈80%

large abscess, and metastatic lesions also influence outcome. Neurologic sequelae develop in 30% to 55% of patients, and in 17% they are incapacitating. Seizures develop in a variable percentage of patients (35% to more than 90%).

■ CRANIAL SUBDURAL EMPYEMA

Subdural empyema, a collection of pus in the space between the dura and arachnoid membranes, accounts for about 20% of all focal CNS infections. The most common predisposing underlying conditions are otorhinologic infections, particularly of the paranasal sinuses. Infection typically develops after spread from sinus or ear to the subdural space via emissary veins or extension of osteomyelitis of the skull in association with an epidural abscess. Subdural empyema may also develop after skull trauma, neurosurgical procedures, or infection of an existing subdural hematoma. Metastatic infections account for only about 5% of the total. The pus may remain localized or spread throughout the subdural space.

Causes
The organisms isolated from patients with subdural empyema are those typically found in patients with chronic otitis or sinusitis (Table 8). The significant number of sterile cultures may reflect difficulties in culturing anaerobic organisms. Subdural empyema typically is caused by a single pathogen that reflects the underlying anatomic focus. Subdural empyemas from otorhinologic infections are most commonly caused by streptococci, and infections after head trauma or surgery are caused by staphylococci and gram-negative bacilli. A variety of pathogens have been reported in patients with distant foci of infection.

Clinical Presentation
Patients present with symptoms related to increased intracranial pressure, meningeal irritation, or focal inflammation. Symptoms may be present for a few days to several weeks. Most patients also display findings of the original infection. A variety of symptoms may be present (Table 9).

Diagnosis
Subdural empyema should be suspected in any patient with focal neurologic findings and meningeal signs. Diagnosis is made by imaging studies with contrast-enhanced CT or MRI. A subdural empyema appears as a crescent-shaped area of hypodensity adjacent to the falx cerebri or below the cranial vault. With contrast enhancement, an intense line can be seen between the subdural collection and the cerebral cortex. MRI is more sensitive in detecting subdural empyemas, particularly at the base of the brain, in the posterior fossa, or along the falx cerebri. MRI can differentiate subdural empyema from sterile collections on the basis of signal intensity. CT is better able to visualize bone and is the technique of choice to detect osteomyelitis or penetrating injury.

Therapy
Successful therapy of subdural empyema requires a combination of surgical and medical approaches. Drainage is useful to relieve mass effect and obtain cultures to guide antimicrobial therapy and is needed as an adjunct to antibiotic treatment. The optimal drainage procedure is still under debate. Although early studies documented lower mortality in patients undergoing craniotomy, studies were not controlled for severity of illness. A larger number of patients who were gravely ill may have undergone burr-hole drainage because it is less invasive.

Antimicrobial therapy should be directed against pathogens revealed by Gram stain of aspirated material and the primary site of infection. The rationale for the choice of appropriate antimicrobials is the same as for treatment of brain abscess. The duration of therapy with parenteral antibiotics should be 3 to 6 weeks, depending on the clinical response.

Prognosis
Prognosis is related to the degree of neurologic impairment at presentation. Mortality is about 7% in patients who are alert and well oriented, 21% in patients who are lethargic or comatose but respond purposefully, and 56% in patients who are unresponsive. Neurologic sequelae in the form of hemiparesis and aphasia are common, and up to 40% of patients may have seizures.

CRANIAL EPIDURAL ABSCESS

An epidural abscess is a localized infection between the dura mater and the overlying skull. Emissary veins cross the dura, so a concomitant subdural empyema is present in up to 81% of cases. Because of this, the causes and pathogenesis are identical to those of subdural empyema.

Symptoms of epidural abscess may initially relate entirely to the primary focus of infection. Patients typically complain of headache but have no other symptoms unless they have subdural empyema. The dura is closely adherent to the skull, preventing rapid expansion of the abscess and sudden neurologic deficit. Neurologic symptoms eventually develop, particularly with a subdural empyema.

Imaging with CT or MRI is the procedure of choice to diagnose cranial epidural abscess. Treatment is the same as for subdural empyema.

SUPPURATIVE INTRACRANIAL THROMBOPHLEBITIS

Suppurative thrombophlebitis occurs intracranially because of the close proximity of the dural venous sinuses to other structures in the skull. Paranasal sinusitis or infection of the soft tissue of the face or mouth may be complicated by cavernous sinus thrombosis. Otitis media or mastoiditis may result in lateral sinus thrombosis or infection of superior and inferior petrosal sinuses. Suppurative thrombophlebitis of the superior sagittal sinus may develop after infection of the face, scalp, or subdural or epidural space or after meningitis. In each, the causative pathogen depends on the site of the original infection (Table 10).

Pathogenesis

The dural venous sinuses and cranial veins are valveless, and blood flow is determined by pressure gradients. Bacteria that enter the facial veins are carried through the cavernous sinuses to the petrosal sinuses and finally the internal jugular vein. Conditions that increase blood viscosity, such as trauma, dehydration, malignancy, and pregnancy, increase the likelihood of developing thrombosis. Predisposing conditions are not identified in every case.

Clinical Presentation

The clinical presentation depends on the location of disease (Table 11). In infection of the cortical venous system, neurologic deficits are determined by the adequacy of collateral blood flow. Patients with inadequate cerebral perfusion may develop depressed consciousness, seizures, signs of increased intracranial pressure, and focal neurologic signs. Patients with cavernous sinus thrombosis present most commonly with fever, periorbital swelling, and headache.

The periorbital swelling seen in cavernous sinus thrombosis must be distinguished from the periorbital edema that may accompany sinusitis, and from the syndromes of periorbital and orbital cellulitis. Periorbital cellulitis is a "preseptal" area of cellulitis that involves the eyelid but spares the orbit. Thus it responds to medical therapy alone. However, orbital cellulitis, suggested by the additional findings of proptosis, diminished visual acuity, and restricted extra-

Table 10 Suppurative Intracranial Thrombophlebitis: Organism by Site of Infection	
Sinusitis	Streptococci Staphylococci Anaerobes
Soft-tissue infections of the face	*Staphylococcus aureus* Streptococci
Otitis, mastoiditis	*Haemophilus influenzae* Gram-negative bacilli Staphylococci

Table 11 Symptoms of Suppurative Thrombophlebitis	
Cavernous sinus thrombosis	Photophobia, ptosis, diplopia, proptosis, chemosis, weak extraocular muscles, papilledema, altered mental status, meningismus, decreased visual acuity
Involvement bilaterally	Same findings in opposite eye
Septic lateral sinus thrombosis	Headache >80%, earache, vomiting, vertigo associated with otitis, fever and abnormal ear findings, increased facial sensation, sixth nerve palsy, facial pain
Superior sagittal sinus	Altered mental status, motor deficits, papilledema, nuchal rigidity, seizures >50%
Inferior petrosal sinus	Gradenigo's syndrome (ipsilateral facial pain and lateral rectus weakness)

ocular movements, often requires surgical drainage of the orbit. A CT scan should be performed immediately if this entity is suspected. Of course, cavernous sinus thrombosis may complicate periorbital or orbital cellulitis.

Diagnosis

MRI is the diagnostic procedure of choice. It demonstrates the difference between thrombosis and normally flowing blood. CT may also be useful but is less sensitive and specific than MRI. Imaging also allows full evaluation of the paranasal sinuses and intracranial structures. If there is a high index of suspicion for septic thrombophlebitis and CT and MRI are negative, carotid angiography with venous phase studies should be performed.

Therapy

Antimicrobial therapy is directed against pathogens responsible for the underlying site of infection. Considerations are the same as for brain abscess and subdural empyema. Surgery plays an important role in patients in whom antimicrobial therapy alone is ineffective. Patients with cavernous sinus thrombosis secondary to sphenoid sinusitis often require surgical intervention.

Recent data suggest that anticoagulation with antimicrobial therapy may reduce mortality, particularly if employed early in disease. The major risk of anticoagulation is intracranial hemorrhage. This risk precludes the use of anticoagulation in septic lateral vein thrombophlebitis because of the increased risk of intracerebral hemorrhage in these patients.

Suggested Reading

Brock DG, Bleck TP: Extra-axial suppurations of the central nervous system, *Semin Neurol* 12:263, 1992.

Chun CH, et al: Brain abscess: a study of 45 consecutive cases, *Medicine* 65:415, 1986.

Enzmann DR: Magnetic resonance imaging update on brain abscess and central nervous system aspergillosis. In Remington JS, Schwartz MN, eds: *Current clinical topics in infectious diseases,* vol 13, Boston, 1993, Blackwell.

Mathisen GE, Johnson JP: Brain abscess, *Clin Infect Dis* 25:763, 1997.

Wispelway B, Dacey RG, Scheld WM: Brain abscess. In Scheld WM, Durack D, Whitley R, eds: *Infections of the central nervous system,* ed 2, Philadelphia, 1997, Lippincott-Raven.

Wispelway B, Scheld WM: Brain abscess. In Mandell GL, Dolin R, Bennett JE, eds: *Principles and practices of infectious diseases,* ed 4, New York, 1995, Churchill-Livingstone.

THE DIAGNOSIS AND MANAGEMENT OF SPINAL EPIDURAL ABSCESS

T. Erik Michaelson
Jeffrey L. Silber
Mark J. DiNubile

Epidural abscess is an uncommon cause of back pain, although several authors have noted a rising incidence in recent years. Because it represents a potentially crippling but treatable condition, early diagnosis and aggressive therapy are mandatory. Unfortunately, this disease is still associated with substantial morbidity, often related to delays in diagnosis and treatment.

Epidural abscesses may be categorized anatomically into those involving the spinal or cranial epidural space. Spinal epidural abscesses can be further subdivided into acute and chronic presentations. Such a classification correlates, albeit imperfectly, with certain clinical and laboratory manifestations, bacteriology, cerebrospinal fluid (CSF) formulas, anatomic details, pathology, and pathogenesis (Table 1).

The nontuberculous bacterial spinal epidural abscess constitutes the major focus of this review. Tuberculous, fungal, and parasitic abscesses of the spinal and cranial epidural spaces are less commonly encountered in the United States. Metastatic carcinoma and lymphoma represent important alternative diagnoses that can masquerade as infections.

■ CLINICAL PRESENTATION

The manifestations of spinal epidural abscess were described by Heusner (1948) as evolving through four overlapping stages: (1) spinal ache, to (2) root pain, to (3) weakness, to (4) paralysis. The actual time between the onset of pain and development of neurologic deficits can be highly variable. The often-rapid evolution from backache to neurologic catastrophe (or even death) forces physicians to consider this entity in the differential diagnosis of all patients with back pain, especially when fever and localized spinal tenderness coexist. Common presenting complaints may also include root pain (sometimes described as "electric" in character), weakness, and paresthesias. Atypical presentations include meningismus (with cervical involvement), acute abdominal pain (with thoracic infection), and hip pain (with lumbar disease).

In patients presenting with an epidural abscess, an inapparent primary focus, such as endocarditis, adjacent osteomyelitis, or a distant visceral abscess, may be present. Such occult infections can require special therapeutic interventions.

■ RISK FACTORS

Patients with a history of back trauma are predisposed to seed the injured area during transient bacteremia and therefore constitute a group at special risk for vertebral osteomyelitis and/or epidural abscess. Suspicion of epidural infection should also be raised when a patient with osteomyelitis or after recent back surgery, epidural anesthesia, or lumbar puncture reports increasingly severe back pain. The development of a cervical epidural abscess following acupuncture in the nuchal area has been reported.

Any patient with bacteremia or candidemia incurs some risk of metastatic seeding. Patients with cutaneous infection, "line sepsis," dental abscess, pharyngitis, decubitus ulcer, urinary tract infection, or endocarditis can develop a secondary epidural focus through hematogenous spread, even in the absence of recognized back injury. The risk appears highest in the aftermath of *Staphylococcus aureus* bacteremia and is not totally eliminated by the 2 to 4 weeks of antibiotic therapy usually given to such patients. Injecting drug users with or without endocarditis may present with infections of the epidural space. Diabetic patients and patients undergoing hemodialysis also appear to be at increased risk of epidural space infection.

Table 1 Characteristic Findings in Acute versus Chronic Spinal Epidural Abscess

	ACUTE	CHRONIC
Duration of symptoms	Less than 2 wk	More than 2 wk
Fever	Often present	Low grade or absent
Systemic toxicity	Sometimes	Infrequently
Source	Hematogenous, often from skin	Local extension from vertebral osteomyelitis
Back pain	Always	Always
Localized spinal tenderness	Very common	Nearly universal
Root weakness	Common	Common
Peripheral leukocytosis	Usually present	Usually absent
Erythrocyte sedimentation rate	Greatly elevated	Greatly elevated
CSF leukocytes* (per cubic millimeter)	Usually 50-1000	Often less than 50
CSF protein above 100 mg/dl	Almost always	Almost always
Anatomic location	Usually posterior to spinal cord	Commonly anterior to spinal cord
Gross pathology	Purulent exudate	Granulation tissue

CSF, Cerebrospinal fluid.
*Frank pus may be encountered if the abscess is entered. If this occurs, the spinal needle must not be further advanced because introducing the needle into the subarachnoid space may induce meningitis. The aspirated purulent material should be sent for appropriate studies, including Gram stain and cultures.

■ BACTERIOLOGY AND PATHOGENESIS

S. aureus is the organism most commonly isolated from epidural abscesses, often resulting from inapparent primary foci. Less common pathogens include streptococci, anaerobes, *Candida* species, *Salmonella, Brucella,* and various gram-negative rods. Vertebral infection with yeast typically is a consequence of catheter-related candidemia and may not be aborted by line removal and short-course antifungal therapy. Gram-negative osteomyelitis, septic arthritis, and epidural infection in young adults are often complications of intravenous drug use. Urinary tract or pelvic infection can spread to the lumbar spine and epidural space through vascular anastomoses in Batson's plexus.

Epidural abscesses of hematogenous origin are most often located in the dorsolateral thoracic or lumbar area, where the epidural space is widest. Abscesses that form secondary to adjacent osteomyelitis usually involve the epidural space anteriorly or circumferentially.

Tuberculous spondylitis (Pott's disease) with chronic epidural abscess may be the first or sole manifestation of reactivation tuberculosis. Although the illness is often clinically and radiologically indistinguishable from that caused by pyogenic bacteria, the course is often protracted. Histopathology typically reveals fibrous connective tissue studded with granulomata containing multinucleated giant cells and caseating necrosis. Acid-fast bacilli (AFB) can often be demonstrated by appropriate stains. Operative intervention is not routinely required for Pott's disease in the absence of neurologic involvement.

Other unusual pathogens isolated from spinal epidural collections have included *Actinomyces, Nocardia, Cryptococcus, Blastomyces, Aspergillus, Rhizopus,* and *Echinococcus.*

Every patient who experiences acute or progressive back pain, fever, and local spine tenderness must be evaluated for the possibility of spinal epidural abscess. Despite its subtle and variable presentation, the diagnosis must be considered promptly after presentation. Not all of the symptoms and signs classically attributed to an epidural abscess are present in every patient—especially children and those with a sub-acute or chronic course. In the latter group, fever and systemic complaints may be minimal. In several large series, 35% to 58% of the patients were given initial diagnoses unrelated to the spine. These patients should be treated with the same degree of urgency accorded patients with cancer and new back pain.

Conventional radiology of the spine may not be helpful because osseous destruction can be absent or inapparent. Although fever may be low grade or nonexistent in patients with chronic epidural abscess, they will have abnormal spine radiographs more commonly than those with acute disease. Bone and gallium scans and computed tomography (CT) often disclose abnormalities, although these are rarely diagnostic and thereby postpone definitive interventions.

Whether acute or chronic, all patients with suspected epidural space infection require magnetic resonance imaging (MRI) of the spine or a CT or conventional myelogram on an urgent basis. MRI is currently the study of choice. If contrast is injected into the subarachnoid space, CSF should first be obtained for stains and cultures, glucose and protein levels, total and differential cell counts, and cytology. Spinal puncture should be performed at a site as far as possible from the area of suspected infection. The needle should be advanced slowly, with frequent aspiration; if pus is encountered, the needle should be withdrawn and the material sent for appropriate tests. CT-guided aspiration of an epidural collection may be necessary to obtain a microbiologic diagnosis if nonsurgical management is planned.

■ TREATMENT

Traditional management of spinal epidural abscess includes a medicosurgical approach, with immediate surgical decompression and prolonged antibiotic therapy. Exposure of the entire abscess, with drainage and irrigation, has been standard practice.

Antibiotics should be begun promptly and often empirically. An antistaphylococcal agent should be included routinely in the initial antibiotic regimen. Agents active against gram-negative organisms and anaerobes should be added to the regimen if these organisms are suspected on clinical grounds. For example, a patient with a lumbar epidural abscess of suspected urinary origin would be given broader coverage if a gram-negative organism is found on Gram stain or culture of the urine. The regimen should be modified once results of stains, cultures, and susceptibility tests from an aspirate or operative specimen are available. Blood cultures, preferably obtained before antibiotic administration, may yield the causative organism.

Ultimately, culture and antimicrobial susceptibility dictate the final choice of antibiotic(s). Staphylococcal infection is usually treated with nafcillin, 2 g IV every 4 hours. Alternatives in penicillin-allergic patients include cefazolin, 1 g IV every 8 hours; clindamycin, 600 mg IV every 8 hours; and vancomycin, 1 g IV every 12 hours. Vancomycin must be used when methicillin-resistant staphylococci are recovered or strongly suspected. There is emerging clinical experience at this time with the use of extended-spectrum quinolones (e.g., levofloxacin) for the treatment of staphylococcal epidural abscesses. In susceptible staphylococcal infections associated with osteomyelitis, an oral regimen of rifampin, 600 to 1200 mg daily, with either ciprofloxacin, 750 mg twice daily, or levoquin, 500 mg once or twice daily, would be a reasonable choice for completion of a prolonged antibiotic course after successful acute management. For susceptible gram-negative infections, trimethoprim-sulfamethoxazole (TMP-SMX), an advanced-generation cephalosporin, or a quinolone may be used. Metronidazole (500 mg orally or intravenously every 8 hours) is the drug of choice for most anaerobic infections. Quinolones, TMP-SMX, and metronidazole should be given orally to patients who can tolerate medication by mouth. The cost in iatrogenic complications (as well as dollars) can be dramatically reduced by removing intravenous catheters.

The optimal duration of antibiotic therapy has not been studied in a systematic fashion; recommendations range from 2 to 8 weeks. Therapy for at least 6 weeks, preferably with a bactericidal regimen, is often required because of coexistent vertebral osteomyelitis.

Wheeler has reviewed 38 cases of epidural abscess managed conservatively (i.e., without surgical intervention). Nearly half had an underlying condition predisposing to epidural abscess; three-quarters involved multiple vertebral levels. Overall, 23 of 38 patients recovered completely. Medical management was more successful in patients who presented with localized back or radicular pain only. Surprisingly, 12 of 15 cases with partial neurologic deficits also improved. However, a few patients with minor neurologic presentations had no change ($n = 2$) or persistent neurologic sequelae ($n = 2$). It is unclear whether those patients would have benefited from prompt surgical intervention.

Controversy remains whether any patient with spinal epidural abscess should be managed without surgery. Medical management alone may be an option for selected patients who have no significant neurologic deficits or a contraindication to surgery (Table 2). Unfortunately, some patients will suffer a neurologic progression despite appropriate antibiotics; sometimes, this will happen suddenly and

Table 2 Possible Indications for Medical Management of Spinal Epidural Abscess without Operative Intervention

Absence of "significant" or progressive spinal cord or cauda equina dysfunction

or

Poor surgical candidate

or

Complete paralysis for more than 72-96 hr

and

Diagnosis is secure and causative organism has been identified

seemingly unpredictably. When this occurs, the deficit may not be reversible, even if surgery is then done promptly. In addition to mass effect, vascular compromise from spinal arterial or venous thrombosis with cord infarction may play a key pathophysiologic role in these tragic cases.

The role of medical therapy in spinal epidural abscess is likely to evolve. Advances in radiologic and microbiologic techniques over the past 20 years make conclusions from earlier studies hard to apply today. Use of serial MRI examinations to follow the patient's course may obviate the need for invasive procedures in some patients, but the natural history of MRI findings is not yet clearly charted. Percutaneous drainage of epidural abscesses may be a useful compromise approach in some patients for both diagnosis and treatment, but the literature provides only anecdotal experiences with this procedure so far. There is concern about the risk of seeding the subarachnoid space and inducing meningitis, although this theoretical complication has yet to be reported.

All patients with epidural abscess, whether managed conservatively or not, must be evaluated in detail at least daily. Acute neurologic decompensation can lead to irreversible changes within hours, even in patients clinically stable up to that point.

■ PROGNOSIS

Spinal epidural abscess was often fatal in the preantibiotic era. With advances in diagnostic and therapeutic modalities, poor outcomes are much less common today. Nevertheless, mortality rates of 10% to 30% continue to be reported. Up to a third of survivors have persistent weakness or paralysis. Khanna and others recently performed a retrospective analysis of factors associated with poor neurologic prognosis and/or mortality in 41 cases. They found presenting symptoms of back pain or radiculopathy to be associated with the best outcome, regardless of symptom duration. For patients presenting with neurologic deficits, duration of symptoms ("acute" versus "chronic" presentations) has been awarded variable prognostic value in the published literature to date. Khanna found that more severe presenting symptoms and signs heralded a poorer prognosis, with a trend to better outcome if treatment is initiated within 72 hours. Other poor prognostic indicators were patient age, "severe" thecal sac compression on imaging studies, operative findings of granulation tissue rather than pus, and lumbosacral involvement, compared with thoracic or cervical sites. There was no attributable prognostic significance to anterior versus posterior location or craniocaudal extent.

■ COMMENTS

Although uncommon, epidural abscess is a potentially devastating infection whose neurologic consequences can often be prevented or reversed by prompt diagnosis and appropriate medicosurgical treatment. Spinal epidural abscess may present as an acute or chronic process. Typical symptoms of acute spinal epidural abscess include fever, backache, and root pain for less than 2 weeks. Pathogenesis often involves hematogenous spread, usually of *S. aureus*, from a distant, often trivial infection. Patients with a more chronic course usually have developed epidural infection by local extension from adjacent vertebral osteomyelitis. Their major complaints are backache and weakness; fever is typically low grade. Early diagnosis and aggressive medicosurgical intervention are essential for optimal results in most patients because neurologic function may deteriorate at an unpredictable rate, often without warning.

Selected Reading

Baker AS, et al: Spinal epidural abscess, *N Engl J Med* 293:463, 1975.

Danner RL, Hartman BJ: Update of spinal epidural abscess: 35 cases and review of the literature, *Rev Infect Dis* 9:265, 1987.

Heusner AP: Nontuberculous spinal epidural infections, *N Engl J Med* 239:845, 1948.

Kaufman DM, Kaplan JG, Litman N: Infectious agents in spinal epidural abscesses, *Neurology* 90:1810, 1980.

Khanna RK, et al: Spinal epidural abscess: evaluation of factors influencing outcome, *Neurosurgery* 39:958, 1996.

Verner EF, Musher DM: Spinal epidural abscess, *Med Clin North Am* 69:375, 1985.

Wheeler D, et al: Medical management of spinal epidural abscesses: case report and review, *Clin Infect Dis* 15:22, 1992.

MYELITIS AND PERIPHERAL NEUROPATHY

Poh-Lian Lim
Newton E. Hyslop, Jr.

■ MYELITIS

Myelitis is infectious or noninfectious inflammation of the spinal cord. It may be divided into processes that directly attack cord structures, or primary myelitis, and those that begin in adjacent structures but progress to alter cord function, or secondary myelitis.

Primary myelitis presents as one of three discrete clinical patterns: (1) anterior poliomyelitis, (2) leukomyelitis, and (3) transverse myelitis. Poliomyelitis is inflammation involving the gray matter, whereas leukomyelitis is confined to the white matter. Transverse myelitis, inflammation of an entire cross-section of the spinal cord, is not necessarily limited to one spinal segment. A number of infectious agents are known to cause or to be associated with myelitis. Postinfectious transverse myelitis, accounting for about one third of all cases, appears most commonly in young patients and is associated with viral infections (e.g., rubeola, varicella, rubella, influenza, mumps, infectious mononucleosis). Myelitis has also been described following vaccinations.

Secondary myelitis is the result of focal inflammatory processes within the cord (intraspinal abscess) or adjacent to the cord (epidural abscess, subdural empyema). Common causes are shown in Figure 1.

There are five cardinal manifestations of spinal cord disease: pain, motor deficits, sensory deficits, abnormalities of reflexes and muscle tone, and bladder dysfunction. The distribution of neurologic deficits depends on the spinal segment(s) affected. Local pain occurs at the site of the lesion and can assume a radicular quality if the nerve roots are involved. Paresthesias have greater localizing value than radicular pain. Weakness is present in virtually all disorders of the spinal cord and, in myelitis, may progress over hours, days, or weeks. Acute paraplegia and spinal shock are characterized by areflexia, atonia, and absent plantar reflexes. More slowly progressive lesions and recovery from acute disease are associated with hyperreflexia and hypertonia. Bladder dysfunction is usually not an early sign of spinal cord disease, although if spinal shock develops, flaccid bladder paralysis ensues with urinary retention and overflow incontinence. Chronic myelopathies cause a small, spastic bladder and result in urgency, frequency, and incontinence.

Acute transverse myelitis of infectious origin must be distinguished from compressive myelopathies (e.g., epidural or intraspinal abscess, tumor) and any other noninfectious cause of myelitis such as multiple sclerosis or systemic lupus erythematosus. Myelography or magnetic resonance imaging (MRI) must be performed early to exclude a compressive lesion.

The general approach to testing is summarized in an algorithm (see Figure 1), starting first with the history and physical examination, including a detailed neurologic examination, and proceeding with radiologic studies and lumbar puncture as indicated. Further investigation involving serologic and neurologic testing may be suggested, depending on

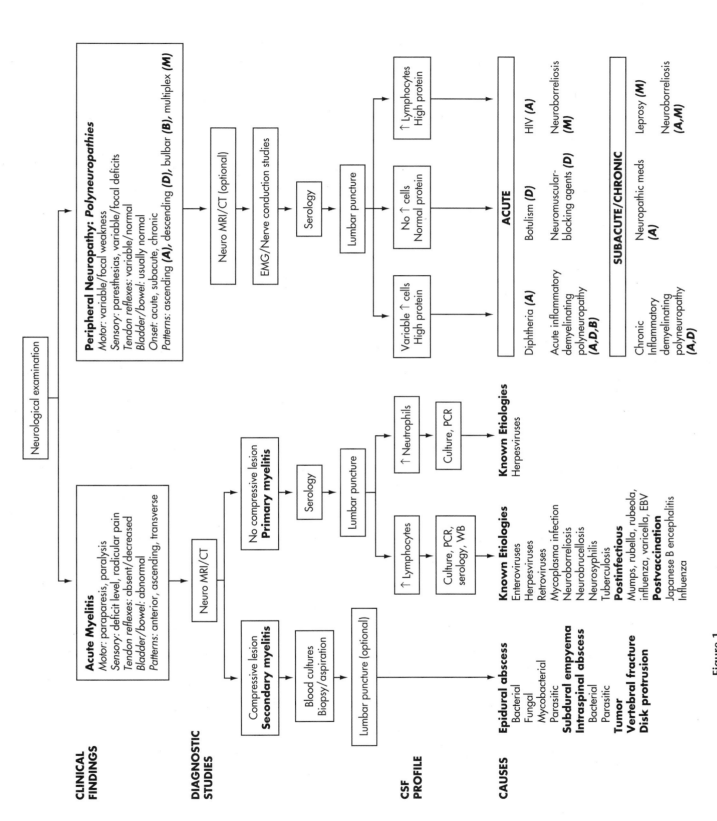

Figure 1

Algorithm for diagnosis and treatment of acute myelitis and peripheral neuropathy.

epidemiologic risk factors and clinical patterns. Cerebrospinal fluid (CSF) samples should be saved for other studies such as culture, protein electrophoresis, and polymerase chain reaction (PCR), which may be helpful in diagnosis of various etiologic agents. For acute transverse myelitis of unknown etiology, some authors advise a 3-day trial of high-dose intravenous steroid "pulse therapy," plus antivirals directed against herpesviruses (see the following).

Human Immunodeficiency Virus

Vacuolar myelopathy is associated with advanced human immunodeficiency virus (HIV) infection and in some series has been found in up to 50% of persons with acquired immunodeficiency syndrome (AIDS) undergoing autopsy. In severe cases, patients develop spastic paraparesis of the lower extremities with or without involvement of the arms. The weakness, which may be asymmetric, evolves over weeks. Coexisting neuropathy is often present. A discrete sensory level is unusual, and sphincter dysfunction occurs later in the course of the disease. It is also often associated with HIV dementia. There is no known effective treatment.

Tropical Spastic Paraparesis/ HTLV-I–Associated Myelopathy

HTLV-I is a retrovirus associated with adult T-cell leukemia and tropical spastic paraparesis/HTLV-I–associated myelopathy (TSP/HAM). It is endemic in the Caribbean basin and southern Japan. In the southeastern United States, seroprevalence may be as high as 2.1%, and HTLV-I/II coinfection with HIV approaches 10%. Because risk factors for HTLV-I infection overlap with those for HIV, patients should also be tested for HIV infection. Intravenous drug users appear to have the highest prevalence of infection.

HTLV-I causes a chronic meningomyelitis with focal destruction of the gray matter and demyelination. The posterior columns and corticospinal tracts of the thoracic cord are primarily affected. The mean age of onset of neurologic disease is 40 to 50 years, with women more commonly affected than men (2.5:1 to 3:1). Patients typically complain of bilateral weakness and stiffness of the lower extremities, but may also have difficulty walking and back pain. Later in the disease, neurogenic bladder may develop. Physical examination shows spastic paraparesis, hyperreflexia, and extensor plantar reflexes. Vibratory sensation and proprioception are reduced. Typically, the disease is slowly progressive, although the upper extremities are usually not affected. The CSF may demonstrate a lymphocytic pleocytosis, elevated IgG, oligoclonal banding, and specific anti–HTLV-I antibodies. Diagnosis is by HTLV-I seropositivity in peripheral blood and abnormal CSF findings. The differential diagnosis includes multiple sclerosis, syphilitic meningomyelitis, and adhesive arachnoiditis. Because the virus is also associated with polymyositis, weakness secondary to myopathy must also be excluded. High-dose steroids (prednisone, 60 mg/day for 4 weeks, then tapered off over 2 weeks) may significantly benefit patients with myositis. There is no established antiretroviral therapy, but immunomodulating agents such as interferon-alpha (3 million units/day for 4 weeks) may provide benefit.

Herpesviruses

Acute transverse myelitis and ascending myelitis are rare manifestations of the herpesviruses, although in the era of AIDS they have increasing causative importance. Herpes simplex virus (HSV) types I and II, varicella-zoster virus (VZV), cytomegalovirus (CMV), and Epstein-Barr virus (EBV) have all been associated with myelitis, usually in immunocompromised patients. The myelitis pattern is often nonspecific and asymmetric, although severe ascending necrosis of the cord appears to be most typical and may begin with plexitis. The skin lesions characteristic of HSV I and II and VZV may suggest these causes, but absence of rash cannot reliably exclude them. Patients usually have fever with rapidly progressive neurologic deficits. The CSF shows both lymphocytic and neutrophilic pleocytosis patterns, elevated protein, and normal or reduced glucose. Early empiric therapy with intravenous acyclovir, ganciclovir, or foscarnet may preserve cord function pending definitive diagnosis, when immunocompromised patients present with acute transverse myelitis of unknown origin.

Herpesvirus simiae (B virus) occurs naturally among primates of the genus *Macaca*, reaching 80% prevalence as animals reach sexual maturity. Viral shedding occurs intermittently from mucosa but is increased during breeding season or illness. B virus was first isolated in 1933 from a researcher who died of rapidly progressive meningoencephalitis after being bitten by a macaque monkey. Subsequently, more than 25 cases have been described in persons who handled monkeys or their tissues. Others at risk include laboratory workers exposed to B virus–contaminated rhesus monkey cell cultures. The incubation period ranges from 5 to 30 days, and infection in untreated persons has a fatality rate of approximately 70%. Early symptoms include vesicular eruptions at the exposure site, often with severe pain and regional lymphadenopathy. Local numbness, weakness, and viremic symptoms may follow. Late manifestations include meningitis and encephalitis, avoidable if therapy begins early. B virus infection, a notifiable disease, is diagnosed by serology and viral culture of wound sites, herpetic lesions, and mucosa, which should be performed at specially designated laboratories. MRI may show enhancing lesions in an ascending pattern. The Centers for Disease Control and Prevention (CDC) recommends that asymptomatic persons with a positive wound site culture should be treated with oral acyclovir (800 mg five times daily). Therapy may be discontinued after 14 days if no seroconversion or continued viral shedding is documented. All symptomatic persons should be hospitalized for treatment and isolation with barrier precautions. Intravenous acyclovir (10 to 15 mg/kg every 8 hours) should be instituted at a dose adjusted for renal function and continue until symptoms resolve and serial viral cultures are negative for 14 days. Long-term suppressive therapy and monitoring for viral shedding are recommended.

Enteroviruses

The enteroviruses are well-known causes of infectious myelitis, of which poliovirus is most common worldwide. In Western developed nations, polio is now unusual, but sporadic cases of myelitis caused by other enteroviruses still occur (e.g., Coxsackie A and B, Echo, hepatitis A, and other enteroviruses). Myelitis caused by the nonpolio enteroviruses, generally less severe than that caused by polio, produces weakness rather than paralysis. In some cases of viral myelitis, it may be difficult to distinguish between postinfectious, immune-mediated cord injury and direct viral invasion. The presence of virus in the CSF is supportive of direct viral invasion. Enteroviruses can be recovered from CSF as well as from blood, pharynx, and stool. Acute and convalescent serologies may also establish acute infection. Treatment is supportive.

Syphilis

Four types of spinal cord disease are associated with *Treponema pallidum* infection: tabes dorsalis, syphilitic meningomyelitis, anterior spinal artery syndrome, and gummas of the meninges and cord. Because of its varied pathogenesis, syphilis should be considered in the differential diagnosis of nearly all diseases of the spinal cord. The CSF usually shows a lymphocytic pleocytosis, elevated protein, and normal glucose. A positive Venereal Disease Research Laboratory test (VDRL) in the CSF is specific but generally insensitive. See the chapter *Syphilis and Other Treponematoses* for treatment guidelines.

Mycoplasma pneumoniae

Central nervous system (CNS) complications of *Mycoplasma pneumoniae* infection are probably the most common extrapulmonary manifestation of this disease. Although encephalitis is the most common neurologic complication, meningitis, polyradiculitis, and myelitis have also been reported. The exact pathogenesis of CNS disease is unknown, but it may be secondary to direct invasion, elaboration of neurotoxins, autoimmune complexes, or vasculitis. A history of recent or concurrent respiratory tract infection, especially in a child or young adult, should suggest the diagnosis. If active infection is present, antibiotic therapy may be effective. Tetracycline penetrates the CNS more effectively than erythromycin but is otherwise contraindicated in young children. Steroids and plasmapheresis have also been advocated but remain controversial. See the chapter *Mycoplasma* for further details of diagnosis and treatment.

Brucellosis

Approximately 2% to 5% of patients with brucellosis have neurologic complications, often with considerable clinical overlap. Neurologic involvement is subacute or chronic, and it encompasses encephalitis, myelitis, and radiculopathy; however, the most common neurologic manifestation is meningitis with cranial nerve palsies and vasculitis. Myelopathy typically involves the corticospinal tracts and produces a pure upper motor neuron syndrome without sensory findings. CSF usually reveals a lymphocytic pleocytosis, elevated protein, and hypoglycorrhachia. CSF cultures are positive in fewer than 50% of cases. Treatment of neurobrucellosis currently consists of multidrug therapy for 2 to 4 months. If there is a symptomatic epidural abscess, surgical exploration and decompression may be advisable. Adjunctive use of steroids early in meningitis may reduce complications resulting from vasculitis. Diagnosis and treatment are further discussed in the chapter *Brucellosis.*

■ NEUROPATHY

Neuropathy refers to injury to one or more nerves at any level along their pathways. Infectious causes of neuropathy often prefer one of four anatomic patterns: mononeuropathy, mononeuropathy multiplex, polyneuropathy, and plexopathy. The polyneuropathies may fall into any of three clinical patterns: ascending, descending, or bulbar. Neuropathies are further classified according to the type of functional nerve involvement: purely motor, sensory, autonomic, or mixed.

Consequently, the approach to the patient with peripheral neuropathy begins with identification of the pattern of illness. Initially, the history should focus on the onset of symptoms and their relation to antecedent or comorbid illnesses. An acute onset is highly suggestive of an inflammatory, immunologic, vascular, or toxic cause, all mechanisms by which infectious pathogens may cause disease. Chronic neuropathies of infectious origin, while less common, do occur, particularly leprosy and Lyme borreliosis. In general, an acute onset suggests a more favorable prognosis and should prompt a timely search for the underlying cause to prevent permanent neurologic sequelae.

In classifying the neuropathy, the physical examination should address the following questions: Does the involvement include more than one type of function? Is involvement symmetric or asymmetric, distal or generalized, ascending or descending? Is there a sensory level on the trunk? Do motor and sensory deficits overlap, and do they match subjective complaints? What are the activity levels of the deep tendon reflexes and other reflexes? Is sphincter function normal? Is there evidence of denervation? Are skin lesions associated with the nerve deficits?

Diagnostic clues to infection may be suggested by risk factors, such as inadequate immunization (tetanus, diphtheria), a recent or current systemic illness (*Campylobacter* gastroenteritis in Guillain-Barré syndrome), insect exposures such as to tick bites (Lyme disease), consumption of home-canned or cured foods (botulism) or of unpasteurized dairy products (brucellosis), high-risk sexual contact (syphilis), injecting drug use (wound botulism, tetanus), and residence history (leprosy).

By establishing the anatomic pattern of illness and its rate of onset, the neuropathic syndrome may be identified and further investigations pursued to diagnose specific etiologic agents. Some of the major infectious causes of peripheral neuropathy are discussed next and summarized in Tables 1 through 4.

Leprosy

Leprosy, or Hansen's disease, is a chronic mycobacterial infection primarily affecting the skin and peripheral nerves. Worldwide, it is one of the most common diseases of the peripheral nerves. Although it is a rare endemic disease in the United States, new cases are still diagnosed, mainly in immigrants from Southeast Asia. Ranging from tuberculoid to lepromatous disease, leprosy is a spectrum of illness

Table 1 Peripheral Neuropathy

SYNDROME/DISEASE	ORGANISM/ETIOLOGY	SYMPTOMS, SIGNS, AND NEUROLOGIC FINDINGS	CN	PN	CORD	OTHER FINDINGS	RISK FACTORS
Polyneuritis: *Acute* Guillain-Barré Landry Miller-Fisher *Chronic* CIDP	1. Idiopathic 2. Infection associated	*Onset:* Acute/subacute and chronic *Common features:* Progressive, symmetric weakness Distal→proximal limbs Truncal→cranial muscles Paresthesias, hypotonia, areflexia *Clinical patterns:* Ascending, descending, bulbar	✓	✓		Variable autonomic dysfunction (ileus, cardiac)	Preceding viral illness or vaccination prior to episode Infection associated: Viral (EBV, HIV, hepatitis) Bacterial (*Campylobacter*) Chlamydia (*C. psittaci*) Mycoplasma (*M. pneumoniae*) Spirochetes (Lyme borreliosis)
Neuropathy due to bacterial toxins	*C. diphtheriae*	*Onset:* Acute/subacute *Clinical patterns:* Bulbar symptoms Ascending peripheral neuropathy	✓	✓		Pharyngitis with pseudomembrane Myocarditis Endocarditis	Absence of protective immunity Epidemic respiratory diphtheria Contaminated wound
	C. botulinum	*Onset:* Acute/subacute (dose related) *Clinical patterns:* Bulbar symptoms Myasthenia-like weakness	✓	✓		Autonomic dysfunction (dry tongue, ileus, urinary retention) Decreased vital capacity	Food sources Contaminated wounds (IDUs) Sinusitis in cocaine snorters
	C. tetani	*Onset:* Acute/subacute (dose related) *Clinical patterns:* Localized, cephalic, generalized	✓	✓	✓	Autonomic dysfunction Hypertensive crises Decreased vital capacity Involuntary muscle group spasms	Absence of protective immunity Puncture/contaminated wounds Infected neonatal umbilical cord stumps
Antiinfectives	Aminoglycosides Polymyxins	*Onset:* Acute (concentration related) *Clinical patterns:* Neuromuscular blockade	✓	✓		Decreased vital capacity Generalized paralysis	Excessive or unadjusted dosage for lean body mass
	Isoniazid ddI, ddC, d4T Chloramphenicol Metronidazole Nitrofurantoin	*Onset:* Subacute (dose and duration related) *Clinical patterns:* Symmetric Distal paresthesias and weakness Progressive loss of distal deep tendon reflexes		✓			Isoniazid: lack of pyridoxine Antiretrovirals: Preexisting neuropathy, Excessive or unadjusted dosage Antibiotics: cumulative dosage
Vasculitis	Polyarteritis nodosa (PAN) Wegener's	*Onset:* Subacute *Clinical patterns:* Mononeuritis multiplex *Common features:* Asymmetric weakness, paresthesias, loss of deep tendon reflexes in affected areas		✓		PAN: asymptomatic microaneurysms Wegener's: sinusitis, pulmonary and renal lesions, ± eosinophilia	PAN: chronic active hepatitis B Wegener's: unknown etiology
Leprosy	*Mycobacterium leprae*	*Onset:* Insidious/but acute if reversal reaction *Clinical patterns:* Mononeuritis multiplex Polyneuropathy *Common features:* Anesthetic lesions, enlarged nerves		✓		Deformity Nerves most commonly affected: median, ulnar, peroneal	General Genetic susceptibility Prior residence in endemic areas Neuropathy Tuberculoid Reversal reaction

Table 2   Polymorphic Neurologic Syndromes Associated with Infections

SYNDROME/ DISEASE	ORGANISM/ ETIOLOGY	SYMPTOMS, SIGNS, AND NEUROLOGIC FINDINGS	CN	PN	CORD	OTHER FINDINGS	RISK FACTORS

HIV-associated	HIV-1	*Onset:* Acute, subacute and chronic
		Clinical patterns:
		Acute:
		  GBS, Bell's palsy, mononeuritis multiplex
		Subacute/chronic:
		  Vacuolar myelopathy: progressive spasticity; Sensory peripheral neuropathy
			✔	✔	✔	*Acute infection:* aseptic meningitis, infectious mononucleosis syndrome
						Late disease: concurrent HIV encephalopathy
							IVDU, sexual transmission, exposure to contaminated blood or body fluids

Mycoplasma associated	*Mycoplasma pneumoniae*	*Onset:* Acute *Clinical patterns:* Ascending myelitis (leukomyelitis), polyradiculitis	✔	✔	✔	Commonly associated with encephalitis	Recent upper respiratory infection in child or young adult
Neurobrucellosis	*Brucella* species	*Onset:* Subacute/chronic *Clinical patterns:* Radiculitis, myelitis, CN palsies	✔	✔	✔	Encephalitis, meningitis, mycotic aneurysm	Unpasteurized milk products, occupational exposure to livestock and cattle parturition
Neuroborreliosis	*Borrelia burgdorferi*	*Onset:* Acute and chronic *Clinical patterns:* *Acute:* Bell's palsy, aseptic meningitis, encephalitis, transverse myelitis *Chronic:* weakness, paresthesias	✔	✔	✔	*Acute:* Erythema chronicum migrans	Tick-bite Travel or residence in endemic areas
Neurosyphilis	*Treponema pallidum*	*Onset:* Acute and chronic *Clinical patterns:* Acute syphilitic meningitis Chronic asymptomatic Chronic symptomatic (meningovascular, behavioral, tabes dorsalis, myelopathy)	✔	✔	✔	Dementia Gumma (cord/meninges) Uveitis, optic atrophy Deafness	Asymptomatic (abnormal CSF only) and symptomatic neurosyphilis occurs after early syphilis, with or without standard antibiotic treatment for primary or secondary syphilis; higher risk with HIV infection
VZV associated	VZV	*Onset:* Acute *Clinical patterns:* Sensory radiculitis (CN and PN) Ascending and transverse myelitis	✔	✔	✔	Dermatomal vesicles Uveitis, corneal ulcer Encephalitis	Immunosuppression

Table 3 Myelitis

SYNDROME/DISEASE	ORGANISM/ETIOLOGY	SYMPTOMS, SIGNS, AND NEUROLOGIC FINDINGS	CN	PN	CORD	OTHER FINDINGS	RISK FACTORS
Anterior poliomyelitis syndrome	Poliovirus 1, 2, 3	*Onset:* Acute *Clinical patterns:* Spinal and bulbar paralysis *Common feature:* Asymmetric flaccid paralysis	✓		✓	"Minor illness" (3–4 days): influenza-like syndrome "Major illness" (5–7 days): aseptic meningitis, myeloencephalitis	Absence of protective immunity and travel in endemic areas Live vaccine in immunodeficiency
	Nonpolio Enterovirus Coxsackie A,B Echovirus	*Onset:* Acute *Clinical pattern:* Similar to polio but milder disease	✓		✓	CNS phase: aseptic meningitis, myeloencephalitis	Seasonal incidence in temperate climates (summer), year-round in tropical climates
Ascending myelitis syndrome (leukomyelitis)	HIV-1	*Onset:* Acute/subacute *Clinical patterns:* Sensory neuropathy, spastic paraparesis	✓	✓	✓		See below
	HTLV-1	*Onset:* Subacute/chronic *Clinical patterns:* Tropical spastic paraparesis		✓			Injecting drug use Prior residence in endemic areas
	Herpesviruses: CMV, EBV, HSV, VZV	*Onset:* Acute *Clinical patterns:* Ascending pattern w/initial plexitis Asymmetric commonly					Advanced immunosuppression
	Herpes B virus (Monkey B)	*Onset:* Subacute (5–30 days) *Clinical patterns:* Aseptic meningitis Ascending encephalomyelitis			✓	Prodromal illness *Early:* (vesicles) *Intermediate:* numbness, weakness, hiccups	Macaque monkey bite or exposure to tissues Laboratory workers exposed to contaminated cell cultures
Transverse myelitis syndrome	*Primary myelitis:* VZV Spirochetes* Schistosomiasis Postmeningococcal	*Onset:* Acute (after prodrome) *Clinical patterns:* Sensory motor level Initial spinal shock Hyperreflexia below level of lesion			✓		Related to epidemiology of primary infection
	Secondary myelitis: Bacteria, fungi, mycobacteria	*Onset:* Acute/subacute *Clinical patterns:* Radicular-spinal cord syndrome Cauda equina syndrome			✓	Related to primary infection and organisms	Injecting drug use Hematogenous osteomyelitis Back surgery: intraoperative contamination

*Spirochetes include *Borrelia* species (*B. burgdorferi*—Lyme, *B. recurrentis*—relapsing fever), *Leptospira* species, and *T. pallidum.*
CMV, Cytomegalovirus; *HSV,* herpes simplex virus; *EBV,* Epstein-Barr virus; *HIV,* human immunodeficiency virus; *VZV,* varicella-zoster virus; *IDUs,* injecting drug users; *IVDU,* intravenous drug use; *GBS,* Guillain-Barré syndrome; *CIDP,* chronic idiopathic demyeleiating polyneuropathy; *CSF,* cerebrospinal fluid; *CNS,* central nervous system.

Table 4 Etiology of Neuropathic Syndromes
in HIV Infection

IMMUNE-MEDIATED RESPONSE TO HIV
Bell's palsy
Acute inflammatory demyelinating neuropathy (Guillain-Barré
    syndrome)
Chronic inflammatory demyelinating neuropathy
VASCULITIS
Bell's palsy
Ataxic dorsal radiculopathy
Mononeuritis multiplex: HBV-associated cryoglobulinemia
OPPORTUNISTIC INVASIVE HERPESVIRUS INFECTIONS
Cytomegalovirus (CMV)
    Polyradiculopathy
    Mononeuritis multiplex
Herpes simplex virus (HSV-2)
    Polyradiculopathy
Varicella-zoster virus (VZV)
    Herpes zoster
    Polyradiculopathy
MENINGITIS
Cryptococcal
Neurosyphilitic
Tuberculous
MALIGNANCY
Lymphoma
NUTRITIONAL
Multiple vitamin deficiencies: folate, pyridoxine, B_{12}
DRUG TOXICITY FROM CONCURRENT ANTIINFECTIVES
Antiretroviral nucleoside analogues:
    Dideoxycytosine (ddC)
    Dideoxyinosine (ddI)
    D4T
Niacin analogs: isoniazid (INH) without B_6
IDIOPATHIC
Predominantly sensory neuropathy of AIDS

resulting from a complex interaction between the organism and the host's immune response. The three cardinal manifestations of leprosy are anesthetic skin lesions, palpably enlarged peripheral nerves, and acid-fast bacilli on slit skin smear. Although skin lesions have a variable appearance, anesthesia of the involved skin is the one characteristic feature in typical leprosy. Lepromatous leprosy usually results in symmetric anesthesia of the colder areas of the body (e.g., pinnae, dorsa of hands and feet), whereas nerve involvement in indeterminate and tuberculoid leprosy is typically asymmetric.

The peripheral nerves most commonly involved are the facial, ulnar, median, common peroneal, and posterior tibial nerves. Superficial nerves, such as the ulnar and posterior auricular nerves, are readily accessible to palpation and are often enlarged and tender. Because neuropathic mutilation of the hands and feet is a significant cause of disability, a complete motor and sensory examination of the hands and feet should be performed before beginning therapy. Slit skin smears are usually positive in lepromatous and borderline lepromatous leprosy but are typically negative in tuberculoid and borderline tuberculoid disease. Where the disease is

rare, such as in the United States, skin biopsy should be performed. Slit skin smears are performed by making small incisions into the dermis at multiple sites. The fluid is then stained for acid-fast bacilli. The organism cannot be cultured in vitro. Skin testing with lepromin is not useful in diagnosis.

Treatment regimens for leprosy are based on the burden of infecting organisms and the host's immune status. After starting chemotherapy, patients must be monitored for neuritis as a complication of reversal reactions and erythema nodosum leprosum (ENL), which may require steroid or thalidomide administration. Specific details about therapy can be found in the chapter *Leprosy*.

HIV-Associated Neuropathy

Neuropathy is one of the most common disorders associated with HIV disease. Occasionally, neuropathy is the initial manifestation of HIV infection itself, such as Bell's palsy or Guillain-Barré syndrome. Late-onset neuropathy is frequently overshadowed by the more striking CNS complications of HIV infection, such as vacuolar myelopathy and AIDS dementia complex, or by opportunistic infections of the CNS such as toxoplasmic encephalitis or progressive multifocal leukoencephalopathy (PML). However, subclinical neuropathy may be nearly universal at the time of death. Many causes of neuropathy have been described in HIV-infected persons (Table 2).

Predominantly sensory neuropathy is the most common neuropathy seen in AIDS and is one of the most debilitating aspects of advanced HIV infection. Its exact cause is unclear, although immune complex vasculitis has been suggested by pathology studies. Patients usually complain of painful paresthesias and burning of the distal extremities, primarily of the soles of the feet. On examination, only patients with progressive HIV neuropathy will exhibit a generalized decrease in sensation in the affected areas and atrophy of the intrinsic muscles of the feet. Deep tendon reflexes of the ankles are eventually lost, but patellar reflexes may be exaggerated by coexisting myelopathy. When reflexes are affected, nerve conduction studies are consistent with distal axonal degeneration. Reversible causes of neuropathy should be excluded.

Mononeuritis multiplex is a simultaneous or sequential neuropathy of noncontiguous nerve trunks evolving over days to years. Mononeuritis multiplex may be seen early in HIV infection, even before immunosuppression has occurred. Isolated cranial neuropathies may also occur at any stage of HIV infection. Acute facial weakness characteristic of Bell's palsy usually occurs early in HIV infection and is often associated with a lymphocytic meningitis. In advanced HIV infection the differential diagnosis of cranial neuropathies includes CNS opportunistic infections, such as cryptococcosis and acute herpes zoster, and meningeal lymphomatosis.

Treatment of HIV predominantly sensory neuropathy is generally unsatisfactory. Highly active antiretroviral therapy (HAART) has no predictable therapeutic effect on established neuropathy. Also, because subclinical disease is probably universal in advanced HIV infection, late-stage patients beginning chronic therapy with antiretroviral agents having dose-dependent neurotoxicity, such as dideoxyinosine (ddI), dideoxycytosine (ddC), and stavudine (d4T), should be regularly evaluated for onset of clinical neuropathy.

Herpesvirus Neuropathies in AIDS

CMV infection of the peripheral nerves, essentially unknown prior to AIDS, is the consequence of reactivation of systemic CMV infection and is often associated with evidence of active CMV infection in other systems, particularly retinitis. The capacity of CMV to invade both endothelial and Schwann cells accounts for its varied clinical manifestations. Polyradiculopathy, the most dramatic of these syndromes, is caused by CMV more often than by other herpesviruses. It is characterized by a subacute onset of ascending motor weakness, areflexia, incontinence or urinary retention, paresthesias, and variable sensory dysfunction. Patients often complain of pain in the back and legs. Intense inflammation of the lumbar nerve roots, dorsal root ganglia, and spinal cord result in characteristic CSF findings mimicking bacterial meningitis: polymorphonuclear predominance (up to 90%), hypoglycorrhachia, and elevated protein. CSF white blood cell counts can vary from fewer than 50 to more than 3000. Diffuse enhancement of the cauda equina on postcontrast MRI has been reported. Specific diagnostic tests may be helpful but are generally insensitive (e.g., CMV culture of CSF) or overly invasive (e.g., biopsy). Cytologic examination of the CSF may demonstrate CMV inclusions. PCR detection of CMV DNA in CSF is diagnostic. Early treatment of CMV polyradiculopathy is undertaken with ganciclovir (GCV) at dosages of 5 mg/kg intravenously (IV) twice a day for 2 weeks, followed by a maintenance dosage of 5 mg/kg/day. Other herpesviruses causing radiculomyelitis in AIDS patients are HSV II and varicella-zoster.

Syphilis in HIV Infection

CNS syphilis may also present as a subacute polyradiculopathy in HIV infection. In contrast to CMV and HSV, the CSF contains lymphocytes, and the CSF VDRL is usually but not always positive. Therefore, if other evidence points to prior syphilis but the CSF VDRL is negative, the patient should be treated empirically with high-dose penicillin G. Because HIV infection, irrespective of CD4 count, may contribute to an unacceptably high number of treatment failures, close follow-up of syphilis serologies and CSF VDRL is warranted.

Inflammatory Demyelinating Neuropathies

Acute inflammatory demyelinating neuropathy, or Guillain-Barré syndrome (GBS), has a well-known association with a variety of infectious diseases such as EBV, CMV, HIV, *Mycoplasma pneumoniae,* psittacosis, Lyme disease, and particularly *Campylobacter jejuni.* In more than half of patients a mild respiratory or gastrointestinal tract illness precedes the onset of the disorder by 1 to 3 weeks. Patients usually have an ascending symmetric weakness that can progress to respiratory failure. Areflexia and a variable degree of sensory loss are also evident. Transient paresthesias and pain in the back and legs are frequent complaints. Constitutional symptoms are unusual. The CSF is typically acellular with elevated protein, but variations occur.

GBS must be distinguished from other neurologic illnesses (e.g., myasthenia gravis) and two uncommon infectious diseases, botulism and poliomyelitis. In botulism the pupillary reflexes are lost early, and there may be significant autonomic dysfunction (e.g., bradycardia, dry mouth, abdominal cramps, urinary difficulty). Polio usually occurs in clusters and manifests as meningeal symptoms, fever, and asymmetric paralysis.

Therapy of GBS consists of respiratory monitoring and support, and early plasmapheresis. Some studies suggest that intravenous immunoglobulin (IVIG) at 0.4 g/kg/day for 5 days is as effective as plasmapheresis. However, plasmapheresis remains the treatment of choice. Steroids have no benefit.

Chronic inflammatory demyelinating polyneuropathy is also seen in patients infected with HIV. Like GBS, it presents primarily as weakness with varying degrees of sensory loss. Physical examination reveals proximal muscle weakness of the upper and lower extremities. Weakness of the neck flexors is particularly suggestive. As in GBS, CSF analysis is remarkable for elevated protein and the absence of cells. The presence of cells raises suspicion of HIV infection. Plasmapheresis is the treatment of choice.

Neuropathies Caused by Bacterial Toxins

Diphtheria is rare in the United States but may still be seen in unimmunized children and in adults with waning immunity. Diphtheria toxin, elaborated in pharynx or contaminated wound, causes a noninflammatory demyelination of the cranial and peripheral nerves. In pharyngeal diphtheria, locally produced toxin paralyzes the pharyngeal and laryngeal muscles, causing the earliest neurologic symptoms. The patient speaks with a nasal voice and complains of dysphagia and nasal regurgitation. As the disease progresses over 1 to 2 months systemic intoxication, loss of ocular accommodation is followed by a generalized ascending or descending sensorimotor polyneuropathy. Specific therapeutic guidelines are discussed in the chapter *Corynebacteria.*

Tetanus and botulism are the other two neurologic disorders caused by elaborated bacterial toxins. Both toxins exert their effects by interrupting normal nerve conduction rather than by directly damaging the nerve. They are discussed further in the chapters *Clostridia* and *Food Poisoning.*

Lyme Borreliosis

Borrelia burgdorferi infection can result in acute and chronic neuropathies. Acute disease occurs within 4 to 12 weeks after tick bite and is usually characterized by peripheral and cranial neuropathies with meningoencephalitis. Acute disease also presents as plexitis, mononeuropathy multiplex, or myelitis. Unilateral or bilateral facial palsies, the most common neurologic manifestations, may be seen in 50% of patients. In endemic areas, facial palsy with a history of tick bite is sufficient to warrant empiric therapy, even in the absence of meningitis.

Months to years after infection, chronic Lyme borreliosis can cause intermittent distal paresthesias and radicular pain. Physical examination may be normal, but nerve conduction studies demonstrate axonal neuropathy. Treatment of Lyme meningitis and other neurologic complications includes intravenous antibiotics for 2 to 3 weeks, but symptomatic response to therapy is slow. Diagnosis and specific antibiotic therapy are discussed in the chapter *Lyme Disease.*

Suggested Reading

Barohn RJ: Approach to peripheral neuropathy and neuronopathy, *Semin Neurol* 18:7, 1998.

Hahn AF: Guillain-Barré syndrome, *Lancet* 352:635, 1998.
Holmes GP, et al: Guidelines for the prevention and treatment of B-virus infections in exposed persons, *Clin Infect Dis* 20:421, 1995.
Hyslop NE, Leach RS: Infectious diseases of the spinal cord and peripheral nervous system. In Gorbach SL, Bartlett JG, Blacklow NR, eds: *Infectious diseases,* Philadelphia, 1998, Saunders.
Pruitt AA: Infections of the nervous system, *Neurol Clin* 16:419, 1998.

REYE'S SYNDROME

Rajiv R. Varma

Reye's syndrome is typically a disease of children, but it also occurs in young adults. It is associated with a wide variety of viral prodromes, especially influenza B and chickenpox. The adverse effects of salicylates in the causation or exacerbation of Reye's syndrome is now generally accepted, and avoidance of their use in children with viral illnesses and subsequent dramatic decline in the incidence has provided further support for the role of salicylates in the pathogenesis. However, Reye's syndrome may occur without salicylate ingestion.

Reye's syndrome usually has a biphasic course. The initial phase is a viral prodrome, usually upper respiratory and associated with fever. This phase may improve for a couple of days. Following this apparent recovery, during the second phase, vomiting usually occurs and is often persistent and protracted, and it is followed by mental changes. There are no localizing signs. Mental function may deteriorate in hours. The staging criteria of Lovejoy and associates have been adopted by the National Institutes of Health for the staging of Reye's syndrome (Table 1). The liver is generally enlarged and smooth, and jaundice is absent except in severe cases. Patients appear well nourished, and edema and ascites are generally absent. The liver chemistries show a hepatocellular pattern and should be measured in children with unexplained mental changes. Blood ammonia determination performed within 24 hours of the mental changes correlates well with severity, and levels greater than five times normal may indicate a poor outcome. Lumbar puncture shows a normal cerebrospinal fluid despite increased opening pressure. Hypoglycemia and decreased spinal fluid glucose are more common in children 4 years of age or younger. Accurate diagnosis cannot be made without liver biopsy, which must include electron microscopy to reveal characteristic mitochondrial changes. Microvesicular fatty change is suggestive but *not* conclusive. Predominantly microvesicular fatty change may occur in several disorders or may follow drug hepatotoxicity (Table 2). Diagnosis remains uncertain if electron microscopy is not performed. Therefore firm diagnosis of Reye's syndrome requires liver histology and electron microscopic studies. Electron microscopy shows characteristic pleomorphic and enlarged mitochondria with loss of dense granules and cristae mitochondrales. Associated electron microscopy changes include proliferation of smooth endoplasmic reticulum and perioxisames. In the Reye-like syndromes liver mitochondria are normal or near normal.

In children with Kawasaki's disease or juvenile rheumatoid arthritis, salicylates are still widely used. In these patients, the risk of Reye's syndrome would still appear to be significant. In these children, one should recognize the risks and have a high index of suspicion for Reye's syndrome. In younger adults who regularly use several doses of aspirin daily or frequently, viral illnesses may carry a higher risk for Reye's syndrome.

Table 1 Staging of Reye's Syndrome					
	STAGE I	**STAGE II**	**STAGE III**	**STAGE IV**	**STAGE V**
Level of consciousness	Lethargic; follows verbal commands	Combative or stuporous; verbalizes in appropriately	Coma	Coma	Coma
Posture	Normal	Normal	Decorticate	Decerebrate	Flaccid
Response to pain	Purposeful	Purposeful	Decorticate	Decerebrate	None
Pupillary reaction	Brisk	Sluggish	Sluggish	Sluggish	None
Oculocephalic reflex (doll's eyes)	Normal	Conjugate deviation	Conjugate deviation	Inconsistent or absent	None

Staging criteria adopted at the NIH Reye's Syndrome Consensus Development Conference held in March 1981.

Table 2   Causes of Predominantly Microvesicular Steatosis
Reye's syndrome
Fatty liver of pregnancy
Jamaican vomiting sickness
L-Asparaginase
Didanosine
Fialuridine (FIAU)
Hepatitis C virus infection*
Acyl-CoA dehydrogenase deficiencies
Long chain
Medium chain
Short chain

*Usually mixed type of steatosis.

■ REYE-LIKE SYNDROMES

Reye's syndrome is an acquired form of mitochondrial disease that follows a variety of viral illnesses. Aspirin exacerbates the acute mitochondrial injury. With the avoidance of aspirin in children, the number of Reye's syndrome cases has dramatically declined, and the likelihood of diseases related to Reye-like syndrome has increased. This further underscores the value of obtaining liver tissue for histology and especially electron microscopy. Without characteristic mitochondrial changes, the diagnosis of Reye's syndrome remains in question. Features favoring Reye-like syndrome include the following: (1) recurrent episodes; (2) presence of similar episodes in siblings; (3) absence of vomiting during episodes; (4) onset before 3 years of age; and (5) frequent hypoglycemia, feeding disorders, cardiac enlargement, and muscle weakness.

This list of mitochondrial hepatopathies is extensive and beyond the scope of this brief review. These hepatopathies resemble Reye's syndrome. Vomiting appears to be less common in Reye-like syndromes. The reader is referred to a number of texts for additional information. Because Reye's syndrome and Reye-like syndromes usually have a mitochondrial defect in common, drugs that adversely affect mitochondrial function would also be expected to increase the severity of both groups of disorders. Some of these drugs include aspirin, valproic acid, barbituates, and alcohol. The tests should be undertaken when the patient is symptomatic and when the metabolic abnormalities are most pronounced. Some of the abnormalities associated with Reye-like syndromes are mild and likely to be missed during asymptomatic stages. Diagnosis of Reye's and Reye-like syndrome should be undertaken at a tertiary care facility with experience in the management of these cases. Management of acutely ill patients in the intensive care setting with house staff availability is recommended.

■ THERAPY

Cerebral edema is the main cause of morbidity and mortality, and adequate control of cerebral edema is the main goal of therapy. A careful correction of metabolic abnormalities, including hypoglycemia, should be attempted. However, 100% replacement fluid and electrolyte imbalance is not necessary; about 80% to 90% correction may be preferable and probably reduces the risk of cerebral edema. Serum osmolality should be maintained between 305 and 310. I prefer the use of 10% dextrose with hypotonic saline. This reduces the chances of hypoglycemia. Hypoglycemia may require additional intravenous 50% dextrose boluses. Protection of airway by intubation and hyperventilation may be needed in severe cases. The head should be elevated. Sedation should be avoided as much as possible, and use of fresh frozen plasma should also be kept to a minimum but may be necessary to do a liver biopsy.

The therapy of Reye's syndrome is best undertaken at a tertiary care facility experienced in the management of severe liver diseases and cerebral edema by a team approach. Several groups have been enthusiastic about exchange transfusion in severe cases, but controlled data are not available. Early recognition and prompt therapy during the initial stages of mental changes is more likely to be followed by a successful outcome without residual neurologic deficit.

■ REYE'S SYNDROME IN ADULTS

Because aspirin is still widely used by adults, the possibility of Reye's syndrome as a cause of unexplained encephalopathy should be kept in mind. With the avoidance of salicylates in children, Reye-like syndromes are now more likely to be seen in adults.

The diagnosis of Reye's syndrome is more difficult in adults because Reye's syndrome is even less likely in adults and drug abuse and other medical problems more common in adults make it more difficult to make a diagnosis. Metabolic disorders mimicking Reye's syndrome are less likely. Therapy is similar. Persons using aspirin repeatedly will appear more at risk.

Suggested Reading

Balistreri WF, Schubert WK: Liver disease in infancy and childhood. In Schiff L, Schiff ER, eds: *Diseases of the liver*, Philadelphia, 1999, Lippincott.

Belay ED, et al: Reye's syndrome in the United States from 1981 through 1997, *N Engl J Med* 340:1377, 1999.

Bove KE, et al: Hepatic lesions in Reye's syndrome, *Gastroenterology* 69:685, 1975.

Meythaler JM, Varma RR: Reye's syndrome in adults: diagnostic considerations, *Arch Intern Med* 147:61, 1987.

Treem WR, et al: Medium chain and long chain acyl CoA dehydrogenase deficiency: clinical, pathologic and ultrastructural differentiation from Reye's syndrome, *Hepatology* 6:1270, 1986.

Treem W, Sokol R: Mitochondrial hepatopathies, *Sem Liver Dis* 18:237, 1998.

Varma RR: Reye's syndrome: handbook of experimental pharmacology. In Cameron REG, Feuer G, de la Igenia FA, eds: *Drug induced hepatotoxicity*, Heidelberg, 1995, Springer-Verlag.

PROGRESSIVE MULTIFOCAL LEUKOENCEPHALOPATHY

Joseph R. Berger

In their seminal report in 1958, Astrom, Mancall, and Richardson described a progressive neurologic syndrome with characteristic neuropathologic findings of demyelination, giant astrocytes, and oligodendrocytes with abnormal nuclei. Although these investigators referenced prior descriptions, they were responsible for crystallizing the entity and naming it *progressive multifocal leukoencephalopathy* (PML). In 1965, Zu, Rhein, and Chou identified for the first time viral particles in glial nuclei, which resembled papovavirus. This family derives its name from the initial letters of the three genuses that form the family, papilloma, polyoma, and vacuolating viruses. Subsequently, Padgett isolated polyoma virus from PML brain in glial cell cultures. This virus proved to be a double-stranded DNA virus of icosahedral symmetry. It appears that almost all cases of PML are caused by the JC virus of the polyoma virus genus. The ability of the virus to hemagglutinate type O erythrocytes has permitted the performance of seroepidemiologic studies that demonstrate that JC virus is present worldwide. By the age of 20 years, most individuals have serologic evidence of exposure to JC virus. Spread of JC virus is believed to be via respiratory secretions. The detection of JC virus in tonsillar tissue is highly suggestive, although not confirmatory, of this route of dissemination. No acute illness has been consistently identified with primary JC virus infection. The infection typically remains latent until a number of events transpire, most importantly the occurrence of impaired cell-mediated immunity. Until the last decade, chronic lymphocytic leukemia and lymphoma were the underlying illnesses most often associated with PML. However, in the last 15 years, the number of cases of PML has risen dramatically as a result of acquired immunodeficiency syndrome (AIDS). It is no longer a rare disease.

As its name implies, the disease is characterized by multiple sites of demyelination with a distinctive microscopic triad of multifocal myelin and oligodendroglial cell loss with minimal inflammatory infiltrate; hyperchromatic enlarged oligodendroglial nuclei; and enlarged and bizarre-appearing astrocytes with irregularly lobulated nuclei (Figure 1). The viral particles may be detected by electron microscopy, immunostaining, or polymerase chain reaction (PCR). The virus appears in three forms: a filamentous form in the nuclei of infected cells, and in spherical or paracrystalline forms in either nucleus or cytoplasm. Virions are visualized mostly in oligodendrocytes and rarely in astrocytes.

Most studies now report an incidence of approximately 5% in patients with AIDS. A 20-fold increase in the prevalence of PML was seen between the years 1980 to 1984 and

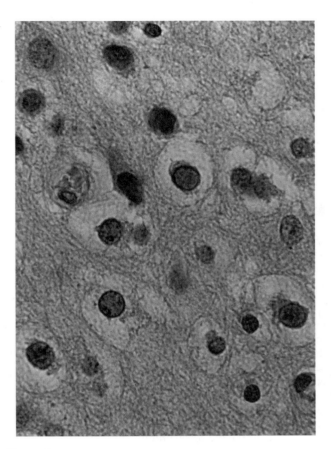

Figure 1
Abnormal infected oligodendrocytes with enlarged nuclei identified by in situ hybridization.

1990 to 1994 in south Florida, with all but 2 of 156 cases of PML in this series occurring in association with human immunodeficiency virus (HIV). AIDS patients with PML generally have significant lymphopenia and low CD4 lymphocyte counts; however, more than 10% of AIDS patients with PML have CD4 counts in excess of 200 cells/mm^3 at the time of presentation. In light of the widespread exposure to JC virus by adulthood, the presence of serum antibodies to JC virus is not a reliable indicator for risk of future development of PML in the AIDS population. JC virus can be detected in the peripheral blood lymphocytes (PBLs) in 0% to 8% of normal persons by PCR but in approximately 40% of HIV-seropositive persons without PML%. Whether the demonstration of JC virus in PBLs is a predictor of an "at-risk" population still remains to be determined.

The JC virus may be found in many extraneural sites, including kidneys, lymph nodes, tonsils, lung, and liver, but it is unlikely that there is replication in these tissues. Urinary excretion of JC virus can be detected.

The numbers of AIDS patients developing PML greatly exceeds that of other illnesses having similar degrees of impaired cell-mediated immunity, suggesting that factors related to HIV infection may be amplifying the frequency of the disease. The upregulation of endothelial adhesion molecules for JC virus–infected B lymphocytes due to cytokines elaborated by HIV-infected macrophages and microglial cells in the brain may contribute to its increased frequency in this condition.

PML probably results from reactivation of a latent JC virus infection. Most newborns have antibodies against JC virus (73.7%), which tend to disappear by 11 months of life (8.3%). Thereafter, an increase in antibodies against JC virus occurs with age: 45% from 1 to 5 years, 65% from 6 to 10, and 65% to 90% in those older than 11 years. Most cases of PML have IgG antibodies to JC virus, not IgM, suggesting reactivation and not reinfection.

■ CLINICAL MANIFESTATIONS AND DIAGNOSIS

The clinical manifestations of PML are multiple and depend on the area of white matter involved. The most common signs and symptoms vary with the population studied. Common abnormalities include weakness, gait disturbance, speech and language disorders, cognitive dysfunction, and visual loss. Weakness, often hemiparesis, is the foremost manifestation of the disease both at onset and time of diagnosis. Ataxia, dysarthria, numbness, headaches, aphasia, seizures, and vertigo are occasionally noted. Rarely, focal cognitive deficits, such as prosopagnosia, apraxia, left-sided neglect, and Gerstmann's syndrome are observed; however, global deficits such as memory disturbances and personality changes are more common. PML is rarely present in the absence of detectable focal findings on careful neurologic evaluation.

The diagnosis of PML is strongly suggested by the typical appearance on imaging studies. On CT, multiple white matter hypodensities are revealed (Figure 2), but MRI is more sensitive. The lesions of PML appear hyperintense on T2 and hypointense on T1 (Figure 3). The scalloped appearance of these areas is caused by subcortical "U" fibers involvement. Although any area can be affected, there is a predilection for the parietooccipital region. About a third of patients have posterior fossa involvement, and 5% have only cerebellar and brainstem lesions. Most patients have bilateral abnormal areas, and basal ganglia may be affected, presumably because of myelinated fibers that course through this area. Enhancement is not typical, but up to 9% of patients can have faint peripheral enhancement around the lesions.

PML must be differentiated from HIV leukoencephalopathy, although this can be difficult on a radiologic basis. The latter has cortical involvement, does not enhance, and is isointense on T1W1. Clinical distinguishing characteristics are its rapid course, focal features, and subcortical involvement. In contrast, HIV encephalopathy or dementia has a more protracted course, is of a cortical nature, and only rarely has focal features.

■ CEREBROSPINAL FLUID

Routine studies on cerebrospinal fluid (CSF) are not particularly helpful in the diagnosis of PML. A mild increase in protein can be detected in some patients, as well as presence

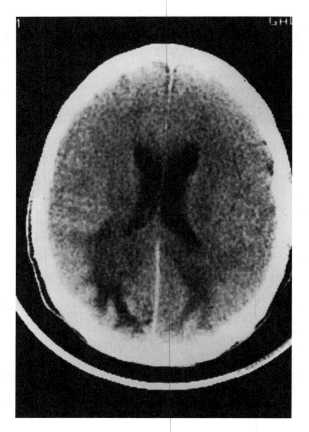

Figure 2
Computed tomography scan shows hypodense abnormalities in bilateral occipital lobes.

of oligoclonal bands and increased IgG synthesis (elevated CSF index). Myelin basic protein may be detected in the CSF. However, PCR for JC virus has become a useful test for diagnosing the disorder in patients with the appropriate clinical and radiographic features. CSF PCR has a specificity of 100%, a high ha-sensitivity, with the capacity to detect between 1 and 10 JC virus DNA copy equivalents per 10 μl of CSF. One laboratory detected 10^5 copies per 10 μl of CSF.

Despite the sensitivity and specificity of CSF PCR for JC virus, tissue examination remains the gold standard for diagnosis of PML. The previously described pathognomonic histopathologic findings are seen by light microscopy, and viral particles may be demonstrated by electron microscopy. Viral DNA can be detected by in situ hybridization and JC virus antigens by immunocytochemistry.

■ PROGNOSIS

The prognosis of PML is typically grim, with death occurring in most patients between 1 and 18 months (mean 4 months) after disease onset. There have been occasional reports of stabilization and improvement, clinically and radiologically, both in HIV and non-HIV cases. Certain features seem to be associated with a greater likelihood of long survival (in excess of 12 months), including PML as the heralding illness of AIDS, lesser degree of immunosuppres-

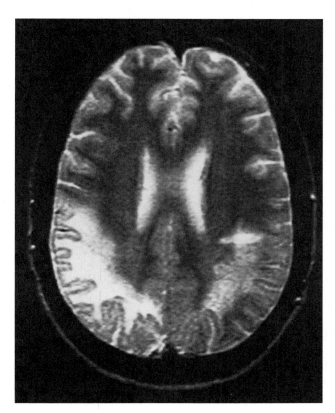

Figure 3
This T$_2$-weighted magnetic resonance imaging image shows extensive hyperintense signal abnormalities in the right parietooccipital white matter and smaller subcortical lesions on the left.

sion (CD4 counts >300 cells/mm^3), enhancement on radiographic imaging, and any evidence of clinical recovery. Low CSF JC viral loads have also correlated with longer survival.

■ TREATMENT

The treatment of PML remains frustrating. To date, there are no unequivocally successful therapeutic modalities. Most of the extant literature consists of anecdotal reports. Zidovudine (AZT) and other antiretrovirals have been proposed as adjunctive therapy for AIDS-associated PML. One patient has been described with an apparent response to zidovudine, and other investigators have commented on similar cases. Zidovudine at 1000 mg or more daily should be attempted in light of its superior ability to cross the blood-brain barrier. Perhaps more exciting have been the small, retrospective series that have strongly suggested the value of highly active antiretroviral therapy (HAART) in HIV-infected patients with PML. The benefit of HAART in AIDS-associated PML has not been universally observed, however.

Nucleoside analogs have been used because they impede the synthesis of DNA. In vitro studies have clearly demonstrated the ability of cytosine arabinoside (Cytarabine, ARA-C), a cytosine analog, to inhibit JC virus replication, and anecdotal reports of intravenous and intrathecal adminis-

tration suggested the value of this therapy in treating PML. However, a carefully conducted clinical trial of AIDS-related PML failed to show any value of either intravenous or intrathecal administration of ARA-C when compared with placebo. Despite anecdotal reports of the value of other nucleoside analogs in PML, such as adenine arabinoside (Vidarabine, ARA-A), none has been convincingly demonstrated the ability to ameliorate the disease course.

Interferons have also had occasional positive results both subcutaneously and intrathecally when used in conjunction with ARA-C. In a pilot study of 17 patients with AIDS and PML treated with alpha 2a interferon and zidovudine, two had long-term clinical stabilization, although none improved. A retrospective study compared patients with AIDS-associated PML receiving a minimum treatment of 3 weeks of 3 million units of interferon-alpha daily with untreated historical controls. Results suggested that interferon-alpha treatment delayed the progression of the disease, palliated symptoms, and significantly prolonged survival. Better-designed trials with this agent are clearly warranted.

The antineoplastic drug camptothecin, a DNA topoisomerase I inhibitor, has been demonstrated to block JC virus replication in vitro when administered in pulsed doses in amounts nontoxic to cells. Its therapeutic usefulness in PML has been entirely anecdotal. Another antineoplastic drug, topotecan, may also inhibit JC virus replication. However, both these drugs display significant systemic toxicity, and their value in the treatment of PML remains open to question.

Cidofovir and its cyclic counterpart have demonstrated selective antipolyomavirus activity. Currently, a well-designed AIDS Clinical Trials Group study is addressing the value of cidofovir.

Increased understanding of the molecular biology of JC virus and new technologies will likely result in novel strategies. One possibility is the use of an antisense oligonucleotide that binds selectively to a targeted region of mRNA. Genetic manipulation of certain proteins that bind to a purine-rich domain may also result in inhibition of transcription and downregulate viral expression.

Suggested Reading

Berger J, Major E: Progressive multifocal leukoencephalopathy. In Merigan T, Barlett J, Bolognesi D, eds: *Textbook of AIDS medicine*, Baltimore, 1999, Williams & Wilkins.

Berger JR, et al: Progressive multifocal leukoencephalopathy in patients with HIV infection, *J Neurovirol* 4:59, 1998.

Clifford DB, et al: HAART improves prognosis in HIV-associated progressive multifocal leukoencephalopathy [see comments], *Neurology* 52:623, 1999.

De Luca A, et al: Response to cidofovir after failure of antiretroviral therapy alone in AIDS-associated progressive multifocal leukoencephalopathy, *Neurology* 52:891, 1999.

Dorries K, Arendt G, Eggers C: Nucleic acid detection as a diagnostic tool in polyomavirus JC induced progressive multifocal leukoencephalopathy, *J Med Virol* 54:196, 1998.

Meylan PR, et al: Monitoring the response of AIDS-related progressive multifocal leukoencephalopathy to HAART and cidofovir by PCR for JC virus DNA in the CSF, *Eur Neurol* 41:172, 1999.

Yiannoutsos CT, et al: Relation of JC virus DNA in the cerebrospinal fluid to survival in acquired immunodeficiency syndrome patients with biopsy-proven progressive multifocal leukoencephalopathy, *Ann Neurol* 45:816, 1999.

CEREBROSPINAL FLUID SHUNT INFECTION

Fred F. Barrett

Table 1 Causative Agents of Shunt Infection*

ORGANISM	NUMBER	PERCENTAGE
Coagulase-negative staphylococci	265	51
Staphylococcus aureus	105	20
Streptococcus sp.	23	4
Other gram-positive bacteria	10	2
Gram-negative bacilli	73	15
Miscellaneous	40	8

*Combined results of several studies.

Although cerebrospinal fluid (CSF) shunts have prolonged the survival and quality of life of hydrocephalic patients, they are associated with significant complications, mainly malfunction and infection. Shunt infection occurs in 1% to 30% of procedures. With careful attention to surgical detail and strict adherence to operative and postoperative protocols, surgery-related infection rates as low as 1% to 2% are now being reported in the literature.

■ PATHOGENESIS

The CSF shunt can become infected via a number of routes. Most surgery-related infections are a result of intraoperative contamination of the wound by microorganisms from the patient's own skin flora. Nonsurgical infection of the ventriculoperitoneal (VP) shunt may be a result of perforation of the bowel or translocation of fecal flora across the intact bowel wall. It is speculated that ventriculoatrial (VA) shunts can become infected as a result of transient asymptomatic bacteremia, but this route has not been conclusively documented. Finally, it is well known that CSF shunts become colonized during systemic infection with the common childhood meningitis pathogens: *Haemophilus influenzae, Streptococcus pneumoniae, Neisseria meningitidis,* and group B streptococci.

Shunt infection occurs more often in young infants, and in some series, the incidence is high in patients with meningomyelocele. Additional factors associated with shunt infection include preexisting skin conditions such as decubiti, concomitant sites of infection (otitis media, pneumonia, urinary tract infection), prolonged operating time, and experience of the neurosurgeon. Infection rates do not differ between primary and revision procedures unless the revision is done for prior infection, in which case rates may be higher. Factors not generally associated with shunt infection include gender, cause and degree of hydrocephalus, number of prior neurosurgical procedures, and type of shunt (VP, VA) or shunt device.

■ CAUSES

Coagulase-negative staphylococci are isolated from more than 50% of cases, and *Staphylococcus aureus* accounts for as many as 25% of infections (Table 1). Coagulase-negative staphylococci isolated from infected shunts often produce glycocalyx (slime) and demonstrate a tendency to adhere or bind to the shunt material. This increased adherence makes eradication of the organism with antibiotics difficult if not impossible. Enteric and nonenteric gram-negative organisms are less commonly isolated but when encountered are more commonly found in infants. Skin flora organisms of low pathogenicity such as *Corynebacterium* and *Propionibacterium* species, as well as a variety of streptococcus species and fungi, have also been isolated.

■ DIAGNOSIS

Diagnosis of shunt infection is based on Gram stain smears and cultures of CSF obtained from the shunt reservoir. The diagnosis is confirmed when the same microorganism is isolated from two or more individual cultures of shunt reservoir CSF or shunt hardware, or the Gram stain reveals an organism that is morphologically compatible with the organism isolated via culture.

■ SHUNT INFECTION SYNDROMES

Clinical and laboratory features of shunt infection depend on the type of shunt and route of infection. Four generally distinct shunt infection syndromes have been described: colonization, infection associated with wound infection, distal infection with peritonitis, and shunt infection associated with bacterial meningitis. Although there is overlap among these syndromes, they are discussed as separate entities.

Colonization

Patients present without evidence of wound infection. Approximately 75% of cases occur within 2 months of surgery, but onset may be delayed for many months—even as long as a year or more. The presenting symptoms of VP shunt colonization usually are those of shunt malfunction (lethargy, headache, vomiting, full fontanelle, increasing head circumference, separated cranial sutures) with low-grade fever and minimal, if any, peritoneal symptoms or signs. In contrast, patients with colonized VA shunts have high fever and varying degrees of toxicity because of the associated bacteremia, but symptoms of shunt malfunction are uncommon.

Laboratory Features

CSF obtained via direct ventricular puncture is sterile in up to 50% of cases, and the causative agent is almost always isolated from shunt reservoir CSF unless the patient has received antibiotic therapy. Even when ventricular CSF is culture positive, especially with coagulase-negative staphylococci, symptoms and signs of ventriculitis are often minimal. Blood cultures are virtually always positive in VA shunt colonization but rarely positive in VP colonization. In the absence of ventriculitis, CSF findings are near normal, with minimal pleocytosis (100 to 200 leukocytes/m/^{3}), normal to slightly decreased glucose, and normal to slightly elevated protein.

Coagulase-negative staphylococci and other skin commensals of low virulence account for most cases of colonization. *S. aureus* and gram-negative bacteria are also isolated, but less often than in other syndromes.

Surgical Therapy

The approach to surgical treatment of shunt colonization (Table 2) depends on the type of shunt and severity of symptoms. Early one-stage replacement of a colonized VA shunt is possible if CSF obtained via direct ventricular puncture is sterile and if bacteremia is easily controlled by a brief course of systemic antibiotic therapy. If CSF obtained by direct ventricular puncture is culture positive or the culture status is unknown, removal and replacement should be delayed until after sterilization of blood and shunt reservoir CSF by appropriate systemic and intrashunt antibiotics.

The distal end of a colonized VP shunt should be exteriorized to allow sterilization of the peritoneal cavity by systemic antibiotic therapy and relief of any associated abdominal symptoms, which if present are usually mild. External ventricular drainage via the externalized shunt allows for control of ventricular pressure while infection is treated with systemic and intrashunt antibiotics. When shunt reservoir CSF cultures are sterile, the shunt can be replaced on the opposite side. Replacement of only the distal catheter following "sterilization" of the shunt has been reported, but the relapse rate is higher than with total replacement.

Wound Infection

The patient usually presents within days to weeks of surgery with obvious wound infection or dehiscence as well as erythema and swelling along the shunt tubing tract. There may be no evidence of shunt malfunction or central nervous system infection early after wound dehiscence, but many patients eventually develop symptoms and signs of ventriculitis (i.e., fever, headache, meningeal signs, and vomiting). This is especially common with *S. aureus* infection.

Laboratory Features

Shunt reservoir CSF is almost always culture positive, and CSF parameters are often typical for ventriculitis with significant pleocytosis, hypoglycorrhachia, and elevated protein. Blood cultures are usually positive in VA wound and shunt infection and may be positive with VP wound and shunt infection.

S. aureus is the most common agent of wound and shunt infection, but enteric and nonenteric gram-negative bacteria are also isolated. Coagulase-negative staphylococci and other skin flora are often isolated in mixed infection, which is common in wound and shunt infection.

Table 2 Outcomes of Various Methods of Treatment of Shunt Infection*

THERAPY	CURE RATE (%)		
	RANGE	MEDIAN	MEAN
Antibiotics† alone, shunt not revised or removed	10-52	30	30
Antibiotics plus partial shunt removal	39-75	44	53
Antibiotics plus immediate shunt replacement‡	48-100	88	78
Antibiotics plus delayed shunt replacement§	95-100	100	98

*Combined results of several studies.
†Systemic, with or without intraventricular antibiotics.
‡VA shunts in most cases.
§VP shunts exteriorized in most instances.

Surgical Therapy

The patient with wound and shunt infection is often acutely ill, with significant toxicity and CNS symptoms. Accordingly, early and aggressive therapy may be life-saving. Almost always the shunt must be completely removed immediately to allow for effective treatment of the wound and central nervous system infection. A new external ventricular drainage catheter should be inserted so that intraventricular antibiotics can be administered and ventricular pressure monitored. When the wound infection has healed and when CSF cultures are sterile, a new shunt can be placed on the opposite side.

Distal Infection

Distal shunt infection with peritonitis should be suspected in any patient with a VP shunt who presents with abdominal symptoms or signs. The patient usually has acute or chronic symptoms simulating appendicitis, cholecystitis, perforated viscus, or other intraabdominal pathology. Manifestations of shunt malfunction are uncommon, fever usually is low grade, and symptoms of central nervous system infection are uncommon. The diagnosis is often discovered at the time of exploratory laparotomy. Most cases develop within 2 months of surgery, but onset can occur many months to over a year later. The postulated routes of distal infection include introduction at surgery, perforation of the bowel by the shunt, and translocation of bacteria across the intact bowel wall.

Laboratory Features

CSF parameters may be normal, but there is often some degree of pleocytosis, with normal to slightly decreased glucose and normal to minimally elevated protein. Blood cultures usually are sterile and shunt reservoir CSF is often culture positive. The diagnosis should be suspected even when shunt reservoir CSF parameters are normal and cultures are sterile. The causative agent is sometimes isolated only from distal shunt CSF or the exteriorized distal shunt tip.

Mixed infection is the rule in distal shunt infection with peritonitis. Gram-negative enteric bacteria predominate,

Table 3 Dosages of Parenteral Antibiotics for Shunt Infection

ANTIBIOTIC	DOSE (mg/kg/day)	ROUTE	INTERVAL (hr)	ADULT DOSE (g/day)
Nafcillin	150-200	IV	6	10-12
Vancomycin	40-60	IV	6-8	2-4
Rifampin	15-20	IV or PO	12-24	0.6
Cefotaxime	150-200	IV	6-8	10-12
Ceftazidime	150-200	IV	8	6-8

but coagulase-negative staphylococci, *S. aureus,* other skin flora organisms, and nonenteric gram-negative bacteria are also isolated.

Surgical Therapy

Optimal treatment includes exteriorization of the distal shunt tubing along with administration of systemic and intrashunt antibiotics. Ventricular pressure is controlled via use of the shunt for CSF drainage. The shunt usually is replaced on the opposite side when shunt reservoir CSF cultures are sterile. As in the case of colonization, there have been reports of success with replacement of only the distal catheter, but the relapse rate is higher than with total replacement.

Bacterial Meningitis

Central nervous system infection with the usual meningitis pathogens of childhood (*H. influenzae, S. pneumoniae, N. meningitidis,* and the group B streptococci) occurs in children with CSF shunts at the same or a greater rate than in normal children. Presenting symptoms are those of bacterial meningitis, and shunt infection is incidental. CSF and blood cultures usually are positive, and CSF findings are typical for bacterial meningitis. Treatment with systemic antibiotics appropriate for the agent is usually sufficient to cure the shunt infection. Intrashunt antibiotics are seldom necessary, and the shunt usually does not require replacement unless there is associated malfunction.

■ ANTIMICROBIAL THERAPY

Antimicrobial therapy of shunt infection (Table 3) is based on accurate identification of the causative agents and careful determination of antibiotic susceptibility. Direct administration of intraventricular (intrashunt) antibiotic (Table 4) is often necessary because of poor penetration of the blood-brain barrier by many systemically administered antimicrobial agents, especially in the absence of significant meningeal inflammation.

Shunt infection caused by methicillin-susceptible *S. aureus* and coagulase-negative staphylococci can be effectively treated with high-dose parenteral antistaphylococcal penicillins combined with intraventricular antibiotic therapy. Penicillins and cephalosporins have been used successfully for intraventricular therapy, but in recent years, vancomycin is preferred by most clinicians. Because of highly variable pharmacokinetics, it is necessary to monitor CSF vancomycin levels when this drug is used for intraventricular therapy.

Table 4 Intraventricular Doses of Antibiotics for Shunt Infection

ANTIBIOTIC	DOSE (mg)*
Gentamicin	2-4
Tobramycin	2-4
Amikacin	5
Vancomycin	5-10

*Dilute in preservative-free saline.

An initial dose of 5 to 10 mg diluted in perservative-free saline is used by most investigators. Trough levels should be maintained above the minimum inhibitory concentration of the infecting organism; acceptable levels are 5 to 10 μg/ml. These levels usually can be maintained by administering intraventricular vancomycin every 24 to 72 hours.

In the case of shunt infection caused by methicillin-resistant *S. aureus* or coagulase-negative staphylococcus, parenteral and intrashunt vancomycin is the mainstay of therapy. Rifampin is added by many clinicians, both in this situation and in the treatment of methicillin-susceptible staphylococcal infection.

Intraventricular vancomycin in combination with oral rifampin and trimethoprim-sulfamethoxazole has been used with success by some investigators in the treatment of staphylococcal shunt infection.

Shunt infections caused by enteric and nonenteric gram-negative bacteria usually can be successfully treated with a combination of parenteral broad-spectrum penicillin or third-generation cephalosporin along with an intraventricular aminoglycoside. As with vancomycin, intraventricular aminoglycoside therapy must be monitored by obtaining CSF levels. The appropriate initial dose of gentamicin and tobramycin is 2 to 4 mg, and for amikacin it is 5 mg. Intraventricular gentamicin has been associated with some toxicity, and CSF levels of aminoglycosides should probably not exceed acceptable peak blood levels.

Nonstaphylococcal gram-positive shunt infections can be effectively treated with a combination of a parenteral penicillin or cephalosporin and intraventricular vancomycin or aminoglycoside. Treatment of anaerobic shunt infection is based on the specific organism and results of susceptibility studies; combined parenteral and intraventricular therapy is almost always required.

The appropriate duration of antimicrobial treatment for shunt infection is arbitrary but is determined to a great extent by the goal of therapy. When the goal is sterilization of the shunt without replacement or with only partial replacement, treatment is prolonged (14 to 21 days). I only occasionally use this approach, but when it is used, I continue parenteral and intraventricular therapy until I have five consecutive negative shunt reservoir CSF cultures, the last being negative for 48 hours before discontinuing therapy. When the goal of therapy is control of infection before total replacement, I continue parenteral and intraventricular therapy until the shunt reservoir CSF culture is negative for at least 48 hours and then replace the shunt on the opposite side, continuing parenteral therapy for several days after surgery.

In the occasional patient with persistently positive reservoir CSF cultures or symptomatic ventriculitis despite adequate antibiotic therapy, it may be necessary to remove the shunt to cure the infection. In this case, a new external drainage catheter is inserted for control of CSF pressure and administration of intraventricular antibiotic.

■ PREVENTION

The efficacy of antibiotic prophylaxis in the prevention of surgery-related shunt infection remains controversial. A meta-analysis of 12 adequately controlled clinical trials identified only one individual study favoring prophylaxis (trimethoprim-sulfamethoxazole). However, in the aggregate, prophylactic antibiotics were associated with significant reduction in these infections. A wide variety of antimicrobial agents, primarily antistaphyloccal penicillins, were used in these studies.

Suggested Reading

Bisno A: Infections of central nervous system shunts. In: *Infections associated with indwelling medical devices*, Washington DC, 1989, American Society for Microbiology.

Gardner P, Leipzig T, Phillips P: Infections of central nervous system shunts, *Med Clin North Am* 69:297, 1985.

Hirsch BE, et al: Instillation of vancomycin into a cerebrospinal fluid reservoir to clear infection: pharmacokinetic considerations, *J Infect Dis* 163:197, 1991.

Kestle JRW, et al: A concerted effort to prevent shunt infection, *Childs Nerv Syst* 9:163, 1993.

Langley JM, et al: Efficacy of antimicrobial prophylaxis in placement of cerebrospinal fluid shunts: metaanalysis, *Clin Infect Dis* 17:98, 1993.

Pople IK, Bayston R, Hayward RD: Infection of cerebrospinal fluid shunts: a study of etiological factors, *J Neurosurg* 77:29, 1992.

Venes JL: Infections of CSF shunt and intracranial pressure monitoring devices, *Infect Dis Clin North Am* 3:289, 1989.

Younger JJ, Barrett FF: Infections of central-nervous-system shunts. In Schlossberg D, ed: *Infections of the nervous system*, New York, 1990, Springer-Verlag.

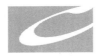

ENVIRONMENTAL RISKS AND CLUES

FEVER IN THE RETURNING TRAVELER

Martin S. Wolfe

A common problem of travelers, either on the trip or after they return, is a febrile illness, usually caused by infection. Fever in a traveler is often caused by disease not specifically related to travel and just as likely to occur at home. These include, among others, such cosmopolitan causes as common cold, influenza, tonsillitis, pyelonephritis, and bacterial or mycoplasmal pneumonia. However, the subject of this chapter is more exotic diseases acquired in developing countries. With the great increase in volume and speed of travel between developed and developing countries, physicians in the United States and other developed countries are seeing more patients with exotic tropical infections. Some of these infections are widespread in developing countries, and others are limited to small areas. Thus a knowledge of geographic distribution may be essential to the correct diagnosis.

The most common tropical fevers in travelers are malaria, enteric fever, hepatitis, amoebic liver abscess, and rickettsial and arboviral infections.

■ MALARIA

A febrile traveler returning from an area of endemic malaria must first and foremost be evaluated for malaria. Most malarial infections occur in travelers who have had inappropriate, irregular, or no chemoprophylaxis. However, all febrile travelers from a malarious area must be examined for malaria because no chemoprophylactic regimen can be considered fully protective. Potentially lethal falciparum malaria usually occurs within 4 weeks after leaving a malarious area. *Plasmodium vivax* and *Plasmodium ovale* malaria may occur up to 3 years after exposure if primaquine has not been taken to eliminate persistent latent parasites in the liver. *Plasmodium malariae,* which does not have a latent liver phase, is the least common species seen in travelers. Typical symptoms are high fever, shaking, chills, sweats, headache, and myalgias. Symptoms may be modified or masked according to the immune status, as in an immune native of an endemic area, or by the use of prophylactic antimalarial drugs. Severe *Plasmodium falciparum* infections can rapidly lead to such lethal complications as cerebral malaria, renal failure, severe hemolysis, and adult respiratory distress syndrome.

Diagnosis is by appropriately prepared and carefully examined Giemsa-stained thin and thick malaria smears. A single negative set of smears cannot rule out malaria; smears should be repeated at 6-hour intervals for at least 24 hours. Specific therapy for malaria is discussed in the chapter *Malaria.*

■ ENTERIC FEVER

Typhoid and paratyphoid fevers can be contracted from contaminated food or water where the prevalence of these bacteria is high. Typhoid vaccines offer protection to no more than 70% of recipients. Enteric fever should be suspected in travelers returning from an endemic area with fever, headaches, abdominal pain, diarrhea, or cough. Symptoms may not develop until several weeks after return. Diagnosis is confirmed by positive blood, stool, or urine culture. Febrile agglutinin (Widal) tests may be useful. *Salmonella typhi* organisms worldwide have developed multiple antibiotic resistance, and a quinoline is the drug of choice. See the chapter *Salmonella* for specific therapy details.

■ HEPATITIS

Travelers to the developing world who have not received immunoglobulin or hepatitis A vaccine run a significant risk of contracting hepatitis A from contaminated water or food. Rare cases of hepatitis E have been contracted in South Asia and elsewhere, and this type of hepatitis may not be prevented by immunoglobulin. Hepatitis B is usually contracted from sexual contact and is uncommon in travelers. In the preicteric phase of acute hepatitis, fever, chills, myalgias, and fatigue may occur, and this syndrome can mimic malaria and other acute tropical fevers. Hepatitis serologic testing can confirm infection, but when these tests are negative in a patient with apparent hepatitis, cytomegalovirus or mononucleosis infection should be considered.

■ AMOEBIC LIVER ABSCESS

A period of acute diarrhea often precedes development of an amoebic liver abscess. A returned traveler with fever and right upper quadrant pain should be suspected of this infection. Sonography or computed tomography (CT) of the liver will show a filling defect, and an amoebic serology test will confirm infection. Needle aspiration is seldom required for diagnosis or treatment. There is very rapid clinical response to metronidazole, 750 mg three times daily for 10 days, followed by a luminal drug such as paromomycin (Humatin), 500 mg three times daily for 7 days.

RICKETTSIAL INFECTIONS

Tick typhus can be contracted in West, East, and South Africa and in the Mediterranean littoral. Infection typically begins with a skin eschar at the tick-bite site, fever, chills, and headache, and in a few days, a diffuse papular rash can develop. Epidemic, scrub, and murine typhus and Q fever are much less commonly contracted by travelers. The Weil-Felix agglutination battery can be used for initial screening, and confirmation can be obtained from indirect fluorescent antibody tests for specific rickettsial organisms. Tetracycline is highly effective and response is generally rapid. A single 200-mg dose of doxycycline may be adequate, but 100 mg twice a day for 5 to 7 days may be required for some *Rickettsia* species.

VIRAL FEVERS

Dengue fever, endemic in most parts of the tropical world, is the most commonly imported arbovirus infection. Symptoms include fever, headache, body ache, and eye pain. Typically, a diffuse rash appears on the third to fifth day as other symptoms abate. Japanese B encephalitis is a rare infection of travelers to rural areas of the Far East. A number of other rarer acute viral illnesses have been imported from endemic areas, including lethal Lassa and Marburg fever viruses from West and Central Africa. Diagnosis is usually confirmed serologically, and treatment is generally supportive.

LESS COMMON FEBRILE ILLNESSES IN TRAVELERS

African trypanosomiasis was contracted by 15 American travelers from 1967 to 1987. Although the risk is low, even short-term travelers to game parks of East and Central Africa should take precautions against tsetse fly bites. Travelers should inform their physician of exposure history if symptoms such as trypanosomal chancre at a bite site, fever, evanescent rash, headache, and lethargy develop up to 4 weeks after returning home.

Tuberculosis remains a threat worldwide. Although travelers uncommonly are infected, any returnee with fever, cough, and chest radiography evidence suggestive of pulmonary disease should be evaluated for tuberculosis. Tuberculin skin testing before and after travel is best.

Brucellosis is contracted from contaminated raw goat or cow milk or soft cheese. Presentation can be with fever, chills, sweats, body aches, headache, monarticular arthritis, weight loss, fatigue, or depression. Diagnosis is by blood culture and/or specific agglutination tests. Treatment is with a tetracycline plus streptomycin or gentamicin.

Leptospirosis is common in the tropics but is rarely contracted by travelers. Infection is acquired through direct or indirect contact with infected animals. Most infections are anicteric and mild. Initial symptoms may include high remittent fever, chills, headache, myalgias, nausea, and vomiting. No more than 10% of patients develop jaundice. Diagnosis is usually made with serology. Early therapy with penicillin or tetracycline is usually beneficial.

Histoplasmosis, a cosmopolitan disease, has rarely infected travelers to Latin America. Visitors to caves contaminated with bat droppings are at particular risk. Consideration should be given to histoplasmosis in a returned traveler with pulmonary, or less likely, disseminated disease. Ketoconazole or itraconazole given for 3 to 6 weeks is effective treatment for acute symptomatic cases.

Visceral leishmaniasis (kala-azar) is extremely rare in American tourists, although European travelers have been infected around the Mediterranean littoral. Symptoms include fever, hepatosplenomegaly, and wasting. Diagnosis is confirmed by demonstrating leishmanial organisms in a biopsy specimen of liver, spleen, or bone marrow. Pentavalent antimonial compounds are the drug of choice for initial treatment.

Lyme disease occurs in Europe and the United States and may also be present in other parts of the world. Hikers in particular should take precaution against tick bites in any recognized endemic area.

Relapsing fever is caused by a spirochetal organism and occurs in a louseborne, primarily epidemic form and in a more widely scattered tickborne endemic form. The latter form is present in the western United States and has been diagnosed in returnees from that area to the eastern United States. Imported relapsing fever is uncommon, but cases have been contracted in West Africa, Spain, and Central America. Diagnosis is by finding the spirochetes in a thick or thin Giemsa-stained blood smear. Treatment is with a tetracycline.

Legionnaires' disease cases in travelers have continued to rise since 1995, and it is believed that travel-related cases are underestimated. Most cases (80%) are associated with travel within Europe. Diagnosis in suspected cases is made from culture, seroconversion, and urinary antigen detection. Initial treatment is with a macrolide or quinolone plus rifampin.

Melioidosis is endemic primarily in Southeast Asia and sporadically occurs in other areas. The majority of imported cases are seen in refugees from southeast Asia, in returned servicemen from that area, and occasionally in tourists. An asymptomatic form of infection is most common, but acute pneumonic and septicemic forms may occur. Chronic suppurative forms may also develop in various organs. These forms can lie dormant for many years and have the capacity to flare into acute fulminant symptoms. Any patient with a pneumonic process who is returning from rural areas of Southeast Asia should be considered to have possible melioidosis. Diagnosis is by special culture techniques or by serology. The most effective treatment is with ceftazidime.

Human immunodeficiency virus (HIV) infection is a particular hazard from sexual contact, blood transfusion, or contaminated needle or syringe contact in highly endemic areas of the tropical world. A number of disposable syringes and needles should be carried by the traveler who may need injection while traveling in areas where only nondisposable products are used. HIV serology screening should be done on any traveler with such exposure.

Most viral and bacterial causes of diarrhea, amebic dysentery, and occasionally *Giardia lamblia,* may also cause fever, which may precede diarrhea by some hours or days. Acute schistosomiasis, acute fascioliasis, and acute bancroftian filariasis are uncommon causes of fever in travelers.

Drugs used for prophylaxis or treatment of travel-related infections may themselves be a cause of fever. These include sulfonamide-containing drugs such as trimethoprim-sulfamethoxazole and pyrimethamine with sulfadoxine (Fansidar) (used for malaria treatment). Quinine and doxycycline may rarely cause fever. Drugs obtained abroad, often in combinations and without prescription, may cause a cryptic fever. It is worthwhile to stop all nonessential medications pending an etiologic diagnosis in febrile travelers.

Suggested Reading

Drugs for parasitic infections, *Med Lett Drugs Ther* 40:1, 1998.

Humar A, Keystone J: Evaluating fever in travellers returning from tropical countries, *BMJ* 312:953, 1996.

Liu LX, Weller PF: Approach to the febrile traveler returning from Southeast Asia and Oceania, *Curr Clin Top Infect Dis* 12:138, 1992.

Strickland GT: Fever in the returned traveler, *Med Clin North Am* 76:1375, 1992.

Wilson ME: *A world guide to infections,* New York, 1991, Oxford University Press.

Wyler DJ: Evaluation of cryptic fever in a traveler to Africa, *Curr Clin Top Infect Dis* 12:329, 1992.

SYSTEMIC INFECTION FROM ANIMALS

David J. Weber
William A. Rutala

More than 200 infectious diseases of animals can be transmitted to humans through bites and scratches, direct contact, aerosols, arthropod vectors, or contamination of food, water, or milk. Strictly speaking, *zoonoses* refer only to those diseases that are transmitted from vertebrate animals to humans. Contact with animals is frequent, even in urban centers. Pets are a major reservoir and source of zoonoses, especially for children. In 1996, 31.6% of households owned a dog, 27.3% owned a cat, and 4.6% owned a pet bird. The total number of animals owned was 52.9 million dogs, 59.1 million cats, and 12.6 million birds. Other common pets include fish, reptiles, rabbits, hamsters, gerbils, and mice. Leisure pursuits such as hunting, camping, and hiking, which are increasingly common, bring people into close contact with wild animals, arthropods, and sometimes contaminated water. Travelers to remote and rural areas may be exposed to diseases rarely acquired in the United States. Finally, occupational exposures to domestic animals or animal products may result in acquisition of a zoonosis. Individuals working with animals, such as livestock farmers, veterinarians, researchers, and handlers, are especially vulnerable through direct animal contact. Persons handling agricultural products, hides, and other products of animal origin are also at high risk for zoonotic diseases. It is important to remember that many of the occupations that bring persons into contact with animals (e.g., farming, fishing, animal control) also result in contact with environmental reservoirs of infectious agents.

■ CLINICAL APPROACH

Zoonoses are caused by a diverse group of microorganisms. Infectious syndromes caused by zoonotic pathogens are equally diverse. Hence, classification of zoonoses is difficult for the clinician. Diseases may be classified by the nature of the pathogen, animal host, mode of transmission from animal to human, geographic range of host, or clinical syndrome (i.e., systemic disease or specific organ system of infection). Although most zoonoses are relatively unusual, they must be included in the differential diagnosis of many clinical syndromes. All patients with an infectious syndrome whose cause is not apparent after a standard history and physical examination should be questioned to assess the possibility of a zoonosis. First, the clinician should question patients about exposure to pets and ask whether they own or have had recent contact with a dog, cat, bird, fish, reptile, or rodent. If contact may have occurred, the clinician should ask about a history of bites or scratches. Second, the patient should be asked about exposure to farm animals (which may also be pets) such as horses, pigs, cattle, and fowl (i.e., chickens and turkeys). The clinician should determine the amount and degree of exposure. Third, patients should be asked about leisure pursuits such as hunting, fishing, hiking, and camping. The clinician should assess specific animal contacts such as dressing or skinning animals, ingestion of water from streams and lakes, and bites by arthropods such as ticks (see also the chapter *Tickborne Disease*). Fourth, the clinician should obtain a careful travel history. Ascertaining whether a patient has had an animal bite or scratch while visiting an area endemic for rabies is particularly important. Because the incubation period for rabies may extend for years, persons bitten or scratched by dogs or other possible rabid hosts should be considered for postinjury prophylaxis. In general, evaluation for specific zoonoses should be based on the possibility of exposure (Table 1).

A brief description of the approach to possible systemic infections caused by animals is provided in subsequent paragraphs. More detailed information may be found in specific chapters in this book or in the references in the suggested reading at the end of this chapter.

■ GENERALIZED SYSTEMIC INFECTIONS

Many zoonoses cause severe systemic symptoms. The range of possible pathogens can often be narrowed if the patient manifests specific organ involvement. Diseases to consider in patients with fever without focal signs on initial history and physical examination include *Aeromonas* sepsis, babesiosis, brucellosis, *Capnocytophaga canimorsus* sepsis, ehrlichiosis, cat-scratch disease, leptospirosis, listeriosis, plague, Q fever, rat-bite fevers, relapsing fever, Rocky Mountain spotted fever (RMSF) and other rickettsial infections, salmonellosis, tularemia, and viral hemorrhagic fevers.

Zoonoses may be associated with skin lesions. A generalized maculopapular rash may occur with cat-scratch fever, Colorado tick fever, ehrlichiosis, leptospirosis, lymphocytic choriomeningitis, psittacosis, RMSF, and other rickettsial infections (exceptions include Q fever and trench fever), rat-bite fever resulting from *Spirillum minus,* relapsing fever, and salmonellosis. Most rashes associated with zoonoses are too nonspecific to be of significant clinical utility. Crepitant or gangrenous lesions may be associated with *Aeromonas, C. canimorsus,* or *Vibrio vulnificus* and related species. Petechial and purpuric lesions may occur with viral hemorrhagic fevers (e.g., dengue, yellow fever, Ebola, Lassa), RMSF, *Rickettsia prowazekii* infection, rat-bite fever resulting from *Streptobacillius moniliformis,* relapsing fever, and *C. canimorsus* sepsis. A local eschar often occurs with rickettsial infections due to *R. conorii, R. australis, R. sibirica, R. akari,* and *R. tsutsugamushi.* Local skin lesions with or without lymphangitis may occur with cat-scratch fever, rat-bite fever resulting from *S. minor,* and tularemia.

The rashes associated with RMSF and Lyme disease are highly characteristic and important to the diagnosis. The rash of RMSF typically appears between the third and fifth days of illness. However, it is absent in 5% to 15% of patients. Initially maculopapular, it begins on extremities, often around the wrist and ankles. As the rash progresses, it spreads centripetally to the trunk and characteristically involves the palms and/or soles. As it evolves, it becomes more clearly defined and more petechial and may rarely progress to skin necrosis or gangrene. The hallmark of Lyme disease is a characteristic skin lesion, erythema migrans, which often occurs at the site of the tick bite after 2 to 20 days. Erythema migrans is characteristically an expanding annular erythematous plaque with central clearing, most commonly seen in the axilla, thigh, and groin. Color varies from pink to violaceous. Erythema migrans may last up to 4 weeks and may recur during the secondary stage of infection.

■ SYSTEMIC INFECTIONS RESULTING FROM ANIMAL BITES

Dog bites account for 70% to 93% of animal bites, and cat bites account for 3% to 15%. Bites from wild animals constitute fewer than 1% of bite wounds. The infection rate from penetrating dog bites is approximately 5% to 15%. Cat bites are more likely to become infected. Approximately 1% of rodent bites become infected.

Although infections following animal bites may be caused by various flora, some generalizations can be made. The most common organism to cause infection following feline bites is *Pasteurella multocida* (see the chapter *Human and Animal Bites*).

The agents of rat-bite fever, *S. moniliformis* and *S. minor,* may be transmitted by several small rodents, including the rat, mouse, and gerbil. Both agents cause a systemic illness. Infections with *Aeromonas hydrophila* may follow bites inflicted in the water or by aquatic animals, such as snakes and alligators. Severe local infection progressing to crepitant cellulitis with systemic toxicity may occur. Although most cases of tularemia follow the handling of rabbits, infection may be transmitted by bites from other animals, including the cat, coyote, pig, and squirrel. *C. canimorsus* is an unusual systemic infection strongly associated with dog bites. More than 50% of patients have reported dog bites before clinical infection, although infection has also been reported following scratches from dogs, cat bites or scratches, and contact with wild animals. Approximately 80% of patients reported in the literature have a predisposing condition, most commonly splenectomy. Other predisposing conditions have included Hodgkin's disease, trauma, idiopathic thrombocytopenia purpura, alcohol abuse, steroid therapy, and chronic lung disease.

■ RESPIRATORY INFECTIONS

Zoonotic pneumonias are community acquired and are usually unaccompanied by expectorated sputum. Thus they are atypical pneumonias that may be mistaken for pneumonia caused by agents such as *Legionella* species, *Mycoplasma pneumoniae,* and *Chlamydia pneumoniae.* Zoonotic pneumonias that may be acquired at home include *P. multocida* (cats and dogs), Q fever (parturient cats), and psittacosis (birds). Hunting or hiking may bring people in contact with animals capable of transmitting Q fever, RMSF, tularemia, plaque, brucellosis, leptospirosis, psittacosis, and anthrax. Persons engaged in the processing of animal products are at risk for brucellosis and anthrax. The hantavirus pulmonary syndrome (HPS), a systemic illness characterized by fever, myalgias, and respiratory failure, results from inhalation of aerosols of excreta from infected rodents (see the chapter *Viral Hemorrhagic Fevers*).

Few zoonotic pneumonias are capable of being transmitted from person to person. However, nosocomial transmission of *M. bovis,* plague, psittacosis, and Q fever has been reported.

Table 1   Infectious Diseases Acquired from Animals

DISEASE	PERSONS AT RISK*	BIRDS, FOWL	CATS, DOGS	FARM ANIMALS	FISH, REPTILES,† WATER	RABBITS	RODENTS‡	ARTHROPOD VECTORS	WILD ANIMALS
VIRAL									
Bovine postular stomatitis	I, III			+					
California encephalitis	I, III, rural, public							+++	
Colorado tick fever	I, II							+++	
Eastern equine encephalitis	III, V, VI, public							+++	
Hantavirus pulmonary syndrome	I, III, public						+++		
B virus (*Herpesvirus simiae*)	IV, V								Macaca monkeys
Lymphocytic choriomeningitis	I, IV, V, public						+++		
Milker's nodule (pseudocowpox)	I, II			+					
Newcastle disease	I, II, IV, V	++							
Orf (contagious ecthyma)	I, II			+					
Powassan encephalitis	I, public							+++	
Rabies	III, VI, public		++	+					
Rotavirus	I, III, IV, public			++					
St. Louis encephalitis	I, public							+++	
Venezuelan encephalitis	II, III, IV							+++	
Western equine encephalitis	III, VI, public							+++	
Yellow fever	II							+++	+++
BACTERIAL									
Aeromonas	III, IV, VIII, public				+++				
Anthrax (wool sorter's disease)	I, II, IV			+++					
Brucellosis	I, II, III, V			+++					
Campylobacteriosis	I–IV	+	++		++		++		
Capnocytophaga canimorsus sepsis	III, IV, IX, public		+++						
Cat-scratch fever	III, IV, IX, public		+++						
Edwardsiella tarda infection	IV, VIII				++				
Ehrlichiosis	I, III, IV, VI, IX, public							+++	
Erysipeloid	I, II, III, VIII	++	+	+	++		++		
Leptospirosis	I–V	++	+	++	+		++		
Listeriosis	IX, public	+	+	+++		+			
Lyme disease	I, III, IV, VI, public							+++	+
Murine typhus	I, III, IV						(vector)	+++	
Mycobacteriosis (*M. marinum*)	VIII				+++				
Pasteurellosis	III, IV, public	+++	+++	+		++			
Plague	III, IV, V, VII						++		++
Plesiomonas infection	VIII				+++				
Psittacosis	I–VI	+++							

Disease	Persons at risk (groups)*
Q fever	I, II, V
Rat-bite fever	I, II, III
Relapsing fever	I, II, IV
Rocky Mountain spotted fever	I, III, IV, IX, public
Salmonellosis	I-IV, VIII, IX
Staphylococcus aureus infection	I, II, IV, IX
Group A streptococcal infection	I, II, IV, public
Tetanus	I-V
Tuberculosis	I, II, IV, V, IX
Tularemia	I, II, V
Vibriosis	III, VIII
Vibrio vulnificus infection	VIII, IX
Yersiniosis	I-V, VIII
FUNGI	
Ringworm	I-VI
PARASITES	
Babesiosis	III, IV, IX
Cryptosporidiosis	I-IV, VI, IX
Cystircercosis	public
Dipylidiasis	IV
Dirofilariasis	III
Echinococcosis	I
Giardiasis	I, III, IV
Toxocariasis	IV
Toxoplasmosis	IV, IX
Trichinosis	public

+, Rare source; ++, occasional source; +++, most-common source; *vector*, not spread directly by animal but always via vector.

*Persons at risk: Group I (*agriculture*), farmers and other people in close contact with livestock and their products; group II (*animal-product processing and manufacture*), all personnel of abattoirs and of plants processing animal products or by-products; group III (*forestry, outdoors*), persons frequenting wild habitats for professional or recreational reasons; group IV (*recreation*), persons in contact with pets or wild animals in the urban environment; group V (*clinics, laboratories*), health care personnel who attend patients and health care workers, including laboratory personnel, who handle specimens, corpses, or organs; group VI (*epidemiology*), public health professionals who do field research; group VII (*emergency*), public affected by catastrophes, refuges, or people temporarily living in crowded or highly stressful situations; group VIII (*fisherman*), people catching or cleaning fish or engaging in recreational activities in the water; group IX (*immunocompromised hosts*), people who are immunocompromised because of immunodeficiency, cancer chemotherapy, organ transplants, immunosuppressive medications, liver and/or renal disease.

†Reptiles include lizards, snakes, and turtles.
‡Rodents include hamsters, mice, and rats.

■ NEUROLOGIC SYNDROMES

Neurologic syndromes that may arise from zoonoses include encephalitis, meningitis, cranial nerve neuropathy, myelopathy, and peripheral neuropathy.

Encephalitis in the United States may result from infection with any of a variety of viral agents transmitted to humans by an insect vector from a vertebrate host. These diseases include California encephalitis (mosquitoes, small mammals), Colorado tick fever (tick, chipmunks, and squirrels), dengue (mosquitoes, humans), Eastern equine encephalitis (mosquitoes, birds), Powassan fever (ticks, medium-size rodents, and carnivores such as woodchucks, badgers, and foxes), St. Louis encephalitis (mosquitoes, unclear host), and Venezuelan equine encephalitis (mosquitoes, passerine birds).

Encephalitis may be the most predominant or the sole manifestation of toxoplasmosis, brucellosis, cat-scratch disease, listeriosis, leptospirosis, Lyme disease, relapsing fever, murine typhus, Q fever, rabies, RMSF, and psittacosis. Meningitis may also result from brucellosis, *C. canimorsus* infection, listeriosis, plague, salmonellosis, tularemia, leptospirosis, Lyme disease, relapsing fever, ehrlichiosis, Q fever, RMSF, psittacosis, and several of the arbovirus diseases.

Suggested Reading

Acha PN, Szyfres B: *Zoonoses and communicable diseases common to man and animals*, ed 2, Scientific Publication No. 503, Washington, DC, 1987, Pan American Health Organization.

Chomel BB: Zoonoses of house pets other than dogs, cats, and birds, *Pediatr Infect Dis* 11:479, 1992.

Elliot DL, et al: Pet-associated illness, *N Engl J Med* 313:985, 1985.

Goldstein EJC: Household pets and human infection, *Infect Dis Clin North Am* 5:117, 1991.

Mushatt DM, Hyslop NE: Neurologic aspects of North American zoonoses, *Infect Dis Clin North Am* 5:703, 1991.

Palmer SR, Soulsby L, Simpson DIH: *Zoonoses*, Oxford, 1998, Oxford University Press.

Weber DJ, Rutala WA: Zoonotic infections, *Occupation Med State Art Rev* 14:247, 1999.

Weinberg AN: Respiratory infections transmitted from animals, *Infect Dis Clin North Am* 5:649, 1991.

Weinberg AN, Weber DJ: Animal-associated human infections, *Infect Dis Clin North Am* 5:1, 1991.

TICK-BORNE DISEASE

J. Thomas Cross, Jr.
Richard. F. Jacobs

Exposure to ticks is an important part of the history of a patient with signs and symptoms of systemic infection. Important factors include tick activity in the area, season of the year, geographic distribution of ticks known to carry specific pathogens, site of exposure, and signs and symptoms at presentation in relationship to the time of exposure. Tests for the diagnosis of tick-borne infections are frequently inadequate. Therefore the physician must understand the epidemiology and symptoms of tickborne infections to make a quick and accurate diagnosis. A high index of suspicion is required for the diagnosis of many tickborne infections. Physicians must consider them during periods of high tick activity; however, cases occasionally are seen during winter. It is helpful to use epidemiologic data from local state health departments and publications such as the *Morbidity and Mortality Weekly Report* to evaluate the risk of tick-related infections.

An embedded tick found 3 days to 2 weeks before symptoms appear should alert the physician to the possibility of tick-related infections. The difficulty with determining the specific infection lies in the fact that most are initially nonspecific in presentation (Table 1). The nonspecific signs and symptoms of most tick-borne diseases include fever, malaise, and flulike symptoms. However, it is useful to consider specific categories of symptoms. For example, Lyme disease has the characteristic rash of erythema migrans, arthritis, and neurologic abnormalities with systemic manifestations. Rocky Mountain spotted fever (RMSF) may be manifested as a classic complex of headache, photophobia, petechial rash on the wrists and ankles, thrombocytopenia, and hyponatremia. The differential diagnosis of RMSF can be quite varied: ehrlichiosis, brucellosis, salmonellosis, Epstein-Barr virus, cytomegalovirus, enterovirus, and many others. It is often helpful to categorize tickborne infections according to the patient's history and presenting signs and symptoms (Table 2).

■ FEVER, HEADACHE, MYALGIAS (FLULIKE ILLNESS)

Infections associated with the triad of fever, headache, and myalgias, or more succinctly, flulike illnesses, include RMSF, other spotted fever rickettsiae, ehrlichiosis, tularemia, relapsing fever, Q fever, and Colorado tick fever. Usually, travel history or residence in an endemic area will suggest the diagnosis. If the fever is persistent with a biphasic or recurring pattern, Colorado tick fever or relapsing fever should be strongly considered. If pneumonia occurs with the triad of symptoms, tularemia, RMSF, and Q fever should be considered.

Table 1   Tick-Related Infections in the United States

DISEASE	ORGANISM	VECTOR	RESERVOIR	GEOGRAPHIC DISTRIBUTION	TYPE OF ILLNESS
Babesiosis	*Babesia microti*	*Ixodes scapularis*	*Peromyscus leucopus* (white-footed mouse)	Islands of Massachusetts, Rhode Island, New York	Malaria-like; fever, anemia, renal failure
Lyme disease	*Borrelia burgdorferi*	*Ixodes scapularis* *Ixodes pacificus*	Rodents, deer	Northeastern, midwestern, and western United States	Fever, erythema migrans, headache, myalgias; multiple stages
Tularemia	*Francisella tularensis*	*Ambylomma americanum,* *Dermacentor andersoni,* *D. variabilis*	Rabbits, dogs, rodents	Southern, southeastern, midwestern United States	Fever, lymphadenopathy, pneumonia
Rocky Mountain spotted fever (RMSF)	*Rickettsia rickettsii*	*Dermacentor variabilis,* *D. andersoni*	Dogs, cats, rodents	Southeastern United States western hemisphere	Fever, headache, rash, toxic appearance
Ehrlichiosis	*Ehrlichia chaffeensis*	*D. variabilis,* *A. americanum*	Dogs	South-centeral and south Atlantic United States	Fever, chills, hematologic abnormalities
	Human granulocytic ehrlichia agent	Same	Same	Northeast, midwestern United States	Fever, chills, hematologic abnormalities
Relapsing fever	*Borrelia hermsii,* *B. turicatae,* *B. parkeri*	*Ornithodoros hermsii, O. turicata, O. parkeri*	Rodents	Grand Canyon, western mountains United States	Fever, chills, relapsing course
Q fever	*Coxiella burnetii*	Inhalation of infected aerosols	Cattle, sheep, cats, ticks	Nova Scotia, Europe, Australia	Fever, headache, pneumonia
Colorado tick fever	Coltivirus	*Dermacentor andersoni*	Squirrels, rabbits, deer	Rocky Montain states	Fever, headache, leukopenia
Tick paralysis	Neurotoxin	*Dermacentor andersoni,* *D. variabilis,* *A. americanum,* *A. maculatum,* *I. scapularis*		Pacific Northwest, Rocky Mountain states	Ascending flaccid paralysis, ataxia

■ FEVER, RASH, MULTISYSTEM INVOLVEMENT

Tickborne infections often have nonspecific rashes that are not helpful in delineating the final diagnosis. However, typical rashes do occur with certain of these infections. RMSF can present 2 or 3 days after the tick bite as blanching erythematous macules on the wrists and ankles. The rash progresses rapidly to a maculopapular or petechial rash concentrated on the distal extremities, usually the palms and soles. The rash is frequently confused with meningococcemia, especially when it progresses to a confluent hemorrhagic infiltration with thrombotic disease similar to purpura fulminans. Lyme disease is classically diagnosed by its rash, erythema migrans. It occurs in about 50% of patients and is diagnostic for the disease; serology is not indicated because with early treatment, the serology will be negative. The classic lesion is an erythematous macule that expands over several days to weeks with a warm, raised, pruritic but usually painless character. In some patients the lesion has a central clearing. Patients will often develop multiple secondary lesions. Ehrlichiosis can cause a rash similar to that of RMSF, but generally it is spotless.

■ FEVER, ADENOPATHY

Tularemia is the classic tickborne disease associated with fever and adenopathy. The site of involvement is usually the neck in children and the groin in adults. This is thought to be related to the site of tick attachment. An ulcerative lesion at the tick-bite site with regional lymphadenopathy is characteristic of the ulceroglandular form of tularemia, the most common form of the disease. Lymphadenopathy has also been described with RMSF, Lyme disease, and ehrlichiosis.

Table 2 Presenting Signs and Symptoms in Tickborne Illnesses

FEVER, HEADACHE, MYALGIAS (FLULIKE ILLNESS)
Rocky Mountain spotted fever (RMSF)
Ehrlichiosis
Tularemia
Relapsing fever
Q fever
Colorado tick fever

FEVER, RASH, MULTISYSTEM INVOLVEMENT
RMSF
Lyme disease
Ehrlichiosis

FEVER, ADENOPATHY
Tularemia
Lyme disease
RMSF
Ehrlichiosis

FEVER, HEMATOLOGIC ABNORMALITIES
Babesiosis
Colorado tick fever
RMSF
Ehrlichiosis

FEVER, NEUROLOGIC MANIFESTATIONS
RMSF
Colorado tick fever
Tick paralysis
Lyme disease

■ FEVER, HEMATOLOGIC ABNORMALITIES

The hematologic manifestations of the tickborne diseases are the most interesting and yet poorly understood presentations. Babesiosis causes hemolytic anemia similar to that of malaria. The diagnosis in endemic areas is made on the organisms using thick and thin blood smears. Leukopenia is described in Colorado tick fever and RMSF. Thrombocytopenia is associated with RMSF and its classic early rash. Ehrlichiosis caused by *Ehrlichia chaffeensis* classically results in pancytopenia without a characteristic rash. It also can be diagnosed by observing the organisms (morulae) in peripheral blood smears or in bone marrow preparations.

■ FEVER, NEUROLOGIC MANIFESTATIONS

Neurologic manifestations in a febrile child with a history of exposure to ticks indicate RMSF, Colorado tick fever, tick-borne encephalitis, or tick paralysis. Lyme disease in its later stages has a high incidence of neurologic deficits, including aseptic meningitis, cranial neuritis, motor and sensory radiculitis, peripheral neuropathies, and myelitis. However, Bell's palsy can occur early in the illness and be the only manifestation of the disease.

■ EMPIRIC THERAPY

The diagnosis of tickborne infections is usually based on presumptive clinical findings at the time of diagnosis. Most specific tests are insensitive to early disease or require the physician to send tests out to a reference laboratory. Therefore empiric therapy is usually undertaken before a specific serologic confirmation is obtained. In these cases, acute serum should be sent for specific diagnostic testing and some saved for later studies if the initial findings are negative. Acute titers that are presumptively positive should be confirmed with convalescent titers. Empiric antibiotics are based upon the most likely diagnosis for the endemic area, the season, and the clinical manifestations of the illness. Tetracyclines are a logical choice in most tickborne infections. For children younger than 8 years of age chloramphenicol can also be used; however, its efficacy is poor or not well established in many tickborne infections (e.g., ehrlichiosis, Lyme disease, relapsing fever). Beta-lactam antibiotics are effective for Lyme disease but are ineffective for most other tickborne infections. For specific treatment and more detail about individual illnesses, see the specific chapters.

Suggested Reading

Cross JT, Jacobs RF: Tularemia: treatment failures with outpatient use of ceftriaxone, *Clin Infect Dis* 17:976, 1993.

Fishbein DB, Dawson JE, Robinson LE: Human ehrlichiosis in the United States, 1985 to 1990, *Ann Intern Med* 120:736, 1994.

Goodpasture HC, et al: Colorado tick fever: clinical, epidemiologic, and laboratory aspects of 228 cases in Colorado in 1973-1974, *Ann Intern Med* 88:303, 1978.

Horowitz HW, et al: Clinical and laboratory spectrum of culture-proven human granulocytic ehrlichiosis: comparison with culture-negative cases, *Clin Infect Dis* 27:1314, 1998.

Horton JM, Blaser MJ: The spectrum of relapsing fever in the Rocky Mountains, *Arch Intern Med* 145:871, 1985.

Jacobs RF, Schutze GE: Ehrlichiosis in children, *J Pediatr* 131:184, 1997.

Lyme disease—United States, 1991-92, *MMWR Morb Mortal Wkly Rep* 42:345, 1993.

Spach DH, et al: Tick-borne diseases in the United States, *N Engl J Med* 329:936, 1993.

Weber DJ, Walker DH: Rocky Mountain spotted fever, *Infect Dis Clin North Am* 5:19, 1991.

RECREATIONAL WATER EXPOSURE

Mary E. Wilson

Many common forms of recreation involve water exposure. Pathogens in water infect susceptible humans by multiple routes: through skin and mucous membranes, via inhalation of aerosols, aspiration, and ingestion. Clinical manifestations of these infections range from superficial skin lesions to fatal, systemic infections. The survival of many water-associated pathogens is influenced by climate, season, other environmental conditions, and the level of sanitation. The types and abundance of organisms vary depending on the salinity, pH, temperature, and other characteristics of the water. Hence, many are found only or primarily in certain geographic regions or during some seasons of the year.

Outbreaks of infections related to recreational water exposures are common. In the United States in 1995 to 1996, for example, 37 such outbreaks in 17 states were reported to the Centers for Disease Control and Prevention (CDC). More than 9000 persons were affected by these outbreaks. Cryptosporidiosis, giardiasis, *Escherichia coli* O157:H7 gastroenteritis, shigellosis, leptospirosis, and pseudomonas dermatitis have been the most commonly reported infections related to recreational water exposures in the United States in recent years. Outbreaks of adenovirus 3 (causing pharyngitis), cercarial dermatitis, hepatitis A (public swimming pool), and Norwalk virus–related diarrhea have also been reported. Chlorinated swimming pools, water parks, lakes, ponds, and whirlpools have been common sources. Outbreaks related to recreational water use are most common in the summer months.

Patients typically do not volunteer specific descriptions of water exposures because they may not recognize their relevance. Table 1 lists some of the kinds of water exposures that have been associated with infections and can be used as a checklist to help the clinician obtain relevant history. Most water-associated infections will become apparent within hours to days (usually <14 days) of exposure. An important exception is schistosomiasis, which may first become manifest months or longer after exposure. Relevant history includes types of exposures; dates, duration, and location of exposures; and type of water (e.g., mountain stream, lake, hot tub, chlorinated pool, salt water). During participation in water sports, people commonly ingest water and inhale aerosols.

Ingestion of contaminated water, whether during swimming, showering, or drinking, often causes infections manifested by diarrhea. Some pathogens have the capacity to cause systemic infection after ingestion. Fecally contaminated water may contain a potpourri of microbes—bacteria,

Table 1   Types of Activities Associated with Water Exposures

Swimming, wading, diving
Near-drowning events
Fishing, hunting
Rafting, boating, sailing, surfing, windsurfing, water-skiing
Water parks (wave pools and water slides)
Sitting in hot tubs, whirlpools
Showering and bathing
Drinking water and water-containing beverages (untreated surface water consumed during hiking, camping)
Care of fish tanks, aquariums

Table 2   Clinical Manifestations of Infections Related to Water Exposures

SKIN AND MUCOSAL SURFACE EXPOSURES
Conjunctivitis
Keratitis
Otitis externa
Dermatitis (including folliculitis)
Mastitis
Cellulitis
Fasciitis
Endometritis (reported after intercourse in water)
Systemic infection
ASPIRATION, INHALATION, INGESTION
Pharyngitis
Sinusitis
Meningoencephalitis
Pneumonitis
Gastroenteritis, colitis
Systemic infection

viruses, protozoa, and helminths—causing a variety of illnesses with differing manifestations and incubation periods. Swimming at beaches near a sewage outlet, for example, leads to increased rates of conjunctivitis, otitis externa, skin and soft-tissue infections, and gastrointestinal infections.

Water recreational activities are often group activities, so contaminated water may be associated with outbreaks, sometimes involving dozens or even hundreds of people. In addition to caring for the acutely ill patient, the clinician must consider the public health issues and alert the appropriate authorities. Early interventions may slow or halt an outbreak and allow early recognition of other cases. In many instances, outbreaks are the result of inadequate operation or maintenance procedures.

The route of entry may influence the clinical findings for several of the water-associated pathogens, with skin penetration causing local wound infections and ingestion causing diarrheal infections. Table 2 lists the range of clinical manifestations of infections that follow water exposure. With some of the more virulent organisms or in the setting of immune compromise, infection may enter the bloodstream after any one of several entry points. Minor trauma, cuts, bites, and breaks in the skin can provide the portal of entry for many water-dwelling microbes. Table 3 summarizes

Table 3   Infections and Infestations Acquired via Percutaneous and Permucosal Water Exposures

PATHOGEN OR DISEASE	SOURCE
BACTERIA	
Aeromonas hydrophila*+	Fresh water streams, lakes, soil
Burkholderia pseudomallei (melioidosis)*+	Fresh water, soil (tropics, subtropics)
Chromobacterium violaceum*+	Fresh water rivers, soil (tropics, subtropics)
Leptospirosis+	Fresh water contaminated with animal urine (especially in tropics, subtropics)
Mycobacterium marinum*	Fish tanks, swimming pools
Pseudomonas aeruginosa*	Hot tubs, whirlpools, swimming pools
Vibrio vulnificus, other vibrios*+	Seawater
Tularemia*+‡	Fresh water contaminated by infected animal; inoculation of skin, conjunctiva, oropharyngeal mucosa
HELMINTHS	
Schistosomiasis*+	Fresh water streams, lakes (focal in Asia, Africa, South America)
Cercarial dermatitis (nonhuman schistosomes)*	Fresh and salt water (worldwide)
PROTOZOA	
Acanthamoeba species (several cause keratitis)+‡	Fresh water, especially stagnant ponds, during hot summers; hot tubs, swimming pools, thermal springs
VIRUSES	
Adenoviruses (swimming pool conjunctivitis)‡	Swimming pools; probably other freshwater sites
Coxsackieviruses+‡	Fresh water
OTHER	
Swimmers itch*	Sea water

Note that *Pseudomonas* dermatitis and *M. marinum* may rarely be associated with systemic infection, primarily in compromised hosts.
*Skin and soft tissue.
+Systemic infection.
‡Conjunctivitis.

infections and infestations that enter through the skin. Table 4 lists specific infections acquired via aspiration, inhalation, and ingestion.

Several water-associated infections can be rapidly progressive or can lead to serious complications. Because some of these are infrequent or rare, they may be unfamiliar to most physicians. The following section provides a brief summary of each. More common infections, such as shigellosis, campylobacteriosis, salmonellosis, and *E. coli* O157:H7, which can be acquired through water exposure, are covered in more detail in other chapters of the book. Table 5 lists the recommended treatment for the less familiar water-associated infections.

■ PENETRATION THROUGH SKIN

Pseudomonas Dermatitis or Folliculitis
Use of hot tubs and whirlpools, and occasionally swimming pools and water slides, has been associated with development of a characteristic diffuse rash caused by *Pseudomonas aeruginosa.* The rash, which is maculopapular or vesiculopustular and usually itchy, develops within 48 hours of exposure and usually resolves within a week. Lesions are more prominent in areas covered by a bathing suit or clothing. Associated findings may include otitis externa, mastitis (in men and women), conjunctivitis, and lymphadenopathy. Infection is typically self-limited in healthy hosts; immunocompromised persons may develop hemorrhagic bullae, pneumonia, and bacteremia. Outbreaks can be large, involving hundreds of persons. Infections can be prevented

if water is maintained at a pH of 7.2 to 7.8 with adequate chlorination (free, residual chlorine levels should be in the range of 2.0 to 5.0 mg/L).

Otitis Externa (Swimmer's Ear)
Infection of the external ear canal, otitis externa, is common in swimmers. Usual symptoms are mild pain and itching around the ear. Pain may become more severe if infection progresses. Common organisms are *Staphylococcus aureus* and *P. aeruginosa;* multiple bacterial species are often recovered from cultures. Purulent drainage and local lymphadenopathy may develop. Occasionally, infections progress to cellulitis that requires systemic antibiotic therapy. Topical therapy can be effective in early infections. (See the chapter *Otitis Media and Externa* for treatment.)

Cercarial (Schistosome) Dermatitis
Cercarial dermatitis, also known as *swimmer's* or *clam digger's itch,* is caused by penetration of skin by cercariae of nonhuman schistosomes (often avian schistosomes). An itchy maculopapular rash develops in water-exposed areas of the body. Lesions appear hours to a day or more after water exposure and are often less prominent in areas covered by a bathing suit or other protective clothing. Papules may become vesicular. Secondary bacterial infection may result from scratching-related skin abrasions. Lesions peak in 2 to 3 days and typically resolve over 1 to 2 weeks without specific therapy. In persons with previous exposures, lesions may develop sooner and may be more severe. Treatment is symptomatic and may include antihistamines and topical steroids. Systemic steroids have been used in severe cases.

Table 4 Specific Infections Acquired via Inhalation, Aspiration, or Ingestion

DISEASE OR PATHOGEN	MAIN CLINICAL FINDING
Acanthamoeba (especially *Naegleria fowleri*)	Meningoencephalitis
Adenovirus 3	Pharyngitis, fever, conjunctivitis
Amebiasis (*Entamoeba histolytica*)	Colitis, liver abscess
Balantidiasis (*Balantidium coli*)	Diarrhea or dysentery
Campylobacteriosis	Diarrhea
Cholera (*Vibrio cholerae*)	Diarrhea, dehydration
Coxsackieviruses	Diarrhea
Cryptosporidiosis	Diarrhea
Cyclospora	Diarrhea
Escherichia coli O157	Bloody diarrhea
Giardiasis	Subacute diarrhea
Hepatitis A	Acute hepatitis
Hepatitis E	Acute hepatitis (can be fatal in pregnancy)
Legionnaires' disease	Pneumonia
Leptospirosis	Fever, protean manifestations; can be hemorrhagic
Melioidosis	Pneumonia, sepsis, skin lesions; protean manifestations
Norwalk virus	Diarrhea
Poliovirus	Nonspecific febrile illness; flaccid paralysis <1%
Pontiac fever	Fever
Primary amebic meningoencephalitis (see Acanthamoeba)	
Rotavirus	Diarrhea
Salmonellosis	Diarrhea; extraintestinal infection if bacteremic
Shigellosis	Diarrhea; dysentery
Toxoplasmosis	Fever, lymphadenopathy, lymphocytosis
Tularemia	Fever, lymphadenopathy, pneumonia
	Manifestations depend on route of transmission
Typhoid fever	Fever
Vibrio parahemolyticus	Watery diarrhea; occasionally dysentery
Vibrio vulnificus	Sepsis, bullous skin lesions
Yersinia enterocolitica	Fever, diarrhea, acute mesenteric lymphadenitis

Nonhuman schistosomes are widely distributed, including in temperate areas, and may contaminate fresh, brackish, and seawater.

Schistosomiasis

Penetration of the skin by human schistosomes (e.g., most often *Schistosoma mansoni, S. haematobium, S. japonicum*) may cause redness, urticaria, and itchy papules, typically less severe than the cercarial dermatitis described. Systemic manifestations of schistosomiasis may develop months or years later. Among 28 travelers who developed schistosomiasis after water exposures in Mali, 36% gave a history of schistosomal dermatitis. Infection can follow even brief water exposures, including river rafting. Attack rates have often been high in travelers who swim, wade, or bathe in infested water. An acute illness characterized by fever, malaise, and eosinophilia (Katayama fever) may develop 2 to 6 weeks after exposure. Neurologic complications (including transverse myelitis) can occur early or late. Clinical findings vary with the species of schistosome.

Seabather's Eruption (also Marine Dermatitis or Sea Lice)

Seabather's eruption is caused by penetration of the skin by *Linuche unguiculata, Edwardsiella lineata,* and other larvae of the phylum Cnidaria. Characteristic findings include an intensely itchy, papular rash that begins 4 to 24 hours after swimming in the ocean. The lesions are found in areas covered by a bathing suit and at points of contact (e.g., flexural areas, wristbands of diving suits). The tiny larvae are entrapped by the bathing suit, which acts as a mechanical stimulus for the release of nematocysts and injection of toxin by the larvae. Outbreaks are sporadic. Persons with extensive involvement may have systemic symptoms, including fever. Lesions usually clear within 10 days. Antihistamines and topical steroids may provide symptomatic relief. Systemic steroids have been used in severe cases.

Legionnaires' Disease

Several outbreaks have been traced to exposures in resort hotels and to whirlpools on cruise ships. Hence, this is an infection to consider in persons with febrile illness and pneumonia after travel. In 1994, an outbreak occurred in cruise ship passengers exposed to a contaminated whirlpool spa. Fifty cases were identified from nine cruises. In addition, several outbreaks of Pontiac fever have been traced to exposures in hot tubs or whirlpools. Pontiac fever results from the aerosolized antigens of *Legionella pneumophila.*

Vibrio Soft-Tissue Infections

Vibrio vulnificus, V. parahemolyticus, V. alginolyticus and other *Vibrio* species can cause soft-tissue infections. Organisms can be introduced by injuries (often on the lower extremity) that break the skin during swimming in the ocean or walking on beaches or can enter via preexisting open skin lesions. After trauma, *V. vulnificus* can cause pustular lesions, lymphangitis, and cellulitis, which may be mild or rapidly progressive, causing pain, myositis, skin necrosis, and gangrene. Surgical debridement (or amputation) in addition to antibiotic therapy and general support may be necessary.

Vibrio soft-tissue infections, including necrotizing fasciitis, can also follow ingestion of contaminated food (commonly raw shellfish). Gastroenteritis may be associated with high-grade bacteremia and high mortality. Large, bullous skin lesions may occur with primary vibrio bacteremia (especially *V. vulnificus*). Severe infections are more common in persons with chronic liver disease or other underlying diseases that compromise immune function.

Vibrios are found in seawater or brackish water and are part of the usual bacterial flora of coastal waters in the United States and elsewhere. They are more abundant in warmer months, and most reported infections occur in the

Table 5   Diagnosis and Treatment of Selected Infections

PATHOGEN/DISEASE	DIAGNOSIS*	TREATMENT
Aeromonas hydrophilia	C	TMP-SMX or FQ; third-generation cephalosporins; aminoglycosides; imipenem
Burkholderia pseudomallei	C	Ceftazidime (imipenem or meropenem; TMP-SMX)
Chromobacterium violaceum	C	Limited clinical data. May be sensitive to FQ, TMP-SMX, tetracyclines, aminoglycosides, extended-spectrum penicillins
Francisella tularensis (tularemia)	S, C	Streptomycin or gentamicin (tetracycline, ciprofloxacin; chloramphenicol)
Leptospirosis	S, C	Penicillin or a tetracycline
Mycobacterium marinum	C (at 30° C)	Minocycline or clarithromycin (TMP-SMX; rifampin plus ethambutol; doxycycline)
Primary amebic meningoencephalitis	Visualization of trophozoites in cerebrospinal fluid; C	Amphotericin IV and intrathecally
Schistosomiasis	Eggs in tissue, urine, or stool; S	Praziquantel
Vibrio vulnificus	C	Doxycycline, ceftazidime, or other tetracycline or ceftazidime (FQ)

TMP-SMX, Trimethoprim-sulfamethoxazole; *FQ,* fluoroquindone.
*Method of diagnosis: culture (C), serology (S).

summer. Many vibrios, in addition to *V. cholerae,* can cause diarrheal illness.

Treatment of soft-tissue and systemic infections following seawater exposure should include coverage for *Vibrio* species.

Aeromonas hydrophila

Aeromonas hydrophila is a non–spore-forming, motile, facultatively anaerobic gram-negative organism found in freshwater lakes, streams, and soil. Puncture wounds or soft-tissue injury in contaminated water may lead to cellulitis that can resemble acute streptococcal infection with lymphangitis and fever. If not treated with effective drugs, it can progress to bullae formation and necrotizing myositis with gas in soft tissues. Findings can mimic gas gangrene.

Ingestion of *Aeromonas* may cause diarrhea. Aspiration of *Aeromonas*-contaminated water may lead to *Aeromonas* pneumonia and bacteremia. Soft-tissue infections may require local debridement along with systemic antibiotic therapy.

Melioidosis (Burkholderia pseudomallei)

This water and soil-associated gram-negative organism found especially in tropical and subtropical areas is a common cause of pneumonia, skin lesions, and sepsis in parts of Southeast Asia. The organism can be acquired through minor skin wounds or via aspiration or ingestion. Infection can be acute, subacute, or chronic and has protean manifestations, including cavitary lung disease, splenic abscesses, and osteomyelitis. The organism can persist silently in the human host and reactivate decades after acquisition.

Acanthamoeba Infections, Including Primary Amebic Meningoencephalitis

Free-living amebae of the genus *Acanthamoeba,* found in soil and freshwater, can enter human tissues and cause local or disseminated infection. Several species of *Acanthamoeba*

have been reported to cause keratitis and granulomatous inflammation, which may be acute or subacute. Soft-tissue infections have also been reported. Minor trauma to the cornea, as may occur in persons who wear contact lenses, predisposes patients to infection. The diagnosis is confirmed by finding *Acanthamoeba* on biopsy, corneal scrapings, or culture. Treatment typically requires both debridement and topical therapy (several agents have been tried: combinations of miconazole nitrate, propamidine isethionate, and Neosporin; and propamidine isethionate and dibromopropamidine, among others).

Acanthamoeba species, usually *Naegleria fowleri,* cause primary amebic meningoencephalitis, typically in young healthy persons. Trophozoites enter the nose during swimming or diving, penetrate the cribriform plate, and invade via olfactory neuroepithelium, causing rapid destruction of gray and white matter. Symptoms usually begin 3 to 7 days after exposure to water. Infection causes high fever, headache, and stiff neck, resembling bacterial meningitis, and is usually fatal. Diagnosis is made by finding trophozoites in the cerebrospinal fluid (CSF) (wet mount, Giemsa staining after fixation, or by culture). Infections have followed exposures in lakes, rivers, stagnant ponds, thermal springs, canals, and hot tubs and are more common during very warm periods.

Chromobacterium violaceum

Chromobacterium violaceum is a gram-negative organism found in abundance in tropical and subtropical freshwater rivers and soils. The rarely reported infections have usually followed penetrating skin injury and are typically bacteremic. Persons with chronic granulomatous disease are at risk for severe infection.

Leptospirosis

Leptospirosis has caused outbreaks in swimmers (lake, creek, other fresh water), kayakers, and white-water rafters (e.g., in Costa Rica). Fresh water becomes contaminated with urine of infected domestic and wild animals. Humans become infected when organisms enter through skin, especially if abraded, or mucous membranes, or after ingestion of contaminated water or food. Infections are more common in tropical and subtropical areas and during warm seasons in temperate regions. In the United States, infections have been especially common in Hawaii. Patients have systemic infection with protean manifestations, sometimes including fever, meningitis, pneumonia, jaundice, and hemorrhage.

Mycobacterium marinum

Mycobacterium marinum usually invades only superficial tissue after local inoculation. Infection manifests as red plaques, papules, or nodules (sometimes with sporotrichoid spread). The infection is sometimes called *swimming pool granuloma* and *fish tank granuloma* because of the associations with fish and water. This subacute infection, most often on the hand or arm, can occur after exposure to fresh or salt water in aquariums and in swimming pools. Because the organism is relatively chlorine resistant, infection can follow exposures in chlorinated pools.

Tularemia

Tularemia, caused by *Francisella tularensis,* an organism that sometimes contaminates water (from an infected animal), can infect via multiple routes, including through conjunctivae, skin, and oropharynx and the gastrointestinal tract. Ticks and other arthropods can transmit infection. It is mentioned in this chapter because infection can be severe, even fatal, but does respond to appropriate therapy.

Giardiasis

Outbreaks of giardiasis have often been traced to ingesting unfiltered, unchlorinated, or inadequately chlorinated surface waters. Many infections in campers and hikers have followed drinking from mountain streams, even in remote wilderness areas.

Suggested Reading

Benenson AS, ed: *Control of communicable diseases manual,* ed 16, Washington, DC, 1995, American Public Health Association.

Levy DA, Bens MS, Craun GF: Surveillance for waterborne-disease outbreaks—United States, 1995-1996. In CDC surveillance summaries, December 11, 1998, *MMWR* 47(No. SS-5):1, 1998.

Schlossberg D: *Infections of leisure,* Herndon, VA, 1999, American Society of Microbiology.

Wilson ME: *A world guide to infections: diseases, distribution, diagnosis,* New York, 1991, Oxford University Press.

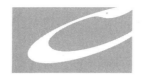

THE SUSCEPTIBLE HOST

EVALUATION OF SUSPECTED IMMUNODEFICIENCY

Thomas A. Fleisher

The need to evaluate immunologic function has become a part of the standard practice of clinical medicine, resulting at least in part from the worldwide pandemic of human immunodeficiency virus (HIV) infection. This chapter presents the general methods available to assess immune function and identifies when to apply them to the clinical situation.

The primary clinical problem that sets the stage for initiating an immunologic evaluation is a history of increased susceptibility to infection. In general, the characteristic features of the recurrent infections provide critical insights into the most likely level of immune dysfunction, serving as a critical guide to the evaluation of immune function.

Defects in lymphoid immunity involving antibody production (humoral immunity) lead to recurrent infections, usually involving the sinopulmonary tract, with high-grade encapsulated bacteria such as *Haemophilus influenzae* or *Streptococcus pneumoniae*. The normal humoral immune response consists of the production of antibodies directed at the capsular carbohydrate antigens present on these organisms, facilitating their elimination. In contrast, the clinical picture of patients with defective T-cell immunity typically consists of recurrent infections with opportunistic organisms, including *Pneumocystis carinii* and *Mycobacterium avium-intracellulare* (MAI). Clearly, functional T cells are required to prevent or clear infection with these intracellular organisms. Abnormalities in phagocytic cell (neutrophil) function, as well as significantly decreased numbers of these cells, result in recurrent cutaneous and deep-seated abscesses, pneumonias, periodontitis, osteomyelitis, and occasionally life-threatening sepsis. Typically, these infections involve bacteria such as *Staphylococcus aureus* and *Serratia marcesens* and fungi such as *Candida albicans* and *Nocardia*

and point to the critical role of mobile phagocytic cells in the normal host defense. Congenital defects in specific complement components can also be associated with recurrent infections, although in many cases, these are also linked to the development of autoimmune disease. Deficiency of the component C3 leads to repeated sinopulmonary infections similar to agammaglobulinemia, whereas deficiencies in the terminal complement components (C6, C7, C8, C9) result in recurrent systemic infections or meningitis with neisserial organisms.

Clinical suspicion of a defect in immune function is primarily generated through a medical history that identifies recurrent infection. Careful attention should be paid to the frequency and sites of infections, the types of organisms involved, and the therapy required. Any patient with a history of increased susceptibility to infection must also be carefully questioned about risk factors for HIV infection. In addition, a careful family history is also important because most defined primary immunodeficiencies are genetically linked. The physical examination can provide clues in the case of specific primary immunodeficiencies (e.g., typical facies in the hyper-lgE syndrome, scars from abscess drainage sites associated with neutrophil defects) and may also provide clues suggesting secondary immunodeficiencies (e.g., oral hairy leukoplakia or Kaposi's sarcoma in HIV infection).

■ EVALUATING B CELL FUNCTION (Table 1)

Clinical findings that suggest an abnormality in antibody production are recurrent or chronic bacterial infections involving the sinopulmonary tract. Gastrointestinal, hematologic, and autoimmune disorders may also be associated with antibody deficiencies.

The clinical screening of antibody-mediated immune function can be accomplished by measuring serum levels of the three major immunoglobulin classes: IgG, IgA, and IgM. The results must be compared with age-matched normal ranges, typically expressed as 95% confidence intervals. The serum immunoglobulin levels are the net of protein production, use, catabolism, and loss.

There are no rigid standards regarding the diagnosis of immunoglobulin deficiency, although an IgG value below 3 g/L (300 mg/dl) requires careful monitoring. When any

Table 1　Evaluation of Suspected Antibody (B-Cell) Immunodeficiency

SCREENING TESTS	SECONDARY TESTS
Quantitative immunoglobulins	B-cell enumeration
Specific antibody	In vitro B-cell function tests
Circulating specific	(primarily research)
antibodies	
Postimmunization	
antibodies	
Protein antigens	
Carbohydrate antigens	
IgG subclasses (± utility)	
HIV testing	

HIV, Human immunodeficiency virus.

Table 2　Evaluation of Suspected T-Cell Immunodeficiency

SCREENING TESTS	SECONDARY TESTS
HIV testing	T-cell enumeration
Lymphocyte count	T-cell proliferation (mitogen,
Delayed-type hypersensitivity	alloantigen, antigen)
skin tests	T-cell cytokine production
	Cytokine receptor generation

HIV, Human immunodeficiency virus.

degree of hypogammaglobulinemia is associated with significant recurrent bacterial infection, it suggests the need for replacement therapy with intravenous immunoglobulin.

Measurement of a functional antibody response is particularly useful when the total immunoglobulin levels are normal or only slightly depressed in the face of a history of recurrent sinopulmonary infection. The simplest method is evaluation for spontaneous antibodies (e.g., anti–blood group antibodies [isohemagglutinins], antibodies to prior immunizations). The definitive method involves immunizing and assessing preimmunization versus 3-week-post-immunization antibody levels using both protein antigens (e.g., tetanus toxoid) and polysaccharide antigens (e.g., Pneumovax). Guidelines for normal responses, which are usually provided by the testing laboratory, typically consist of at least a fourfold increase in antibody level to a protein antigen and at least a twofold increase and/or protective levels of antibody following exposure to a polysaccharide antigen.

Despite the preponderance of recurrent opportunistic infections resulting from HIV infection, appropriate testing to rule out this diagnosis should be considered even in the face of recurrent bacterial infection. This type of clinical presentation is particularly common among HIV-infected children. Special testing may be needed to rule out HIV infection in the setting of absent or diminished antibody production because the screening tests depend on detecting anti-HIV–specific antibodies (enzyme-linked immunosorbent assays [ELISA] and Western blot assays).

An additional and readily available test is quantitation of IgG subclass levels, which has particular utility in evaluating the IgA-deficient patient with significant recurrent bacterial infections. However, in most settings, detection of an IgG subclass deficiency still requires the demonstration of an abnormality in functional antibody production before therapy such as intravenous immunoglobulin is indicated.

The secondary tests of humoral immunity are generally performed in centers specializing in immune testing and fall into two general categories: evaluation of B-cell number and testing of in vitro B-cell function. The former assesses circulating cell numbers and is usually performed by flow cytometry comparing the results with age-matched controls. The latter involves studies directed at B-cell proliferation and in vitro immunoglobulin biosynthesis.

■ EVALUATING T-CELL FUNCTION (Table 2)

A clinical history of recurrent opportunistic infections strongly suggests an abnormality in T-cell function. Immunodeficiency of T cells is found most commonly accompanying HIV infection, and initial screening assays should always include testing for HIV infection. In addition, the absolute lymphocyte count (i.e., white blood cell count with differential) and cutaneous delayed-type hypersensitivity (DTH) response to recall antigens should be performed. The significance of the former relates to the fact that T cells normally constitute approximately three fourths of the circulating lymphocytes. The DTH response provides an in vivo window of T-cell function in response to previously encountered antigens. Failure to respond may reflect T-cell dysfunction (T-cell anergy), or it may indicate that the host has not been exposed (sensitized) to the test antigen. Consequently, it is prudent to use more than one antigen for DTH testing. Clinical correlates of a DTH response include the cutaneous response to poison ivy and other contact hypersensitivity reactions.

The screening tests for T-cell function are often followed by additional testing to complete the assessment of cellular immunity. This parallels that of B cells with quantitation of T cells by flow cytometry together with in vitro functional testing (e.g., proliferation assays, cytokine production, cytokine receptor generation). Recent data demonstrate that abnormalities of the interferon gamma receptor on monocytes may be associated with recurrent or persistent infections with *Mycobacterium avium* complex organisms. This new information establishes a molecular basis for a more limited form of immunodeficiency manifested as recurrent or chronic infection with a specific organism despite conventional, multiagent, antimicrobial therapy. Thus specific defects in the inflammatory response can also produce a more limited form of immune deficiency.

■ EVALUATING NATURAL KILLER CELL FUNCTION

The third arm of the lymphoid system consists of circulating cells distinct from B and T cells, the natural killer (NK) cells. Deficiency in NK-cell function has been described in one patient with recurrent herpes infections. In addition, experimental models point to a role for the NK cell in allograft and tumor rejection. Testing of NK cells includes quantitating the cells by flow cytometry and assaying killing activity with standard in vitro assays.

Table 3 Evaluation of Suspected Neutrophil Deficiency

SCREENING TESTS	SECONDARY TESTS
Multiple neutrophil counts	CD11, CD18 assessment
Review neutrophil	Respiratory burst assessment
morphology	Nitroblue tetrazolium test
	Flow cytometric test
	Specific enzyme testing
	Chemotaxis evaluation
	Rebuck skin window
	In vitro chemotaxis
	Boyden chamber
	Soft agar assay

■ EVALUATING NEUTROPHIL FUNCTION (Table 3)

The clinical features of neutrophil dysfunction usually include recurrent bacterial and fungal infections of the skin, periodontal tissue, lymph node, lung, liver, and bone. This clinical presentation is most commonly observed with neutropenia resulting from decreased production, altered localization, or increased destruction of the neutrophil. In addition, some primary and secondary abnormalities of neutrophil function also demonstrate patterns of increased susceptibility to infections.

The clinical pattern of infection often can help to discriminate the underlying problem. Patients with neutropenia and those with the leukocyte adhesion deficiency (LAD) tend to have recurrent cellulitis, periodontal disease, otitis media, pneumonia, and rectal or gastrointestinal abscesses. Although LAD is accompanied by a persistent granulocytosis, there is in effect a tissue neutropenia because of the underlying defect that renders the granulocytes incapable of moving to sites of infection. In contrast, patients with chronic granulomatous disease (CGD) have significant problems with liver and bone abscesses as well as pneumonias. Furthermore, they tend to have less difficulty with cellulitis or otitis media and lower frequency of beta-strep and *Escherichia coli* infections than patients with neutropenia.

Screening studies directed at the evaluation of neutrophil function should start with the leukocyte count, differential, and cell morphology. If neutropenia and morphologic abnormalities are ruled out, the evaluation should be directed at assays that provide functional information about neutrophils. Included are the flow cytometric assessment of the neutrophil adhesion molecules, CD11 and CD18, on the cell surface, which are absent or depressed in LAD patients. The neutrophil oxidative burst pathway can be screened using either the nitroblue tetrazolium test (NBT) or a flow cytometric assay, both of which are abnormal in patients with CGD. Finally, evaluation of neutrophil-directed movement (chemotaxis) can be performed in vivo using the Rebuck skin window technique as well as in vitro with a Boyden chamber or a soft agar system. Abnormalities of chemotaxis have been observed secondary to certain pharmacologic agents as well as the leukocyte adhesion deficiency, Chediak Higashi syndrome, Pelger-Huet anomaly, and juvenile periodontitis. A hallmark clinical feature of significantly abnor-

Table 4 Evaluation of Suspected Complement Abnormality

SCREENING TEST	SECONDARY TESTS
CH50	Component immunoassays
	Component functional assays

mal chemotaxis is diminished neutrophil infiltration with decreased inflammation at sites of infection.

Functional testing of neutrophils has its greatest yield when evaluating patients with recurrent infections associated with a genetic neutrophil abnormality. Many patients with histories of recurrent cutaneous abscesses fail to demonstrate abnormalities in the aforementioned tests. This likely is related to the very specific measurement provided by certain tests and the relative insensitivity of the other tests in discerning mild functional abnormalities.

■ EVALUATING THE COMPLEMENT SYSTEM (Table 4)

The clinical features of complement deficiencies vary, with many early component defects being associated with autoimmune disease and C3 deficiency with both glomerulonephritis and recurrent bacterial sinopulmonary infection. Deficiencies of the membrane attack complex (C6, C7, C8, C9) result in increased susceptibility to neisserial infections.

The best screening test for the classical complement pathway is the total hemolytic complement activity (CH50) assay. Assuming correct handling of the serum sample (because of the lability of the complement system), a markedly depressed CH50 result strongly suggests a complement component deficiency. This can be followed with selected component immunoassays that are available in larger laboratories, and component functional testing that is available only in specialized complement laboratories.

■ RECOMMENDATIONS

The clinical pattern of recurrent infections remains the single most useful clue in determining the likelihood of immune deficiency and identifying the best approach for evaluation. HIV infection has become the most likely cause of immune deficiency, and appropriate diagnostic testing for HIV is critical, particularly in the setting of recurrent opportunistic infection. When the history identifies repeated bacterial infections involving the sinopulmonary tract, abnormalities in antibody production and C3 deficiency (extremely rare) should be considered. Opportunistic infections suggest T-cell dysfunction, and bacterial and fungal infections of the skin, lungs, and bone strongly suggest decreased neutrophil numbers or defective neutrophil function. All of these possibilities must be tempered by the fact that the range of infections between normal individuals can vary significantly, and the line distinguishing normal from abnormal is not always clear. More limited immune dysfunction with recurrent MAI has been recognized, and in some patients, this results from defects in the interferon gamma receptor. Other similar patients have undefined defects, and it is likely that other, more limited, immune disorders presenting with recurrent infections will be characterized in the future. The definition of these may prove valuable in devising novel approaches to the therapy of serious and persistent infections.

Laboratory studies are essential for evaluating the status of immune function. However, the optimal use of these tests requires that they be used in an orderly fashion, starting with the simpler screening tests chosen based on the clinical clues provided by the history and physical examination. Furthermore, the results of these tests are relatively easy to interpret when they are either clearly normal or absolutely abnormal. The difficulty arises in determining the actual degree of immune dysfunction when the results fall in an intermediate range. To address this, prudent use of a combination of tests often clarifies the status of immune function or dysfunction.

Suggested Reading

Figueroa JE, Densen P: Infectious diseases associated with complement deficiencies, *Clin Microbiol Rev* 4:359, 1991.

Fleisher TA, Tomar R: Introduction to diagnostic laboratory immunology, *JAMA* 278:1823, 1997.

Frank MM: Detection of complement in relation to disease, *J Allergy Clin Immunol* 89:641, 1992.

Holland SM, Gallin JI: Evaluation of the patient with recurrent bacterial infections, *Ann Rev Med* 49:185, 1998.

Lehrer RI, et al: Neutrophils and host defense, *Ann Intern Med* 109:127, 1988.

Primary immunodeficiency diseases: report of a WHO scientific-group, *Clin Exp Immunol* 109(suppl 1):1, 1997.

Shearer WT, et al: Laboratory assessment of immune deficiency disorders, *Immunol Allergy Clin North Am* 14:265, 1994.

INFECTION IN THE NEUTROPENIC PATIENT

Clarence B. Sarkodee-Adoo
William G. Merz
James D. Dick
Judith E. Karp

> **Table 1** Principles of Empiric Antibiotic Therapy During Finite Chemotherapy-Induced Neutropenia
>
> Recognition of commonly occurring pathogens, commonly infected sites, link between specific pathogens and specific sites, drug- and/or tumor-related barrier breakdown
> Broad coverage directed against the most common pathogenic organisms arising in the specific clinical setting and at the specific timing during intensive chemotherapy
> Prevention of development of multiply resistant organisms
> Hold the fort until the underlying lesion is corrected by the return of neutrophils

Various cellular and humoral surveillance mechanisms protect the host from overwhelming infections by microorganisms. Although humoral mechanisms neutralize and prepare microbes for eventual destruction, the final arbiter of microbial eradication is the phagocytic cell with microbicidal capabilities. It is not surprising, therefore, that the severely granulocytopenic (or neutropenic) host has highly compromised ability to contain infectious pathogens, even those of the normal flora. Furthermore, the risk is directly proportional to the depth and duration of neutropenia.

Nowhere is the critical role of the granulocyte in host surveillance so clearly demonstrable as in patients with acute leukemia with resultant profound bone marrow failure. The lessons learned from these patients have contributed in a major way to the ability to design and deliver curative therapies not only to leukemia patients but also to patients with other types of malignancies as well. Indeed, the principles guiding empiric antibiotic therapy for fever and infection in the neutropenic host have remained constant since they were formulated more than two decades ago (Table 1). In such patients, the absence or impairment of a localizing inflammatory response resulting from neutropenia plus the lack of rapid diagnostic tests to identify causative organisms necessitate the prompt empiric implementation of broad-spectrum antibiotics against potential pathogens.

Today, there are new options thanks to advances in several major areas: an expanding armamentarium of both broad and targeted coverage, an increasing capacity to define the specific drug susceptibility profiles of diverse organisms, the advent of hematopoietic and immune system biomodulators, and innovative methods of drug delivery. Counterbalancing this progress is the continuing emergence of resistant microbes, which require new agents with novel mechanisms implemented in innovative approaches. In addition, the current health care climate places greater-than-ever economic pressures on the delivery of care to patients with febrile neutropenia.

■ ANTIBACTERIAL APPROACHES

Gram-Negative Infections

Gram-negative (GN) bacterial infections arising from the gastrointestinal (GI) tract have been a major cause of morbidity and mortality in persons with neutropenia. Mucosal destruction from cytotoxic drugs permits dissemination of the indigenous bacterial flora, in particular *Escherichia coli, Klebsiella* species, and *Pseudomonas aeruginosa*. Life-threatening infections by these bacteria early in the course of profound cytotoxic drug-induced marrow aplasia led to the concept of oral GI prophylaxis to prevent early-onset GI-based infection and inhibit late-onset GI colonization with drug-resistant pathogens. Initial studies were limited by host intolerance and emergence of resistant bacteria. More recently, the oral fluoroquinolones have been shown to provide broad-spectrum activity against aerobic GN pathogens, including *P. aeruginosa*. Their mechanism of action, inhibition of bacterial DNA gyrase, may prevent acquisition of plasmid-mediated resistance to other agents. Randomized, controlled trials involving adult leukemia and bone marrow transplant (BMT) patients have demonstrated that prophylactic use of quinolones is effective in reducing the incidence of GI-based aerobic GN infections, as compared with placebo or trimethoprim-sulfamethoxazole. Good results have been obtained with oral norfloxacin, which, although not well absorbed, provides high concentrations locally within the GI tract while preserving the anaerobic flora and thus colonization resistance against fungal overgrowth or acquisition of new aerobic pathogens. Other quinolones, such as ciprofloxacin, which are more completely absorbed, have been used for systemic treatment of both local and disseminated infections. Such use in both neutropenic and nonneutropenic individuals has led to the emergence of quinolone-resistant organisms in some studies.

Fever without obvious precipitating causes in the neutropenic host must be interpreted as a sign of infection, even in the absence of other localizing or systemic symptoms, and must prompt the empiric institution of antibacterial antibiotics. Numerous trials continue to validate this concept using agents directed against aerobic and facultative GN bacteria, especially *P. aeruginosa*. To this end, the noncross-resistant combination of aminoglycoside and an antipseudomonal penicillin provides noncompetitive mechanisms of action and potential antibacterial synergy. However, the renal, auditory, and vestibular toxicity that may be associated with prolonged aminoglycoside use is substantial. Nephrotoxicity is a particular concern in the setting of cyclosporin after allogeneic BMT. Therapeutic drug level monitoring, which is necessary to limit aminoglycoside toxicity, adds to the cost of therapy.

The role of single-agent antibiotics in infection management in neutropenic patients continues to be assessed. Several beta-lactam antibiotics (e.g., aztreonam, ceftazidime, imipenem, cefepime) offer broad-spectrum activity against GN bacteria, including *P. aeruginosa*. These drugs are resistant to beta-lactamase hydrolysis, and with their potentially wide range of activity, they offer an attractive alternative to aminoglycoside-containing regimens. In addition, imipinem and cefepime are efficacious against some gram-positive (GP) organisms and anaerobic organisms. The postantibiotic effect associated with imipinem is particularly useful in the setting of profound neutropenia. Newer fluoroquinolones, including levofloxacin, sparfloxacin, and trovafloxacin, show activity against anaerobic bacteria while preserving the broad-spectrum activity of the traditional

Table 2 Increased Incidence of Gram-Positive and Fungal Infection Complications During Induced Neutropenia

Effective empiric antibacterial coverage of potentially life-threatening gram-negative infections at the time of first infectious fever

Heightened ability to deliver dose-intensive therapies, with resultant increase in skin, oropharyngeal, and gastrointestinal mucosal cytotoxicity

Increased use of indwelling catheters, leading to increased skin barrier breakdown

Increased use of parenteral hyperalimentation

Development of beta-lactam antibiotic resistance and vancomycin resistance by gram-positive organisms

Concurrent immune suppression, particularly important with fungal infections

Graft-versus-host disease in bone marrow transplant patients

fluoroquinolones toward GN and GP bacteria. This, coupled with their ease of administration and favorable toxicity profile, makes them attractive candidates for empiric treatment of febrile neutropenia. Unfortunately, studies indicate that bacteria that have acquired resistance to other fluoroquinolones may be less susceptible to these newer agents.

Gram-Positive Infections

Recently, there has been an increasing prevalence of GP infections, resulting in substantial morbidity. Factors underlying this increase are delineated in Table 2. In addition to skin invasion by indwelling catheters, chemotherapy-induced cytotoxicity to skin and mucosal barriers is a significant factor in development of first fever from GP infection. The dissemination of GP organisms from any of these possible sites of barrier breakdown can be suppressed by effective prophylactic therapy. The recent recognition of overwhelming infections caused by *Streptococcus mitis* in association with high-dose chemotherapy-induced and/or radiation therapy–induced oropharyngeal mucositis further supports a prophylactic approach.

Vancomycin, a cell wall–acting glycopeptide antibiotic, is efficacious against a broad range of GP organisms, including many isolates of *Staphylococcus, Corynebacterium* species, and other bacteria that are resistant to beta-lactam antibiotics. In prospective clinical trials at centers where GP infections are prevalent, vancomycin therapy begun empirically at the time of first infectious fever results in prompt fever resolution, rapid clearance of local and/or disseminated GP infections, and prevention of late-onset GP infections in acute leukemia patients with indwelling venous catheters and chemotherapy-induced neutropenia. In centers where GP infections have been less prevalent, the role for early empiric vancomycin is less clear. In these settings, vancomycin has been effective in treating and eradicating established infection in a timely fashion, suggesting that the drug can be added selectively and nonempirically in some instances. The use of vancomycin either prophylactically or therapeutically for GP infections prolongs the length of indwelling catheter life in the deeply aplastic host and prevents the occurrence and/or propagation of infection-related thrombophlebitis. A number of small studies have demonstrated the feasibility of less-strict therapeutic drug level monitoring during vancomycin therapy. This would be of advantage in reducing the costs associated with vancomycin use. Teicoplanin, which exhibits a profile of antibacterial activity that is similar to vancomycin, has the advantage of once-daily administration.

Since 1986, vancomycin-resistant enterococci (VRE) have emerged as an increasingly visible clinical problem, with a more than 20-fold increase in resistance noted for all enterococci associated with nosocomial infections since 1989. Various isolates of VRE exhibit different patterns of resistance, with the van A phenotype, often expressed by strains of *E. faecalis* and *E. faecium,* being the most common and best studied. In these strains, an inducible plasmidborne genetic transposition results in synthesis of cell wall peptide residues incapable of binding to peptidoglycan antibiotics, thus avoiding cell wall disruption. These enterococci are also intrinsically resistant to many antibiotics, including beta-lactams (because of the presence of penicillin-binding proteins with decreased affinity), aminoglycosides, and cephalosporins. Quinolone resistance has also been the rule with these strains; thus therapeutic options for patients infected with these multiply resistant enterococci are limited. This problem has spawned a vigorous search for newer antibiotic agents that might provide some activity against VRE. Unfortunately, in vitro activity against VRE isolates identified in several classes of drugs has not readily translated into effectiveness in clinical VRE infection. Thus the establishment and maintenance of vigorous infection control procedures remains the cornerstone of dealing with this group of organisms, not only to limit their dissemination but also to prevent glycopeptide resistance in other more virulent GP pathogens such as *Staphylococcus aureus.* Indeed, recent studies have documented vancomycin resistance in *S. aureus* in the setting of prolonged vancomycin treatment for methicillin-resistant *S. aureus,* although in these reports vancomycin resistance could be overcome by beta-lactams or gentamicin in combination with vancomycin. A combination of careful and innovative antibiotic use and strict adherence to appropriate infection control procedures are the only means for dealing with the expanding problems of antibiotic resistance in GP bacteria in the compromised host.

Infection control procedures are also important in limiting the spread of the GP-bacillus *Clostridium difficile.* This organism is associated with colitis and diarrhea in patients with prolonged exposure to broad-spectrum antibiotics or some forms of chemotherapy, notably cisplatin. Diarrhea in a patient with chemotherapy-induced marrow aplasia and fever presents special problems: bloody stool from thrombocytopenia and/or chemotherapy-induced mucositis, as well as the absence of stool leukocytes because of neutropenia, limit the value of diagnostic stool examination. Moreover, the fevers associated with *C. difficile* are often mistaken for (or obscured by) those of concurrent bacterial, viral, or fungal infection. In addition to compromising their fluid, electrolyte, and nutritional status, *C. difficile* colitis may predispose patients to the dissemination of GI tract–based organisms, which, although not ordinarily pathogenic, contribute to illness upon bloodstream invasion. Dissemination of VRE is a particular problem in this setting. Unfortunately,

the discontinuation of antibiotics, clearly important in the treatment of *C. difficile* diarrhea, is not feasible in patients with febrile neutropenia. Recent research has focused on methods for the more rapid and accurate diagnosis of these infections, including antigen detection tests that detect bacterial toxin in stool samples, polymerase chain reaction (PCR)-based assays, and newer methods for increasing the yield from stool culture. Anticlostridial antibodies are also being investigated for the prevention and treatment of this disease.

Among neutropenic patients who develop fever, there may be a clinically identifiable subset who are at lower risk of developing overwhelming or life-threatening infections. Outpatients with responding tumors and no concurrent medical illnesses, who account for approximately 40% of febrile neutropenic episodes in some centers, appear to belong to this low-risk group. Other favorable factors may include shorter expected duration of neutropenia, absence of mucositis and of indwelling venous access catheters, and the prophylactic use of oral quinolones or hematopoietic growth factors. However, patients who are bacteremic, have obvious sites of infection, or are known to have a history of fungal infection do not belong to the low-risk group, regardless of the presence of favorable characteristics. Recent studies have evaluated a number of treatment options for low-risk patients, such as outpatient management, early discharge, or the use of oral antibiotics. In some of these limited studies, outpatient management of carefully selected low-risk febrile neutropenic adults and children has been shown to be safe; however, the widespread adoption of such a treatment strategy, although attractive in expected cost savings, must await further validation in larger trials.

■ FUNGAL INFECTIONS

Fungal infection is an increasingly common cause of morbidity and mortality among patients compromised by neutropenia, especially those with acute leukemia and prolonged, therapy-induced bone marrow aplasia. Ironically, this increase is in part caused by the higher rate of survival during early aplasia resulting from improved control of overwhelming bacterial infections. Additional factors include therapy-induced mucosal toxicity, hyperalimentation, iron overload, and the prolonged use of broad-spectrum antibiotics, which leads to imbalance in GI flora. The use of indwelling catheters is also associated with fungal infections, notably *Candida parapsilosis,* and with cardiac involvement by disseminated fungal infections. Fungal infections are particularly problematic in patients who, in addition to being neutropenic, are also immunocompromised. Such impairment of cellular or humoral immune function may arise as a result of the underlying disease (e.g., Hodgkin's disease, lymphoma, multiple myeloma, lymphocytic leukemia) or as a result of treatment with glucocorticoids, cyclosporin or newer immunosuppressants, or BMT. In BMT patients, graft-versus-host disease and the consequent need for immunosuppressive therapy represent further risk factors for the development of fungal infections (see Table 2).

Several studies have examined the role of antifungal agents given prophylactically to patients with acute leukemia or undergoing BMT. Although most cases of hematogenous or invasive candidal infections are preceded by colonization of mucosal surfaces, trials of local polyene or azole antifungals to control oropharyngeal, sinonasal, or disseminated candidiasis have produced variable results. Moreover, even when decreases in systemic candidal infections have been detected, these agents have not reduced the incidence or severity of infections caused by filamentous fungi. Trials of low-dose systemic amphotericin B prophylaxis (0.1 to 0.3 mg/kg/day) in acute leukemia and BMT patients yield data varying from major decreases in incidence and mortality of fungus infections, including invasive aspergillosis, to no effect whatsoever.

The triazole antifungal agents fluconazole and itraconazole have also been examined for efficacy in preventing fungal infection during profound therapy-induced bone marrow aplasia. Fluconazole suppresses *Candida albicans* and *Candida tropicalis* colonization and superficial infections, which can predispose patients to hematogenous spread and invasive infections. Prophylactic dosages of 400 mg/day of fluconazole have been associated with significant reductions in the incidence of fungal colonization, hematogenous candidiasis, and mortality in prospective trials of patients undergoing BMT, and were as effective and less toxic than amphotericin B (0.5 mg/kg three times weekly) in leukemia patients. However, fluconazole prophylaxis may predispose to acquisition and superinfection with drug-selected pathogens (e.g., *Candida krusei* and *C. glabrata*). Fluconazole has had no demonstrable prophylactic effect against infections caused by filamentous fungi, particularly *Aspergillus* species. In contrast, itraconazole has activity against filamentous fungi, including *Aspergillus* species. However, azoles lack any activity against zygomycoses. There are also some concerning data from animal studies suggesting that previous exposure to azole antifungals may compromise the therapeutic efficacy of amphotericin B, although this has not been shown in clinical studies.

Antifungal Therapy

Data from autopsy series indicate that mortality from fungal infection has increased in cancer patients along with developments in dose-intensive chemotherapy and BMT. Tissue and/or bloodstream fungal invasion has been found in 25% to 40% of persistently febrile persons with neutropenia, and a high incidence of mortality is associated with delaying treatment until the time of specific diagnosis. This problem is compounded by the lack of sensitive laboratory tests providing rapid identification of pathogenic fungi or of generally available methods for fungal drug susceptibility testing. Tests based on the detection of specific *Candida* or *Aspergillus* antigens, metabolites, and nucleic acids, which would be expected to produce a more rapid diagnosis, remain in development. Early clinical trials using PCR-based assays are promising. Invasive procedures to establish the diagnosis are often contraindicated in the clinical setting of deep marrow aplasia and may be unreliable in establishing a specific diagnosis. The significance of positive fungal cultures obtained noninvasively from the GI or urinary tract with respect to colonization versus infection is controversial. Although radiographic studies with computed tomography (CT) are useful in the early detection as well as the follow-up

of deep-tissue invasion, particularly pulmonary aspergillosis, these studies do not provide absolute or specific identification of the responsible pathogen. For these reasons, amphotericin B is advocated for the empiric treatment of persistently febrile neutropenic patients, an approach that has been shown to result in clinical responses, including a reduction in mortality. Empiric amphotericin B at moderate dosages (0.5 mg/kg/day) has produced responses in 50% to 70% of patients so treated and provides good antifungal therapy for common yeast pathogens (e.g., *C. albicans* and *C. glabrata*). However, breakthrough infection with *C. tropicalis*, *C. krusei*, and *Trichosporon* species occur with moderate-dose amphotericin B. High-dose empiric therapy may be initiated in patients colonized with non-*albicans* species who have refractory fever.

A critical determinant of survival following disseminated fungus infections during profound marrow aplasia is prompt and aggressive therapy with amphotericin B. Investigators at several centers have demonstrated that prompt detection and institution of aggressive fungicidal therapy with high-dose (1 to 1.25 mg/kg/day) amphotericin B alone or in combination with 5-fluorocytosine (5-FC) results in enhanced survival in infections caused by filamentous organisms such as *Aspergillus* and *Fusarium* species and non-*albicans* yeasts. *Candida lusitaniae*, which is resistant to amphotericin B, may remain sensitive to fluconazole, giving fluconazole a special role in the treatment of *C. lusitaniae* infections. The impact of prompt amphotericin use is most clearly seen in documented infection caused by filamentous fungi; the survival rate decreases from above 80% when amphotericin B is instituted before definitive diagnosis to 44% when amphotericin B institution is delayed. The timing of such empiric intervention may not differ from a late prophylaxis approach, in which antifungal treatment is started before there is clear clinical evidence of infection on the basis of nonspecific clinical findings. Although late prophylaxis may be inadequate to prevent overt infection in the absence of granulocytes and/or the presence of damaged barriers, it may result in a reduced microbial burden even when only moderate dosages of amphotericin B (0.5 mg/kg/day) are used initially.

The isolation of candidal organisms from blood cultures is evidence of disseminated infection and should prompt the institution of amphotericin B. In other patients, fungal infection may be evidenced by specific tissue or organ involvement without demonstrable fungemia (e.g., esophageal or hepatosplenic candidiasis) and invasive pulmonary aspergillosis. In the case of esophagitis, endoscopy may be useful to establish the diagnosis and exclude drug-induced mucositis or infection with herpes simplex, cytomegalovirus, or bacteria. Nonetheless, the prompt clinical response of candidal esophagitis to fluconazole or amphotericin has led some clinicians to reserve endoscopy for refractory cases.

Prolonged neutropenia (>2 to 4 weeks) is a risk factor for the development of hepatosplenic candidiasis, although in most cases the diagnosis is not made until after neutrophil count recovery. Fever that persists after recovery from prolonged neutropenia, especially if associated with abdominal pain, hepatomegaly, and an elevated serum alkaline phosphatase level, should lead to a suspicion of hepatosplenic candidiasis. Noninvasive imaging with contrast-enhanced

CT or magnetic resonance imaging (MRI) is an important aid to the diagnosis. Ultrasonography, although not as sensitive, may be useful for serial monitoring. Blood cultures and cultures of percutaneously obtained liver lesions are often falsely negative, and in some cases, biopsies may need to be obtained by laparoscopy or minilaparotomy. Periodic acid–Schiff and methenamine silver stains may demonstrate budding candidal forms, sometimes with pseudohyphae. Confirmation of the diagnosis is important because of the need for prolonged treatment with amphotericin B, usually lasting weeks and therefore associated with significant toxicity and costs. Lipid-based preparations of amphotericin B have been shown to be especially effective in treating hepatic candidiasis and result in less renal toxicity.

Invasive pulmonary aspergillosis remains an important cause of morbidity and mortality in the neutropenic patient. Many cases result from the reactivation of previously dormant infection, and patients who have survived invasive pulmonary aspergillosis in the context of chemotherapy-induced neutropenia have a 50% risk of recrudescence during a subsequent neutropenic cycles. These patients benefit from amphotericin B initiated before the development of neutropenia with further cycles of chemotherapy. However, aspergillosis may also be acquired nosocomially, with construction sites, ventilation systems, and perhaps indoor plants as the sources of infection. High-efficiency particulate air (HEPA) filters may reduce the incidence of nosocomially acquired aspergillosis. *A. fumigatus* and *A. flavus* are most commonly responsible for these infections, and their isolation from respiratory secretions or by bronchoalveolar lavage is predictive of true pulmonary infection. Bronchoscopic biopsy may provide a definitive tissue diagnosis, although a negative result should not be taken to indicate the absence of fungal disease. Treatment requires the prompt institution of higher dosages of amphotericin B, in the range of 1 to 1.5 mg/kg/day. Chest and sinus CT scans are important in the diagnosis and follow-up of invasive aspergillosis.

Central nervous system infection by invasive fungi, including *Aspergillus,* should be considered in the differential diagnosis of sudden-onset strokes or seizures with or without fever in the neutropenic patient. Unfortunately, even in patients in whom the diagnosis was suspected early, treatment results with amphotericin B with or without 5-FC have been unsatisfactory, and almost all patients have died. New treatment approaches are urgently needed for this fortunately uncommon problem.

Innovations in Antifungal Therapy

Ergosterol, an essential component of fungal cell membranes, is the target of both the polyenes, which include amphotericin B, and the azoles such as fluconazole, ketoconazole, and itraconazole. While amphotericin B disrupts the fungal cell membrane by binding to intact ergosterol, the azoles exert their action through the inhibition of ergosterol synthesis. Newer azoles under development are expected to have increased activity against *C. krusei* and *C. lusitaniae* relative to fluconazole and amphotericin B. Like the azoles, the allylamines inhibit ergosterol synthesis, although at a different enzymatic step. Unfortunately, terbinafine, the only member of that class that is currently available, is

limited to the treatment of dermatophytic infections, partly because of its pharmacokinetic profile. Because of these competing mechanisms of action it is, at least in theory, difficult to combine azoles with polyene antifungals to extend their spectrum of activity, analogously to what has been done with antibacterials. Other antifungal agents under development target other fungal components and may act synergistically with currently available antifungals. Notably, the pneumocandins and echinocandins inhibit synthesis of the fungal cell wall glucan and are active against diverse selected pathogens (e.g., *Candida* species, *Aspergillus* species, *Cryptococcus neoformans,* and *Pneumocystis carinii*). Potentiation of the activity of both fluconazole and amphotericin B against *C. neoformans* by a pneumocandin has recently been demonstrated in vitro. Other potential targets for antifungal drug activity include chitin, an essential component of the fungal cell wall absent from mammalian systems, and fungal DNA topoisomerase. Future studies may also evaluate humanized monoclonal antibodies directed against fungal surface antigens in combination with fungicidal agents and lactoferrin, which may exert an antifungal effect through blockade of fungal iron metabolism.

Attempts to improve the therapeutic index of amphotericin B have resulted in the development of lipid-based formulations for aerosolized or intravenous delivery and an oral aqueous suspension for oropharyngeal candidiasis. Currently, three preparations of lipid-based amphotericin B have been approved by the U.S. Food and Drug Administration: amphotericin B lipid complex, amphotericin B cholesteryl sulfate, and liposomal amphotericin B. Early experience with these formulations, reported mainly in case series and open label studies, demonstrates efficacy at least equivalent to traditional amphotericin B, including responses in some patients with infections, notably hepatosplenic candidiasis, in whom conventional amphotericin B had failed. Unfortunately, central nervous system aspergillosis does not appear to be responsive to at least one of these agents. More recently, prospective trials, some randomized, have confirmed the efficacy of lipid-complex formulations in the prophylaxis and treatment of fungal infections in neutropenic patients. Importantly, they have been associated with much less nephrotoxicity than conventional amphotericin B, even when given concurrently with cyclosporin. Infusion-related side effects, such as fever and chills, also appear to be reduced in frequency with the use of these formulations. To date, the major barrier to widespread use of these newer preparations appears to be their cost relative to traditional amphotericin B.

■ ADJUNCTIVE ROLE OF BIOMODULATION IN INFECTION MANAGEMENT

Several clinical trials have evaluated the adjunctive role of recombinant human hematopoietic growth factors (cytokines) such as the colony-stimulating factors (CSF) in the management of neutropenia. Although the administration of granulocyte (G) or granulocyte-macrophage (GM) colony-stimulating factor during cytotoxic chemotherapy with or without BMT for diverse malignancies was associated with modest improvements in the duration and depth of neutropenia in some studies, the impact on mortality or infection-related mortality could not be reproducibly demonstrated. G-CSF and GM-CSFs have also been used with or without chemotherapy to mobilize hemopoietic stem cells for collection from the peripheral blood (peripheral blood stem cells [PBSCs]). Recent studies demonstrate that the use of PBSCs for autotransplantation leads to faster marrow engraftment, reduction in the duration of profound neutropenia ($<100/mm^3$), and a decrease in overall antibiotic use.

Mucosal defense systems are of prime importance in protecting the neutropenic host from infection. In addition to cellular factors, mucosal integrity in mammals is also a function of the secretion of various chemical substances, including immunoglobulins, lysozymes, lactoferrins, and recently described peptides such as defensins, protegrins, tachyplesins, and magainin II, which possess broad antibacterial and antifungal properties. The effects of chemotherapy on the secretion and function of these substances and their role in chemotherapy-induced microbial dissemination remain to be elucidated and applied therapeutically. Still, it is clear that in addition to direct cytotoxic effects on mucosal cells, chemotherapy and radiation therapy also initiate a complex series of cytokine-mediated processes whose net effect is cell death. Tumor necrosis factor (TNF) alpha, a major effector in this process, is a target for innova-

tive therapies directed at attenuating therapy-related mucositis. Clinical trials of pentoxifylline, an inhibitor of TNF synthesis, have yielded disappointing results. Ketoconazole is also known to be a potent inhibitor of TNF production but has not been evaluated systemically for this indication. Thalidomide, another inhibitor of TNF synthesis, is of particular interest because it has been shown to promote healing of oral aphthous ulcers in patients with HIV disease. Soluble TNF receptor also remains to be studied for a potential effect on mucositis through inhibition of TNF activity. Other cytokines may have a direct beneficial effect on mucositis. For example, interleukin-11 is a multifunctional cytokine that exhibits cytoprotective effects on GI epithelium in preclinical models of radiation and chemotherapy-induced mucositis and improves survival in neutropenic rats with *Pseudomonas aeruginosa* gut colonization when given at the onset of fever. Similarly, strategies to mitigate graft-versus-host disease in BMT patients might prevent GI mucosal destruction and thus might be expected to reduce the incidence and severity of neutropenic infections in that setting.

■ FUTURE DIRECTIONS

The strategies for prevention, diagnosis, and therapy of infections in the neutropenic host are continually being

---

Table 3   Guidelines for the Prevention and Management of Infections in Neutropenic Hosts

Prophylaxis	Norfloxacin, 400 mg orally q12h, for prevention of GN sepsis
Started at day 0 or at day of granulocytes <500 ×10⁹/L; maintain throughout granulocytopenia	Acyclovir, 250 mg/m² IV q8h, for prevention of herpes simplex virus reactivation
Additional options	Addition of GP coverage (e.g., vancomycin, 500 mg IV q12h if GP infection rate is high)
	Addition of antifungal prophylaxis (e.g., low-dose amphotericin B, azoles)
	Addition of cytokines (e.g., G- or GM-CSF, IL)
First infectious fever	Antipseudomonal penicillin (e.g., ticarcillin, 270 mg/kg/24 hr) (continuous infusion) provides GN, anaerobic, and some GP coverage, and aminoglycoside (e.g., gentamicin, 2 mg/kg IV q6h) provides broad-spectrum coverage and synergistic effect with penicillins
	Single-agent imipenem-cilastin, 500 mg q6h, or cefepime, 2 g q8h
Progressive disease	With clinical suspicion of smoldering bacterial infection substitute TMP-SMX for gentamicin
No response within 48-72 hr of starting first fever coverage	Add vancomycin if not already started
	Clinical evidence of more rapidly deteriorating condition: substitute amikacin, 8 mg/kg IV q6h and piperacillin, 270 mg/kg/24 hr (continuous infusion)
	With clinical suspicion of fungal infections (~5%-10% of first fever), add amphotericin B, 0.5 mg/kg/day IV
Recrudescent fever >72 hr after starting first fever coverage without microbial documentation	Add amphotericin B (0.5 mg/kg/day) if not started already
	Switch to amikacin-piperacillin if bacterial sepsis suspected
Specific treatment of microbiologically documented infection	Bacterial-specific antibiotic or combinations of antibiotics
	Fungal species dependent:
	amphotericin B, 0.5 mg/kg/day
	amphotericin B, 1.0-1.25 mg/kg/day, plus 5-FC, 25 mg/kg orally q6h,* for more refractory yeast species and all filamentous mycoses
	Lipid-based amphotericin B for special situations—renal insufficiency, hepatosplenic candidiasis

GN, Gram-negative; *GP,* gram-positive; *G,* granulocyte; *GM,* granulocyte-macrophage; *IL,* interleukin; *TMP-SMX,* trimethoprim-sulfamethoxazole; *5-FC,* 5-fluorocytosine.
*To achieve serum level of 30-60 µg/ml to avoid 5-FC related toxicity.

refined, with the realistic possibility of tailoring such interventions to the particular infecting pathogen and the specific host determinants (Table 3). New antibiotics with unique mechanisms of action and novel delivery systems are designed to provide pathogen-directed toxicity while sparing host tissues. Emerging modalities to reconstitute or augment elements of host surveillance can, in turn, protect against the establishment or extension of infection. Combinations of these agents may afford a multitargeted approach. These innovative strategies may modify and improve the overall scheme aimed at preventing and eradicating infections in these compromised hosts. Yet the emergence of resistant pathogens, exemplified by VRE, vancomycin-resistant staphylococci, and amphotericin-resistant fungi, continues to challenge the therapeutic armamentarium and the ability to eradicate and prevent infections in compromised hosts. Such challenges will be addressed through the development of structurally and functionally novel antibiotics and antifungal agents that target molecular pathways that are critical to survival of the offending organism, coupled with innovative approaches to antibiotic use and rigorous adherence to methods that physically limit the spread of these pathogens among patients and caregivers.

Suggested Reading

Ellis M, et al: An EORTC international multicenter randomized trial (EORTC number 19923) comparing two dosages of liposomal amphotericin B for treatment of invasive aspergillosis, *Clin Infect Dis* 27:1406, 1998.

Greene JN: Catheter-related complications of cancer therapy, *Infect Dis Clin North Am* 10:255, 1996.

Karp JE, Merz WG, Charache P: Response to empiric amphotericin B during antileukemic therapy-induced granulocytopenia, *Rev Infect Dis* 13:592, 1991.

Karp JE, Merz WG, Dick JD: Management of infections in neutropenic patients: new opportunities and emerging challenges, *Curr Opin Infect Dis* 7:430, 1994.

Walsh TJ, et al: Liposomal amphotericin B for empirical therapy in patients with persistent fever and neutropenia. National Institute of Allergy and Infectious Diseases Mycoses Study Group, *N Engl J Med* 340:764, 1999.

HIV INFECTION: INITIAL EVALUATION AND MONITORING

Aaron E. Glatt

Ahmed Rabbat

Human immunodeficiency virus (HIV) infection is a major catastrophic event in a patient's life, bringing fear, frustration, and challenge to the physician and society. More than 1 million people in the United States are infected with HIV, with hundreds of thousands more expected to become infected during the next few years. Worldwide, 40 million people are infected.

Primary care physicians will care for most of these patients, especially in the earliest stages of infection. Thus they need to know which elements of the history and physical examination hold particular importance, which screening and diagnostic studies are necessary, when and how to begin antiretroviral therapy, which preventive measures should be offered, and how to provide appropriate counseling on many other important issues. Therefore a major goal of initial evaluation is to assess what level of immune compromise is present.

■ HIV SEROCONVERSION

Patients may present with an acute illness shortly after primary infection with HIV-1 or HIV-2. Individuals may have nonspecific symptoms characterized by lymphadenopathy, malaise, fever, anorexia, diarrhea, headache, and rash; rarely, opportunistic infections have been reported. Many persons do not seek medical attention. An estimated date of initial HIV infection may be helpful to assess disease progression. This is possible to document when there has been an isolated known exposure such as an occupational injury, short period of substance abuse, or a single new sexual partner.

Establish the route and risks for acquisition of HIV with open, nonjudgmental questions because this is important for reducing further transmission and recognizing complications.

■ HISTORY AND PHYSICAL EXAMINATION

HIV disease causes and predisposes to multiple organ disease; evaluation should be systematic and comprehensive. After a detailed chief complaint and history of present illness are obtained, a thorough review of systems on all patients is necessary. Detailed physical examination with careful documentation of baseline observations is essential for early recognition of new problems. It is important to recognize that highly active antiretroviral therapy (HAART) may significantly alter the natural history of HIV infection. In addition, HAART may be associated with side effects such as lipodystrophy and other signs and symptoms.

Review of Systems
General
Fever, weight loss, malaise, fatigue, shaking chills, night sweats, and loss of appetite can be initial findings of significant illness. They are less common in early HIV infection. They may signify worsening immunosuppression. Weight and nutritional assessment should be recorded at each visit.

Skin
The skin of nearly all HIV-infected persons will eventually be affected secondary to infectious and noninfectious dermatologic disorders. Skin or nail pigmentation and rashes of all varieties can occur in disseminated or sporadic fashion, and they may be clues to underlying serious illness, coinfection, or worsening immunosuppression (Table 1).

Lymph Nodes
Nonspecific small, symmetric, mobile nodes, commonly seen in patients with HIV infection, often reflect nonspecific reactive hyperplasia. Acute generalized lymphadenopathy can be seen during seroconversion. Non-Hodgkin's lymphoma (NHL) and infectious pathogens can present as single or multiple nodes.

At each visit, lymph node groups should be assessed for size, quantity, texture, and tenderness. Biopsy is not helpful unless nodes are rapidly enlarging or are associated with fever and weight loss.

Head, Eyes, Ear, Nose, and Throat
Candida and herpes simplex virus often cause painful cheilitis, stomatitis, or pharyngitis and can manifest at any stage of HIV infection. Cytomegalovirus (CMV), Epstein-Barr virus (EBV; oral hairy leukoplakia), varicella-zoster virus, mycobacterial infection, *Cryptococcus neoformans, Histoplasma capsulatum,* Kaposi's sarcoma, squamous cell carcinoma, and NHL may be visible on oral examination, and idiopathic aphthous ulcers are a significant cause of troublesome oral pain. Toothache and dental tenderness may indicate periodontal disease or abscess and may cause both fever and headache. Gingival and periodontal infection are particularly aggressive in patients with HIV infection.

Facial pain, nasal obstruction, postnasal drip, and headache can be caused by sinusitis, which occurs frequently in HIV infection. Atopy may coexist.

Blurred vision, scotoma, or decreased visual acuity suggests CMV retinitis. Complete eye examinations at baseline and when retinitis is a consideration is essential, especially in hosts with CD4 cell count below 50/ml and if HAART is not successful.

Headache of new onset or changing character may be an early manifestation of a central nervous system opportunistic process.

Table 1 Commonly Seen Cutaneous Manifestations in HIV Patients	
ETIOLOGY	**CLINICAL FEATURES**
BACTERIAL INFECTION	
Bacillary angiomatosis	Numerous angiomatous nodules associated with fever, chills, and weight loss
Staphylococcus aureus	Folliculitis, ecthyma, impetigo, bullous impetigo, furuncles, and carbuncles
Syphilis	May occur in different forms (primary, secondary, or tertiary); chancre may become painful due to secondary infection
FUNGAL INFECTION	
Candidiasis	Mucous membranes (oral, vulvovaginal), less commonly *Candida intertrigo* or *paronychia*
Cryptococcoses	Papules or nodules that strongly resemble molluscum contagiosum; other forms include pustules, purpuric papules, and vegitating plaques
Seborrheic dermatitis	Scaling and erythema in the hair-bearing areas such as the eyebrows, scalp, chest, and pubic area
ARTHROPOD INFESTATIONS	
Scabies	Pruritus with or without rash; usually generalized but can be limited to a single digit
VIRAL INFECTION	
Herpes simplex	Vesicular lesion in clusters; perianal, genital, orofacial, or digital; can be disseminated
Herpes zoster	Painful dermatomal vesicles that may ulcerate or disseminate
HIV	Discrete erythematous macules and papules on the upper trunk, palms, and soles are the most characteristic cutaneous finding of acute HIV infection
Human papilloma virus	Genital warts (may become unusually extensive)
Kaposi's sarcoma (herpesvirus)	Eythematous macule or papule, enlarge at varying rates, violaceous nodules or plaques, occasionally painful
Molluscum contagiosum	Discrete umbilicated papules commonly on the face, neck, and intertriginous site (axilla, groin, or buttocks)
NONINFECTIOUS	
Drug reactions	More common and severe in HIV patients
Nutritional deficiencies	Mainly seen in children and patients with chronic diarrhea; diffuse skin manifestations, depending on the deficiency
Psoriasis	Scaly lesions; diffuse or localized; can be associated with arthritis
Vasculitis	Palpable purpuric eruption (can resemble septic emboli)

HIV, Human immunodeficiency virus.

Cardiopulmonary

Precise baseline pulmonary and cardiovascular examinations are important because of increasing pulmonary and cardiac complications in advancing HIV disease. Shortness of breath at rest or with exertion, its duration and progression, whether a cough is dry or productive, sputum color, amount, and odor may help with the differential diagnosis. Hemoptysis can be caused by tuberculosis, thrombocytopenia, bacterial pneumonia, or other lung pathology. Chest pain can be caused by pneumonia, spontaneous pneumothorax (often *Pneumocystis*-related), pericarditis, herpes zoster, or HIV-related cardiomyopathy. Palpitation and postural hypotension suggest symptomatic anemia.

Gastrointestinal

Gastrointestinal diseases are increasingly frequent as HIV disease progresses. Odynophagia, dysphagia, retrosternal chest pain, nausea, anorexia, and weight loss are commonly associated with esophagitis due to *Candida*, herpes simplex, CMV, or more rarely, lymphoma. Hepatic or splenic enlargement may be an early manifestation of HIV-related complications; the baseline size should be documented.

Right upper quadrant pain associated with fever and elevated alkaline phosphatase may indicate viral or drug-induced hepatitis, cholelithiasis, or acalculous cholecystitis related to *Mycobacterium avium* complex (MAC) or cryptosporidiosis.

Epigastric or left upper quadrant pain may indicate pancreatitis. Abdominal distension, tenderness, masses, constipation, or fecal incontinence may be caused by Kaposi's sarcoma, lymphoma, carcinoma, gastrointestinal opportunistic infections (CMV, histoplasmosis, tuberculosis), or parasitic infestation. Diarrhea occurs in 30% to 66% of adults with HIV. *Salmonella, Cryptosporidium, Isospora,* CMV, microsporidia, and other enteric pathogens commonly occur. Constipation is commonly seen in patients taking methadone, heroin, or opioids, as well as other medicines.

Painful defecation or rectal pain can be caused by trauma, perirectal abscess, herpes, or other sexually transmitted diseases. Careful sexual and social histories may help identify the pathogens. Perirectal areas should be carefully examined for lesions, abscess, fissures, proctitis, and ulcerations. Stool should be tested for occult blood.

Genitourinary, Obstetric, and Gynecologic Manifestations

Painful, frequent urination may indicate urinary tract infection, sexually transmitted disease, or vulvovaginitis. The latter are more common and possibly more difficult to treat in HIV infection. Recurrent or severe vaginitis, vaginal discharge, and pruritus are common and may not be related solely to sexual practices. Prompt evaluation of all genital discharges, ulcers, and lesions will allow correct identification of any sexually transmitted disease.

Women should be queried regarding menstrual history, fertility, method of birth control, and numbers and dates of pregnancies and abortions. Menstruation may become irregular in worsening HIV infection, and fertility declines as well. Prior tubal scarring from salpingitis or pelvic inflammatory disease predisposes to ectopic pregnancy and infertility. An external genital, rectal, and complete pelvic examination (speculum and bimanual), including Pap tests and appropriate cultures and stains, should be performed initially and at least annually.

Neurologic

Neuropsychiatric complications eventually occur in up to 80% of patients, yet symptoms may go unrecognized because of coping strategies and the large reserve available until significant deterioration is noted. Subtle neurologic deterioration, memory loss, and poor concentration may be the only early signs of HIV dementia. Central and peripheral neurologic complications may be caused by HIV infection, opportunistic infections, medications, or malignancy. Illness can occur at any stage of HIV infection, albeit with different manifestations. Symptoms depend greatly on the location of the abnormality and the pathophysiology involved. Progressive encephalopathy or peripheral neuropathy can occur years or even decades after seroconversion; intracranial mass lesions are usually a late complication of HIV disease.

Distal predominantly sensory polyneuropathy, chronic inflammatory demyelinating polyneuropathy, mononeuropathy, herpesvirus and CMV radiculitis, and neuropathies of vitamin deficiency are commonly seen. Neurologic evaluation and appropriate diagnostic testing may differentiate treatable from less responsive pathology. A carefully documented baseline neurologic examination, including mental status assessment, cranial nerve testing, and evaluation of sensation, strength, coordination, and reflexes, should be part of an initial and yearly comprehensive evaluation. Mini-mental status test results should be clearly documented.

Musculoskeletal

Myalgia and proximal muscle weakness, tenderness, and wasting may be manifestations of primary HIV or drug-related myositis. Severe, persistent oligoarthritis, primarily affecting the large lower limb joints with exquisite pain, psoriatic arthritis with erosive changes and crippling deformities, and septic arthritis caused by *Staphylococcus aureus,* especially in substance abusers, are not uncommon. Changes in fat distribution secondary to HAART may also be present.

Medical History

A clear history of prior HIV-related events, CD4 cell counts, viral load complications, opportunistic infections, and malignancies will help stage HIV infection, provide prognostic information, and clarify therapeutic options. Opportunistic infections signify marked immunocompromise and are discussed at length in a subsequent chapter.

HIV infection significantly increases the risk of tuberculosis. Purified protein derivative (PPD) status, previous exposure to tuberculosis, and previous prophylaxis or treatment (date, duration, and medications) are critical. Noncompliance, prior hospitalizations, and geographic and social factors play major roles in development of drug resistance and empiric management.

Medications

Polypharmacy, with prescription agents and vitamin, mineral, and herbal supplements, and alternative medications are very common. They can cause or change disease manifestations and be associated with adverse effects and toxicity, which can be confused with symptoms of HIV-related disease. For example, vitamin overdosing may cause diarrhea, abdominal cramps, peripheral neuropathy, increased intracranial pressure, headache, anorexia, nausea, and vomiting. Drug interactions are also common and must be diligently sought for both prescription and nonprescription medicines.

Allergy

The physician should differentiate between allergic reaction and intolerance, which is commonly misinterpreted as allergy. The specific reaction, duration, and resolution of toxicity for each medication should be noted. Rash and fevers are the most common type of adverse drug manifestations.

Social History

Particular attention must be given to all aspects of the psychosocial history, especially residence status, occupational history, substance abuse, and sexual history. A complete sexual history should be obtained, including orientation, practices, lifetime number of partners, prostitution, and any previous sexually transmitted diseases. Dietary habits and water sources are important for certain pathogens.

Travel History

Because certain opportunistic infections occur predominantly in particular geographic regions, place of birth and travel history are particularly useful in formulating a differential diagnosis (e.g., southwestern United States for coccidiomycosis, Ohio River Valley for histoplasmosis). History of travel to developing or tropical countries may raise suspicion of travelers' diarrhea, malaria, leishmania, kala-azar, strongyloidiasis, *Penicillium* infection, HIV-2, and so on.

Pets

Certain opportunistic infections have been associated with particular animals. Patients should be queried regarding exposure to animals and advised about methods of avoiding zoonoses. *Bartonella* (formerly *Rochalimea*) species have been associated with cat-scratch disease and bacillary angiomatosis, and exposure to cats may be associated with toxoplasmosis.

■ LABORATORY STUDIES

Laboratory testing, although invasive, uncomfortable, and expensive, is often the only way to establish or confirm a diagnosis. Laboratory studies should be individualized, but several general principles apply (Tables 2 and 3).

A complete blood count may reveal mild normocytic, normochromic anemia, which often develops as HIV progresses. Macrocytosis develops on zidovudine and can help assess compliance. Pancytopenia may suggest bone marrow involvement or infiltration, isolated thrombocytopenia may be an early finding of HIV infection, and leukopenia and/or a blunted neutrophil response to infection is a common finding. Neutropenia often becomes more pro-

Table 2   Purposes of Laboratory Testing in HIV Infection

1. Establish baseline parameters.
2. Identify underlying disease.
3. Determine appropriate therapy.
4. Estimate the likelihood and rate of disease progression.
5. Monitor response to therapy.
6. Monitor adverse reactions and toxicities.
7. Screen for common/preventable illnesses.

HIV, Human immunodeficiency virus.

nounced with various drug therapies (e.g., zidovudine, trimethoprim-sulfamethoxazole, pentamidine).

Assessment of chemistries and liver function and hepatitis tests are useful in diagnosing concurrent illness and as a guide to monitoring drug toxicities or development of new illness.

A nonspecific syphilis test (RPR) or the venereal disease research laboratory (VDRL) tests, with confirmatory fluorescent treponemal antibody absorbed (FTA-abs) tests, should be performed initially and repeated annually in patients at risk. Lumbar puncture may be indicated for patients with reactive serologies of uncertain duration and/or symptoms.

A PPD should be placed on initial evaluation and at least annually except in patients with a history of tuberculosis or reactive PPD. Baseline chest radiography is recommended regardless of PPD status.

Baseline antitoxoplasma IgG antibodies may influence prophylaxis decisions and help with the evaluation and empiric treatment of central nervous system mass lesions. CMV and EBV serologies, and baseline cryptococcal antigen testing, have no value. Cholesterol and lipid evaluation may be very important in patients on HAART.

Viral load testing and CD4 lymphocyte counts, useful markers of immune status, should be obtained every 3 months as a guide for treatment and prophylactic interventions. CD4 monitoring should be discontinued when clinical decisions are no longer based on the results. There is significant variability in CD4 cell counts; the aggregate picture over weeks or months is more useful than a single reading for major therapy decisions.

Viral load testing is essential for monitoring the efficacy of HAART and the most ultrasensitive assays, capable of detecting as low as 20 viral particles per ml should be used.

■ VACCINATIONS

Patients should receive immunizations as early as possible in the course of HIV infection to optimize response (Table 4), although clinical efficacy is difficult to assess.

Pneumococcal vaccine should be given. The merit of a booster in 5 years is controversial. It is unknown if *Haemophilus influenzae* vaccination is indicated for HIV-infected adults.

Patients without serologic evidence of hepatitis B exposure or immunity should be given hepatitis B vaccine. It is unknown when and if booster is necessary, but a single booster is often given to health care workers and others between 5 and 10 years after initial vaccination.

Table 3 Routine Laboratory Studies Guidelines for HIV-Infected Adults

TEST	INDICATION	INTERVAL
Antitoxoplasma antibody (IgG)	Screening for previous exposure	Baseline
	Guide diagnostic and empiric management	? yearly in patients with negative results
Chemistry and liver functions	Evaluation of baseline renal and liver function, and nutritional status	Baseline
	Diagnosis of concurrent hepatitis	Every 6-12 mo
	Monitoring of drug toxicities	More frequently in patients with advanced disease, baseline abnormalities, or with drug toxicity
	Monitoring of efficacy of therapy	
Chest radiograph	Screening for disease	Baseline
	Diagnosis of active disease	If pulmonary disease suspected
Complete blood count	Evaluation of anemia, leukopenia, or thrombocytopenia	Baseline
	Monitoring of drug toxicities	Every 6 mo
	Monitoring of efficacy of therapy	More frequently in patients with abnormalities or those taking marrow suppressing agents
	Assessment of compliance	
Hepatitis profile	Diagnosis of viral hepatitis	Baseline
	Evaluation for vaccination	During potential acute infection
	Response to vaccination	Postvaccination
Lymphocyte subset testing (CD4 cells)	Guiding initiation of prophylactic and/or antiretroviral therapy	Baseline
	Prognostic information	Every 6 mo if >500
	Monitoring of efficacy of therapy	Every 3 mo if <500
		Discontinue when <50
RNA polymerase chain reaction	Monitoring of HIV activity	Baseline
	Monitoring of efficacy of therapy	Every month until antiretroviral therapy efficacy is established
		Every 3 mo if truly stable clinical
RPR or VDRL	Screening for syphilis	Baseline
	Monitoring of response to therapy	Yearly (at least) in patients at risk/prior infection
	Use of specific test (i.e., FTA) for, confirmation and/or false-negative specimen	Monthly for 6 mo, and at 9 and 12 mo after therapy
		During new symptoms
Tuberculosis skin test (purified protein derivative)	Screening for infection or previous exposure	Baseline, if negative history
	Identification of new converters	Yearly, if negative history
		More frequently if at greater risk

HIV, Human immunodeficiency virus.

Table 4 Vaccination Guidelines for HIV-Infected Adults

VACCINE	FREQUENCY
Pneumococcal vaccine	Once (booster at 5 yr)
Hepatitis B vaccine series	Series of three (0, 1, and 6 mo) (booster in 5 yr)
Influenze	Yearly (in autumn)
Inactivated polio vaccine	As per standard published guidelines
Diphtheria/tetanus	As per standard published guidelines
Measles (MMR)	As per standard published guidelines
Haemophilus influenzae vaccine	Once?

HIV, Human immunodeficiency virus.

Influenza vaccine is recommended annually.

Inactivated polio vaccine, standard childhood vaccinations, and booster diphtheria and tetanus immunizations can be given as per published guidelines. Hepatitis A vaccine may also be indicated among selected at-risk populations.

GUIDELINES FOR FOLLOW-UP

Patients receiving HAART need to be followed closely to ensure compliance, efficacy, and optimal management. Once fully stable, asymptomatic HIV patients should be examined and reevaluated every 1 to 3 months, and usually much more frequently if immunocompromise worsens. Follow-up of symptomatic patients should be individualized. Most patients have numerous psychosocial needs that also must be addressed; referral to the appropriate staff is essential for complete and compassionate care.

Suggested Reading

Ann Intern Med 128(pt 2):1057, 1998.
Centers for Disease Control and Prevention: 1993 Revised classification system for HIV infection and expanded surveillance case definition for AIDS among adolescents and adults, *MMWR* 41:1, 1992.
Ong K, Iftikhar S, Glatt A: Medical evaluation of the adult with HIV infection, *Infect Dis Clin North Am* 8:289, 1994.
USPHS/IDSA Prevention of opportunistic infection working Group: 1997 USPHS/IDSA guidelines for the prevention of opportunistic infections in persons infected with human immunodeficiency virus, *MMWR* 46(RR-12):1, 1997.

HIV INFECTION: ANTIRETROVIRAL THERAPY

Frank Palella

John P. Phair

In the United States, by mid-1999, fifteen approved antiretroviral agents are available for treatment of human immunodeficiency virus type-1 (HIV-1) infection; six nucleoside analogs reverse transcriptase inhibitors (NRTIs), three nonnucleoside reverse transcriptase inhibitors (NNRTIs), and six protease inhibitors (PIs). Current guidelines recommend combining two NRTIs and a PI, two NRTIs and a NNRTI, or two PIs plus two reverse transcriptase inhibitors (Table 1). These potent combinations generally result in suppression of viral replication and CD4 cell repletion, especially in treatment naive individuals. In addition to effects on plasma HIV-RNA copy and CD4+ lymphocyte number, highly active antiretroviral therapy (HAART) produces a reduction in morbidity resulting from opportunistic diseases and decreased mortality. These results have been replicated in several cohorts and have consistently followed increasing use of combinations using PIs.

Measurement of plasma HIV-RNA has enhanced the ability to establish a prognosis and monitor therapy. Initiation of HAART should be followed by a significant decrease in HIV-RNA copy number within 4 weeks when treating naive patients. By 16 to 24 weeks, HIV-RNA levels are below the limit of detection (<20 or 50 copies) using the third-generation ultrasensitive methods in 40% to 70% of treated patients. Failure to achieve undetectable levels of viral-associated RNA within the first several months of therapy suggests either that drug-resistant virions have been selected, that the pharmacokinetics of the chosen agents are unfavorable in the individual patient, or that the patient has been unable to comply with the complex treatment regimen.

Opinions differ as to the optimal time to initiate antiretroviral therapy. It is generally agreed that patients with symptomatic HIV infection and persons with fewer than 500/mm^{3}CD4+ lymphocytes should be treated. Randomized clinical trials and analyses of observational databases support these recommendations. There is less consensus about beginning treatment in asymptomatic patients with more than 500/mm^3 T-helper cells and plasma copy numbers below 20,000/ml. It is clear that an asymptomatic patient cannot be made to feel better with treatment, but antiretroviral therapy can make an individual feel worse. The argument favoring initiation of therapy cites the continuing effects of even low levels of viral replication on immunocompetence and the increased risk of mutations, potentially leading to selection of antiviral-resistant variants or an earlier appearance of quasispecies that use both the chemokine receptors CXCR4 and CCR5, variants associated with more rapid progression. Current guidelines also recommend that patients manifesting the acute viral syndrome be offered therapy. The rationale is based on the possibility of preserving HIV-specific immune responses resulting in a greater chance of nonprogression. No double-blind randomized trials demonstrating the clinical efficacy of this strategy are available.

The choice of the initial combination of agents in naive patients should be based on a plan that preserves options for a second or third regimen if necessary. In treatment-experienced individuals, the choice of an effective combination requires a complete history of previous antiretroviral therapy because persistence of plasma HIV-RNA above the limits of detection implies that drug-resistant virions predominate. Genotypic and phenotypic assays are becoming increasingly available and may play a larger role in the choice of both initial as well as subsequent therapies.

The fifteen FDA-approved agents and the one drug available through expanded access are listed in Table 2. All interfere with one of two viral enzymes, reverse transcriptase or protease. The former is responsible for the initial step of intracellular viral replication, the transcription of proviral DNA from the viral RNA; the latter proteolytically cleaves the polyprotein product of the gag-pol genes into the structural proteins p17, which lines the envelope bilayer, and p24, the core protein that is polymerized to form a core containing the viral genome. Failure to complete this terminal step of viral replication renders the virus noninfectious.

■ NUCLEOSIDE ANALOG REVERSE TRANSCRIPTASE INHIBITORS

The NRTIs have been in use since 1987, when zidovudine (ZVD, AZT, RetrovirR) was released. Additional NRTIs include didanosine (ddI, VidexR), zalcitabine (ddC, HividR), lamivudine (3TC,EpivirR), stavudine (d4T ZeritR), and the most recent addition, abacavir (ZiagenR). These agents require intracellular phosphorylation; the resultant triphosphate is incorporated into the lengthening strand of proviral DNA and act as a chain terminator preventing addition of more nucleic acids to the proviral DNA.

Monotherapy with AZT or ddI was associated with a transient clinical benefit that can be extended by switching to alternative nucleoside monotherapies. Combinations of NRTIs, AZT plus ddI, AZT plus ddC, AZT plus 3TC, and d4T plus ddI provided more convincing evidence of clinical benefit in randomized clinical trials and currently form the backbone of HAART, which also includes either a PI or NNRTI. Each NRTI has associated toxicities that can preclude use in patients with underlying bone marrow, liver, pancreatic, or neurologic disease. The adverse effects of the NRTIs are listed in Table 3.

Abacavir, the most recently approved NRTI, has been used successfully in a variety of combination therapies with other NRTIs, NNRTIs, or PIs. It is a potent agent providing effective treatment for viral isolates resistant to 3TC and, to some extent, AZT. Its use is associated with a 3% to 5% incidence of hypersensitivity reactions manifest by fever, malaise, gastrointestinal symptoms, and/or rash. When this reaction is recognized and abacavir discontinued, reintroduction of the agent is associated with more serious adverse effects, including hypotension and occasionally death. Therefore it is imperative that abacavir not be reintroduced

Table 1 Recommended Antiretroviral Agents for Treatment of Established HIV Infection

Preferred	Strong evidence of clinical benefit and/or sustained suppression of plasma viral load column A and column B. Drugs are listed in random, not priority, order:	One choice each from
	Column A	Column B
	Indinavir	ZDV + ddl
	Nelfinavir	d4T + ddl
	Ritonavir	ZDV + ddC
	Saquinavir-SGC[a]	ZDV + 3TC[b]
	Ritonavir + saquinavir-SGC or HGC[c]	d4T + 3TC
Alternative	Less likely to provide sustained virus suppression 1 NNRTI − 2 NRTIs (column B)[d]	
Not generally recommended	Strong evidence of clinical benefit but initial virus suppression is not sustained in most patients 2 NRTIs (column B) Saquinavir-HGC + 2 NRTIs (column B)[e]	
Not recommended	Evidence against use, virologically undesirable, or overlapping toxicities All monotherapies[f] d4T + ZDV[g] ddC + ddl[g] ddC + d4T[g] ddC + 3TC[g]	

3TC, Lamivudine; *d4T,* stavudine; *ddC,* zalcitabine; *ddl,* didanosine; *HGC,* hard-gel capsule; *NNRTI,* nonnucleoside reverse transcriptase inhibitor; *NRTI,* nucleoside analog reverse transcriptase inhibitor; *SGC,* soft-gel capsule; *ZDV,* zidovudine.

[a]Virologic data and clinical experience with saquinavir-SGC (Fortovase) are limited in comparison with those of other protease inhibitors.

[b]High-level resistance to 3TC develops within 2 to 4 weeks in partially suppressive regimens; optimal use is in three-drug antiretroviral combinations that reduce viral load to <500 copies/ml.

[c]Use of ritonavir, 400 mg bid with saquinavir-SGC (Fortovase), 400 mg bid, results in similar drug exposure and antiretroviral activity as when using 400 mg bid of saquinavir-HGC (Invirase) in combination with ritonavir. However, the combination with Fortovase has not been extensively studied, and gastrointestinal toxicity may be greater when using Fortovase.

[d]The only combinations of 2 NRTIs + NNRTI that have been shown to suppress viremia to undetectable levels in the majority of patients remaining on treatment for more than 28 weeks are ZDV + ddl + nevirapine and ZDV + 3TC + delavirdine. Use of nevirapine or delavirdine may result in resistance that precludes efficacy of new NNRTIs, such as efavirenz.

[e]Use of saquinavir-HGC (Invirase) is generally not recommended, except in combination with ritonavir.

[f]Zidovudine monotherapy may be considered for prophylactic use in pregnant women with low viral load and high CD4 T-cell counts to prevent perinatal transmission.

[g]The combination of NRTIs is not recommended on the basis of lack of clinical data on the combination and/or overlapping toxicities.

Table 2 Antiretroviral Drugs and Dosage

ANTIRETROVIRAL DRUG	GENERIC NAME	ABBREVIATION	TRADE NAME	USUAL DOSE
NRTIs	Abacavir	ABC	Ziagen	300 mg bid
	Didanosine	ddI	Videx	200 mg bid or 400 mg qd
	Lamivudine	3TC	Epivir	150 mg bid
	Stavudine	d4t	Zerit	40 mg bid, <60 kg 30 mg bid
	Zalcitabine	ddC	Hivid	0.75 mg tid
	Zidovudine	AZT/ZVD	Retrovir	300 mg bid
NNRTIs	Delavirdine	DLV	Rescriptor	400 mg tid
	Efavirenz	EFV	Sustiva	600 mg qd
	Nevirapine	NVP	Viramune	200 mg qd ×14 days then 200 mg bid or 400 mg qd
Protease Inhibitors	Amprenavir	VX478/141W94	Agenerase	1200 mg bid
	Indinavir	IDV	Crixivan	800 mg q8h
	Nelfinavir	NLF	Viracept	750 mg q8h or 1250 bid
	Ritonavir	RTV	Norvir	600 mg bid increase from 300 mg bid to 400 mg bid 500 mg bid q3days
	Saquinavir mesylate	SQV	Invirase	600 mg q8h
	Saquinavir soft-gel cap	SQV SGC	Fortovase	1200 mg q8h
Nucleotide Analog RTI	Adefovir*	Bis-Pom, PMEA	Preveon	120 mg qd ×4 weeks then 60 qd

NRTIs, Nucleoside reverse transcriptase inhibitors; *NNRTIs,* nonnucleoside reverse transcriptase inhibitors; *RTI,* reverse transcriptase inhibitor.

*Available through expanded access.

Table 3   Common Adverse Effects of Antiretroviral Drug

ANTIRETROVIRAL DRUG	COMMON ADVERSE EFFECTS
Abacavir	Nausea, vomiting, hypersensitivity (no rechallenge)
Didanosine	Peripheral neuropathy, pancreatitis, diarrhea
Lamivudine	Anemia, gastrointestinal upset
Stavudine	Peripheral neuropathy
Zalcitabine	Peripheral neuropathy, oral ulcers
Zidovudine	Bone marrow suppression, gastrointestinal upset, headache, myopathy
Delavirdine	Rash
Efavirenz	Rash, dizziness, light-headedness, nausea
Nevirapine	Rash, hepatic transaminase increase
Amprenavir	Rash, headache, nausea
Indinavir	Renal colic from drug precipitation, hyperbilirubinemia
Nelfinavir	Diarrhea
Ritonavir	GI upset, diarrhea, circumoral paresthesias
Saquinavir	Low bioavailability
Saquinavir sgc	Diarrhea
Adefovir	Gastrointestinal upset, Fanconi syndrome, must take with carnitine, 500 mg/day

into a therapeutic regimen if discontinued because of the hypersensitivity reaction.

■ NONNUCLEOSIDE REVERSE TRANSCRIPTASE INHIBITORS

NNRTIs bind directly to the reverse transcriptase downstream from the active catalytic site, thus inhibiting enzymatic function. These agents do not require intracellular phosphorylation and rapidly begin to block viral replication. However, the first two NNRTIs introduced, nevirapine and delavirdine, selected resistant mutants within 2 to 4 weeks of initiation of therapy when given as monotherapy. Thus NNRTIs, including the most recently approved agent, efavirenz (SustivaR) are in use in triple-drug combinations. Often, two NRTIs are combined with an NNRTI in a PI-sparing regimen. Such combinations have been used successfully as initial therapy, especially in patients with higher CD4+ lymphocyte counts and lower viral loads. NNRTIs are also used as part of salvage therapy combinations.

The NNRTIs generally are well tolerated, except for an associated rash, manifest most commonly in the first 2 to 4 weeks of therapy. Severe, grade 3 or 4, rashes are uncommon, and the overwhelming majority of patients can continue use of the NNRTI. Nevirapine has been associated with increases in hepatic transaminases, and approximately half of patients beginning efavirenz will complain of light-headedness, headache, or nightmares. Unlike the NRTIs, nevirapine and efavirenz induce hepatic cytochrome P-4503A4 enzyme system, lowering the bioavailability of agents metabolized by this system, including other antiviral drugs such as the PIs. Delavirdine can suppress this

enzyme system, resulting in higher plasma concentrations of coadministered agents that are metabolized by this enzyme.

■ PROTEASE INHIBITORS

Administration of PIs as monotherapy results in dramatic decreases in plasma HIV-RNA copy number and a rapid increase in CD4+ lymphocyte counts. However, monotherapy in time again selects resistant viral strains. Therefore PIs, which were introduced into the clinic in late 1995, have become the core of HAART regimens. Currently, approved PIs include indinavir (CrixivanR), nelfinavir (ViraceptR) ritonavir (NorvirR), saquinavir, hard-gel capsules (InviraseR), saquinavir soft-gel capsules (FortovaseR) and amprenavir (AgeneraseR).

All available PIs are peptidomimetic molecules, and therefore cross-resistance is a problem. Differing requirements as to frequency of ingestion and dosing in relation to meals must be considered in deciding on the appropriate PI for use in a specific patient. For example, indinavir and saquinavir are administered every 8 hours, but indinavir must be taken on an empty stomach or following a fat-free or protein-free light meal. In addition, indinavir therapy requires maintenance of a high fluid intake to prevent precipitation of the drug in the renal tubules.

The most important decision that the physician must make is whether the patient is committed to the complicated regimen necessitated by HAART. Failure to adhere to the dosing schedule can and does result in suboptimal plasma concentrations of the PI, favoring selection of resistant mutants. It is better to await a patient's commitment to HAART rather than to lose the benefit of this class of drugs by attempting to force acceptance of a complex treatment program. In addition, a thorough discussion of what is possible in terms of a patient's lifestyle can avoid nonadherence. For example, avoiding an every 8-hour dosing schedule may be the most appropriate approach for persons with a busy work schedule.

All of the PIs can produce some diarrhea. Patients with chronic active hepatitis B or C often have hepatic enzyme increases with use of any of the PIs. Other adverse effects are more agent specific. Thus indinavir is associated with nephrolithiasis in persons who can not maintain an adequate fluid intake and causes an asymptomatic hyperbilirubinemia; ritonavir produces circumoral paresthesias during the initial weeks of therapy.

A major concern when administering PIs is the effect of these agents on the hepatic cytochrome P450 system. All PIs inhibit the metabolism of other agents by this system, with ritonavir being the most potent. As a result clearance of many medications, including antihistamines, tricyclic antidepressants, and opiates, is decreased, leading to elevated drug concentrations and, often, serious adverse effects (Tables 4 to 6). Conversely, the inhibition of this enzyme system by ritonavir has been used to enhance the concentration of other PIs. The most widely studied dual protease combination is that of ritonavir and saquinavir. Reduced daily doses of ritonavir, 400 mg every 12 hours, enables saquinavir to be given at lower dosages, 400 mg, at less frequent intervals, every 12 hours. This combination results

Table 4   Drugs That Should Not be Used with Protease Inhibitors*

DRUG CATEGORY	INDINAVIR	RITONAVIR	SAQUINAVIR (GIVEN AS INVIRASE OR FORTOVASE)	NELFINAVIR	ALTERNATIVES
Analgesics	(None)	Meperidine Piroxicam Propoxyphene	(None)	(None)	Aspirin Oxycodon Acetaminophen
Cardiac	(None)	Amiodarone Encainide Flecainide Propafenone Quinidine	(None)	(None)	Limited experience
Antimycobacterial	Rifampin	Rifabutin†	Rifampin Rifabutin	Rifampin	For rifabutin (as alternative for *Mycobacterium avium-intracellulare* treatment): clarithromycin, ethambutol (treatment, not prophylaxis), or azithromycin
Ca† channel blocker	(None)	Bepridil	(None)	(None)	Limited experience
Antihistamine	Astemizole Terfenadine	Astemizole Terfenadine	Astemizole Terfenadine	Astemizole Terfenadine	Loratidine
Gastrointestinal	Cisapride	Cisapride	Cisapride	Cisapride	Limited experience
Antidepressant	(None)	Bupropion	(None)	(None)	Fluoxetine Desipramine
Neuroleptic	(None)	Clozapine Pimazide	(None)	(None)	Limited experience
Psychotropic	Midazolam	Clorazepate Diazepam Estazolam Flurazepam Midazolam Triazolam Zolpidem	Midazolam Triazolam	Midazolam Triazolam	Temazepan Lorazepam
Ergot alkaloids (vasoconstrictor)	Dihydroergotamine (D.H.E. 45) ergotamine‡ (various firm)	Dihydroergotamine (D.H.E. 45) ergotamine‡ (various firm)	Dihydroergotamine (D.H.E. 45) ergotamine‡ (various firm)	Dihydroergotamine (D.H.E. 45) ergotamine‡ (various firm)	Limited experience

*The contraindicated drugs listed are based on theoretical considerations. Thus drugs with low therapeutic indexes yet with suspected major metabolic contribution from cytochrome P450CA, Cyp2D5, or unknown pathways are included in this table. Actual interactions may or may not occur in patients.
†Reduce rifabutin dosage to one quarter of standard dose.
‡This is likely a class effect.

in a dramatic increase in the plasma concentrations of saquinavir and provides a potent durable double PI regimen. Similar findings with the combination of ritonavir and indinavir have been reported. Amprenavir, the newest PI, appears to be as potent as the other PIs when used in combination with two NRTIs. Use of this PI is associated with a rash in 5% of patients. Nausea and headache, not uncommonly, also are reported.

Use of all PIs is associated with an increased prevalence of hypertriglyceridemia and hypercholesterolemia. A subset of patients also manifest fat redistribution with peripheral fat wasting, breast enlargement, and central fat deposition with development of a paunch, which results from increased visceral abdominal fat and occasionally a dorsocervical fat pad or "buffalo hump" in the absence of alteration in cortisol secretion. A smaller group of patients manifest overt insulin resistance with hyperglycemia and, less commonly, diabetes. All of these findings have been recognized in HIV-1–infected patients not receiving PIs but have been more commonly reported since the introduction of these agents. The mechanism of these changes currently is not known.

■ NEW CLASSES OF DRUGS

Adefovir (bis-POM, PMEA, PreveonR), a nucleotide analog that inhibits reverse transcriptase, was available through a

Table 5   Drug Interactions between Protease Inhibitors and Other Drugs

		DRUG INTERACTIONS REQUIRING DOSE MODIFICATIONS		
	INDINAVIR	**RITONAVIR**	**SAQUINAVIR***	**NELFINAVIR**
Fluconazole	No dosage change	No dosage change	No data	No dosage change
Ketoconazole and itraconazole	Decrease dosage to 600 mg q8h	Increases ketoconazole >3-fold; dosage adjustment required	Increases saquinavir levels 3-fold; no dosage change	No dosage change
Rifabutin	Reduce rifabutin to half dose: 150 mg qd	Consider alternative drug or reduce rifabutin dose to one quarter	Not recommnended with either Invirase or Fortovase	Contraindicated
Oral contraceptives	Modest increase in Ortho-Novum levels: no dosage change	Ethinyl estradiol levels decreased: use alternative or additional contraceptive method	No data	Ethinyl estradiol and norethindrone levels decreased; use alternative or additional contraceptive method
Miscellaneous	Grapefruit juice reduces indinavir levels by 26%	Desipramine increased 145%; reduce dosage Theophylline levels decreased; increase dosage	Grapefruit juice increases saquinavir levels†	

*Several drug interaction studies have been completed with saquinavir given as Invirase or Fortovase. Results from studies conducted with Invirase may not be applicable to Fortovase.
†Conducted with Invirase.

compassionate use protocol. It requires only two phosphorylation steps to become the active moiety that is effective in diverse cell populations. No cross-resistance to NRTIs has been documented. It is given once daily because of its long intracellular half-life, which favors patient adherence. It is also active against herpes virus and hepatitis B, common coinfections in HIV-1–infected patients. However, 40% of patients receiving this agent for 6 months or more develop evidence of a renal tubular deficit resembling Fanconi syndrome. These renal effects usually are reversible with discontinuation of therapy or dosage reduction. The company does not plan on further development of this agent.

With the evidence that establishment of HIV-1 infection requires interaction of the virus with a chemokine receptor in addition to CD4, interest in blocking adherence of the virus to cells has resurfaced. Early attempts to block viral attachment with administration of soluble CD4 failed. However, use of altered chemokines, the natural ligands for the chemokine receptors, inhibits the interaction of the virus with these receptors and may prove to offer an additional form of antiviral therapy. The transmembrane viral envelope protein, gp41, mediates fusion of the virus with the target cell and is responsible for entry of the viral RNA into the cell. The peptide T-20 blocks this interaction and is currently in phase 1 trials and appears to inhibit viral replication.

■ USE OF ANTIRETROVIRAL AGENTS AS PROPHYLAXIS

Chemoprophylaxis following occupational exposure is recommended by the Centers for Disease Control and Prevention. No trials have been completed to support these recommendations; however, a retrospective case-control study reported that administration of zidovudine after exposure was associated with an 80% reduction in risk of infection. The current recommendations are based on the concept that the risk of transmission varies with the clinical status of the infected patient.

The choice of agents used in prophylaxis should take into account the possibility of resistance. Specific recommendations are detailed in the chapter *Percutaneous Injury: Risks and Management*. At present, trials of chemoprophylaxis for sexual exposure are in progress but no findings are available. It may be prudent to provide prophylaxis to sexually exposed patients similar to that provided after a needlestick.

■ FURTHER PROBLEMS

A major problem with the currently available potent drug combinations is that they are less effective in patients who have received NRTI monotherapy or dual NRTI treatment for prolonged periods. Patients who have developed toxicities or have comorbidities that limit the use of some of the available agents also pose a challenge to the physician. Thus the clinician often must seek a therapy that is both effective and tolerated using agents from each of the three classes. One potentially promising new approach uses hydroxyurea. Hydroxyurea is a ribonucleotide reductase inhibitor, which depletes the intracellular substrate of the enzyme reverse transcriptase, enhancing the intracellular concentration of triphosphorylated ddI, the active form of the drug. Addition of hydroxyurea, 500 mg every 12 hours, is a strategy that appears to salvage ddI as a useful agent in some patients who have extensive experience with this agent.

Table 6 Drug Interactions: Protease Inhibitors and Nonnucleoside Reverse Transcriptase Inhibitors Effect of Drug on Levels/Dosage

DRUG AFFECTED	INDINAVIR	RITONAVIR	SAQUINAVIR*	NELFINAVIR	NEVIRAPINE	DELAVIRDINE	EFAVIRENZ
Indinavir (IDV)		No data	Levels: IDV no effect SQV 4-7× Dosage: no data	Levels: IDV 50% Dosage: No data	Levels: IDV↓ 28% Dosage: IDV, 1000 mg q8h	Levels: IDV↓ 150% Dosage: IDV, 600 mg q8h	Levels: IDV↓ 31% Dosage: IDV 1000 mg q8h
Ritonavir (RTV)	No data		Levels: RTV no effect SQV 20× Dosage: Invirase or Fortovase, 400 mg bid, + RTV, 400 mg bid	Levels: RTV no effect NFV 1.5× Dosage: no data	Levels: RTV↓ 11% Dosage: standard	Levels: RTV 70% Dosage: no data	Levels: RTV 18% Dosage: RTV, 600 mg bid (500 mg bid for intolerance)
Saquinavir (SQV)	Levels: SQV 4-7× IDV no effect Dosage: no data	Levels: SQV 20× RTV no effect Dosage: Invirase or, Fortovase, 400 mg bid, + RTV, 400 mg bid		Levels: SQV 3-5× NFV 20% Dosage: standard NFV Fortovase, 800 mg tid	Levels: SQV↓ 25% Dosage: no data	Levels: SQV 5× Dosage: standard for Invirase (monitor transaminase levels)	Levels: SQV ↓ 60% Coadministration not recommended
Nelfinavir (NFV)	Levels: NFV 80% IDV 50% Dosage: no data	Levels: NFV 1.5× RTV no effect Dosage: no data	Levels: NFV 20% SQV 3-5× Dosage: no data		Levels: NFV 10% Dosage: standard	Levels: NLV 2× DIV↓ 50% Dosage: standard (monitor for neutropenic complications)	Levels: NFV ↑ 26% Dosage: standard
Nevirapine (NVP)	Levels: IDV↓ 28% Dosage: standard	Levels: RTV↓ 11% Dosage: standard	Levels: SQV↓ 25% Dosage: no data	Levels: NFV 10% Dosage: standard		Do not use together	Coadministration not recommended
Delavirdine (DEV)	Levels: IDV 40% Dosage: IDV 600 q8h	Levels: RTV 70% Dosage: no data	Levels: SQV 5× Dosage: standard for Invirase; monitor transaminase levels	Levels: NFV 2× DIV↓ 50% Dosage: standard (monitor for neutropenic complications)	Do not use together		Coadministration not recommended
Efavirenz (EFV)	Levels: EFV no effect Dosage: standard	Levels: EFV 21% Dosage: standard	Levels: EFV↓ 2% Coadministration not recommended	Levels: EFV no effect Dosage: standard	Coadministration not recommended	Coadministration not recommended	

*Several drug interaction studies have been completed with saquinavir given as Invirase or Fortovase. Results from studies conducted with Invirase may not be applicable to Fortovase.

■ COMMENTS

Routine use of HAART has produced clinical benefit but is challenging for the patient and clinician. The increasing complexity of treatment regimens has required physicians to be more aware of drug-drug interactions, unusual adverse effects, and the need to monitor closely the virologic effectiveness of the treatment. The physician embarking on therapy with potent antiretroviral combinations must involve the patient in a thorough discussion of the necessity for adherence, possible adverse effects, and the potential benefits of treatment.

Suggested Reading

Carpenter CJ, et al: Antiretroviral therapy for HIV infection in 1998; recommendations of the IAS-USA panel, *JAMA* 280:78, 1998.

Detels R, et al: Effectiveness of potent antiretroviral therapy on time to AIDS and death in men with known HIV infection duration, *JAMA* 280:1497, 1998.

Henderson K: Postexposure chemoprophylaxis for occupational exposures to the human immunodeficiency virus, *JAMA* 281:931, 1999.

Lori F, et al: Long-term suppression of HIV-1 by hydroxyurea and didanosine, *JAMA* 1437, 1997.

Mellors JW, et al: Plasma viral load and CD4+ lymphocytes as prognostic markers of HIV-1 infection, *Ann Intern Med* 126:946, 1997.

Miller V, et al: Clinical experience with non-nucleoside reverse transcriptase inhibitors, *AIDS* 11(suppl A):S946, 1997.

Palella FJ Jr, et al: Declining morbidity and mortality among patients with advanced human immunodeficiency virus infection, HIV outpatient study investigation, *N Engl J Med* 338:853, 1998.

AIDS: THERAPY FOR OPPORTUNISTIC INFECTIONS

Tze Shien Lo

Harry Rosado-Santos

Merle A. Sande

This chapter discusses therapy of opportunistic infection in acquired immunodeficiency syndrome (AIDS). Recommendations for primary and secondary prophylaxis of opportunistic infection are found in a subsequent chapter.

■ *PNEUMOCYSTIS CARINII*

Pneumocystis carinii pneumonia (PCP) is a major cause of morbidity and mortality in AIDS patients. However, its incidence has been decreasing as a result of highly active antiretroviral therapy (HAART) as well as effective prophylaxis and therapy for PCP itself. The clinical manifestations of *P. carinii* infection are changing; extrapulmonary involvement and atypical pneumonitis are becoming more common.

For patients with mild to moderate disease or Pao_2 greater than 70 mm Hg, oral trimethoprim-sulfamethoxazole (TMP-SMX) remains the drug of choice (Figure 1). The major disadvantage of this regimen is its high incidence of adverse reactions in patients with AIDS. These reactions include fever, rash, nausea, azotemia, hepatitis, leukopenia, and thrombocytopenia. Rechallenge treatment with TMP-SMX may be attempted in patients who have mild adverse reactions. However, this drug should not be given to patients with a history of Stevens-Johnson syndrome, exfoliative dermatitis, or anaphylaxis caused by sulfa drugs. Concurrent use of TMP-SMX with another myelotoxic drug such as zidovudine or ganciclovir may cause severe bone marrow suppression. Complete blood counts (CBCs) and absolute neutrophil counts should be closely monitored if TMP-SMX is used concurrently with other myelotoxic drugs. Dapsone-trimethoprim and clindamycin-primaquine work about as well as TMP-SMX. These two combination regimens are contraindicated in patients with glucose-6-phosphate dehydrogenase (G6PD) deficiency. Dapsone and primaquine may cause methemoglobinemia, and monitoring of methemoglobin levels is required, especially in patients with marginal oxygenation. Other adverse effects of clindamycin-primaquine include rash, *Clostridium difficile* colitis, and diarrhea. Atovaquone is a well-tolerated oral drug; however, its variable absorption keeps response rates lower than those of TMP-SMX, and relapses are more common. Aerosol pentamidine may be useful in some cases. Aerosol pentamidine is not effective against extrapulmonary *P. carinii* infection, and parenteral administration may be necessary.

For patients with moderate to severe disease or Pao_2 less than 70 mm Hg or P(A-a) (arterial-alveolar gradient) greater than 35 mm Hg, intravenous TMP-SMX and pentamidine are therapeutic options (Figure 2). The administration of TMP-SMX requires a large volume of fluid (1 L/day) that may worsen respiratory distress. However, concurrent use of diuretics may alleviate volume overload. Pentamidine is comparable in efficacy with TMP-SMX.

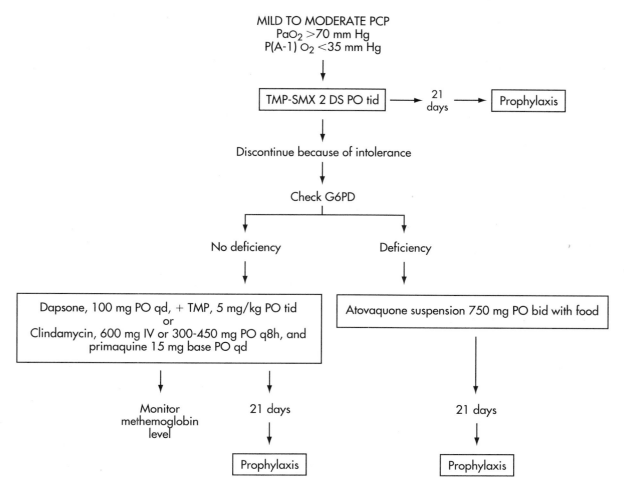

Figure 1
Algorithm for the treatment of mild to moderate *Pneumocystis carinii* pneumonia (PCP).

However, it is associated with more serious side effects such as nephrotoxicity, alteration of glucose metabolism, pancreatitis, neutropenia, thrombocytopenia, and hypotension. Thus its use is usually limited to patients who cannot tolerate TMP-SMX. Pentamidine is generally given via slow intravenous infusion because a more rapid rate may cause hypotension and arrhythmia. Alteration in glucose metabolism may result in either hyperglycemia or hypoglycemia, which are commonly seen in patients who develop concomitant renal toxicity. Blood glucose monitoring is required during therapy and for 2 weeks afterward. Clindamycin-primaquine and trimetrexate-leucovorin are alternative therapies for patients with moderately severe PCP.

A course of treatment for PCP is generally 21 days for any regimen. Survival and response of the patients depend on the severity of pulmonary dysfunction and tolerance to treatment. Clinical response to therapy generally occurs at the end of the first week. Treatment should not be considered to have failed unless there is no improvement after day 7 to day 10 or there is continued worsening after 5 days of treatment. Adverse drug reactions, which are common in

AIDS patients, tend to appear in the second week of therapy. If therapy must be changed, switching the regimen is preferred because adding a new drug is no more effective than using a single-drug regimen. During the first 5 days of treatment, patients with moderate to severe disease often deteriorate clinically or develop respiratory failure, presumably because of the inflammatory response to the damaged organisms in the lung. Adjunctive corticosteroid therapy has been shown to reduce this inflammatory response and to decrease mortality and the number of patients requiring respiratory support. Corticosteroid therapy should begin at the same time or within 1 or 2 days of initiation of treatment in patients with PCP who have PaO_2 less than 70 mm Hg or the A-a gradient greater than 35 mm Hg. Delaying corticosteroid therapy until after 72 hours has no clinical benefit and may be associated with an increased risk of other opportunistic infections. The recommended dosage of prednisone is 40 mg twice daily for 5 days, then 40 mg daily for 5 days, and 20 mg daily for 11 days. Adverse effects of corticosteroid use in this clinical setting are surprisingly few, but there is an increased incidence of thrush and reactivation of localized herpetic lesions.

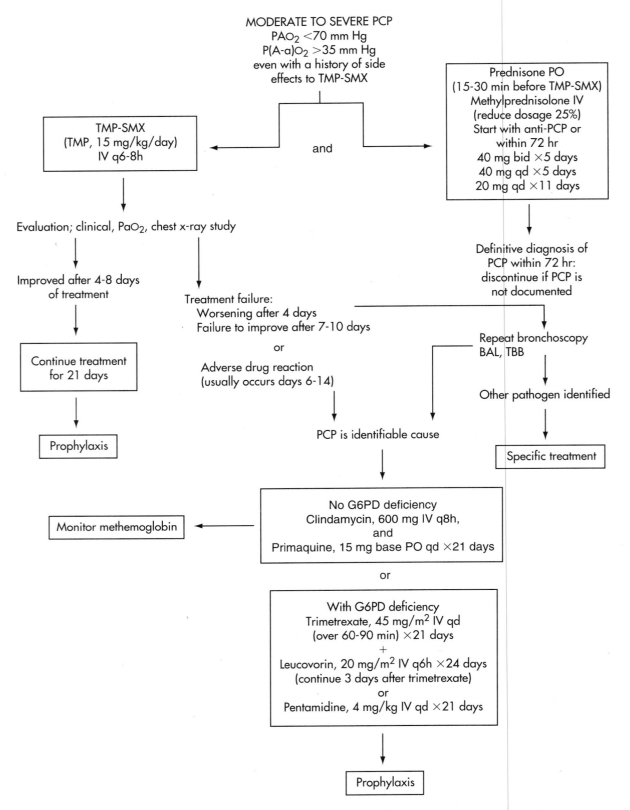

Figure 2
Algorithm for the treatment of moderate to severe PCP. *CXR,* Chest x-ray; *BAL,* bronchoal-veolar lavage; *TBB,* transbronchial biopsy; *PCP, Pneumocystis carinii* pneumonia.

■ TOXOPLASMOSIS

Toxoplasma gondii is the most common cause of central nervous system (CNS) infection in AIDS patients. The incidence is high in the Caribbean, Haiti, France, Germany, and the developing world. Toxoplasmosis is usually reactivation of infection. Positive *Toxoplasma* serology and a low CD4 count strongly predict a potential to develop *Toxoplasma* encephalitis. Infection may be acquired by exposure to a cat or by eating undercooked pork, mutton, or beef contaminated by the organisms. A presumptive diagnosis consists of the characteristic computed tomography (CT) or magnetic resonance imaging (MRI) findings, multiple enhancing mass lesions in more than one location, and a positive IgG antitoxoplasma titer above 1:64. Nevertheless, a solitary mass lesion on MRI study or a negative serology for antitoxoplasma antibody should not be used as an exclusion criterion. In suspected cases, a trial of antitoxoplasma treatment should be considered. Most patients show clinical improvement within 7 to 10 days. A patient who fails to respond or deteriorates after 1 week of therapy is a candidate for brain biopsy to rule out lymphoma or another infectious process.

Ninety percent of patients respond to the combination of pyrimethamine and sulfadiazine. The major disadvantage of this regimen is dose-related bone marrow suppression, which requires concomitant use of folinic acid. Folic acid must not be given because it will inhibit pyrimethamine activity. Patients who receive other myelosuppressive agents (i.e., zidovudine or ganciclovir) should have dosage modification and hematologic monitoring. Other adverse effects, including fever, rash, crystalluria, and hepatitis, usually develop within 7 to 10 days. An alternative regimen with comparable efficacy is pyrimethamine and folinic acid (as in primary regimen), plus either clindamycin, 600 mg orally or intravenously (PO/IV) every 6 hours; clarithromycin, 1 g PO twice a day; azithromycin, 1.2 to 1.5 g/day PO; dapsone, 100 mg/day PO. Although this regimen is associated with gastrointestinal disturbance, it has less hematologic toxicity than sulfadiazine plus pyrimethamine. Initial treatment should be continued for 6 weeks, then maintenance therapy should be continued indefinitely. Patients who present with seizures should also receive anticonvulsant drugs, at least during the initial treatment period. Patients with intracranial hypertension and impending herniation may need a short course of dexamethasone, 10 mg every 6 hours.

■ *MYCOBACTERIUM AVIUM* COMPLEX

Disseminated *Mycobacterium avium* complex (MAC) infection usually develops late in the course of human immunodeficiency virus (HIV) disease, when the CD4 cell counts are less than $100/mm^3$. MAC may be acquired via a gastrointestinal or respiratory route, as the organisms are ubiquitous in food, water, and soil. MAC infection usually accompanies other opportunistic infections; thus the patient's symptoms may be nonspecific.

The initial treatment regimens for MAC infection should include clarithromycin or azithromycin with ethambutol

Table 1 Treatment for Disseminated MAC
Clarithromycin, 500 mg PO bid
or
Azithromycin, 500 mg PO qd
plus
Ethambutol, 15-25 mg/kg/day PO
plus
Rifabutin, 300 mg PO qd
One or more of the following agents are recommended by some authorities to be added to the above three drugs:
Ciprofloxin, 750 mg PO bid
Amikacin, 7.5-15 mg/kg IV qd

and rifabutin (Table 1). Ciprofloxacin or amikacin may be added as a fourth drug. The goals of treatment are to reduce the symptoms and improve the quality of life. Effective MAC therapy may be needed for life because disseminated infection cannot be eradicated.

■ TUBERCULOSIS

The increasing incidence of tuberculosis (TB) is probably related to both reactivation of latent infection and rapid progression to symptoms after acquiring a new infection in HIV-infected patients. TB can spread rapidly through casual contact and respiratory droplets. The emergence of multidrug-resistant (MDR) organisms and an increased risk of nosocomial transmission have intensified the problem, and aggressive efforts are being made to control these outbreaks. Reinfection during treatment with MDR organisms is also reported. Purified protein derivative (PPD) skin tests in patients with early-stage HIV disease are likely to be reactive, and reaction of more than 5 mm of induration may indicate infection with *Mycobacterium tuberculosis*. In patients with advanced immunosuppression, anergy is more common, and a negative PPD skin test does not rule out TB. MDR TB is likely to be diagnosed in foreign-born patients, patients from areas where MDR TB has become a problem (New York, Florida), and patients who have a history of inadequate treatment. Patients with cavitary lesions also have a high frequency of MDR organisms because they harbor greater numbers of mycobacteria.

An initial four-drug regimen consisting of isoniazid (300 mg/day), rifampin (600 mg/day), pyrazinamide (15 to 25 mg/kg/day), and ethambutol (15 mg/kg/day) is recommended for the first 2 months. Isoniazid and rifampin should then be continued for a total of 9 months or at least 6 months beyond culture conversion. With an effective drug regimen and an adequate duration of chemotherapy, nearly all patients can be cured. Nevertheless, treatment may fail, usually because of noncompliance with the treatment regimen. Treatment may be complicated by frequent adverse drug reactions and drug interactions. Both isoniazid and rifampin may lower the serum levels of ketoconazole and fluconazole. Ketoconazole can interfere with the absorption of rifampin.

Treatment of MDR TB requires a five- or six-drug regimen based on the prevailing patterns of resistance. These regimens usually include the fluoroquinolones (ciprofloxacin or sparfloxacin or levofloxacin) and amikacin. See the chapter *Tuberculosis* for more details on therapy.

■ FUNGAL DISEASES

Cryptococcus neoformans

Cryptococcus neoformans is a common cause of life-threatening meningitis in AIDS patients. The disease is global because the fungus is ubiquitous in soil and bird excrement (pigeon droppings.) Cryptococcal infection is generally acquired via the respiratory route but may cause infection in any organ. The most common sites of infection are the meninges and brain. The mortality of patients diagnosed with cryptococcal meningitis is great in the first 2 to 6 weeks of therapy. Altered mentation (confusion, lethargy, obtundation), cranial nerve deficits, cerebrospinal fluid (CSF) cryptococcal antigen (CRAg) titers above 1:1024, and CSF white blood cell (WBC) counts below 20/mm^3 are risk factors associated with poor outcome.

Initial treatment for high-risk patients is slow intravenous infusion of amphotericin B, 0.7 to 1 mg/kg/day. The total dosage and length of amphotericin B depend on the clinical response of the patient. Generally, at least 1 to 2 weeks of administration is required. If there is definite clinical improvement after that, therapy may be switched to fluconazole, 400 mg/day for 8 to 10 weeks, or amphotericin may be continued to a total dose of 1.5 to 2.5 g over 6 to 8 weeks. Flucytosine (5-FC), 25 mg/kg every 6 hours, can be given in combination with amphotericin B for 2 weeks or until the patient is clinically stable, after which fluconazole may be given. This combined regimen is associated with an increase in myelosuppression, especially in patients with impaired renal function. Its value has yet to be clearly demonstrated. Adverse effects of amphotericin B include reversible impairment of renal function, hypokalemia, hypomagnesemia, anemia, fever with chills, nausea, and vomiting. Adequate hydration with saline and dosage modification of amphotericin B may alleviate renal toxicity. Amphotericin B should be discontinued if serum creatinine (Cr) is greater than 2.5 mg/dl and can be restarted after Cr drops below 1.5 mg/dl. Premedication with acetaminophen, antiemetics, potassium, and magnesium supplements may also be needed.

Fluconazole can be used as initial treatment in patients with moderate disease and normal mentation. The drug is well absorbed and penetrates well into the CSF. The recommended dosage is 400 mg/day orally for 6 to 10 weeks. Adverse effects of fluconazole are mainly gastrointestinal intolerance, rash, and impaired hepatic function. Fluconazole increases serum level of phenytoin, warfarin, and sulfonylureas, and its serum level may be lowered by rifampin and raised by thiazide. Fluconazole can be given in conjunction with flucytosine, 37.5 mg/kg every 6 hours orally for 10 weeks, as an alternative therapy.

Increased intracranial pressure may develop as an early or late complication of cryptococcal meningitis. Shunt placement should be considered in patients with noncommunicating hydrocephalus. Daily repeated lumbar puncture with removal of 15 to 30 ml of CSF may be required and is successful in reducing elevated intracranial pressure.

Serum and CSF CRAg titers often increase after initiation of antifungal treatment; however, the increased titers do not correlate with treatment failure. The serum CRAg titers often stabilize in the second month; thus the CRAg titer may be useful for monitoring the response of therapy. A stable or declined CRAg titer may indicate quiescent disease and a rise in titer with clinical evidence of disease, recrudescence of infection.

Fluconazole, 200 mg/day, is an effective and convenient regimen for maintenance therapy. Amphotericin B as a maintenance therapy has a high relapse rate and is associated with a significantly higher rate of drug toxicity and central venous catheter infections.

Figure 3 is an algorithm for the diagnosis and management of cryptococcal meningitis.

■ *CANDIDA* INFECTION

Oral and vaginal candidiasis are often seen as the CD4 count drops down to the 200 to 300/mm^3 range. Oral candidiasis (thrush) may indicate progression to AIDS and herald other opportunistic infections. Treatment with topical nystatin or clotrimazole troches for 10 to 14 days may be initially adequate. Recurrent infection is common, especially in patients who receive prolonged antibiotic medication. Oral fluconazole or itraconazole is used in recurrent cases or cases that fail to respond to topical therapy. Fluconazole is more effective and less toxic than ketoconazole and provides a longer disease-free period than clotrimazole. However, candidiasis that is unresponsive to fluconazole increases with prolonged azole use, especially in patients with very low CD4 counts. The correlation between in vitro resistance and fluconazole unresponsiveness is imperfect.

Candida esophagitis in AIDS patients may or may not accompany oral thrush. Empiric treatment with fluconazole, 200 mg PO on the first day, then followed by 100 mg/day for 14 days, or itraconazole oral solution, 200 mg PO/day or 100 mg PO twice a day for 14 days, may be given. If the patient improves with these regimens, chronic suppression with fluconazole, 100 mg PO per day or 100 to 150 mg PO per week, should be considered. If no clinical improvement occurs after 1 week, endoscopy should be performed to rule out other causes. If endoscopic findings confirm *Candida* infection while the patient is receiving oral drug therapy, parenteral amphotericin B, 0.5 mg/kg/day, or amphotericin B oral solution, 100 mg/ml (5 ml) PO four times a day, may be useful. Maintenance therapy consists of fluconazole, 100 mg PO per day or 100 mg to 150 mg PO per week for life, to prevent relapse.

Invasive *Candida* infection, or candidemia, is rare. It is associated with iatrogenic causes such as an indwelling catheter, prolonged use of broad-spectrum antibiotics, and drug-induced neutropenia. Amphotericin B is the drug of choice for systemic *Candida* infection. The dosage and duration of amphotericin B should match the immune status of the patients and the severity of the infection. Removal of the catheter is necessary in catheter-related candidemia. Fluconazole may be effective therapy in hepatosplenic and renal candidiasis in patients without neutropenia. A recent study has shown that fluconazole and amphotericin B are not significantly different in their effectiveness

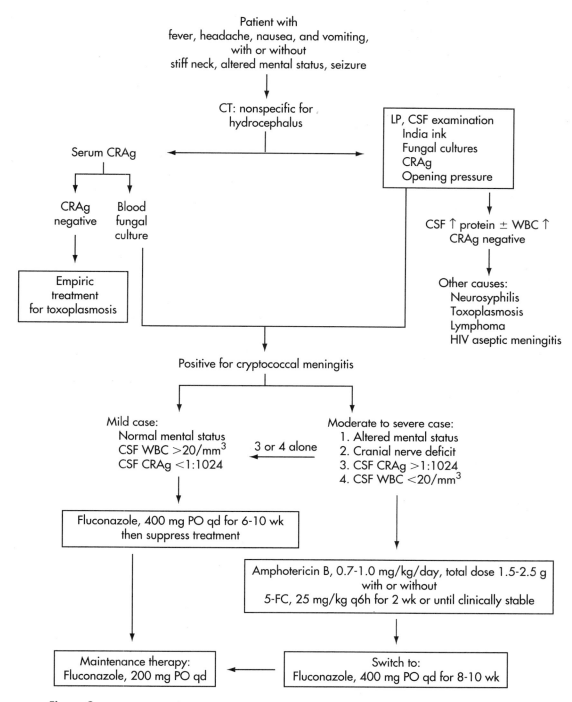

Figure 3
Algorithm for the diagnosis and treatment of cryptococcal meningitis. *CT,* Computed tomography; *CRA,* cryptoccal antigen; *LP,* lumbar puncture; *CSF,* cerebrospinal fluid; *WBC,* white blood cell count.

in treating candidemia of patients with neither neutropenia nor major immunodeficiency.

■ HISTOPLASMOSIS

The endemic areas of histoplasmosis are the Mississippi and Ohio River valleys, Puerto Rico, the Dominican Republic,

and Central and South America. AIDS patients who reside in or travel to the endemic areas may acquire the infection via inhalation of organisms from soil containing droppings of birds and bats.

Amphotericin B is the optimal initial therapy. The recommended regimens are parenteral amphotericin, B 0.5 to 1.0 mg/kg/day for 7 days, followed by a reduction to 0.8 mg/kg every other day (or three times a week). The goal of

Table 2 Treatment of Cytomegalovirus Infection

DRUG	ADVERSE EFFECTS	COMMENTS
Ganciclovir	Neutropenia, thrombocytopenia CNS: confusion, convulsion, psychosis, headache, dizziness GI: nausea, vomiting, diarrhea Others: abnormal LFT, rash, phlebitis	More convenient to administer during induction Avoid other myelotoxic drugs, e.g., AZT (consider ddI or d4T) Ganciclovir-resistant CMV may develop after 3 months of ganciclovir monotherapy
Foscarnet	Nephrotoxicity Electrolyte imbalance ↓ Ca, Mg, K ↓ or ↑ PO_4 (phosphate) Anemia Penile ulcer	Rapid IV infusion may cause fatal hypocalcemia, arrhythmia and seizure (need infusion pump); requires electrolyte supplement; Cr should be ≤2 mg/dl to start foscarnet; avoid other nephrotoxic drugs (e.g., amphotericin B, aminoglycoside, pentamidine)

CNS, Central nervous system; *GI,* gastrointestinal; *LFT,* liver function test; *AZT,* zidovudine; *ddI,* didanosine; *d4T,* stavudine; *CMV,* cytomegalovirus; *Cr,* creatinine.

amphotericin treatment is to reach a total dose of 10 to 15 mg/kg as rapidly as the patient can tolerate and then switch to therapy with itraconazole. Recent studies suggest that itraconazole may be as effective as amphotericin B as initial therapy. Maintenance therapy with itraconazole, 200 mg/day indefinitely, is necessary to prevent relapse.

■ COCCIDIOIDOMYCOSIS

Coccidioides immitis is an agent of mycosis endemic to the southwestern United States. A fungus, it exists in the soil and causes primary pulmonary infection via inhalation. Acquired or reactivated coccidioidal infection may develop early in the course of HIV disease. The treatment of choice is parenteral amphotericin B, 0.5 to 1.0 mg/kg/day for 7 days, followed by 0.8 mg/kg every other day, to reach a total dose of at least 2.5 g. Fluconazole, 400 to 800 mg PO per day for at least 9 months, also provides a good response in patients with coccidioidal meningitis. Itraconazole alone (200 mg PO twice a day) for 12 to 18 months appears to be effective for nonmeningeal coccidioidomycosis. Indefinite maintenance therapy is necessary with fluconazole, 400 mg/day, to prevent relapse (see the chapter *Coccidioidomycosis*).

■ VIRAL INFECTIONS

Cytomegalovirus

The clinical manifestations of cytomegalovirus (CMV) infection generally occur late in the course of HIV disease. Retinitis usually responds well to therapy; however, if left untreated, the disease may cause irreversible blindness. Response of other CMV infected sites is less predictable. CMV can be isolated from blood, urine, pulmonary secretions, and lung tissue in AIDS patients with other opportunistic infections such as PCP. These patients usually respond to therapy of PCP alone. CMV pneumonitis is extremely rare. Ganciclovir and foscarnet are the drugs of choice for treatment of CMV infection (Table 2). In addition to anti-CMV activity, both ganciclovir and foscarnet are active against herpes simplex virus (HSV) and varicella-zoster virus (VZV). Foscarnet is effective against ganciclovir-resistant CMV and has anti-HIV activity.

Initial treatment for CMV retinitis (Figure 4) consists of ganciclovir, 5 mg/kg infused over 1 hour twice a day; the dosage should be reduced in patients with impaired renal function. Ganciclovir is more convenient to administer than foscarnet and is therefore the first line of treatment for CMV disease. The major adverse effect of ganciclovir is myelosuppression. The dosage should be reduced when the absolute neutrophil count (ANC) falls below 1000/mm³ or discontinued when the ANC is less than 500/mm³ and platelet counts are less than 25,000/mm³. The drug can be restarted when the ANC rises above 750/mm³. Granulocyte colony–stimulating factor (G-CSF), 300 mg subcutaneously three times per week, may reverse ganciclovir-induced neutropenia. Concurrent use of other myelotoxic drugs (i.e., zidovudine, TMP-SMX) should be temporarily discontinued. Other adverse effects of ganciclovir include confusion, dizziness, headache, convulsion, nausea, vomiting, diarrhea, and abnormal liver function tests.

Foscarnet must be delivered by an intravenous infusion pump over a minimum of 1 hour. Rapid infusion of foscarnet may reduce the serum ionized calcium level because the drug chelates calcium. The initial dosage of foscarnet is 90 mg/kg every 12 hours for 14 to 21 days; again, the dosage should be reduced in patients with impaired renal function. Foscarnet, although generally free of myelotoxicity, is associated with renal and electrolyte disorders, especially in dehydrated patients. The drug may lower calcium, magnesium, and potassium levels and may cause hypophosphatemia or hyperphosphatemia. Thus it requires frequent monitoring of renal function and serum electrolytes. To minimize nephrotoxicity, prehydration or concurrent administration of isotonic saline should be given daily during therapy. Other nephrotoxic drugs (i.e., amphotericin B, aminoglycosides, pentamidine) should be interrupted if serum Cr is greater than 2.9 mg/dl and restarted if serum Cr is less than 2 mg/dl.

Duration of induction therapy for CMV retinitis is 14 to 21 days. The initial response rate for retinitis is approximately 80% to 90% with either ganciclovir or foscarnet therapy. Decrease in visual acuity caused by edema of the macula may improve with treatment, but visual-field deficits from damaged retina are not reversible. Relapse rates are extremely high. Because the drugs are virustatic against CMV, infection may continue to progress, and patients must receive long-term maintenance therapy. CMV esophagitis

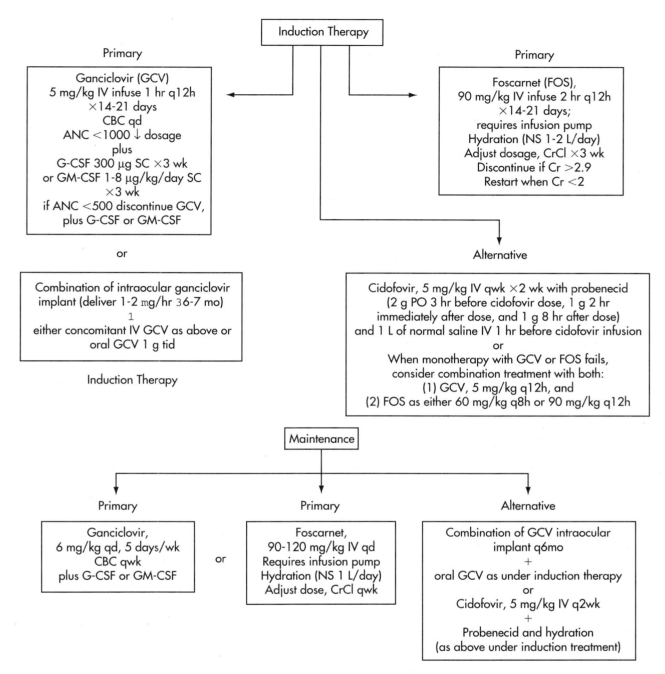

Figure 4

Algorithm for the treatment of cytomegalovirus retinitis. *CBC,* Complete blood count; *ANC,* absolute neutrophil count; *G-CFS,* granulocyte colony–stimulating factor; *GM-CSF,* granulocyte–macrophage colony stimulating factor; *Plt,* platelet count; *NS,* normal saline; *CrCl,* creatinine clearance.

and enterocolitis may or may not respond to ganciclovir or foscarnet treatment. CMV disease that is refractory to single-drug treatment with either ganciclovir or foscarnet may respond to a combination of these drugs. Toxicities between the two drugs do not overlap; lowering the dosages of these two agents may be possible, and associated toxicities may be reduced.

Maintenance therapy (see Figure 4) requires permanent installation of a central venous catheter to administer the drug. Maintenance therapy can be ganciclovir, 5 mg/kg/day 7 days a week or 6 mg/kg/day 5 days a week, or foscarnet, 90 to 120 mg/kg/day with 1.7 L/day of oral or intravenous hydration. Recent data have shown that foscarnet is effective and less toxic than ganciclovir, and it is the drug of choice for maintenance therapy. Oral ganciclovir is well tolerated, but its bioavailability is low. Ganciclovir-resistant CMV may develop, often after 3 months of continuous ganciclovir therapy; foscarnet is the drug of choice in this situation.

Table 3	Treatment of Herpes Simplex Infections
Mild mucocutaneous infection	ACV, 400 mg PO tid, *or* famciclovir, 250 mg PO tid, *or* valacyclovir, 1 g PO bid, all for 5-10 days
Severe mucocutaneous infection	ACV, 5.0 mg/kg q8h IV for 5-10 days, *or* foscarnet, 40 mg/kg q8h IV for 21 days, *or* ganciclovir, 5 mg/kg IV q12h for 5-10 days
Visceral organ infection	ACV, 10 mg/kg IV (1 h) q8h for at least 10 days, *or* foscarnet, 40 mg/kg q8h IV for 1 days, *or* ganciclovir, 5 mg/kg q12h for 5-10 days
Chronic prophylaxis	ACV, 400 mg PO bid or 200 mg PO tid, *or* foscarnet, 40 mg/kg IV qd, *or* famciclovir, 250-500 mg PO bid, *or* valacyclovir, 500 mg PO qd, all indefinitely

ACV, Acyclovir.

Table 4	Treatment of Varicella Virus
Shingles	ACV, 800 mg PO 5 times/day, *or* famciclovir, 500 mg PO tid, *or* valacyclovir, 1 gr PO tid, all for 7 days
Disseminated infection	ACV, 10-12 mg/kg IV (1 hr) q8h for 7-14 days
Primary infection	ACV, 10-12 mg/kg IV (1 hr) q8h for 7 days
ACV-resistant HSV	Foscarnet, 60 mg/kg IV bid for 14-26 days, *or* 40 mg/kg tid (2 hr) for 14-26 days

ACV, Acyclovir; *HSV,* herpes simplex virus.

Maintenance therapy may be indefinite but with immune reconstitution from HAART, some authorities now favor discontinuing viral suppression.

■ HERPES SIMPLEX VIRUS

HSV infection in HIV-infected patients commonly presents as recurrent orolabial, genital, and anorectal lesions. The frequency and severity of the disease depend on the degree of immunosuppression. In AIDS patients, reactivation of HSV is frequent and is associated with severe symptoms, including disseminated infections. HSV encephalitis is rare.

Mild HSV mucocutaneous infection is treated with acyclovir (ACV), 400 mg orally three times a day; famciclovir, 250 mg PO three times a day; or valacyclovir, 1 g PO two times a day for 5 to 10 days (Table 3). Local care of the lesion and topical antibiotic application are important for comfort and prevention of secondary infection. Clinical improvement should be observed within 1 to 2 weeks after therapy in ACV-sensitive HSV infection. However, recurrence often develops shortly after ACV is discontinued; thus oral ACV, 400 mg twice a day or 200 mg three times a day, may be required for maintenance. Oral ACV occasionally causes mild toxicities such as nausea, vomiting, and headache. In severe cases, ACV, 5 mg/kg intravenously (IV), may be infused over 1 hour every 8 hours for 5 to 10 days. A serious infection such as retinitis, esophagitis, or CNS infection may require a dosage of up to 10 mg/kg IV every 8 hours for at least 10 days. Most patients can tolerate intravenous ACV treatment, but phlebitis, nausea, hematuria, nephropathy, hypotension, and encephalopathy may develop. These toxicities are generally associated with renal insufficiency and high drug level in the plasma. Dosage adjustment is necessary for patients with impaired renal function. Other rare adverse effects of ACV that may be serious include CNS symptoms, confusion, tremor, delirium, psychosis, seizure,

and coma. Ganciclovir, 5 mg/kg IV every 12 hours for 5 to 10 days, can be given as an alternative in severe or extensive cases.

ACV-resistant HSV can emerge during ACV treatment, especially in large fungating anal ulcers, and can cause lesions refractory to therapy. These ACV-resistant HSV are usually sensitive to foscarnet. Foscarnet IV, 40 mg/kg every 8 hours for 21 days, can be given in ACV-resistant cases.

■ VARICELLA-ZOSTER VIRUS

HIV-infected patients are at increased risk for shingles or recurrent dermatomal varicella (VZV) infection at any time in the course of HIV disease. As with HSV, most adult AIDS patients usually have had primary VZV infection (chickenpox) and are not susceptible to primary infection. Primary infection disease may be more severe and complicated by disseminated visceral organ infection.

Shingles that are limited to one dermatome can be treated with ACV, 800 mg PO five times daily; famciclovir, 500 mg PO three times a day; or valacyclovir, 1 g PO three times a day for 7 days (Table 4). Patients with disseminated infection should be treated with ACV, 10 to 12 mg/kg IV infused over 1 hour every 8 hours for 7 to 14 days. Acyclovir treatment has been shown to reduce the duration of viral shedding, new lesion formation, and disseminated infection. ACV-resistant VZV may have characteristic findings of hyperkeratotic or nodular lesions that respond poorly to adequate doses of ACV therapy. ACV-resistant VZV calls for intravenous foscarnet (infuse over 2 hours), 40 mg/kg three times daily or 60 mg/kg twice daily for 14 to 26 days or until the lesions are completely healed. Primary VZV infection (chickenpox) can be treated with acyclovir, 10 to 12 mg/kg IV infused over 1 hour every 8 hours for 7 days.

Suggested Reading

Cohen PT, Sande MA, Volberding PA: *The AIDS knowledge base,* ed 3, Boston, 1999, Little, Brown.

Sande MA, Gilbert DN, Moellering RC: *The Sanford guide to HIV/AIDS therapy,* Hyde Park, 1999, Antimicrobial Therapy.

Sande MA, Volberding PA: *The medical management of AIDS,* ed 6, Philadelphia, 1999, Saunders.

THE PROPHYLAXIS OF OPPORTUNISTIC INFECTIONS IN HIV DISEASE

Evelyn J. Fisher

The use of infection prophylaxis has been a major advance in HIV disease. The Centers for Disease Control and Prevention (CDC) has recently published the 1999 update of the United States Public Health Service/Infectious Diseases Society of America guidelines for opportunistic infection prophylaxis in human immunodeficiency virus (HIV) disease. Currently, a major issue is the possibility of discontinuing prophylaxis if a sustained rise in CD4+ cell count has occurred in response to antiretroviral therapy. There are very little good data on this issue; some data are available for primary *Pneumocystis, Mycobacterium avium,* and to a lesser extent, secondary cytomegalovirus prophylaxis.

Primary prophylaxis is that given before development of an infection. The best known and most effective is trimethoprim-sulfamethoxazole (TMP-SMX) prophylaxis against *Pneumocystis carinii* pneumonia (PCP). TMP-SMX is 90% or more effective and is estimated to add a year to survival in late HIV disease. Other prophylaxes that are highly effective ($\geq$70% efficacy) have now become standard of care in HIV disease: prophylaxis against tuberculosis (TB) if there has been exposure or a positive tuberculin skin test, and against disseminated *Mycobacterium avium* (MAC) infection and toxoplasmosis.

Secondary prophylaxis is that given after acute treatment of an opportunistic infection to prevent or reduce the incidence of relapse. For some difficult-to-treat infections, this is more accurately called *maintenance* or *chronic suppressive therapy.* A common error of clinicians not experienced in HIV is to omit secondary prophylaxis. Secondary prophylaxis is optional only if (1) the infection is non–life-threatening, such as mucocutaneous herpes simplex or *Candida* esophagitis; (2) the patient refuses it; or (3) the patient cannot tolerate any prophylaxis regimen.

An outline of major primary prophylaxis decision points is presented in Table 1. Tables 2 and 3 list major primary and secondary prophylactic drugs, their indications, efficacy status, and dosages. Table 4 presents the major toxicities, drug interactions, and status of use in pregnancy.

■ *PNEUMOCYSTIS CARINII* PNEUMONIA

Primary and Secondary Prophylaxis

TMP-SMX is the drug of choice. TMP-SMX also is effective prophylaxis for toxoplasma and certain bacterial infections, particularly pneumonia. Dose-limiting toxicity (mainly rash

Table 1 Outline of Major Primary Prophylaxis Decision Points

All patients	TB prophylaxis if indicated (see Table 2 and text)
	Pneumococcal vaccine q5yr
	Hepatitis A (HAV) vaccine if HAV susceptible and hepatitis C (HCV)+
	PCP prophylaxis if indicated (see indications 2-5 in Table 2)
CD4 <200	Above plus add:
	PCP prophylaxis for all patients
CD4 <100	Toxoplasma prophylaxis if indicated (see Table 2)
CD4 <50	MAC prophylaxis

CD4, CD4+ T lymphocytes/μl; *TB,* tuberculosis; *PCP, Pneumocystis carinii* pneumonia; *MAC,* disseminated *Mycobacterium avium* complex.

or fever) occurs in 25% of patients taking one double-strength (DS) tablet daily, and in 10% of those taking one DS tablet three times weekly. Patients having mild reactions to TMP-SMX may sometimes be treated through the reaction with antihistamines. Patients who have had mild- to moderate (non–life-threatening) reactions to higher dosages of TMP-SMX can be rechallenged with a lower dosage—one single-strength (SS) tablet daily or one DS tablet three times per week—after the reaction has resolved; about 70% will tolerate the lower dosage. Because TMP-SMX is significantly more effective than the alternative PCP prophylaxes, oral desensitization to TMP-SMX may be considered (see Suggested Reading).

Efficacy is approximately equal for all the alternative PCP prophylaxis agents but is less than that of TMP-SMX. Dapsone (a sulfone used in leprosy treatment) is the cheapest and most convenient. It is tolerated by up to two thirds of those allergic to TMP-SMX. It should be avoided, however, if the patient has had a severe TMP-SMX reaction (exfoliation or erythema multiforme). Ideally, the clinician should test for glucose-6-phosphate-dehydrogenase (G6PD) deficiency before dapsone use, although severe hemolysis is rare in North American populations. Dapsone requires gastric acid for absorption; hence attention to drug interactions is critical. The value of attempting to increase the efficacy of dapsone by adding a second drug (particularly if breakthrough PCP has occurred) is as yet unproved but may be tried. Second drugs being added to dapsone include atovaquone, pyrimethamine, trimethoprim, or aerosol pentamidine.

Atovaquone suspension has the advantages of a lack of cross-reactivity with sulfas and dapsone, and efficacy for toxoplasmosis prophylaxis. Disadvantages include the inconvenience of a liquid and high cost.

Aerosolized pentamidine is rarely used these days except in patients who cannot tolerate any of the oral drugs. Its disadvantages include expense, inconvenience, lack of prevention of toxoplasmosis or extrapulmonary pneumocystis, and risk of TB transmission (as a result of cough during treatment). About half of patients require pretreatment and sometimes posttreatment bronchodilator therapy (e.g., inhaled albuterol) to prevent bronchospasm and cough. Patients with negative toxoplasma IgG antibodies should be

Table 2 Primary Prophylaxis

INFECTION	INDICATION	EFFICACY STATUS	REGIMENS DRUG/DOSAGE
Pneumocystis carinii pneumonia (PCP)	1. CD4 <200 µl 2. Thrush 3. Chemotherapy 4. Consider for CD4 percent <14% 5. Consider if prior AIDS-defining illness	Proved—standard of care	Trimethoprim-sulfamethoxazole (TMP-SMX) DS 160/800 mg/day or three times/week TMP-SMX SS, 80/400 mg/day
		Proved	Dapsone, 100 mg/day Atovaquone suspension, 1500 mg/day Aerosolized pentamidine, 300 mg q1mo
		Possible	IV pentamidine, 4 mg/kg q2-4wk
Tuberculosis (TB)	1. Positive tuberculin skin test (PPD) 2. History of positive PPD without prior prophylaxis 3. Recent exposure to active TB	Proved—standard of care	Isoniazid (INH), 300 mg, with pyridoxine, 50 mg/day for 9 mo (or for directly observed prophylaxis: INH, 900 mg with pyridoxine, 100 mg two times per week) Rifampin suspension, 600 mg/day plus pyrazinamide (PZA), 20 mg/kg/day for 2 mo
	Alternative for INH intolerance, or exposure to INH-resistant, but rifampin-sensitive, TB	Probable	Rifabutin, 300 mg/day plus pyrazinamide (PZA), 20 mg/kg/day for 2 mo Rifampin suspension, 600 mg/day for 4 mo
	Alternative: For exposure to TB resistant to both INH and rifampin	Unknown Unknown	Rifabutin, 300 mg/day for 4 mo Two- or three-drug regimen for 6 mos: Pyrazinamide (PZA), 1.5 g/day, *plus* ethambutol, 15-25 mg/kg/day, ± *either* ofloxacin, 400 mg bid *or* ciprofloxacin, 750 mg bid
Disseminated *Mycobacterium avium* (MAC)	CD4 <50/µl	Proved—standard of care	Azithromycin, 1200 mg qwk Clarithromycin, 500 mg PO bid
		Proved	Rifabutin, 300 mg/day
Toxoplasma	CD4 <100/µl and *Toxoplasma* IgG antibody positive	Proved—standard of care	TMP-SMX DS, 160/800 mg/day
		Probable	TMP-SMX SS, 80/400 mg/day or TMP-SMX DS three times/weekly Dapsone, 50-100 mg/day *plus* pyrimethamine, 50 mg weekly, with leukovorin, 25 mg/wk
		Possible	Atovaquone suspension, 1500 mg/day, pyrimethamine, 25 mg/day, with leukovorin, 10 mg/day
Cytomegalovirus (CMV)	CD4 <50/µl and CMV IgG antibody positive	Uncertain—not routinely recommended	Oral ganciclovir, 1 g tid

CD4, CD4+ cell count; *DS*, double-strength; *SS*, single-strength.
*Do not use rifampin if patient is using a protease inhibitor or nonnucleoside reverse transcriptase inhibitor; substitute a rifabutin-containing regimen, with appropriate rifabutin dosage modification (see footnote to Table 4).

retested when their CD4+ cell count falls below 100 cells/µl so that toxoplasmosis prophylaxis can be added if they have seroconverted.

Discontinuation of primary PCP prophylaxis may be considered for patients whose CD4+ cell count has risen to greater than 200 cells/µl and remained in that range for at least 3 to 6 months. Sustained reduction in viral load for that time would be an additional criterion. Resumption of prophylaxis is currently recommended when the CD4+ cell count falls to less than 200 cells/µl. Data are inadequate at this time regarding any discontinuation of secondary PCP prophylaxis.

Table 3   Secondary Prophylaxis = Chronic Maintenance/Suppression

INFECTION	INDICATED INDEFINITELY	EFFICACY	DRUG/DOSAGE
PCP	Yes*	Proved	Same as primary
Disseminated *Mycobacterium avium* complex (MAC)	Yes*	Proved	Continue acute treatment indefinitely; for example, clarithromycin, 500 mg PO bid, *plus* ethambutol, 15-25 mg/kg/day, *with or without* rifabutin, 300 mg/day, or fluoroquinolone
Toxoplasma	Yes	Proved	Sulfadiazine, 500 mg q6h, *plus* pyrimethamine, 50 mg/day, with leucovorin, 10 mg/day (also covers PCP prophylaxis)
		Probable, somewhat less effective	Clindamycin, 300-450 mg qid, *plus* pyrimethamine, 50 mg/day, with leucovorin, 10 mg/day
		Possible	Atovaquone, 750 mg bid-qid, with or without pyrimethamine, 50 mg/day, with leucovorin, 10 mg/day
Herpes simplex	Only if frequent/severe recurrences	Proved	Acyclovir, 400 mg bid, or famciclovir, 500 mg bid
		Probable	Valacyclovir, 500 mg bid
Candida esophagitis	Only if frequent/severe recurrences	Proved	Fluconazole, 100-200 mg/day
		Probable	Itraconazole oral solution, 200 mg/day (use if fluconazole resistance is suspected); itraconazole capsule, 200-400 mg/day; or ketoconazole, 200-400 mg/day
Cryptococcus	Yes	Proved	Fluconazole, 200-400 mg/day
		Proved, but less effective	Itraconazole, 200 mg bid
Cytomegalovirus (CMV)	Yes for retinitis,* need unpredictable for other CMV disease	Proved	Ganciclovir IV, 5 mg/kg/day; foscarnet IV, 90-120 mg/kg/day (120 mg more effective); or oral ganciclovir, 1-1.5 g tid
		Proved for retinitis	Ganciclovir eye implant intravitreally q6-9 mo with oral ganciclovir, 1-1.5 g tid
		Alternative for retinitis	Cidofovir, 5 mg/kg IV q2wk, with probenecid, 2 g 2 hr before dose and 1 g at 2 hr and 8 hr after the dose
Histoplasma	Yes	Proved	Itraconazole capsule, 200 mg bid
Coccidioides	Yes	Probable	Fluconazole, 400 mg/day
Aspergillus	Yes	Probable	Itraconazole capsule, 200 mg bid
Salmonella bacteremia	Often—use for at least several months	Probable, drug of choice	Ciprofloxacin, 500 mg bid
		Alternative	Trimethoprim-sulfamethoxazole DS, 160/180 mg PO bid

PCP, Pneumocystis carinii pneumonia; *DS,* double-strength.
Note: All drugs are oral unless otherwise stated.
*See text for discussion of possible discontinuation during period of CD4+ cell rebound.

■ TOXOPLASMA (TOXO)

Primary Prophylaxis

Patients with CD4 cells less than 100/μl and IgG toxo antibodies run a one-third risk of developing cerebral toxoplasmosis. About 15% to 30% of HIV-infected persons in North America are toxo seropositive. Toxo prophylaxis is now a standard of care for these people. TMP-SMX DS, one tablet daily, has been shown effective; the efficacy of TMP-SMX DS three times per week or once SS daily is likely. Alternatives to TMP-SMX include (1) dapsone plus pyrimethamine and (2) atovaquone. Dapsone should be avoided after life-threatening sulfa reactions. If toxoseropositive patients are receiving aerosolized pentamidine, toxo coverage must be added in the form of atovaquone with or without pyrimethamine.

Table 4 Major Toxicities, Drug Interactions, and Use in Pregnancy

ANTIMICROBIAL AGENT	MAJOR ADVERSE REACTIONS	MAJOR DRUG INTERACTIONS: EFFECT ON DRUG ACTIVITY	USE IN PREGNANCY*
Acyclovir	GI + renal at high dosage		Yes (C)
Atovaquone	Rash, often clearing on treatment, diarrhea	Decreased by rifampin and metoclopramide	No data (C)
Azithromycin	GI upset, rarely hepatitis,	See *Clarithromycin* (azithromycin interacts less than clarithromycin)	Yes, preferred over clarithromycin (B)
Cidofovir (given with probenecid)	Major nephrotoxicity; neutropenia, metabolic acidosis, ocular hypotony Probenecid: rash, nausea, fever	Cidofovir: increased nephrotoxicity with other drugs causing same Probenecid: increases AZT, ACE inhibitors, acetaminophen, NSAIDs, benzodiazepines, theophylline, and others	Avoid if possible, teratogenic at low dosages in animals (C)
Ciprofloxacin	GI upset, photosensitivity	Increases theophyllin Absorption decreased by antacids, ddI, sucralfate, iron, magnesium, zinc	Probably safe (no human arthropathy reported) (C)
Clarithromycin	GI upset, rarely hepatitis	Increases cisapride (potential cardiac arrhythmias), rifabutin (increased uveitis), and carbamazepine	No data, animal teratogen (C)
Clindamycin	GI upset, *Clostridium difficile* colitis, rash in 20% of HIV patients (often can treat through)		Yes (B)
Dapsone	Rash, fever, hepatitis, anemia, especially with G6PD deficiency; methemoglobinemia	Decreased by rifampin and antacid drugs (H_2 blockers, ddI buffer)	Yes (C)
Ethambutol	GI upset, optic neuritis, elevated uric acid	Decreased by aluminum antacids—give 2 hr apart	Yes (B)
Famciclovir	Nausea, headache		Yes, but acyclovir preferred because of greater experience (B)
Fluconazole	GI upset, rash, rarely hepatitis	Decreased by rifampin, increases cisapride (cardiac arrhythmias), rifabutin (uveitis), carbamazepine, phenytoin, sulfonylurea hypoglycemics, warfarin	Avoid if possible: a few cases of fetal abnormalities reported after prolonged use at dosages ≥400 mg/day (C)
Foscarnet	Nephrotoxicity; decreased calcium, potassium, magnesium; nausea, anemia; rarely mucosal ulcers	Increased nephrotoxicity with other drugs causing same; increased hypocalcemia with pentamidine	If absolutely necessary (C)
Ganciclovir	Neutropenia, fatigue, some decrease in renal function	Increased neutropenia with other drugs causing same; increases ddI levels	No (marked embryo toxicity in animals) (C)
INH	Peripheral neuropathy, hepatitis, CNS effects	Increases carbamazepine (and vice versa), disulfiram, phenytoin, absorption decreased by aluminum antacids	Yes (N/A)
Itraconazole	GI upset, rash, rarely hepatitis; occasional hypertension and hyperkalemia with high dosages	Absorption decreased by antacids, ddI, and sucralfate; see *Fluconazole* for other important interactions	Avoid if possible, based on fluconazole data (C)
Ketoconazole	Adrenocortical and sex hormone suppression, with high dosages; rarely hepatitis	Absorption decreased by antacids, ddI, and sucralfate; see *Fluconazole* for other	Avoid if possible, based on fluconazole data (C)

Table 4 Major Toxicities, Drug Interactions, and Use in Pregnancy—cont'd

ANTIMICROBIAL AGENT	MAJOR ADVERSE REACTIONS	MAJOR DRUG INTERACTIONS: EFFECT ON DRUG ACTIVITY	USE IN PREGNANCY*
Ofloxacin: See *Ciprofloxacin*			
Pentamidine, aerosol	Bronchospasm, cough		Yes: no data, but systemic absorption minimal
Pentamidine IV	Hypoglycemia, nephrotoxicity, hypotension, pancreatitis, hypocalcemia	Increased nephrotoxicity with other drugs causing same; increased hypocalcemia with foscarnet	No animal data (C)
Pyrazinamide (PZA)	Hepatitis, elevated uric acid	Decreased markedly by zidovudine (AZT)	Avoid if possible: no animal data (C)
Pyrimethamine	GI upset, neutropenia, anemia, hemolysis with G6PD deficiency	Increased bone marrow suppression when used with other antifolates	Yes‡ (C)
Rifabutin	Uveitis, neutropenia, orange urine	Increased by protease inhibitors (PIs), clarithromycin and fluconazole (leading to more uveitis)—reduce dosage with PI†; decreased by certain NNRTI—may need to increase dosage†; decreases NNRTI delavirdine—avoid concomitant use	Yes (B)
Rifampin	Hepatitis, rash, orange urine	Markedly decreases protease inhibitor, NNRTI, and atovaquone—avoid rifampin, substitute rifabutin; decreases oral azoles, contraceptives, hypoglycemics, dapsone, methadone, phenytoin, warfarin	Yes (C)
Trimethoprim-sulfamethoxazole (TMP-SMX) and sulfadiazine	Nausea, rash, fever, hepatitis, neutropenia, photosensitivity, nephrotoxicity; hemolysis with G6PD deficiency	TMP-SMX increases warfarin	Yes (C)

GI, Gastrointestinal; *ACE,* angiotensin-converting enzyme; *NSAIDs,* nonsteroidal antiinflammatory drugs; *ddI,* didanosine; *HIV,* human immunodeficiency virus; *G6PD,* glucose-6-phosphate-dehydrogenase; *CNS,* central nervous system; *NNRTI,* nonnucleoside reverse transcriptase inhibitor (nevirapine, efavirenz, delavirdine).

*FDA Pregnancy category: B, Animal studies indicate no fetal risk but there are no human studies, *or* animal studies show fetal risk, but adequate studies in pregnant women have shown no adverse effects, including in the first trimester. C, Animal studies demonstrate fetal risk but there are no human trials, *or* neither human nor animal studies are available. D, Evidence exists for fetal risk in humans, but benefit may outweigh risk.

N/A, Not available (drug approved before requirement for such testing).

Yes, Category B; or Category C where there has been sufficient experience to say that if fetal risk exists, it must be very low. *If necessary,* Insufficient experience, but drug is theoretically safer than alternative. *No data,* Insufficient experience; may need to be used if disease is serious.

†Reduce rifabutin dosage to 150 mg/day for use with the protease inhibitors (PIs) amprenavir, indinavir, nelfinavir, or saquinavir; use rifabutin 150 mg qod with the PI ritonavir. Rifabutin dosage is increased to 450 mg/day when used with the nonnucleoside reverse transcriptase inhibitor (NNRTI) efavirenz, and possibly also with the NNRTI nevirapine.

‡Consider deferral of pyrimethamine for primary toxoplasma patients until after pregnancy.

Secondary Prophylaxis

About half of the full treatment dose of sulfadiazine and pyrimethamine is most commonly used, and this regimen also provides PCP prophylaxis. For sulfa-intolerant patients, clindamycin at higher dosages plus pyrimethamine is usually effective but does not cover PCP. There are considerably fewer data for high-dose atovaquone suspension with or without pyrimethamine; this regimen would provide PCP prophylaxis.

■ FUNGAL INFECTIONS

Primary Prophylaxis

Primary prophylaxis of *Candida* esophagitis and cryptococcal disease (mainly meningitis) is not recommended, despite efficacy, because of concerns about drug resistance, drug interactions, lack of survival benefit, and cost. *Candida* strains resistant to the oral azole antifungal drugs, seen mainly in patients with CD4+ cells less than 100/µl, are difficult to treat. In areas highly endemic for histoplasma or coccidioides, disseminated disease resulting from these soil fungi may account for 25% of opportunistic infections. In such areas, the possibility of prophylaxis should be discussed with patients. Itraconazole is used for histoplasma, and fluconazole is used for coccidioides.

Secondary Prophylaxis

For cryptococcus suppression, fluconazole is more effective than amphotericin B. For patients intolerant to fluconazole, itraconazole, 400 mg/day, can be used, although it is probably less effective. *Candida* suppression may be considered if recurrences are very frequent or severe, but Candida resistance remains a threat. For histoplasma suppression, itraconazole, 200-mg capsule twice daily is used; for coccidioides suppression, fluconazole, 400 mg/day.

■ *MYCOBACTERIUM AVIUM* COMPLEX

Primary Prophylaxis

Disseminated MAC occurs in 30% or more of persons with AIDS, almost always when the CD4+ cell count is less than 50/μl. It causes extreme fever, rigors, drenching night sweats, anemia, and severe wasting. Weekly azithromycin is most commonly used because of the low pill burden and lower likelihood of drug interactions. If there is gastrointestinal (GI) intolerance to the single 1200-mg dose of azithromycin, the drug may be given as 600 mg twice daily once a week. In the face of severe nausea, some clinicians are giving 500 or 600 mg three times per week or even 250 mg daily, but only anecdotal data exist for this dosing. Clarithromycin is the second choice; rifabutin is generally used only if the azalides cannot be used. It is important to rule out active MAC or TB infection before starting these drugs in symptomatic individuals.

Two recent trials indicated that in patients experiencing CD4 rebound while receiving anti-HIV therapy, primary MAC prophylaxis can be withheld so as long as CD4+ cells remain greater than 100/μl.

Secondary Prophylaxis

Treatment is continued for life with clarithromycin (alternative, azithromycin) and ethambutol, preferably with a third drug. Rifabutin is generally used as the third drug; alternatively, fluoroquinolones, such as ciprofloxacin, may be used. Clofazimine is no longer used.

■ TUBERCULOSIS

Primary Prophylaxis

There is no other medical condition that so predisposes to the development of active TB as does HIV infection. In tuberculin-positive patients, the risk of active TB is 5% to 10% per year for HIV-positive patients versus 5% to 10% per lifetime for HIV-negative persons.

Indications include the following:

- Positive tuberculin skin test (PPD ≥5 mm)
- History of positive tuberculin test

- Recent contact with active TB case (social or nosocomial) (Note: Prophylaxis must be given after any significant exposure, even if patient has previously received TB prophylaxis, because TB reinfection can occur.)

Either 9 months of isoniazid (INH) or 2 months of two drugs (rifampin or rifabutin plus pyrazinamide) is used. The short course is less often used in HIV-infected persons because of the drug interaction potential with antiretroviral therapy. Rifampin cannot be used with protease inhibitors or nonnucleoside reverse transcriptase inhibitors; the rifabutin dosage must be altered with these drugs. INH can be used twice weekly in a directly observed prophylaxis setting.

The value of prophylaxis for high-risk anergic persons (e.g., institutionalized persons, persons from developing countries) has not been established.

It is critical to rule out active TB before starting prophylaxis. Chest radiographs are sufficient for asymptomatic patients. If chest x-ray results show parenchymal infiltrate, intrathoracic nodes, or fibrotic scarring, three sputum cultures should be obtained. If there is no other explanation for infiltrate, the clinician should start the patient on full four-drug treatment for TB. After 2 months of treatment, if cultures are negative and chest radiographic findings are unchanged, the drugs may be discontinued. If the patient has received rifampin (or rifabutin) plus pyrazinamide for 2 months, the patient will have completed the short-course prophylaxis regimen and needs no further prophylaxis.

Secondary Prophylaxis

After a full course of therapy for TB, no chronic suppressive therapy is needed. Treatment of TB in HIV patients results in very high cure rates *if* the organism is drug sensitive and the patient compliant. However, when TB treatment is suboptimal, relapse rates are significantly higher in HIV than non-HIV patients. Therefore, it is critical that all HIV-infected persons receive directly observed therapy for tuberculosis.

■ VARICELLA-ZOSTER

No prophylaxis has been shown effective for zoster. Varicella-zoster virus (VZV)–susceptible persons (those who have not had chickenpox or shingles or who lack VZV antibodies) should receive VZV immunoglobulin (VZIG) within 4 days after close contact with a person who has chickenpox or shingles.

■ HERPES SIMPLEX

Primary Prophylaxis

Technically, primary prophylaxis is not used for herpes simplex because chronic suppression is used only in patients who have a history of herpes outbreaks.

Secondary Prophylaxis

The options for secondary prophylaxis are suppression versus re-treating each episode. Acyclovir is preferable because of its relatively low cost. Famciclovir and valacyclovir offer no dosing advantage in the usual twice-daily prophylaxis regimens. Valacyclovir at very high dosages in a trial of CMV prophylaxis was associated with an unexplained trend to increased mortality. In very late disease, chronic suppression is usually necessary, often at higher dosages. Large, partially treated mucocutaneous herpetic ulcers promote development of acyclovir-resistant herpes. Efforts should be made to avoid this situation by giving dosages of acyclovir high enough to keep ulcers healed. Acyclovir dosages of up to 800 mg five times per day may be used. If these dosages do not work, acyclovir resistance is likely, necessitating therapy with intravenous cidofovir or foscarnet.

■ CYTOMEGALOVIRUS

Primary Prophylaxis
CMV disease, mainly retinitis and gastrointestinal, is diagnosed in about 10% to 25% of AIDS patients, almost always when the CD4+ cell count is less than $50/\mu l$. Those with CMV IgG antibodies are at risk. Prophylaxis with oral ganciclovir is not routinely recommended for several reasons, including conflicting reports of efficacy, drug toxicity, pill burden, and cost.

Secondary Prophylaxis
Our current CMV drugs slow down, but do not halt, progression of CMV retinitis. Higher dosages of ganciclovir or foscarnet may be needed later in the course of disease. For ganciclovir, maintenance dosages of up to 7.5 mg/kg day, or 5 to 7.5 mg/kg every 12 hours, have been used, generally with granulocyte colony–stimulating factor support. With foscarnet, single daily maintenance doses of greater than 120 mg/kg/day cannot be used, but the induction doses of 90 mg/kg every 12 hours can be maintained if tolerated. The combination of ganciclovir and foscarnet is synergistic. Dosages of both these drugs must be altered if renal function is abnormal. In other forms of CMV disease, such as GI, "CMV wasting syndrome" (viremia, fever and weight loss), hepatitis, and pneumonia, some clinicians discontinue suppression if there has been a good response to acute treatment because apparent spontaneous remissions may occur. Cidofovir is less often used because of nephrotoxicity.

Initial studies suggest that oral ganciclovir is effective for suppression of CMV retinitis, with no significant difference between intravenous (IV) and oral administration. Because blood levels are lower with oral administration, the theoretical concern remains that the oral drug may prove in the long run to be less effective or lead to more resistance than with the IV route. Nevertheless, oral administration is clearly more convenient and avoids the risks of indwelling IV access. Use of the ganciclovir ocular implant should also be considered.

Discontinuation of secondary prophylaxis (chronic suppression) for CMV retinitis is sometimes possible in patients experiencing CD4 cell rebound if the following conditions are met: CD4 cell count greater than 100 to $150/\mu l$ for more than 3 to 6 months, durable HIV viral load suppression, non–sight-threatening lesion, adequate vision in the other eye, and ability to undergo regular ophthalmologic examinations.

■ BACTERIAL INFECTIONS

Primary and Secondary Prophylaxis
The administration of pneumococcal vaccine as soon as feasible after HIV diagnosis is recommended. Revaccination every 5 years is currently suggested. Because vaccine efficacy is less when CD4 cells are low, revaccination may be given to patients initially vaccinated when CD4 were less than $200/\mu l$ who are now experiencing a CD4 count rebound to greater than 200 as a result of anti-HIV therapy. Although the use of TMP-SMX (for PCP prophylaxis) and azithromycin or clarithromycin (for MAC prophylaxis) may reduce bacterial respiratory infections, they are not used solely for such purposes because of concerns about drug resistance. Patients with severe neutropenia may be treated with granulocyte colony–stimulating factors; prophylactic antibiotics are not used for neutropenia in HIV disease.

Suggested Reading
Centers for Disease Control and Prevention: 1999 USPHS/IDSA guidelines for the prevention of opportunistic infections in persons infected with human immunodeficiency virus: U.S. Public Health Service (USPHS) and Infectious Diseases Society of America (IDSA), *MMWR* 48 (RR19):i, 1, 1999. Web site at www.hivatis.org.

INFECTIONS IN PATIENTS WITH NEOPLASTIC DISEASE

Donald Armstrong

Patients with neoplastic disease and suspected infection come to the physician with two main factors to be considered in their evaluation: their epidemiologic background and their immune defect or defects. The febrile cancer patient raises the question whether the fever is caused by the neoplasm. After evaluation, the next question is whether to treat empirically. In this chapter, I outline an approach to these patients, stressing the individuality of each patient along with the complexity of the evaluation.

■ EPIDEMIOLOGY

People may be exposed to a variety of organisms through travel, work, habits, or hobbies; in the home; or in other hospitals. The right questions must be asked about their background. A person with children at home is likely to be exposed to a number of infectious agents such as respiratory syncytial virus, varicella-zoster virus, and cytomegalovirus (CMV). Hospitals are a rich source of antibiotic-resistant organisms such as methicillin-resistant *Staphylococcus aureus* and vancomycin-resistant *Enterococcus,* and it is important to know where an individual has been hospitalized and what resistance patterns are known to inhabit that hospital.

With a thorough knowledge of the epidemiologic background of the patient, and therefore clues to possible causes of fever, the physician can direct investigation or start empiric therapy accordingly. The next step is to turn to the immune defect or defects (Table 1) to direct further evaluation or empiric therapy. The organisms that must be considered in empiric therapy are listed in Table 1, but with hospitalized patients, the organisms may be specific to the hospital. A regimen appropriate for one hospital may not be appropriate for another.

■ NEUTROPHIL DEFECT

The most common neutrophil defect encountered in patients with malignancy is an absolute neutropenia following cytotoxic chemotherapy. When doing the history and physical examination and evaluating laboratory (e.g., x-ray examination) results, keep in mind that neutropenic patients do not make pus. Physical signs may be absent or altered, as may x-ray findings. After careful evaluation, if there is no obvious site of infection, such as cellulitis or pneumonia, assume the infection is arising from the gastrointestinal

tract. Thus empiric therapy should be effective against the organisms to be anticipated in that patient's intestinal flora at that time. This will vary according to the hospital the patient is in or has been in, previous courses of antibiotics, and other epidemiologic factors (see the chapter *Infection in the Neutropenic Patient*).

■ HELPER T-LYMPHOCYTE DEFECTS

T4 lymphocyte-mononuclear phagocyte defects are seen regularly in patients with underlying lymphomas, such as Hodgkin's disease, and those with leukemias, such as acute lymphoblastic and hairy cell leukemia. These patients are prey to an entirely different group of opportunistic pathogens (see Table 1). Some of these, such as *Mycobacterium tuberculosis, Nocardia asteroides,* and CMV, produce subacute as well as acute disease, and immediate empiric therapy may not be necessary. In other instances, however, optimal specimens should be collected and empiric therapy instituted for a subacute infection that can become acute and produce rapidly fatal disease in the severely immunocompromised host. Examples are tuberculosis, histoplasmosis, and pneumocystosis. If a patient with a severe T-cell defect does have fever and looks toxic without specific signs or symptoms and if there is any question about a B-lymphocyte defect, an empiric therapy that covers pneumocystosis (even with negative chest radiographic findings), salmonellosis, and pneumococcus should be used. A reasonable regimen for this is ceftriaxone plus trimethoprim-sulfamethoxazole.

■ SPLENIC AND B-CELL DEFECTS

Patients without a spleen develop extraordinarily severe infections caused by *Streptococcus pneumoniae*. They may also develop generally less severe infections caused by *Haemophilus influenzae* and *Neisseria meningitidis*. These must be treated early and intensively. With the emergence of penicillin-resistant pneumococci, an empiric regimen should contain ceftriaxone and vancomycin. Infections with these same organisms are seen in patients with B-cell defects, especially those caused by multiple myeloma and chronic lymphocytic leukemia. In all of these patients, the disease resulting from these encapsulated organisms can be especially severe, with accompanying bacteremias, often with no obvious source. The most rapidly progressive disease I have seen was caused by the pneumococcus in splenectomized patients with underlying leukemia or lymphoma. The defect may last for years.

In summary, evaluation of infections in the patient with neoplastic disease depends on multiple factors, which include (1) the epidemiologic background of the patient, (2) the immune defect or defects, (3) the resident organisms in a given hospital that could be responsible, and (4) clinical judgment. The first three can be estimated easily. The last requires considerable bedside experience, and in general, it is prudent to err on the side of treatment rather than observation.

Table 1 Immune Defects and the Infecting Organisms to Be Anticipated in the Patient with Malignancy

IMMUNE DEFECT	EXAMPLES	BACTERIA	FUNGI	PARASITES	VIRUSES
Interrupted integument	Indwelling IV catheters or chemotherapy-induced gastrointestinal ulcers	Streptococci Staphylococci Enterobacteriaceae Pseudomonas aeruginosa Corynebacterium spp.	Candida spp. Mucoraceae Aspergillus spp. Fusarium spp. Rhodotorula spp.		Herpes simplex
Surgical procedure	Tracheostomy Respiratory assistance Endoscopies Gastrointestinal or gyne- cologic surgery	Streptococci Staphylococci Enterobacteriaceae P. aeruginosa Bacteroides fragilis	Candida spp.		Herpes simplex
Neutrophil dysfunction	Acute leukemia Chemotherapy	Streptococcus spp. Staphylococcus aureus Enterobacteriaceae P. aeruginosa Enterococci	Candida spp. Aspergillus spp. Mucoraceae Trichosporon spp. Fusarium spp. Pseudallescheria boydii		
T-lymphocyte dysfunction	Hodgkin's disease Hairy cell leukemia	Listeria monocytogenes Salmonella spp. Nocardia asteroides Mycobacterium spp. Legionella spp. Rhodococcus equi	Cryptococcus neoformans Candida spp. Histoplasma capsulatum Coccidioides immitis Penicillium marneffei	Pneumocystis carinii Toxoplasma gondii Strongyloides stercoralis Cryptosporidium Isospora belli Microsporidia	Measles Varicella-zoster Cytomegalovirus Adenovirus Respiratory syncytial virus HHV6 Echovirus
Globulin dysfunction	Multiple myeloma Chronic lymphocytic leukemia	Streptococcus pneumoniae Haemophilus influenzae Neisseria meningitidis		P. carinii Giardia lamblia	
Splenic dysfunction	Staging laparotomy for Hodgkin's lymphoma	H. influenzae S. pneumoniae		Plasmodium spp. Babesia spp.	

HHV6, Human herpes virus-6.

Suggested Reading

Armstrong D: Empiric therapy for the immunocompromised host, *Rev Infect Dis* 13:S763, 1991.

Brown AE, White MH: Controversies in the management of infections in immunocompromised patients, *Clin Infect Dis* 17(suppl 2):317, 1992.

Freifeld AC: The antimicrobial armamentarium, *Hematol Oncol Clin North Am* 7:813, 1993.

Quie PG, Solberg CO: Infections in the immunocompromised host. In Armstrong D, Cohen J, eds: *Infectious diseases*, London, 1999, Mosby.

CORTICOSTEROIDS, CYTOTOXIC AGENTS, AND INFECTION

Jenny K. Lee
Robert L. Murphy

Iatrogenic immunosuppression typically involves the use of corticosteroids and/or cytotoxic agents. Recent advances in immunosuppressive therapy have greatly decreased morbidity and mortality secondary to transplantation rejection and autoimmune diseases. However, with these powerful immunosuppressive agents comes the risk of life-threatening opportunistic infections.

The specific type of agent, the dosage used, the length of therapy, and the underlying disease process all affect the incidence and type of infectious complication likely to occur with immunosuppressive therapy. Understanding the mechanism of action of these agents will aid in choosing the appropriate empiric therapy in patients with signs of infection.

■ MECHANISM OF ACTION OF CORTICOSTEROIDS

Corticosteroids are powerful antiinflammatory agents capable of significantly suppressing immune function. In the case of an overaggressive immunologic response to antigenic stimuli, corticosteroids may benefit patients by decreasing the inflammatory response.

Corticosteroids suppress immunity by blocking lymphocyte proliferation through inhibition of the production of interleukins 1 and 6 (IL-1 and IL-6) in macrophages. They also reduce formation of other cytokines such as IL-2, IL-4, interferon gamma, leukotrienes, tumor necrosis factor (TNF), and prostaglandins. In addition, corticosteroids reduce adhesion molecules on endothelial cells and inhibit the migration of granulocytes to the site(s) of infection. Antibody formation and turnover are also affected, especially at high dosages and with prolonged use of corticosteroids.

Collectively, this leads to an inhibition of T-cell proliferation, cytotoxic T-cells response, and antigen-specific immune responses. This subsequently increases the likelihood of acquiring an opportunistic intracellular pathogen, decreases the response to delayed skin test hypersensitivity, blocks the normal febrile response, reduces the polymorphonuclear inflammatory responses, and decreases the lymphocyte, monocyte, basophil, and eosinophil counts in the peripheral blood. There is essentially no bone marrow suppression.

Corticosteroids and the Risk of Infection

Myriad pathogens are associated with impaired cellular immunity and corticosteroid use (Table 1). Most of the organisms listed rarely cause significant or life-threatening disease in the immunocompetent patient. Some, such as *Pneumocystis carinii*, cause disease only in the immunocompromised individual. In addition, the rate of infection varies by underlying disease process. For instance, patients with

---

Table 1   Pathogens Commonly Associated with Corticosteroid Use

BACTERIA
Legionella pneumophila
Listeria monocytogenes
Mycobacterium tuberculosis
Nocardia species
Salmonella species

FUNGI
Blastomyces dermatitidis
Candida species
Coccidioides immitis
Cryptococcus neoformans
Histoplasma capsulatum

HELMINTHS
Strongyloides stercoralis

PROTOZOA
Cryptosporidium parvum
Pneumocystis carinii
Toxoplasma gondii
Plasmodia species

VIRUSES
Cytomegalovirus
Epstein-Barr virus
Herpes simplex
Varicella-zoster
Influenza

acquired immunodeficiency syndrome (AIDS) or childhood acute lymphocytic leukemia have higher rates of *Pneumocystis carinii* pneumonia (PCP) than patients without these diseases but receiving chronic corticosteroid therapy. For patients requiring chronic corticosteroid therapy, the infection rate for many of the pathogens listed in Table 1 is actually quite low overall. Except for tuberculosis, varicella, and recurrent herpes simplex infections, there is almost always a concurrent underlying impairment of cellular immunity separate from the iatrogenic impairment secondary to steroid use.

In relatively short-term controlled studies, the overall risk of developing an infection is approximately 50% higher in subjects taking corticosteroids than in those taking placebos. Furthermore, infection is more likely in patients with underlying neurologic disorders and less likely in those with intestinal, hepatic, or renal diseases. Infection is also more likely in those taking more than 10 mg of corticosteroids daily and taking more than 700 mg total. Thus cumulative dose, daily dose, and underlying disease all affect the likelihood of opportunistic infection in patients receiving corticosteroid therapy. The evidence is less clear regarding risk of infectious complications in patients taking a chronic low-dose corticosteroid.

Therapy with Corticosteroids

In certain disease states, the immunologic and/or inflammatory response itself can damage tissue. There is considerable evidence that certain inflammatory cytokines, such as TNF, IL-1, and interferon gamma, can cause significant damage in a site often distant from the initiating infection. The effectiveness of corticosteroid therapy in a variety of infections such as bacterial meningitis has been hotly debated for years. In other cases, such as PCP, corticosteroids have clearly improved outcomes and clearance of infection. Table 2 outlines the disease processes for which there is moderate to good evidence that steroids are useful.

■ MECHANISM OF ACTION OF CYTOTOXIC AGENTS

Cytotoxic agents can be primarily divided into three groups: immunophilin-binding agents, antiproliferative agents, and anti–T-cell biologic products (Table 3).

Two of the most common antirejection agents in transplantation are the immunophilin-binding agents, cyclosporin (Sandimmune), and tacrolimus (FK-506). Cyclosporin is a cyclic polypeptide that inhibits T-lymphocyte activation by inhibiting the production of IL-2 and other cytokines. It binds to cytoplasmic immunophilin. This drug-immunophilin complex blocks the action of the enzyme calcineurin, thereby inhibiting growth and proliferation of T lymphocytes. The advantages include both lack of bone marrow suppression and sparing of suppressor cell function. Cyclosporin has relatively low rates of infection when used alone; however, it is commonly combined with agents such as prednisone because of their synergistic immunosuppressive activity. Tacrolimus also binds an immunophilin and inhibits the production of IL-2 in T lymphocytes.

The antiproliferative agents are drugs that are primarily cancer chemotherapeutic drugs used to treat metastatic disease. However, they are increasingly used in transplantation and in autoimmune diseases such as systemic lupus erythematosus and rheumatoid arthritis. These agents inhibit both DNA and RNA synthesis and are bone marrow suppressive. Antiproliferative agents act against both B and T lymphocytes. The oldest class of these drugs are the alkylating agents, such as cyclophosphamide and chlorambucil. Other classes include antimetabolites, such as methotrexate and actinomycin D, and purine antagonists such as azathioprine (Imuran). Mycophenolate mofetil (Cellcept) is the prodrug of mycophenolic acid. It is commonly used for antirejection in solid organ transplantation.

Anti–T-cell biologic products such as OKT3 (muromonab-CD3 or Orthoclone OKT3) and antilymphocyte globulin (ALG) therapy (Atgam) are also important agents against rejection in solid organ transplantation. OKT3 is a monoclonal antibody that reacts with CD3 receptors on lymphocytes. Within minutes of infusion, circulating T lymphocytes become virtually undetectable. ALG is obtained from horses, rabbits, or goats immunized with human

---

Table 2 Infections with Moderate to Good Evidence That Adjuvant Corticosteroids Use Has Benefit

INFECTION	CORTICOSTEROID THERAPY
Bacteria meningitis in children with *Haemophilus influenzae* type B	Dexamethasone, 0.15 mg/kg q6h ×4 days
Pneumocystis carinii pneumonia, Po_2 <70 mm Hg	Prednisone, 40 mg bid ×5 days, then 40 mg qd ×5 days, then 20 mg qd ×11 days
Acute severe laryngotracheobronchitis (croup)	Dexamethasone, >0.3 mg/kg qd ×3-4 days
Allergic bronchopulmonary aspergillosis	Prednisone, 45-60 mg qd until infiltrate clears, then taper
Typhoid fever, critically ill	Dexamethasone, 3 mg/kg ×2-3 days
Tetanus	Prednisolone, 40 mg qd ×10 days
Tuberculous pericarditis and meningitis	Prednisone, 40-80 mg qd

---

Table 3 Commonly Used Cytotoxic Agents in Transplantation

IMMUNOBINDING AGENTS
Cyclosporin (Sandimmune)
Tacrolimus (FK-506 or Prograf)
ANTIPROLIFERATIVE AGENTS
Azathioprine (Imuran)
Mycophenolate mofetil (Cellcept)
Methotrexate
Actinomycin D
Cyclophosphamide
Chlorambucil
ANTI–T-CELL BIOLOGIC PRODUCTS
OKT3 (muromonab-CD3 or Orthoclone OKT3)
Antilymphocyte globulin (Atgam)

lymphoid cells. It results in elimination of T lymphocytes and a decrease in proliferation of newly formed lymphocytes. After discontinuation of ALG therapy, the quantity of circulating T lymphocytes gradually returns to normal, but the proliferative response of lymphocytes remains impaired.

Cytotoxic Agents and the Risk of Infection

A common adverse effect of many of the cytotoxic chemotherapeutic agents is bone marrow suppression. The inhibition of proliferating cell types is directly related to the immunosuppressive effect. Decreased lymphocytes, monocytes, and granulocytes all increase the risk of a variety of infections.

There is some variation in effects of these agents. Cyclosporin therapy, which blocks T-lymphocyte activation and inhibition of cell-mediated immunity, is likely to result in infection with an intracellular pathogen. Likewise, treatment with OKT3, ALG, tacrolimus, methotrexate, and azathioprine are also likely to inhibit cell-mediated immunity and increase the risk of infection with an intracellular pathogen. Therefore empiric therapy should be aimed against the pathogens listed in Table 1.

Special consideration for *Mycobacterium tuberculosis*, endemic fungi, cryptococcus, PCP, and the herpivirdiae should be given. Treatment with the alkylating agents cyclophosphamide and chlorambucil have a stronger effect on B-lymphocyte production and primary antibody responses. Infections with extracellular bacteria are commonly seen with these agents, as well as with those that result in granulocytopenia for long periods, and empiric therapy should be against the pathogens listed in Table 4. Fungal and parasitic infections are not typically associated with humoral deficiencies. However, in granulopenic patients, special consideration should be made to include fungal pathogens such as *Aspergillus* and *Candida* species.

With the advent of powerful immunosuppressive agents such as corticosteroids and cytotoxic agents in transplantation, cancer chemotherapy, and treatment of autoimmune diseases, there has been an emergence of a wider spectrum of infections. Understanding the effects of these agents on the immune system will help in successfully treating the iatrogenically immunosuppressed patient.

Table 4 Pathogens Common in Patients with Deficiencies in Humoral Immunity and/or Granulocytopenia

GRAM-NEGATIVE BACILLI
Escherichia coli
Klebsiella species
Pseudomonas aeruginosa
Enterobacter cloacae
Haemophilus influenzae
Serratia species
Proteus species
Salmonella species

GRAM-POSITIVE COCCI
Staphylococcus aureus
Staphylococcus epidermidis
Streptococcus pneumoniae
Streptococcus pyogenes
Enterococcus faecalis

ANAEROBES
Bacteroides species
Clostridium species
Fusobacterium species

PARASITES
Giardia lamblia

FUNGI
Candida species
Aspergillus species

Suggested Reading

Barbuto JAM, Akporiaye ET, Hersh EM: Immunopharmacology. In Katzung BG, ed: *Basic and clinical pharmacology,* Stamford, CT, 1998, Appleton & Lange.

Ho M, Dummer JS: Infections in transplant patients. In Mandell GL, Bennett JE, Dolin R, eds: *Mandell, Douglas, and Bennett's principles and practice of infectious diseases,* New York, 1995, Churchill Livingstone.

Meunier F: Infections in patients with acute leukemia and lymphoma. In Mandell GL, Bennett JE, Dolin R, eds: *Mandell, Douglas, and Bennett's principles and practice of infectious diseases,* New York, 1995, Churchill Livingstone.

Schimpff SC: Infections in the cancer patient—diagnosis, prevention, and treatment. In Mandell GL, Bennett JE, Dolin R, eds: *Mandell, Douglas, and Bennett's principles and practice of infectious diseases,* New York, 1995, Churchill Livingstone.

INFECTION IN TRANSPLANT PATIENTS

Rima Abu-Nader

Carlos V. Paya

Despite continued progress in reducing both rejection and infection rates in transplant recipients, infections remain the leading cause of morbidity and mortality in this subset of immunocompromised patients. Adequate preventive measures, aggressive diagnostic pursuits, and timely treatment interventions have all been effective in reducing the frequency, severity, and poor outcome of infections in the posttransplant period. However, the continuous introduction of more powerful immunosuppressive drugs perpetuates the risk of infection.

In general, different types of infections occur at different times from the date of transplantation, depending on the immune status of the host to a specific pathogen, comorbidities, and environmental exposures. Also, the type, frequency, and severity of infection all depend on the organ being transplanted.

Conventionally, a timetable for various infections, originally developed by Rubin, has been adapted to clinical practice. Posttransplant infections are grouped, according to a chronologic table, under one of three time periods: infections that characteristically occur from 0 to 1 month after transplantation (0 to 30 days), from 2 to 6 months after transplantation, and thereafter (Table 1).

This chapter reviews the characteristic infections in each of the aforementioned time periods and focuses on specific treatments directed against the causative pathogens. Pertinent information related to organ-specific infections is discussed and treatment recommended.

■ EARLY INFECTIOUS COMPLICATIONS

This period, which spans from the day of transplantation to 1 month afterward, is characterized by infections stemming from surgical complications. Fever, in this context, should always raise suspicion for infection, keeping in mind that many pathogens do not always cause pyrexia, such as cryptococcus and *Pneumocystis carinii*; also, fever may be absent when there is severe organ failure and vigorous steroid use for rejection. Allograft rejection and drug reactions are additional possible sources for fever. For instance, acute lung rejection is known to cause fever as opposed to heart allograft rejection, which normally does not. Renal and liver allotransplantation have an intermediate risk of causing fever when rejecting. A description of the major infections that can occur with different types of organ transplants soon after surgery is outlined next.

| **Table 1** Chronologic Sequence of Common Posttransplant Pathogens in Solid Organ Transplant Recipients* ||
TIME FROM TRANSPLANTATION	**PATHOGEN**
Early period (0-1 mo)	Bacteria
	Candida spp.
	Herpes simplex virus
Middle period (2-6 mo)	*Listeria monocytogenes*
	Nocardia spp.
	Mycobacterium tuberculosis
	Herpesviruses (e.g., CMV, EBV, HHV6 and 7)
	Candida species
	Aspergillus species
	Endemic fungi
	Cryptococcus neoformans
	Pneumocystis carinii
	Toxoplasma gondii
	Strongyloides stercolaris
Late period (beyond 6 mo)	CMV (retinitis)
	EBV (PTLD)
	VZV
	Papovaviruses
	Endemic fungi
	Community acquired pathogens

CMV, Cytomegalovirus; *EBV,* Epstein-Barr virus; *HHV,* human herpesvirus; *PTLD,* posttransplantation lymphoproliferative disease; *VZV,* varicella-zoster virus.
*The categorization in this timetable is not absolute and exceptions may apply.

Solid Organ Transplant
Bacterial Infections
Infections, in the first month after solid organ transplantation, are usually related to surgical complications. Bacterial or candidal wound infections, intravenous devices and drainage catheter–related sepsis are not uncommon. Specifically, in renal transplant recipients, especially cadaveric kidney and combined kidney-pancreas recipient groups, urinary tract infections (UTIs) tend to occur more frequently than in other types of solid organ transplants. In addition to the usual causative agents of UTIs, organisms such as *Enterococcus, Staphylococcus,* and *Pseudomonas aeruginosa* may be implicated. It should be emphasized that a UTI can be totally asymptomatic with no evidence of pyuria in transplant patients, which makes surveillance urine cultures a useful diagnostic tool in this situation.

Intraabdominal infections occur more often after liver, pancreas, or intestinal transplantation; the incidence is proportional to the length and technical difficulties of the operative procedure. In the case of liver transplantation, abscesses tend to form within the graft in the event of biliary or vascular obstruction. Biliary leak with secondary peritonitis or cholangitis may also occur. The bacterial flora for these abdominal infections normally involves enterococci, with vancomycin-resistant enterococci (VRE) becoming increasingly reported, as well as anaerobic and gram-negative enteric rods. In the case of pancreas transplantation, perigraft infections in the form of abscess or perigraft fluid collection are not uncommon.

By far, pulmonary infections are the most common type of infection in heart and lung transplant patients because of the surgical anatomy, and they are usually ventilator associated, whereas mediastinitis predominates more in heart transplant patients. Most pulmonary infections are caused by *Klebsiella* species, *P. aeruginosa*, *Enterobacter* species, and *Haemophilus influenzae*. *Burkholderia cepacia* colonization poses a particular problem in cystic fibrosis patients undergoing lung transplants.

Viral Infections

Herpes simplex virus (HSV) reactivation is not organ specific but rather common to all HSV-seropositive transplant patients in this early period. The advent of acyclovir prophylaxis soon after transplant surgery has significantly reduced oral and genital mucocutaneous lesions in HSV-seropositive individual recipients. Pneumonia, complicating orolabial lesions in intubated solid organ transplant patients, carries a high mortality rate. Esophagitis may be a sequel of HSV mucositis but, interestingly, encephalitis from HSV is rarely seen in the transplant population. OKT3, which is a monoclonal antibody that depletes T cells and that is being used as an immunosuppressant, seems to trigger HSV reactivation.

Fungal/Mycobacterial and Parasitic Infections

The fact that pancreas transplants drain into the gallbladder, thereby causing both enzymatic digestion of the bladder wall and change in urinary pH, allows *Candida* species to grow more liberally. Candidal abdominal infections should be included in the differential diagnoses of abdominal symptoms in the early period after liver transplantation. An approach to circumvent this problem was made possible with oral selective bowel decontamination. The latter regimen contains a nonabsorbable antifungal agent that decreases *Candida* colonization in the gut.

Bone Marrow Transplant

In the first month after bone marrow transplantation, neutropenia usually prevails and the patient is susceptible to HSV reactivation. This stems from the fact that the mucosal barrier is disrupted from the conditioning regimens administered in preparation for bone marrow transplantation. HSV reactivation can manifest as either mucocutaneous lesions or as limited or disseminated skin disease. Aside from neutropenia, other predisposing factors to infections in bone marrow transplant patients in this early period include indwelling vascular catheters.

Also common in this early period are pneumonia, UTIs, and line-related infections. The prophylactic use of antibiotics such as fluoroquinolones, although reducing the incidence of serious gram-negative infections, promotes gram-positive organisms, such as staphylococci, enterococci, and more recently, viridans streptococci and *Candida* species.

Bloodstream infections with bacteria or *Candida* may complicate the clinical picture; *Candida* may disseminate to the liver, spleen, kidneys, eyes and lungs, blossoming hematogenously when the leukocyte count is restored. Fever may be the sole clinical manifestation, and blood cultures may remain negative. Physical signs such as retinal exudates or nodular skin lesions may be the first clues to candidemia. Computed tomography (CT) scan of the abdomen shows typical "bull's-eye lesions" in the liver of patients with hepatosplenic candidiasis. Systemic antifungal treatment for deep-seated infection is warranted at this point.

The use of antifungal prophylaxis with fluconazole has reduced the number of *Candida albicans* isolates. However, this practice may have led to the emergence of relatively more infections with non-*albicans Candida* species known to be resistant to fluconazole, such as *Candida krusei*.

Other fungal infections may appear at any stage after transplantation. *Aspergillus* species are a major concern in this period. Invasive disease is common after inhalation of conidia, leading to nodular cavitary pneumonia. Diagnosis is made either clinically or by biopsy of involved tissue because blood cultures are routinely negative. Invasive fungal sinusitis with aspergillus or zygomycetes, although rarely observed in solid organ transplant recipients, is often seen in bone marrow transplant recipients. Central nervous system abscesses or infarction may develop with progression of disease.

Pulmonary infections constitute a major proportion of infections in the preengraftment period; nosocomial pathogens are the main offenders. Neutropenic enterocolitis, also known as typhlitis, has a less common but consistent association with profound neutropenia. It involves a necrotizing process of the gastrointestinal tract that is manifested clinically by fever and abdominal pain. Surgical intervention may be required if medical therapy fails.

■ INFECTIONS IN THE MIDDLE PERIOD (2 TO 6 MONTHS)

By this time, the intensity of immunosuppression is greater and opportunistic infections increase in frequency. Pathogens to consider in this period include viruses such as cytomegalovirus (CMV) and Epstein-Barr virus (EBV), fungi such as *Pneumocystis carinii*, *Aspergillus* species, and *Cryptococcus neoformans*, and parasites such as *Toxoplasma gondii*.

Transplant candidates from endemic areas are usually screened for the presence of any of the geographically restricted fungal infections such as *Histoplasma*, *Blastomyces*, and *Coccidioides* species.

Solid Organ Transplant
Bacterial Infections

An important cause of opportunistic bacterial infection in solid organ transplant patients is *Listeria monocytogenes*, especially in the first 2 months after transplantation. This organism is acquired by ingestion of contaminated food, and diarrhea may be the initial clinical feature. The organism spreads hematogenously, and meningitis often ensues.

Viral Infections

By far, the single most common viral infection in all types of transplants is CMV infection. CMV is in its usual latent state in monocyte-derived macrophages until it reactivates and causes disease in the seropositive recipient. It can cause a primary infection in a seronegative transplant recipient of an organ from a seropositive donor. Reactivation of CMV in seropositive recipients is fairly common, especially when certain predisposing factors are present. Superinfection with a new CMV strain contained in the transplanted organ is also possible in seropositive individuals. Risk groups for developing CMV disease have been stratified according to the percent incidence among each type of organ transplant. For instance, lung transplants rank as the high-risk group, whereas liver, heart, and pancreas transplants fall in the intermediate-risk group. Renal transplants belong to the low-risk group. Also, several risk factors have been considered as major contributors to development of CMV disease, such as donor CMV status, antilymphocyte (e.g., OKT3) use, retransplantation, and fulminant hepatitis before transplantation. CMV infection has a wide spectrum of clinical manifestations, ranging from asymptomatic to severe disease. CMV disease is further divided into CMV syndrome (fever, leukopenia, thrombocytopenia, arthralgia or even frank arthritis) or specific organ involvement. The latter corresponds to the transplanted organ (e.g., CMV hepatitis in liver transplant recipients and CMV pneumonitis in lung transplant recipients). CMV infection has been associated with other opportunistic infections and implicated in allograft rejection of kidneys, hearts, and possibly livers.

Several diagnostic methods are available to detect CMV. The conventional culture method, which takes 2 to 3 weeks before a cytopathic effect is apparent, remains the gold standard. The advent of the shell vial assay method has made results possible within 24 hours. The antigenemia test is even more rapid and more sensitive than the shell vial assay and can be used as a marker for active infection. Molecular-based techniques, such as polymerase chain reaction (PCR) and reverse transcription-PCR (RT-PCR), have also been developed as a means to improve detection sensitivity.

Available antiviral agents that are active against CMV include ganciclovir and foscarnet. Ganciclovir is most commonly used for treatment of established CMV disease. However, in an effort to prevent CMV disease, both prophylactic and preemptive strategies have been proposed for the high-risk groups. The reader is referred to recent reviews listed at the end of this chapter.

Primary infection with EBV in the transplant recipient causes a mononucleosis syndrome but can also first become apparent in the form of allograft dysfunction, bowel perforation, weight loss, or pulmonary process. The most devastating complication of EBV replication in organ transplant recipients is the development of polyclonal or monoclonal B-cell proliferative syndromes, collectively termed *post-transplantation lymphoproliferative disease* (PTLD). The incidence of PTLD ranges from 1% (in renal transplants) to 14% (in small-bowel transplants) depending on the transplanted organ. Risk factors include EBV seronegative status before transplantation, use of OKT3, CMV mismatch, and tacrolimus-based immunosuppression. Acyclovir or ganciclovir, initiated for CMV prophylaxis, may control EBV viral shedding, but treatment with antiviral agents is no longer effective when PTLD is well established, and measures such as reduction of immunosuppression, chemotherapy, or radiation therapy may be attempted. More recently, EBV was implicated in the development of leiomyosarcoma, T-cell lymphoma, Hodgkin's disease, carcinoma of the stomach and colon, and squamous cell carcinomas.

Fungal Infections

Fungal infections are more commonly seen in liver transplant patients and are encountered most frequently in the first 2 months of transplantation. The most serious fungal infection in the solid organ transplant patient is aspergillosis. Four species of this mycelial fungus cause invasive disease: *Aspergillus fumigatus, A. flavus, A. niger,* and *A. terreus.* Aspergillosis tends to occur in the first 3 months of transplantation, and almost all affected patients, treated or not, have a fatal outcome. The conidia usually gain entry into the respiratory system through inhalation and proceed to invade the blood vessels after bypassing the dysfunctional neutrophils and alveolar macrophages in the lungs. Invasive pulmonary disease as well as metastatic disease to the brain or other foci are common. Diagnosis of aspergillosis usually requires a tissue biopsy because recovery is rare from blood cultures.

As for endemic dimorphic fungi, a primary infection or reactivation of an old infection can occur, and high suspicion for such infection needs to be entertained when a patient lives in an endemic area.

Pneumocystis carinii affects close to 10% of solid organ transplant patients when prophylaxis is not administered for the first 6 months after transplantation. Pneumonia is a common feature, often complicated by spontaneous pneumothorax. *Pneumocystis* is commonly isolated with CMV.

Parasitic Infections

Most cases of *Toxoplasma gondii* occur in the first 2 months after transplantation, but the risk of clinical infection can be as long as 7 years. Seronegative heart transplant recipients of a seromismatched heart are most susceptible to primary infection. Seropositive heart transplant patients are also predisposed to reactivation of the latent parasite because of its tropism to muscle tissue, but reactivation can also be seen in other types of transplants. Clinical presentations include pericarditis or myocarditis, pneumonia, meningoencephalitis, brain abscess formation, and retinochoroiditis, among others. Depending on the disease manifestations, diagnosis can be obtained by examination of tissue biopsy, bronchoalveolar lavage specimens, cerebrospinal fluid (CSF), or vitreous fluid.

Strongyloides stercolaris has a unique autoinfective cycle within the gastrointestinal tract that enables it to persist for decades without causing symptoms. In the immunocompromised host, however, a hyperinfestation syndrome may develop and lead to hemorrhagic pneumonia and enterocolitis within the parasite's normal migratory path (i.e., the gastrointestinal tract and lungs). Dissemination of larvae to extraintestinal foci, such as central nervous system (CNS) and heart, can be devastating.

Bone Marrow Transplant

By the end of the first month, the transplanted marrow has engrafted but the lymphocytes are still dysfunctional. Here the risk of acute graft-versus-host disease (GVHD) is at its highest; when it sets in, the incidence of interstitial pneumonia increases markedly. CMV pneumonia accounts for the majority of interstitial pneumonitis cases in that setting. Two risk factors directly linked to CMV pneumonia are the use of antithymocyte globulins and allogeneic transplantation. As opposed to solid organ transplants, CMV reinfection here does not exist. CMV infection, demonstrated by either seroconversion or viral shedding, may be asymptomatic or accompanied by constitutional symptoms. Organ involvement can develop in up to 40% of patients, usually in the form of pneumonia, which carries a mortality rate of up to 50% despite therapy. The gastrointestinal tract may also be involved, with resultant enterocolitis, gastritis, or esophagitis. *Aspergillus* species replace *Candida* as the major fungal pathogen during this period.

■ LATE INFECTIOUS COMPLICATIONS

The fourth to sixth month usually marks the beginning of maintenance immunosuppression. Beyond the 6-month period, most transplant patients (70% to 80%) resemble the general community with regard to infection, except in certain situations. These include patients with chronic rejection in whom immunosuppression was augmented and patients with chronic viral infections such as CMV chorioretinitis or EBV-induced lymphoproliferative disorders.

Community-acquired viral infections such as influenza virus and respiratory syncytial virus (RSV) infections can be severe in patients who maintain good allograft function. Contact avoidance or early identification of exposure is essential.

Solid Organ Transplant
Bacterial Infection
Aside from the risk of acquiring respiratory infections, community exposure to bacterial foodborne pathogens may occur at this stage and cause a protracted illness. Renal transplant patients are particularly susceptible to nontyphoidal *Salmonella,* which can present as a febrile illness with bacteremia, UTI, or gastroenteritis; relapses are common. Factors such as corticosteroid use and prolonged hemodialysis increase the risk for salmonella infections.

Viral Infection
Unlike other manifestations of CMV disease, CMV retinitis predictably occurs in the period beyond 6 months. Patients present with blurring of vision, scotomata, or decreased visual acuity. Diagnosis is made by funduscopy, and treatment initiated with ganciclovir.

Bone Marrow Transplant
In the period from 3 to 6 months and beyond, chronic GVHD, if present, prevents the full recovery of B- and T-cell function, constantly making the host vulnerable to infections. Also, GVHD may require immunosuppressive therapy, further increasing the risk of acquiring opportunistic infections. One of the manifestations of GVHD, the sicca syndrome, affects the mucociliary clearance of the respiratory epithelium and thus increases the risk for pneumonia. In addition, humoral immunity is not fully recovered and thus pneumonia caused by encapsulated bacteria may still occur during this period.

Pathogens with potential for reactivation posttransplantation and pathogens with specific association to the type of host defense mechanism defect are outlined in Tables 2 and 3.

Selected Pathogens
Mycobacterium tuberculosis
Reactivation of *Mycobacterium tuberculosis* can occur particularly if the patient is from an endemic region or had inadequate prophylaxis or treatment or a recent skin test conversion. Primary infection can also occur but is rarely transmitted in the allograft. Overall, *M. tuberculosis* has a higher propensity for dissemination and a lower response rate to treatment in transplant patients compared with the general population. Cavitary lung lesions still can occur, as can exudative pleural effusions. Fever is more common than night sweats or weight loss, and PPD may be falsely negative.

Atypical mycobacteria should always be considered in the differential diagnosis of a skin lesion, tenosynovitis, or joint infection late after a solid organ transplantation. Typically, a painful, erythematous subcutaneous nodule develops insidiously, after a local skin injury and may evolve into an abscess. Cyclophosphamide therapy in heart transplant patients seems to be a predisposing factor. Medical treatment accompanied by surgical debridement are often necessary.

Nocardia species
Nocardial infection is notably absent in the first month after transplantation but assumes tremendous importance from the second month on. Heart and renal transplant patients are particularly susceptible to nocardial infections. The latter typically causes pneumonia but can also involve the joints, skin, and brain. Besides the risk conferred by immunosuppressive therapy, factors such as rejection, neutropenia, and azathioprine-based immunosuppression play an important role in the pathogenesis of nocardial infection. The widespread use of trimethoprim-sulfamethoxazole as a prophylactic agent in the first 3 to 6 months after transplantation, although originally aimed at preventing *Pneumocystis carinii* pneumonia (PCP), has lowered the incidence of nocardia and listeria as well as bacterial UTIs. Prolonged treatment with trimethoprim-sulfamethoxazole is the rule once diagnosis of nocardiosis is established.

Legionella
Infection with *Legionella* can occur at any time and as early as several weeks after transplantation. It can be a community-acquired or a nosocomial infection and has a propensity to solid organ transplants and to an episode of rejection. Pneumonia inevitably develops.

Human Herpesvirus 6
Human herpesvirus 6 (HHV-6) was first isolated from patients with lymphoproliferative disorders. It is closely related to CMV and has been associated with febrile illnesses in renal transplant patients. In addition, some reports have attributed to HHV-6 an entity of interstitial pneumonitis, skin rash, and fever occurring in bone marrow transplant patients. A delay in bone marrow engraftment has also been observed in association with HHV-6 infection in vivo. It has been considered, together with HHV-7, to worsen the clinical presentation of CMV disease.

Cryptococcus neoformans
Infections caused by *Cryptococcus neoformans* can occur at any time after transplantation. A subacute or chronic men-

Table 2 Pathogens with Potential for Reactivation after Organ Transplantation

VIRUSES	FUNGI	MYCOBACTERIA	PARASITES
Herpes simplex virus Cytomegalovirus Epstein-Barr virus Varicella-zoster virus Human herpesvirus 6 Hepatitis B or C Papovavirus (JC, BK)	*Blastomyces dermatitides* *Coccidioides immitis* *Histoplasma capsulatum*	*Mycobacterium tuberculosis*	*Strongyloides stercoralis* *Toxoplasma gondii*

Table 3 Time Sequence of Defects That Occur in Host Defense Mechanisms after Transplantation and Associated Pathogens

HOST DEFENSE MECHANISM	TIME AFTER TRANSPLANTATION	PATHOGEN ASSOCIATED WITH DEFECT
Local defenses (skin, mucous membranes, gastrointestinal tract, and so on)	Early period	Bacteria Herpes simplex virus
Neutrophil/phagocytic function	Early period	Bacteria *Candida* spp. *Aspergillus* spp. Zygomycetes
Cell-mediated immunity	Middle period	*Listeria monocytogenes* *Nocardia* spp. Mycobacteria Herpesviruses *Pneumocystis carinii* *Aspergillus* spp. and other fungi *Cryptococcus neoformans* *Toxoplasma gondii* *Strongyloides stercolaris*
Humoral immunity	Mid to late period	Encapsulated bacteria *Aspergillus* spp. *Pneumocystis carinii* Varicella-zoster virus

ingitis manifesting with headaches, fever, or mental status changes is the rule. A CSF examination or even a serum evaluation for cryptococcal antigen is sensitive enough to make the diagnosis. Of note, cryptococcuria, when present, is pathognomonic of systemic infection. The mainstay treatment for cryptococcal meningitis is amphotericin B alone or in combination with flucytosine. Maintenance therapy with oral fluconazole is instituted thereafter.

Varicella-Zoster Virus

Varicella-zoster virus (VZV) gains priority over CMV in the late period after transplantation (beyond 6 months) and within the first year of bone marrow transplantation (with a median onset of 5 months). Reactivation causes herpes zoster in the seropositive recipients, who constitute 90% of the total transplant population. It manifests as pain with or without a rash along a dermatome and may involve other dermatomes at distant sites. Primary VZV infection has more serious sequelae in the remaining 10% of the transplant population, where dissemination, characterized by pneumonia, skin lesions, encephalitis, pancreatitis, hepatitis, and disseminated intravascular coagulation are frequent. Primary VZV infection may also present in the form of the classical chickenpox syndrome.

Papovaviruses

Human papillomaviruses are known to cause anal infection with secondary neoplasia in solid organ transplants, as well as urinary papillomatous lesions and cervical squamous tumors in women with renal allografts. Several reports of JC virus–induced progressive leukoencephalopathy have been described in the transplant literature. Moreover, BK polyoma virus infection is commonly seen after bone marrow transplantation as a causative agent of hemorrhagic cystitis. The same virus has been implicated in few cases of ureteral strictures in renal transplant patients.

Treatment recommendations for specific pathogens are summarized in Table 4.

■ COMMENTS

A high index of suspicion for infection should always be present in bone marrow or solid organ transplantation, particularly in the first 6 months. Careful assessment of the risk factors surrounding a posttransplant patient, the judicious interpretation of microbiologic data, and the awareness of hazardous interactions between a variety of drugs should all lead to the ultimate treatment approach. Prophy-

Table 4 Treatment Recommendations for Specific Pathogens

ORGANISM	DISEASE	PREFERRED TREATMENT/ALTERNATIVE TREATMENT*
Aspergillus spp.	Invasive, pulmonary or extrapulmonary	Amphotericin B (lipid formulations are equally efficacious) 1-1.5 mg/kg/day IV for a total of 2.5 g and at least for 2-3 wk or longer if no clinical improvement; then itraconazole, 200 mg PO bid
Burkholderia cepacia	Pneumonia	TMP-SMX, 15-20 mg/kg/day ± inhaled aminoglycoside
	Septicemia	Alternative: ceftazidime or imipenem
Candida spp.	Mucocutaneous candidiasis	Clotrimazole troches or nystatin pastilles ×7-14 days
	Esophagitis	Fluconazole, 200 mg PO ×1 day, then 100 mg PO qd ×14-21 days
	Candidemia	Amphotericin B, 0.5-0.7 mg/kg/day IV, then switch to fluconazole or start fluconazole, 800 mg ×1 day, then 400 mg/day ×14 days
Cryptococcus neoformans	Pneumonia	Amphotericin B, 0.5-1.0 mg/kg/day IV, ±5-FC, 100 mg/kg/day ×2 wk, then maintenance with fluconazole, 400 mg/day ×10 wk
	Meningitis	Alternatively: fluconazole, 400 mg PO qd ×10 wk
Cytomegalovirus (CMV)	See text for manifestations	Ganciclovir, 5 mg/kg IV q12h ×14-21 days
	CMV pneumonia in bone marrow transplant	Induction: GCV, 5 mg/kg IV q12h ×14 days + IVIG, 500 mg/kg IV qod, or CytoGam, 150 mg/kg IV ×14 days
		Maintenance: GCV, 5 mg/kg IV qd 5 d for 4 wk + IVIG, 500 mg/kg, or CytoGam, 150 mg/kg IV once per week for 4 wk
Epstein-Barr virus	PTLD	No antiviral agent
Herpes simplex	Mucocutaneous	Acyclovir, 200 mg PO (or equivalent) 5 times/day ×7 days
	Disseminated	Acyclovir, 5-10 mg/kg IV q8h ×7-14 days
Legionella	Pneumonia	Erythromycin, 1 g IV q6h, ± rifampin or levofloxacin, 500 mg/day, ± rifampin for 3 wk
Listeria	Meningitis	Ampicillin, 2 g IV q4h, + gentamicin, 2 mg/kg IV loading dose, then 1.7 mg/kg IV q8h
		Alternative: TMP-SMX, 15-20 mg/kg/day IV
Mycobacterium tuberculosis	Pulmonary or extra-pulmonary	At least two bactericidal agents (INH, rifampin or pyrazinamide) for 12 mo
		Alternative: INH, 300 mg/day for 9 mo, rifampin, 600 mg/day for 6 mo, and PZA, 2 mg/kg/day for 3 mo
Nocardia	Pneumonia	TMP-SMX, 15 mg/kg/day for 6 mo
	Metastatic abscesses	Alternatives: minocycline, 200 mg PO bid ×6 mo
		Ceftriaxone or imipenem if acutely ill
Pneumocystis carinii	Pneumonia	TMP-SMX, 15-20 mg/kg/day IV/PO ×14-21 days
		Alternative: Pentamidine, 4 mg/kg/day IV ×14-21 days
Salmonella	Abdominal, pulmonary, urinary and vascular infections	Ceftriaxone, 1-2 g IV q24h
		Alternative: fluoroquinolone
Toxoplasma gondii	Meningoencephalitis	Pyrimethamine, 50-100 mg PO bid on first day, then 25 mg PO qd, + folinic acid, 10 mg/day, + sulfadiazine, 1-1.5 g PO qid
	Brain abscess	
	Myocarditis/pericarditis	Alternative: clindamycin + pyrimethamine + folinic acid
	Hepatitis/chorioretinitis	
Varicella-zoster virus (VZV)	Localized zoster	Acyclovir (or equivalent), 10 mg/kg IV q8h ×7 days, or 800 mg PO 5 times daily ×7-10 days
	Primary VZV infection or disseminated infection	Acyclovir 500 mg/m² IV q8h ×7-14 days (+VZIG for primary VZV infection)

TMP-SMX, Trimethoprim-sulfamethoxazole; *5-FC,* fluorocytosine or flucytosine; *GCV,* ganciclovir; *IVIG,* intravenous immunoglobulin; *CytoGam, CMV* immunoglobulins; *INH,* isoniazid; *PZA,* pyrazinamide; *PTLD,* posttransplantation lymphoproliferative disease; *VZIG,* varicella-zoster immunoglobulin.

*All suggested treatment regimens should be adjusted according to susceptibility testing results when applicable. Also, dosage adjustments should be made based on renal and/or hepatic function, when indicated.

lactic regimens directed against different organisms have decreased the severity, if not the incidence, of infections caused by those pathogens.

Suggested Reading

Bowden RA, Ljungman P, Paya CV, eds: *Transplant infections,* 1998, Philadelphia, Lippincott-Raven.

Fishman JA, Rubin RH: Infection in organ-transplant recipients, *N Engl J Med* 338:1741, 1998.

Patel R, Paya CV: Infections in solid-organ transplant recipients, *Clin Microbiol Rev* 10:86, 1997.

Sable CA, Donowitz GR: Infections in bone marrow transplant recipients, *Clin Infect Dis* 18:273, 1994.

INFECTION IN THE BURN-INJURED PATIENT

Roger W. Yurt

The diagnosis of infection in the patient with major burn injury is especially problematic because the signs of infection are the same as those of the response to injury. The tissue injury that occurs with a major burn and the associated inflammatory response to it cause one of the greatest perturbations of homeostasis that occurs in any disease state. Thus the greatest challenge in developing a differential diagnosis in the burn-injured patient is to distinguish between the injury state and infection. That the manifestation of infection may be blunted by diminished immune response further complicates evaluation of the patient while also contributing to an increased susceptibility to infection. The challenge posed in the clinical and laboratory evaluation of the burn-injured patient is summarized in the outline of injury related changes in Table 1.

■ INJURY PATHOPHYSIOLOGY AND SUSCEPTIBILITY TO INFECTION

The initial approach to the burn-injured patient is oriented toward limiting the progression of the injury by stabilization of the patient and maintenance of blood flow to the wound. The zone of coagulative necrosis consists of tissue that has been irreversibly damaged, whereas the surrounding zone of stasis contains areas of potentially reversible injury. Adjacent areas, known as the *hyperemic zone,* may also evolve to become necrotic if blood flow is not maintained. For this reason, the primary goal of early burn therapy is to ensure adequate delivery of oxygen, nutrients, and circulating cells to the wound. In addition to prevention of progression of injury, immediate burn care focuses on maintenance of a viable tissue interface at which both specific and nonspecific defenses against infection can be mounted.

The depth of burn injury is categorized as partial or full thickness. Full-thickness injuries will heal only by contraction, ingrowth of surrounding epidermis, or grafting of tissue because all epidermis in the wound has been destroyed. These wounds are leathery and dry, contain thrombosed vessels, and are insensate. Partial-thickness wounds contain residual epidermis, which can close the wound if blood flow is maintained and infection does not supervene. They are erythematous and moist, and pain is elicited by touch. Deep partial-thickness wounds contain only epithelial elements associated with organelles of the skin. They take longer to heal (2 to 3 weeks) than superficial partial thickness wounds, and there is greater functional and cosmetic deformity if they are allowed to heal primarily. These

Table 1 Clinical and Laboratory Signs Related to Injury That Complicate the Evaluation of the Patient with Burn Injury

SIGN	ABNORMALITY
General condition	Lethargy-electrolyte imbalance
	analgesic effects
	Hyperventilation
	pain, topical agents
	Tachycardia
	pain, volume depletion, hyper-metabolism
Fluid balance	Hypovolemia
	initial injury
	delayed-evaporative loss
Fluid composition	Hypernatremia
	free water loss
	inadequate fluid replacement
	Hyponatremia
	excessive free water
	effects of topical silver nitrate
	Hyperglycemia
	stress
Temperature	Hypothermia
	heat loss to environment
	large fluid requirement
	Hyperthermia
	hypermetabolism
	endotoxin from wound
Neutrophil response	Neutrophilia
	acute
	5-7 days after injury
	Neutropenia
	2-3 days after injury

wounds are difficult to differentiate by clinical evaluation from superficial partial-thickness injuries, which usually heal within 10 days to 2 weeks.

The dynamic aspect of burn wounds is dramatically seen when partial-thickness wounds convert to full-thickness wounds during a difficult resuscitation of a patient. Although this is rarely seen with current methods of resuscitation, resuscitation that is delayed or performed on patients at extremes of age occasionally will show this progression. Any agent that causes cellular death can lead to a deeper wound. With this in mind, caustic topical agents and vasopressors are avoided, the wound is not allowed to desiccate, and the patient is kept warm.

Both mortality and susceptibility to infection correlate directly with the extent of surface area injury. Distribution of surface area varies with age, so a chart is used to plot accurately the extent and depth of surface area burned. The rule of nines may be used to estimate the extent of injury as follows: torso—back and front each 18%, each leg 18%, each arm 9%, and head 9%. Calculation of the extent of injury is helpful in estimating fluid requirements and prognosis. Patients with greater than 25% to 30% total body surface area burn exhibit the pathophysiologic features already described.

■ PREVENTION OF INFECTION

Current data do not support the general use of prophylactic systemic antibiotics in the inpatient population. Frequent evaluation of the wound and surrounding tissue allows early and appropriate therapy of cellulitis while sparing a majority of patients exposure to unnecessary antibiotics. However, it is common practice to give systemic antibiotics (penicillin) to outpatients with burns because it is not possible to observe closely and ensure appropriate care of the wound. The use of systemic antibiotics in these patients is individualized such that those who are likely to follow up with their care and recognize changes in their wounds are not given antibiotics. The one time that prophylactic systemic antibiotics are used in inpatients is at the time of surgical manipulation because this may cause bacteremia. Antibiotics are administered immediately before and during burn wound excision. The choice of antibiotics is dictated by knowledge of the current flora in the burn center or more specifically by the burn wound flora of the individual patient.

The mainstay of prevention of burn wound infection is aggressive removal of the necrotic tissue and closure of the wound with autograft. In the interim, topical antimicrobial prophylaxis will decrease the incidence of conversion of partial-thickness to full-thickness wound by local infection, and these agents may prolong the sterility of the full-thickness burn wound. Silver sulfadiazine is the most commonly used topical and is a soothing cream with good activity against gram-negative organisms. Because it does not penetrate the wound, it is used only as a prophylactic antimicrobial. Bacterial resistance to silver sulfadiazine has been reported, and it has been reported to cause neutropenia. Silver nitrate in a 0.5% solution is an effective topical agent when used before wound colonization. This agent does not penetrate eschar, and therefore its broad-spectrum gram-negative effectiveness is diminished once bacterial proliferation has occurred in the eschar. Additional disadvantages of this agent include the need for continuous occlusive dressings, which limit evaluation of wounds and restrict range of motion. The black discoloration of the wound, as well as the environment, contribute to a decrease in use of silver nitrate. Mafenide acetate (Sulfamylon) cream has a broad spectrum of activity against gram-negative organisms but little activity against staphylococci. A significant advantage of this agent is that it penetrates the burn eschar and therefore is effective in the colonized wound. The disadvantages of Sulfamylon are a transient burning sensation, an accentuation of postinjury hyperventilation, and inhibition of carbonic anhydrase activity. Recent experience with a new silver-impregnated dressing that does not have to be changed daily suggests that this agent is a good alternative for prophylaxis against infection in partial-thickness wounds.

The goal of burn therapy is to prevent burn wound infection by permanent closure of the wound as rapidly as possible. Early removal of necrotic tissue and wound closure has the advantages of removal of eschar before colonization, which typically occurs 5 to 7 days after injury, and of reduction of the overall extent of injury. A drawback of early excisional therapy is the possibility that burned tissue that may heal if left alone over a 2 to 3 week period may be unnecessarily excised.

Advances in resuscitation have led to the ability to salvage an increasing number of patients from the shock phase immediately after injury and have resulted in a greater number of patients surviving to the time (2 to 3 days after the injury) when the effects of inhalation injury become clinically prominent. In patients without inhalation injury but with large burns, postinjury hyperventilation and subsequent decreases in tidal volume may lead to atelectasis and subsequent pneumonia. Diminished mucociliary functions and destruction of airways by inhalation of products of combustion lead to airway obstruction and infection. Frequent diagnostic and therapeutic bronchoscopy are necessary in this group of patients. Attempts at specific prophylaxis of the sequelae of inhalation injury, such as nebulization of antibiotics and treatment with steroids, have failed to show any benefit.

Nosocomial infections are of even greater concern in the burn intensive care setting than other units because of the large open colonized wounds. Cross-contamination is avoided by use of gowns, gloves, and masks by nurses, medical staff, and visitors. The patient is not touched except with a gloved hand, and each patient is restricted to his or her own monitoring and diagnostic equipment. If adequate nursing care can be provided, it is preferable to isolate patients who have large open wounds in individual rooms. Cohort patient care has been shown to be effective in eliminating endemic infections.

■ DIAGNOSIS AND TREATMENT OF INFECTION

Wound Infection

Because the full-thickness burn wound is at high risk for infection, routine clinical and laboratory surveillance of the wound is an absolute necessity. Daily observation of the wound for discoloration, softening or maceration of the eschar or the development of cellulitis provides early detection of wound-associated infection. Although surface cultures of the burn wound provide insight into the organisms that are colonizing the wound, evaluation of a biopsy of the burn wound is the only way to obtain an accurate assessment of the status of the wound. Systematic evaluation of burn wounds with quantitative culture of biopsies of all areas of wound change documents the clinical diagnosis of wound infection and provides identification and antimicrobial sensitivity of the involved organism. Routine biopsy of full-thickness burn wounds on an every-other-day schedule provides evidence of advancing wound infection and serves as a basis for initiating therapy. A rapid fixation technique allows histologic diagnosis of invasive infection within 3 hours, whereas quantitative counts and identification of the organism is available within 24 hours.

This combined use of histologic and culture techniques provides early diagnosis as well as the identity of the organism and its sensitivity to antimicrobials. When the findings are consistent with invasive infection (greater than or equal to 10^5 organisms per gram of tissue), aggressive surgical therapy is instituted to excise the involved wound. In preparation for surgery or in patients who require stabilization before general anesthesia is given, a penetrating topical agent is used (Sulfamylon). The choice of antibiotic is based on previous biopsy sensitivity data or data accumulated on sensitivities of the current flora in the patient population.

A growing number of patients appear to be presenting with primary nonsuppurative gram-positive infections. These infections are often caused by methicillin-resistant *Staphylococcus aureus* (personal observation), and whether diminished neutrophil response or a change in the nature or virulence of such organisms may explain this phenomenon is unknown.

Pulmonary Infection

From a practical standpoint, inhalation injury is diagnosed by history, physical examination, and bronchoscopy. A history of exposure to fire in a closed space along with findings of carbonaceous sputum, singed nasal vibrissae and facial burns are associated with a high incidence of inhalation injury. Bronchoscopy reveals upper airway edema and erythema while bronchorrhea, carbon in the bronchi and mucosal slough suggest lower airway and parenchymal injury. Carboxyhemoglobin levels may be elevated, but with a half-life of 45 minutes on 100% oxygen the level may be normal. Chest x-ray studies are of little value in making the diagnosis of inhalation injury because they are often normal for the first 72 hours after injury. Xenon ventilation-perfusion lung scan reveals trapping of xenon in the ventilation phase and is supportive of a diagnosis of small airway obstruction secondary to injury of distal airways and parenchyma. Although hematogenous pneumonia is less common than in the past, it remains a significant problem in the patient with burns. When it occurs, the source (most commonly wound or suppurative vein) must be defined and eradicated. Prophylactic antibiotics are not used for either bronchopneumonia or hematogenous pneumonia; specific therapy is based on knowledge of previous endobronchial culture, and sensitivity is substantiated by repeat cultures at the time of diagnosis.

Suppurative Thrombophlebitis

Suppurative thrombophlebitis is mentioned in particular in relation to the patient with burn injury because it is the most common cause of repeatedly positive blood cultures in the presence of appropriate antibiotics in this population. These findings alone should lead to a presumptive diagnosis of a suppurative process in a previously cannulated vein. The process may be insidious, with only minimal clinical findings. Because this complication is common, venous cannulation should be minimized, but when necessary, catheters should be changed every 3 days. Treatment consists of surgical excision of the entire involved vein to the level of normal bleeding vessel. In this setting the differential diagnosis should include endocarditis.

Suggested Reading

Yurt RW: Burns. In Polk HC, Gardner B, Stone HH, eds: *Basic surgery,* St Louis, 1993, Quality Medical Publishing.
Yurt RW: Burns. In Mandell GL, Gennett JE, Dolin R, eds: *Mandell, Douglas, and Bennett's principles and practice of infectious diseases,* New York, 1995, Churchill Livingstone.

DIABETES AND INFECTION

Stefan Bughi
Francisco L. Sapico

Diabetes mellitus is a prevalent disorder, affecting more than 16 million Americans, with a larger population of about 20 million people having glucose intolerance. More than 90% of diabetic patients have type 2 diabetes. Microvascular and macrovascular complications are related to blood glucose control and disease duration and are more commonly seen in the elderly.

Diabetic patients are also at risk for infections, and uncontrolled diabetes has a negative effect on infection control. There is a common belief among clinicians that diabetic patients are more susceptible to infections. Studies have shown that polymicrobial soft-tissue infections persist longer in the diabetic mouse model than in nondiabetic counterparts. Moreover, review of the literature reveals that certain infections are overpresented in the diabetic population.

■ PREDISPOSING FACTORS TO INFECTION

The abnormalities in host defense mechanisms in diabetic patients are related to the presence of metabolic imbalance associated with diabetes. Hyperglycemia has been implicated in disorders of immune function, such as alteration of polymorphonuclear leukocyte (PML) chemotaxis, phagocytosis, and decreased intracellular bactericidal activities. The effect of hyperglycemia on phagocytic activity was recently associated with an increase in cytosolic calcium and is reversible with the improvement of blood glucose level.

Defects in humoral immunity have been described with decreased opsonization of certain organisms and deficiency in the fourth component of complement (Table 1). Defective cellular immunity has also been shown, with decreased response to phytohemaglutinins and poor skin test reactivity. Poor granuloma formation has also been reported in diabetic patients. All these changes are aggravated by microcirculatory failure, which alters the diffusion of both cellular

Table 1 Impaired Defense Mechanisms in Diabetic Patients

WHITE CELL FUNCTION
Decreased chemotaxis
Decreased phagocytosis and intracellular killing
Decreased number of phagocytizing monocytes
Decreased in vitro killing of *Staphylococcus aureus, Escherichia coli,* and *Candida* by neutrophils

HUMORAL IMMUNITY
Decreased antibody response to the bacterial antigens
Deficiency of the fourth component of the complement

CELL-MEDIATED IMMUNITY
Altered T-lymphocyte function
Decreased lymphoblastic proliferation after exposure to antigens
Poor granulation formation

and humoral factors, as well as antibiotics, to the affected site. Development of peripheral and autonomic neuropathy and progression of macrovascular changes further increase the diabetic patient's risk of infection.

■ RESPIRATORY INFECTIONS

Diabetic patients are prone to aspiration pneumonia, especially in the presence of gastroparesis, a complication that occurs in 40% to 60% of those with diabetes. The risk of aspiration also increases with impairment of consciousness associated with hypoglycemia or the hyperosmolar state. Diabetic patients also have a higher risk of developing *Klebsiella* staphylococcal pneumonia and pneumonitis following influenza.

Diabetic patients are known to more frequently develop clinical tuberculosis (TB) if infected and also to have atypical locations and appearance of the disease. The incidence of tuberculosis is 16 times higher in the diabetic population than in the nondiabetic population. For this reason, the presence of a positive purified protein derivative (PPD) skin test, even with a normal chest radiograph, requires isoniazid (INH) prophylaxis for a minimum of 6 months, regardless of age.

■ MUCORMYCOSIS

More than three fourths of cases of rhinocerebral mucormycosis occur in diabetics. Most of the patients have diabetic ketoacidosis. Mucormycosis is caused by a group of fungi known as *Mucorales,* the most common genera being Rhizopus, Absidia, and *Rhizomucor.* These fungi invade nasal and paranasal membranes, as well as blood vessels, resulting in thrombosis and tissue infarction. Local spread of infection results in ophthalmoplegia, blindness, cavernous sinus thrombosis, meningoencephalitis, and brain abscesses, leading to rapid death in untreated cases. Patients with mucormycosis may develop periorbital edema and chemosis. Diagnosis is made by biopsy of the necrotic black eschars and demonstration of nonseptate thick-walled hyphae with special staining. Computed tomography (CT) scan or magnetic resonance imaging (MRI) can be helpful in assessing the

extent of disease and aid the surgeon in debridement. Treatment with intravenous amphotericin B, 1 mg/kg/day, or liposomal amphotericin B, 5 mg/kg/day, should be started as soon as possible and should be given up to a total of 2 to 4 g of regular amphotericin B. Even with early diagnosis and treatment, mortality with mucormycosis can be as high 50%. Those who survive may require reconstructive surgery and long-term psychologic counseling.

■ INVASIVE OTITIS EXTERNA

Invasive otitis externa is an invasive infection usually caused by *Pseudomonas aeruginosa.* It starts in the external auditory canal and progresses to the surrounding subcutaneous tissue. Rarely, the etiologic agent is *Aspergillus, Klebsiella pneumoniae,* or other organisms. More than 90% of patients have diabetes, often with poor metabolic control. Characteristically, the disease begins with periauricular cellulitis and granulation tissue at the junction of the cartilaginous and osseous portions of the external auditory canal. Infection spreads along the cartilage cleft, resulting in parotitis; mastoiditis; osteomyelitis of the temporomandibular joint, skull base, and cervical vertebrae; septic thrombophlebitis; cranial nerve palsy; and meningitis. Facial nerve (VII) palsy occurs in 30% to 40% of cases and does not necessarily carry a poor prognosis. However, development of palsies of cranial nerves IX and XII implies deep infection sometimes complicated by sigmoid sinus thrombosis and central nervous system (CNS) infection, which results in death in 30% of patients. The extent of tissue involvement can be determined accurately with the use of CT scan or MRI, which also helps the surgeon in performing extensive debridement.

Four weeks of parenteral antipseudomonal antibiotic therapy is generally recommended. Frequently, combination therapy of beta-lactam agents (piperacillin, ceftazidime, cefipime, or aztreonam) with an aminoglycoside are used. Other regimens used a combination of two antipseudomonal beta-lactams, or even a single agent such as ciprofloxacin. If oral quinolones are used, longer therapy (3 months) is recommended by some authorities.

■ GASTROINTESTINAL INFECTIONS

Candida esophagitis has been reported to occur with increased frequency in diabetic patients. The most common presentation is retrosternal pain or dysphagia after the ingestion of cold or hot drinks. This disorder occurs more often in diabetic patients who receive broad-spectrum antibiotics. Oral thrush can be absent. Endoscopic examination and biopsy are the preferred diagnostic procedures. Treatment with oral fluconazole (400 mg initial dose, followed by 200 mg/day) is necessary for a minimum of 3 weeks, or at least for 2 weeks after resolution of symptoms.

Emphysematous cholecystitis is a surgical emergency, characterized by gas production in or around the gallbladder. The infection is highly virulent and often induced by multiple pathogens; among the most common are *Clostridia* (50% to 70%) and gram-negative bacilli such as *Escherichia coli* and *Klebsiella.* This infection is predominantly seen in diabetic male patients (70%) and is associated with gallbladder gangrene (74%) and perforation (21%). There is high mortality even with early diagnosis (15% to 25%). Half of the patients have gallstones. Diagnosis requires serial x-ray examinations or CT scan.

Treatment requires high-dose parenteral broad-spectrum antibiotics aimed at both anaerobic and gram-negative bacteria (imipenem or piperacillin-tazobactam), together with prompt surgical intervention.

■ URINARY TRACT INFECTIONS

Diabetic female patients have a two-fold to fourfold higher incidence of bacteriuria and nosocomial urinary tract infection (UTI), and higher risk of developing upper UTI (pyelonephritis). Among the predisposing factors are the presence of neurogenic bladder, uncontrolled diabetes and glycosuria, recurrent vaginitis, renal disease, and urologic instrumentation. Neurogenic bladder makes single-dose or 3-day course of antibiotic treatment less effective, and patients may require a longer course of therapy for cystitis (i.e., 5 to 7 days). In the presence of recurrent infection, 10 to 14 days of therapy may be necessary.

Emphysematous cystitis is often the result of infection with *E. coli* or other Enterobacteriaceae. More than 80% of cases are in diabetic patients, who may present with pneumaturia and gas in the urinary bladder wall and the collection system, seen on either plain x-ray or CT scan studies. The disease usually responds to antibiotics targeting the Enterobacteriaceae.

Emphysematous pyelonephritis is a life-threatening suppurative infection of the renal and perirenal tissue. It occurs predominantly in diabetic patients (70% to 90%), more often in women than in men. The disease is usually unilateral, more often affecting the left kidney. More than 40% of cases have underlying urinary tract obstruction. *E. coli* is the predominant isolated organism (>70%). Patients present with fever, chills, flank pain, confusion, and often sepsis. Occasionally, patients present with fever of unknown origin. The diagnosis is made by demonstration of gas on plain x-ray film or CT scan of the abdomen. Treatment usually requires a combination of surgical intervention (unilateral nephrectomy) and antibiotic therapy. Survival rate is more than 90% in patients who have both surgical and antibiotic treatment versus 25% in cases treated with antibiotics alone.

Papillary necrosis can occur as a complication of emphysematous pyelonephritis or as an isolated entity. More than 50% of cases are described in diabetic patients, with other cases being seen in patients with analgesic abuse, sickle cell disease, and urinary tract obstruction. Many patients present acutely with fever, ureteral colic, microscopic or macroscopic hematuria, and pyuria. Half of the patients develop renal failure. Some patients have an indolent presentation and may pass sloughed papillary tissue in the urine. Diagnosis can be made by renal ultrasound. However, the test of choice is retrograde pyelography. For patients who present with obstruction and do not pass the detached papilla spontaneously, surgical removal is indicated through cystoscopy with ureteral instrumentation. Antibiotic therapy for a minimum of 2 weeks may be required, as in pyelonephritis.

Perinephric abscess should be suspected in patients who present with "pyelonephritis" but who have a poor response to 4 or 5 days of intravenous antibiotic therapy. One third of cases are described in diabetic patients who present with pyuria, moderate fever, and abdominal of flank mass in the affected kidney (50% of cases). Among the gram-negative organisms, *E. coli* is the most common isolate, and ascending infection is the usual route of spread. The diagnosis requires use of renal ultrasound, CT, or MRI studies, which also can help exclude ureteral obstruction. Surgical drainage is mandatory (open surgery or percutaneous catheter placement) in combination with 4 weeks of parenteral antibiotic therapy.

Fungal UTIs occur with increased frequency in the diabetic population, especially after long-term broad-spectrum antibiotics or Foley catheter placement. Most of the patients have asymptomatic candiduria and are afebrile. However, severe infections complicated with fungus ball formation, obstruction, and sepsis have been seen. For this reason, all asymptomatic (presumably colonized) patients should be carefully observed for any signs of deterioration. Development of fever or azotemia must be investigated for possible ureteral obstruction, renal involvement, or disseminated fungal disease. Quantitative colony counts of only 10,000/ml of yeast in the urine may be sufficient to cause disease. Among the most common isolates are *C. albicans, C. tropicalis,* and *C. glabrata.* Because fluconazole is excreted in the urine, either intravenous or oral route of administration are effective forms of therapy. As an alternative therapy, amphotericin B can be used intravenously in patients with renal involvement or as bladder irrigations in patients with cystitis. Patients who have evidence of obstruction will require surgical intervention.

■ SKIN AND SOFT-TISSUE INFECTIONS

Superficial infections are often caused by *Staphylococcus aureus,* which commonly colonizes the nasal mucosa and the skin of diabetic patients. Recurrent abscesses require drainage and antibiotic therapy. Elimination of the *S. aureus* carrier state can be achieved by application of bacitracin ointment to the nares and oral administration of rifampin, bactrim, or minocycline (two drugs in combination for 10 to 14 days). Diabetic patients also have a higher incidence of postoperative clean wound infections.

Necrotizing infections may be superficial (infection external to deep fascia without myonecrosis) or deep. Crepitant (anaerobic) cellulitis is a superficial process. It is produced by multiple organisms, most often anaerobes. Infection is seen more frequently in diabetic patients with chronic, nonhealing lower-extremity ulcers. Crepitus is present on palpation because of subdermal and subcutaneous gas dissection. Treatment of this infection requires appropriate parenteral antibiotics and surgical debridement. Necrotizing fasciitis occurs when infection spreads along the superficial fascial planes without muscle involvement. This is a mixed infection caused by both aerobes and anaerobes (e.g., *Bacteriodes* species, *Enterococcus* species, Peptostreptococcus, *E. coli, Proteus*); however, occasionally *Streptococcus pyogenes* can be the single pathogen incriminated. Dermal necrosis follows thrombosis of skin vessels. In the later stages of the infection, destruction of the small nerve fibers results in patchy area of skin anesthesia. Management requires broad-spectrum coverage antibiotics to cover both aerobic and anaerobic flora (e.g., Zosyn, imipenem) and thorough debridement and drainage, using the "filleting procedure." The subcutaneous tissue is left open, and irrigation with normal saline or Ringer's lactate solution is performed. Many patients require repeated debridement. Infection produced by *S. pyogenes* is often complicated by toxic shock syndrome (see the chapter *Staphylococcal and Streptococcal Toxic Shock and Kawasaki Syndromes*).

Deep Necrotizing Infections

Necrotizing cellulitis (nonclostridial myonecrosis) is produced by the same bacteria responsible for necrotizing fasciitis; however, infection progresses to deeper layers and involves the muscle. This form of infection occurs most commonly in diabetic patients (75%) and often involves the lower extremities. Infection can also affect the abdominal wall or perineum, especially after surgery, penetrating trauma, or instrumentation. Treatment requires coverage of both aerobic and anaerobic pathogens, and should cover *S. aureus*, gram-negative enteric organisms, *E. coli*, *Proteus*, *Bacteroides fragilis*, and Enterococcus species. All patients need to have aggressive debridement and resection of the necrotic muscle. Hyperbaric oxygen therapy may be considered, if available.

Diabetic patients are also at risk for clostridial myonecrosis, including *C. septicum*. Aggressive surgical removal of the affected muscles (or amputation) with appropriate antimicrobial therapy, as well as hyperbaric oxygen therapy, may be administered.

Foot infections in diabetic patients are responsible for 20% of their hospital admissions. The most important predisposing factors are peripheral neuropathy, vascular disease, immunopathy, and history of a previous ulcer. The severity of diabetic foot infection can vary from mild and superficial (often monobacterial, caused by *S. aureus* or *S. epidermidis*) to moderate or severe deep infection. Tissue gangrene is usually induced by polymicrobial (mixed aerobic and anaerobic) infections. The presence of deep tissue abscess or bone involvement can be determine by use of MRI. Evaluation of vascular supply, in any patient with diminished or absent peripheral pulses, requires arterial Doppler (with both pressure and wave forms studies) and measurement of transcutaneous oxygen tension.

Mild infections without systemic symptoms can be treated with oral antibiotics (Augmentin, quinolones, or first-generation cephalosporins) and require close follow-up at 48 to 72 hours. If parenteral therapy is considered, cefazolin or cefuroxime may be used for presumed monobacterial infection. Moderate non–limb-threatening infections can be managed with local debridement and parenteral antibiotic therapy with a broader coverage. The empiric therapy can be altered based on culture results. For soft-tissue infection, duration of therapy should be 10 to 14 days based on the clinical outcome. Limb-threatening infections (extensive cellulitis, deep ulcer, plus lymphangitis, and/or osteomyelitis) may require broad coverage (piperacillin-tazobactam, imipenem, or meropenem) empirically, which should be altered based on culture results. Surgical debridement, drainage of any abscess collection, and excision of necrotic tissue should be done promptly. Bone infection may require extirpation of the affected bone or amputation, dictated by the extent of bone involvement, the status of vascular supply, and the extent of soft-tissue infection. Preservation of the ambulatory capacity should be considered. If infected bone is not totally removed, 10 weeks of antibiotic therapy (4 weeks IV plus 6 weeks PO) may be necessary based on the bone biopsy and culture results. When cultures are not available, empiric therapy with levofloxacin IV plus metronidazole PO, cepepime IV plus metronidazole PO, or imipenem, for a total of 10 weeks may be given. For patients with complicating factors such as extensive osteomyelitis, multiple recurrent infections, and poor vascular supply whose infected bone cannot be surgically removed, indefinite oral suppressive therapy may be considered.

Suggested Reading

Boulton AJM: The pathogenesis of diabetic foot problems: an overview, *Diabetic Med* 13:S12, 1996.

Lipsky BA, Pecoraro RE, Larson SA: Outpatient management of uncomplicated lower-extremity infections in diabetic patients, *Arch Intern Med* 150:790, 1990.

Sapico FL, Bessman AN: Infections in the diabetic patient, *Infect Dis Clin Prac* 1:339, 1992.

TRAUMA-RELATED INFECTION

John D. Brownlee
Mark A. Malangoni

Table 1 Potential Pathogens and Their Anatomic Locations

Staphylococcus epidermidis	Skin, oropharynx
Staphylococcus aureus	Skin, oropharynx, upper gastrointestinal tract
Beta-hemolytic streptococci	Oropharynx
Streptococcus pneumoniae	Oropharynx
Anaerobic streptococci	Oropharynx, vagina
Enterobacteriaceae (e.g., *Escherichia coli*, *Klebsiella*, *Enterobacter*)	Gastrointestinal tract, vagina, perineum
Candida albicans	Oropharynx, gastrointestinal tract
Clostridium perfringens	Skin, perineum
Bacteroides fragilis	Distal gastrointestinal tract
Bacteroides species (non-*fragilis*)	Oropharynx, gastrointestinal tract

Infection is a relatively common complication of trauma. Although hemorrhage and central nervous system injury are more common causes of early mortality, most patients who die more than 48 hours after injury usually succumb to the consequences of infectious complications.

Trauma-related infection represents either infection at an original site of injury or infection that occurs as a direct result of the injury. Examples of the former are an infected soft-tissue laceration or osteomyelitis at the site of an open fracture. The latter include empyema after a penetrating wound to the chest and an intraabdominal abscess that follows a gunshot wound to the colon. Infection also may occur at sites remote from the area of injury; however, these infections usually result from invasive monitoring devices or lifesaving treatments such as mechanical ventilation.

Injury can lead to infection by (1) direct contamination of a sterile site with exogenous microorganisms; (2) disruption of a natural epithelial barrier of the gastrointestinal, respiratory, or gynecologic tract, with contamination from endogenous microorganisms; (3) impairment of local antimicrobial clearance mechanisms by direct damage to tissue and the introduction of substances such as foreign bodies or hematomas that act as adjuvants to promote infection; and (4) impairment of systemic antimicrobial defenses through secondary effects related to the consequences of injury.

Various preexisting conditions also may contribute directly to the development of trauma-related infections. Examples include diabetes mellitus, obesity, malnutrition, advanced age, alcoholism, and renal failure. Invasive and diagnostic interventions such as the placement of endotracheal tubes, intravascular catheters, and urinary catheters provide direct access to sterile body sites, bypassing the normal defenses to infection and providing a portal of entry for pathogens. These microorganisms may cause infection at the site of entry or may cause a distant infection following hematogenous contamination.

Trauma-related infection occurs either from the introduction of small numbers of pathogenic bacteria or following contamination from a large inoculum of less pathogenic organisms. Several potential pathogens are found consistently throughout the body (Table 1). Improper treatment can predispose to infection by impairing the clearance of subpathologic concentrations of bacteria. Importantly, the adequacy of the blood supply to the area of injury can affect the propensity to develop infection, and impairments of perfusion because of preexisting disease or the injury per se will increase the risk of developing a trauma-related infection.

Efforts to prevent infection should begin immediately after injury. Initial management includes wound examination to determine the depth of injury and to identify recesses, foreign bodies, hematomas, and devitalized tissue. Wounds should be covered with a sterile dressing as soon as possible to prevent further contamination. In traumatic wounds associated with fractures, there is a direct relationship between the risk of infection and the severity of soft-tissue injury. Early immobilization of the fracture helps reduce additional soft-tissue damage and can help decrease the risk of infection by preventing dissemination of contaminating bacteria. Foreign material must be removed manually or by irrigation. Bleeding should be controlled by the application of direct pressure or by identification and ligation of bleeding points. Hematomas should be evacuated and gentle blunt dissection used to identify and assess the injury to specialized tissues such as muscle, tendon, nerve, and vascular structures. Debridement of all devitalized soft tissues is essential to proper wound management.

After appropriate cleansing, the type and technique of wound closure can be addressed. In general, the simplest appropriate technique is preferred over more elaborate ones. Clean wounds with low risk for infection should undergo primary closure. Heavily contaminated wounds or wounds that are at high risk for infection should not be closed initially. In this situation, it is more prudent to repeat cleansing and debridement of the site of injury and delay closure until the wound is cleaned and can be sutured safely. Unless the wound environment can be treated sufficiently to allow for closure with a low risk of infection, it should be allowed to heal by secondary intention.

Missile track wounds of the extremities are best managed by early debridement and irrigation of entrance and exit sites and coverage with sterile dressings. These tracks are usually contaminated and often cannot be adequately cleansed and debrided. They should be left open, cleansed two to three times daily, and allowed to heal by secondary intention. Complex wounds with extensive areas of soft-tissue devitalization are best managed by debridement and irrigation with loose approximation of the skin. Any remaining areas of exposed soft tissue can be managed with wet-to-dry dressing changes to promote a healthy granulating bed that can be covered later with a split-thickness skin graft or full-thickness skin or can be allowed to heal by secondary intention.

Antibiotic therapy is not a substitute for sound clinical judgment, excellent local wound care, aseptic technique, and careful handling of tissues. For uncomplicated minor wounds with minimal contamination and a low risk of infection, antibiotic therapy is unnecessary. Empiric antibiotic therapy may be beneficial when there is heavy bacterial contamination, an open fracture or joint space, major soft-tissue injury, or a delay of initial management for greater than 6 hours and for patients who are predisposed to infections. Cultures of contaminated wound sites usually add little to treatment decisions. Tetanus toxoid and tetanus immunoglobulin should be administered in accordance with established guidelines for contaminated wounds. Empiric antibiotic therapy should be directed against gram-positive bacteria in most wounds. When fecal contamination has occurred, such as with a farm injury or a human bite, anaerobes and gram-negative enteric bacteria must also be included in the antimicrobial spectrum. Treatment should be continued only for 24 hours in wounds with a minor or moderate degree of contamination because longer periods of drug use are not associated with better results. Recommended antibiotic choices are listed in Table 2.

Intraabdominal infection after penetrating abdominal trauma is an important paradigm that defines risk factors for trauma-related infection in a body cavity. The patient's age, number of organs injured, units of blood products transfused, and presence of a severe contaminating injury such as a colon injury define a group of patients at high risk for infection after penetrating abdominal trauma. These factors are indicators of decreased physiologic reserve, impairments as a result of the systemic effects of injury, the effects of hemorrhagic shock, and the contribution of heavy bacterial contamination to the risk of infection. Because these risk factors cannot be completely defined before operation, empiric treatment with a broad-spectrum cephalosporin such as cefotetan or cefoxitin is indicated. Patients with a low risk of infection need only a single dose of antibiotic, but those with a high risk of infection, such as colon injury, should be treated for 24 hours. Treatment longer than 24 hours is of no added value.

Traditionally, antibiotic therapy for established intraab-

Table 2 Antibiotic Therapy for Traumatic Wounds

Minor lacerations	No antibiotics recommended
Heavily contaminated lacerations	Cefazolin, 1-2 g IV q8h Amoxicillin-clavulanate, 500 mg PO q12h, or 250 mg q8h, or cephalexin, 500 mg PO q6h
Farm injuries and human bites	Cefoxitin, 2 g IV q6h, or Ampicillin-sulbactam, 1.5-3.0 g IV q6h, or Piperacillin-tazobactam, 3.375 g IV q16h, or Amoxicillin-clavulanate, 500 mg PO q12h, or 250 mg q8h (see the chapter *Human and Animal Bites*)
Penetrating abdominal wounds	Cefotetan, 2 g IV q12h, or Cefoxitin, 2 g IV q6h, or Piperacillin-tazobactam, 3.375 g IV q6h (≤24 hr duration)

dominal infection after penetrating trauma included an aminoglycoside combined with either clindamycin or metronidazole. Because of the risks of nephrotoxicity and difficulty achieving appropriate serum concentrations using aminoglycosides, single-agent regimens such as imipenem-cilastatin or meropenem are preferred. For patients who are allergic to these drugs, ciprofloxacin plus metronidazole is a useful alternative.

Bullets or pellets that penetrate the gastrointestinal tract and lodge in soft tissues can result in soft-tissue infections. This usually occurs because of concomitant soft-tissue injury and bacterial contamination. In this situation, the contaminating foreign body should be removed, debridement done, and the area drained.

Suggested Reading

Fabian TC, et al: Duration of antibiotic therapy for penetrating abdominal trauma: a prospective trial, *Surgery* 112:789, 1992.

Nichols RL, et al: Risk of infection after penetrating abdominal trauma, *N Engl J Med* 311:1065, 1984.

Polk HC: Factors influencing the risk of infection after trauma, *Am J Surg* 165:2S, 1993.

INFECTIOUS COMPLICATIONS IN THE INJECTION DRUG USER

Carlo Contoreggi

Vivian E. Rexroad

John S. Lambert

Intravenous drug abuse is a widespread public health problem. Medical complications associated with injecting drugs are commonly infectious as a result of frequent septic parenteral insults or the transmission of bloodborne infectious agents.

■ ENDOCARDITIS

Endocarditis, a life-threatening infection of the heart vales and/or endocardium, is associated with septic parenteral injections. Right-sided valvular infections commonly occur in injection drug users (IDUs) as a result of septic inoculations. Intravenous injection with low-pressure venous return increases the susceptibility of right-sided structures to endocarditis. Concurrent pulmonary hypertension caused by drug adulterants, such as talc, may also predispose to right-sided valvular disease.

Despite the high prevalence of endocarditis, the offending pathogens are not specific to injectors. *Staphylococcus aureus* is the most commonly identified organism, but other pathogens, including *Pseudomonas, Serratia,* groups A and B streptococcus, and *Streptococcus viridans,* are found. Increasingly, fungal pathogens are seen with immunodeficiency.

The clinical diagnosis of endocarditis in the drug abuser can be difficult, with many nonspecific signs and symptoms. The hallmark finding is fever. Other constitutional symptoms such as chills, sweats, and arthralgia are less specific and are commonly observed in opiate-dependent patients during withdrawal. The physical signs associated with left-sided endocarditis are seldom present.

Initial antimicrobial therapy should cover penicillinase-resistant staphylococci. Antibiotic coverage with nafcillin or oxacillin plus gentamicin is usually initiated. Once the organism is identified and sensitivies are available, medication choices may be modified. If methicillin-resistant staphylococcus is suspected, nafcillin or oxacillin should be replaced with vancomycin (see the chapter *Endocarditis* for specifics of therapy).

The IDU is often not compliant with prolonged hospitalization and the long therapy that endocarditis may require. A recent preliminary study has shown efficacy of a 7-day course of oral ciprofloxacin, 750 twice daily, and rifampin, 300 every 12 hours, as combination therapy for uncomplicated right-sided endocarditis. Patient compliance is still a concern even with short-term therapy of endocarditis.

Right-sided endocarditis generally carries a good prognosis when a full course of antibiotic therapy sterilizes the infecting pathogens. Serious complications are uncommon, but septic pulmonary emboli may cause clinically evident ventilatory and perfusion mismatch and pneumonia. Right-sided endocarditis has a mortality rate of less than 5% compared with up to 25% mortality seen with left-sided endocarditis. Inflammatory myocarditis seen with endocarditis is often multifactorial in substance abusers, with cocaine abuse, human immunodeficiency virus (HIV) infection, and injection drug use as contributing factors.

■ BONE AND JOINT INFECTIONS

Gram-positive bacteria and *Pseudomonas aeruginosa* are the most commonly isolated organisms in bone and joint infections. Osteomyelitis most commonly affects the fibrocartilaginous joints such as the vertebral, sternoarticular, and sacroiliac joints. Optimal therapy involves isolation of the pathogen by culture or biopsy before initiation of antimicrobial medications. Given the wide variety in the susceptibility of the infecting organism(s) in immunosuppressed patients, bone or joint cultures are often necessary for accurate diagnosis. In addition to bacterial infections, fungal infections are increasingly described in both immunodeficient and immunocompetent hosts.

■ SKIN AND SOFT-TISSUE INFECTIONS

Septic parenteral injections often lead to skin and soft-tissue infections. Infectious and chemical thrombophlebitis, abscesses, and cellulitis are all common venous insults.

Life-threatening cutaneous infections seen in this population include fasciitis, myonecrosis, and gangrene. Tissue crepitance, extensive cellulitis, evidence of systemic toxicity, and severe pain are highly suggestive of deep infection. Plain radiographs may be helpful in identification of extensive tissue destruction and gas production associated with gangrene.

Injected drugs and their adulterants are often damaging to veins, resulting in progressive sclerosis. With the loss of peripheral venous access, the IDU often attempts more dangerous injection sites such as the femoral, axillary, jugular, penile, and mammary veins. Serious infections and thrombotic events, such as jugular and axillary thrombosis, penile gangrene, and mammary and inguinal fasciitis, can result from injections at these sites.

Once intravenous access is not available, many substance abusers will administer drugs subcutaneously; this is known as skin popping. Staphylococci and streptococci are the most common pathogens. The IDU often shows signs of immunosuppression, and in this setting, other bacterial pathogens are encountered, including *Escherichia coli, Klebsiella, Bacteroides, Clostridia,* and mixed flora consisting of aerobic, anaerobic, and fungal organisms.

Self-limited infections usually can be treated with local care and may not require systemic antibiotics. Severe infections should be managed with surgical debridement and inpatient antibiotic therapy.

■ VIRAL HEPATITIS

The epidemiology of hepatitis A has changed dramatically in the past decade, with drug abuse being recognized as a significant transmission risk. Hepatitis A is associated with fecal-oral transmission. Contaminated marijuana has been reported as a transmission agent for hepatitis A.

Hepatitis B, C, D, and G (HBV, HCV, HDV, and HGV, respectively) are associated with parenteral transmission. The incidence of HBV and HCV in IDU populations is very high worldwide, with a significant proportion infected with both HBV and HCV.

Chronic HBV infection is associated with persistent hepatitis B surface antigen (HBsAg) and hepatitis Be antigen (HBeAg), although hepatic inflammation varies widely. HBeAg is associated with increased infectivity, more severe disease, and eventual cirrhosis. The HBV virion is not cytotoxic but mediates a host cytotoxic T-cell response that causes hepatocellular inflammation and necrosis. Coinfection with HIV-1 with its associated cellular immune deficiency reduces the severity of the host cytotoxic response. Progressive HIV-associated cellular immunodeficiency manifests with reduced hepatic inflammation and lower serum transaminase concentrations. Other serologic measures of HBV infection in HIV are not diminished.

HDV, or delta particle infection, is common in IDUs. This infection, which requires coinfection with HBV, imparts a more severe course than HBV alone. Coinfection with HBV and HDV is associated with increased incidence of fulminant hepatic failure. Vaccination with HBV vaccine will also prevent HDV infection.

Though less well characterized than HBV, HCV appears to be heterogenous, with significant genetic and immunologic variability. Parenteral transmission is better established than other routes of HCV transmission (i.e., familial, sexual, or maternal-fetal). Most cases are traced to parenteral exposures, either through blood or blood-product transfusion or injection drug use. In IDU populations, there is evidence that HBV and HCV coinfection increases the severity of clinical hepatitis and the persistence of transaminase elevation.

A recently isolated flavivirus known as HGV has been detected in the individuals at high risk for parenteral transmission, including the IDU, hemophiliacs, transplant recipients, and homosexuals. Preliminary studies in IDUs did not find an association between the markers of HGV infection and markers for liver inflammation (elevated ALT, AST, and γ-glutamyl transferase). Also, HGV RNA was found more frequently in the serum of younger IDUs with a shorter duration of drug use, and it is hypothesized that these individuals contract HGV infection and may later clear the virus. These studies require confirmation once reliable antibody tests are available for HGV components. However, these initial findings suggest that HGV does not cause significant chronic liver disease.

The development of progressive hepatitis and end-stage liver failure from HBV, HCV, and HDV in the IDU population is likely to increase as this population ages. Effective therapy for chronic HBV and HCV remains limited, but studies have shown efficacy of agents such as alpha-interferon. (See the chapter *Chronic Hepatitis.*)

■ HUMAN T-CELL LEUKEMIA/LYMPHOMA VIRUS

The incidence of non-HIV retroviral infections is lower than that of HBV, HCV, or HDV among IDUs in Europe, North America, and Australia. Human T-cell leukemia/lymphoma virus (HTLV)-II infection is more frequently reported than HTLV-I in IDUs. Viral transmission primarily occurs parenterally and sexually, and maternal-fetal transmission is less frequent than with HIV. Endemic pockets of HTLV-II infection exist in Asia and the Caribbean basin. With increased injection drug use and high-risk sexual exposures, the prevalence of HTLV-II infection may increase.

HTLV-I causes cancers, chiefly leukemia and lymphoma, and a neurologic disorder, tropical spastic paraparesis. HTLV-II causes hairy-cell leukemia and T-cell lymphoma. The clinical sequelae of HTLV-II infection are less well defined than those of HIV-1. It appears that the incidence of disease from HTLV-II infection alone is low, about 0.5%.

HTLV-II infection causes subtle immune dysfunction that is mild compared with that of HIV-I infection. Coinfection with HIV-1 and HTLV-II causes more severe immune dysfunction than HIV-1 infection alone. Coinfection with HIV has also been associated with acquired T-cell depletion ichthyosis in the IDU. The long-term clinical effects of HTLV-II infection and the pace of its continued penetration into drug-abusing populations remains to be seen.

■ IMMUNOLOGIC ABNORMALITIES

IDUs have subtle abnormalities in immune function independent of HIV and other retroviral infections. Abnormal circulating immune factors include elevated plasma immunoglobulins, especially the immunoglobulins IgM and IgG; false-positive rheumatoid factor and syphilis serology; and the presence of febrile agglutinins and complement fixation tests. Cellular immunity has also been demonstrated to be abnormal in the IDU. HIV-1–antibody-negative parenteral opiate abusers may have elevated total T-lymphocyte counts as well as increased T-helper and T-suppressor cells. Measures of cellular immunity show diminished function. Natural killer (NK) cell function is diminished, and cytotoxic T-lymphocyte (CTL) function may also be impaired. Cellular immune functions are essential for host recognition of pathogens and for immune stimulants such as those in vaccines. It is possible that without intact cellular immunity, future HIV-1 vaccine effectiveness may be compromised in the active IDU.

Effective substance abuse treatment with discontinuation of septic injections may restore immunocompetence. Immune studies of patients maintained with methadone show that immune dysfunction improves after discontinuation of injection drug use.

■ TUBERCULOSIS

Mycobacterium tuberculosis, which is endemic in drug abusers, is a highly virulent bacteria that infects both immunocompetent and immunodeficient individuals. Coinfection of tuberculosis (TB) and HIV is found in a significant number of new TB cases. In those infected with HIV, TB primarily shows pulmonary involvement early. With progressive immunosuppression, disseminated extrapulmonary TB is common.

All HIV-infected patients should be tested for TB with purified protein derivative (PPD) skin test. The PPD should be administered as early in the course of their disease as possible and every 12 months or if clinical symptoms suggest new infection.

Untreated individuals with exposure to TB as evidenced by positive PPD are at high risk for recurrence of latent infection; especially patients with advanced immunodeficiency. Immunocompromised hosts recently exposed to TB should receive prophylaxis, as should anergic individuals with known environmental exposure and patients who are at high risk (i.e., the IDU and other substance abusers).

■ SEXUALLY TRANSMITTED DISEASES

Epidemiologic studies find that sexually transmitted diseases (STDs) are commonly found in IDUs. Providers who serve the IDU should be vigilant in screening for asymptomatic STD. Screening for syphilis may be problematic in IDU populations. The IDU is often reported to have false-positive test results with rapid plasma reagin (RPR) tests of 1:4 or greater and negative results for fluorescent treponemal antibody absorption (FTA-ABS) tests. However, changes in titer should be seen with serial screening. Practitioners should have a low threshold for repeating the FTA-ABS because some syphilis-infected patients may show transients elevations in RPR with or without reactivity in the FTA-ABS.

Drug-injecting women show high rates of STDs. These risks are clearly associated with the number of sexual partners, failure to use condoms, and commercial sex work. The STDs seen in this population include primary and recurrent genital herpes, recurrent genital warts, gonorrhea, trichomoniasis, chlamydia, and recurrent vaginal candidiasis. In addition to their significant morbidity, comcomitant STD will increase the incidence of sexual transmission of HIV and possibly other infectious agents (including hepatitis B and C and the HTLV retroviruses).

■ CONSIDERATIONS FOR THE HIV-1– INFECTED SUBSTANCE ABUSER

Pneumocystis carinii Pneumonia

Pneumocystis carinii is a ubiquitous organism that colonizes the respiratory tract early in life and becomes a pathogen in the setting of moderate to severe immunodeficiency. *P. carinii* pneumonia (PCP) occurred in nearly 90% of New York City IDUs evaluated in a recent study and was the most frequent acquired immunodeficiency syndrome (AIDS)-defining illness.

Bacterial Infections

An important aspect of the clinical management of opportunistic complications in the IDU is the early recognition, treatment, and prevention of potentially life-threatening bacterial infections. Bacterial infections involve those sites common in nonimmunocompromised hosts. Bacterial pneumonia, bronchitis, sinusitis, endocarditis, and sepsis are more common in HIV-positive IDUs. *Streptococcus pneumoniae* and *Haemophilus influenzae* are common pathogens in HIV-1–infected drug abusers. These organisms are highly virulent, and severe infections may occur early in the course of immunodeficiency. In addition to injection drug use, smoking and other constitutional factors such as nutrition and stress increase susceptibility to infection.

Prevention of primary infection with pneumococcal polysaccharide and *H. influenzae* type b vaccination has been shown to be effective in HIV-infected hosts. (See the chapter *HIV Infection: Initial Evaluation and Monitoring.*)

Toxoplasmosis

Toxoplasma gondii is a ubiquitous protozoal parasite found in soil. It is often ingested in raw meat. Activation of infection usually occurs with severe immunosuppression. Serologic testing early in the course of HIV infection to determine exposure is indicated, with prophylaxis as discussed in the chapter *Prophylaxis of Opportunistic Infections in HIV Disease.*

Fungal Infections

These pathogens are seen in the setting of both moderate (CD4 counts of 200 to 500 mm^3) and profound (CD4 counts <100 mm^3) immunosuppression. Invasive *Candida* infections commonly present as vaginitis, esophagitis, and oropharyngeal mucositis in mild to moderate immunosuppression.

Other fungal infections are commonly seen in more severe immunosuppression. These pathogens cause disseminated and invasive tissue disease, with osteomyelitis, pneumonia, meningitis, and other central nervous system lesions commonly seen. *Histoplasmosis* (endemic in the Ohio Valley), *coccidioidomycosis* (prevalent in the Southwestern states), and *cryptococcosis* (endemic throughout North America) are ubiquitous fungal pathogens.

Opportunistic Viral Infections

Herpes simplex virus (HSV), varicella-zoster virus (VZV), cytomegalovirus (CMV), and Epstein-Barr virus (EBV) are common viral pathogens seen in the setting of severe to profound immunosuppression. Clinical manifestations of HSV are primarily mucocutaneous and may affect the genital, urinary, and gastrointestinal tracts. VZV causes localized dermatomal cutaneous lesions with disseminated disease seen in severe immunosuppression. The clinical presentation of CMV is variable, with neurologic, ocular, and gastrointestinal disease common in the setting of severe to profound immunosuppression.

Once CMV was identified, lifelong therapy was thought to be necessary; however, with the advent of effective antiretroviral regimens prolonged therapy may not be necessary.

■ BEHAVIORAL CONSIDERATIONS

The integration of substance abuse treatment with primary care for immunodeficiency can impact both clinical outcome and cost of care. It is essential for the health care provider to realize that this population is notoriously non-compliant and difficult to reach. Access to clearly identifiable care providers who can coordinate complex social services for patients will greatly aid in the management of the medically ill substance abuser. Compliance, although difficult to manage, may be aided with the use of specific contingencies for continued illicit drug use, medical non-compliance, and failure to keep scheduled appointments.

The use of methadone maintenance therapy in opiate-dependent HIV-1–infected patients slows the rate of progression of HIV disease when compared with non–methadone-maintained opiate-dependent individuals. In addition, the use of methadone or other opiate agonist therapy (i.e., buphrenorphine, LAAM [levo-alpha-acetyl methadol]) or the opiate antagonist naltrexone, in combination with behavioral therapy, can substantially improve the medical compliance of HIV-1–positive patients.

Direct-observed therapy (DOT) has been shown effective in the treatment of tuberculosis and in the prophylaxis of opportunistic infections. Until recently, the pharmacokinetics of most antiretroviral medication was such that once-daily dosing regimens were not possible. However, it has been shown that some current antiretroviral medications, such as nucleoside analogue didanosine (ddI) and the non-nucleoside reverse transcriptase inhibitor nevirapine, may be administered once daily with acceptable antiviral effect. New protease inhibitors with once-daily dosing profiles are currently in clinical trials. Thus it is likely that DOT will be effective for newer antiretroviral medication regimens, and the use of opiate replacement therapy has been used to improve medication adherence. It is clear that improved medication adherence and compliance with medical care will better control HIV and prolong life. This strategy should also improve outpatient clinic attendance, thus avoiding more expensive emergency and inpatient medical care.

■ PREVENTION OF INFECTIOUS COMPLICATIONS IN DRUG USERS

Perhaps the most important consideration for health care providers working with substance abusers is the recognition that it is possible to influence behaviors and enable drug users to choose less dangerous routes of drug use. Risk reduction may avert the substance abuser from contracting new infectious diseases. Effective syringe-cleaning methods for injectors or preferably the provision of clean injection equipment can prevent transmission of HIV-1 and other parenterally transmitted diseases such as hepatitis. The use of condoms will protect both the drug user and their sexual partners from HIV-1, hepatitis, and STD.

Suggested Reading

Bennett CL, et al: Medical care costs of intravenous drug users with AIDS in Brooklyn, *J Acquir Immun Defic Syndr* 5:1, 1992.

Lee HH, et al: Patterns of HIV-1 and HTLV-I/It in intravenous drug abusers from the middle Atlantic and central regions of the USA, *J Infect Dis* 162:347, 1990.

Levine DP: Infectious endocarditis in intravenous drug abusers. In Levine DP, Sobel JD, eds: *Infections in intravenous drug abusers*, New York, 1991, Oxford University Press.

INFECTION IN THE ALCOHOLIC

Laurel C. Preheim
Martha J. Gentry-Nielsen

Acute and chronic alcohol ingestion exert direct and indirect effects on host defenses against infection (Table 1). Recent studies suggest that the immunotoxic effects of ethanol result from direct cytotoxicity and from a shift in the balance of cytokines produced from the proinflammatory to more immunoinhibitory products. However, the adverse effects of ethanol itself may be indistinguishable from those caused by concomitant cirrhosis, malnutrition, poor hygiene, adverse living conditions, and abuse of tobacco and other drugs. This discussion includes infections associated with increased frequency or severity in patients who abuse alcohol (Table 2). The suggested antibiotic dosages are for adult patients with normal renal function. Therapeutic decisions always should be made with the knowledge that alcoholic liver disease can interfere with the metabolism and excretion of certain antiinfective agents and that some antimicrobials can cause or exacerbate hepatic dysfunction.

■ PNEUMONIA

Bacterial pneumonia usually follows aspiration of oropharyngeal flora into the lungs. Consequently, the most commonly reported causes of pneumonia in this setting include *Streptococcus pneumoniae*, anaerobes, aerobic gram-negative bacilli, and *Haemophilus influenzae*. Standard diagnostic approaches are used to evaluate alcoholic patients who exhibit signs or symptoms of pneumonia. Organisms seen on sputum Gram stain often can help guide empiric antibiotic therapy. In addition to obtaining sputum and blood cultures, any significant pleural fluid visible on chest roentgenogram should be sampled for appropriate stains as well as cultured for aerobic and anaerobic organisms. Because

Table 1 Immunodefects and Alcoholism
MECHANICAL DEFECTS
Diminished cough reflex
Impaired glottal closure
Lung atelectasis caused by ascites
Decreased ciliary function
HUMORAL IMMUNITY
Increased serum immunoglobulins
Decreased alveolar IgG subclasses
Decreased complement activity
Decreased serum bactericidal activity
CELL-MEDIATED IMMUNITY
Decreased skin test reactions
Decreased numbers of T-lymphocytes
Alterations in T-lymphocyte subsets
Altered cytokine production
Decreased suppressor cell activity
Decreased lymphocyte mitogenic response
Decreased natural killer cell function
PHAGOCYTES
Granulocytopenia (rare)
Decreased granulocyte chemotaxis
Decreased granulocyte bactericidal activity
Decreased macrophage phagocytosis
Decreased macrophage bactericidal activity

Table 2 Infections in Alcoholics
Bacterial pneumonia
Streptococcus pneumoniae
Anaerobes
Klebsiella pneumoniae
Haemophilus influenzae
Tuberculosis
Spontaneous bacterial peritonitis
Escherichia coli
K. pneumoniae
S. pneumoniae
Bacteremia
E. coli
S. pneumoniae
Group A streptococcus
Clostridium perfringens
Non-01 *Vibrio cholerae*
Vibrio vulnificus
Salmonella sp.
Bartonella quintana
Endocarditis
Gram-negative bacilli
S. pneumoniae
Diphtheria
Pancreatic abscess
Hepatitis B and C
HIV infection and AIDS

HIV, Human immunodeficiency virus; *AIDS,* acquired immunodeficiency syndrome.

the severity of bacterial pneumonia is increased in alcoholics, hospitalization for parenteral antibiotic therapy is usually indicated. The length of hospital stay and the need for intensive care units are likely to be higher, and the expected mortality rate is greater than twice that for nonalcoholic patients.

Pneumococcal Pneumonia

S. pneumoniae, or the pneumococcus, remains the most common cause of both community-acquired bacterial pneumonia and bacterial meningitis in adults. Outbreaks of pneumococcal pneumonia have occurred among residents of men's shelters and prisons, where close proximity enhances the risk of transmission for oropharyngeal organisms. Alcoholic patients have the usual signs and symptoms of pneumococcal pneumonia, including sudden onset, often with a single shaking chill, fever, and subsequent productive cough. Secondary complications, including empyema and bacteremia, are common in ethanol abusers, particularly those with liver disease.

Despite appropriate therapy, the reported overall mortality for adult bacteremic pneumococcal pneumonia increases from approximately 20% to greater than 50% in patients with cirrhosis. The Advisory Committee on Immunization Practices recommends pneumococcal polysaccharide vaccine for all alcoholics. However, the antibody responses may be blunted, and the efficacy of the vaccine has been questioned in this high-risk population.

Parenteral penicillin G, 6 to 12 million units intravenously daily in divided doses, is the treatment of choice for pneumococcal pneumonia caused by penicillin-sensitive strains (minimum inhibitory concentration [MIC] ≤ 0.06 μg/ml). For patients who are allergic to penicillin, alternative agents would include cefazolin, 1 to 2 g intravenously every 8 hours; erythromycin, 0.5 to 1 g intravenously every 6 hours; levofloxacin, 500 mg intravenously or orally every 24 hours; or gatifloxacin, 400 mg intravenously or orally every 24 hours. Cephalosporins should be avoided in patients with penicillin allergy manifested as hives, urticaria, or anaphylaxis. Higher dosages of penicillin G (8 to 12 million units intravenously daily); ceftriaxone, 1 to 2 g intravenously or intramuscularly daily; levofloxacin; gatifloxacin or moxifloxacin are effective therapy for severe infections caused by pneumococci with intermediate resistance to penicillin (MIC, 0.1 to 1 μg/ml). Levofloxacin, gatifloxacin, moxifloxacin, linezolid, or vancomycin, 1 g intravenously every 12 hours, are effective against pneumonia caused by pneumococci with high-level resistance to penicillin (MIC, ≥ 2 μg/ml).

Anaerobic Pneumonia

Anaerobic oropharyngeal bacteria, including peptostreptococci, *Fusobacterium* species, and *Prevotella melaninogenicus* are commonly involved in aspiration pneumonia and can cause lung abscess and empyema. Intoxication interferes with several host defenses against aspiration of oropharyngeal contents. Alcoholics often have severe periodontal disease, which can increase the number of anaerobic organisms in the aspirated inoculum. Clinical signs and symptoms commonly progress slowly over weeks or months before patients present with malaise, low-grade fever, cough producing foul-smelling sputum, and/or weight loss. Parenteral therapy with penicillin is usually effective. Clindamycin, 600 to 900 mg intravenously every 8 hours, is indicated for anaerobic pleuropulmonary infections in patients who are allergic to penicillin or who respond poorly to penicillin therapy.

Gram-Negative Pneumonia

Gram-negative bacilli such as *Klebsiella pneumoniae* and *Enterobacter* species are more likely to colonize the oropharynx and cause pneumonia in alcoholics than in nonalcoholics. The combination of bloody sputum and an upper lobe infiltrate with a bulging fissure that has been classically associated with *Klebsiella* pneumonia is rarely seen today. Mortality with gram-negative bacillary pneumonia exceeds that of pneumococcal pneumonia and increases further if neutropenia is also present. Combination therapy with an aminoglycoside plus an expanded-spectrum beta-lactam antibiotic, such as cefepime, 1 to 2 g intravenously every 12 hours; cefotaxime, 1 to 2 g intravenously every 8 hours; or piperacillin, 4 g intravenously every 6 hours, is recommended. Ciprofloxacin, 200 to 400 mg intravenously every 12 hours; levofloxacin; gatifloxacin; and moxifloxacin may also be effective.

The coccobacillus *H. influenzae* frequently causes pneumonia in alcoholics. Most patients will respond to ampicillin, 2 g intravenously every 6 hours. Ampicillin-sulbactam, 1.5 to 3 g intravenously every 6 hours, or cefuroxime, 750 mg intravenously every 8 hours is effective therapy for patients infected with ampicillin-resistant strains. Levofloxacin and azithromycin, 500 mg intravenously every 24 hours are additional alternatives.

■ TUBERCULOSIS

Historically, tuberculosis (TB) has been strongly associated with ethanol abuse, and alcoholics have 15 to 200 times the TB incidence rates of control populations. After decades of steady decline, the number of new cases of tuberculosis in the United States rose in 1985 and continued to climb into the early 1990s. Because of renewed control efforts, the number of new cases has again declined annually since 1992. Most cases occur in urban areas, where the incidence is especially high among the homeless and patients with acquired immunodeficiency syndrome (AIDS). Outbreaks of TB have occurred among indigent alcoholics housed in shelters. Most individuals remain asymptomatic early in the disease. Later, they may note malaise, fatigue, anorexia, weight loss, afternoon fevers, or night sweats. Cough is frequent, generally producing mucopurulent sputum that may be tinged with blood. The most common abnormality on chest roentgenogram is a multinodular cavitary infiltrate in the apical or subapical posterior areas of the upper lobes or in the superior segment of a lower lobe. Pleural effusions may be present. Roentgenographic findings of TB are confined to the lower lung fields in up to 18% of patients.

Hospitalized patients suspected of having active pulmonary TB should be placed in respiratory isolation. Tuberculin skin testing is useful, but false-negative reactions occur in up to 20% of persons with known TB on first testing.

The diagnosis of TB depends on isolation of *Mycobacterium tuberculosis* from clinical specimens. Sputum smears reveal acid-fast bacilli in 50% to 80% of patients with pulmonary TB. Susceptibility testing should be performed on *M. tuberculosis* isolates from any clinical specimen. Although there is no convincing evidence that alcohol abuse is associated with increased risks of extrapulmonary infection, miliary TB should remain in the differential diagnosis of fever of unknown origin in an alcoholic patient.

Alcoholic patients are less likely than nonalcoholic patients to be compliant with therapy for TB and thus are more likely to relapse. Current treatment guidelines with special emphasis on directly observed therapy should be followed to reduce risks of both therapeutic failure and emergence of drug-resistant strains (see the chapter *Tuberculosis*).

■ PERITONITIS

Up to 30% of patients with alcoholic liver disease and ascites develop spontaneous bacterial peritonitis (SBP). In this condition, bacterial cultures of ascitic fluid are positive, the fluid contains more than 300 neutrophils/mm^3, and there is no evident intraabdominal source of infection. SBP usually results from hematogenous seeding of ascitic fluid. Patients with severe acute or chronic liver disease have decreased serum complement levels, diminished serum bactericidal activity, and reduced bacterial clearance by macrophages of the reticuloendothelial system. Because the ability of ascitic fluid to opsonize bacteria and thus facilitate phagocytosis correlates closely with total protein concentration, patients with low ascitic fluid protein levels are at particular risk for SBP.

Many patients exhibit other findings of end-stage liver disease, such as hepatorenal syndrome, encephalopathy, and variceal bleeding. Other clinical features include fever, vomiting, abdominal pain, and physical signs of peritonitis. However, signs or symptoms of infection are absent in approximately one third of patients with SBP, so diagnostic paracentesis is indicated for all alcoholic patients with ascites. Fluid should be submitted to the laboratory for chemistry tests, cell count and differential, and microbiologic stains and cultures. Centrifugation of ascitic fluid and Gram stain of the sediment will reveal organisms in 25% to 68% of patients with SBP. Some authorities recommend that a portion of ascitic fluid be inoculated directly into blood culture bottles at the bedside. Peripheral blood cultures should be performed if SBP is suspected.

Most cases of SBP are caused by gram-negative bacilli, especially *Escherichia coli* and *K. pneumoniae*. Possible gram-positive pathogens include *S. pneumoniae*, enterococci, and staphylococci. Anaerobes cause only 6% of SBP cases, presumably because of the relatively high pO$_2$ of ascitic fluid. Empiric therapy should be directed against the likely pathogens. Suitable choices include ampicillin-sulbactam, 1.5 to 3 g intravenously every 6 hours, or cefotaxime, 1 to 2 g intravenously every 8 hours. (See the chapter *Peritonitis*.)

TB peritonitis can occur in patients with alcoholic liver disease. Clinical findings resemble those of bacterial peritonitis, and acid-fast stains of ascitic fluid are usually negative. The diagnosis is best made with stains and cultures of peritoneal tissue, especially when obtained by peritoneoscope-directed biopsy. The treatment regimen is the same as for pulmonary tuberculosis.

■ BACTEREMIA

The liver plays a major role in clearing bacteria from the bloodstream. Alcoholic cirrhosis adversely affects hepatic reticuloendothelial system function. Both intrahepatic and extrahepatic arteriovenous shunts divert blood from macrophages that line liver capillary beds. In addition, both acute intoxication and cirrhosis interfere with bactericidal activity of these tissue phagocytes. Hypocomplementemia, neutropenia, and reduced serum bactericidal activity also may contribute to bacteremia in these patients. Neutropenia is strongly associated with increased mortality, and treatment with granulocyte colony-stimulating factor may be warranted for neutropenic patients.

E. coli is the most common cause of spontaneous bacteremia in alcoholic and cirrhotic patients. Additional organisms causing bacteremia or sepsis include other gram-negative bacilli, S. pneumoniae, group A streptococci, and Clostridium perfringens. Alcoholics with cirrhosis are particularly susceptible to sepsis caused by non-01 Vibrio cholerae and Vibrio vulnificus, an opportunistic pathogen found in marine waters. Bacteremia can follow ingestion of contaminated shellfish, or exposure to seawater can result in a cutaneous infection. The latter may progress from erythematous or ecchymotic patches to bullae formation, subcutaneous necrosis, and bacteremia. V. vulnificus infections are associated with high mortality rates. Appropriate antibiotic therapy includes ceftazidime, 2 g intravenously every 8 hours, plus doxycycline, 100 mg intravenously or orally every 12 hours; cefotaxime, 2 g intravenously every 8 hours; or ciprofloxacin, 400 mg intravenously or 750 mg PO every 12 hours. Nontyphoidal salmonella septicemia, especially that caused by Salmonella typhimurium and Salmonella choleraesuis, also has been associated with alcoholic liver disease. Homeless people and alcoholics also are at increased risk for bacteremia caused by Bartonella quintana, and the seroprevalence for this organism is high among homeless people in both the United States and Europe.

■ ENDOCARDITIS

Alcoholism is one of the strongest risk factors for pneumococcal endocarditis, and a few reports link cirrhosis with increased frequency and severity of endocarditis caused by other bacteria. It remains an uncommon complication of cirrhosis, however, seen in only 1% to 14% of cirrhotic patients. The aortic valve is most likely to be involved. Many patients have no demonstrable underlying cardiac valvular abnormalities. Compared with that in nonalcoholics, endocarditis in cirrhotic patients is more likely to involve gram-negative bacilli such as E. coli and less likely to be caused by alpha-hemolytic streptococci.

■ OTHER INFECTIONS

Diphtheria
The lifestyle and poor hygiene of many alcoholics can predispose them to Corynebacterium diphtheriae infection. Cutaneous rather than pharyngeal diphtheria was reported in most cases from three outbreaks from the Skid Row district of Seattle. Many skin lesions were secondarily infected with group A streptococci. Erythromycin remains the treatment of choice. Routine immunization with combined tetanus and diphtheria toxoid is highly recommended for all patients in high-risk groups.

Pancreatic Abscess
Alcohol abuse is a common cause of acute pancreatitis, and pancreatic abscess is a rare but potentially catastrophic complication. Primary abscesses characteristically evolve rapidly and culminate in severe sepsis. Secondary abscesses, which may present weeks after the acute inflammation, commonly involve infection of a pancreatic pseudocyst. The cardinal signs of abscess are high fever, septicemia, a rapidly enlarging abdominal mass, and multisystem organ failure in severe cases. Early surgical drainage is important. Initial empiric antibiotic therapy should be aimed at the most common pathogens, including E. coli, other enteric aerobes, and anaerobic gram-negative bacilli.

Viral Hepatitis
Hepatitis viruses and alcohol abuse are the two main causes of liver cirrhosis. Alcoholic patients have a higher rate of nonresponsiveness to the hepatitis B envelope vaccine compared with nonalcoholic patients, and ethanol may adversely affect the cellular immune responses to the virus. Nonetheless, several studies have detected a high prevalence of serum markers for hepatitis B infection in patients with alcoholic cirrhosis, suggesting that hepatitis B virus may exacerbate chronic liver disease and cirrhosis in alcoholics. Likewise, hepatitis C virus is found at a high incidence in alcoholic patients, and 20% to 30% of patients infected with hepatitis C will progress to cirrhosis. Furthermore, alcohol ingestion may accelerate liver damage and hasten the clinical progression of hepatitis C infection. The nature of the relationship between these two viral infections and alcoholic liver disease requires further study.

Human Immunodeficiency Virus Infection
Studies in a population of alcoholics in New York found a relatively high prevalence of human immunodeficiency virus (HIV) infections, and conversely, there is a high prevalence of alcoholism in the HIV-positive population. It is not clear whether alcohol abuse predisposes to HIV infection at the time of exposure, although intoxication does have a disinhibiting effect on risk-taking behavior. It also is unclear whether alcohol consumption increases the rate of HIV replication within the host, although ethanol intake has been shown in some studies to increase HIV replication in isolated human blood mononuclear cells. It is likely that the well-described adverse effects of ethanol on cell-mediated immune function may reduce host defenses against HIV infection. Finally, the effect of ethanol ingestion

on progression from asymptomatic HIV infection to AIDS-defining opportunistic infections has not been clearly established. In a retrospective human study, progression to AIDS was not abbreviated by the use of ethanol, but chronic alcohol ingestion by CD4 depleted mice enhanced persistence of *Pneumocystis carinii*. Aside from the direct effects of acute alcohol ingestion, the concomitant malnutrition and liver disease seen with chronic alcoholism may amplify the immunosuppressive effects of ethanol and hasten the progression from asymptomatic HIV infection to manifestations of AIDS.

Suggested Reading

Cook RT: Alcohol abuse, alcoholism, and damage to the immune system—a review, *Alcoholism: Clin Exp Res* 22:1927, 1998.

Davis CC, Mellencamp MA, Preheim LC: A model of pneumococcal pneumonia in chronically intoxicated rats, *J Infect Dis* 163:799, 1991.

MacGregor RR, Louria DB: Alcohol and infection, *Curr Clin Top Infect Dis* 17:291, 1997.

Sternbach GL: Infections in alcoholic patients, *Emerg Med Clin North Am* 8:793, 1990.

INFECTIONS IN THE ELDERLY

Kent Crossley

Although virtually all significant types of infections that occur in the elderly are discussed elsewhere in this book, certain aspects of infectious diseases in older individuals need to be emphasized. This chapter stresses the unique aspects of the etiology and therapy of infections in the elderly (defined here as older than 65 years of age). Infections that occur in long-term care institutions are only briefly discussed.

For several reasons, infections in the elderly are an important area of concern for medicine. The number of individuals older than 65 is increasing dramatically. Although representing only 13% of the U.S. population at present, the elderly consume 25% of all prescription medications and a similarly disproportionate amount of other health care services. Moreover, with few exceptions (some viral infections and venereal diseases), most common infections occur more often in older individuals.

Although the mortality associated with many infections is increased in the elderly, age alone is now seen as a relatively unimportant risk factor for infection-related death or serious morbidity. Rather, it is the variety of comorbid conditions that are increasingly common with advancing age that appear to be closely associated with greater morbidity and mortality from infection.

It has become clear in the last decade that there is a general hyporesponsiveness of the immune system in elderly individuals. This is the most likely explanation for the muted symptoms and signs that are a common denominator of infections in the aged. It is well documented in a number of types of infectious illnesses that maximum temperatures, white blood cell count elevations, and the overtness of clinical signs and symptoms are all less pronounced in older individuals than in younger adults. In clinical terms, this means that an elderly patient may have a serious bacteremic infection without chills, fever, or leukocytosis. This is one of the most important things to remember about infections in the aged.

■ PRINCIPLES OF ANTIBIOTIC USE

Table 1 summarizes current recommendations for treatment of common infections in the elderly. Important points to note include the following:

1. Aminoglycoside antibiotics may be best avoided in older individuals because of their potential toxicity. It is possible that the once-daily administration of these drugs may be associated with more side effects in older individuals. Although probably appropriate in neutropenic, immunocompromised elderly or in the presence of documented *Pseudomonas* infection, I would try to use other agents when possible. The number of indications for aminoglycosides has been dramatically reduced by the availability of broad-spectrum beta-lactams and the quinolones.
2. Because most antibiotics are excreted by renal routes and because of the decline in renal function with increasing age, higher dosages may be potentially more problematic in the elderly.
3. Broad-spectrum therapy is appropriate initially in the treatment of serious infection if the cause is unclear. Older individuals lack much of the physiologic reserve of younger adults and usually have one or more comorbid diseases. In the presence of a serious infection, the elderly can rapidly become very unstable. Using drugs that are active against most of the likely causes of the infection (with the least possible toxicity) is most appropriate.

■ URINARY TRACT INFECTION

Urinary tract infection (UTI) is increasingly common with increasing age. This reflects obstruction as a result of prostatic enlargement in males and a variety of changes in the

Table 1   Antibiotics Recommended for Initial (Empiric) Therapy for the Elderly

INFECTION	ANTIBIOTICS	COMMENTS
Acute fever, unidentified source	Imipenem, 0.5 g q6h IV, or meropenem, 0.5-1.0 q8h IV	Broad spectrum, limited toxicity
Urinary tract infection	*Gram-negative organisms:* Third-generation cephalosporin (e.g., ceftazadime, 1.0 g q8-12h), broad-spectrum penicillin with beta-lactamase inhibitor (e.g., ticarcillin clavulanate, 3.1 g IV q4-6h), imipenem, meropenem, or quinolone (e.g., ciprofloxacin, 400 mg IV q12h)	Consider imipenem-meropenem if in LTCF or a recurrent infection; use in combination with low-dose aminoglycoside (e.g., gentamicin, 40-60 mg/day) if resistant organisms are probable Oral quinolone (e.g., ciprofloxacin, 250 mg bid, or norfloxacin, 400 mg bid) appropriate if not seriously ill
	Gram-positive organisms: Vancomycin, 10-15 mg/kg q12h IV	Active against enterococci, staphylococci, and streptococci
Pneumonia	Third-generation cephalosporin (cefotaxime, 1.0-2.0 g q8-12h IV, or ceftriaxone, 1 g IM or IV q12h) plus a macrolide (e.g., azithromycin, 0.5 g/day IV)	Consider using ceftazidime or imipenem for nosocomial pneumonia Macrolide (preferably azithromycin, 500 mg on day 1, then 250 mg on days 2-4), quinolone with antipreumococcal activity (gatifloxacin, 400 mg/day, or levofloxacin, 500 mg/day) for oral therapy in less seriously ill patients
Pressure sores	Broad-spectrum beta-lactam agent with beta-lactamase inhibitor (e.g., ticarcillin-clavulanate)	Other treatment regimens active against Bacteroides, enteric gram-negative organisms, and staphylococci may be used
Infective endocarditis	Vancomycin with gentamicin	Modify as appropriate after results of cultures and antibiotic susceptibility testing are available
Infectious (bacterial) diarrhea	Ciprofloxacin (500 mg PO bid) or other quinolone	
Meningitis	Third-generation cephalosporin (e.g., ceftraxone, 2 g IV q12h) plus ampicillin, 50 mg/kg q8h IV	*Listeria monocytogenes* is not susceptible to cephalosporins
Septic arthritis	Nafcillin (2.0 g IV q4-6 h) or vancomycin	Consider addition of ceftazidime pending Gram stain results

LTCF, Long-term care facility.
NOTE: Therapy should be modified as appropriate after results of Gram stain, culture, and antibiotic susceptibility testing are available.

defense mechanisms of the female urinary system. The risk of instrumentation and catheterization, procedures often associated with development of infection, also increases in the elderly population.

Asymptomatic bacteriuria is more common in both elderly men and women than in younger subjects. Multiple studies have demonstrated that treatment of this infection is without value, primarily because it usually rapidly relapses after treatment is completed.

Escherichia coli accounts for the bulk of UTIs in young women. In older individuals, the bacteriology is more complex. Infecting organisms are usually from other genera (e.g., *Serratia, Pseudomonas*) and are often resistant to multiple antibiotics. For this reason, urine culture and sensitivity should always be done before initiating therapy in an elderly individual.

A 10-day course of treatment is most appropriate for the clinical lower UTI (i.e., cystitis) in elderly women. Although 1- or 3-day therapy with trimethoprim-sulfamethoxazole (TMP-SMX) or a quinolone antibiotic is well studied in younger women, there is little information on the effectiveness of this regimen in older women. In men, because the focus of infection may be within the prostate, a minimum of 14 days of treatment is recommended. TMP-SMX or a quinolone would also be appropriate initial choices. Because of convenience of twice-daily dosing and the need to use only a small dose (because these antibiotics concentrate in the urine), I would prefer to use norfloxacin (400 mg twice daily) or ciprofloxacin (250 mg twice daily).

For patients thought to have upper tract infection and for those who are seriously ill, therapy should be initially parenteral. Selection should be guided by Gram stain of the urine. If gram-negative organisms are present, a broad-spectrum beta-lactam agent with activity against *Pseudomonas aeruginosa* (e.g., imipenem, ticarcillin-clavulanate, or ceftazidime) or a quinolone would be appropriate initial choices. If a gram-positive organism is present in the Gram stain (nearly always representing staphylococci or enterococci), vancomycin would be the most appropriate antibiotic to start pending culture and susceptibility results. Multiply-resistant gram-negative organisms may cause infection in patients with previous UTIs, those who have recently been taking antibiotics, and immunosuppressed patients. In these situations (and in documented *Pseudomonas* infections), an agent such as imipenem, meropenem, or another broad-spectrum beta-lactam should be given with an aminoglycoside.

Infections in individuals with chronic indwelling urinary catheters should be treated only when symptomatic. Virtually all catheterized patients will have asymptomatic bacteriuria. Treatment in catheterized patients with symptomatic infection needs to be based on culture and sensitivity results. Although there is not good evidence that catheter removal is important, it is often done before initial therapy for these infections.

■ PNEUMONIA

Pneumonia is an increasingly common problem with increasing age. *Streptococcus pneumoniae* is the single most common cause in the elderly. The importance of pneumococcal polysaccharide vaccine (which is protective against most all of the penicillin-resistant strains identified to date) cannot be overstressed. Gram-negative organisms (e.g., *Haemophilus influenzae, Moraxella,* and *E. coli*) are also commonly recovered. In contrast to traditional teaching, nonbacterial organisms such as *Mycoplasma pneumoniae* and *Chlamydia pneumoniae* are now recognized as important causes of pneumonia in older adults. *M. pneumoniae* and *C. pneumoniae* may each account for up to 10% of episodes of acute pneumonia in the elderly. Respiratory synctial virus (RSV) is also recently recognized as a significant cause of pneumonia in the aged. Although RSV-associated illness is similar to clinical influenza, bronchospasm appears to be more common. Rhinoviruses can also occasionally cause pneumonia in older individuals.

Because of the variety of agents that may cause pneumonia in the elderly, attempts to document the etiology of the infection by sputum cultures (and blood cultures if the patient is seriously ill) need to be made. Sputum cultures after initiation of therapy are usually of no value; appropriate cultures need to be obtained before starting therapy.

In an otherwise healthy elderly adult living in the community, initial therapy for pneumonia could be with either a macrolide or one of the newer quinolones. The newer quinolones (e.g., gatifloxacin, amifloxacin, levofloxacin) have activity against many gram-negative organisms, atypical agents such as *Mycoplasma*, and *S. pneumoniae* (including those strains resistant to penicillin). Because of this, and other broad-spectrum and once-daily dosing, these agents may become increasingly popular in the outpatient therapy of pneumonia in elderly individuals. Gatifloxacin is the most active of this group against *S. pneumoniae*.

For patients with community-acquired pneumonia who are hospitalized, empiric treatment should be broad spectrum and effective against gram-positive and gram-negative bacteria as well as atypical agents. Broad-spectrum parenteral beta-lactams such as a third-generation cephalosporin (e.g., ceftriaxone), a penicillin and beta-lactamase inhibitor combination (e.g., ticarcillin-clavulanate) in conjunction with a parenteral macrolide (azithromycin or erythromycin) probably represents optimal therapy. Although only limited data are available, in a patient with a functioning gastrointestinal tract, oral therapy with gatifloxacin or levofloxacin may be a possible option. Although parenteral therapy is most often appropriate in patients who are ill enough to be hospitalized, the nearly complete absorption of the quinolones after oral dosing and their broad spectrum suggest this may become a convenient and cost-effective approach.

■ TUBERCULOSIS

About one quarter of tuberculosis cases in the United States occur in individuals older than 65. This is a special problem for nursing homes because the incidence in long-term care is about four times that in the community. Older individuals with a positive tuberculin skin test who have one of a number of additional risk factors (e.g., gastrectomy or steroid therapy) or who have recently converted their skin test need to be treated with isoniazid, 300 mg/day for 1 year. Managing clinical tuberculosis in an elderly individual is similar to that for younger patients, except that the drugs that are potentially ototoxic and nephrotoxic (e.g., streptomycin) should be avoided. Monitoring for hepatic toxicity when using isoniazid is also important.

■ PRESSURE ULCERS

Efforts to attempt to prevent pressure-associated ischemia are extremely important. Once an ulcer develops, infection often follows. Topical antimicrobials are ineffective in the management of these lesions. Systemic antimicrobials should be used if clinical cellulitis is evident at the margin of a pressure ulcer or if there is evidence of deep infection or osteomyelitis. Therapy needs to be effective against anaerobic bacteria and both gram-negative and gram-positive organisms. Oral therapy might include a combination of an oral cephalosporin and metronidazole, or amoxicillin-clavulanate. Appropriate parenteral therapy might include imipenem, ticarcillin-clavulanate, or one of the broader-spectrum cephalosporins (e.g., ceftriaxone, cefotaxime) or a quinolone combined with metronidazole or clindamycin for anaerobic coverage. If material can be obtained for culture (usually best done by needle aspiration), therapy can be modified once results are available.

Most of the other skin and soft tissue infections in the aged, as in younger individuals, are caused by group A beta-hemolytic streptococci or *Staphylococcus aureus*. Treatment of these infections is not significantly different in older individuals.

■ BACTEREMIA

In one recent study, nearly 15% of the cases of community-acquired bacteremia were in individuals older than 84 years of age. Usual primary sites of infection include the urinary tract, intraabdominal sites, the lower respiratory tract, and skin and soft tissue. Appropriate empirical therapy would be that for the underlying infection. Especially in patients with bacteremia that does not promptly resolve, evaluation should rule out presence of an abscess or obstruction.

■ MENINGITIS

S. pneumoniae remains the most common cause of meningitis in older adults. The second most common cause is *Listeria monocytogenes.* This is important to know when selecting therapy because this organism is not killed by cephalosporin antibiotics. Initial therapy of meningitis of unknown cause in an elderly individual must include ampicillin, which is active against *L. monocytogenes.*

■ INFECTIONS IN RESIDENTS OF LONG-TERM CARE FACILITIES

All of the types of infections that may occur in older individuals may develop in residents of long-term care facilities (LTCFs). Methicillin-resistant *S. aureus* (MRSA) and, in some areas of the United States, vancomycin-resistant enterococci (VRE), have a strong association with LTCF residency. Residents are also especially prone to epidemic respiratory or gastrointestinal disease, which are particularly common in winter months. Selecting antibiotic therapy for patients who reside in LTCFs requires an awareness that resistant gram-negative organisms, MRSA, and VRE are possible causes of the infection.

Suggested Reading

Crossley K, Peterson PK: Infections in the elderly—new developments. In Remington JS, Swartz MN, eds: *Current clinical topics in infectious diseases,* vol 18, Malden, MA, 1999, Blackwell Science.

Hocking TL, Choi C: Tuberculosis: a strategy to detect and treat new and reactivated infections, *Geriatrics* 52:52, 1997.

Nicolle LE, Strausbaugh LJ, Garibaldi RA: Infections and antibiotic resistance in nursing homes, *Clin Microbiol Rev* 9:1, 1996.

NEONATAL INFECTION

Robert S. Baltimore

■ EPIDEMIOLOGY

Neonatal infections are usually classified according to time and mode of onset in three categories: (1) prenatal, (2) perinatal, (early onset), and (3) nursery-acquired (late onset). The division in time between early and late onset is usually 2 to 5 days of age (Table 1). Infections that begin within the first month of life are considered neonatal, but many intensive care units for neonates provide continuing care for infants several months of age with complex problems that are the result of prematurity and complications of neonatal disorders. Therefore neonatal nursery-associated infections may occur in infants up to 1 year of age. Bacterial infections caused by rapidly dividing high-grade pathogens that set in substantially before birth usually result in a stillbirth. Generally, it is impossible to distinguish infections acquired shortly before birth from those acquired as a result of contact with maternal vaginal, fecal, or skin flora during delivery.

Neonatal sepsis occurs in approximately 2 to 4 per 1000 live births in the United States. Worldwide reports vary from 1 to 10 per 1000 live births. Risk factors noted in Table 1 have a strong predictive influence on infection rates. Term infants born without incident have a low incidence of infection, lower than any other population of hospitalized patients. Infants susceptible to early-onset postnatal infections are primarily those born prematurely. Premature infants born to mothers with an infection or whose membranes rupture more than 6 hours before delivery may have an infection rate of 20% or more. In profoundly premature infants, extra vigilance is required for early recognition and treatment of infection. Premature infants are much more likely to develop sepsis as a consequence of the amnionitis caused by ascending infection than are term infants. Similarly, premature infants are at a greater risk for developing an invasive infection if born to a mother with peripartum infection than are term infants.

Nosocomial infection in the nursery is an important and growing problem, and today most infections in neonatal units are nosocomial. As the technology for treating very premature and very sick infants has increased, so too has the population of surviving immunocompromised infants who require life support equipment such as ventilators, intravascular catheters, total parenteral nutrition, extracorporeal membrane oxygenation, and surgical drains, each of which carries a substantial risk of infection (see Table 1). The liberal use of broad-spectrum antibiotics in neonatal care units increases the risk of acquisition of pathogens by interfering with the development of normal flora in these infants who have no normal flora at birth. In contrast, the risk of acquiring nosocomial *viral* infections appears to depend mostly on the chances of contact with the virus and not preexisting disease in the infant. Therefore community activity of respiratory and gastrointestinal viruses and defects in the barriers to prevent spread, especially handwashing, within the unit appear to be the most important risk factors for viral infection.

■ MICROBIOLOGY

Table 1 lists the major bacterial organisms responsible for early and late postnatal sepsis. The organisms that cause meningitis in the neonate are the same as for sepsis.

Table 1   Characteristics of Prenatal, Early-Onset, and Late-Onset Neonatal Infections

	PRENATAL ONSET	EARLY-ONSET INFECTIONS	LATE-ONSET INFECTIONS
Age at onset	Before birth	Birth to 2-5 days	2-5 to 30 days
Transmission	Transplacental or ascending	Maternal flora transmitted peripartum	Nosocomial
Risk factors	Maternal infection	Prolonged premature rupture of membranes	Contact with hands of colonized personnel
	Prolonged premature rupture of membranes	Septic or traumatic delivery	Contact with aerosols of bacteria
		Maternal infection: especially urogenital	Contaminated equipment: (e.g., isolettes, ventilators, IV lines)
		Fetal anoxia	Debilitating illness
		Male sex	Congenital anomalies
		Maternal factors (poverty, preeclampsia, cardiac disease, diabetes)	Surgery (including necrotizing enterocolitis)
			Treatment for early onset infection
Most common pathogens	Cytomegalovirus	*Escherichia coli*	Those causing early onset infections
	Syphilis	Group B streptococci	*Staphylococcus aureus*
	Toxoplasma	*Klebsiella* spp.	Coagulase-negative staphylococci
	Maternal vaginal flora	*Enterococcus* spp.	*Pseudomonas aeruginosa*
		Listeria monocytogenes	*Candida* spp.
		Other Enterobacteriacae *(Proteus, Citrobacter, Enterobacter)*	

Escherichia coli and group B streptococci have accounted for about 80% of early-onset sepsis and meningitis in the past. With perinatal prophylaxis using penicillin having been recommended since 1996, the rate of group B streptococcus appears to be declining. In the past 15 years, the microbiology of late-onset sepsis has shifted, with an increase of coagulase-negative staphylococci and *Candida* species that appears to be caused by the increased survival of extremely premature infants and use of parenteral alimentation and broad-spectrum antibiotics. Empiric therapy is guided by this information on the microbiology of neonatal infections.

■ ANTIMICROBIAL THERAPY

Empiric Therapy for Early-Onset Sepsis

Antibiotics for early-onset infections are generally commenced before the identification of the infecting organism. Neonates, especially premature ones, typically fail to manifest classic signs and symptoms of infection. Thus many schemata have been developed for empiric antibiotic treatment of infants with multiple epidemiologic risks alone or nonspecific signs and laboratory test abnormalities plus epidemiologic risk factors. The common features of these schemata are recognition of the risk factors listed in Table 1; the possibility that severe infection may present as temperature instability or other vital sign changes, unexplained hyperbilirubinemia, vomiting, or changes in feeding; and the recognition that a very short delay in treatment may result in overwhelming sepsis and death. Such schemata vary from hospital to hospital according to the population served, the type of hospital, and resources for screening. Screening tests may also include hematologic findings such as white blood cell count, the ratio of immature to mature cells of the granulocyte series, and acute phase reactants such as erythrocyte sedimentation rate, C-reactive protein, and concentrations of certain lymphokines such as IL-6, and each has been reported to have moderate positive and negative predictive values.

Treatment is designed to provide adequate antimicrobial activity against the organisms listed in Table 1. Often, the focus of infection is unknown initially, but therapy is directed against bacteremia and meningitis because experience demonstrates that these are the most likely foci. Approximately one fourth of infants with bacterial sepsis also have meningitis. If pneumonia or a urinary tract infection is present, physical examination or screening tests, chest radiograph, and urinalysis will demonstrate these foci. Tables 2 and 3 list the antibiotics found to be safe and effective and commonly used for neonatal infections. The recommended dosing (see Table 3) takes into consideration the absorption, metabolism, distribution, and excretion, which differ from older children and change rapidly during early life.

Empiric treatment is generally a broad-spectrum penicillin with an aminoglycoside antibiotic or with an extended-spectrum (third-generation) cephalosporin (see Table 2). Most pediatric infectious disease practitioners continue to use an extended-spectrum penicillin, usually ampicillin, with an aminoglycoside, usually gentamicin. The advantages of this combination are low cost, considerable experience, and known low toxicity. The advantages of the extended-spectrum cephalosporins are greater activity on a weight basis against many of the pathogens and excellent central nervous system penetration in the presence of inflammation. There is concern, however, about the development of resistant flora if these agents are used routinely in a large number of infants in a hospital unit, and rapid development of resistance to these agents has been reported. Also, *Listeria* and *Enterococcus* species are resistant to the cephalosporins. If gram-negative bacillary meningitis is diagnosed on the basis of examination of the cerebrospinal fluid, it is reasonable to use ampicillin plus an extended-spectrum cephalosporin as a first choice.

If *Pseudomonas aeruginosa* is a likely pathogen, tobramycin is a better aminoglycoside choice than gentamicin because it has higher activity against this species. Extended-spectrum beta-lactam agents such as ceftazidime and piperacillin are also used for *Pseudomonas* species. If infections

Table 2 Empiric Antibiotic Treatment for Presumed Neonatal Sepsis (with or without Meningitis)

AGE AND LOCATION OF INFANT AT ONSET	ANTIBIOTIC REGIMEN	ALTERNATIVE REGIMENS
Early-onset sepsis	Ampicillin *plus* gentamicin*	Ampicillin *plus* cefotaxime
Late-onset sepsis (up to 1 mo)		
Readmission from the community	Ampicillin *plus* cefotaxime (or ceftriaxone†)	Ampicillin *plus* gentamicin* *with or without* cefotaxime (or ceftriaxone†)
In the hospital, with no intravenous catheter(s)	Ampicillin *plus* gentamicin*	Ampicillin *plus* cefotaxime (or ceftriaxone†)
In the hospital, with intravenous catheter(s)	Oxacillin *or* vancomycin* *plus* gentamicin*	Vancomycin* *plus* cefotaxime (or ceftriaxone†)

*Adjust dosage according to concentration of the antibiotic in the blood once a steady state has been achieved.
†Ceftriaxone can displace bilirubin from albumin, thus intensifying hyperbilirubinemia, and may also cause deposition of sludge in the gallbladder, so it should be used with caution in newborns.

Table 3 Dosage Schedules of Commonly Used Parenteral Antibiotics for Neonatal Infections

| ANTIBIOTIC AGENT | ≤7 DAYS OF AGE | | >7 DAYS OF AGE | |
	DOSAGE (mg/kg/day)	DOSES/DAY	DOSAGE (mg/kg/day)	DOSES/DAY
PENICILLINS				
Penicillin G	50,000-100,000 units*	2-3†	100,000-200,000 units	3-4
Ticarcillin	150-225 mg	2-3	225-300 mg	3-4
Mezlocillin, piperacillin	150-225 mg	2-3	225-300 mg	3-4
Penicillinase-resistant penicillins (oxacillin, methicillin, nafcillin)	50-100 mg	2	100-200 mg	3-4
Ampicillin	50-150 mg	2-3	100-200 mg	3-4
AMINOGLYCOSIDES				
Amikacin‡	15-20 mg	2	22.5-30 mg	3
Gentamicin‡	5 mg	2	7.5 mg	3
Tobramycin‡	4-5 mg	2	6 mg	3
CEPHALOSPORINS				
Cefotaxime	100 mg	2	150 mg	3
Ceftazidime	60-100 mg	2-3	90-150 mg	3
Ceftriaxone	50 mg	1	75 mg	1
MISCELLANEOUS ANTIBIOTICS				
Clindamycin	10-15 mg	2-3	15-20 mg	3-4
Vancomycin‡	20-30 mg	2	30-45 mg	3
Chloramphenicol‡	25 mg	1	25-50 mg	1-2
Aztreonam	60-90 mg	2-3	90-120 mg	3-4
ANTIFUNGAL AGENTS				
Amphotericin B	0.25-1.0 mg	1	0.25-1.0 mg	1
Flucytosine§	150 mg	4	150 mg	4
Fluconazole¶	3-6 mg	1	3-6 mg	1
ANTIVIRAL AGENTS				
Acyclovir	20-45 mg	2-3	20-45 mg	2-3
Ribavirin (by aerosol)	6 g	1	6 g	1

*Where there is a dosage range, the higher figure is used for treatment when meningitis is present. For sepsis without meningitis, the higher end of the dosage range is recommended for more severe infections or when the measured serum antibiotic concentration is lower than the therapeutic range.
†Where there is a range of number of doses/day, the greater number and larger dose is used for neonates with a birth weight over 2 kg and the lower number doses with a smaller daily dose is for neonates with a birth weight under 2 kg.
‡Dosing should be guided by laboratory determination of serum antibiotic concentrations once a steady state has been reached.
§Limited data on dosing neonates. Dosage indicated is from cases in the literature.
¶Limited data in neonates. Child dosage is listed.

caused by gentamicin-resistant gram-negative bacilli have recently been encountered in the unit, amikacin or netilmicin are the aminoglycosides of choice.

Empiric Therapy for Late-Onset Sepsis

The infants most likely to have late-onset infections are ill residents of an intensive care nursery. Ideal empiric antibiotic therapy takes into consideration the resident flora of the nursery, especially isolates from previously infected neonates and the particular risk factors of the patient. If intravascular cannulae have not been used, if the infant has not been treated for a previous infection, and if there have not been isolates of gentamicin-resistant gram-negative aerobic bacilli, it is appropriate to use the same empiric treatment as for early-onset sepsis (see Table 2). In fact, this is usually not the case, and another regimen is often more appropriate. Ill infants often have one or more intravascular catheters in place, and these may be the focus of infection. The most common bacterial species causing catheter-associated infections are coagulase-negative staphylococci and *Staphylococcus aureus*. Although penicillinase-resistant semisynthetic penicillins (oxacillin, nafcillin, methicillin) are usually the agents of choice against staphylococci, resistance to this class, commonly called *methicillin resistance*, is rising in many institutions. In addition, coagulase-negative staphylococci appear to have a higher incidence in very-low-birthweight infants, and these pathogens are more likely to show methicillin resistance. Therefore, in institutions with substantial methicillin resistance of staphylococci, it is reasonable to use vancomycin for empiric treatment of late-onset catheter-associated infections. Generally, an aminoglycoside is added. If an infant develops new symptoms of infection while receiving gentamicin, either amikacin or third-generation cephalosporin is substituted.

Once the results of culture and susceptibility tests are available, empiric treatment is changed to definitive treatment. Penicillin is used for group B streptococci, and ampicillin or ampicillin plus gentamicin are used for *Enterococcus* species or *Listeria*. Oxacillin, nafcillin, or vancomycin are used for staphylococci, depending on susceptibility of the isolate. For gram-negative bacillary infections, ampicillin or ampicillin plus an aminoglycoside or third-generation cephalosporin (depending on susceptibility) is used and continued for 7 to 10 days unless there is an additional focal infection that requires a longer duration of treatment. When peritonitis caused by necrotizing enterocolitis is present, the addition of clindamycin to the regimens recommended for sepsis may be of value for treatment of staphylococci and gram-negative anaerobes.

■ ADJUNCTIVE THERAPY OF SEPSIS

In addition to antibiotic therapy, infants with sepsis require intensive care. Intravenous fluid management and treatment for shock and respiratory failure should be carried out in appropriate neonatal units.

The use of agents to support or enhance the immune system has been studied but continues to be controversial. A number of small studies suggest that exchange transfusion, transfusion of concentrated white blood cells when there is severe neutropenia and bone marrow failure, specific immunoglobulin preparations, and commercial intravenous immunoglobulin preparations reduce mortality resulting from neonatal sepsis. Unfortunately, many studies show these modalities to be either ineffective or only slightly better than placebo. Recent meta-analyses suggest that intravenous immunoglobulin, 500 to 750 mg/kg as a single dose, may be beneficial in the treatment of neonatal sepsis. Immune system enhancers and cell transfusion have not been widely adopted, and if any adjunct is used in the treatment of overwhelming sepsis, the one with which a facility has the most experience may be the best because complications are known to occur with each agent.

■ THERAPY AND MANAGEMENT OF OTHER FOCAL INFECTIONS

Meningitis

The dosages of some antibiotics are increased when treating meningitis. This is to allow for the lower antibiotic concentrations in central nervous system tissue and cerebrospinal fluid (CSF) than in blood. Antibiotics that are bactericidal are preferred over those that are bacteriostatic because the latter work less well in the central nervous system. Intrathecal or intraventricular administration of antibiotics has not been associated with improvement in outcome. Intraventricular instillation may occasionally be warranted when treating resistant organisms if they have not been eradicated using conventional antibiotic dosing.

Ampicillin plus gentamicin or cefotaxime are recommended for empiric treatment of neonatal meningitis. Complications and delayed sterilization are more common with gram-negative bacillary meningitis in the newborn than with childhood meningitis beyond the neonatal period caused by the usual organisms for that age group. In evaluating the infant being treated for bacillary meningitis, the clinician should repeat the lumbar puncture every 48 hours until the CSF is sterile and at the end of therapy to monitor antibiotic efficacy. Continued positive cultures may signal the need to change antibiotics or look for a focus, such as a brain abscess, with cranial imaging. Assuming no complications, antibiotics are usually continued for 3 weeks. For group B streptococcal meningitis, repeat lumbar puncture has little value when the clinical response is good and no late complications occur. Length of treatment is 2 to 3 weeks. Hydrocephalus is an unfortunately common complication of neonatal meningitis, and it is important to monitor the head circumference during therapy and later. Infants who develop an increase in ventricular size should be evaluated by a neurosurgeon for placement of a CSF shunt. At this time, there are no data to suggest that adjunctive steroid treatment is either safe or beneficial for neonatal meningitis.

Pneumonia

Neonatal pneumonia can have a prenatal onset, can be in association with early-onset sepsis, as a complication of a noninfectious respiratory condition such as respiratory distress syndrome or meconium aspiration, or as a nosocomial pneumonia associated with mechanical ventilation. Rarely is diagnostic lower lung tissue or sputum of good quality available for definitive microbiologic diagnosis. Thus there is little information on optimal therapy for pneumonia as an isolated infection. In general, the bacterial pathogens are the same as for early- and late-onset sepsis, and empiric antimicrobial treatment is the same. Antibiotic therapy is usually for 10 to 14 days and extended to 21 days for the rare cases of staphylococcal pneumonia. In addition, organisms of maternal origin, such as *Chlamydia trachomatis,* which can be treated with erythromycin or sulfisoxazole, and genital mycoplasmas, such as *Mycoplasma hominis* and *Ureaplasma urealyticum,* for which there is no proven treatment in the neonate, may be encountered. There are reports of treatment of *U. urealyticum* with erythromycin but little convincing evidence of efficacy.

Urinary Tract Infection

Percutaneous bladder puncture is the best method of culture to avoid contamination. Bladder catheterization is acceptable but is more likely to result in contamination of the urinary tract. If the same organism is recovered from the urine and the blood, it may not be clear whether the urinary tract was the initial focus of infection or was seeded from blood, unless there is an obvious urinary tract anatomic abnormality. Late-onset urinary tract infections may either be associated with a congenital malformation or urinary tract instrumentation or be spontaneous, with no discoverable underlying cause. Initial antibiotic treatment should be similar to the approach to the neonate with sepsis according to Table 2 and following identification of the pathogen continued with one of the agents listed in Table 3 according to the susceptibility of the isolate. Because of the unpredictable absorption of oral antibiotics, the treatment is generally with parenterally administered drug. Although treatment for 10 to 14 days with an agent that has renal concentration and excretion is conventional, the neonate, like older individuals, may have a poor response or relapse in the presence of obstruction, a foreign body, or incomplete voiding. Because of the high rate of congenital malformations in neonates with urinary tract infections, imaging studies such as renal ultrasound should be part of the management.

Skeletal Infections

Septic arthritis and osteomyelitis in the neonate are generally secondary to bacteremia. Although neonatal osteomyelitis is not common, *S. aureus* is the most commonly isolated organism, and group B streptococci and gram-negative aerobes, especially *E. coli,* are also encountered. *S. aureus* skeletal infections in the neonate are often severely destructive and associated with later disabilities, and they have a tendency to be associated with multiple foci and rupture through the incompletely formed epiphyseal plate. Empiric therapy is similar to that for sepsis but an agent active against *S. aureus,* such as oxacillin or nafcillin, should be added. Management includes aspiration of infected bone or septic joint, with open drainage considered if aspiration is insufficient to drain the focus. Length of treatment is generally at least 3 weeks for septic arthritis and at least 4 weeks for osteomyelitis. A longer course may be necessary if there is delayed sterilization, late appearance of a second focus, or other complications. There is too little experience with oral agents for skeletal infections in the neonate to recommend this route.

■ VIRAL INFECTIONS

Herpes Simplex Infections

Herpes infections of the newborn are transmitted from the mother's genital tract to the infant, usually at delivery. The incidence is approximately 1 in 4000 deliveries. The infants of mothers with primary genital herpes lesions at the time of delivery rather than recurrent herpes are at highest risk, but many mothers of infants with herpes infection are unaware of ever having had genital herpes. The incubation period is generally from 3 or 4 days to a month. Most neonatal herpes infections are caused by herpes simplex type 2. The presentation of neonatal herpes may include (1) only cutaneous, eye, and mucous membrane manifestations (vesicles); (2) only central nervous system infection; or (3) disseminated visceral infection. Combinations of the three may occur as well. Severity and prognosis are worst for disseminated visceral disease and best for cutaneous disease.

Acyclovir is the antiviral agent of choice. Moderately ill infants who are treated early in the course of manifest infection appear to benefit the most from treatment. The usual dose in a term infant is 30 to 45 mg/kg/day divided every 8 hours. The optimal duration of treatment is unknown, but although early studies used a duration of 10 days, most practitioners extend the course to 14 to 21 days because of reports of recurrences with the shorter regimen, and even longer courses are being investigated.

Varicella-Zoster Virus

Infants born of mothers who have active varicella are in danger of developing overwhelming infection from varicella-zoster virus (VZV) if the mother's lesions appear in the period between 5 days before delivery and 2 days after delivery. The rationale is that infants exposed during this period may have received a large dose of VZV intravenously by transplacental exposure. Infants exposed earlier in utero receive antibody transplacentally from the mother and generally develop a mild infection. Infants exposed after birth also develop mild varicella. If an infant is exposed to VZV during the critical perinatal period described, treatment with varicella-zoster immunoglobulin (VZIG), 125 units (one vial of 1.25 ml), given as soon as possible after delivery or exposure is recommended.

Viral Pneumonia

Respiratory syncytial virus, influenza viruses, parainfluenza viruses, and adenoviruses can cause severe respiratory disease in neonates, and the diagnosis is made by viral culture or rapid antigen tests. In general, antimicrobial treatment is not available. Ribavirin by aerosol, which in earlier studies appeared to shorten the course of respiratory syncytial virus–associated bronchiolitis in infants, may be used, but there is little information concerning efficacy in neonates. Recent studies cast doubt on the efficacy of ribavirin, even for older infants. If given, ribavirin is delivered via a special ultrasonic nebulizer. The dosage is aerosolization of one 6-g vial per day independent of age, and special expertise is required for use with intubated patients on assisted ventilation.

Suggested Reading

Baltimore RS: Perinatal bacterial and fungal infections. In Jenson HB, Baltimore RS, eds: *Pediatric infectious diseases: principles and practice,* Norwalk, CT, 1995, Appleton & Lange.

Peter G, ed: *1997 Red Book: report of the committee on infectious diseases,* ed 24, Elk Grove Village, IL, 1997, American Academy of Pediatrics.

Remington JS, Klein JO: *Infectious diseases of the fetus and newborn infant,* ed 4, Philadelphia, 1995, Saunders.

Sáez-Llorens X, McCracken GH Jr: Perinatal bacterial diseases. In Feigin RD, Cherry JD, eds: *Textbook of pediatric infectious diseases,* ed 4, Philadelphia, 1998, Saunders.

PREGNANCY AND THE PUERPERIUM: INFECTIOUS RISKS

Raul E. Isturiz
Jorge Murillo

Infectious diseases that occur during pregnancy and the puerperium pose special risks to the mother and fetus. Furthermore, therapeutic and preventive measures often must be modified during pregnancy because of the potential for serious adverse effects.

With the premise that the efficacy of every diagnostic and therapeutic option must be individually weighed against the possible side effects, this chapter discusses problems that are common or severe.

■ URINARY TRACT INFECTIONS

Asymptomatic bacteriuria and symptomatic infection of the upper and lower urinary tracts are associated with significant risks to mother and fetus. Recommendations include (1) routine, semiquantitative culturing of a properly collected urine specimen (or at least dipstick or nitrites) at the first prenatal visit; (2) prescribing safe antibiotic treatment; (3) surveying for recurrent or persistent bacteriuria; (4) retreating and performing urologic evaluation of those with recurrent or persistent disease; and (5) using suppressive therapy until delivery in selected cases (Figure 1).

Patients with cystitis can be treated orally pending the results of the urine culture. Oral cephalosporins, beta-lactam plus beta-lactamase inhibitor, or nitrofurantoin except at term can be used for 7 to 10 days. The oral cephems may be especially useful if found safe during pregnancy (Table 1).

When pyelonephritis is the working diagnosis, we prefer to admit pregnant patients to the hospital and support them with fluids, perform blood and urine cultures, evaluate renal function, and treat with intravenous (IV) antibiotics guided by the urine Gram stain. Renal ultrasonography is also performed in the hospital in the first 72 hours. When deterioration occurs, management in the intensive care unit, low exposure IV pyelogram, and helical computed tomography (CT) are options.

Third-generation cephalosporins and beta-lactam plus beta-lactamase inhibitor are appropriate initial antibiotics. We avoid aminoglycosides when possible and favor aztreonam, ceftazidime, imipenem, cilastatin, or meropenem for resistant gram-negative organisms (Table 2).

■ PREMATURE RUPTURE OF MEMBRANES

Premature rupture of the membranes (PROM) can occur at any time before uterine contractions and labor start. The most important predictor of neonatal infection among infants born to patients with PROM are maternal colonization with group B streptococci and clinical chorioamnionitis. Subclinical infection or inflammation of the chorioamniotic membranes causes an important proportion of the cases. The overall incidence of positive amniotic fluid cultures in patients with PROM is estimated at 28% and increases to as much as 39% with preterm labor. The microorganisms found routinely in the lower genital tract are frequently isolated from the amniotic fluid or cervical os of patients with PROM. They include *Mycoplasma,* group B streptococcus, *Fusobacterium,* and *Gardnerella vaginalis.* Cultures are polymicrobial in about 32% of cases.

Hospitalization and treatment should not be delayed. For preterm PROM, we recommend IV ampicillin and erythromycin for 48 hours, followed by oral treatment with the same drugs or amoxicillin-clavulanate and erythromycin estearate for 5 to 7 additional days when delivery does not occur.

■ INTRAAMNIOTIC INFECTION

Maternal fever and fetal tachycardia are common initial manifestations of amniotic fluid infection; foul amniotic fluid and uterine tenderness are late and sometimes absent. When other sources of fever can be excluded, especially when membranes are ruptured, a specimen of amniotic

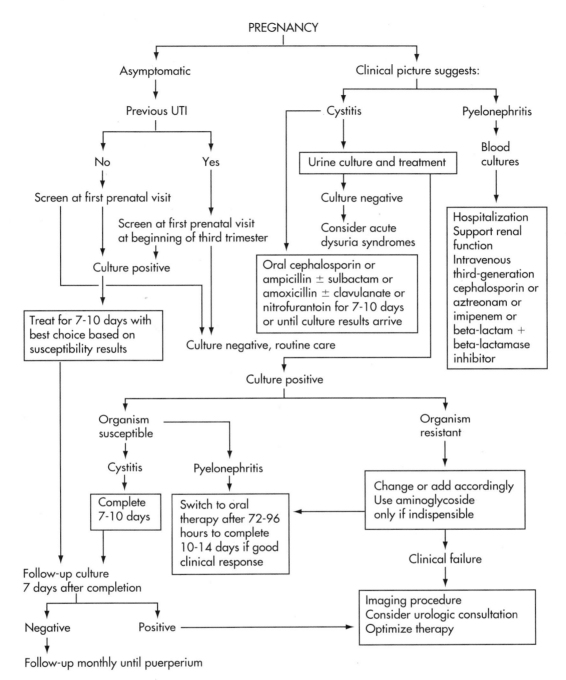

Figure 1
Management of urinary tract infection during pregnancy.
*Not advised near term.
†Ticarcillin not advised in first trimester.

fluid is obtained for aerobic, anaerobic, and *Mycoplasma* cultures as well as rapid tests such as Gram stain (48% sensitivity, 99% specificity), glucose (highly sensitive when <14 mg/dl), white blood cell count (about 50/mm^3), and interleukin-6 assay. A recent study has shown that the results of Gram stain combined with amniotic fluid glucose level are superior to any single test. Because antibiotics can prevent spread of this infection to mother and fetus, they are used immediately afterward. Initial therapy includes IV ampicillin, 2 g every 6 hours, plus clindamycin, 900 mg every 8 hours, plus gentamicin, 2 mg/kg loading dose, then 1.5 mg/kg every 8 hours. Ampicillin-sulbactam, 1.5 to 3 g every 6 hours, and in late pregnancy ticarcillin-clavulanate, 3.1 g every 6 hours, are newer alternatives. Aztreonam, ceftriaxone, ceftazidime, or imipenem can substitute for the aminoglycoside. However, in patients in labor, aggravated by chorioamnionitis, and undergoing cesarean section, the postoperative dosage of clindamycin and gentamicin has not reduced the risk of endometritis.

Table 1 Treatment of Asymptomatic Bacteriuria and Cystitis in Pregnancy

ORAL ANTIMICROBIAL	DOSAGE ×7 DAYS	COMMENTS
Ampicillin or amoxicillin	250 mg tid	Extensive experience Resistant bacteria encountered
Ampicillin-sulbactam or amoxicillin-clavulanate	250 mg tid	Less experience, more expensive Resistant bacteria less frequent
Cephalexin	250 mg tid	Single dose probably less effective
Cephradine	250 mg tid	
Cefadroxil	500 mg bid	
Cefixime	400 mg bid	For resistant gram negative; little experience
Nitrofurantoin	100 mg qid 25 mg qid or 100 mg qd	Therapy Suppression Not for *Staphylococcus saprophyticus* Rule out G6PD deficiency Do not use near term

G6PD, Glucose-6 phosphate-dehydrogenase.

■ MYCOBACTERIAL INFECTION IN PREGNANCY

Because tuberculosis (TB) often follows an unfavorable course during pregnancy and in the puerperium and because the disease can be transmitted to others, the isolation and treatment of the pregnant woman with active TB is never postponed. Isoniazid, 5 mg/kg/day, maximum 300 mg/day, causes no special untoward effect if pyridoxine is given (50 mg/day). Ethambutol, 15 mg/kg/day, is also considered safe. Data are less complete with rifampin, 600 mg/day, but suggest that it can be used as well. If no multidrug resistance (MDR) is known or suspected, treatment with isoniazid and ethambutol is appropriate in the first trimester and for mild disease, but for moderate to severe disease, especially after the first trimester, the three drugs are used together. Therapy for 9 months is advised. The use of pyrazinamide is controversial because the data on teratogenicity are inadequate, and streptomycin should be avoided because of the risk of toxicity to the fetal eighth nerve. MDR is addressed in the chapter *Tuberculosis*; drugs can be chosen with consideration of mother and fetus. Isoniazid prophylaxis can be given as soon as the indication arises or after delivery, always with pyridoxine. Pregnant women with TB infection or disease must be screened for human immunodeficiency virus (HIV). In pregnant patients with acquired immunodeficiency syndrome (AIDS), the treatment of disseminated disease caused by *Mycobacterium avium* complex is difficult because agents such as ciprofloxacin, clofazimine, and amikacin may not be suitable. More data on clarithromycin and azithromycin are awaited. (See the chapters *Tuberculosis* and *Nontuberculous Mycobacteria*).

Table 2 Treatment of Upper Urinary Tract Infections

PARENTERAL ANTIMICROBIAL	DOSAGE	COMMENTS	FDA CATEGORY
Ampicillin-sulbactam	1.5-3 g q6h	*	B
Amoxicillin-clavulanate	1-2 g q8h	*	B
Ticarcillin-clavulanate	3.1 g q6h	†	B
Piperacillin-tazobactam	3.4-4.5 g q8h		B
Methicillin, nafcillin, and oxacillin	1-2 g q4-6h		B
Cefotaxime	1-2 g q8-12h	Maximum, 12 g/day	B
Ceftriaxone	1-2 g q24h	Maximum, 4 g/day	B
Ceftazidime	1-2 g q8-12h		B
Cefoperazone	2-4 g q6-12h		B
Aztreonam	1-2 g q6-8h	Maximum, 8 g/day	B
Imipenem-cilastatin			B
Gentamicin and tobramycin	Loading: 2 mg/kg		C
	Maintenance: 1.7 mg/kg q8h Single daily dose: 5.1 mg/kg		D
Amikacin	Loading: 10 mg/kg Maintenance: 7.5 mg/kg q12h Single daily dose: 15 mg/kg		D
Vancomycin	0.5-1 g q6-12h		B

Pseudomonas aeruginosa, Enterobacter, Morganella, Providencia, Serratia, and *Citrobacter freundii* are predictably resistant.
†Do not use in first trimester.

■ MALARIA AND PREGNANCY

Pregnant women, especially primigravidae, are vulnerable to high parasitemia and severe infection; fetuses are vulnerable to low birth weight, prematurity, stillbirth, and congenital disease. Hence, efforts should be directed at preventing exposure to malarial parasites and treating clinical episodes promptly. All of the antimalarial agents have some potential for untoward effects on the fetus, but chloroquine phosphate, the blood schizonticide of choice for oral prophylaxis (500 mg, 300 mg base once a week before the potential exposure and continued for 4 weeks afterward) and therapy (1 g, 600 mg base stat, then 500 mg in 6 hours, then 500 mg/day for two doses) for all plasmodium species except for chloroquine-resistant *Plasmodium falciparum,* has proved well tolerated and remarkably free of side effects in obstetric patients. Primaquine phosphate, the exoerythrocitic hepatic schizonticide of choice for preventing relapses of *Plasmodium vivax* infection, is generally contraindicated during pregnancy because of the high risk of hemolysis in glucose-6-phosphate-dehydrogenase (G6PD)–deficient patients, but it can be given postpartum, and once a week chloroquine may be substituted. Pyrimethamine-sulfadoxine, three tablets orally as a single dose, can be used for mild to moderate infections caused by chloroquine-resistant *P. falciparum* or when drug sensitivity is questionable. Quinine sulfate, two capsules three times a day for 7 to 10 days, with or without clindamycin, 450 mg orally four times a day, is reserved for more severe infections. Patients unable to take oral drugs can be given IV quinidine gluconate (1) 10 mg/kg over 4 hours followed by 0.02 mg/kg/min by continuous pump infusion for 72 hours or until the patient is able to take oral quinine sulfate, or (2) 15 mg/kg over 4 hours followed by 7.5 mg/kg over 4 hours every 8 hours plus clindamycin, 10 mg/kg followed by 5 mg/kg every 8 hours. Extremely close follow-up with special attention to hypoglycemia is advised. Data on the fetal side effects of mefloquine are controversial. Artemether and artesunate have not been adequately tried during pregnancy in humans.

■ TOXOPLASMOSIS

The rationale for early treatment of toxoplasmosis acquired during gestation is to decrease the incidence and severity of fetal infection. When the maternal diagnosis is established during pregnancy, spiramycin, a macrolide antibiotic with an antibacterial spectrum similar to erythromycin, 1 g orally three times a day, reduces the rate of transmission of infection to the fetus by approximately 60%. The drug, available in the United States through the Food and Drug Administration (1-888-463-6332), is continued until delivery, assuming fetal infection has been excluded. If fetal infection is confirmed (the diagnostic method of choice is amniotic fluid polymerase chain reaction (PCR) examination at 18 weeks of gestation), oral pyrimethamine, 25 mg/day plus sulfadiazine, 4 g/day, is superior and therefore should be started together with folinic acid, 10 mg/day, as soon as the diagnosis is established.

Serologic screening is to be performed before pregnancy or at the first prenatal visit, before gestational week 22, and finally near term in previously seronegative women. If the tests are or become positive, acute IgM (requires confirmation in a reference laboratory, i.e., Palo Alto Medical Foundation Research Institute, 650-853-4828), IgA, or IgE can prove recent infection and mandate therapy. HIV-infected women are treated with pyrimethamine-sulfadiazine, 100 mg twice a day on day 1, followed by 50 to 75 mg daily (pyrimehomine), and 8 to 4 g daily (sulfadiazine) and suppressed for life with 50 mg daily and 2 g daily. Maintenance trimethroprim-sulfamethoxazole (TMP-SMX) for *Pneumocystis carinii* pneumonia (PCP) prophylaxis may prevent toxoplasmosis.

■ HERPES SIMPLEX VIRUS INFECTION OF THE GENITAL TRACT

Preventing neonatal disease in babies born to mothers with genital infection is controversial. If no active disease is present, vaginal delivery appears safe, but if active lesions are apparent at parturition and membranes are intact, a cesarean section is considered safer. However, in the presence of ruptured membranes and especially after 4 hours, the decision can be rapid delivery by either route. A high index of suspicion and immediate isolation and treatment of infants with early infections are warranted.

■ HEPATITIS B AND C

Because of the serious consequences of perinatal transmission, screening of all pregnant women for active hepatitis B infection and administration of vaccine and/or specific immunoglobulin prophylaxis to infants of mothers with positive serology are recommended. Interferon and/or ribavirin have not been studied during pregnancy.

■ HIV INFECTION AND ACQUIRED IMMUNODEFICIENCY DISEASE

We manage most aspects of HIV infection and AIDS in the pregnant patient as in nonpregnant females. In addition, zidovudine, antepartum 100 mg orally five times a day; intrapartum, 2 mg/kg IV over 1 hour, then 1 mg/kg/hour until delivery to the mother, and 2 mg/kg every 6 hours orally for 6 weeks to the newborn, is established therapy for prevention of vertical transmission. Shorter and simpler regimens (300 mg every 12 hours initiated at 36 weeks' gestation and 300 mg every 3 hours during labor) given to non–breast-feeding women have shown a 50% decline in vertical transmission rates. Elective cesarean section can further reduce the risk of fetal infection and should be considered individually.

■ POSTPARTUM ENDOMETRITIS

Infection of the uterine cavity is a significant cause of postpartum fever. Predisposing factors include PROM, prolonged labor, numerous vaginal examinations, internal fetal monitoring, poor nutrition, lack of prenatal care, and cesarean section. Fever and tachycardia, foul lochia, uterine tenderness, and purulent cervical drainage are characteristic findings. A biopsy of the decidual lining and a specimen from the fundus of the uterus should be obtained for aerobic and anaerobic cultures, which must include *Mycoplasma, Ureaplasma,* and *Chlamydia*. When a mass is palpated, ultrasonography and CT can establish its characteristics and guide decisions about aspiration and/or further procedures. Therapy is draining the uterus and aggressively administering IV broad-spectrum empiric antimicrobials. Clindamycin, 900 mg IV every 8 hours, plus gentamicin, 2 mg/kg loading dose IV, then 1.5 mg/kg every 8 hours, has had a response rate of up to 95%. The recent increased incidence of enterococcal infection may partially explain the increase in failure rates; this organism should be kept in mind. Newer beta-lactam antibiotics such as aztreonam, ceftazidime, ceftixoxime, cefotetan, ampicillin-sulbactam, and ticarcillin-clavulanate offer equivalent and often superior coverage (Table 3). The treatment is continued until the patient is afebrile for 24 to 48 hours, and no oral antibiotic follow-up is usually necessary.

■ PUERPERAL MASTITIS

Acute breast infections, although not life-threatening, may produce significant discomfort and serious sequelae. High fever followed by localized symptoms or signs is the common clinical sequence. Blood cultures are useful; ultrasonography and needle aspiration may help establish the diagnosis in selected patients. *Staphylococcus aureus* and *Staphylococcus epidermidis* account for most cases. Many patients with mild to moderate infection can be treated as outpatients with oral or parenteral antibiotics. Oral cloxacillin and dicloxacillin, 250 to 500 mg every 6 hours; cephalexin or cephradine, 500 mg every 6 hours; or cefadroxil, 0.5 to 1 g every 12 hours, have been used with success and minimal side effects. Women with severe infections are treated with IV therapy with oxacillin or nafcillin, 1 to 2 g every 4 to 6 hours; cefazolin, 2 g every 8 hours; cefuroxime, 750 to 1500 mg every 8 hours; or vancomycin, 1 g every 12

hours, depending on the penicillin allergy status. Breast abscesses occur in 4% to 10% of women despite antimicrobial therapy, and when they are present, surgical drainage is indicated. Antianaerobic coverage can be added pending microbiologic findings. Continuation of lactation is encouraged during therapy.

■ CESAREAN SECTION AND EPISIOTOMY WOUND INFECTIONS

The rate of infection after cesarean section is higher than after episiotomy, and the risk factors are different; however, both are polymicrobic, and both carry the potential for severe complications. Early recognition of simple infection, necrotizing fasciitis, synergistic gangrene, and clostridial myonecrosis can be lifesaving. Antibiotic combinations such as ampicillin plus clindamycin plus gentamicin at the dosages described earlier, drainage, and excision of all necrotic and pale tissue are essential. High-dose penicillin is used for *Clostridium perfingens* myonecrosis with radical surgery. Adjunctive hyperbaric oxygen is used when available.

Suggested Reading

Carpenter CCJ, et al: Antiretroviral therapy for HIV infection in 1998. Updated recommendations of the International Aids Society—USA panel, *JAMA* 280:78, 1998.

Connor EM, et al: Reduction of maternal-infant transmission of human immunodeficiency virus type 1 with zidovudine treatment, *NEJM* 331:1173, 1994.

Hussey MJ, et al: Evaluating rapid diagnostic tests of intra-amniotic infection: Gram stain, amniotic fluid glucose level, and amniotic fluid to serum glucose level ratio, *Am J Obstet Gynecol* 179:650, 1998.

The International Perinatal HIV Group: The mode of delivery and the risk of vertical transmission of human immunodeficiency virus type 1, *N Engl J Med* 340:977, 1999.

McCormack W: Pelvic inflammatory disease, *N Engl J Med* 330:115, 1994.

Patterson TF, Andriole VT: Detection, significance, and therapy of bacteriuria in pregnancy. Update in the managed care era, *Infect Dis Clin North Am* 11(3):593, 1997.

Turnquest M, et al: Chorioamnionitis: Is continuation of antibiotic therapy necessary after cesarean section? *Am J Obst Gynecol* 179:1261, 1998.

DIALYSIS-RELATED INFECTION

Peter Mariuz

Roy T. Steigbigel

The overall incidence and prevalence of patients treated for end-stage renal disease (ESRD) continually increase in the United States. Data from the U.S. Renal Data System (USRDS) 1998 Annual Report show that for 1996, 283,932 patients were treated for ESRD and 73,091 new patients started ESRD treatment. Prevalence is actually higher because the USRDS does not contain data on non-Medicare patients. According to the USRDS, after cardiovascular disease, infections are the second most common cause of death of patients receiving long-term dialysis, and they are a leading cause of hospitalization. Data on the mortality of patients on dialysis followed for 16 years, a longer period than in the USRDS, show that infections account for 36% of deaths versus 14.4% for cardiovascular disease. Abnormalities of cellular immunity, neutrophil function, and complement activation are associated with chronic renal failure and cited as risk factors for the increased susceptibility to infection. Most dialysis-related infections are caused by common microorganisms rather than by opportunistic pathogens and are related to vascular and peritoneal dialysis access. This chapter focuses on the treatment of infections related to dialysis access devices.

■ TYPES OF ACCESS DEVICES FOR DIALYSIS

The wide variety of catheters available for hemodialysis (Table 1) differs according to the duration of use (acute versus chronic) and intraperitoneal versus extraperitoneal designs. The peritoneal catheters for acute use (<3 days) have the same basic design, a relatively stiff length of straight or slightly curved nylon or polyethylene tubing with side holes at the distal portion. This is placed at the bedside over a guidewire. These catheters lack cuffs to protect against bacterial migration from the skin along the outer surface of the catheter, so they have a high infection rate when used for more than 3 days. Peritoneal access devices for chronic use are made of silicone rubber or polyurethane, usually with one or two Dacron cuffs and side holes at the distal end. They can be placed by use of guidewire and dilators or peritoneoscopy. The silicone rubber or polyurethane surface elicits growth of squamous epithelium in the subcutaneous tunnel and at the catheter's entry and exit sites. The Dacron cuffs provoke a local inflammatory response resulting in the formation of fibrous and granulation tissues within 4 weeks. Both epithelial and fibrous tissues prevent bacterial migration along the tunnel. In addition, the fibrous tissue anchors the catheter. Examples of peritoneal catheters for chronic use include the straight or curled Tenckoff catheter widely used in the United States, Oreopoulos-Zellerman, Lifecath, and Toronto Western II. It is not known whether these newer catheters provide any advantage over the Tenckoff design.

■ INFECTIOUS COMPLICATIONS OF VASCULAR ACCESS DEVICES

Local infections occur at the exit site or in the tunnel of percutaneously inserted silicone catheters. The clinical presentations of exit-site infection include pain, erythema, tenderness, induration, and purulent discharge surrounding the site. Tunnel infections are associated with pain, erythema, tenderness, or induration involving the subcutaneous tract of the catheter. Infection of autologous arteriovenous (AV) fistulas and prosthetic polytetrafluoroethylene (PTFE) grafts can manifest as cellulitis, perifistular abscess, false aneurysm, draining sinus, and in PTFE shunts, bleeding when the grafts' suture lines are involved. Fever, leukocytosis, or left shift in the differential leukocyte count may be present. All local access device infections may be complicated by concomitant bacteremia, sepsis, and suppurative

Table 1 Vascular Access Devices for Hemodialysis	
TEMPORARY VENOUS ACCESS (USUALLY LESS THAN 2-3 WEEKS)	**PERMANENT ACCESS FOR ESRD**
Single- or double-lumen (Mahurkar type) catheter into the subclavian vein	Arteriovenous fistula using autogenous saphenous vein or PTFE, Teflon
Silastin-Teflon shunt for CAVH or CAVHD	Dacron cuffed double-lumen silicon catheter (Permcath); rarely used; surgically inserted into the subclavian or internal jugular vein through a subcutaneous tunnel
Twin wide-bore femoral catheter for CAVH or CAVHD	Scribner arteriovenous shunt, now used infrequently
Temporary venous access in ESRD: single- or double-lumen venous catheter inserted over guidewire into the subclavian, femoral,* or internal jugular vein	

ESRD, End-stage renal disease; *PTFE*, polytetrafluoroethylene; *CAVH*, continuous arteriovenous hemofiltration; *CAVHD*, continuous arteriovenous hemodialysis.

*Femoral vein placement is associated with high rate of infection, so it is usually removed by 72 hours.

Table 2   Microbiology of Access Device Infections

HEMODIALYSIS	PERITONEAL DIALYSIS
Staphylococcus aureus (50%-80%)	*Staphylococcus epidermidis* and *S. aureus* (50%)
Other gram-positive bacteria (*S. epidermidis*, streptococci, including enterococci, diphtheroides), gram-negative organisms (*Escherichia coli, Pseudomonas aeruginosa, Acinetobacter* spp., and other enteric gram-negative bacteria) (15%-30%)	Other gram-positive bacteria (streptococci, including enterococci, diphtheroides)
	Gram-negative organisms (*E. coli, P. aeruginosa, Acinetobacter* spp., and other enteric gram-negative bacteria)
Occasionally fungi	Occasionally fungi

Percentages in parentheses are approximate proportional incidence from numerous references.

Table 3   Treatment of Hemodialysis Access-Site Infections

TYPE OF INFECTION	THERAPY
Exit-site infection in a temporary access device with or without bacteremia	Catheter removal and vancomycin, 1 g IV; subsequent doses based on serum levels; aminoglycosides or broad-spectrum beta-lactam antibiotics if gram-negative organisms suspected
Tunnel infection	Catheter removal and antibiotics as above
Catheter-related sepsis	Catheter removal; empiric broad-spectrum antimicrobial therapy with vancomycin and gentamicin, 1.5 mg/kg IV in a single dose; subsequent antimicrobial therapy based on pathogen and sensitivity pattern
Suppurative thrombophlebitis	Catheter removal, antimicrobial therapy based on pathogen and sensitivity pattern; surgical consultation for possible exploratory venotomy
Arteriovenous fistula infection	Vancomycin and gentamicin as above; incision and drainage of abscess; ligation or removal of prosthetic arteriovenous fistulas for occlusion or tunnel infection or if response to treatment is not prompt; surgical repair of a malfunctioning infected shunt may be possible
	10-14 days of therapy commonly used for exit and tunnel infections with catheter removal; if the catheter remains in place, 2-3 weeks of antimicrobials

---

thrombophlebitis. Bacteremia may lead to metastatic foci of infection, including septic arthritis, septic pulmonary emboli, endocarditis, osteomyelitis, brain abscess, and splenic abscess. Bacteremia and sepsis may be present without signs or symptoms of infection at the access site.

Microbiology

A specific microbiologic diagnosis of access-related infection can frequently be made by Gram stain and culture of purulent material from the cannula exit site or with AV fistulas from needle exit sites, fistulas, or abscess fluid. In addition, blood cultures drawn from the access device and other peripheral sites should be obtained. The organisms responsible for access device infection are shown in Table 2.

Therapy

Therapy is ultimately based on the results of cultures from infected sites and blood. Initial management plans are shown in Table 3. Relative indications for removal of the access device include tunnel infections, suppurative thrombophlebitis, septicemia, and bacteremia with metastatic foci of infection, infections caused by gram-negative organisms and fungi, lack of response to medical therapy within 24 to 48 hours, recurrent infection in a catheter with the same pathogen, and involvement of the suture lines of PTFE grafts. Any associated fluid collections should be drained. Intravenous (IV) vancomycin is often used in initial therapy for access device infections because staphylococci are the most common pathogens. Depending on the type of dialyzer used, therapeutic blood levels of vancomycin may be achieved for 5 to 10 days. After a 1-g IV dose of vancomycin, serum levels should be monitored after 5 to 7 days to ensure adequate trough levels. To avoid overuse of vancomycin with induction of vancomycin-resistant bacteria, methicillin-sensitive staphylococci should be treated with IV nafcillin, 1 to 2 g every 4 to 6 hours or cefazolin, 1 g every 24 to 48 hours supplemented with 1 g after dialysis. Fifteen to thirty percent of infections are caused by gram-negative bacilli. If gram-negative organisms are suspected, an aminoglycoside, cefepime, or aztreonam should be used in combination with vancomycin. The initial choice of antimicrobials should be influenced by the sensitivity of organisms prevalent in the patient's geographic region.

■ INFECTIONS ASSOCIATED WITH PERITONEAL DIALYSIS CATHETERS

Continuous ambulatory peritoneal dialysis (CAPD) has a relatively high incidence of exit-site and tunnel infections (0.6 to 0.7 per dialysis year). Thirty percent of patient transfers from peritoneal to hemodialysis are a consequence of catheter complications and peritonitis. CAPD catheter exit-site and particularly tunnel infections may result in peritonitis and catheter loss. Diagnosis of exit-site infection is based on erythema, tenderness, induration, and/or puru-

Table 4   Treatment of Peritoneal Dialysis Access Device Infections

TYPE OF INFECTION	THERAPY
Exit-site infection with minimal erythema without purulent discharge	Topical mupirocin, chlorhexidine, hydrogen peroxide, or povidone iodine bid; avoid mupirocin with polyurethane catheter.
Gram-positive exit-site infection	Dicloxacillin, 250-500 mg PO q6h, or cephalexin, 250-500 mg PO q6h, or trimethoprim-sulfamethoxazole, 160/800 mg PO bid. Clindamycin may also be used. IV or IP route can be used. For methicillin-resistant staphylococci: vancomycin, 1 g/wk IV. Rifampin, 600 mg PO qd, can be added for possible synergistic effect. Ultrasound to rule out tunnel or cuff involvement; 2-3 weeks of therapy generally recommended; shave external cuff and explore tunnel if infection persists; if this fails, catheter removal.
Gram-negative exit-site infection	*Pseudomonas aeruginosa* should be suspected pending culture results. Ciprofloxacin, 500 mg PO bid; not to be taken concomitantly with phosphate binders or antacids; alteration of therapy based on culture results. Therapy should be continued for 2-3 weeks. Catheter removal if infection persists beyond 2-3 weeks; early catheter removal should be considered if *Pseudomonas* or *Stenotrophomonas* isolated.
Tunnel infection	Antimicrobials as for exit-side infections with removal of catheter.

lent discharge from the exit site. Pericatheter erythema without purulent drainage may be an early sign of infection. Crusting caused by a small amount of exudate at the exit site may not be indicative of infection. Erythema, tenderness, induration, pain, and abscess in the area between the catheter cuffs suggests tunnel infection. This can be confirmed by ultrasonography, which will reveal an area of hypoechogenicity (fluid collection) between the tube or the cuff of the catheter and surrounding tissues. Indications for tunnel sonography include presence of exit-site infection (to assess the efficacy of therapy and prognosis of tunnel infections) and recurrent peritonitis. A specific microbiologic diagnosis can be made by performing a Gram stain and culture of purulent exudate. The organisms responsible for CAPD catheter infections are shown in Table 2.

■ THERAPY

Therapy is ultimately based on the results of microbiologic culture data. Initial management plans are shown in Table 4. Therapy should be continued until the exit site appears normal. Indications for catheter removal, shown in Table 5, include peritonitis, bacteremia, and sepsis. Relative indications for catheter removal are tunnel infections (particularly if there is no response to therapy noted on serial ultrasound examinations), involvement of the deep cuff (which often leads to peritonitis), chronic exit-site infections (no cure after 2 to 4 weeks of therapy), and exit-site infections associated with involvement of the superficial cuff as noted on ultrasound, and infections caused by fungi. Ultrasonographic evidence of tunnel involvement is associated with frequent catheter loss (50%) because of refractory or recurrent peritonitis. The use of serial ultrasound examinations may also be useful to monitor the efficacy of antimicrobial therapy of tunnel infections. A 30% or greater decrease in the size of the fluid collection after 2 weeks of therapy is often associated with catheter salvage. Prolonged courses of antimicrobial therapy, although sometimes necessary, should be avoided given the growing problem of antimicrobial resistance. Infections with vancomycin-resistant enterococci (VRE) and, more ominously, vancomycin-resistant

Table 5   Indications for Peritoneal Dialysis Catheter Removal

Peritonitis
Bacteremia
Sepsis
Tunnel infections
Chronic exit-site infections
? Infections caused by fungi

strains of *Staphylococcus aureus* and *S. epidermidis* reported in dialysis patients receiving prolonged (months) treatment make the judicious use of this drug imperative. In chronic exit-site infections, adjunctive surgical therapy may help control infection and result in catheter salvage. Surgical procedures that have been used include cuff shaving (removal of the external cuff), debridement and curettage of the exit-site and sinus tract, incision, and debridement along the subcutaneous tunnel with exteriorization of the superficial cuff and relocation of the exit site. It is not known which of these is most effective. Among gram-positive organisms *S. aureus* is more commonly associated with poor response to medical therapy, tunnel infections, and catheter loss.

■ PERITONITIS ASSOCIATED WITH CAPD INFECTIONS

Peritonitis is a common complication of CAPD. Although the incidence varies from center to center, the overall incidence is 1.3 episodes per patient per year. Peritonitis may be less common in continuous cycle–assisted peritoneal dialysis (CCPD) and nocturnal intermittent peritoneal dialysis (NIPD) than in other forms of CAPD. An additional, modest reduction in the incidence of peritonitis has been achieved with use of Y-set transfer kit (particularly infections from skin flora). Bacteria gain entry to the peritoneum through the lumen of the catheter, often after improper technique in connecting the transfer set to the dialysate bag or the catheter to the transfer set, from the outside surface of the catheter, complicating an exit-site or tunnel infection, or by hematogenous spread and from the bowel or pelvis. Clinical manifestations include abdominal pain, fever, chills, malaise, nausea, vomiting, constipation, or diarrhea with abdominal tenderness, rebound tenderness, and leukocytosis. The peritoneal fluid may appear cloudy and will almost always contain more than 100 polymorphonuclear leukocytes per cubic millimeter of fluid. In any suspected CAPD infection, including those that appear to be localized to the exit site, a Gram stain and culture of the peritoneal fluid should be obtained with cell count and differential.

Bacteriology

A single pathogen is usually involved. Polymicrobial infection suggests a perforated viscus or other intraabdominal or pelvic pathologic process. Most cases of peritonitis (70%) are caused by gram-positive bacteria. Collectively, *S. aureus* and *S. epidermidis* account for almost 50% of infections. *Pseudomonas aeruginosa* and other enteric gram-negative bacilli constitute 20% to 30%, and fungi, mostly *Candida albicans,* fewer than 1 to 10 percent. Some 5% to 20% of cases are culture negative.

Therapy

No clinical trials establishing the optimal antibiotic drugs and route of administration have been done. Antibiotics may be given by the IV, oral, or intraperitoneal (IP) route. The IP route is preferred because of its convenience. There is no therapeutic advantage to IV therapy. Helpful information for the initial choice of antimicrobials includes peritoneal fluid Gram stain results, history of microbe-specific peritonitis, coexistent exit-site infection, and intraabdominal pathology. Given the increasing prevalence of vancomycin-resistant gram-positive bacteria, the routine use of this drug for empiric therapy can no longer be justified. If the Gram stain suggests gram-positive bacteria, gram-negative bacteria, or is negative or unavailable, empiric therapy should be initiated; IP cefazolin or cephalothin, 500 mg/L loading dose then 125 mg/L in each exchange with an aminoglycoside such as gentamicin, 0.6 mg/kg body weight in one daily exchange. Alternatives to cefazolin or cephalothin include nafcillin, clindamycin, vancomycin, and ciprofloxacin in order of preference.

Fluconazole, 200 mg PO or IP daily, should be used for yeast infections. If clinical improvement is noted, therapy should be continued for 4 to 6 weeks. If there is no clinical improvement after 3 to 5 days, the clinician should remove the catheter and treat for 10 more days; immediate catheter removal is advocated for patients who appear septic. Amphotericin B is an alternative to fluconazole for patients who are not responding or who have organisms insensitive to fluconazole such as *Candida krusei* and filamentous fungi.

After 24 to 48 hours, 70% to 90% of dialysate fluid cultures will yield a specific pathogen, and therapy should be modified accordingly. For *S. aureus* or *S. epidermidis* sensitive to nafcillin, the clinician should administer this drug at 125 mg/L in each exchange or the first-generation cephalosporin may be continued. The aminoglycoside should be stopped. Rifampin, 600 mg/day PO, may be added for patients responding slowly to the initial regimen. If the patient does not improve, the clinician should evaluate for tunnel infection. For staphylococci resistant to methicillin,

nafcillin or the cephalosporin and aminoglycoside should be discontinued. Vancomycin, 2 g (30 mg/kg) IP every 7 days, or if the organism is sensitive, clindamycin, 300 mg/L loading dose and then 150 mg/L maintenance is used. Rifampin should be added as stated previously. For enterococci sensitive to ampicillin, the cephalosporin should be discontinued and ampicillin started at 125 mg/L in each exchange: the clinician should consider continuing the aminoglycoside. In penicillin-allergic patients, vancomycin, 2 g IP per week, should be used. Treatment of VRE depends on the antimicrobial sensitivities of the specific organism. Enterococci are part of the intestinal flora; therefore intraabdominal pathology must be considered. For other gram-positive organisms, therapy should be based on antibiotic sensitivity results. For gram-negative organisms other than *Pseudomonas* and *Stenotrophomonas maltophilia,* a first-generation cephalosporin may suffice, and the aminoglycoside can be discontinued. If the microbe is resistant to cefazolin, the choice of another cephalosporin should be based on sensitivity testing.

Fourteen days of therapy are usually adequate. If multiple gram-negative organisms are isolated, evaluation for intraabdominal pathology should be undertaken. For *Pseudomonas aeruginosa* or *Stenotrophomonas maltophilia,* the clinician should consider use of two agents (one being an aminoglycoside) chosen based on sensitivity testing results and continue for at least 3 weeks. Eighth nerve toxicity may complicate aminoglycoside use, particularly after 2 to 3 weeks of therapy. If the infection is catheter related, the clinician should remove the catheter and continue antibiotics for 1 week.

For polymicrobial or anaerobic infections, the clinician should consider surgical intervention, continue the aminoglycoside, continue or change the cephalosporin based on sensitivity testing, and add metronidazole, 500 mg every 8 hours IV or PO.

Most patients demonstrate significant clinical improvement within 2 to 4 days. Patients who fail to respond to therapy should be reevaluated. Peritoneal fluid should be examined with cell counts, Gram stains, and culture. In addition, intraabdominal or gynecologic pathology requiring surgical intervention and unusual pathogens (fungi, mycobacteria) must be considered. The clinician should remove and culture the catheter of patients whose original cultures are negative but who remain symptomatic after 2 to 4 days.

■ LESS COMMON PATHOGENS

There are conflicting data regarding the intrinsic risk of dialysis patients for developing tuberculosis. It is likely that any predisposition of these patients to tuberculosis is related more to the prevalence of tuberculosis in the community than to host factors. However, there is a higher incidence of extrapulmonary tuberculosis in this population than in the community. Treatment is the same as for patients without ESRD except that dosing of some agents must be adjusted for renal failure and others should be avoided. Isoniazid is given at 150 mg/day orally with a supplemental dose after dialysis. Rifampin requires no dosage adjustment. The dosage of ethambutol is 5 mg/kg/day orally with a supplemental dose after dialysis. Some authorities believe that pyrazinamide use should be avoided if possible; ethionamide is given at 250 to 500 mg/day orally.

Listeria monocytogenes septicemia, meningitis, and endocarditis have been rarely described in patients with ESRD, usually as a complication of iron overload or during immunosuppressive therapy. Yersiniosis complicating iron overload has also been reported. Disseminated or rhinocerebral phycomycosis in nondiabetic patients receiving hemodialysis may have a link to deferoxamine use. The treatment includes amphotericin B and surgical debridement of all infected sites.

Suggested Reading

Bander SJ, Schwab ST: Central venous angioaccess for hemodialysis and its complications, *Sem Dialysis* 5:121, 1992.

Goldman M, Vanherweghem J-L: Bacterial infections in chronic hemodialysis patients: epidemiologic and pathophysiologic aspects, *Adv Nephrol* 19:315, 1990.

Keane WF, et al: Peritoneal dialysis-related peritonitis treatment recommendations, 1996 update, *Perit Dial Int* 16:557, 1996.

Piraino B: Management of catheter-related infections, *Am J Kidney Dis* 27:754, 1996.

Steigbigel RT, Cross AS: Infections associated with hemodialysis and chronic peritoneal dialysis. In Remington JS, Swartz MN, eds: *Current clinical topics in infectious diseases,* vol 5, New York, 1984, McGraw-Hill.

Twardowski ZJ, Prowant BF: Current approach to exit-site infections in patients on peritoneal dialysis, *Nephrol Dial Transplant* 12:1284, 1997.

U.S. Renal Data System: *USRDS 1998 Annual Data Report,* Bethesda, MD, 1998, National Institutes of Health, National Institute of Diabetes and Digestive and Kidney Diseases.

Vychytil A, et al: New criteria for management of catheter infections in peritoneal dialysis patients using ultrasonography, *J Am Soc Nephrol* 9:290, 1998.

INFECTED IMPLANTS

Gilberto Rodriguez
Gordon Dickinson

This chapter addresses infections associated with artificial devices of a specialized nature. Optimal treatment requires participation of surgical specialists experienced in the management of these difficult infections. This is especially the case for pseudophakic endophthalmitis, in which therapy includes intraocular injections.

■ INTRAOCULAR LENS–ASSOCIATED INFECTIONS (PSEUDOPHAKIC ENDOPHTHALMITIS)

Cataract surgery is one of the most commonly performed operations in the United States. More than 1 million intraocular lenses are implanted each year. Fortunately, the incidence of pseudophakic endophthalmitis is very low. Pseudophakic endophthalmitis is thought to occur as a consequence of contamination with flora of the conjunctival sac or lid margin at the time of surgery. There also have been reports of infections arising from contamination of lenses and neutralizing and storage solutions.

The differential diagnosis of endophthalmitis following cataract extraction includes sterile inflammation as well as bacterial and fungal infection. The most common presenting signs and symptoms include pain in the involved eye, decreased visual acuity, red eye, lid edema, hypopyon, and absent or poor red reflex. A single bacterial strain is usually isolated; the most common pathogen is a coagulase-negative staphylococcus (approximately 50% in one large series) followed by *Staphylococcus aureus*. Virtually any microorganism can be implicated. Delayed-onset pseudophakic endophthalmitis has been reported after uncomplicated initial cataract surgery. This entity presents one or more months after the surgery and is manifest by waxing and waning ocular inflammation. The leading cause of delayed-onset pseudophakic endophthalmitis is *Propionibacterium acnes*. Diagnostic evaluation requires aqueous and vitreous samples for Gram stain and culture. Vitrectomy may have therapeutic as well as diagnostic value.

Patients should be seen by an ophthalmologist immediately. Antimicrobials administered intraocularly and topically are the mainstay of treatment for this localized infection. Because of unpredictable antibiotic penetration, systemic antibiotics are of secondary importance and generally unnecessary. (See also the chapter *Endophthalmitis.*)

■ BREAST IMPLANT–ASSOCIATED INFECTIONS

Breast implants are used in reconstruction of the breast following mastectomy or for cosmetic purposes. The implants typically consist of silicone shells filled with saline or silicone gel. They are implanted in a subglandular or submuscular pocket through inframammary, periareolar, or transaxillary approaches. Infections following breast implant placement is uncommon with an incidence of less than 2%. Endogenous flora of human breast tissue are similar to skin flora and account for most infections. The most common pathogen found in breast implant–associated infection is *S. aureus,* followed by coagulase-negative staphylococcus and *Propionibacterium* species. Other less common organisms include *Lactobacillus,* diphtheroids, *Bacillus,* and alpha-streptococcus. Signs and symptoms of infection include pain, tenderness, swelling, drainage, warmth, and erythema around the wound margin and the prosthesis. Occasionally, the implant may be extruded by the infection.

Clusters as well as sporadic infections caused by *Mycobacterium fortuitum* complex have been reported. The source of the pathogen is usually not identified, and the route of infection is unknown. The onset of this infection is usually more subtle than those caused by other pathogens and may range from 1 week to a few months after implantation. Initial signs and symptoms include breast swelling, tenderness, warmth, and discharge of an odorless, serosanguineous, or purulent exudate. Gram stain of the fluid usually reveals no organisms but many polymorphonuclear leukocytes. Stain for acid-fast bacilli are sometimes positive. A definitive diagnosis is established by culture of the organism.

Breast implant–associated infections are treated with systemic antibiotics against the most common pathogens. Recommended initial empiric therapy may include beta-lactamase–resistant penicillin, first-generation cephalosporin, or for penicillin-allergic patients, vancomycin. Duration of therapy ranges from 2 to 4 weeks, depending on the severity of the infection and the clinical response. Removal of the implant is not always necessary, and a trial of systemic antibiotics is recommended. However, infection from atypical mycobacterium always requires removal of the implant, with debridement of the wound in addition to systemic antibiotic therapy. Most organisms of the *M. fortuitum* complex are sensitive to amikacin, cefoxitin, fluoroquinolones, clarithromycin, and azithromycin, but susceptibility studies should be obtained.

■ PENILE IMPLANT–ASSOCIATED INFECTION

The first artificial penile prosthesis was implanted in the early 1970s. Since then, several penile prostheses have been developed, and they are an accepted treatment for male impotence. An infectious complication after placement of a penile prosthesis is a disastrous event with an incidence rate between 0.8 and 8.3%. Many risk factors for infections have been mentioned, including diabetes mellitus, duration of surgery, immunosuppression, reoperation for technical failures, and inadequate prophylactic antibiotic coverage, but the type of prostheses or incision does not appear to influence the risk of infection. Most penile prosthesis–associated infections likely originate in the operating room at the time of implantation. Common sources of infections include the skin, colorectal, and perianal flora, urine, and operating room environment. Late infections are more likely caused by hematogenous spread or urethral infection. The most commonly isolated pathogen is coagulase-negative staphylococcus; other bacteria include *S. aureus* and gram-negative enteric bacteria such as *Escherichia coli, Pseudomonas aeruginosa, Klebsiella,* and *Proteus.* Gonorrheal and fungal infections have been reported. Signs and symptoms of infections include new onset of pain, swelling, tenderness, erythema, induration, fluctuance, erosion, and extrusion of prostheses. Infections caused by *S. epidermidis* are often subtle and may present with dysfunction of the prostheses or pain upon manipulation of the device.

Empiric antibiotic treatment should be directed at both gram-positive bacteria and gram-negative coliform bacteria, pending isolation of the causative pathogen. Most authors recommend removal of a prosthesis that is surrounded by grossly purulent exudate and irrigation of the compartments that were occupied by prosthetic devices. Treatment should be continued for a week or more after all signs of infection have resolved.

Suggested Reading

Blum MD: Infections of genitourinary prostheses, *Infect Dis Clin North Am* 3:259, 1989.

Carlson AN, Tetz MR, Apple DJ: Infectious complications of modern cataract surgery and intraocular lens implantation, *Infect Dis Clin North Am* 3:339, 1989.

Clegg HW, et al: Infection due to organisms of the *Mycobacterium fortuitum* complex after augmentation mammoplasty. Clinical and epidemiologic features, *J Infect Dis* 147:427, 1983.

Endophthalmitis Vitrectomy Study Group: Results of the endophthalmitis vitrectomy study, *Arch Ophthalmol* 113:1479, 1995.

Freedman AM, Jackson IT: Infections in breast implants, *Infect Dis Clin North Am* 3:275, 1989.

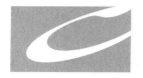

NOSOCOMIAL INFECTION

PREVENTION OF NOSOCOMIAL INFECTION IN STAFF AND PATIENTS

John E. McGowan, Jr.

Nosocomial infections—those acquired in the hospital or other health care facility—affect more than 1.6 million patients annually (Table 1). Adverse consequences of these infections are formidable, with overall annual cost of about $4.5 billion in the United States. Because of their high cost, these infections and attempts to minimize them are a major focus for today's health care facility (HCF). Preventive efforts are especially important in the integrated health care systems that characterize many areas of the United States. This chapter describes strategies and resources to decrease such infections.

The main focus of efforts to minimize nosocomial infections are early recognition and description of the pattern of infection in the HCF, analysis of the epidemiologic features, and action to control and prevent these infections by interventions targeted to the epidemiologic features. Attention must be directed to all aspects of care provided by the integrated health care system. This requires strategies for preventing infection in acute-care hospitals, extended-care facilities, ambulatory care settings such as same-day surgery, and home care settings where infection risk is present, such

as those involving administration of parenteral antimicrobial agents or other intravascular therapy. Infection control efforts originally were focused on the acute care hospital. Given the wide range of settings where care is provided today, a broader definition is essential, as given at the beginning of this chapter.

Spread of infection within an HCF traditionally requires three elements: a source of infecting organisms, a susceptible host, and a mode of acquisition. These factors interact with each other. For example, the classic way a patient and organism meet is by exogenous transfer: here, the infected person acquires organisms in the HCF. After transfer of an organism, the likelihood that it will cause nosocomial infection is determined in part by the potential victim's ability to resist infection. This in turn is influenced by preexisting illness, such as diabetes or acquired immunodeficiency syndrome (AIDS); treatments such as corticosteroids; and use of instruments and procedures (e.g., catheters, surgery). These factors all are more prominent in today's HCF than ever before. As a result, resistance of the patient may be reduced to such a degree that infection can develop from organisms of the patient's own flora and transfer from an exogenous source no longer is required. Even so, transfer from other persons or the hospital environment remain important sources of infecting organisms in the HCF setting.

When exogenous nosocomial infection occurs, pathogens are transmitted by several routes, and the same organism may be spread by more than one of these pathways. The most important today is contact transmission by a direct exchange between the body surface of an infected or colonized person (the source) to the body surface of one who is not. Contact transmission through indirect transfer occurs via an intermediate person (patients, personnel, visitors, volunteers) or object (e.g., food, water, medication, instrument, dressing, glove). Less common is spread by droplets or by airborne transmission of infecting organisms in droplet nuclei or dust. Transmission by vectors such as mosquitoes, flies, rats, and other vermin is significant in some parts of the world but virtually absent in the United States.

Knowing the infecting organism, the likely victim (patient, health care worker, volunteer, visitor), the source (reservoir) of the organism, and the mode of acquisition is essential to design of control measures. These efforts focus on eliminating the organism, removing the reservoir, blocking spread from reservoir to victim, or strengthening the

Table 1 Impact of Nosocomial Infections		
	YEAR	
	1975	**1995**
Hospital admissions	38 million	36 million
Hospital patient days	299 million	190 million
Average length of stay	7.9 days	5.3 days
Nosocomial infections	2.1 million	1.9 million

Adapted from Weinstein RW: *Emerg Infect Dis* 4:416, 1998.

potential victim against the organism's weapons. A study by the Centers for Disease Control and Prevention (CDC) in 1983 suggested that only about 9% of nosocomial infections were being prevented. It has been estimated that about a third of all nosocomial infections are preventable with available techniques.

Minimizing nosocomial infections depends on two crucial activities: (1) recognizing and analyzing new problems as they arise so that appropriate control measures can be instituted and (2) maintaining continuous attention to a series of measures that have been proved to minimize the occurrence of endemic infections. Each is considered in turn.

■ NEW AND CONTINUING PROBLEMS

Dealing with a new or continuing problem of nosocomial infection in an HCF, whether epidemic or endemic, requires several steps (Table 2). Perhaps the most important phase in the investigation is the initial step of realizing that a problem exists and defining its features. Epidemics are rare today, so in most HCFs, a rise in endemic infection will be the problem. Often, the patient's physician or the HCF laboratory may provide the first report of a problem. On occasion, infection control personnel may become aware of the problem through their contact with and surveillance of clinical services in the hospitals, clinics, and home care settings or through another HCF in the region. The next step is careful definition of the problem under consideration. Even a rough case definition will allow initial control measures to be taken and enable all persons involved to agree on the nature of the problem.

Once a definition has been made, attempts to identify all possible cases begin. This effort at complete case finding is crucial because the more cases that are available for analysis, the better the chance of determining the process involved. Case finding has three major aspects. The first activity is ascertaining the reliability of clinical and laboratory information. For example, can a case of the entity under investi-gation be identified by its clinical characteristics? Are laboratory facilities available to make the diagnosis? Next, the completeness of reporting must be considered. Most nosocomial infections manifest themselves while the afflicted patient is still in the HCF, but some appear only after the patient has been discharged. In some studies, up to half of all surgical wound infections become manifest after the patient has left the hospital. Other infections may involve a clinical setting where microbiologic testing is rarely employed. Thus laboratory results cannot be used as the sole basis for surveillance, and this is likely to become even more important as integrated health care systems continue to evolve. A caution is appropriate: infections with onset during HCF stay sometimes have been acquired in the community and have been incubating since HCF admission. Thus not all infections with onset during HCF stay are nosocomial.

When as many cases as possible have been identified, the degree to which this episode is an important deviation from usual occurrence can be considered. Certain situations or types of infection are so dramatic or uncommon that even a single case may be recognized as a problem requiring immediate attention. In other settings, the cost to deal with the infections may be higher than the gain from eliminating the problem. Assuming the decision is made to continue the evaluation, the next step is framing the problem in terms of its location, time course, persons involved, common procedures and instruments employed, and other features. Confirming the identity of the responsible organism often is important in this characterization.

Forming postulates about the reasons for the outbreak, defining the reservoir of the organisms, and identifying the mode of acquisition by the victim (e.g., patient, health care worker, visitor) comes next. These features usually point to specific control measures to check the progress of the problem. Usually, several control measures will be considered, so it is appropriate to decide which factor or factors will be most practical to alter. When one or more actions are taken, follow-up data must be collected to make sure the control measures achieved the desired effect.

■ SPECIFIC MEASURES AND PROGRAMS

Infection control faces many challenges today. Increasing populations of immunocompromised patients and the growing presence of antimicrobial-resistant bacteria are prominent features of health care infection. To combat these changes, infection control requires a structured management process staffed by dedicated personnel to influence behavior of doctors, nurses, and other health care workers. This is similar to quality control in industry, and infection control in HCFs is one of the best examples of quality management in action. A recent task force recommended three principal goals for infection control programs in health care institutions. These are (1) protect the patient; (2) protect the health care worker, visitors, and others in the health care environment; and (3) accomplish the previous two goals in a cost-effective manner, whenever possible. These goals are relevant to patient-care activities in any health care setting, including acute-care hospitals, skilled nursing facilities, nursing homes, rehabilitation units, urgent-care centers, same-day surgery facilities, ambulatory

---

Table 2 Steps in Investigation of a Health Care Institution Outbreak

Recognize the problem (surveillance, early warning from patient's physician).
    Case definition
Complete case finding.
    Reliability of reporting (search database for other cases; review laboratory methods)
    Completeness of reporting
    Additional data
Define occurrence.
Characterize the outbreak (demography, location, time).
Form hypotheses about causes (mode of acquisition, reservoirs, vectors).
Initiate control activities, with procedural changes as required.
Do follow-up surveillance to make sure control measures work.

Adapted in part from McGowan JE Jr, Metchock B: Infection control epidemiology and clinical microbiology. In Murray PR, Baron EJ, Pfaller MA, et al, eds: *Manual of clinical microbiology,* ed 7, Washington, DC, 1999, American Society for Microbiology.

care centers and home care programs. The success or failure of the infection control program is defined by its effectiveness in achieving these goals.

To deal with endemic nosocomial infections, the HCF must have a defined intervention system with clear goals for changing behavior and practice and for maintaining these improvements. Both *direct* actions to change behavior (e.g., choosing a handwashing agent that minimizes skin drying) and *indirect* methods (e.g., education to tell why handwashing is important) are essential. Because it is not clear how to deal with most patient and organism factors, the major focus must be on nosocomial infections that are preventable. Thus major attention is given to proper patient care practices aimed at reducing microbial reservoirs and limiting spread of organisms from person to person (Table 3). The CDC has published Guidelines for the Prevention and Control of Nosocomial Infections, including the following: (1) guideline for prevention of catheter-associated urinary tract infections, (2) guideline for handwashing and hospital environmental control, (3) guideline for infection control in hospital personnel, (4) guideline for prevention of intravascular infections, (5) guideline for isolation precautions in hospitals, (6) guideline for prevention of nosocomial pneumonia, and (7) guideline for prevention of surgical wound infections. These are available on the Internet (see Suggested Reading).

Handwashing addresses the most common mode of spread of many nosocomial pathogens, carriage on the hands of health care workers. Most of the microorganisms that cause HCF-related infections are present only transiently on the hands and are easily removed by a brief handwashing. Because this procedure plays such a pivotal role in control of infection, groups such as the CDC have published detailed recommendations for the practice. Unfortunately, handwashing after each patient contact is not practical. In addition, the agents dry the skin, which reduces incentive. Therefore guidelines focus on handwashing after touching a patient or environmental object likely to be contaminated with microorganisms rather than demanding a rote response of washing after entering any patient's room. Plain soap and water are sufficient for general purposes, although in critical care units, some authorities recommend using an antiseptic preparation.

Table 3 Patient Care Areas of Focus to Reduce Nosocomial Infection in Patients and Health Care Workers

Handwashing
Barrier precautions (isolation)
    Standard precautions (universal precautions, body substance isolation)
    Transmission-based precautions (airborne, droplet, contact)
Control and prevention of device- and procedure-related infections in patients
    Surgery (asepsis, perioperative antimicrobial prophylaxis)
    Disinfection and sterilization of supplies and equipment
    Closed drainage systems for indwelling urinary catheters
    Intravascular catheters and their delivery systems (e.g., bottles, tubings)
    Ventilators, nebulizers, other respiratory therapy equipment
Immunization
    Patients and potential patients (e.g., pneumococcal vaccine)
    Health care workers (e.g., hepatitis B vaccine)

Barrier precautions (isolation) are intended to prevent organisms present on one patient from reaching another. The CDC guidelines for isolation in hospitals are based on two levels of performance. First are standard precautions, designed for care of all patients in the hospital regardless of diagnosis or whether they are thought to have infection. This includes universal blood and body fluid precautions and procedures to reduce risk of acquisition of pathogens from moist body substances. A second level, transmission-based precautions, are used for patients documented or suspected to be infected or colonized with highly transmissible or epidemiologically difficult pathogens. This latter group contains measures that vary according to the way the target organism spreads: airborne, droplet, or contact. Of particular use are lists of specific clinical syndromes that are highly suspicious for infection, with the appropriate transmission-based empiric precautions for each, until a diagnosis can be made.

Control of device- and procedure-related infections is a major focus because the four most common types of nosocomial infection—postoperative wound infection, bacteriuria, bacteremia, and pneumonia—are all closely associated with procedures and instruments. Several guidelines and critical pathways have been developed by the CDC and others to minimize infections associated with them. Among the most important are those for surgery. Avoiding long preoperative hospital stays, having preoperative treatment of active infections, avoiding shaving of the operative site the night before the procedure, limiting traffic in the operating room, providing appropriate perioperative antimicrobials, and ensuring proper air flow in the operating room all can help reduce infections. The most important determinant of infection risk after surgery is the technical skill of the surgeon and operative team. Length of surgery, amount of trauma to tissues, degree of contamination of surgical fields, and several other factors contribute to likelihood of postoperative infection. It is perhaps for this reason that feeding individual infection rates back to surgeons has been found to lead to decreased rates of surgical wound infection.

Invasive devices penetrate anatomic barriers of the patient. The physician must be especially careful in the use of urinary catheters, intravascular catheters, and ventilators because these invasive devices are key risk factors for urinary tract, bloodstream, and respiratory infections that arise in an HCF. Fortunately, guidelines and critical pathways for proper use have been developed for each of these devices, and infection control plans for most HCFs where these are used include measures to ensure proper implementation. Individual physicians contribute best to reducing the infection risk from these devices by considering and reconsidering whether the devices are needed for their patients. "When in doubt, leave it out" is still a good philosophy when it comes to using these implements because their use carries an increased risk of infection in all cases.

A final way to minimize infections in HCFs is strengthening those in the institution against infection. For patients, proper nutrition, control of underlying diseases that predispose to infection, and proper immunization are all important elements. For example, the recent rise of strains of *Streptococcus pneumoniae* that are resistant to penicillin and, in some cases, to the newer cephalosporins makes treatment of infections caused by this organism much more difficult.

This means that the role of immunization against this organism must be advanced for adults. Likewise, immunization against hepatitis B virus is crucial for protection of the health care worker, and immunization against viral agents that may be transmitted in the HCF, such as measles virus, should be considered as well.

■ MAINTAINING CONTROL MEASURES

Design and implementation of infection control practices is important but perhaps easier than maintaining these practices after they are introduced. It is possible that in an established program, the next administrative problem or the next inservice talk will not be greeted by the same enthusiasm as the previous one. Likewise, new occurrences of problems may not respond to the measures taken to deal with these issues, even when they have worked time and time again in the past. A fresh approach and fresh enthusiasm may be required to make sure that time-tested remedies are still the appropriate ones and that they are carried out as

well as in the past. For practicing physicians, this enthusiasm can be generated easily by remembering that each control measure is a proven way to avoid nosocomial infections in their patients.

Suggested Reading

Abrutyn E, Goldmann DA, Scheckler WE: *Saunders infection control reference service,* Philadelphia, 1998, WB Saunders.

Bennett JV, Brachman PS, eds: *Hospital infections,* ed 4, Boston, 1998, Little, Brown.

Centers for Disease Control and Prevention: The CDC Guidelines for the Prevention and Control of Nosocomial Infections consists of several documents, which are available at a CDC Web site: http://www.cdc.gov/ncidod/hip/Guide/overview.htm.

Goldmann DA, Platt R, Hopkins CC: Control of nosocomial infections. In Gorbach S, ed: *Infectious diseases,* ed 2, Philadelphia, 1998, WB Saunders.

Mayhall CG, ed: *Hospital epidemiology and infection control,* Baltimore, 1998, Williams & Wilkins.

Scheckler WE, et al: Requirements for infrastructure and essential activities of infection control and epidemiology in hospitals: a consensus panel report, *Infect Control Hosp Epidemiol* 19:114, 1998.

Weinstein RA: Nosocomial infection update, *Emerg Infect Dis* 4:416, 1998.

PERCUTANEOUS INJURY: RISKS AND MANAGEMENT

Bradley N. Doebbeling

One of the major risks to a health care worker's health and career is development of an occupational bloodborne infection. Although many different infectious agents have been transmitted via blood exposure, three viruses are the most important causes of occupational bloodborne infection: hepatitis B virus (HBV), hepatitis C virus (HCV), and the human immunodeficiency virus (HIV). The most efficient mode of bloodborne pathogen transmission to health care workers is percutaneous or "sharps" injury because a large volume of blood (or infectious dose) may be inoculated in a single exposure. Despite considerable progress in the development and implementation of safer "needleless" devices and systems, percutaneous injuries will continue to occur and thus appropriate postexposure prophylaxis (PEP) of injuries will be required.

■ EXPOSURE ASSESSMENT

To determine the need for PEP, an assessment must be made to estimate the risk of transmission from the exposure. The first step in evaluating a sharps injury is determining whether the exposure was clinically significant (see "Expo-

sure Code" in Figure 1). There is a broad spectrum of risk of transmission, ranging from no risk for injury from a sterile needle without prior body fluid contact to high risk associated with an injury caused by a large, hollow-bore needle just removed from a blood vessel of a patient with an active bloodborne infection. Higher volumes of blood are transmitted in a needlestick from a hollow-bore needle than from a solid needle; similarly, larger-bore needles transmit larger volumes of blood. In addition, passage of a needle through a rubber glove decreases the volume of blood transmitted and thus the transmission risk. Use of double-gloves reduces the amount of blood transmitted even further. Because the risk of infection increases with the amount of infected blood (thus the number of infectious particles) in a needlestick, these data provide useful information in assessing the risk of a given injury.

If the sharp device was in contact with blood prior to the injury, the second assessment is whether the source patient either is at risk for or has a known bloodborne infection (see "HIV Status Code" in Figure 1). To evaluate the source's likelihood of being infectious, a careful review of his or her clinical and epidemiologic risk factors for infection from an important bloodborne pathogen, such as HBV, HCV, or HIV, should be performed.

■ SEROLOGIC TESTING

Serologic testing of the source, if possible, should be performed for a clinically significant exposure to determine whether a bloodborne infection is present. Baseline serologic testing of the exposed health care worker should also be performed to document seronegativity, should an occupationally related infection occur. After informed consent is obtained, both the source patient and the injured health care

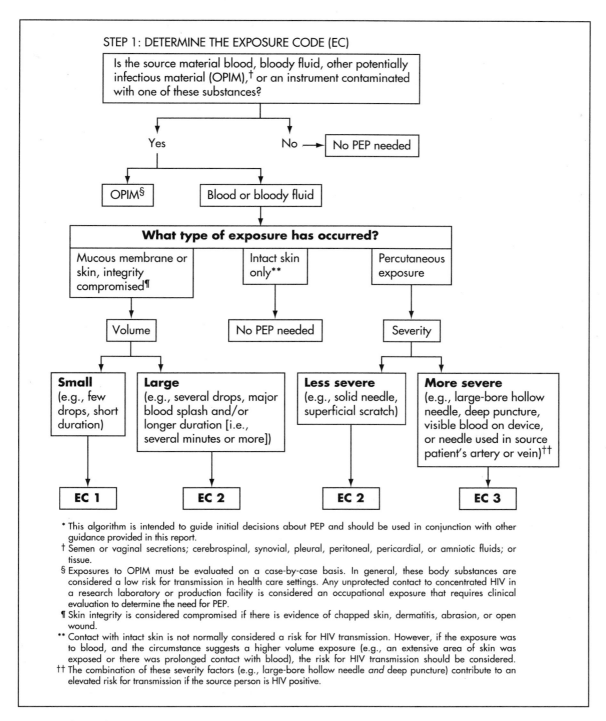

STEP 1: DETERMINE THE EXPOSURE CODE (EC)

Is the source material blood, bloody fluid, other potentially infectious material (OPIM),† or an instrument contaminated with one of these substances?

Yes   No ⟶ No PEP needed

OPIM§   Blood or bloody fluid

What type of exposure has occurred?

Mucous membrane or skin, integrity compromised¶   Intact skin only**   Percutaneous exposure

Volume   No PEP needed   Severity

Small (e.g., few drops, short duration)   **Large** (e.g., several drops, major blood splash and/or longer duration [i.e., several minutes or more])   **Less severe** (e.g., solid needle, superficial scratch)   **More severe** (e.g., large-bore hollow needle, deep puncture, visible blood on device, or needle used in source patient's artery or vein)††

EC 1   **EC 2**   **EC 2**   **EC 3**

* This algorithm is intended to guide initial decisions about PEP and should be used in conjunction with other guidance provided in this report.

† Semen or vaginal secretions; cerebrospinal, synovial, pleural, peritoneal, pericardial, or amniotic fluids; or tissue.

§ Exposures to OPIM must be evaluated on a case-by-case basis. In general, these body substances are considered a low risk for transmission in health care settings. Any unprotected contact to concentrated HIV in a research laboratory or production facility is considered an occupational exposure that requires clinical evaluation to determine the need for PEP.

¶ Skin integrity is considered compromised if there is evidence of chapped skin, dermatitis, abrasion, or open wound.

** Contact with intact skin is not normally considered a risk for HIV transmission. However, if the exposure was to blood, and the circumstance suggests a higher volume exposure (e.g., an extensive area of skin was exposed or there was prolonged contact with blood), the risk for HIV transmission should be considered.

†† The combination of these severity factors (e.g., large-bore hollow needle *and* deep puncture) contribute to an elevated risk for transmission if the source person is HIV positive.

Figure 1
Determining the need for HIV postexposure prophylaxis after an occupational exposure. *(Reprinted from* MMWR Morbid Mortal Wkly Rep *47[RR-7]:1, 1998.)*   *Continued*

worker should be tested for evidence of infection with HIV, HBV, and HCV. These tests include a hepatitis B surface antigen (HBsAg), hepatitis C antibody (anti-HCV), and an HIV antibody (anti-HIV-1) test. If the worker has been previously vaccinated for HBV and the immune response is unknown, a hepatitis B surface antibody (anti-HBs) test would be helpful. Some authors have recommended obtaining liver transaminases on both the donor and injured

worker to assess for evidence of hepatitis. Instead of obtaining a baseline anti-HIV-1 test on all exposed workers, another reasonable option is to save serum from the injured worker for testing later if needed. Subsequently, follow-up care should be dictated by the likelihood of transmission and the need for ongoing counseling; follow-up testing is recommended at 6 weeks, 3 months, 6 months, and optionally at 1 year.

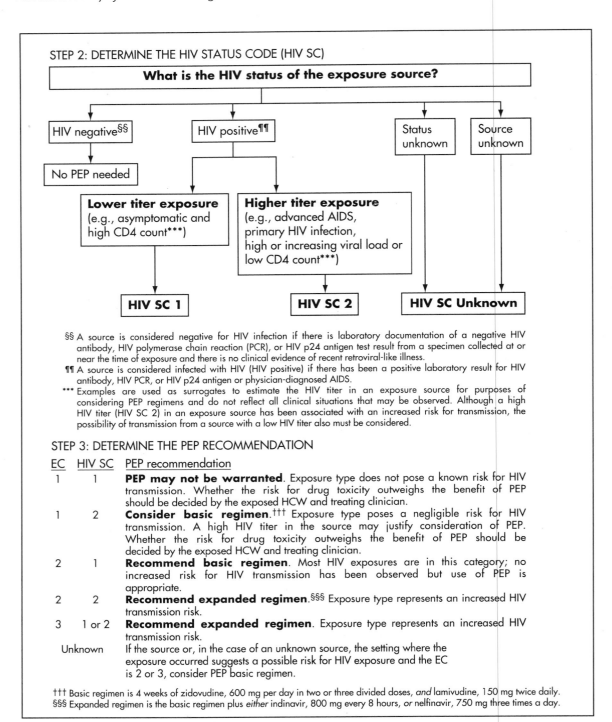

STEP 2: DETERMINE THE HIV STATUS CODE (HIV SC)

What is the HIV status of the exposure source?

HIV negative§§ → No PEP needed

HIV positive¶¶

Status unknown

Source unknown

Lower titer exposure
(e.g., asymptomatic and high CD4 count***)

Higher titer exposure
(e.g., advanced AIDS, primary HIV infection, high or increasing viral load or low CD4 count***)

HIV SC 1   **HIV SC 2**   **HIV SC Unknown**

§§ A source is considered negative for HIV infection if there is laboratory documentation of a negative HIV antibody, HIV polymerase chain reaction (PCR), or HIV p24 antigen test result from a specimen collected at or near the time of exposure and there is no clinical evidence of recent retroviral-like illness.

¶¶ A source is considered infected with HIV (HIV positive) if there has been a positive laboratory result for HIV antibody, HIV PCR, or HIV p24 antigen or physician-diagnosed AIDS.

*** Examples are used as surrogates to estimate the HIV titer in an exposure source for purposes of considering PEP regimens and do not reflect all clinical situations that may be observed. Although a high HIV titer (HIV SC 2) in an exposure source has been associated with an increased risk for transmission, the possibility of transmission from a source with a low HIV titer also must be considered.

STEP 3: DETERMINE THE PEP RECOMMENDATION

EC	HIV SC	PEP recommendation
1	1	**PEP may not be warranted**. Exposure type does not pose a known risk for HIV transmission. Whether the risk for drug toxicity outweighs the benefit of PEP should be decided by the exposed HCW and treating clinician.
1	2	**Consider basic regimen**.††† Exposure type poses a negligible risk for HIV transmission. A high HIV titer in the source may justify consideration of PEP. Whether the risk for drug toxicity outweighs the benefit of PEP should be decided by the exposed HCW and treating clinician.
2	1	**Recommend basic regimen**. Most HIV exposures are in this category; no increased risk for HIV transmission has been observed but use of PEP is appropriate.
2	2	**Recommend expanded regimen**.§§§ Exposure type represents an increased HIV transmission risk.
3	1 or 2	**Recommend expanded regimen**. Exposure type represents an increased HIV transmission risk.
Unknown		If the source or, in the case of an unknown source, the setting where the exposure occurred suggests a possible risk for HIV exposure and the EC is 2 or 3, consider PEP basic regimen.

††† Basic regimen is 4 weeks of zidovudine, 600 mg per day in two or three divided doses, *and* lamivudine, 150 mg twice daily.

§§§ Expanded regimen is the basic regimen plus *either* indinavir, 800 mg every 8 hours, *or* nelfinavir, 750 mg three times a day.

Figure 1—cont'd
For legend see p. 403.

■ BLOODBORNE PATHOGENS

Hepatitis B Infection

Before the hepatitis B vaccine was available, health care workers with frequent blood contact developed definite HBV infection at a rate of 1% per year, compared with 0% among those with infrequent blood exposure. Hepatitis B is transmitted at the highest rate of any of the bloodborne pathogens following percutaneous exposure to an infected patient. The risk of transmission is related to the viral titer and ranges from as low as 10%, up to 40%, depending on the absence or presence of hepatitis B e antigen (HBeAg), respectively. The greatest risk of transmission occurs with exposure to blood, although it may occur with exposure to other body fluids, particularly those containing blood. As with other bloodborne infections, the most effective route of

Table 1 Management of Percutaneous, Permucosal, or Nonintact Skin Exposure of Health Care Workers to Blood or Body Fluids, or Other Potentially Infectious Material

EXPOSED HCW
Initial Steps
    Assess clinical significance of exposure.
    If clinically significant, test source if possible for HBsAg, anti-HCV, anti-HIV-1.
    Review hepatitis B vaccination history.

UNVACCINATED HCW OR KNOWN NONRESPONDER
Unknown Source
    Test HCW for HBsAg, anti-HBs, anti-HCV, anti-HIV-1 (or save serum).*
    If HBsAg and anti-HBs negative, give HBIG 0.06 ml/kg IM within 24-48 hr.†
    If HBsAg negative, initiate HBV vaccine series; if nonresponder, modify risks,‡ revaccinate.
    Consider HIV postexposure prophylaxis per protocol (see Figure 1).
Known Source
    Test HCW for HBsAg, anti-HCV, anti-HIV1 (or save serum).
    If HCW HBsAg negative, initiate HBV vaccine series; if nonresponder, modify risks,‡ revaccinate.
    Consider HIV postexposure prophylaxis per protocol (see Figure 1).
    Proceed according to source serology.
Source HBsAg Positive
    If HCW HBsAg and anti-HBs negative, give HBIG, 0.06 ml/kg IM within 24-48 hr.†
    Complete HBV vaccine series.
Source HBsAg Negative
    Complete HBV vaccine series.

VACCINATED HCW WITH PROTECTIVE LEVELS OF ANTIBODY (ANTI-HBs >10 mIU/ml) DOCUMENTED PREVIOUSLY OR NATURAL IMMUNITY
Unknown Source
    Test HCW for anti-HCV, anti-HIV-1 (or save serum).*
    Consider HIV postexposure prophylaxis per protocol (see Figure 1).
Known Source
    Test HCW for anti-HCV, anti-HIV-1 or save serum.*
    Consider HIV postexposure prophylaxis per protocol (see Figure 1).

VACCINATED HCW WITH UNDOCUMENTED HEPATITIS B VACCINE RESPONSE
Unknown Source
    Test HCW for anti-HCV, anti-HBs, anti-HIV-1 (or save serum).*
    If HBsAg and anti-HBs negative, give HBIG, 0.06 ml/kg IM within 24-48 hr.†
    If HCW anti-HBs <10 mIU/ml, give HBV vaccine dose.
Known Source
    Test HCW for anti-HCV, anti-HBs, anti-HIV-1 (or save serum).
    If HCW anti-HBs <10 mIU/ml, give HBV vaccine dose.
    Consider HIV postexposure prophylaxis per protocol (see Figure 1).
    Proceed according to source serology.
Source HBsAg Positive
    If HCW prior serologic response (anti-HBs) not checked, give HBIG, 0.06 ml/kg IM within 24-48 hr.†
Source HBsAg Negative
    No further prophylaxis needed.

FINAL STEPS
    Retrain worker in standard precautions and safe performance of invasive procedures.
    Arrange follow-up testing, counseling and management per schedule.‖
    Observe for signs, symptoms of viral hepatitis or retroviral illness.

HCW, Health care worker; *HBsAg*, hepatitis B surface antigen; *anti-HCV*, hepatitis C antibody; *anti-HIV-1*, human immunodeficiency virus 1 antibody; *anti-HBs*, hepatitis B surface antibody.

*Blood may be stored by institution for testing for anti-HIV-1 if HCW develops HIV infection or the donor patient is HIV positive. Administration of HBIG should not be delayed beyond 48 hours awaiting serologic testing because efficacy decreases over time.

†Modifiable risks for nonresponse include intradeltoid administration, discontinuation of smoking, weight loss (or administration with 2-inch needle if obese), use of fresh vaccine, use of an alternative brand of vaccine.

‖Follow-up testing is recommended at 6 weeks, 3 months, 6 months, and (optional) 12 months.

exposure to HBV is percutaneous, because of direct exposure to high concentrations of the virus. Occasionally, inapparent transmission occurs when no obvious exposure is recalled; this likely results from mucous membrane or nonintact skin exposure to blood. In addition, human bites can transmit HBV, so postbite prophylaxis is just as important as following any other percutaneous injury.

One of the most important primary preventive measures for occupational bloodborne infection is the hepatitis B vaccine. Despite long-term evidence demonstrating the safety and efficacy of the vaccine, many workers remain unvaccinated. The vaccine not only prevents clinical HBV infection and cirrhosis but also protects against hepatitis D infection, an incomplete viral infection that requires prior or concurrent HBV infection to replicate. If administered appropriately, the three–vaccine dose series induces immunity in approximately 95% of adults. Serologic response may be checked 1 to 6 months after the third dose; a level of 10 mIU/ml is considered protective. Risk factors for poor response include obesity, increased age, smoking, presence of immunocompromise, administration in other than the deltoid muscle, incorrect storage, and the specific recombinant vaccine formulation. If the health care worker is not immune following the three-dose series, modifiable risk factors should be changed (smoking, weight loss, administration site, commercial manufacturer) and the patient reimmunized. The duration of protection is unknown; however, clinically evident acute infection or chronic viral hepatitis has not been reported in initial vaccine responders, and booster doses are not recommended.

If the worker has been previously immunized, prophylaxis of clinically significant occupational exposures to blood (percutaneous, permucosal or cutaneous) is recommended only if the worker's serologic response to the vaccine was not checked or was known to be inadequate. If the exposed worker was previously immune after vaccine, it is no longer recommended to check for persistence of protective levels of antibody. If serologic response was not checked after immunization, it should be obtained (target anti-HBs titer, >10 mIU/ml).

For the previously unimmunized or nonimmune, hepatitis B hyperimmunoglobulin (HBIG) should be given for initial passive immunity, and the vaccine administered at a separate site. Based on clinical trials of HBV perinatal prophylaxis, combination HBIG and hepatitis B vaccine appears to be most efficacious in preventing transmission. The optimal dose of HBIG is uncertain; however, an intramuscular dose of 0.06 ml/kg should be protective. Because the efficacy of HBIG decreases markedly with time following exposure, it should be given expeditiously, within 24 hours after exposure. If there has been no response to vaccine previously, a repeat dose of HBIG should be given at 1 month.

Postexposure follow-up should occur at 1 to 6 months after vaccination, with serologic testing to document development of protective antibody. However, if HBIG is given, testing should wait until 4 to 6 months after exposure because anti-HBs has been administered passively. Reinforcement of key standard precautions concepts should occur following exposure to decrease the likelihood of transmission to others.

Hepatitis C Infection

Hepatitis C virus has been found to be the major cause of non-A, non-B hepatitis and is currently the major cause of posttransfusion hepatitis. Most seroprevalence studies demonstrate a slightly higher seroprevalence among health care workers than in the general population, although the likelihood of occupational infection appears to be relatively low. The risk of transmission from percutaneous injury has not been well quantified but ranges from 3% to 10% after exposure to seropositive blood, based on initial studies. Transmission via other routes, including close personal or sexual contact, occurs infrequently.

Postexposure testing should occur soon after exposure to

document no prior infection, and again 6 and 12 months later to determine whether transmission has occurred. Nearly all persons who develop HCV infection will have measurable antibody by 1 year. The relatively low risk of sexual transmission of HCV suggests that no special precautions other than counseling for sexual contacts are likely necessary. If seroconversion occurs, it is important to follow the patient's liver function tests to determine whether chronic HCV infection occurs. Chronic HCV infection has been shown to respond to treatment. New tests are now available to confirm the presence of the virus and assess the genotype, which is related to the likelihood of response to treatment.

Controversy has existed over the role of serum immunoglobulin (IG) after percutaneous blood exposure. Current data suggest the likelihood of benefit of IG is low, and it is not routinely recommended. Similarly, based on the response of some chronic HCV infections to interferon, some providers have offered it as prophylaxis after exposure. However, interferon is not recommended as PEP until data are available regarding its efficacy in this setting.

Human Immunodeficiency Virus Infection

Percutaneous exposure to HIV-infected blood is much less likely to transmit infection than exposure to either HBV- or HCV-infected blood. Estimates of the risk for transmission by percutaneous exposure from prospective, longitudinal studies are 0.31%, with a 95% confidence level of 0.20 to 0.57. Transmission via mucous membrane or nonintact skin exposure to HIV-infected blood or body fluids has been reported; the risk is quite low but is difficult to estimate. However, exposure to HIV-infected blood often elicits considerably more serious concern from health care workers because of the consequences of HIV infection.

A variety of potential risk factors have been suggested as possibly contributing to the risk of HIV transmission following percutaneous exposure. Data from a case-control study of HIV seroconversion after percutaneous exposure suggests that the following are independent risk factors: visible blood on the object, a "deep" parenteral exposure, and failure to take zidovudine after exposure. Data from this study and a clinical trial demonstrating the protective effect of zidovudine prophylaxis in pregnancy argue for the use of antiretroviral prophylaxis after significant exposure.

Institutional policy outlining the routine management of such exposures should be developed and made available to all health care workers. A number of authors have recommended washing the wound with soap and water and encouraging the wound to bleed freely, although no data are available to support this practice. The injured health care worker should be seen as soon as possible after the injury and appropriate serologic testing performed. Counseling regarding the risks of the exposure, needed follow-up, recommended prophylaxis, and emotional support are all extremely important.

The decision regarding whether to recommend PEP involves a number of factors. The risks and benefits of antiretroviral chemoprophylaxis should be discussed. Minor side effects, including gastrointestinal symptoms (nausea, vomiting), headache, myalgia, and fatigue, are relatively common. The failure of zidovudine for PEP has been documented in a number of cases. The decision to offer antiretroviral prophylaxis after a parenteral exposure is a judgment that should carefully weigh the risks of the specific injury, risks versus potential benefits of prophylaxis, and the attitude of the exposed health care worker based on the best available data.

Public Health Service Guidelines have outlined the recommended management of parenteral exposures to HIV-infected blood (see Figure 1). Recommendations for PEP have been modified to include a 4-week regimen of two drugs (zidvudine and lamivudine) for most HIV exposures. An expanded regimen is recommended for exposures with an increased risk for transmission or if resistance to one or more of the antiretroviral agents recommended is known or suspected.

Dosages recommended for these first-line drugs include zidovudine (AZT or Retrovir), 300 mg twice daily or 200 mg three times daily; lamivudine (3TC or Epivir), 150 mg twice daily; or ZDV plus 3TC (Combivir), 1 tablet twice daily. Protease inhibitors include Indinavir (IDV or Crixivan), 800 mg every 8 hours (on an empty stomach), and nelfinavir (Viracept), 750 mg three times daily (with meals or a light snack).

Suggested Reading

Cardo DM, Bell DM: Postexposure management. In DeVita VT Jr, Hellman S, Rosenberg SA, ed: *AIDS: biology, diagnosis, treatment and prevention*, ed 4, Philadelphia, 1997, Lippincott-Raven.

Cardo DM, et al: A case-control study of HIV seroconversion in health care workers after percutaneous exposure, *N Engl J Med* 337:1485, 1997.

Centers for Disease Control and Prevention: Public Health Service guidelines for the management of health-care worker exposures to HIV and recommendations for postexposure prophylaxis, *MMWR Morbid Mortal Week Report* 47(RR-7):1–28, 1998. (see http:///www.cdc.gov/epo/mmwr/preview/mmwrhtml/00052722.htm)

Centers for Disease Control and Prevention: Recommendations for preventing transmission of human immunodeficiency virus and hepatitis B virus to patients during exposure-prone invasive procedures, *MMWR Morbid Mortal Week Report* 40:1, 1991.

Centers for Disease Control and Prevention: Protection against viral hepatitis: recommendations of the Immunization Practices Advisory Committee (ACIP), *MMWR Morbid Mortal Week Report* 39:17, 1990.

Department of Labor Occupational Safety and Health Administration: Occupational exposure to blood-borne pathogens: final rule, *Fed Reg* 56:C29-CFR Part 1910.1030:64175, 1991.

Doebbeling BN, Wenzel RP: Nosocomial viral hepatitis and infections transmitted by blood and blood products. In Mandell GL, Bennett JE, Dolin R, *Principles and practice of infectious diseases*, ed 4, New York, 1995, Churchill Livingstone.

Hospital Infection Control Practices Advisory Committee (HICPAC): Guidelines for infection control in health care personnel, Centers for Disease Control and Prevention, *Infect Control Hosp Epidemiol* 19:407, 1998.

HOSPITAL-ACQUIRED FEVER

Arthur E. Brown

While the development of fever in a patient who is hospitalized may be the clinical expression of a community-acquired infection that has completed its incubation period, this chapter deals only with the possible causes that are related to hospitalization. The reader, however, should keep other diagnoses in mind and inquire about the patient's history of travel, pet and animal exposure, hobbies, sexual activity, dietary preferences and exposures, occupational exposures, recent immunizations, drug ingestion within the past month (including corticosteroids), recent exposure to febrile or ill individuals, and other epidemiologic factors such as season of the year.

Sources of fever in the hospitalized patient may be infectious and/or noninfectious, and they may occur alone or together. Infectious causes of fever in a hospitalized patient most likely are nosocomial or hospital-acquired infections.

Nosocomial infections include bloodstream infections, lower respiratory tract infections (pneumonia), wound infections (surgical site infections), and urinary tract infections (Table 1). Clues as to the source of fever are best found by obtaining a thorough history, reviewing the medical record, and performing a complete physical exam. A history of previous placement of prosthetic devices, ranging from orthopedic to intravascular, must be obtained. Disorders of immune function, valvular heart disease, prior illness and/or allergies, and history of transplantation should be reviewed with the patient. The physical examination should be complete but focus on vital signs, general appearance, signs of toxicity, skin rash, presence and location of adenopathy, pulmonary examination, presence of cardiac murmur or rub, presence of genital, mucosal, and/or conjunctival lesions, hepatic tenderness, hepatosplenomegaly, costovertebral angle tenderness, arthritis, neck stiffness, meningismus, spinal tenderness, and/or neurologic dysfunction. Obviously, the postoperative patient will have special attention given to the operative site and wounds. Consultation with the surgeon regarding the operative findings, technical difficulties, and complications is essential. Similarly, conferring with the endoscopist after bronchoscopy, endoscopic retrograde cholangiopancreatography, colonoscopy, or cystoscopy may reveal information regarding the etiology of postendoscopic fever in such a patient. The patient with cancer may receive a significant amount of blood products over time and may develop transfusion- or infusion-related infections (see the chapter *Transfusion-Related Infection*). Infections found in the alcoholic, drug abusing, thermally

Table 1 Infectious Causes of Hospital-Acquired Fever

BLOODSTREAM INFECTIONS
Sepsis
  Bacteremia
  Fungemia
Intravascular device-related
  Hickman-Broviac-Port
  Central line
LOWER RESPIRATORY TRACT INFECTIONS
Pneumonia
  Aspiration
  Ventilator-related
URINARY TRACT INFECTIONS
Catheter-related
After instrumentation, cystoscopy, and so on
SURGICAL SITE INFECTIONS
Wounds
Deep space
Abscess
OTHER
Transfusion-related (bacterial, fungal, viral, parasitic)
Prosthetic device infection
Meningitis/epidural abscess
Intensive care unit–related
Pseudomembranous colitis (*Clostridium difficile*)

Table 2 Noninfectious Causes of Hospital-Acquired Fever

Drug, anesthetic agent, biologicals (e.g., vaccines, cytokines)
Pulmonary
  Atelectasis, pulmonary embolism
Thrombophlebitis
Nonviral hepatitis
Cardiac
  Myocardial infarction, pericarditis
Cancer—tumor fever
Neurologic
  Subarachnoid hemorrhage
  Subdural hematoma
  Intracranial hemorrhage
  Seizure (postictal)
Transfusion reactions
Factitious fever

injured, diabetic, elderly, or immunocompromised patient require special consideration (see the chapters covering these topics). The immunocompromised patient with cancer in particular may have a variety of possible infectious etiologies to consider (see the chapter *Malignancy and Infection*).

The evaluation of hospital-acquired fever should take into consideration the possible foci of infection. A complete blood count, urinalysis, chest radiograph, and cultures of blood, urine and sputum (if indicated) are essential. Appropriate cultures of wound sites and drainage are also important. In patients with diarrhea, stool specimens should be obtained and tested for the *Clostridium difficile* toxin. When a rash is present, a biopsy of the skin should be obtained for both histological and microbiological examination. Most important, a Gram stain can be very revealing and enable the physician to prescribe a more specific antimicrobial regimen until the culture results are available. It is important that the specimens are obtained correctly and are transported to the microbiology laboratory quickly. This aids in the recovery of fastidious organisms, particularly anaerobic bacteria. The quality of the specimen must also be ascertained, especially in specimens of sputum. The Gram stain will reveal whether sputum or saliva has been obtained. Similarly, it is essential to obtain fresh material from a drainage site rather than the material which has been dwelling in the collection apparatus.

The febrile patient in the intensive care unit most likely has multiple vascular access devices—any of which may be a source of infection. Generally, these should be removed and the tips sent for culture. Such a patient may also be intubated and dependent on mechanical ventilation. An endotracheal or tracheal specimen of sputum obtained by suction should be Gram stained and sent for culture. Appropriate computed tomography (CT) scans should be conducted to locate a deep (i.e., pelvic) source of fever in a postoperative patient who underwent abdominal surgery. Ultrasonographic studies help in evaluating the liver and spleen. Sometimes, gallium scans or indium labeled white blood cell scans may assist in locating occult foci of infection. Once located, radiographically guided drainage or open drainage of the abscess can be achieved.

Noninfectious etiologies make up 20% to 25% of causes of fever in hospitalized patients (Table 2). These noninfectious causes of fever are no less important than infectious causes. Determining the cause of fever in hospitalized patients can be very challenging because of the multiplicity of possible etiologies.

Suggested Reading

Armstrong D: Empiric therapy for the immunocompromised host, *Rev Infect Dis* 13:S763, 1991.

Kernodle DS, Kaiser AB: Postoperative infections and antimicrobial prophylaxis. In Mandell GL, Bennett JE, Dolin R, eds: *Mandell, Douglas, and Bennett's principles and practice of infectious diseases*, ed 4, New York, 1995, Churchill Livingstone.

McGowan, JE, et al. Fever in hospitalized patients, *Am J Med* 82:580, 1987.

Weber DJ, Cohen MS: The acutely ill patient with fever and rash. In Mandell GL, Bennett JE, Dolin R, eds: *Mandell, Douglas, and Bennett's principles and practice of infectious diseases*, ed 4, New York, 1995, Churchill Livingstone.

POSTOPERATIVE WOUND INFECTIONS

E. Patchen Dellinger

Postoperative wound infection is the archetypal surgical infection because it follows a surgical procedure and requires surgical intervention for resolution. As with many infections, best results are obtained by prompt diagnosis and treatment, which is facilitated by understanding the risk factors. The most obvious factor influencing risk of infection is the density of bacterial contamination of the incision. This was recognized several decades ago in the wound classification system that divides all surgical wounds into the four categories: clean, clean-contaminated, contaminated, and dirty. Clean wounds result from an elective procedure without break in technique that does not involve any area of the body other than skin normally colonized by resident bacteria. Clean-contaminated wounds result from a procedure such as elective bowel resection that intentionally opens the gastrointestinal (GI) tract or other colonized region such as the female genital tract but does not result in grossly visible spill of contents during the procedure. Contaminated procedures are those with gross spill from the GI tract or trauma and emergency procedures in which a wound has been created without normal antisepsis and sterile technique. A dirty wound is one that results from an operation in an area of active infection or previous bowel injury and leak. Among these categories, infection risk ranges historically, before modern understanding and practice of perioperative antibiotic prophylaxis, from 2% for clean wounds to 30% to 40% for dirty wounds when the skin is closed primarily.

Studies done many decades ago demonstrate that essentially all surgical incisions, even in clean operations, have some bacteria in the wound at the end of the procedure. Clinicians have recognized that the nature of host defenses and the extent to which the operative procedure or preexisting disease impairs these defenses also influences the risk of wound infection. Modern wound classifications that include underlying risk as well as the risk of bacterial contamination predict infection more accurately. The most widely used system now assigns 1 point each for wound classification of contaminated or dirty, an operation lasting longer than the 75th percentile for that procedure, and an American Society of Anesthesiology physical status classification of 3 or 4. In this system, the risk of postoperative wound infection for patients with risk points of 0, 1, 2, or 3 is 1.5%, 2.9%, 6.8%, and 13.0%, respectively (Table 1). These data reflect modern use of perioperative prophylactic antibiotics, as discussed in the chapter *Surgical Prophylaxis*.

■ DIAGNOSIS

The diagnosis of postoperative wound infection is obvious when the wound opens and discharges pus. However, the diagnosis is ideally made earlier and prompt therapeutic intervention undertaken. It is rare for a postoperative wound infection to be clinically evident before the fourth or fifth postoperative day. The sole exceptions to this are infections caused by beta-hemolytic streptococci and by histotoxic *Clostridium* species and, more rarely, wound toxic shock. These infections can be clinically evident within fewer than 24 hours, and although they are rare, they tend to be devastating. The wound of any patient with severe systemic signs of infection during the first few days after an operation should be inspected for signs of infection (Figure 1). Streptococcal infections are marked by local signs of inflammation and at times an exudate containing white blood cells (WBCs) and gram-positive cocci. Clostridial infections lack signs of inflammation and produce a thin exudate lacking WBCs because of the action of the exotoxins, but gram-positive rods without spore formation are evident on Gram smear. Thirteen cases of wound toxic shock were confirmed by the Centers for Disease Control and Prevention (CDC) during an 18-month period, representing less than 1% of all cases of toxic shock reported during that period. More than half of these cases presented within 48 hours of an operation. The earliest signs were fever, diarrhea, and vomiting. Profuse watery diarrhea,

---

Table 1   Comparison of NRC Wound Classification with NNIS Risk Index for Prediction of SSI Risk

| NRC CLASS | NNIS RISK INDEX | | | | | MAXIMUM RATIO (NRC)* |
	0	1	2	3	ALL	
Clean	1.0	2.3	5.4	—	2.1	5.4
Clean-contaminated	2.1	4.0	9.5	—	3.3	4.5
Contaminated	—	3.4	6.8	13.2	6.4	3.9
Dirty	—	3.1	8.1	12.8	7.1	4.1
All	1.5	2.9	6.8	13.0	2.8	—
Maximum ratio (NNIS)*	2.1	1.7	1.8	1.0	—	—

Modified from Dellinger EP, Ehrenkranz NJ: Surgical infections. In Bennett JV, Brachman PS, eds. *Hospital infections,* ed 4, Philadelphia, 1998, Lippincott-Raven.
*Ratio of the lowest to the highest infection rate in wound class or risk index. Note that the highest maximum ratio for any of the NNIS indices is 2.1, whereas the lowest maximum ratio for any of the NRC wound classes is 3.9. Clearly, the NNIS index more accurately describes the infection risk of operative procedures.

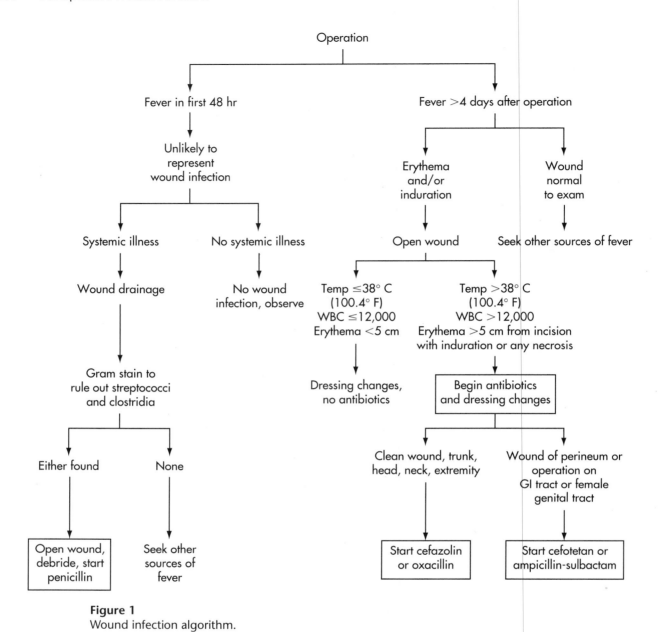

Figure 1
Wound infection algorithm.

erythroderma, and hypotension were also characteristic. Initially local signs of wound infection were often absent. Drainage and irrigation of the wound in combination with a systemic antistaphylococcal antibiotic is recommended. Although most wound infections are diagnosed between 5 and 15 days after the procedure, in some cases, diagnosis may be delayed considerably. This is more likely with wounds with a significant amount of tissue overlying the area such as abdominal wounds in morbidly obese patients and wound infections under chest wall musculature following a posterolateral thoracotomy.

Because most patients have some fever in the first several days after a major operative procedure such as abdominal exploration or thoracotomy, fever is not a specific sign of postoperative infection (Figure 2). It is tempting for the surgeon to continue prophylactic antibiotics or to restart antibiotics if the patient shows early postoperative fever, but this impulse should be resisted because these infections cannot be resolved without opening the wound. When antibiotics are given early without a commitment to open the wound, the most likely results are a delay in diagnosis and definitive treatment, a consequent increase in morbidity, and risk of additional complication such as wound dehiscence or herniation. A few surgical wounds exhibit erythema adjacent to the incision, either concentrated around skin sutures or staples or diffusely. In the absence of marked induration and/or drainage, this erythema usually does not indicate wound infection. The average clinician will be sorely tempted to prescribe antibiotics for a patient with such a wound, but most resolve without any specific treatment, and no data suggest that administration of antibiotics in such a situation will prevent the need to open the wound.

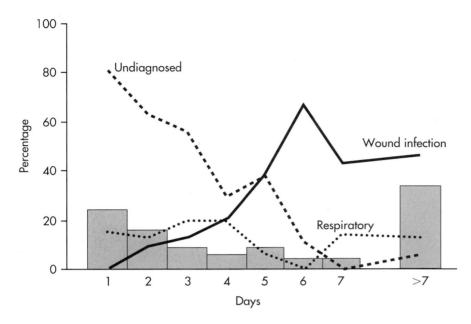

Figure 2
Bars represent the percent of all post-operative fevers occurring on the indicated day following an operative procedure. Lines indicate the percent of fevers occurring on each day attributable to the cause indicated. *(From Dellinger EP: Approach to the patient with postoperative fever. In Gorbach S, Bartlett J, Blacklow N, eds: Infectious diseases, ed 2, Philadelphia, 1998, WB Saunders.)*

■ THERAPY

Incisional Drainage

The primary treatment for a wound infection is to open the wound and evacuate the infected material. Antibiotics are used as adjunctive treatment only for patients who exhibit signs of significant systemic response to the infection or in whom there is evidence of invasive soft tissue infection beyond the boundaries of the surgical incision. The evidence for infection may be most prominent in a portion of the incision, but in most cases, the entire incision will be involved under the skin and will have to be opened. If necrotic tissue is found in the wound, some preliminary debridement may be helpful, but the small shreds of involved tissue will separate by themselves over time if the wound is left open and subjected to gauze dressing changes two to three times daily, decreasing in frequency as the wound clears. The importance of dressing changes is greater if the wound is deep, as in patients with severe obesity or in posterolateral thoracotomy wounds in muscular patients. If the wound is undermined, it is important to place the dressing so that gauze is in contact with all areas of the wound, but the dressings should not be put in forcefully or under pressure because this causes pain, inhibits drainage of exudate, and stimulates excess scar formation and slows wound closure, which occurs through the normal mechanism of contracture of granulation tissue.

When an incision is opened initially, it should be inspected by a physician who understands the procedure and the underlying anatomy. If the procedure was a celiotomy or a thoracotomy, the integrity of the closure of the abdominal or chest wall should be verified and evidence sought for purulent fluids originating deep to the abdominal or chest wall. In some cases, the incisional infection is not the primary event but is a signal of more severe and more extensive infection at a deeper level (see the chapters *Abdominal Abscess* and *Peritonitis*).

Antibiotics

Antibiotics should be administered empirically at the time of diagnosis and opening of the wound only when there are signs of a significant systemic reaction with temperature above 38° C (100.4° F), elevated pulse rate, or absolute WBC count above 12,000 or when inspection of the wound reveals invasive infection in the subcutaneous space or at the fascial level or when surrounding erythema and induration extend more than 5 cm from the line of incision. The agent chosen should be guided by Gram smear of the wound exudate and the nature of the procedure. Infections following clean operations that have not entered the GI tract and that involve the head and neck, trunk, or extremities tend to be caused by *Staphylococcus aureus* or less commonly streptococcal species. If Gram smear confirms gram-positive cocci, treatment is appropriate with an initial parenteral dose of cefazolin or oxacillin, 1 g IV. For patients allergic to penicillin and cephalosporins, clindamycin, 900 mg, or vancomycin, 1 g IV is acceptable. If the patient can take oral fluids and is not thought to have bacteremia, subsequent treatment can be with oral cephalexin or cephradine, 500 mg, or clindamycin, 450 mg four times daily. Antibiotic treatment should be continued only as long as systemic signs of infection or local cellulitis continue to be present, usually 3 days or less.

For infections that follow operations in the axilla, gram-negative enteric bacilli are more commonly causative, and after operations on the perineum or involving the GI tract or the female genital tract both facultative and obligate anaerobic bacilli and cocci are often involved. In these cases, if antibiotic treatment is thought necessary, initial treatment can be cefotetan, 1 g IV every 12 hours, cefoxitin, 1 g IV every 6 hours, or ampicillin-sulbactam, 3 g IV every 6 hours. Patients allergic to penicillin and cephalosporins can receive ciprofloxacin, 400 mg IV every 12 hours, combined with either clindamycin, 900 mg IV every 8 hours, or metronidazole, 1 g IV every 12 hours, or they can take aztreonam, 1 g

IV every 8 hours, plus clindamycin, 900 mg IV every 8 hours. Again, the treatment should usually be 3 days or less, and if the patient is able to take oral agents, switching to an oral regimen of amoxicillin-clavulanate, 500 mg every 6 hours, once daily; or ciprofloxacin, 500 mg every 12 hours, combined with either clindamycin, 450 mg, or metronidazole, 500 mg every 6 hours, should be considered.

In the rare patient who has an invasive wound infection caused either by beta-hemolytic streptococci or by a histotoxic *Clostridium* species diagnosed in the first 48 hours after operation, aggressive antimicrobial therapy is necessary in addition to opening the wound and inspecting it in the operating room under general anesthesia, with the option of aggressive soft-tissue debridement if evidence of spreading soft-tissue invasion and necrosis is found. Penicillin G, 4 million units IV every 4 hours, is appropriate if the diagnosis of streptococcal or clostridial infection is firm. If in doubt, cefazolin or vancomycin provides treatment for staphylococcal infections in addition to streptococcal and clostridial infections, but the addition of metronidazole for anaerobic coverage may be prudent.

■ WOUND CLOSURE

The most reliable method for handling an infected wound that has been opened is to continue dressing changes and allow the wound to close spontaneously by secondary intention. In straightforward wound infections, this results in a very satisfactory result in many cases. In a minority of wounds, the incision can be reclosed, usually with tapes, after the incision has cleared up and is lined by healthy granulation tissue. The failures that occur at this time are as often caused by the geometry of the wound as they are by the bacterial content.

Suggested Reading

Culver, DH, Horan TC, et al: Surgical wound infection rates by wound class, operative procedure, and patient risk index *Am J Med* 91(Suppl 3B): 152S, 1991.

Dellinger, EP: Perioperative infection. In Meakins JL ed: *Surgical infections: diagnosis and treatment,* New York, 1999, Scientific American.

Dellinger EP: Approach to the patient with postoperative fever. In Gorbach S, Bartlett J, Blacklow N, editors: *Infectious diseases in medicine and surgery,* Philadelphia, 1998, WB Saunders.

Garibaldi, RA, Brodine S, et al: Evidence for the noninfectious etiology of early postoperative fever, *Infect Control* 6:273, 1985.

Horan, TC, Gaynes RP, et al: CDC definitions of nosocomial surgical site infections, 1992: a modification of CDC definitions of surgical wound infections, *Am J Infect Control* 20:271, 1992.

National Academy of Sciences, National Research Council, et al: Postoperative wound infections: the influence of ultraviolet irradiation on the operating room and of various other factors, *Ann Surg* 160 (suppl 2):1, 1964.

TRANSFUSION-RELATED INFECTION

Virginia R. Roth
William R. Jarvis

The transfusion of blood and blood components is associated with a very low but ever-present risk of infection. It is estimated that 1 in every 2000 units of blood may carry an infectious agent and that about 4 in 10,000 recipients develop a chronic disease or die as a result of receiving contaminated blood. A wide variety of viral, bacterial, and parasitic agents have been associated with blood transfusion (Table 1). Concerns have also been raised about the potential for transmission of Creutzfeldt-Jakob disease (CJD) and its new variant (nv-CJD) through blood products. However, no human cases of CJD or nv-CJD have been causally liked to blood transfusion, and case-control studies have not found blood transfusion to be a risk factor for CJD. The risk of viral transmission has been markedly reduced with improved screening. The risk is now estimated to be 1 in 676,000 units for human immunodeficiency virus (HIV), 1 in 63,000 units for hepatitis B virus (HBV), and 1 in 41,000 to 1 in 103,000 units for hepatitis C virus (HCV). Because the risk of viral or parasitic infection is very low and blood is screened for HCV, HBV, HIV, and human T-cell lymphoma/leukemia virus (HTLV) 1, the remainder of this chapter focuses on bacterial complications of blood transfusion, which can be diagnosed and treated.

Although the rate of bacterial contamination of blood products is unknown, the rate of bacterial infection associated with blood products is estimated to be similar to that of viral infection. The fatality rate associated with transfusion-related sepsis has been estimated to be 1 in 6 million transfused units. However, more common nonfatal episodes of transfusion reaction, which may result from bacterial contamination of blood or blood components, are often assumed to be an immune response to transfused leukocytes and are not fully investigated for contamination.

■ WHOLE BLOOD AND ERYTHROCYTES

After collection, whole blood may be maintained at room temperature for up to 8 hours before being stored at 1° to 6° C (33.8° to 42.8° F) up to 35 or 42 days, depending on the additives used (Table 2). Erythrocytes may be prepared from whole blood at any point during the normal storage period of the whole blood. The erythrocytes then may be stored at 1° to 6° C up to the expiration date of the whole blood unit from which they were prepared. The growth of psychrophilic organisms, such as *Yersinia enterocolitica* and *Pseudomonas* species, is favored by these storage conditions, accounting for most erythrocyte transfusion-related sepsis episodes (Table 3). These episodes tend to occur with units that have been stored for more than 14 to 25 days, which reflects a growth lag of about 7 to 14 days

followed by exponential growth of the organism; levels of 10^9 organisms/ml are reached by 38 days, and 315 ng of endotoxin/ml (approximately 4,000 EU/ml) by 28 to 34 days. Transfusion of such units can lead to both septic and endotoxic shock.

■ PLATELETS

Platelets are stored in oxygen-permeable containers with agitation at 20° to 24° C (68° to 75.2° F) for up to 5 days. Platelet transfusion-related sepsis usually involves common skin organisms, such as *Staphylococcus epidermidis, S. aureus*, or other aerobic bacteria that can grow rapidly at room temperature (see Table 3). Sepsis episodes related to platelet transfusion also tend to occur with units that are late in the storage period (around 4 to 5 days), when there may be a higher titer of organisms than early in the storage period. In addition, sepsis episodes occur more frequently with pooled platelet units than with single-donor apheresis units. A pooled platelet unit is prepared by combining 6 to 10 random donor platelet concentrates up to 4 hours before transfusion. In contrast, an apheresis unit is prepared by separating platelets from the whole blood of a single donor and returning other blood components to the donor. The higher rate of sepsis associated with pooled platelets is seen primarily because, on average, pooled platelets are stored longer than apheresis platelets. With pooled platelets, there also is a higher risk of contamination associated with the exposure to multiple donors or with the manipulation of the concentrates.

■ PLASMA AND PLASMA-DERIVED PRODUCTS

Plasma is either collected by apheresis or prepared from whole blood and is stored at below −18° C (−0.4 ° F) within 6 hours of collection. It can be thawed in a water bath using a plastic overwrap or in a microwave and subsequently stored at 1° to 6° C up to 24 hours before transfusion. The survival of bacteria is not supported by these storage conditions. However, equipment may carry contamination; for example, one reported case of sepsis associated with a plasma transfusion was attributed to a contaminated water bath used for thawing the unit.

Table 1   Infections Transmissible by Blood Transfusion
VIRUS
Hepatitis
Hepatitis A virus (HAV)
Hepatitis B virus (HBV)
Hepatitis C virus (HCV)
Hepatitis D virus (HDV)
Hepatitis G virus (HGV)
Cytomegalovirus (CMV)
Epstein-Barr virus (EBV)
Nonhepatitis
HIV-1 and 2
HTLV-1 and 2
Human herpes virus 8 (HHV-8)*
Parvovirus
Colorado tick fever virus
BACTERIA
Yersinia
Pseudomonas
Staphylococcus
Other gram-positive and gram-negative bacteria
Rickettsia
Spirochetes
Syphilis
Recurrent fever
Lyme disease*
Ehrlichia*
PROTOZOA
Plasmodium (malaria)
Babesia
Trypanosoma (Chaga's disease)
Toxoplasma
Leishmania
Nematode (loasis, other microfilaria)

HIV, human immunodeficiency virus; *HTLV*, human T-cell lymphoma/leukemia virus.
*Potential risk only, no reported case.

Table 2   Blood Component Storage Conditions and Estimated Contamination Rates

COMPONENT	STORAGE CONDITIONS	ESTIMATED CONTAMINATION RATE
Whole blood	≤8 hours at room temp	0.03%
CPDA-1	≤35 days at 1°-6° C	
CPD plus AS	≤45 days at 1°-6° C	
Packed red blood cells		≤0.5%
CPDA-1	≤35 days at 1°-6° C	
CPD plus AS	≤45 days at 1°-6° C	
Platelets	≤5 days at 20°-24° C	Single donor, ≤2.5%
		Pooled, ≤10%
Plasma	Frozen, stored ≤18° C	≤0.1%
	For use, thawed and stored ≤24 hours at 1°-6° C	

CPDA, Citrate-phosphate-dextrose-adenine (additives); *CPD*, citrate-phosphate-dextrose; *AS*, adenine saline (additives).

Table 3   Reported Episodes of Transfusion-Associated Sepsis

PATHOGEN	PERCENTAGE	DURATION IN DAYS FROM COLLECTION TO TRANSFUSION	
		MEDIAN	RANGE
ERYTHROCYTES			
Yersinia enterocolitica	49.0	24	7-41
Pseudomonas fluorescens	23.5	24	16-32
Serratia liquefaciens	7.8	21	17-26
Treponema pallidum	2.0	<1	—
Pseudomonas putida	2.0	—	—
Other species	15.7	23	20-26
PLATELETS			
Staphylococcus epidermidis	33.3	4	3-5
Salmonella cholerasuis	11.7	<1	—
Serratia marcescens	8.3	2	1-3
Staphylococcus aureus	5.0	5	3-6
Bacillus cereus	5.0	—	—
Streptococcus viridans group	3.3	3	1-6
Salmonella enteriditis	3.3	5	3-5
Other species	23.3	4	2-6

Contamination of plasma-derived products also is thought to be rare. They are prepared from plasma stored under very stringent conditions, and many of the products also undergo viral inactivation procedures. However, contamination may still occur, as demonstrated by outbreaks of HCV infections associated with the administration of contaminated intravenous immunoglobulin and (HAV) associated with plasma-derived products.

■ SOURCES OF CONTAMINATION

Contamination of blood or blood components may occur intrinsically if a donor is bacteremic or viremic at the time of donation; it also may occur extrinsically from the skin during phlebotomy or from containers and other equipment used during processing and storage. The infecting organism may reflect the source of contamination. With *Y. enterocolitica*–contaminated erythrocytes, the implicated source is often an asymptomatic episode of gastrointestinal (GI) illness within the previous month. Because the GI illness is usually mild, the donor may not recall or may neglect to report the episode.

■ CLINICAL MANAGEMENT

Although these contamination episodes are rare, it is important to consider the possibility of blood and blood component contamination when a patient develops a fever during or soon after a transfusion (Figure 1). If bacteremia cannot be ruled out, the transfusion should be stopped immediately. Any residual blood product and administration set should immediately be quarantined and refrigerated. A Gram-stained and/or acridine orange–stained smear of the blood product should be performed. Stain and/or culture of blood component segments usually are negative, even when the unit itself is positive; this may reflect low-level contamination of the unit at the time of donation. Cultures of the blood product, the patient's blood before antimicrobials are begun, and any intravenous solution used during transfusion should be obtained promptly. Information about the donor should be reviewed completely. If organisms are recovered from the recipient and blood product, molecular typing of patient and donor isolates may prove causality.

After appropriate cultures are obtained, broad-spectrum empiric antimicrobial therapy should be started. Empiric treatment of suspected sepsis associated with blood products must be based on the component. Because most reported sepsis episodes associated with erythrocyte transfusion have been caused by *Y. enterocolitica* or *Pseudomonas* species, particularly *P. fluorescens*, initial therapy may include trimethoprim-sulfamethoxazole or an antipseudomonal beta-lactam and an aminoglycoside. Because infectious complications associated with platelets are usually caused by aerobic bacteria such as coagulase-negative staphylococci or *S. aureus* and occasionally gram-negative organisms, initial empiric therapy may include a penicillinase-resistant penicillin and an aminoglycoside. Empiric therapy should be narrowed as soon as an infecting pathogen and antimicrobial susceptibility are identified.

■ PREVENTION

Sensitive, rapid diagnostic tests for detecting bacterial contamination are not yet available. Therefore minimizing the risk of transfusion-associated sepsis depends on appropriate donor screening, donor site inspection and preparation, and proper handling of the blood components (Table 4). Detection of infectious complications associated with blood products may be increased by educating the medical and blood bank staff about the signs and symptoms of patients with transfusion reactions, the importance of immediately reporting transfusion reactions to the blood bank, promptly culturing the blood of the recipient, promptly performing stains and culture of the blood component, and ensuring quarantined refrigerated storage of the unit and administra-

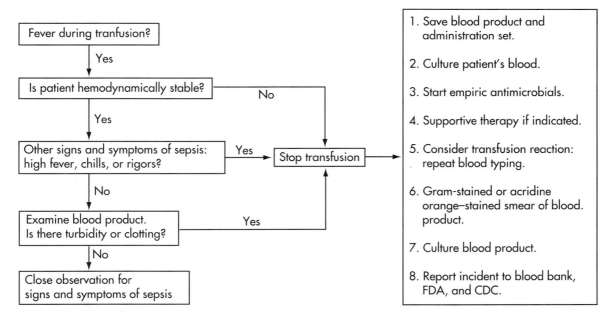

Figure 1
Algorithm for the evaluation of fever associated with transfusion.

Table 4   Prevention of Transfusion-Associated Sepsis
DONORS
Screen for infectious diseases (health questionnaire); inquire about travel, behaviors, dental work, signs and symptoms of recent illness.
PHLEBOTOMY
Inspect site; avoid dimpled areas of the skin.
Prepare site properly.
Use aseptic techniques.
BAG AND COMPONENT PREPARATION
Use aseptic techniques.
Perform proper cleaning and disinfection of processing equipment; use plastic overwraps in water baths for thawing.
Use appropriate storage conditions.
Visually inspect contents before transfusion.

tion set unit contamination has been excluded. The Centers for Disease Control and Prevention (CDC), American Red Cross, American Association of Blood Banks, and Department of Defense are coordinating a national effort to improve reporting and workup of transfusion-related sepsis through the Bacterial Contamination of Blood Products (*BaCon*) Study. Any culture-confirmed episodes of transfusion-related sepsis should be reported to the blood bank from which the unit was obtained, to the Food and Drug Administration (301-827-6220), and to the CDC *BaCon* Study coordinator (404-639-6420).

Acknowledgment
The authors acknowledge the work of Dr. Ann Do in the first edition, upon which this revised chapter is based.

Suggested Reading

BaCon Study Web site: http://www.cdc.gov/ncidod/hip/bacon/.

Blajchman MA: Bacterial contamination and proliferation during the storage of cellular blood products, *Vox Sang* 74 (suppl 2):155, 1998.

Goodnough LT, et al: Transfusion medicine: blood transfusion, *N Engl J Med* 340:438, 1999.

Schreiber GB, et al: The risk of transfusion-transmitted viral infections, *N Engl J Med* 334:1685, 1996.

Wagner SJ, Friedman LI, Dodd RY: Transfusion-associated bacterial sepsis, *Clin Microbiol Rev* 7:290, 1994.

INTRAVASCULAR CATHETER–RELATED INFECTIONS

Claude Afif

Issam Raad

Intravascular catheters are widely used in the management of chronic and critically ill patients. It is estimated that more than 200,000 nosocomial bloodstream infections (BSIs) occur each year, most of which are intravascular device related. The national nosocomial infection surveillance system reported that the rate of catheter-related bloodstream infection (CRBSI) ranges from 2.1 to 30.2 BSIs per 1000 vascular catheter days. In the initially ill patient, the direct implication of CRBSI is an extension of hospital stay by an average of 6 to 7 days and an increased cost to around $30,000 per survivor.

■ PATHOGENESIS

Most indwelling vascular catheters become colonized by microorganisms within 24 hours after their insertion. Electron microscopy studies of catheter surfaces show that adherent microorganisms can be found in either a free-floating form or sessile form embedded in a biofilm.

The dynamic process of adherence is the result of the interaction of three factors: the intrinsic properties of the catheter, microbial factors, and host-derived proteins. The physical characteristics of the catheter, such as surface irregularities and charge difference, facilitate bacterial adherence. Furthermore, some microorganisms adhere better to polyvinyl chloride, silicone, and polyethylene surfaces than to Teflon polymers and polyurethane. Concomitantly, in reaction to the foreign nature of the catheter, a thrombin sheath forms on the internal and external surfaces of the catheter. This newly formed sheath results from the deposition of host-derived proteins such as fibrinogen, fibronectin, lamimin, and thrombospondin.

Microorganisms colonize vascular catheters through different sources: for short-term catheters, the skin of the site of insertion is the major source for colonization; bacterial skin flora migrate along the external surface of the catheter. The hub of the vascular device is the most common source of colonization for long-term catheters. Microorganisms are introduced from the hands of medical personnel. In this case, colonizing bacteria migrate along the internal surface of the catheter. Hematogenous seeding and contamination of the infusate are rare causes of colonization and infection of vascular devices.

Colonizing microorganisms enhance their adherence by producing a microbial factor, the extracellular slime, or glycocalyx, which acts as a protective barrier against op-sonization, phagocytosis, and antimicrobials. Skin flora such as *Staphylococcus epidermidis, Staphylococcus aureus, Bacillus* species, and *Corynebacterium* species remain the predominant source of CRBSI, followed by microorganisms that contaminate the hands of medical personnel, such as *Pseudomonas, Acinetobacter, S. maltophilia,* and *Candida.* Emerging pathogens such as *Achromobacter,* rapidly growing mycobacteria (*M. chelonae* and *M. fortuitum*), and fungal elements such as *Fusarium, Malassezia furfur,* and *Rhodotorula* species have been described in specific conditions (i.e., hyperalimentation, interleukin-2 therapy).

■ CLINICAL MANIFESTATIONS

The clinical presentation of CRBSI consists of nonspecific systemic manifestations, such as fever and chills, and local manifestations at the skin insertion site, such as erythema, edema, tenderness, and occasionally, purulent discharge. Septic thrombophlebitis complicates CRBSI, especially with coagulase-producing organisms (e.g., *S. aureus* and *Candida*) and presents as a right-side endocarditis. The suggested definitions of catheter infections by the Centers for Disease Control and Prevention (CDC) are as follows:

1. Catheter colonization

- The isolation of 15 or more colony-forming units (CFU) of any microorganism by semiquantitative culture (roll-plate method) or 10^3 or more CFU by quantitative culture (e.g., sonication technique), from a catheter tip or subcutaneous segment in the absence of simultaneous clinical symptoms.

2. Local catheter-related infection

- *Exit-site infection:* purulent drainage from the catheter exit site, or erythema, tenderness, and swelling within 2 cm of the catheter exit site, and colonization of the catheter if removed
- *Port-pocket infection:* erythema and/or necrosis of the skin or subcutaneous tissues either over or around the reservoir of an implanted catheter, and colonization of the catheter if removed
- *Tunnel infection:* erythema, tenderness, and induration of the tissues above the catheter and more than 2 cm from the exit site and colonization of the catheter if removed

■ DIAGNOSIS

The diagnosis of catheter-related infection is challenging and often difficult to perform. A definite diagnosis often requires catheter removal and culture and is thus retrospective (Table 1).

The current available laboratory diagnostic techniques are as follows:

1. After catheter removal

- *Semiquantitative culture of catheter tip:* Catheter colonization is defined by a growth of 15 CFU or greater of a catheter tip culture by the roll-plate technique. Al-

Table 1 Diagnosis of Catheter-related Bloodstream Infection (CRBSI)

PROBABLE CRBSI
1. Common skin organism,* *Staphylococcus aureus*, or *Candida* isolated from one or more blood cultures
2. Clinical manifestations of infection (fever and chills)
3. No apparent source of sepsis other than the catheter

DEFINITE CRBSI
All three criteria listed above plus any of the examples of clinical or microbiologic evidence listed below

CLINICAL EVIDENCE
1. Purulent discharge at the catheter insertion site
2. Clinical sepsis that responds to antibiotic therapy upon catheter removal after being refractory to therapy in the presence of the catheter

MICROBIOLOGIC EVIDENCE
1. Differential quantitative blood cultures with 5 : 1 ratio of the same organism isolated from blood drawn simultaneously from the catheter and peripheral vein
2. Differential positivity time whereby the time differential for blood cultures drawn simultaneously through the catheter and peripheral vein respectively exceeds 120 minutes
3. Positive quantitative skin culture whereby the organism isolated from an infected insertion site is identical to that isolated from blood
4. Isolation of the same organism from the peripheral blood and from a semiquantitative or quantitative culture of a catheter segment or tip

*Coagulase-negative staphylococci, micrococci, *Bacillus* and *Corynebacterium* species.

Table 2 Risk Factors Associated with Infections of Intravascular Catheters

DEFINITE	POSSIBLE
1. Violation of aseptic technique during catheter insertion and maintenance	1. Site of catheter insertion
2. Contaminated antiseptic skin solutions	2. Triple-lumen catheters
3. Frequent manipulation of catheters	3. Transparent occlusive plastic dressing
4. Cut downs to insert catheters	4. Neutropenia
5. Prolonged placement of catheters	5. Catheter-related thrombosis
6. Total parenteral nutrition through catheter	
7. Interleukin-2 therapy	

Table 3 Measures to Decrease Risk of Colonization of Central Venous Catheters

SHORT-TERM PLACEMENT (<10 DAYS)
To prevent colonization of external surface of catheter:
Maximum sterile barrier (handwashing, sterile gloves, large drape, sterile gown, mask, and cap)
Infusion therapy team
Cutaneous antimicrobial or antiseptic agents (mupirocin, chlorhexidine)
Subcutaneous silver cuff
Antimicrobial coating of catheter
LONG-TERM PLACEMENT (>10 DAYS)
To prevent colonization of catheter lumen:
Maximum sterile barrier (handwashing, sterile gloves, large drape, sterile gown, mask, and cap)
Infusion therapy team
Antimicrobial flush or lock
Tunneling

though commonly used, this method is limited by recovering microorganisms only from the external surface of the catheter.

· *Quantitative culture of catheter segments:* This method consists in culturing both external and internal surfaces of the catheter by sonication, centrifugation, and vortexing of two segments: the subcutaneous tunneled segment and the catheter tip. This method has proved helpful for long-term catheters. A cut-off value of 10^2 to 10^3 CFU is indicative of catheter colonization depending on the used technique.

· *Catheter staining:* Consists of Gram or acridine orange staining of the catheter tip, with identification of the microorganisms under direct microscopy. However, this technique is time-consuming and operator dependent, which limits its usefulness.

2. Before catheter removal

· *Endoluminal brush technique:* A wire brush is used to culture the endoluminal surface in situ, then Gram or acridine orange staining of the blood drawn through the catheter. However, this method is associated with a 6% risk of transient bacteremia.

· *Paired quantitative blood cultures:* CRBSI is suspected when a blood culture drawn simultaneously through a vascular catheter lumen grows fivefold to tenfold higher CFU compared with blood cultures drawn from a peripheral vein.

· *Differential positivity time:* A recent study has suggested that time to positivity of a culture is closely related to

the inoculum size of microorganisms. Blood cultures are drawn simultaneously from a venous catheter and a peripheral vein. A time differential of 120 minutes or greater favors the site more heavily colonized as the potential source of the infection.

■ PREVENTIVE STRATEGIES

Several preventive measures have shown efficacy in decreasing the risk of catheter-related infection. Risk factors and beneficial preventive interventions are listed in Tables 2 and 3, respectively.

The routine exchange of central venous catheters (CVC) over guided wire at fixed intervals of time is not recommended. Two clinical trials failed to demonstrate a prevention benefit from frequent exchanges of vascular catheters. Others have suggested an increased risk of bloodstream infection. The CDC does not recommend routine guidewire-assisted catheter exchange. However, the guidewire may be used to (1) replace a malfunctioning catheter, (2) convert an existing catheter to a different type, and

(3) determine the source of the bloodstream infection, allowing culture of the exchanged catheter.

Recent developments in catheter coating with antiseptics and antimicrobials seem promising. A meta-analysis of 12 clinical trials showed better efficacy of antiseptic impregnated vascular catheters with chlorhexidine and sulfadiazine in preventing CRBSI when compared with nonimpregnated catheters.

More recent studies with catheters coated with the antibiotics minocycline and rifampin demonstrated a lower rate of catheter colonization and CRBSI when compared with uncoated catheters. Furthermore, when compared with antiseptic impregnated catheters, antibiotic-coated catheters lowered the rate of infection twelvefold.

■ THERAPY (Table 4)

The management of catheter-related infections involves confirming the source of infection; the choice of antimicrobials and duration of therapy; and the decision regarding the need for catheter removal. To confirm the infection, microorganisms recovered from different cultures (i.e., blood through a venous catheter, a peripheral vein, catheter tip, and if applicable, skin insertion site) must be the same. The duration of therapy is extended if the CRBSI is judged to be complicated (i.e., associated with septic thrombophlebitis, endocarditis, or metastatic infection). Most of the CRBSIs will be treated for a period of 7 to 14 days, depending on the isolated microorganisms. However, in cases of complicated CRBSI, the vascular catheter should be removed and the infection treated with parenteral antibiotics for at least 4 weeks.

Coagulase-Negative Staphylococci

The optimal duration of therapy of CRBSI with coagulase-negative staphylococci has not been defined. However, a 7-day course of antimicrobials should be adequate if the patient responds within 48 to 72 hours. Because most coagulase-negative staphylococci are nosocomially acquired and are resistant to penicillinase-resistant penicillins, the choice of a glycopeptide (i.e., vancomycin) is recommended pending susceptibility results.

Although catheter removal was previously considered essential, recent data have shown that the rates of acute mortality and morbidity of CRBSI with coagulase-negative staphylococci were independent of catheter removal.

Staphylococcus aureus

Serious infectious complications arise from *S. aureus* CRBSI. Failure to remove the catheter is associated with persistent bacteremia, relapses, and increased mortality. Uncomplicated episodes of *S. aureus* CRBSI are usually treated for 10 to 14 days with no risk of relapse, whereas complicated episodes with septic thrombophlebitis or endocarditis require therapy for at least 4 weeks.

Candida

Endophthalmitis complicates *Candida* BSI in 15% of untreated cases; thus systemic antifungal therapy is recommended for all cases of catheter-related candidemia. Catheter retention was shown to be an independent risk factor for the persistence of candidemia and higher mortality rate. Furthermore, breakthrough candidemia during adequate therapy is predictive of vascular catheter–related infection. Early catheter removal is indicated for patients with catheter-related candidemia in the absence of other apparent sources of BSI. Therapy with fluconazole at 400 mg/day for 14 days is equivalent to amphotercin B at 0.5 mg/kg/day in this setting and is recommended even in neutropenic patients, unless the isolated organism is resistant to fluconazole (e.g., *C. krusei* or *C. glabrata*).

Gram-Positive Bacilli

Vancomycin remains the antibiotic of choice in the treatment of CRBSI caused by gram-positive bacilli such as *Bacillus* and *Corynebacterium* species. Removal of the catheter is recommended.

Gram-Negative Bacilli

Enteric gram-negative bacilli such as *E. coli, Enterobacter,* and *Klebsiella* are rare causes of CRBSI. However, for *Pseudomonas* species and *S. maltophilia,* the catheter was reported to be a common source of infection. Catheter removal is recommended in addition to therapy with an appropriate antimicrobial for 7 to 10 days.

Mycobacterial Disease

Catheter removal is recommended, and surgical intervention may be needed in long-term catheters infected with *M. chelonae* or *M. fortuitum*. A 14-day course of antimicrobial is suggested. However, longer duration of therapy is required in complicated cases.

Suggested Reading

Blot F, et al: Early positivity of central venous versus peripheral blood cultures is highly predictive of catheter related sepsis, *J Clin Microbiol* 36:105, 1998.

Darouiche RO, et al: A comparison of two antimicrobial-impregnated central venous catheters, *N Engl J Med* 340:1, 1999.

Pearson ML: Guideline for prevention on intravascular device-related infections. Part I: Intravascular device related infections: an overview. Part II: Recommendations for the prevention of nosocomial intravascular device related infections. Hospital Infection Control Practices Advisory Committee, *Am J Infect Control* 24:262, 1996.

Raad I: Intravascular catheter related infections, *Lancet* 351:893, 1998.

Veenstra DL, et al: Efficacy of antiseptic impregnated central venous catheters in preventing catheter related bloodstream infection: a meta analysis, *JAMA* 281:261, 1999.

Table 4   Management of Catheter-Related Infections

MICROORGANISM	DURATION OF THERAPY	CATHETER REMOVAL ADVISABLE
Coagulase-negative staphylococci	7 days	No
Staphylococcus aureus		
Uncomplicated	10-14 days	Yes
Complicated	4 weeks	Yes
Gram-positive bacilli	7 days	Yes
Gram-negative rods	7-10 days	Yes
Candida species	14 days	Yes
Mycobacterium	14 days	Yes

INFECTIONS ASSOCIATED WITH URINARY CATHETERS

Lindsay E. Nicolle

Urinary tract infections (UTIs) are a common and clinically important outcome of the use of any urinary catheter. Urinary catheter use may be considered as follows:

· Short-term indwelling urethral catheters
· Long-term indwelling urethral catheters
· Intermittent catheterization

A catheter is considered a short-term indwelling catheter when the duration of catheterization is less than 30 days, and a long-term indwelling catheter when the catheter remains in situ more than 30 days. Considerations for indwelling suprapubic catheters are similar to those for indwelling urethral catheters. These different types of catheterization are used in different populations and have different risks for the occurrence of infection (Table 1).

■ PATHOGENESIS

Acquisition of urinary infection with catheter use is virtually always through ascending infection (Table 2). With intermittent catheterization, organisms are repeatedly introduced into the bladder at catheterization. Individuals managed with intermittent catheterization virtually always have a neurogenic bladder with incomplete bladder emptying, so organisms, once introduced, may persist in the bladder. The infecting organisms are usually present as colonizing bacteria in the periurethral area but may also contaminate the hands of the individual performing catheterization or the catheter itself.

For indwelling urethral catheters, bacteria introduced at the time of catheterization account for fewer than 5% of infections (see Table 2). More commonly, bacteria ascend into the bladder on the mucous sheath on the external surface of the catheter, or from the drainage tubing or drainage bag in the urine column or with bacterial biofilm on the inner surface of the tubing. Organisms colonizing the periurethral area ascending on the external surface of the catheter are a source of bacteriuria more often in women with indwelling catheters, and organisms gaining access through the tubing occurs more often in men. Disruption of the closed drainage system from the bladder to the drainage bag also introduces bacteria and is associated with a high occurrence of urinary infection within 24 hours of such a break in the system.

■ BACTERIOLOGY

Urinary infection identified in the setting of urethral catheterization falls within the diagnostic grouping of complicated UTI. While *Escherichia coli* remains an important pathogen in these infections, other organisms are frequently isolated. These include other Enterobacteriaceae such as *Klebsiella pneumoniae*, *Citrobacter* species, *Enterobacter* species, and, *Serratia marcesens*. For long-term indwelling catheters in particular, infections with urease-producing organisms such as *Proteus mirabilis*, *Morganella morganii*, or *Providencia stuartii* are common. *Pseudomonas aeruginosa* and other gram-negative nonfermenters such as *Acinetobacter* species are also frequently isolated, as are grampositive organisms, particularly enterococci and coagulase-negative staphylococci. *Candida albicans* and other yeast species also occur, usually isolated from subjects receiving antimicrobials. The high frequency of recurrent infections and subsequent repeated courses of antimicrobials mean resistant organisms occur with increased frequency.

Polymicrobial bacteriuria is a characteristic of infection in subjects with long-term indwelling catheters but may occur with other types of catheterization. For long-term indwelling catheters, infection is usually present with two to five organisms at any time. Long-term indwelling catheters also usually have a bacterial biofilm present, primarily on

Table 1 Types of Catheter Use and Frequency of Urinary Infection in Catheterized Populations

CATHETER	USUAL POPULATION	INFECTION RATE
Indwelling urethral		
Short term	Acute-care facility · Output monitoring · Postsurgical · Acute retention	5% per day Women > men
Long term	Long-term care: 5%-10% of residents · Chronic retention—men · Incontinence—women	100% prevalence
Intermittent catheter	Neurogenic bladder · Spinal cord injury · Multiple sclerosis · Flaccid incontinence	1%-3% per catheterization

Table 2 Methods by Which Organisms Gain Access to the Bladder in Catheter-Acquired Urinary Infection

Ascending infection
  Introduced at catheterization
  Ascending from periurethral area on mucous sheath on external catheter surface
  Intraluminal from drainage bag with urine reflux or bacterial biofilm
  Introduced with breaks in closed drainage
Other (uncommon)
  Hematogenous from another body site

the inner surface of the catheter. Urine specimens obtained for culture through the biofilm-laden catheter may have a bacteriologic profile that differs from that in bladder urine in both quantity and type of organisms isolated.

■ MORBIDITY AND MORTALITY

Most catheter-acquired urinary infections are asymptomatic. However, symptomatic infection does occur frequently in catheterized subjects and may be associated with significant morbidity. Pyelonephritis, fever, and bacteremia may require hospitalization or may result in extended hospitalization when nosocomially acquired. Acute urinary infection in subjects with spinal cord injury or other neurologic diseases may further impair function through autonomic hyperreflexia or increased lower limb spasticity. Urinary infection in residents with chronic indwelling urethral catheters is the most frequent cause of bacteremia in long-term care facilities. Occasionally, acute urosepsis associated with catheterization may lead to death. Mortality is uncommon, however, relative to the high frequency of urinary infection with catheter use.

■ DIAGNOSIS

The diagnosis of urinary infection in a catheterized patient is microbiologic. Clinical findings will then determine whether infection, if present, is symptomatic or asymptomatic. Culture of an appropriately collected urine specimen is essential for the microbiologic diagnosis. The specimen should be collected directly at the time of catheterization for intermittent catheter use, from a newly placed catheter in subjects with long-term indwelling urethral catheters, or by aspiration from the catheter port of a short-term indwelling catheter. The specimen must be collected before antimicrobials for treatment are initiated. Criteria for the microbiologic diagnosis of urinary infection are shown in Table 3. For short-term indwelling urethral catheters, lower quantitative counts of 10^3 CFU/ml or more will usually progress to 10^5 CFU/ml or more over 24 to 48 hours, unless the catheter is removed or antimicrobial therapy is given.

A diagnosis of symptomatic urinary infection should not be made without a positive urine culture. However, patients with short-term indwelling catheters or maintained on intermittent catheterization often have positive urine cultures, and virtually all individuals with chronic long-term indwelling catheters are persistently bacteriuric. Thus a positive urine culture is common at any time in catheterized patients and, although necessary for diagnosis of urinary infection, is not sufficient to identify symptomatic infection in the absence of symptoms localized to the genitourinary tract.

Clinical presentations consistent with urinary infection are listed in Table 4. Although the occurrence of acute pyelonephritis with fever, flank pain and tenderness, or fever with an obstructed catheter may allow a diagnosis of symptomatic urinary infection with a high degree of confidence, there are many potential presentations where a urinary source for symptoms is less definite. A frequent clinical scenario is fever and a positive urine culture, but no localiz-

Table 3 Microbiologic Diagnosis of Urinary Infection in Subjects with Catheter

CLINICAL PRESENTATION	QUANTITATIVE COUNT OF BACTERIA
Asymptomatic	>10^5 CFU/ml on two specimens
Symptomatic	
Lower tract symptoms*	≥10^2 CFU/ml
Systemic symptoms	≥10^2 CFU/ml

*Usually subjects with intermittent catheterization.

Table 4 Clinical Presentations of Acute Urinary Infection in Subjects with Bladder Catheters

Asymptomatic
Symptomatic:

Systemic	• Acute pyelonephritis
	• Fever with catheter obstruction
	• Fever with acute hematuria
	• Bacteremia with urinary isolate
	• Increased lower leg spasms or autonomic hyperreflexia in spinal cord injury
	• Fever with no genitourinary localizing findings (<50% urinary source)
Local*	• Urethritis
	• Epididymitis
	• Urethral abscess
	• Bladder stones
	• Catheter obstruction
	• Prostatitis
	• Scrotal abscess

*Local complications are primarily seen with long-term indwelling urethral catheters.

ing findings referable to the genitourinary tract to support a diagnosis of urinary infection or symptoms elsewhere to identify an alternate source. Urinary infection may be the diagnosis in this situation, but usually, an alternative diagnosis is responsible. In one study of subjects with long-term indwelling catheters, only 33% of such episodes were due to a urinary source. Thus in the absence of localizing findings to the genitourinary tract or bacteremia with the urinary isolate, symptomatic urinary infection is a possible but not definite diagnosis in the febrile catheterized patient with a positive urine culture.

■ TREATMENT

Treatment of asymptomatic bacteriuria is not indicated for subjects managed by intermittent catheterization or while an indwelling urethral catheter, either short- or long-term, remains in place. Pyuria usually accompanies bacteriuria in catheterized subjects, so pyuria is not a marker to identify otherwise asymptomatic individuals who should receive treatment.

Antimicrobial therapy should be given to subjects with asymptomatic bacteriuria before an invasive genitourinary

Table 5 Oral Antimicrobials for Treatment of Urinary Tract Infection in Catheterized Patients with Normal Renal Function

ANTIMICROBIAL	DOSAGE
PENICILLINS	
Amoxicillin	500 mg tid
Amoxicillin-clavulanic acid	500 mg tid
CEPHALOSPORINS	
Cephalexin	500 mg qid
Cefaclor	500 mg qid
Cefadroxil	1 g od or bid
Cefuroxime axetil	250 mg bid
Cefixime	400 mg od
Cefpodoxime proxetil	100-400 mg bid
FLUOROQUINOLONES*	
Norfloxacin	400 mg bid
Ciprofloxacin	250-500 mg bid
Ofloxacin	200-400 mg bid
Fleroxacin	400 mg od
Lomefloxacin	400 mg od
Levofloxacin	250 mg od
OTHER	
Nitrofurantoin	50-100 mg qid
Trimethoprim	100 mg bid
Trimethoprim-sulfamethoxazole	160/800 mg bid

*Recommended for oral empiric therapy.

Table 6 Parenteral Antimicrobials for Treatment of Urinary Tract Infection in Individuals with Normal Renal Function

ANTIMICROBIAL	DOSAGE
AMINOGLYCOSIDE	
Amikacin	5 mg/kg q8h or 15 mg/kg q24h
Gentamicin*	1-1.5 mg/kg q8h or 4-5 mg/kg q24h
Tobramycin*	1-1.5 mg/kg q8h or 4-5 mg/kg q24h
PENICILLIN	
Ampicillin	1-2 g q6h
Piperacillin	3 g q4h
Piperacillin/tazobactam	4 g/500 mg q8h
Ticarcillin/clavulanic	50 mg/kg q6h
CEPHALOSPORINS	
Cefazolin	1-2 g q8h
Cefoxitin	1 g q8h
Cefotetan	1 g q12h
Cefotaxime	1-2 g bid or tid
Cefepime	2 g q12h
Ceftazidime	0.5-2 g q8h
OTHER	
Aztreonam	1 g q6h
Imipenem/cilastatin	500 mg q6h
Vancomycin	500 mg q6h or 1 g q12h

*Recommended for initial empiric therapy with ampicillin if renal function is normal.

procedure where there is a high likelihood of mucosal trauma such as transurethral prostatic resection or stone extraction. Antimicrobial therapy is given immediately before the surgical procedure and is conceptually "prophylaxis" to prevent bacteremia and sepsis, rather than treatment of asymptomatic bacteriuria. Antimicrobial therapy is not indicated before a chronic indwelling urethral catheter change because this is not a high-risk procedure. For women, if bacteriuria persists for 48 hours after removing a short-term indwelling catheter, treatment may be indicated. This clinical question has not been addressed for men, and no definitive recommendation can be given.

When symptomatic infection is clinically diagnosed, a urine specimen for culture should be obtained in every case before initiation of antimicrobial therapy. For individuals with long-term indwelling catheters, the catheter should be replaced before initiating antimicrobial therapy. A urine specimen on which the treatment decision will be based should be obtained immediately from the newly placed catheter. For short-term indwelling catheters, where biofilm formation is less likely, routine catheter replacement is not recommended.

Specific antimicrobial therapy is selected on the basis of the urine culture if a result is available. Oral antimicrobials appropriate for treatment of urinary infection are listed in Table 5, and parenteral antimicrobials are listed in Table 6. The decision with respect to oral or parenteral therapy will be determined by the patient's clinical status and the likelihood of resistant organisms. Parenteral therapy should be initiated in patients who are hemodynamically unstable, are vomiting, have impaired gastrointestinal absorption, or have

a high likelihood of being infected with an organism resistant to oral agents.

Empiric antimicrobial therapy should be initiated pending urine culture results where a patient is significantly ill with fever or other systemic symptoms or when the patient has severe irritative symptoms. The selection of initial empiric therapy is assisted, in some cases, by knowledge of bacteriology of previous urine cultures in the patient or resistance patterns of endemic flora in an institution. An aminoglycoside, with or without ampicillin for enterococci, is usually appropriate for initial empiric parenteral therapy. In the presence of moderate to severe renal failure, an extended-spectrum beta-lactam antimicrobial or fluoroquinolone may be preferred, rather than an aminoglycoside. When there is a concern about resistant organisms, alternative empiric therapy specific for expected susceptibilities should be chosen. Once urine culture and susceptibility results from the pretherapy urine specimen are available, usually 48 to 72 hours after initiation of therapy, antimicrobial therapy can be reassessed and, if appropriate, changed to alternative specific therapy. This will often include a change to oral therapy for patients in whom parenteral therapy was initiated.

If the patient continues to require an indwelling catheter, the treatment duration should be for as short a period as possible, (5 to 7 days). Longer courses of therapy will promote the emergence of organisms of increasing resistance and may potentially increase the difficulty in treating future episodes of symptomatic infection. If the catheter is removed, 7 to 14 days of therapy should be given. For subjects managed with intermittent catheterization, 7 days is recommended for lower tract symptoms and 10 to 14 days for systemic infection.

■ PREVENTION

The most effective means of preventing catheter-associated infection is not to use a catheter or, if there is a compelling clinical indication for use, to limit the duration of catheterization to as short a period as possible (Table 7). For short-term indwelling catheters, the maintenance of a closed drainage system is key to delaying acquisition of infection. Antimicrobial therapy given during the first 3 days of catheterization or at the time of catheter removal are also both associated with a decreased frequency of infection. However, these antimicrobial strategies are not recommended because they lead to infection with more resistant organisms. Other interventions that have been systematically evaluated, such as daily periurethral cleaning with either soap or a disinfectant, addition of disinfectants to the drainage bag, and the coating of the catheter with antibacterial substances, are not effective in decreasing the frequency of infection.

It is not clear that any interventions will decrease the frequency of urinary infection with chronic indwelling urethral catheters. Preventive strategies in these patients must be focused to preventing systemic infection, such as by early identification of catheter obstruction or prevention of trauma of the genitourinary mucosa by the catheter.

For patients managed with intermittent catheterization, use of prophylactic antimicrobials may decrease the frequency of infection in the early catheterization period but is not effective in the long term. When used for the short term, infection with organisms of increased antimicrobial resis-

tance will occur. Thus prophylactic antimicrobials are not recommended in this population. Maintenance of bladder volumes of less than 500 ml in subjects managed with intermittent catheterization also likely decreases the frequency of infection. For nursing home patients, rates of infection with intermittent catheterization are similar if either clean or sterile catheter technique is used. Thus clean technique is recommended because it is less costly.

Table 7 Prevention of Catheter-Acquired Urinary Tract Infection

EFFECTIVE
- Limit duration of catheter use
- Aseptic insertion (for indwelling catheter)
- Maintain closed drainage system
- Antibiotics first 4 days (not recommended)*
- Antibiotics at removal (not recommended)*

NOT EFFECTIVE
- Bladder irrigation with antimicrobial
- Periurethral care with soap or disinfectant
- Disinfectant in drainage bag
- Coating of catheter with antimicrobial substances

*Not recommended because of emerging antimicrobial resistance.

Suggested Reading
Cardenas DD, Hooton TM: Urinary tract infection in persons with spinal cord injury, *Arch Phys Med Rehab* 76:272, 1995.
Stamm WE: Catheter-associated urinary tract infection: epidemiology, pathogenesis, and prevention, *Am J Med* 91:65S, 1991.
Warren JW: Catheter-associated urinary tract infection, *Infect Dis Clin North Am* 11:609, 1997.

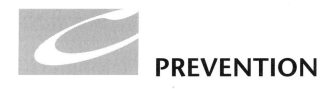

PREVENTION

NONSURGICAL ANTIMICROBIAL PROPHYLAXIS

James P. Steinberg
Mitchell A. Blass

Chemoprophylaxis is the use of an antimicrobial agent to prevent infection. Prophylaxis is often administered after exposure to a virulent pathogen or before a procedure associated with risk of infection. Chronic prophylaxis is sometimes administered to persons with underlying conditions that predispose to recurrent or severe infection. Antibiotics can also be used to prevent clinical disease in persons infected with a microorganism such as *Mycobacterium tuberculosis*. This chapter discusses the specific areas where antimicrobial prophylaxis is generally accepted. For information on prophylaxis of bacterial endocarditis, see the chapter *Endocarditis of Natural and Prosthetic Valves;* for information on prophylaxis in persons infected with the human immunodeficiency virus (HIV), see the chapter *Prophylaxis of Opportunistic Infections in HIV Disease;* for malaria prophylaxis, see the chapter *Malaria;* and for surgical prophylaxis, see the chapter that follows this one.

Several concepts are important in determining whether chemoprophylaxis is appropriate for a particular situation. In general, prophylaxis is recommended when the risk of infection is high or the consequences significant. The nature of the pathogen, type of exposure, and immunocompetence of the host are important determinants of the need for prophylaxis. The antimicrobial agent should eliminate or reduce the probability of infection or if infection occurs, reduce the associated morbidity. The ideal agent is inexpensive and orally administered in most circumstances and has few adverse effects. The ability to alter the normal microbial flora and select for antimicrobial resistance should be limited, so duration of prophylaxis as well as choice of agents is critical. The emerging crisis of antibiotic-resistant bacteria underscores the importance of rational and not indiscriminate use of antimicrobial agents. In addition, the development of antibiotic-resistant pathogens necessitates reassessment of many of the established prophylactic regimens.

The efficacy of chemoprophylaxis is well established in situations such as perioperative antibiotic administration, exposure to invasive meningococcal disease, prevention of recurrent rheumatic fever, and prevention of tuberculosis. Chemoprophylaxis is accepted in other situations without supporting data. When the risk of infection is low, such as with bacterial endocarditis following dental procedures, randomized clinical trials of prophylaxis are not feasible. However, the consequences of infection may be catastrophic, providing a compelling argument for chemoprophylaxis despite the low risk of infection. When prophylaxis is advocated without data confirming efficacy, there should be a scientific rationale to support the use of a particular antimicrobial agent.

Table 1 lists the situations in which antimicrobial prophylaxis is indicated after exposure to certain pathogens. Because the duration of exposure is usually brief, the duration of chemoprophylaxis is short, which helps limit adverse reactions, minimizes the potential for resistance, and limits cost. Some of these pathogens are virulent and can produce serious disease in normal hosts. With exposure to pathogens that cause meningitis, the decision whether to use prophylaxis can be complicated. Because of fear and anxiety provoked by these illnesses there is a tendency to provide prophylaxis to persons outside the high-risk populations. Table 1 also includes microorganisms that have gained notoriety as possible agents of biologic warfare or terrorism.

Persons with an underlying predisposition to infection may benefit from prophylactic antimicrobial agents (Table 2). In contrast to short-term prophylaxis administered after exposures, chronic prophylaxis is often required. Because of the duration of antibiotic administration, the complications of chemoprophylaxis, including alteration of the microbial flora and antibiotic resistance, are major considerations. The emergence of antibiotic-resistant *Streptococcus pneumoniae* may force reassessment of the standard chemoprophylactic recommendations when pneumococcus is a prominent pathogen, as with anatomic or functional asplenia and recurrent otitis.

Chemoprophylaxis for tuberculosis is generally administered to those already infected with *Mycobacterium tuberculosis* (i.e., have a positive tuberculin, or PPD, skin test), in an

Table 1 Prophylaxis Following Selected Exposures

EXPOSURE	PATHOGEN	PROPHYLAXIS*	COMMENTS
Meningitis, meningococcal bacteremia	*Neisseria meningitidis* (see Chapters *Meningococcus and Miscellaneous Neisseriae* and *Bacterial Meningitis*)	Rifampin, 600 mg (10 mg/kg for children) q12h for 4 doses Ciprofloxacin, 500 mg (single dose) (adults only) Ceftriaxone, 250 mg IM one dose (125 mg for children <15 yr old)	Recommended for close contacts only (e.g., family members, roommates, day-care contacts); prophylaxis not recommended for health care workers unless very close contact such as mouth-to-mouth resuscitation occurred: secondary cases reported with meningococcal pneumonia, but role of prophylaxis is uncertain; sulfonamide resistance precludes routine use of sulfadiazine
Meningitis	*Haemophilus influenzae*	Rifampin, 600 mg (20 mg/kg for children) daily for 4 days	Recommended for children < 4 yr old after exposure at home or day care: when such a child is present, prophylaxis should be given to all exposed individuals regardless of age: index case should receive prophylaxis to eradicate nasopharyngeal colonization
Human bite	Viridans and other streptococci, oral anaerobes, *Staphylococcus aureus, Eikenella corrodens*	Amoxicillin-clavulanic acid, 875 mg bid or 500 mg tid for 3-5 days For penicillin allergy, consider clindamycin, 300 mg qid, plus either ciprofloxacin, 500 mg bid, or TMP-SMX, 1 double-strength tablet bid	Risk of infection high: *Eikenella* is resistant to clindamycin and first-generation cephalosporins: clenched-fist injuries often require parenteral antibiotics
Cat bite	*Pasteurella multocida, S. aureus,* streptococci	Amoxicillin-clavulanic acid, 875 mg bid or 500 mg tid for 3-5 days; for penicillin allergy, consider doxycycline, 100 mg bid, or cefuroxime axetil, 500 mg bid	A high percentage of cat bites become infected without prophylaxis First-generation cephalosporins not as active as penicillin against *P. multocida*, which is present in oral flora of 50%-70% of cats
Dog bite	Viridans streptococci, oral anaerobes, *S. aureus, P. multocida, Capnocytophaga canimorsus* (formerly DF-2)	Amoxicillin-clavulanic acid, 875 mg bid or 500 mg tid for 3-5 days; for penicillin allergy, consider doxycycline, 100 mg bid or clindamycin, 300 mg qid, plus either ciprofloxacin, 500 mg bid, or TMP-SMX, 1 double-strength tablet bid	Infection less common than with cat or human bites; need for routine prophylaxis for all bites uncertain; persons without spleens at risk of overwhelming *Capnocytophaga* sepsis, should receive prophylaxis following any dog bite
Sexual assault	*Trichomonas vaginalis, Chlamydia trachomatis, Treponema pallidum, Neisseria gonorrhoeae,* human immunodeficiency virus	Ceftriaxone, 250 mg IM single dose, plus doxycycline, 100 mg bid for 7 days, plus metronidazole, 2 g single dose; may substitute single dose azithromycin, 1 g, for doxycycline	For pregnant victim, erythromycin, 500 mg qid for 7 days, in place of doxycycline or azithromycin; metronidazole acceptable after first trimester; consider use of antiretroviral agents following selected high-risk exposures
Sexual contacts	*T. pallidum*	Benzathine penicillin G, 2.4 million units IM	Treat if exposed within the previous 90 days
Sexual contacts	*N. gonorrhoeae*	Single dose of ceftriaxone, 125 mg IM, or cefipime, 400 mg, or ciprofloxacin, 500 mg, or levofloxacin, 500 mg	Because of possibility of concomitant chlamydial infection, contacts of persons with gonorrhea should also receive azithromycin or doxycycline
Sexual contacts	*C. trachomatis*	Azithromycin, 1 g single dose, or doxycycline, 100 mg bid for 7 days	Erythromycin, 500 mg qid for 7 days, recommended for pregnant women; this regimen is less effective, however

Table 1   Prophylaxis Following Selected Exposures—cont'd

EXPOSURE	PATHOGEN	PROPHYLAXIS*	COMMENTS
Sexual contacts	*T. vaginalis*	Metronidazole, 2 g, single dose	No satisfactory alternatives are available in the United States
Influenza	Influenza A	Amantadine or rimantadine, 100 mg bid for 5-7 wk or for 2 wk if given concurrently with vaccination: use 100 mg daily for those >65 yr old	Recommended for high-risk individuals (elderly, immunocompromised) during outbreaks; usually given to unvaccinated individuals but provides additive protection for the vaccinated; consider for unvaccinated health care workers; two agents have equal efficacy but fewer neurologic side effects with rimantadine; both agents contraindicated in pregnancy
Whooping cough	*Bordetella pertussis*	Erythromycin, 500 mg qid (50 mg/kg qid in children) for 14 days	Secondary attack rate is often >50%; erythromycin prophylaxis, although not 100% effective, reduces transmission and is important in aborting outbreaks
Anthrax	*Bacillus anthracis*	Ciprofloxacin, 500 mg bid for 60 days; alternatives include doxycycline, 100 mg bid, and amoxicillin, 500 mg tid	Inhalational anthrax is considered one of the major threats associated with bioterrorism
Plague	*Yersinia pestis*	Doxycycline, 100 mg bid for 7 days or for duration of exposure	Incubation period for pneumonic plague is short (2-3 days); for established infection, streptomycin IM or gentamicin remain the agents of choice
Tularemia	*Francisella tularensis*	Tetracycline, 500 mg qid for 14 days	Can produce disease following inhalation or percutaneous exposure

*All regimens are administered orally unless otherwise specified.

Table 2   Chronic Prophylaxis in Specific Clinical Settings

UNDERLYING CONDITION/ RECURRENT INFECTIONS	PATHOGENS	PROPHYLAXIS*	COMMENTS
Acute rheumatic fever (prevention of recurrences)	*Streptococcus pyogenes*	Penicillin G, 1.2 million units IM every 3-4 wk; alternatives include penicillin V, 250 mg bid; erythromycin, 250 mg bid; sulfadiazine, 1 g daily (0.5 g if weight <60 lb)	Risk diminishes with increasing age and time since initial attack; optimal duration unknown but continue prophylaxis at least until the early 20s or for 5 yr after most recent attack; some authorities advocate lifelong prophylaxis, especially after rheumatic carditis; risk of prophylaxis failure may be greater with 4 week dosing of penicillin compared to 3 week dosing
Recurrent urinary tract infection	Gram-negative bacilli	TMP-SMX, ½ single-strength tablet (40 mg, 200 mg) daily, or trimethoprim 100 mg, or nitrofurantoin, 50 mg daily	For selected patients with more than three infections yearly; consider prophylaxis for 6-12 mo; alternative strategy is postcoital TMP-SMX, 1 tablet or ciprofloxacin, 500 mg

TMP-SMX, Trimethoprim-sulfamethoxazole.
*All regimens are administered orally unless otherwise specified.

Continued

Table 2   Chronic Prophylaxis in Specific Clinical Settings—cont'd

UNDERLYING CONDITION/ RECURRENT INFECTIONS	PATHOGENS	PROPHYLAXIS*	COMMENTS
Chronic bronchitis, bronchiectasis	*Steptococcus pneumoniae, Haemophilus influenzae, Moraxella catarrhalis*	Amoxicillin, 500 mg tid, or TMP-SMX, 1 double-strength tablet bid, or erythromycin, 250 mg qid, or tetracycline, 500 mg qid	May be useful in selected patients with frequent exacerbations (>4/yr); some authorities prefer antibiotics at first sign of infection
Asplenia, including sickle cell disease	Predominantly *S. pneumoniae*, also *H. influenzae*, meningococci	Penicillin V, 250 mg bid (125 mg bid for children <5 yr old), or benzathine penicillin G, 1.2 million units IM every 4 wk; prophylaxis generally continued 2 yr after splenectomy; for children with sickle cell disease, prophylaxis continued at least until age 5 yr	Efficacy of chemoprophylaxis clearly established for children with sickle cell disease; some authorities recommend amoxicillin or TMP-SMX for children <5 yr old because of risk of *H. influenzae* infection; however, this risk has been dramatically reduced because of immunization; chemoprophylaxis generally not recommended for adults (lower risk); penicillin-resistant pneumococcus diminishes attractiveness of antibiotic prophylaxis and increases the importance of vaccination
Recurrent otitis media	*S. pneumoniae, H. influenzae,* and *M. catarrhalis*	Sulfisoxazole, 50 mg/kg, or amoxicillin, 20 mg/kg daily, or azithromycin, 10 mg/kg qwk	Recommended for children with more than three infections in 6 mo; increasing antibiotic resistance has decreased the efficacy of this strategy and has led some experts to abandon it
Lymphedema with recurrent cellulitis	*Streptococcus pyogenes*	Benzathine penicillin G, 1.2 million units IM monthly	Given only to patients with frequent episodes of cellulitis; efficacy is limited in patients with significant underlying disease
Spontaneous bacterial peritonitis (SBP) in cirrhotic ascites	*Escherichia coli, S. pneumoniae, K. pneumoniae*	Norfloxacin, 400 mg daily, or TMP-SMX, 1 double-strength tablet 5 days/wk	Recent cost analysis showed prophylaxis with either agent cost effective especially in persons with ascites protein concentration of <1 g/dl and in persons with previous SBP (secondary prophylaxis)

TMP-SMX, Trimethoprim-sulfamethoxazole.
*All regimens are administered orally unless otherwise specified.

attempt to prevent the development of active tuberculosis. The criteria for administering chemoprophylaxis listed in Table 3 take into account the following: (1) the risk of developing active tuberculosis is greatest in the first 2 years following PPD conversion, (2) the risk of isoniazid (INH) hepatitis in those older than 35 years of age is greater than the risk of developing tuberculosis except in high-risk individuals including recent skin test converters, (3) the recognition that PPD skin testing may result in false-positive and false-negative test results. Consequently, different diameters of induration are used depending on the prevalence of *M. tuberculosis* infection in the population tested.

Current recommendations call for 6 to 12 months of INH, 300 mg daily (10 mg/kg/day in children). However, 6 months of INH is not as effective as longer courses, and subsequent recommendations will likely increase the minimum duration of prophylaxis to 9 months. The revised recommendations for INH prophylaxis in persons coinfected with HIV have made this change to a 9-month course (to be given daily or twice weekly when directly ob-

Table 3   Criteria for Preventive Therapy for Persons with Positive PPD Skin Tests

SITUATION	PPD SIZE (5 TU)	AGE GROUP
Recent PPD converter (negative PPD within the previous 2 yr, excluding booster phenomenon)	PPD ≥10 mm except ≥5 mm after exposure to active tuberculosis	All ages
Identified risk factors, including HIV infection, immunosuppressive illnesses, abnormal chest radiograph, silicosis, intravenous drug abuse	PPD ≥10 mm except ≥5 mm if HIV seropositive or if radiograph shows fibrotic disease suggestive of old tuberculosis	All ages
Normal hosts from high-incidence groups: indigent patients, residents of extended-care facilities, immigrants from endemic areas	PPD ≥10 mm	Age <35
Normal hosts from low-incidence groups	PPD ≥15 mm	Age <35
Exposure to tuberculosis	HIV seropositive and anergic	All ages
	Initial PPD nonreactive*	Age 0-5 yr

PPD, Purified protein derivative (tuberculin test); *HIV,* human immunodeficiency virus.
*Repeat PPD in 3 months; if negative, stop chemoprophylaxis.

Table 4   Controversial Areas Regarding the Use of Prophylactic Antibiotics*

CONDITION	COMMENTS
Prosthetic device infections	Routine chemoprophylaxis before dental work, or other procedures that cause transient bacteremia in patients with prosthetic joints or vascular prostheses may not be warranted although it is commonly used; prosthetic joint infections caused by oral flora, including α-streptococci, are uncommon, with rate approaching that of endocarditis in patients with mitral valve prolapse without regurgitation, for which chemoprophylaxis is not recommended; coronary stents do not appear to be prone to infection
Travelers' diarrhea	Most authorities do not recommend antibiotic prophylaxis for travelers' diarrhea because of possible adverse reactions, potential for development of resistance, and cost; preferable strategy is judicious use of antimotility agents and empiric fluoroquinolone (ciprofloxacin, 500 mg bid, levofloxacin, 500 mg daily, or norfloxacin, 400 mg bid for 3-5 days) for moderate diarrhea; prophylactic bismuth subsalicylate 2 tablets qid is an alternative
Lyme disease	Risk of Lyme disease following bite by an *Ixodes* tick <3% even where Lyme disease endemic; routine chemoprophylaxis is not recommended; to transmit Lyme spirochete, *Ixodes* tick must be attached >24 hr
Catheter-associated UTI	Systemic antibiotics reduce incidence of UTI during initial 4-5 days after Foley catheter insertion; with prolonged catheterization antibiotic-resistant bacteria appear in urine with increasing frequency, dissuading most authorities from routine use of prophylaxis; prophylactic antibiotics possibly useful in selected high-risk patients during short-term catheterization
Intravenous catheter–associated infections	Flushing central venous catheters with an antibiotic solution, usually vancomycin (antibiotic lock) proposed to reduce catheter-associated bacteremia, vancomycin-resistant enterococci led most authorities, including Centers for Disease Control and Prevention, to oppose this strategy

UTI, Urinary tract infection.
*See also *Infection of Native and Prosthetic Joints.*

served therapy is used). Pyridoxine, 50 g/day, is usually given with INH to prevent peripheral neuropathy. Short-course (2 months) chemoprophylaxis with rifampin, 600 mg/day, plus pyrazinamide, 25 mg/kg/day, appears to be equally efficacious as 12 months of INH. This regimen is an alternative to INH prophylaxis in persons with or without HIV coinfection. In clinical trials, compliance was better with the short-course regimen. The short-course regimen can also be used when infection with INH-resistant *M. tuberculosis* is suspected. In the setting of suspected infection with multidrug- resistant *M. tuberculosis* the decision to provide chemoprophylaxis and the choice of regimen should

be made by experienced health care professionals. For immunocompromised persons, including those with HIV infection, the prophylactic regimen should be based on the susceptibility pattern of the prevalent multiresistant strain.

Chemoprophylaxis has been advocated for other situations, but at this time, it cannot be considered standard practice (Table 4). Although data are limited, it is likely that cost-benefit analyses would not favor routine prophylaxis in these settings or that the benefits of prophylaxis in the short term would be outweighed by long-term consequences such as the development of antibiotic-resistant organisms.

Suggested Reading

Centers for Disease Control and Prevention: Prevention and treatment of tuberculosis among patients infected with human immunodeficiency virus: principles of therapy and revised recommendations, *MMWR* 47 (RR-20):18, 36, 1998.

Centers for Disease Control and Prevention: 1998 guidelines for treatment of sexually transmitted diseases, *MMWR* 47 (RR-1):1, 1998.

DuPont HL, Ericsson CD: Prevention and treatment of traveler's diarrhea. *N Engl J Med* 328:1821, 1993.

Franz DR, et al: Clinical recognition and management of patients exposed to biological warfare agents, *JAMA* 278:399, 1997.

Lurie P, et al: Postexposure prophylaxis after nonoccupational HIV exposure: clinical, ethical, and policy considerations, *JAMA* 280:1769, 1998.

Shapiro GD, et al: A controlled trial of antimicrobial prophylaxis for Lyme disease after deer tick bites, *N Engl J Med* 327:1769, 1992.

SURGICAL PROPHYLAXIS

Joseph Solomkin

The prevention of surgical site infection (SSI) remains a focus of attention because even with application of strict asepsis and antiinfective prophylaxis, wound infections remain a major source of expense, morbidity, and mortality. The Centers for Disease Control and Prevention (CDC) refers to postoperative wound infections as "surgical site infection" and divides these into superficial (involving skin and subcutaneous tissue) and deep (involving the fascia and muscle) incisional infections, and organ/space infections. It is important to note that administration of systemic antiinfectives is only part of a broad program of infection control involving adequate operating room ventilation, sterilization, barrier usage, and delicate surgical technique.

Surgical site infections are the third most commonly reported nosocomial infection, accounting for 14% to 16% of nosocomial infections in hospitalized patients. Approximately 40% of nosocomial infections occurring among surgical patients are surgical site infections, two thirds of which affect the incision and one third involve organ/space infection. Three quarters of deaths of surgical patients with SSI are attributed to that infection, nearly all of which are organ/space infections.

■ RISK FACTORS FOR SURGICAL SITE INFECTION

Information on appropriateness of antimicrobial prophylaxis is of considerable significance because of the cost of infection that *might* have been prevented had prophylaxis been given and, conversely, the cost of providing antimicrobial therapy to a very large number of patients if the yield is only the prevention of a relatively small number of infec-

tions or even the prevention of *no* infection. The costs of providing therapy extend far beyond the acquisition and administration charges. They include costs of treating adverse reactions and the more ominous potential cost of dealing in future times with drug-resistant bacteria. Therefore enormous effort has been expended to identify factors that increase the risk of infection and would, at least potentially, suggest providing antimicrobial prophylaxis.

In 1964, the National Research Council (NRC) sponsored the development of a wound classification scheme (Table 1). A clear connection between the contaminating flora at various surgical sites and subsequent infecting pathogens was established. This microbiologic correlation included recognition of the role of anaerobes in postoperative wound infection and abscess formation. Other experimental work investigated the critical issue of the proper timing for such treatment.

It is assumed that at least three categories of variables serve as predictors of SSI risk: those that estimate the intrinsic degree of microbial contamination of the surgical site as (e.g., the NRC wound class), those the measure the duration of the operation and other less quantifiable elements of the procedure, and those that serve as markers for host susceptibility.

Two subsequent CDC efforts, the Study of the Efficacy of Nosocomial Infection Control (SENIC) project and National Nosocomial Infection Surveillance (NNIS) sought to examine these other variables as predictors of infection. These showed that even within the category of clean wounds, the SSI risk varied from 1.1% to 15.8% (SENIC) and from 1.0% to 5.4% (NNIS), depending on the presence of other risk factors.

The variables that were significantly and independently associated with subsequent surgical site infection included (1) an abdominal operation, (2) an operation lasting more than 2 hours, (3) a surgical site with a wound classification of either contaminated or dirty/infected, and (4) an operation performed on a patient having three or more discharge diagnoses. Each of these variables contributes one point when present, and the risk index varies from 0 to 4. This means that each variable has the same significance as any other. Using this index predicted surgical site infections about twice as well as relying on wound classification. With

Table 1   Surgical Wound Classification

CLASS I/CLEAN

An uninfected operative wound in which no inflammation is encountered, and the respiratory, alimentary, genital, or uninfected urinary tract is not entered. In addition, clean wounds are primarily closed and, if necessary, drained with closed drainage. Operative incisional wounds that follow nonpenetrating (blunt) trauma should be included in this category if they meet the criteria.

CLASS II/CLEAN CONTAMINATED

An operative wound in which the respiratory, alimentary, genital, or urinary tracts are entered under controlled conditions and without unusual contamination. Specifically, operations involving the biliary tract, appendix, vagina, and oropharynx are included in this category, provided no evidence of infection or major break in technique is encountered.

CLASS III/CONTAMINATED

Open, fresh, accidental wounds. In addition, operations with major breaks in sterile technique (e.g., open cardiac massage) or gross spillage from the gastrointestinal tract, and incisions in which acute, nonpurulent inflammation is encountered are included in this category.

CLASS IV/DIRTY/INFECTED

Old traumatic wounds with retained devitalized tissue and those that involve existing clinical infection or perforated viscera. This definition suggests that the organisms causing postoperative infection were present in the operative field before the operation.

the simplified index, a subgroup, consisting of half the surgical patients, can be identified in whom 90% of the surgical wound infections will develop. By the inclusion of factors measuring the risk based on the patient's susceptibility as well as that based on the level of wound contamination, the simplified index predicts surgical wound infection risk about twice as well as the traditional classification of wound contamination.

The problem with this system is that it is not operation specific and depends on variables collected after the operation (at discharge). A second study was then performed through the NNIS system from 44 hospitals from January 1987 through December 1990. A risk index was developed to predict a surgical patient's risk of acquiring an SSI. The risk index score, ranging from 0 to 3, is the number of risk factors present among the following: (1) a patient with an American Society of Anesthesiologists preoperative assessment score of 3, 4, or 5; (2) an operation classified as contaminated or dirty-infected; and (3) an operation lasting more than T hours, where T depends on the operative procedure being performed. The SSI rates for patients with scores of 0, 1, 2, and 3 were 1.5, 2.9, 6.8, and 13.0, respectively. The risk index is a significantly better predictor of surgical wound infection risk than the traditional wound classification system and performs well across a broad range of operative procedures.

It is known that approximately half of surgical site infections occur after discharge, with most occurring within 21 days after operation. Although SSIs occurring after hospital discharge cause substantial morbidity, their epidemiology is not well understood, and methods for routine postdischarge surveillance have not been validated.

ACCEPTED INDICATIONS FOR ANTIINFECTIVE PROPHYLAXIS

There is a wide consensus on specific procedures that warrant antimicrobial prophylaxis. Controlled trials of antimicrobial prophylaxis in minimally invasive procedures have recently been reported. In low-risk laparoscopic cholecystectomy and arthroscopic surgery, routine prophylaxis is not indicated. In contaminated procedures, such as high-risk cholecystectomy and bowel surgery, it is probably safest to apply the standards for similar open procedures in the absence of well-conducted studies.

Generally, elective surgery on the stomach or duodenum for ulcer disease is often not included in those procedures requiring prophylaxis. The highly acidic environment results in a very low endogeneous bacterial density, and rates of postoperative infection without prophylaxis are low. High-risk procedures include operations for cancer, gastric ulcer, bleeding, obstruction, and perforation, as well as operation in the presence of acid-reducing medical or surgical therapy. Prophylaxis is also recommended for gastric procedures for morbid obesity.

CHOICE OF ANTIINFECTIVES FOR PROPHYLAXIS

It is certainly not necessary to cover the entire spectrum of contaminants of a surgical wound. The anticipated pathogens from various operative sites are detailed in Table 2, and recommended regimens are listed in Table 3.

Little work has been done on appropriate dosing. In general, doses of the selected agent that would be used for treatment of established infection are recommended. An important issue concerns the need for repetitive dosing for lengthy procedures. This is in part a function of the half-life of the agent selected and is an additional argument in favor of agents such as cefazolin that have half-lives approaching 2 hours. A current recommendation is to redose the patient at intervals of twice the half-life of the agent provided. It is important to note that increasing the dose of an agent provides less benefit than shortening the dosing interval because drug clearance is logarithmic.

The optimal duration of perioperative antimicrobial prophylaxis is one dose given immediately before initiation of the procedure. A large number of studies document effective prophylaxis with no further dosing after the patient leaves the operating room.

Head and Neck Procedures

For procedures entailing entry into the oropharynx or esophagus, coverage of aerobic cocci is indicated. Prophylaxis has been shown to reduce the incidence of severe wound infection by approximately 50%. Either penicillin-based or cephalosporin-based prophylaxis is effective. Cefazolin is commonly used. Prophylaxis is not indicated for

Table 2   Most Common Likely Pathogens According to Surgical Site

OPERATIONS	LIKELY PATHOGENS
Placement of all grafts, prostheses, or implants	*Staphylococcus aureus;* coagulase-negative staphylococci
Cardiac	*S. aureus;* coagulase-negative staphylococci
Neurosurgery	*S. aureus;* coagulase-negative staphylococci
Breast	*S. aureus;* coagulase-negative staphylococci

Ophthalmic
    Limited data; however, commonly used in procedures such
    as anterior segment resection, vitrectomy, and scleral buckles
	S. aureus; coagulase-negative staphylococci; streptococci gram-
	    negative bacilli

Orthopedic
    Total joint replacement
    Closed fractures/use of nails, bone plates, other internal
        fixation devices
    Functional repair without implant/device
    Trauma
	S. aureus; coagulase-negative staphylococci; gram-negative bacilli

Noncardiac thoracic
    Thoracic (lobectomy, pneumonectomy, wedge resection, other
        noncardiac mediastinal procedures)
    Closed tube thoracostomy
	S. aureus; coagulase-negative staphylococci; *Streptococcus pneu-
	    moniae;* gram-negative bacilli

Vascular	*S. aureus;* coagulase-negative staphylococci
Appendectomy	Gram-negative bacilli; anaerobes
Biliary tract	Gram-negative bacilli; anaerobes
Colorectal	Gram-negative bacilli; anaerobes
Gastroduodenal	Gram-negative bacilli; streptococci; oropharyngeal anaerobes (e.g., peptostreptococci)

Head and neck (procedures with incision through oropharyngeal
    mucosa)
	aurm streptococci; oropharyngeal anaerobes (e.g.,
	    peptostreptococci)

Obstetric and gynecologic	Gram-negative bacilli; enterococci; group B streptococci; anaerobes
Urologic May not be beneficial if urine is sterile	Gram-negative bacilli

Table 3   Pathogens Causing Surgical Site Infections and Antimicrobial Drugs of Choice for Prophylaxis

PROCEDURE	PATHOGEN(S)	DRUG/DOSING	FOR HISTORY OF ANAPHYLACTOID REACTIONS

Clean procedures for which pro-
phylaxis is accepted*
	Staphylococcus aureus and
	    epidermidis
		Cefazolin, 1 g	Clindamycin, 600 mg, or
			    vancomycin, 1 g

Head and neck procedures enter- ing the oropharynx; esophageal procedures	Streptococci and oral anaerobes	Cefazolin, 1 g	Clindamycin, 600 mg, or vancomycin, 1 g

High-risk gastroduodenal and
biliary
	Enterobacteriaceae and
	    streptococci
		Cefazolin, 1 g	Ciprofloxacin, 400 mg, and
			    clindamycin, 600 mg

Nonperforated appendicitis
Colorectal
Abdominal hysterectomy
High-risk caesarean section
Vaginal hysterectomy
	Enterobacteriaceae and *Bacteroi-
	    des fragilis*
		Cefazolin, 1 g, plus metronida-
		    zole, 500 mg, or cefotetan, 1 g
			Ciprofloxacin, 400 mg, and
			    clindamycin, 600 mg

*Includes cardiac and other procedures via median sternotomy, other thoracic, craniotomy, and insertion of vascular and articular prostheses.

dentoalveolar procedures, although prophylaxis is warranted in immunocompromised patients undergoing these procedures.

Neurosurgical Procedures
Studies evaluating the efficacy of antibiotic prophylaxis in neurosurgical procedures have shown variable results. Nonetheless, prophylaxis is currently recommended for cra-

niotomy, laminectomy, and shunt procedures. Coverage targets *Staphylococcus aureus* or *Staphylococcus epidermidis*.

General Thoracic Procedures
Prophylaxis is routinely used for nearly all thoracic procedures. This is particularly true given the likelihood of encountering high numbers of microorganisms during the procedure. Pulmonary resection in cases of partial or com-

plete obstruction of an airway is a procedure in which prophylaxis is clearly warranted. Likewise, prophylaxis is strongly recommended for procedures entailing entry into the esophagus. Although the range of microorganisms encountered in thoracic procedures is extensive, most are sensitive to cefazolin, which is the recommended agent.

Cardiac Procedures

Prophylaxis against *S. aureus* and *S. epidermidis* is indicated for patients undergoing cardiac procedures. Although the risk of infection is low, the morbidity of mediastinitis or a sternal wound infection is great. Numerous studies have evaluated antibiotic regimens based on penicillin, first-generation cephalosporins, second-generation cephalosporins, or vancomycin. Cardiopulmonary bypass reduces the elimination of drugs, so additional intraoperative doses typically are not necessary.

Colorectal Procedures

Colorectal procedures have a very high intrinsic risk of infection and warrant a strong recommendation for prophylaxis. Several studies have demonstrated efficacy with rates of infection decreasing from more than 50% to less than 9%. Antibiotic spectrum is directed at gram-negative aerobes and anaerobic bacteria. All strategies are based on the use of mechanical bowel preparation with purgatives such as polyethylene glycol, mannitol or magnesium citrate, given orally, and enemas. Such pretreatment decreases fecal bulk but does not decrease the concentration of bacteria in the stool. In fact, the risk of infection with mechanical preparation alone is still 25% to 30%. One recommended regimen consists of erythromycin base and neomycin given at 1 PM, 2 PM, and 11 PM (1 g of each drug per dose) the day before a procedure scheduled for 8 AM. Times of administration are shifted according to the anticipated time of starting the procedure, with the first dose given 19 hours before surgery. Metronidazole can be substituted for erythromycin.

Prophylaxis is also recommended for appendectomy. Although the intrinsic risk of infection is low for uncomplicated appendicitis, the preoperative status of the patient's appendix is typically not known. Cefotetan and cefoxitin are acceptable agents. Metronidazole combined with an aminoglycoside or a quinolone is also an acceptable regimen. For uncomplicated appendicitis, coverage need not be extended to the postoperative period. Complicated appendicitis (e.g., with accompanying perforation or gangrene) is an indication for antibiotic therapy, thereby rendering any consideration of prophylaxis irrelevant.

The recommendations for antibiotic prophylaxis for procedures of the biliary tract depend on the presence of specific risk factors. In general, prophylaxis for elective cholecystectomy (either open or laparoscopic) may be regarded as optional. Risk factors associated with an increased incidence of bacteria in bile and thus of increased risk for postoperative infection include age over 60 years, disease of the common duct, diagnosis of cholecystitis, presence of jaundice, and previous history of biliary tract surgery. Only one factor is necessary to establish the patient as high risk. In most cases of symptomatic cholelithiasis meeting high-risk criteria, cefazolin is an acceptable agent. Agents with theo-retically superior antimicrobial activity have not been shown to produce a lower postoperative infection rate.

Obstetric and Gynecologic Procedures

Prophylaxis is indicated for cesarean section and abdominal and vaginal hysterectomy. Numerous clinical trials have demonstrated a reduction in risk of wound infection or endometritis by as much as 70% in patients undergoing cesarean section. For cesarean section, the antibiotic is administered immediately after the cord is clamped to avoid exposing the newborn to antibiotics. Despite the theoretic need to cover gram-negative and anaerobic organisms, studies have not demonstrated a superior result with broad-spectrum antibiotics compared with cefazolin. Therefore cefazolin is the recommended agent.

Urologic Procedures

The range of potential urologic procedures and intrinsic risk of infection varies widely. In general, it is recommended to achieve preoperative sterilization of the urine if clinically feasible. For procedures entailing the creation of urinary conduits, recommendations are similar to those for procedures pertaining to the specific segment of the intestinal tract being used for the conduit. Procedures not requiring entry into the intestinal tract and performed in the context of sterile urine are regarded as clean procedures. However, prophylaxis for specific urologic procedures has not been fully evaluated.

Orthopedic Procedures

Antibiotic prophylaxis is recommended for certain orthopedic procedures. These include the insertion of a prosthetic joint, ankle fusion, revision of a prosthetic joint, reduction of hip fractures, reduction of high-energy closed fractures, and reduction of open fractures. Such procedures are associated with a risk of infection of 5% to 15%, reduced to less than 3% by the use of prophylactic antibiotics. *S. aureus* and *S. epidermidis* predominate in wound or joint infections. Cefazolin provides adequate coverage. The additional use of aminoglycosides and extension of coverage beyond the operative period is common but lacks supportive evidence.

Noncardiac Vascular Procedures

Available data support the recommendation for coverage of procedures using synthetic material, those requiring groin incisions, and those affecting the aorta. Cefazolin is the recommended agent because most infections are caused by *S. aureus* or *S. epidermidis*. Prophylaxis is not recommended for patients undergoing carotid endarterectomy.

■ THE USE OF SYSTEMIC ANTIINFECTIVE PROPHYLAXIS FOR CLEAN PROCEDURES

Perioperative antibiotic prophylaxis has been demonstrated to prevent postoperative wound infection after clean surgery in a majority of clinical trials with sufficient power to identify a 50% reduction in risk. The low risk of infection after many clean procedures requires studies of more than 1000 procedures (sometimes many more) to detect such reductions reliably. This is a serious obstacle to performing conclusive tests of efficacy, and it all but precludes use of conventional clinical trials to identify optimal regimens. Regimens that have been shown to be effective have usually been those with efficacy against *S. aureus* and other pathogens that may be carried in the nares or on the skin. In addition, relatively long half-life in the serum and low cost are important considerations. Cefazolin is a good prophylaxis agent for many clean surgical procedures, although special characteristics of the procedure, increased likelihood of antimicrobial resistance, or antibiotic use concerns may make other agents more suitable in specific situations. The decision to use perioperative antibiotic prophylaxis for clean surgical procedures depends not only on its efficacy but also on the cost of preventing infection. Few cost-benefit analyses have been performed.

To justify use of prophylaxis for clean procedures at a single institution, an accurate assessment of infection rates must be available. This requires a considered effort at postdischarge follow-up. When these data are available, the risk-to-cost benefit ratio can be more knowledgeably assessed. Without accurate information on infection rates by procedure, known risk factors described above may serve as guides. Extremes of age, poor nutritional status, diabetes, and obesity are recognized as significant additional risk factors.

■ ANTIINFECTIVE PROPHYLAXIS FOR COLORECTAL OPERATION

Most surgeons in the United States provide an oral antibiotic bowel preparation such as neomycin plus erythromycin beginning the day before the operation. This has become more difficult because most patients now must receive their bowel preparation at home. The gastrointestinal side effects of the osmotic mechanical preparations now used complicate oral administration of antibiotics. Most surgeons in the United States also provide an intravenous regimen in the intraoperative period.

Recently, an extensive meta-analysis concluded that a single dose or short-term use of an antimicrobial agent is as efficacious as multiple doses. The review also found that there was no convincing evidence suggesting that second- and third-generation cephalosporins are more efficacious than the first two generation agents. No additional benefit was observed in six trials that compared parenteral antiinfectives alone with parenteral plus topical. Several trials showed extra benefit of oral antibiotics if inadequate parenteral antibiotics such as metronidazole alone or piperacillin alone were used. Oral or topical application of antibiotics in addition to the parenteral administration of appropriate antiinfectives is of no benefit. Antibiotics selected for prophylaxis in colorectal surgery should be active against both aerobic and anaerobic bacteria. Administration should be timed to make sure that the tissue concentration of antibiotics around the wound area is sufficiently high when bacterial contamination occurs. Guidelines should be developed locally to achieve a more cost-effective use of antimicrobial prophylaxis in colorectal surgery.

Suggested Reading

Dellinger EP, et al: Quality standard for antimicrobial prophylaxis in surgical procedures. Infectious Diseases Society of America, *Clin Infect Dis* 18:422, 1994.

Nichols RL, et al: Risk of infection after penetrating abdominal trauma, *N Engl J Med* 311:1065, 1984.

Platt R, et al: Prophylaxis against wound infection following herniorrhaphy or breast surgery, *J Infect Dis* 166:556, 1992.

Sheridan RL, Tompkins RG, Burke JF: Prophylactic antibiotics and their role in the prevention of surgical wound infection, *Adv Surg* 27:43, 1994.

Stellato TA, Danziger LH, Gordon N: Antibiotics in elective colon surgery. A randomized trial of oral, systemic, and oral/systemic antibiotics for prophylaxis, *Am Surg* 56:251, 1990.

Woods RK, Dellinger EP: Current guidelines for antibiotic prophylaxis of surgical wounds, *Am Fam Physician* 57:2731, 1998.

IMMUNIZATIONS

Elaine C. Jong

Long-lasting immunity against many serious infectious diseases can be elicited through active immunization, the administration of specific antigens (killed or attenuated microorganisms; purified polysaccharides, proteins, or other components; or recombinant antigens produced by genetic engineering) that stimulate the recipient host's production of protective antibodies. Vaccine doses may be given orally or administered by injection using intradermal, subcutaneous, or intramuscular routes. Passive immunization is the process by which protective immunity is obtained through transfer of performed antibodies from an immune host to a nonimmune recipient, either as immunoglobulin or antibody-specific immunoglobulin.

Protective efficacy resulting from active immunization with a vaccine depends on several factors: the age of the host, with decreased efficacy of certain vaccines observed in the very young and very old; the immune status of the host, with decreased efficacy observed in persons with compromised immune status because of disease or therapy; and the characteristics of the vaccine product itself.

In active immunization, protective levels of specific antibodies usually develop within 2 to 4 weeks on completion of the primary immunization regimen. The antibody response can be recalled and boosted when the immune system is challenged by additional "booster" doses of the vaccine antigen(s) or by exposure to the naturally occurring pathogen. Passive immunization can confer rapid protection, but serum levels of protective antibodies in recipients are highest immediately after receipt, decreasing with the passage of time, and there is no immune recall upon challenge.

Active or passive immunization may be used for preexposure protection against certain diseases, and in some cases, the two forms may be administered simultaneously at different sites. Tetanus, hepatitis A, hepatitis B, and rabies are examples of infections for which active and passive immunizations might be administered at the same time, usually after a high-risk exposure, to invoke rapid immunity as well as the longer-lasting antibody response.

Several different vaccines may be administered concomitantly at separate sites without decreased efficacy, although the timing and sequence of vaccines have to be taken into account. For example, when immunoglobulin is given for passive immunization against hepatitis A, antibodies against several common infections may be present in sufficient amounts to interfere with the response to certain other vaccines. Vaccines against measles, mumps, and rubella (MMR) and varicella may be given on the same day, but immunoglobulin should not be given for 3 months before or 3 weeks after MMR vaccine, and not for 2 months after varicella vaccine (chickenpox). However, vaccines against tetanus, diphtheria, yellow fever, typhoid fever, hepatitis B, rabies, and meningococcal meningitis can be given on the same day as immunoglobulin. If immunoglobulin is given on the same day as hepatitis A vaccine, the vaccine is still efficacious, although the resulting peak antibody titer is lower than when the vaccine is given alone.

The current standard of practice requires that potential vaccine recipients be informed of the potential benefits and adverse side effects of each vaccine. The Vaccine Information Statements (VISs) prepared by the national Immunization Action Coalition (IAC) can be downloaded and copies made for use in patient education from the Web site, http://www.immunize.org/vis/index.htm. All VISs are available in English and up to 17 additional languages. Tolerance to minor adverse effects associated with each vaccine and the potential for more serious vaccine-associated symptoms must also be taken into account in the person who is a candidate for multiple vaccine doses on the same day.

■ CHILDHOOD IMMUNIZATIONS

The routine immunizations recommended during childhood and adolescence prevent nine communicable diseases of public health importance: diphtheria, pertussis (whooping cough), tetanus, polio, *Haemophilus influenzae* type b, hepatitis B, measles, mumps, and rubella (German measles). Table 1 shows the immunization schedules for these diseases according to recommendations from the Centers for Disease Control and Prevention (CDC) Advisory Committee on Immunization Practices (ACIP) and the American Academy of Pediatrics. This table is available on the CDC Web site, http://www.cdc.gov.

New recommendations are emerging for the use of varicella virus (chickenpox) vaccine and hepatitis A virus vaccine, licensed in the United States in 1990s. Varicella vaccine is highly recommended at 12 months of age or older and can be integrated into the schedule of routine childhood immunizations. Varicella vaccine may be administered at the same time as the MMR vaccine. Both vaccines are injected live virus vaccines. If the two vaccines are not given simultaneously on the same day at different sites, the ACIP recommends that the vaccine doses be separated by 28 days if possible to reduce or eliminate possible interference of the vaccine given first with the vaccine given second.

Hepatitis A vaccine is recommended for children 24 months of age or older residing in certain areas within the United States where there is a high incidence of hepatitis A and also before international travel to countries where hepatitis A is highly endemic. In addition, the following groups of children ages 2 through 18 years are considered at high risk and should be immunized with hepatitis A vaccine: foster children, Native American and Alaskan Native, homeless, street teens, male teens who have sex with males, illicit drug users, and those with clotting factor disorders or chronic liver disease.

A consideration of meningococcal vaccine for college-bound students is now recommended following the autumn 1999 meeting of the ACIP, during which the results of two 1998 CDC studies were presented. Freshman dormitory

Table 1   Recommended Childhood Immunization Schedule[a]

VACCINE	BIRTH	2 MO	4 MO	6 MO	12[b] MO	15 MO	18 MO	4-6 YR	11-12 YR	14-16 YR
Hepatitis B[c]	HB-1	HB-2		HB-3						
Diphtheria-tetanus pertussis (DTP)[d]		DTP	DTP	DTP	DTP or DTaP at ≥ 15 mo			DTP or DTaP	Td	
Haemophilus influenzae type b (Hib)[e]		Hib	Hib	Hib	Hib					
Poliovirus		OPV	OPV	OPV				OPV		
Measles-mumps-rubella[f]					MMR			MMR or MMR		

From Advisory Committee on Immunization Practices, American Academy of Pediatrics, and American Academy of Family Physicians.

[a]Recommended vaccines are listed under the routinely recommended ages. Shaded bars indicate range of acceptable ages for vaccination. Although no changes have been made to this schedule since publication in *MMWR* (weekly) in January 1995, this table has been revised to more accurately reflect the recommendations.

[b]Vaccines recommended for administration at 12-15 months of age may be administered at either one or two visits.

[c]Infants born to hepatitis B surface antigen (HBsAg)-negative mothers should receive the second dose of hepatitis B vaccine between 1 and 4 months of age, provided at least 1 month has elapsed since receipt of the first dose. The third dose is recommended between 6 and 18 months of age. Infants born to HBsAg-positive mothers should receive immunoprophylaxis for hepatitis B with 0.5 ml hepatitis B immune globulin (HBIG) within 12 hours of birth, and 5 µg of either Merck, Shape, & Dohme (West Point, Pennsylvania) vaccine (Recombivax HB) or 10 µg of SmithKline Beecham (Philadelphia) vaccine (Engerix-B) at a separate site. For these infants, the second dose of vaccine is recommended at 1 month of age and the third dose at 6 months of age. All pregnant women should be screened for HBsAg during an early prenatal visit.

[d]The fourth dose of DTP may be administered as early as 12 months of age, provided at least 6 months have elapsed since the third dose of DTP. Combined DTP-Hib product may be used when these two vaccines are administered simultaneously. Diphtheria and tetanus toxoids and acellular pertussis vaccine (DTaP) is licensed for use for the fourth and/or fifth dose of DTP in children aged ≥15 months and may be preferred for these doses in children in this age group.

[e]Three *H. influenzae* type b conjugate vaccines are available for use in infants: (a) oligosaccharide conjugate Hib vaccine (HbOC) (HibTITER, manufactured by Praxis Biologics, Inc. [West Henrietta, New York] and distributed by Lederle-Praxis Biologicals [Wayne, New Jersey]); (b) polyribosylribitol phosphate–tetanus toxoid conjugate (PRP-T) (ActHIB, manufactured by Pasteur Mérieux Sérums & Vaccins, S.A. [Lyon, France] and distributed by Connaught Laboratories, Inc. [Swiftwater, Pennsylvania] and OmniHIB, manufactured by Pasteur Mérieux Sérums & Vaccins, S.A. and distributed by SmithKline Beecham) and (c) *Haemophilus* b conjugate vaccine (Meningococcal Protein Conjugate) (PRP-OMP) (PedvaxHIB, manufactured by Merck, Sharp, & Dohme). Children who have received PRP-OMP at 2 and 4 months of age do not require a dose at 6 months of age. After the primary infant Hib conjugate vaccine series is completed, any licensed Hib conjugate vaccine may be administered as a booster dose at age 12-15 months.

[f] The second dose of MMR vaccine should be administered EITHER at 4-6 years of age or at 11-12 years of age. Children who are HIV positive may receive MMR unless they are severely immunocompromised.

residents appear to be at threefold increased risk for meningococcal disease, relative to other persons their age. A single dose of the available polysaccharide vaccine offers protection against serogroups A, C, Y, and W-135. Although the vaccine does not cover serogroup B, approximately 70% of cases among college students in 1998 to 1999 in the United States were caused by serogroups C and Y. The primary immunization consists of a single dose given by injection subcutaneously and confers immunity for at least 3 years in persons 4 years of age and older. There is no official recommendation for booster doses.

Table 2 provides a summary of vaccine regimens and schedules. Consult the CDC Web site, http://www.cdc.gov, for additional details on the vaccines, indications, and dosing.

■ COMBINATION VACCINES

The number of recommended early childhood immunizations creates issues of compliance and scheduling for parents, patients, and health care providers. Depending on the use of existing combination vaccines and new vaccines presently under development, the number of immunization injections per clinic visit can be decreased. The approved use of vaccine combinations (different vaccines combined and administered through the same syringe) depends on efficacy and safety data from clinical trials. Several commercially prepared combination vaccines are available for pediatric use (Table 3), and in some cases, compatible vaccines from a single vaccine manufacturer supplier are available and may be combined according to package insert instructions. New combination vaccines include hepatitis A plus hepatitis B vaccine (Twinrix, SmithKline Beecham) available in Canada, with licensure in the United States anticipated in the near future.

■ ADULT IMMUNIZATIONS

Recommendations for adult immunizations are based on the history of immunizations received in the past and on the need to give booster doses of certain vaccine series where immunity has been shown to wane over a given period. A

Table 2   Vaccine Trade Names for Identification

VACCINE	TRADE NAME	MANUFACTURER
DIPHTHERIA, TETANUS, PERTUSSIS FOR PEDIATRIC USE		
DTP	DTP adsorbed	Connaught
DTP	Tri-Immunol adsorbed	Lederle
DTaP	Acel-immune	Lederle
DTaP	Infanrix	SmithKline Beecham
DTaP	Tripedia	Connaught
DTP-HbOC	Tetramune	Lederle
HAEMOPHILUS INFLUENZAE B		
HbOC	Hib TITER	Lederle
PRP-D	Pro-HIBIT	Connaught
PRP-OMP	PedvaxHIB	Merck
PRP-T*	ActHIB	Connaught
PRP-T†	OmniHIB	SmithKline Beecham
HEPATITIS A		
Hepatitis A	Havrix	SmithKline Beecham
Hepatitis A	Vaqta	Merck
HEPATITIS B		
Hepatitis B	Engerix-B	SmithKline Beecham
Hepatitis B	Recombivax HB	Merck
HUMAN IMMUNOGLOBULIN (INTRAMUSCULAR ROUTE)		
Immunoglobulin	Gammar	Armour
Immunoglobulin		Michigan Department of Public Health (1-517-335-8120)
INFLUENZA		
Influenza	Fluzone	Connaught
Influenza, trivalent, types A and B	FluShield	Wyeth-Ayerst
MEASLES, MUMPS, RUBELLA		
Measles	Attenuvax	Merck
Mumps	Mumpsvax	Merck
Rubella	Meruvax	Merck
Measles, Mumps	Biavax II	Merck
Measles, rubella	M-R-Vax II	Merck
Measles, mumps, rubella	M-M-R II	Merck
MENINGOCOCCUS		
Meningococcus	Menomune-A/C/Y/W-135	Connaught
PNEUMOCOCCUS		
Pneumococcus	Pneumovax 23	Merck
Pneumococcus	Pnu-Immune 23	Lederle
Poliovirus, inactivated, trivalent types 1, 2, 3	IPOL poliovirus	Connaught
Poliovirus, live oral, trivalent, types 1, 2, 3	Orimmune	Lederle
TETANUS, DIPHTHERIA (FOR ADULT USE)		
Tetanus	TE Anatoxal Berna	Berna
Tetanus	Tetanus toxoid adsorbed	Lederle
Tetanus	Tetanus toxoid adsorbed	Wyeth-Ayerst
Tetanus	Tetanus toxoid fluid	Wyeth-Ayerst
Td	Tetanus & diphtheria toxoids adsorbed	Connaught
Td	Tetanus & diphtheria toxoids adsorbed	Lederle
Td	Tetanus & diphtheria toxoids adsorbed	Wyeth-Ayerst
VARICELLA (CHICKENPOX)		
Varicella, live attenuated	Varivax	Merck

Td, Adsorbed tetanus and diphtheria toxoids.
*May be reconstituted with DTP vaccine (Connaught) in the same vial.
†ActHIB and OmniHIB are the same vaccine, manufactured by Pasteur Mérieux, and may be used interchangeably.

detailed review of immunizations is indicated for international travelers, health care workers, and others who have risks of exposure related to occupational activities, individuals 65 years of age and older, and persons with compromised immune status due to disease (human immunodeficiency virus [HIV]), medications, cancer, or other chronic medical conditions.

The adult immunization history should be updated, and documented at the time of initial intake into a primary care practice, during interim health maintenance visits, on em-

Table 3   Schedules for Routine Immunizations of Older Children and Adults

Hib	1 dose	≥15 mo of age or for splenectomized host
Influenza	1 dose	Annually, for indicated risk group.
MMR*	1 dose† SC at age 12-15 mo or older	Boost measles vaccine at 10-12 yr old routinely or give dose 2 at least 1 mo after first; second measles vaccine dose should be given before international travel for people born after 1956 and before 1980.
eIPV (killed vaccine, safe for all ages)	Doses† 1 and 2 SC or IM 4-8 wk apart; dose 3 6-12 mo after dose 2; give dose 4 children aged 4-6 yr	One lifetime booster, before travel in areas of risk.
OPV (attenuated live virus)*	Doses† 1 and 2 PO 6-8 wk apart; dose 3 6 wk-12 mo after dose 2; dose 4 to children 4-6 yr of age	One booster dose to people ≤18 yr old or to previously immunized adults 19 yr or older prior to travel in areas of risk.
Td (for persons over age 7)	3 doses (0.5 ml SC or IM), doses 1 and 2 4-8 wk apart, dose 3 6-12 mo later	Routine booster dose every 10 yr; booster dose after 5 yr for prophylaxis of a dirty wound.
Pneumococcus polysaccharide 23-valent	1 dose (0.5 ml SC or IM)	Consider booster dose at 3-5 yr for highest risk groups.
Varicella (chickenpox) (live attenuated virus)†	0.5 ml SC 12 mo-12 y of age; 2 doses (0.5 ml SC) 4-8 wk apart for persons at least 13 yr of age	May be given concurrently with measles, mumps, and rubella, using separate sites and syringes; may also be given with diphtheria, tetanus, and polio. Lower antivaricella titers when given concomitantly with DTaP or PedvaxHIB

Hib, Haemophilus influenzae type b; *MMR,* measles, mumps, and rubella; *eIPV,* enhanced, inactivated poliomyelitis; *OPV,* oral poliomyelitis; *Td,* adsorbed tetanus and diphtheria toxoids.
*Caution: may be contraindicated in patients with any of the following conditions: pregnancy, leukemia, lymphoma, generalized malignancy, immunosuppression due to human immunodeficiency virus infection or treatment with corticosteroids, alkylating drugs, antimetabolites or radiation therapy.
†See package insert for recommendations on dosage.

ployment in one of the health care or social services professions, and/or prior to international travel. Travel immunizations will be covered in the chapter *Advice for Travelers.* If the immunization history of the person is uncertain or unknown, a conceptual framework of the prevalent practices pertaining to childhood, school, military service, and occupational immunization programs and standards will be helpful for assessing the current immunization status.

■ ROUTINE IMMUNIZATIONS FOR ADULTS

Tetanus/Diphtheria Vaccine and Pertussis Vaccine

The primary series of tetanus and diphtheria vaccines are given in childhood, often as a part of the diphtheria/tetanus/ acellular pertussis (DTaP) vaccine series. A booster dose of the adult formulation of the tetanus/diphtheria (Td) vaccine should be used in persons 7 years of age or older, and booster doses should be given every 10 years throughout adult life.

Health Care Workers

Health care workers exposed to patients with confirmed pertussis infections may warrant antimicrobial prophylaxis and should consult the facility's infection control or occu-

pational health consultant. The use of an acellular pertussis vaccine among adults is currently under clinical investigation.

Measles, Mumps, and Rubella

The measles, mumps, and rubella vaccines are usually given as a combination vaccine (MMR) in early childhood, at 12 to 15 months of age. However, up to 5% of vaccine recipients may fail to respond to primary immunization and have inadequate or waning immunity to measles by adulthood. For this reason, the ACIP and AAP recommend that a second dose of measles vaccine (as a component of MMR) be given in childhood, on school entry. In many American colleges and universities, documentation of receipt of a second dose of measles vaccine or of immunity as evidenced by serum testing for measles antibodies is required for registration. There is no contraindication to using the MMR vaccine to boost measles immunity, even if the recipient is already immune to mumps and rubella. Monovalent measles and rubella vaccines are commercially available but are not commonly recommended or used in vaccine immunization programs.

Potential vaccine adverse reactions include the rare occurrence of usually transient but occasionally prolonged arthralgias and arthritis attributed to the rubella component of the MMR vaccine in nonimmune women of reproductive age—the very group most likely to benefit from immunization against rubella. As with any vaccine, the potential risks versus benefits of immunization with MMR vaccine should be discussed with potential vaccine recipients.

Contraindications
MMR vaccine is a live virus combination vaccine. Women of childbearing age should not be pregnant at the time of receiving MMR vaccine and should defer pregnancy for 3 months after MMR immunization.

HIV-Infected Persons
MMR immunization is recommended for use in susceptible persons with asymptomatic HIV infection, as the potential benefits of immunization appear to outweigh the serious course of natural measles infections in this population.

Health Care Workers
People born before 1957 were generally considered immune to measles, mumps, and rubella by virtue of having had the natural infectious diseases in the pre-MMR vaccine era. However, because a small percentage in this group did not acquire immunity through natural infection, health care workers at hospitals are required to have documentation of serum antibodies to measles and rubella and immunization with MMR if not immune prior to reporting to work.

Varicella Vaccine
Varicella (chicken pox) infections are more likely to result in severe disease, often accompanied by complications such as varicella pneumonia in adults than in children. A live attenuated viral vaccine against varicella (chickenpox) was released in the mid 1990s. The primary series for young people 12 years of age or older and adults consists of two doses given by injection 1 month apart, in contrast to the single dose of this vaccine used in pediatric populations younger than 12 years of age.

Contraindications
The vaccine is a live virus vaccine and is contraindicated in pregnant women. Women of childbearing age should not be pregnant at the time of receiving varicella vaccine and should defer pregnancy for 3 months after varicella immunization. Varicella vaccine is contraindicated in persons with compromised immunity, including individuals with HIV infection.

Health Care Workers
Current occupational health recommendations for health care workers include documentation of varicella immunity or varicella immunization as a condition for working in certain clinics and hospitals.

Polio Vaccine
Immunization against polio is a part of the childhood immunization program, and booster doses are not given routinely in adulthood in the Western Hemisphere (North and South America) and Western Europe, where polio is considered eradicated. Although current pediatric regimens include the use of a combination of the enhanced inactivated polio vaccine (IPV) administered by injection followed by doses of the live attenuated oral polio vaccine (OPV), or a regimen of all IPV doses, a single dose of IPV is recommended as a booster dose in adults.

Hepatitis B Vaccine
Hepatitis B immunization has been included as one of the regular immunizations covered by childhood immunization programs in the United States since 1991. Hepatitis B vaccine should be considered as a "catch-up" immunization among young adults born before the hepatitis B vaccine was incorporated into the routine childhood immunization programs. Hepatitis B immunization should also be recommended to individuals at risk of exposure to hepatitis B virus through occupational risk; treatment with blood products; contact with infected family, friends, or others; or international travel.

The primary series for hepatitis B immunization consists of three doses given by intramuscular injection into the deltoid muscle at 0, 1, and 6 months (Recombivax B, Merck; Engerix B, Smithkline Beecham). An accelerated schedule consisting of three doses of hepatitis B vaccine given at 0, 1, and 2 months, with a booster dose at 12 months has FDA approval (Engerix B).

Health Care Workers
Hepatitis B immunization or immunity is required for work in certain occupations, including health care workers, policemen, firemen, morticians, and others who are likely to have work-related contact with human blood and other bodily substances.

Pneumococcal Vaccine
Pneumococcal vaccine is recommended for all adults 65 years of age and older and for younger adults with chronic cardiopulmonary conditions or chronic diseases. A single dose given by injection of the purified polysaccharide 23-valent pneumococcal vaccine results in protective immunity. A booster dose after a 5-year interval may be recommended in geriatric populations. The release of a new conjugate pneumococcal vaccine is anticipated in the near future.

Viral Influenza Vaccine
The vaccine against viral influenza is reformulated annually based on the current worldwide epidemiology of influenza viruses. Thus annual immunization with the "flu" vaccine is recommended for persons 65 years of age and older, persons with cardiopulmonary conditions and debilitating diseases, and international travelers.

Because the flu vaccine distributed for a given season may not be totally protective against all strains of influenza viruses in circulation in the months following the annual flu vaccine formulation, medications against the flu may be considered in certain high-risk persons. Prophylaxis with or prompt initiation of treatment after onset of symptoms with amantidine (Symmetrel) or rimantidine (Flumadine) during outbreaks of influenza A, or with ambinovir (Relenza) during outbreaks of influenza A or B may prevent or ameliorate a breakthrough attack of the flu.

Hepatitis A Vaccine
The conditions allowing transmission of hepatitis A are ubiquitous, although the relative risk appears to be highest

in countries where sanitation and hygiene are suboptimal, and there is widespread fecal contamination of food and water supplies. In areas of low endemicity for hepatitis A (HAV), outbreaks of the disease are related to contamination of food during preparation by infected food handlers, and to ingestion of fresh or frozen fruits and vegetables imported from areas highly endemic for hepatitis A, contaminated during cultivation or processing. Shellfish from sewage-contaminated beds are another source of foodborne transmission.

In the United States, groups identified by the CDC as being at increased risk for hepatitis A or severe outcomes include travelers, men who have sex with men, users of injecting and noninjecting drugs, persons who have clotting-factor disorders, persons working with nonhuman primates, and persons with chronic liver disease.

Children can serve as a significant reservoir of HAV in outbreaks and in endemic communities. Hepatitis A infections are mild and often anicteric in young children, so infected children are not detected. Fecal-oral transmission to other children and family members, as well as adult teachers or caretakers can easily occur in household, day-care, and institutional settings, especially if children in diapers are present. It is important to note that HAV case fatality rates in healthy individuals rise with age, so although the rate is 0.1% from less than 1 to 14 years of age, it is 0.4% from 15 to 39 years of age, 1.1% in those older than 40 years of age, and 2.7% in persons older than 49 years of age.

Several safe and highly efficacious inactivated hepatitis A vaccines have become available commercially since the 1994 release of Havrix (Smithkline Beecham, Philadelphia, PA; Rixensart, Belgium), the first inactivated HAV vaccine, derived from the HM-175 viral strain, and given by injection. The others include VAQTA (Merck Vaccine Division, West Point, NJ), an inactivated parenteral HAV vaccine derived from the CR-326F strain; AVAXIM (Pasteur Merieux MSD, Paris), an inactivated parenteral HAV vaccine derived from the GBM viral strain; and Epaxal Berna (Swiss Serum Research Institute, Bern), an inactivated parenteral virosomal HAV vaccine derived from the RG-SB viral strain. Havrix and VAQTA are available in the United States and Canada, as well as worldwide. The other vaccines are distributed mostly in western Europe.

The immunization schedules for all the hepatitis A vaccines listed above consist of a single primary dose given by intramuscular (IM) injection into the deltoid muscle, resulting in protective antibody titers within 4 weeks that confer protection for 6 months up to 1 year. The first vaccine dose is followed by a booster dose 6 to 12 months later, producing levels of antibody predicted to give protection up to 10 years or more by mathematical modeling.

Vaccine interchangeability, that is, when one of the inactivated hepatitis A vaccines is used for the primary dose, and then a hepatitis A vaccine made by a different manufacturer is used for the booster dose, has been studied among several of the vaccines listed previously. Although not a recommended or officially approved practice at the time of writing, it appears from the preliminary results of clinical studies that Havrix and VAQTA may be used interchangeably without significant loss of protective antibody levels elicited (data on file, Merck Vaccine Division, West Point, NJ).

Immunoglobulin

Immunoglobulin (IG) purified human immunoglobulin is used to provide protection against hepatitis A virus infection through the passive transfer of preformed antibodies against HAV present in the IG (at least 100 IU/µl). IG is recommended for prevention of hepatitis A following known exposure to a confirmed case of HAV (0.02 ml/kg) and in nonimmune travelers going to HAV endemic areas when there is less than 2 weeks remaining before departure (0.02 ml/kg to 0.06 ml/kg).

Lyme Disease Vaccine

Most Lyme disease cases in the United States have been reported from the Northeast, upper Midwest, and Pacific Coastal areas, but infections have been reported in almost all states. Transmission of the infection from animal reservoirs (rodents and deer) to humans by *Borrelia burgdorferi*–infected *Ixodes* ticks may occur throughout the year and varies by region depending on local climactic conditions. Although residents of endemic areas who spend time outdoors in woodlands, meadows, or even grassy residential yards are at greatest risk of exposure, Lyme disease has been reported in travelers whose exposure consisted of vacationing in an endemic area and in field workers performing certain occupational activities.

A new vaccine against Lyme disease (LYMErix, SmithKline Beecham, Philadelphia) received FDA approval in 1999 and is a recombinant vaccine developed against the *B. burgdorferi* bacteria causing Lyme disease in North America. Lyme disease vaccine (recombinant OspA) contains the lipoprotein OspA, an outer surface protein of *B. burgdorferi* sensu stricto 257, as expressed by *Escherichia coli*.

The vaccine is recommended for individuals aged 15 to 70 years who anticipate exposure in endemic areas. The primary immunization series consists of a 30 µg/0.5 ml dose of the Lyme disease vaccine given at 0, 1, and 12 months as an IM injection into the deltoid area of the upper arm. The duration of protective immunity is not known. Vaccine efficacy against definite Lyme disease was 78% after the complete three-dose series, and 50% after the first two vaccine doses in a randomized, double-blind, multicentered, placebo-controlled trial conducted in highly endemic areas in the United States. An accelerating dosing schedule is pending completion of clinical studies and then approval of the FDA.

The Lyme disease vaccine is contraindicated in persons who have a history of hypersensitivity to any component of the vaccine (kanamycin or aminoglycoside antibiotics, tissue culture media components, aluminum hydroxide). Adverse side effects reported among vaccine recipients include injection site pain (<22%), and generalized "flulike" symptoms, joint and/or muscle aches, headache, fever, chills, rash, dizziness, and stiffness in less than 1%. Clinical studies on vaccine safety and efficacy in pediatric populations younger than 15 years old are currently being conducted. The safety of use in pregnant and lactating women is unknown. Immunization with the Lyme disease vaccine will result in a positive IgG ELISA test for anti-OspA antibodies. If Lyme disease is suspected in a vaccine recipient, Western blot testing is necessary for diagnostic confirmation.

■ SPECIAL CONSIDERATIONS

Attenuated live viral or bacterial vaccines are generally contraindicated for pregnant women and patients with compromised immunity. Exceptions are the recommendations for giving the MMR vaccine to children with HIV infection, and giving the yellow fever vaccine and oral polio vaccines to a pregnant woman traveler with imminent departure to a high-risk destination in a foreign country. In these cases, the theoretical risk of serious adverse vaccine complications may be outweighed by the anticipated benefits of vaccine-elicited protection.

Limited data suggest that administration of toxoid, killed virus, and purified derivative vaccines to HIV patients as appropriate may elicit protective immunity in the vaccine recipient if the CD4 count is greater than $200/mm^3$. An observed rise in viral loads in some HIV patients following vaccination has been of some concern, but the phenomenon is thought to be frequently transient. The current consensus is that a severe infection with a given vaccine-preventable pathogen is more likely to be associated with a more detrimental rise in viral load than that seen secondary to the corresponding immunization.

Annual doses of influenza vaccines are recommended for persons 65 years of age or older and for persons with cardiovascular or pulmonary disease. The vaccines against encapsulated bacteria (*H. influenzae* type b, pneumococcal, and meningococcal vaccines) are recommended for persons who have a history of functional asplenia or of splenectomy because of the risk of overwhelming sepsis associated with infections from these agents.

Vaccine efficacy can be affected by various conditions and therapies that lead to compromise of the immune system. In patients receiving hemodialysis, the suboptimal immune response to hepatitis A and B vaccines may necessitate higher-than-standard antigen doses, given as a special vaccine formulation or as additional doses after the standard series has been administered.

■ TRAVEL IMMUNIZATIONS

The patient seeking vaccine advice for international travel presents an opportunity to review and update routine immunizations as well as assess the risk of exposure to exotic diseases during the trip (see the chapter *Advice for Travelers*).

Suggested Reading

American College of Physicians: *Guide for adult immunization,* ed 3, Philadelphia, 1994, American College of Physicians.

Centers for Disease Control and Prevention: Diphtheria, tetanus, and pertussis: recommendations for vaccine use and other preventive measures. Recommendations of the Immunizations Practices Advisory Committee (ACIP), *MMWR* 40(RR-10):1, 1991.

Centers for Disease Control and Prevention: Hepatitis B virus: A comprehensive strategy for eliminating transmission in the United States through universal childhood vaccination: recommendations of the Immunization Practices Advisory Committee (ACIP), *MMWR* 40:1, 1991.

Centers for Disease Control and Prevention: Update on adult immunization: recommendations of the Immunization Practices Advisory Committee (ACIP), *MMWR* 40(RR-12):1, 1991.

Centers for Disease Control and Prevention: Pertussis vaccination: Acellular pertussis vaccine for reinforcing and booster use—supplementary ACIP statement. Recommendations of the Immunization Practices Advisory Committee (ACIP), *MMWR* 41(RR-1):1, 1992.

Centers for Disease Control and Prevention: Committee on Immunization Practices. Use of vaccines and immune globulins in persons with altered immunocompetence. *MMWR* 42(RR-4):1, 1993.

Centers for Disease Control and Prevention: Standards for pediatric immunization practices recommended by the National Vaccine Advisory Committee, approved by the U.S. Public Health Service. *MMWR* 42(RR-5):1, 1993.

Centers for Disease Control and Prevention: Prevention of hepatitis A through active or passive immunization. Recommendations of the Advisory Committee on Immunization Practices (ACIP), *MMWR* 48(RR-12):1, 1999.

Jong EC, McMullen R: *The travel and tropical medicine manual,* ed 2, Philadelphia, eds: 1995, WB Saunders.

ADVICE FOR TRAVELERS

Phyllis E. Kozarsky

Jay S. Keystone

Studies show that 50% to 75% of short-term travelers to the tropics or subtropics develop some health impairment. Fortunately, most problems are minor, with only 5% requiring medical attention and fewer than 1% requiring hospitalization. Valuable sources of information for travel health advisers are found in Table 1.

All travelers should be encouraged to carry a travel health kit, which should always remain with the traveler and never be stowed with baggage (Table 2).

■ IMMUNIZATIONS

Immunizations may be divided into those of worldwide importance and those of special importance to certain travelers. Those of worldwide importance should be considered by physicians not only for travelers but also the for the general public who are at risk. Examples of those having worldwide importance include diphtheria; tetanus; polio; measles, mumps, and rubella (MMR); influenza; pneumococcus; and hepatitis B vaccines (see the chapter *Immunizations*). Immunizations of special importance for certain travelers include yellow fever, typhoid, cholera, rabies, meningococcal meningitis, Japanese B encephalitis, and hepatitis A. Two vaccines rarely indicated are plague and tickborne encephalitis, the latter of which is not available in the United States. Immunizations should always be recommended according to risk of disease and not according to the country visited.

Most vaccines may be administered simultaneously. A notable exception is measles vaccine, which should be administered at least 2 weeks before or 6 weeks after the receipt of immunoglobulin for hepatitis A protection. In addition, if measles and yellow fever vaccines are not administered simultaneously, they should be separated by an interval of at least 30 days. When both cholera and yellow fever vaccines are indicated, antibody levels have been highest when their administration was separated by at least 3 weeks. Table 3 lists the immunizations of special importance and their schedules.

Immunizations of Worldwide Importance
Diphtheria and Tetanus
Diphtheria continues to be a problem worldwide, with recent outbreaks affecting areas in eastern and northern Europe. Serosurveys have shown that tetanus titers are lacking in many Americans, particularly in women and in adults older than 50. A diphtheria-tetanus booster should be administered at 10-year intervals. Physicians may encourage frequent high-risk travelers to receive a tetanus booster alone every 5 years because a tetanus-prone wound does not necessitate a booster, or tetanus immunoglobulin if tetanus toxoid has been given within 5 years.

Polio
Studies in the United States have found varying levels of immunity to polio in the general population, with recent data revealing 12% of adult American travelers unprotected against at least one serogroup. The Centers for Disease Control and Prevention (CDC) recommends that all adults complete a primary series if they have never received one and also receive a booster dose of polio vaccine once only before travel to an endemic area. If time permits, infants and children younger than 2 years of age should receive at least three doses of polio vaccine. Intervals between doses may be reduced to 4 weeks to maximize immunization status before departure.

Countries considered free of endemic wild poliovirus circulation are the United States, Canada, Japan, Australia, New Zealand, and most of eastern and western Europe. The western hemisphere has been declared polio free; there have been no reported cases of paralytic disease caused by wild poliovirus in the Americas in several years.

Table 1   Sources of Information for Travel Health Advisers

Health Information for International Travel. Published by the U.S. Department of Health and Human Services (CDC) 1999-2000. Available to health care professionals through the Public Health Foundation website: www.phf.org/. An updated book reviewing malaria chemoprophylaxis, immunization requirements, and recommendations for international travel.

Centers for Disease Control and Prevention Voice Information System, Atlanta. A computer-assisted telephone information hotline for worldwide travel health advice. Telephone 877-394-8747; fax 888-232-3299. Web site: www.cdc.gov.

International Association for Medical Assistance to Travelers (IAMAT), 736 Center Street, Lewiston, NY 14092. Telephone 716-754-4883. Provides information on tropical diseases, climate charts, list of English-speaking physicians.

Travel Medicine Advisor. Published by American Health Consultants, Atlanta, GA. This comprehensive looseleaf text, continually revised, provides bimonthly updates and alerts. Telephone 404-262-7436.

Health Hints for the Tropics, 12th Edition, 1998. Published by the American Society of Tropical Medicine and Hygiene (ASTM&H) and written by several of its members. Authoritative source of information for the travel health adviser and for the traveler. Available from ASTM&H Headquarters, 60 Revere Drive, Suite 500, Northbrook, IL 60062. Telephone 847-480-9592; fax 847-480-9282.

International Society of Travel Medicine (ISTM). An association of travel health advisers. The ISTM sponsors biennial meetings. Members receive a quarterly journal and newsletter. For information, fax to 770-736-6732 or visit their Web site: www.istm.org.

Shoreland, Inc. Company providing multimedia tools for travel health advisors and for corporations. Telephone 800-433-5256; Web site: www.shoreland.com.

Rose S: *International travel health guide,* ed 10, Travel Medicine, Inc. 800-872-8633 or through their website: www.travmed. com. Annually updated travel health book for health care workers and the public.

Measles, Mumps, and Rubella

Measles continues to be a major cause of morbidity and mortality in the developing world. Outbreaks of measles in the United States have been linked to cases of imported measles. In the 1980s, it was estimated that over 25% of cases of measles in the United States could be attributed directly or epidemiologically to importations. Because the rate of primary failure with the vaccine was somewhat greater in persons born after 1956 and vaccinated before 1980, the CDC recommends that travelers in this group be revaccinated. A recent serosurvey found that almost 10% of American travelers born after 1956 were seronegative for measles. Immunization may be given at 6 months of age if necessary for travel, followed by a booster injection at 15 months.

Mumps and rubella are less of a health threat to travelers, though both diseases may have serious complications. A report of aseptic meningitis caused by mumps in an American returning from Kenya and reports of rubella outbreaks in the late 1980s in the Pacific reawaken the need to consider protection for all travelers against these illnesses.

Pneumococcus and Influenza

The pneumococcus and influenza vaccines should be administered to those at risk for severe illness from these infections. Bear in mind that influenza may occur year round, depending on the traveler's destination, and that the largest travel-related outbreak of influenza occurred in the "nonflu" season of late summer in Alaska and the Canadian Yukon in 1998.

Hepatitis B

Hepatitis B vaccine has typically been reserved for persons such as health care workers in contact with blood or body fluid secretions in developing countries and for long-term travelers to countries with a high prevalence of infection. Ideally, however, everyone should be immunized against this most important cause of acute and chronic liver disease. In Asia and Africa, up to 20% of children and adults are

---

Table 2   Travel Health Kit
Usual prescription drugs
Aspirin (Tylenol, NSAID)
Bismuth subsalicylate
Sunscreen
Antihistamine, decongestant
Insect repellent
Rehydration solution packets
Steroid cream
Loperamide
Codeine tablets
Mild sedative
High-altitude sickness prophylaxis
Antimalarial chemoprophylaxis
Digital thermometer
Bandages, gauze, adhesive
Antiseptic solution
Antacid
Anti–motion sickness medication
Laxative
Cough preparation
Topical antifungal, antibacterial cream or ointment
Antibiotic for self-treatment of travelers' diarrhea

NSAID, Nonsteroidal antiinflammatory drug.

Table 3   Immunizations for Foreign Travel

VACCINE	ADULT DOSAGE	DURATION OF EFFICACY
LIVE ATTENUATED		
Yellow fever	1 (0.5 ml) SC 10 days to 10 yr before travel	Booster q10yr
Typhoid	1 enteric-coated capsule taken on alternate days for 4 doses with cool liquid 1 hr before a meal	Booster series q5yr
INACTIVATED		
Typhoid	1 dose (0.5 ml) IM	Booster q2yr
Cholera	2 doses (0.5 ml) SC or IM 1 wk to 1 mo or more apart and at least 6 days before travel	Booster q6mo
Rabies preexposure* (HDCV, RVA, or PCEC)	3 doses (1.0 ml) IM (deltoid) on days 0, 7, and 21 or 28 (HDCV may be administered ID 0.1 ml days 0, 7, and 21 or 28)	1 dose (1 ml) IM (deltoid)† (or HDCV 0.1 ml ID) q2yr
Meningococcal (quadrivalent A/C/Y/W-135)	1 dose (0.5 ml) SC	Duration of immunity unknown; booster recommended q3yr
Japanese B encephalitis	3 doses (1 ml) SC days 0, 7, 30	Duration of immunity unknown; booster recommended at 3 yr
Hepatitis A	2 doses, at 0 and 6-12 mo	Unknown
PASSIVE PROPHYLAXIS		
Immunoglobulin for protection against hepatitis A	0.02 ml/kg for travel <3 mo 0.04 ml/kg for travel 4-6 mo	Repeat dose q4-6mo

SC, Subcutaneous; *IM,* intramuscular; *HDCV,* human diploid cell vaccine; *ID,* intradermal.
*If traveler is taking chloroquine or mefloquine for malaria chemoprophylaxis, the series must be completed before initiation of antimalarial treatment. If not possible, IM dosing must be used.
†If risk is high and continuous, serology should be checked every 6 mo. Acceptable antibody level is ≥1.5 titer by rapid fluorescent focus inhibition test.

hepatitis B carriers. As of November 1991, the vaccine has been recommended in the United States for all infants. A combined hepatitis A and B vaccine will become available in the United States in 2000.

Immunizations of Special Importance for the Traveler

Yellow Fever

Yellow fever is a viral illness transmitted by mosquitoes in tropical Africa and South America. It is rare in travelers, but because of its high mortality, individuals journeying to endemic areas require protection. Some countries require evidence of vaccination from all entering travelers and even from individuals whose destination is a noninfected area but who will be crossing the yellow fever zone. The vaccine can be administered only at an approved yellow fever vaccination center. State and local health departments may administer the vaccine or can advise where it can be obtained. Documentation of yellow fever vaccination should be placed on the International Certificate of Vaccination card, which may be obtained from any U.S. government bookstore, and which should be carried with the passport. Individuals for whom the vaccine is contraindicated must carry a waiver on a physician's letterhead to prevent the possibility of requiring an injection at a border.

Typhoid

Though *Salmonella typhi* is prevalent in many countries in Africa, Asia, and Central and South America, typhoid fever is not common in travelers. The oral Ty21a (Berna) vaccine, or the injectible Vi polysaccharide (Pasteur Mérieux) vaccine, the products of choice, should be used by travelers to endemic areas who are going off tourist routes or who are particularly adventuresome with regard to their food and beverage intake. In addition, long-term and frequent short-term travelers to developing countries should receive vaccine.

Cholera

Cholera is caused by ingestion of food or beverage contaminated with *Vibrio cholera,* an organism found in raw sewage. The risk of cholera to travelers is extremely low, estimated to be about 1 case per 500,000 journeys to endemic regions. Most cases occur in travelers returning from visits to family, relatives, and friends in endemic countries. These groups tend to have a greater likelihood of dietary indiscretion. Drinking safe beverages and eating well-cooked food, especially seafood, is the best prevention.

The vaccine, available in the United States, requires two injections for a maximum protection of 30% to 50% for only 3 to 6 months. Because of its poor efficacy, the vaccine is not cost effective for most travelers, even those who will be in endemic areas for long periods. Those for whom the vaccine may be appropriate are those living and working in an epidemic, travelers with achlorhydria, and those who have had a gastrectomy. A new live oral vaccine with greater efficacy is available in parts of Western Europe and Canada.

Rabies

The preexposure rabies vaccine series should be administered to those spending more than 30 days where rabies is a constant threat. The risk is highest where dog rabies is highly endemic, such as Mexico, El Salvador, Guatemala, Peru, Colombia, Ecuador, India, Nepal, the Philippines, Sri Lanka, Thailand, and Vietnam. Of the 20 cases reported in the United States between 1980 and 1997, 12 were acquired outside the country. Travelers should avoid contact with domestic animals and, if bitten, should wash the wound immediately with soap and water and seek medical care. Even if a preexposure rabies series has been administered, postexposure prophylaxis with rabies immunoglobulin and vaccine must be given. For assistance with problems or questions, contact your health department or the Division of Viral and Rickettsial Diseases of the CDC at 404-639-1075.

Meningococcal Meningitis

The meningococcal meningitis vaccine is very protective against disease due to *Neisseria meningitis* serogroups A, C, Y, and W-135. The vaccine is recommended for long-term travelers to the meningitis belt in sub-Saharan Africa and for short-term travelers during the dry season. It is also recommended for travelers to areas where outbreaks have occurred in the past decade and is required for those attending the Haj.

Japanese Encephalitis

Japanese encephalitis (JE) occurs in Asia during the summer and autumn in temperate regions and primarily during the rainy season in the tropics. It is transmitted by night-biting mosquitoes in rural rice-growing, pig-farming areas. Most infections are asymptomatic, but those who do develop clinical illness have a high mortality and 50% or greater likelihood of neurologic sequelae. Since 1981, 11 U.S. residents have been infected, eight of whom were military personnel or their dependents. The risk of JE is about 1 per 5000 per month of rural travel in endemic areas. The risk to short-term urban travelers is quite low. Adventuresome travelers to rural areas and long-term travelers are at greatest risk and should therefore consider immunization.

Hepatitis A and Immunoglobulin

Hepatitis A is the most common immunizable infection in travelers. In contrast to other serious foodborne illnesses, many travel-related cases have occurred with standard tourist itineraries. In fact, the estimated incidence of symptomatic hepatitis A in travelers to the developing world per month of stay abroad is as high as 20 per 1,000 in some destinations. The hepatitis A vaccine is available in the United States and is strongly recommended for all travelers. Immunoglobulin is less available and protects immediately, but only for short duration. It is important to recognize that the mortality from hepatitis A increases with age, and approaches 3% in those older than 50.

Malaria

For prevention of malaria, see the chapter *Malaria.*

Travelers' Diarrhea

Prevention of diarrhea requires careful selection of food and beverages while traveling in the developing world. Foods that are well cooked and still hot or steaming are safest. Fruits peeled by the traveler are safe. Because vegetables such as lettuce and tomatoes grow in areas where human fertilizer may be used and because they cannot be peeled, salads should be avoided unless washed carefully with purified water. Commercially bottled carbonated beverages, alcohol, hot tea, and coffee are also safe. The purity of plain bottled water is not regulated, so this is best avoided. Ice cubes should also be avoided because they are often made with tap water. Milk and dairy products should be pasteurized, cooked, or avoided. Disinfection requires brief boiling or the use of halogens (e.g., chlorine, iodine), although the protozoan cysts of *Giardia lamblia* and *Entamoeba histolytica* are resistant to the latter. Many inexpensive portable purifiers that contain effective iodination are available from camping stores.

Prophylaxis of diarrhea with a daily dose of a quinolone antibiotic (e.g., 500 mg ciprofloxacin) may be appropriate for few short-term travelers who are at very high risk of illness or of serious complications of diarrhea. For more detail, see the chapter *Travelers' Diarrhea.*

Schistosomiasis

Schistosomiasis is caused by infection with a blood fluke, *Schistosoma mansoni, Schistosoma haematobium,* or *Schistosoma japonicum,* which in one part of its life cycle can penetrate the human skin without causing symptoms. A subacute illness similar to serum sickness may occur about 6 weeks after exposure, and chronic problems such as portal hypertension, urinary obstruction, and bladder cancer may result. In recent years, reports of American travelers contracting schistosomiasis and developing unusual central nervous system findings such as transverse myelitis from aberrant egg deposition have heightened the awareness of this disease. Travelers to endemic areas put themselves at risk when they wade, swim, or bathe in freshwater lakes, streams, or rivers containing the reservoir snails.

If exposure to possibly infected water sources is unavoidable, towel-drying the skin immediately after contact may be protective. Screening for exposure involves a serologic test best performed by the Division of Parasitic Diseases at the CDC.

■ MISCELLANEOUS CONSIDERATIONS

The traveler infected with human immunodeficiency virus (HIV) confronts several potential problems. The live oral polio vaccine is generally contraindicated because of the theoretic risk of infection from the vaccine strains of these viruses. The enhanced inactivated polio vaccine may be substituted. A physician may give a waiver if the yellow fever vaccine is required by the destination, but if the traveler will be in an area of high endemicity and if he or she is asymptomatic with a CD_4 lymphocyte above $200/mm^3$, it may be reasonable to give the vaccine. When it was inadvertently administered to HIV-infected military personnel, no adverse events occurred. The new inactivated typhoid vaccine may be used if *Salmonella typhi* exposure is a possibility. Bacillus Calmette-Guérin (BCG) is contraindicated because of the possibility of disseminated disease. Protection against measles is important, and thus immunization with MMR should be considered, although complications have been reported. Some countries have regulations preventing the entry of HIV-infected individuals, including tourists.

Even the most experienced travelers suffer jet lag. It is estimated that the body takes about 1 day to adjust for each time zone crossed. Adequate hydration while traveling, resting after arrival, and judicious use of short-acting benzodiazepines assist the adjustment. Many other maneuvers may be helpful as well. Bright light can reset the internal clock. For travel eastward, it is recommended that travelers seek bright light in the early morning, and for westward travel, they should be in bright light in the late afternoon. Artificial light sources with the appropriate lux intensity may also be used. The use of melatonin is controversial. Melatonin tablets available in health food stores may not contain standardized amount of hormone and therefore cannot be recommended.

With more children, senior citizens, and disabled persons traveling, it is becoming more important to consider the ability of the traveler to withstand the environment and special challenges that destinations offer. For example, travel involving high altitude, difficult terrain, scuba diving, and even commercial flying may be inappropriate for those who have certain underlying medical problems or who may not be fully prepared for hardships they could encounter. For in-depth counseling and/or evaluation, a travel health specialist should be consulted.

Suggested Reading

Centers for Disease Control and Prevention: *Health information for international travel* 1999-2000, 1999, DHHS. Atlanta.

Freedman D, ed: Travel medicine, *Infect Dis Clin North Am* 12:2, 1998.

Lobel H, Kozarsky P: Update on prevention of malaria for travelers, *JAMA* 278:1767, 1997.

Human rabies prevention—United States, *MMWR* 48(RR1):6, January 8, 1999.

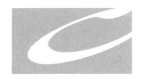

SPECIFIC PATHOGENS AND INFECTIONS

ACTINOMYCOSIS

Thomas A. Russo

■ ETIOLOGIC AGENTS

Actinomycosis is an infectious syndrome caused by anaerobic or microaerophilic bacteria, primarily from the genus *Actinomyces*. It is most commonly caused by *Actinomyces israelii;* however, *A. naeslundii, A. odontolyticus, A. viscosus, A. meyeri, A. gerencseriae,* and *Propionibacterium propionicum* are less common causes of infection. Nearly all of actinomycotic infections are polymicrobial. *Actinobacillus actinomycetemcomitans, Eikenella corrodens, Fusobacterium, Bacteroides, Capnocytopaga, Staphylococcus, Streptococcus,* and *Enterobacteriaceae* are commonly coisolated ("companion organisms") with the agents of actinomycosis in various combinations, depending on the site of the infection. Recently, a variety of bacterial species isolated from human clinical specimens have been reclassified as *Actinomyces* (e.g., *A. europaeus, A. radingae, A. turicensis, A. neuii*). Although their role in disease has not always been defined, these bacteria appear to be uncommon and often opportunistic human pathogens. However, the nature of infections described to date do not clearly establish them as causes of the typical syndrome of actinomycosis, and as a result, the more intensive treatment regimens needed to cure actinomycosis are probably not necessary (see the following).

■ EPIDEMIOLOGY AND PATHOGENESIS

The etiologic agents of actinomycosis are members of the normal oral flora and are often present in bronchi and the gastrointestinal and female genital tracts. Disruption of the mucosal barrier is the critical step for the development of actinomycosis. Subsequently, local infection may ensue and once established, if untreated, spreads contiguously, ignoring tissue planes, in a slow, progressive manner. Although acute inflammation may initially occur at the site of infection, the hallmark of actinomycosis is the characteristic chronic, indolent phase. This stage is manifested by lesions that usually appear as single or multiple indurations. Central necrosis develops, which consists of neutrophils and sulfur granules (a characteristic finding diagnostic in this disease). The walls of the mass are fibrotic and characteristically described as "wooden." Over time, sinus tracts to the skin, adjacent organs, or bone may develop. Rarely, distant hematogenous seeding occurs. Foreign bodies appear to facilitate infection. This occurs most often with intrauterine devices. The contribution of the non-*Actinomyces* coisolates or "companion organisms" to the pathogenesis of actinomycosis is uncertain.

■ INFECTIOUS SYNDROMES

Clinical presentations are myriad. Once common in the preantibiotic era, today the incidence of actinomycosis is diminished, and as a result, so is its timely recognition. It has been called "the most misdiagnosed disease," and it has been stated that "no disease is so often missed by experienced clinicians." Actinomycosis remains a diagnostic challenge. An awareness of the full spectrum of disease will expedite diagnosis and treatment and minimize unnecessary surgical interventions and the morbidity and mortality that all too often occurs with this disease. Three clinical presentations in particular warrant consideration of this unique infection. The combination of chronicity, progression across tissue boundaries, and masslike features mimics malignancy, with which it is often confused. Second, cure of established actinomycosis requires prolonged treatment. Short courses of therapy with active agents usually result in only transient improvement. Therefore actinomycosis should be thought of with refractory or relapsing infections. Last, development of a sinus tract, which may spontaneously resolve and recur, should prompt consideration of this disease.

Oral-Cervicofacial Disease

This is the most common site for infection. The usual presentation is a soft-tissue swelling, abscess, or mass lesion, which is often mistaken for a neoplasm. The angle of the jaw is the most common location, but actinomycosis should be considered with any mass lesion or relapsing infection in the head and neck. Rarely, otitis, sinusitis, and canniculitis can also occur. Pain, fever, and leukocytosis are variably present. Contiguous spread to the cranium, cervical spine, or the thorax and the attendant complications are potential sequelae.

Thoracic Disease

The usual presentation is an indolent, progressive course that involves the pulmonary parenchyma and/or the pleural space. Chest pain, fever, and weight loss are common. A cough, when present, is variably productive. The most common radiographic appearance is either a mass lesion or pneumonitis. Cavitary disease or hilar adenopathy may develop. Many cases have pleural thickening, effusion, or empyema. Pulmonary disease that crosses fissures or pleura; involves the mediastinum, contiguous bone, or the chest wall; or is associated with a sinus tract should suggest actinomycosis. Mediastinal infection is uncommon. The structures within the mediastinum and the heart, including heart valves, can be involved in various combinations, resulting in a variety of presentations. Isolated disease of the breast occurs rarely.

Abdominal Disease

Abdominal actinomycosis is often unrecognized. Months to years usually pass from the inciting event (e.g., appendicitis, diverticulitis, peptic ulcer disease, foreign body perforation, bowel surgery, or ascension from intrauterine contraceptive devices [IUCD] associated pelvic disease) to diagnosis. Because of the flow of peritoneal fluid, and/or direct extension of primary disease, virtually any abdominal organ, region, or space can be involved. The usual presentation is either an abscess or a mass lesion that is often fixed to underlying tissue and mistaken for a tumor. Sinus tracts to the abdominal wall or perianal region may develop. Hepatic infection usually presents as single or multiple abscesses or masses. Isolated disease is presumably via hematogenous seeding from cryptic foci. All levels of the urogenital tract can be infected. Bladder involvement, usually resulting from extension of pelvic disease, may result in obstruction or fistulas to bowel, skin, or uterus. Renal disease usually presents as pyelonephritis and/or renal and perinephric abscess.

Pelvic Disease

Actinomycotic involvement of the pelvis is strongly associated with IUCDs. Although the magnitude of risk is unclear, it would appear to be small. Disease rarely occurs when an IUCD has been in place for less than 1 year; however, the risk of infection increases with time and is often seen in the setting of the "forgotten" IUCD. Symptoms are typically indolent, with fever, weight loss, abdominal pain, and abnormal vaginal bleeding or discharge being most common. Endometritis, if untreated, may progress to a pelvic mass or a tuboovarian abscess. Unfortunately, diagnosis is often delayed, and a "frozen pelvis" mimicking malignancy or endometriosis will develop by the time of recognition.

Central Nervous System

Central nervous system infection is rare. Single or multiple brain abscesses are most common, usually appearing on computed tomography (CT) as a ring-enhancing lesion with a thick wall that may be irregular or nodular.

Musculoskeletal Infection

Osteomyelitis is usually caused by adjacent soft-tissue infection but may be associated with trauma (e.g., fracture of the mandible) or hematogenous spread. The uncommon infection of the extremities is usually a result of trauma. Skin, subcutaneous tissue, muscle, and bone are involved alone or in various combinations. Cutaneous sinus tracts often develop.

Disseminated Disease

Hematogenous spread of infection from any location may rarely result in multiorgan involvement, with the lungs and liver most commonly affected. The presentation of multiple nodules may mimic disseminated malignancy.

■ DIAGNOSIS

The diagnosis of actinomycosis is rarely considered. Most often, the first mention of actinomycosis is from the pathologist after extensive surgery. Because medical therapy alone is often sufficient for cure, the challenge for the clinician is to consider actinomycosis so that this uncommon and unusual infection can be diagnosed in the least invasive fashion and unnecessary surgery can be avoided. CT-guided or ultrasound-guided aspirations or biopsies are being successfully used to obtain clinical material for diagnosis, although surgery may be required. The diagnosis is most commonly made by microscopic identification of sulfur granules (an in vivo matrix of bacteria and host material) in pus or tissues, although occasionally sulfur granules can be grossly identified from draining sinus tracts or pus. Microbiologic identification is less common because of either prior antimicrobial therapy or omission. To optimize yield, the avoidance of even a single dose of antibiotics is mandatory. Because these organisms are normal oral and genital tract flora, their identification in the absence of sulfur granules, from sputum, bronchial washings, and cervicovaginal secretions is of little significance.

■ TREATMENT

Antimicrobial Therapy

Controlled trials evaluating either antimicrobials or studies designed to define duration of therapy in the treatment of actinomycosis have not been performed and will never be done. Therefore treatment decisions are primarily based on the collective clinical experience of the last 50 years. Two principles of therapy have evolved. It is necessary to treat this disease both with high dosages and for a prolonged period. Presumably this is because of the difficulties of antimicrobials penetrating the thick-walled masses that commonly occur with this infection and/or the sulfur granules themselves.

Although therapy should always be individualized, 18 to 24 million units of penicillin intravenously (IV) for 2 to 6 weeks, followed by oral therapy with penicillin or amoxicillin for 6 to 12 months, is a reasonable guideline. Cases with less extensive disease, particularly in the head and neck region, may require less intensive therapy. If the duration of therapy is extended beyond the resolution of measurable disease, relapses, one of the clinical hallmarks of this infection, will be minimized. CT and magnetic resonance imaging (MRI) studies are generally the most objective modalities to accomplish this goal. MRI scans are often more sensitive than CT scans for detecting residual infection and should be used if possible, particularly in areas where the consequences of relapse are particularly significant (e.g., central nervous system). For penicillin-allergic patients, tetracycline has been used most extensively with success. Erythromycin, doxycycline, and clindamycin are other suitable alternatives (Table 1). In the pregnant, penicillin-sensitive patient, erythromycin is a safe alternative. Remarkably, little clinical information is available on the newer antimicrobial agents. Anecdotal successes have been reported with imipenem, ceftriaxone, and ciprofloxacin. Available data suggest that oxacillin, dicloxacillin, cephalexin, metronidazole, and aminoglycosides should be avoided (see Table 1).

Home Therapy

For home IV therapy, the ease of once-a-day dosing makes ceftriaxone appealing in certain circumstances; however, a greater body of literature; supporting its efficacy would be desirable. The availability of portable infusion pumps for home therapy allows for both the appropriate dosing and practical administration of IV penicillin. For infections in critical sites (e.g., central nervous system) this approach remains the safest until more information is available on other agents. The pharmacokinetic properties, availability of oral and parenteral formulations, and potential efficacy of

---

Table 1   Antibiotic Therapy for Actinomycosis*

ANTIMICROBIAL
GROUP 1: EXTENSIVE SUCCESSFUL CLINICAL EXPERIENCE†
Penicillin (18-24 million units/day IV q4h or 1-2 g/day PO q6h)
Erythromycin (2-4 g/day IV q6h or 1-2 g/day PO q6h)
Tetracycline (1-2 g/day PO q6h)
Doxycycline (200 mg/day IV or PO q12-24h)
Minocycline (200 mg/day IV or PO q12h)
Clindamycin (2.7 g/day IV q8h or 1.2-1.8 g/day PO q6-8h)
GROUP 2: ANECDOTAL SUCCESSFUL CLINICAL EXPERIENCE
Ceftriaxone (1-4 g/day IV/IM q12-24h)
Ceftizoxime (2-12 g/day IV/IM q8-12h)
Imipenem (2 g/day IV q6h)
Ciprofloxacin (800-1200 mg/day IV q12h)
GROUP 3: AGENTS THAT SHOULD BE AVOIDED
Metronidazole
Aminoglycosides
Oxacillin
Dicloxacillin
Cephalexin

*Additional coverage for concomitant "companion" bacteria may be required.
†Controlled evaluations have not been performed. Dosing regimens need individualization depending on the site and extent of infection. In general, a maximum antimicrobial dose for 2 to 6 weeks of parenteral therapy followed by oral therapy for a total duration (6 to 12 months) is required for most infections.

---

azithromycin make it appealing. Unfortunately, little in vitro and no clinical data exist on their use to treat actinomycosis.

Treatment of Coisolates

It is unclear whether other bacteria frequently coisolated with the etiologic agents of actinomycosis require treatment; however, many of them are pathogens in their own right. Designing a therapeutic regimen that includes coverage for these organisms during the initial treatment course is reasonable. If microbiology is not available, it is important to consider the site of infection when designing empiric coverage. For example, *Actinobacillus actinomycetemcomitans, Eikenella corrodens, Fusobacterium,* and *Capnocytopaga* are more likely to be coisolates in head and neck infection, whereas the Enterobacteriaceae are more commonly coisolated in abdominal infection.

Surgery or Percutaneous Drainage

In the preantibiotic era, surgical removal of infected tissue was the only beneficial treatment. Despite the availability of effective antimicrobial therapy, combined surgical therapy is still advocated by some authorities. However, an increasing body of literature now supports the approach of initially attempting a cure with medical therapy alone. Successes have been reported in cases of extensive disease that initially appeared to be incurable using antibiotics alone. CT and MRI should be used to monitor the response to therapy. In most cases, either surgery can be avoided or a less extensive procedure will be necessary. This approach is particularly important when the possibility of sparing critical organs is involved, such as the bladder or reproductive organs in women of childbearing age. In a patient with disease in a critical location (e.g., epidural space, selected central nervous system disease) or if suitable medical therapy fails, surgical intervention may be appropriate.

In the setting of actinomycosis presenting as a well-defined abscess, percutaneous drainage in combination with medical therapy is a reasonable approach.

Treatment of the Immunocompromised Host

It is unclear which host defense components are most critical in affording protection against actinomycosis and whether certain hosts are more susceptible to infection. Actinomycosis has been described in association with human immunodeficiency virus (HIV) infection, steroid use, and lymphoproliferative tumors. Whether these infections were caused by disease-associated disruptions of mucosa (e.g., cytomegalovirus infection with HIV infection), host defense abnormalities, immunosuppressive therapy, or some combination of these is unclear. From a treatment perspective, it is reasonable to initially use the same approach as that for noncompromised hosts. Aggressive treatment directed against HIV (e.g., highly active antiretroviral therapy [HAART]) and minimizing immunosuppressive therapy is also desirable if possible. There are no data on the use of immunomodulatory therapy (e.g., interferon-gamma or immunoglobulins).

Refractory Disease

Usually, actinomycosis responds well to medical therapy. However, refractory or perceived refractory disease has been described in HIV-infected individuals as well as apparently normal hosts. In this setting, basic principles of infectious disease apply. The clinician should exclude infection elsewhere (e.g., line-related, *C. difficle* colitis) and/or noninfectious causes (e.g., drug fever, unrelated disease) as being responsible. The clinician should then confirm that high-dose parenteral therapy is being used for initial treatment. Significant purulent collections associated with the actinomycotic infection should be identified and drained. The clinician should consider the possibility that untreated coisolates ("companion organisms") may be responsible. Although penicillin-resistant strains or evolution of resistance during therapy has not yet been clearly documented in vivo, this possibility should be considered when other more likely scenarios are excluded. Finally, surgery should be considered when infection is refractory to medical therapy, although as stated, this usually can be avoided, at least initially.

Actinomyces-Like Organisms

An unresolved issue is whether screening cervical or endometrial specimens for *Actinomyces*-like organisms (ALO) or their detection by immunofluorescence (IF) can predict/prevent IUCD-associated disease. Furthermore, a Papanicolaou smear may fail to detect ALOs even in the presence of active actinomycosis. Although the risk appears to be small, the consequences of infection are significant. Therefore, until more quantitative data become available, in the presence of symptoms that cannot be accounted for, regardless of whether ALOs or IF-positive organisms are detected, it would appear prudent to remove the IUCD and, if advanced disease is excluded, empirically treat for 14 days for possible early pelvic actinomycosis. The detection of ALOs or IF-positive organisms in the absence of symptoms warrants patient education and close follow-up, but not removal of the IUCD, unless an equally suitable means of contraception can be agreed upon.

Suggested Reading

Bennhoff DF: Actinomycosis: diagnostic and therapeutic considerations and a review of 32 cases, *Laryngoscope* 94:1198, 1984.

Brown JR: Human actinomycosis. A study of 181 subjects, *Hum Pathol* 4:319, 1973.

Goodman HM, Centeno BA: Case records of the Massachusetts General Hospital, Case 10-1992, *N Engl J Med* 326:692, 1992.

Russo, TA: Actinomycosis. In Mandell GL, Bennett JE, Dolin R, eds: *Principles and practice of infectious diseases,* ed 5, Philadelphia, 2000, Churchill Livingstone, p. 2645.

Weese WC, Smith IM: A study of 57 cases of actinomycosis over a 36-year period, *Arch Intern Med* 135:1562, 1975.

ANAEROBIC INFECTIONS

Sydney M. Finegold
Hannah M. Wexler

Anaerobic infections are common and some are serious, with a high mortality rate. They are easily overlooked because special precautions are needed for specimen collection and transport to do good bacteriologic studies and because some clinical laboratories fail to grow many or most anaerobes.

Treatment of anaerobic infections may be difficult. Failure to treat for anaerobes in mixed infections may lead to poor or no response. Many antibacterial agents have poor activity against many or most anaerobes, particularly aminoglycosides, the older quinolones, trimethoprim-sulfamethoxazole, and monobactams. Resistance of anaerobes to antimicrobials is increasing.

The most important anaerobes clinically are six genera of gram-negative rods. *Bacteroides*, especially the *B. fragilis* group made up of 10 species (including *B. fragilis*), is particularly important. The other gram-negative genera are *Prevotella*, *Porphyromonas*, *Fusobacterium*, *Bilophila*, and *Sutterella*. Among the gram-positive anaerobes are cocci (primarily *Peptostreptococcus*) spore-forming *(Clostridium)*, and non–spore-forming bacilli (especially *Actinomyces* and *Propionibacterium*) (Table 1).

■ SOURCE OF ANAEROBIC INFECTION

Virtually the only source of anaerobes causing infection is the indigenous flora of mucosal surfaces and to a much lesser extent the skin (Table 2). The major exception is *Clostridium difficile*, the principal cause of antimicrobial agent–associated colitis, which has caused nosocomial infections. Anaerobes outnumber aerobes by 10:1 in the oral and vaginal flora and by 1000:1 in the colon. Factors

---

Table 1   Anaerobes Most Commonly Encountered in Infection*

Bacteroides fragilis group, especially *B. fragilis*
Pigmented and nonpigmented *Prevotella*
Fusobacterium nucleatum
Peptostreptococcus
Clostridium perfringens, Clostridium ramosum

*These five groups together account for about two thirds of anaerobes from clinically significant infections involving anaerobes.

---

predisposing to anaerobic infection include disruption of normal mucosal or cutaneous barriers by disease, surgery, or trauma; tissue injury, which reduces oxidation-reduction potential, favoring growth of anaerobes; impaired blood supply; obstruction of a hollow viscus; and foreign body. Other important factors include the numbers of organisms that get into deeper tissues (the inoculum size), various virulence factors (toxins, enzymes, and other substances) produced by anaerobes, and whether the host's defense system is intact.

■ TYPES OF INFECTION INVOLVING ANAEROBES

In terms of overall frequency, there are four major sites of anaerobic infection: pleuropulmonary, intraabdominal, female genital tract, and skin and soft tissue with or without involvement of underlying bone. Other infections, seen less commonly, primarily involve anaerobic bacteria; examples are brain abscess and bite-wound infections. Virtually all types of infection occurring in humans may involve anaerobic bacteria, and no organ or tissue of the body is immune to infection with these organisms. Table 3 lists infections commonly involving anaerobic bacteria. Abscess formation and tissue destruction are common characteristics of anaerobic infection. Synergy between various anaerobes or between anaerobes and aerobes is often important in mixed anaerobic infections.

Some anaerobic infections are unique (e.g., lung abscess, actinomycosis) and are readily suspected clinically. Major clues to anaerobic infection are listed in Table 4. Only the foul or putrid odor of a lesion or its discharge is specific; the other clues nonetheless may be highly suggestive. The Gram stain is useful because many anaerobes are unique morphologically. Information as to the relative numbers of various organisms may be extremely useful in directing empiric therapy.

■ COLLECTION AND TRANSPORT OF SPECIMENS

Proper collection and transport of specimens is crucial for recovery of anaerobes in the laboratory. Because anaerobes are normal flora, the clinician should be certain not to contaminate the specimens with such flora; this may be difficult at times. A good example of the problem is the patient with suspected aspiration pneumonia. Expectorated sputum is unsuitable because of the large numbers of anaerobes and other organisms present in saliva as indigenous flora; it is necessary to bypass the normal flora. If an empyema is present, thoracentesis provides a good specimen and is indicated therapeutically. In the absence of pleural fluid, bronchoalveolar lavage, a plugged double-lumen catheter with a protected bronchial brush, or percutaneous transtracheal aspiration should be used.

Proper transport requires placing the specimen under anaerobic conditions in a nonnutritive holding medium (in an oxygen-free glass tube) for the trip to the laboratory.

Table 2 Incidence of Various Anaerobes as Normal Flora in Humans

| | GRAM-POSITIVE | | | | | | | GRAM NEGATIVE | | | |
	CLOSTRI-DIUM	ACTINO-MYCES	BIFIDO-BACTERIUM	EUBAC-TERIUM	LACTO-BACILLUS*	PROPIONI-BACTERIUM	COCCI	B. FRAGILIS GROUP	FUSO-BACTERIUM	OTHER GNR	COCCI
Skin	0	0	0	+/-	0	2	1	0	0	0	0
Upper respiratory tract†	0	1	0	+/-	0	1	1	0	1	2	1
Mouth	+/-	1	1	1	1	+/-	2	0	2	2	2
Intestine	2	+/-	2	2	1-2	+/-	2	2	1	2	1
External genitalia	0	0	0	U	0	U	1	+/-	+/-	1	0
Urethra	+/-	0	0	U	+/-	0	+/-	+/-	+/-	1	U
Vagina	+/-	+/-	+/-	+/-	2	+/-	2	+/-	+/-	1	+/-
Endocervix	+/-	0	0	+/-	1	+/-	2	+/-	+/-	1	+/-

GNR, gram-negative rod; U, unknown; 0, not found or rare; +/-, irregular; 1, usually present; 2, usually present in large numbers.

*Includes anaerobic, microaerophilic, and facultative strains.

†Includes nasal pasages, nasopharynx, oropharynx, and tonsils.

Table 3   Infections Commonly Involving Anaerobic Bacteria

Brain abscess
Subdural empyema
Endophthalmitis, panophthalmitis
Periodontal disease
Root canal infection
Odontogenic infections
Chronic sinusitis
Chronic otitis media, mastoiditis
Peritonsillar abscess
Neck space infections
Aspiration pneumonia
Lung abscess
Pleural empyema
Pyogenic liver abscess
Peritonitis
Intraabdominal abscess
Appendicitis
Wound infection after bowel or female genital tract surgery
Endometritis
Salpingitis, tuboovarian abscess
Human and animal bite infection
Infected foot ulcers, especially in diabetics
Infected decubitus ulcer
Anaerobic cellulitis
Clostridial myonecrosis (gas gangrene)
Synergistic nonclostridial myonecrosis
Anaerobic streptococcal myositis
Necrotizing fasciitis
Chronic osteomyelitis
Actinomycosis
Antimicrobial-induced colitis and pseudomembranous colitis

Table 4   Major Clues to Anaerobic Infection

Foul-smelling discharge
Infection close to mucosal surface
Tissue necrosis, gangrene
Gas in tissues or discharges
Infection associated with malignancy
Infection secondary to human or animal bite
Infection related to the use of aminoglycosides, quinolones, trimethoprim-sulfamethoxazole, monobactams, or cephalosporins with poor activity against anaerobes (e.g., ceftazidime)
Classic clinical picture such as gas gangrene, actinomycosis
Infections that are classically of anaerobic origin (e.g., brain abscess, lung abscess)
Septic thrombophlebitis
Unique morphology on Gram stain of exudate
No growth on routine culture; sterile pus

■ THERAPY

The two key approaches to treatment are surgery and antimicrobial therapy. Debridement and drainage usually are essential. Failure to carry out prompt and thorough surgical therapy may lead to lack of response to appropriate antimi-

Table 5   Usual Flora in Anaerobic Pleuropulmonary Infections*

Anaerobes
　Peptostreptococcus (P. micros, P. anaerobius, P. magnus)
　Pigmented *Prevotella (P. denticola, P. melaninogenica,*
　　　P. intermedia, P. nigrescens, P. loescheii)
　Nonpigmented *Prevotella (P. oris, P. buccae, P. oralis)*
　Fusobacterium nucleatum (subsp. *nucleatum, polymorphum)*
　Bacteroides fragilis group
　Non–spore-forming gram-positive rods (*Actinomyces,*
　　　Eubacterium, Lactobacillus)
Viridans streptococci

*In hospital-acquired infections (e.g., aspiration pneumonia), various nosocomial pathogens, such as *Staphylococcus aureus*, Enterobacteriaceae, and *Pseudomonas,* may be involved in addition to the indigenous flora listed above.

Table 6   Usual Flora in Intraabdominal Infection*

Predominant anaerobes
　Bacteroides fragilis
　Bacteroides thetaiotaomicron
　Bilophila wadsworthia
　Peptostreptococcus (especially *P. micros*)
　Clostridium
Predominant aerobes and facultatives
　Escherichia coli
　Streptococcus (viridans group and group D)
　Pseudomonas aeruginosa
Biliary tract infection
　Uncomplicated
　　Escherichia coli, Klebsiella, Enterococcus, and *Clostridium*
　　　perfringens
　Complicated (e.g., prior surgery, malignancy)
　　Bacteroides fragilis group may also be involved

*In hospital-acquired infections, nosocomial pathogens, such as *Staphylococcus aureus* and various Enterobacteriaceae, may also be involved.

crobial agents. Some abscesses are amenable to percutaneous drainage under guidance of ultrasound or computed tomography.

Hyperbaric oxygen (HBO) may have value in selected circumstances, such as gas gangrene, to help demarcate the infection; for example, it may indicate where amputation should be done in the case of an extremity infection. There has never been clear-cut clinical evidence of significant benefit from HBO, however; surgical therapy should never be delayed to administer HBO.

Initial antimicrobial therapy is necessarily empiric; it takes some time to get definitive information on the infecting flora because it is usually complex. Rational empiric therapy is based on the clinician's assessment of the nature of the infectious process, knowledge of the usual infecting flora in such infections (Tables 5 to 9), and patterns of resistance to antimicrobial drugs in the particular hospital. Also the clinician take into account how the usual flora may

Table 7   Usual Flora in Female Genital Tract Infections

Anaerobes
  Peptostreptococcus
  Bacteroides fragilis group
  Prevotella (especially *P. bivia, P. disiens* pigmenters)
  Clostridium (especially *C. perfringens*)
  Actinomyces, Eubacterium (in intrauterine contraceptive
    device–associated infections)
Aerobes
  Streptococcus (groups A, B, others)
  Escherichia coli
  Klebsiella
  Gonococcus (in sexually active patients)
  Chlamydia (in sexually active patients)
  Mycoplasma hominis (in postpartum patients)

Table 8   Usual Flora in Diabetic Foot Ulcers

Anaerobes
  Peptostreptococcus (especially *P. magnus, P. prevotii,*
    P. anaerobius, P. asaccharolyticus)
  Bacteroides fragilis group (especially *B. fragilis* and
    B. thetaiotaomicron)
  Other *Bacteroides*
  Pigmented *Prevotella*
Aerobes
  Enterococcus
  Staphylococcus aureus
  Streptococci (especially group B)
  Proteus mirabilis
  Escherichia coli
  Other Enterobacteriaceae
  Pseudomonas aeruginosa

Table 9   Predominant Flora of Skin and Soft-Tissue Abscess

IN INTRAVENOUS DRUG ABUSERS
Anaerobes
  Fusobacterium nucleatum
  Peptostreptococcus micros
  Actinomyces odontolyticus
  Pigmented *Prevotella*
Aerobes
  Staphylococcus aureus
  Streptococcus (*S. milleri* group, viridans group, group A)
IN NON–INTRAVENOUS DRUG ABUSERS
Anaerobes
  Peptostreptococcus (*P. magnus, P. micros, P. asaccharolyticus*)
  Pigmented *Prevotella*
  Actinomyces
  Fusobacterium nucleatum
Aerobes
  Staphylococcus aureus
  Streptococcus (*S. milleri* group, group A, viridans group)

Table 10   Principal Beta-Lactamase–Producing Anaerobes

Bacteroides fragilis group
Bacteroides splanchnicus, B. capillosus
Pigmented *Prevotella, Porphyromonas*
Prevotella oralis group
Prevotella: P. oris, P. buccae
Prevotella: P. bivia, P. disiens
Bilophila wadsworthia
Fusobacterium nucleatum
Fusobacterium: F. mortiferum, F. varium
Clostridium ramosum
Clostridium clostridioforme
Clostridium butyricum

have been modified by pathophysiology or disease and by prior antimicrobial therapy. Careful analysis of the Gram stain of the specimen may also suggest the need to modify the empiric approach. In certain situations, the pharmacologic properties of the drugs and whether they are bactericidal are important considerations. In central nervous system infections, for example, the drug must cross the blood-brain barrier well. In such infections and in endocarditis, bactericidal activity is important. A good clinician will be in close contact with the microbiology laboratory, particularly in the case of a very sick patient. Ideally, such contact begins before the specimen is submitted and is maintained until full culture results are available. The microbiologist may take advantage of information from the clinician to use special selective or other media in setting up the culture and can often look at cultures more often than with routine cultures, using an anaerobic chamber or other device to examine the culture without exposing it to oxygen. Preliminary culture information may dictate modification of the initial empiric antimicrobial regimen.

Antimicrobial resistance is an increasing problem with anaerobic bacteria. Various mechanisms for such resistance are known; they are the same as with aerobes. Beta-lactamase production is one of the most common mechanisms of such resistance; fortunately, this can be overcome to some extent by combinations of beta-lactam drugs with beta-lactamase inhibitors such as clavulanic acid, sulbactam, or tazobactam. Table 10 lists the more common beta-lactamase–producing anaerobes. Unfortunately, hyperproduction of beta-lactamases and production of metalloenzyme beta-lactamases may render some of our better drugs inactive.

Tables 11 and 12 summarizes the activity of various antimicrobials against the major anaerobes encountered clinically, as found in the Wadsworth Anaerobic Bacteriology Laboratory experience. Testing was done by the Wadsworth agar dilution method. Antimicrobials not listed in the table are not approved by the Food and Drug Administration or are generally not recommended for therapy of anaerobic infections. In most cases, clinical data support the use of these agents for management of infection with the organisms indicated. Patterns of susceptibility vary among geographic locations and even among hospitals in the same city, primarily because of the patterns of usage of antimicro-

Table 11 Susceptibility of Gram-Positive Anaerobic Bacteria

% SUSCEPTIBLE[a,b]	PEPTOSTREPTOCOCCUS	C. DIFFICILE[c]	C. RAMOSUM	C. PERFRINGENS	OTHER CLOSTRIDIUM SPECIES	NSF-GPR[d]
>95	Penicillin G Piperacillin Amoxicillin + clavulanate Ampicillin + sulbactam Piperacillin + tazobactam Ticarcillin + clavulanate Cefoperazone Cefoperazone + sulbactam Cefotetan Cefoxitin Ceftazidime Ceftizoxime Ceftriaxone Biapenem Imipenem Meropenem Chloramphenicol Clinafloxacin Satifloxacin Sparfloxacin Trovafloxacin Metronidazole	Ampicillin Piperacillin Ticarcillin Amoxicillin + clavulanate Ampicillin + sulbactam Piperacillin + tazobactam Ticarcillin + clavulanate Cefotetan Imipenem Meropenem Clinafloxacin Satifloxacin Trovafloxacin Metronidazole	Amoxicillin + clavulanate Piperacillin + tazobactam Ticarcillin + clavulanate Ceftizoxime Imipenem Clinafloxacin Satifloxacin Metronidazole	Ampicillin Piperacillin Ticarcillin Ampicillin + sulbactam Amoxicillin + clavulanate Piperacillin + tazobactam Ticarcillin + clavulanate Cefotetan Ceftizoxime Biapenem Imipenem Chloramphenicol Ciprofloxacin Clinafloxacin Satifloxacin Fleroxacin Sparfloxacin Trovafloxacin Metronidazole Azithromycin Clarithromycin Erythromycin Roxithromycin	Amoxicillin Ampicillin Carbenicillin Penicillin G Piperacillin Ticarcillin Ampicillin + sulbactam Amoxicillin + clavulanate Biapenem Imipenem Chloramphenicol Clinafloxacin Satifloxacin Trovafloxacin Metronidazole Minocycline	Penicillin G Piperacillin Amoxicillin + clavulanate Ampicillin + sulbactam Piperacillin + tazobactam Ticarcillin + clavulanate Cefotaxime Ceftizoxime Biapenem Imipenem Meropenem Chloramphenicol Clindamycin Clinafloxacin Satifloxacin Levofloxacin Minocycline

Percent susceptible						
85–95	Levofloxacin Clindamycin Minocycline	Ceftriaxone Biapenem Chloramphenicol	Ampicillin Piperacillin Ampicillin + sulbactam Chloramphenicol; Trovafloxacin Clindamycin	Lomefloxacin Clindamycin	Moxalactam	Cefotetan Cefoxitin Ceftriaxone Cefoperazone + sulbactam; Trovafloxacin Azithromycin Clarithromycin Erythromycin Roxithromycin
70–84		Ciprofloxacin Ofloxacin Azithromycin Clarithromycin Erythromycin Fleroxacin Tetracycline Roxithromycin	Cefoxitin Clindamycin	Minocycline	Levofloxacin Ofloxacin Sparfloxacin Clindamycin Tetracycline	Cefoperazone Moxalactam Sparfloxacin Tetracycline
50–69		Clindamycin Minocycline Tetracycline Azithromycin Clarithromycin Erythromycin Roxithromycin	Sparfloxacin Minocycline Tetracycline	Tetracycline	Cefoperazone Cefotaxime Cefoxitin Ceftizoxime Ceftriaxone Ciprofloxacin Azithromycin Clarithromycin Erythromycin Roxithromycin	Ciprofloxacin Ofloxacin Metronidazole
<50	Lomefloxacin	Cefoxitin Ceftizoxime Ciprofloxacin Fleroxacin Lomefloxacin Sparfloxacin	Ciprofloxacin Fleroxacin Lomefloxacin Azithromycin Clarithromycin Erythromycin Roxithromycin		Ceftazidime Fleroxacin Lomefloxacin	Fleroxacin Lomefloxacin

[a] The order of listing of drugs within percent susceptible categories is not significant.
[b] According to the NCCLS-approved breakpoints (M11-A3), using the intermediate category as susceptible.
[c] Breakpoint is used only as a reference point. C. *difficile* is primarily of interest in relation to antimicrobial-induced pseudomembranous colitis. These data must be interpreted in the context of level of drug achieved in the colon and impact of agent on indigenous colonic flora.
[d] Non–spore-forming, gram-positive rod.

Table 12   Susceptibility of Gram-Negative Anaerobic Bacteria

% SUSCEPTIBLE[a,b]	B. FRAGILIS	OTHER B. FRAGILIS GROUP[d]	OTHER BACTEROIDES	C. GRACILIS	PREVOTELLA
>95	Piperacillin Amoxicillin + clavulanate Ampicillin + sulbactam Cefoperazone + sulbactam Piperacillin + tazobactam Ticarcillin + clavulanate Cefoxitin Biapenem Imipenem Meropenem Chloramphenicol Clinafloxacin Satifloxacin Levofloxacin Ofloxacin Trovafloxacin Metronidazole	Ampicillin + sulbactam Cefoperazone + sulbactam Piperacillin + tazobactam Ticarcillin + clavulanate Biapenem Imipenem Meropenem Chloramphenicol Clinafloxacin Satifloxacin Trovafloxacin Metronidazole Minocycline	Piperacillin Amoxicillin + clavulanate Ampicillin + sulbactam Ticarcillin + clavulanate Cefoperazone Cefoperazone + sulbactam Cefotaxime Cefoxitin Ceftizoxime Biapenem Imipenem Chloramphenicol Clinafloxacin Satifloxacin Levofloxacin Trovafloxacin Metronidazole Clindamycin	Piperacillin Amoxicillin + clavulanate Piperacillin + tazobactam Ticarcillin + clavulanate Cefoxitin Ceftizoxime Ceftriaxone Biapenem Imipenem Meropenem Chloramphenicol Ciprofloxacin Clinafloxacin Satifloxacin Fleroxacin Lomefloxacin Sparfloxacin Trovafloxacin Metronidazole Azithromycin Clindamycin Erythromycin Roxithromycin Minocycline Tetracycline	Piperacillin Amoxicillin + clavulanate Ampicillin + sulbactam Piperacillin + tazobactam Ticarcillin + clavulanate Cefoxitin Ceftizoxime Biapenem Imipenem Meropenem Chloramphenicol Clinafloxacin Satifloxacin Trovafloxacin Metronidazole Clindamycin
85-95	Cefotetan Ceftizoxime Clindamycin Minocycline	Amoxicillin + clavulanate Piperacillin Cefoxitin Ceftizoxime	Cefotetan Ceftazidime Ceftriaxone Clarithromycin Erythromycin Roxithromycin Minocycline		Ceftriaxone Azithromycin Clarithromycin Erythromycin Roxithromycin

[a]The order of listing of drugs within percent susceptible categories is not significant.
[b]According to the NCCLS-approved breakpoints (M11-A3), using the intermediate category as susceptible.
[c]NCCLS approved breakpoint is 4 µg/ml. However, the breakpoint should probably be lowered to 1 µg/ml, which will considerably lower the values for percent susceptible. For example, at 1 µg/ml, no strains of the *B. fragilis* group were susceptible.
[d]Excluding *B. fragilis*.

PORPHYROMONAS	SUTTERELLA WADSWORTHENSIS	F. NUCLEATUM	F. MORTIFERUM AND F. VARIUM	OTHER FUSOBACTERIUM	B. WADSWORTHIA
Piperacillin	Amoxicillin + clavulanate	Piperacillin	Piperacillin	Penicillin G	Piperacillin
Amoxicillin + clavulanate	Ticarcillin + clavulanate	Amoxicillin + clavulanate		Ampicillin + sulbactam	
Cefoxitin	Cefoxitin	Piperacillin + tazobactam	Piperacillin + tazobactam	Piperacillin + tazobactam	Ticarcillin
Ceftizoxime	Ceftriaxone	Ticarcillin + clavulanate	Ticarcillin + clavulanate		Amoxicillin + clavulanate
Ceftriaxone		Cefoxitin	Cefoxitin	Cefoxitin	Ampicillin + sulbactam
Biapenem	Imipenem	Ceftizoxime	Biapenem	Biapenem	Cefotetan
	Meropenem		Imipenem	Imipenem	
Imipenem	Ciprofloxacin Fleroxacin	Ceftriaxone Biapenem	Meropenem	Meropenem	Cefoxitin Ceftizoxime
Meropenem		Imipenem	Chloramphenicol	Chloramphenicol	Imipenem
Chloramphenicol		Meropenem	Clinafloxacin		
Clinafloxacin DU 6859A		Chloramphenicol	DU 6859A Trovafloxacin	Clinafloxacin DU 6859A Metronidazole	Chloramphenicol Ciprofloxacin
Sparfloxacin Trovafloxacin Metronidazole Azithromycin		Clinafloxacin Satifloxacin Levofloxacin Ofloxacin	Metronidazole Minocycline	Clindamycin Minocycline Tetracycline	Satifloxacin Fleroxacin Lomefloxacin Sparfloxacin
Minocycline		Sparfloxacin Trovafloxacin Clindamycin Metronidazole Minocycline Tetracycline			Trovafloxacin Metronidazole Minocycline Tetracycline
Ciprofloxacin	Piperacillin		Amoxicillin + clavulanate	Piperacillin	Clindamycin
Clarithromycin	Piperacillin + tazobactam	Azithromycin	Ceftizoxime	Amoxicillin + clavulanate	
Clindamycin	Ceftizoxime		Ceftriaxome	Ticarcillin + clavulanate	
Erythromycin				Cefoperazone + sulbactam	
Roxithromycin	Trovafloxacin			Cefotaxime Cefotetan Ceftizoxime Ceftriaxone	

Continued

Table 12 Susceptibility of Gram-Negative Anaerobic Bacteria—cont'd

% SUSCEPTIBLE[a,b]	B. FRAGILIS	OTHER B. FRAGILIS GROUP[d]	OTHER BACTEROIDES	C. GRACILIS	PREVOTELLA
70-84	Moxalactam Ceftriaxone Clarithromycin	Levofloxacin Clarithromycin Clindamycin	Penicillin G Moxalactam Ofloxacin Sparfloxacin Azithromycin		Ciprofloxacin Oflaxacin Sparfloxacin Minocycline
50-69	Cefoperazone Cefotaxime Ceftazidime Sparfloxacin	Cefoperazone Cefotetan Moxalactam Ofloxacin Sparfloxacin	Ciprofloxacin Tetracycline		Tetracycline
<50	Penicillin G[c] Ciprofloxacin Fleroxacin Lomefloxacin Azithromycin Erythromycin Roxithromycin Tetracycline	Penicillin G Cefotaxime Ceftazidime Ceftriaxone Ciprofloxacin Fleroxacin Lomefloxacin Azithromycin Erythromycin Roxithromycin	Fleroxacin Lomefloxacin		Fleroxacin Lomefloxacin

[a]The order of listing of drugs within percent susceptible categories is not significant.
[b]According to the NCCLS-approved breakpoints (M11-A3), using the intermediate category as susceptible.
[c]NCCLS approved breakpoint is 4 µg/ml. However, the breakpoint should probably be lowered to 1 µg/ml, which will considerable lower the values for percent susceptible. For example, at 1 µg/ml, no strains of the B. fragilis group were susceptible.
[d]Excluding B. fragilis.

bial agents. Four drugs or groups of drugs are active against most clinically significant anaerobic bacteria. These are metronidazole; carbapenems, such as imipenem; chloramphenicol; and combinations of beta-lactam drugs with a beta-lactamase inhibitor. Non–spore-forming anaerobic gram-positive bacilli (e.g., *Actinomyces* and *Propionibacterium*) are commonly resistant to metronidazole. There are disturbing reports of resistance in small numbers of strains of the *B. fragilis* group to all of the above agents. Three other drugs or groups of drugs have good activity but are less active than the four groups just mentioned. These are cefoxitin, clindamycin, and broad-spectrum penicillins such as ticarcillin and piperacillin. Some 15% to 25% of strains of the *B. fragilis* group are resistant to these latter compounds in many hospitals in the United States and elsewhere. Cefoxitin and clindamycin are relatively weak in activity against clostridia other than *C. perfringens* (20% to 35% of such strains are resistant), and some anaerobic cocci are resistant to clindamycin.

Some cephalosporins, such as ceftizoxime and cefotetan, have sufficient antianaerobic activity to be useful in treating certain anaerobic infections and are comparable with cefoxitin and clindamycin plus gentamicin in double-blind comparative studies. These cephalosporins clearly have been shown to be effective in three types of infections: appendicitis with no more than localized complications, female genital tract infections such as pelvic inflammatory disease and endometritis, and infected foot ulcers or similar soft-tissue infection with or without underlying bone infection. One may save on drug costs with these cephalosporins; this also saves the more potent drugs for serious infections. However, they not be prescribed for severely ill patients.

Because most anaerobic infections are mixed, involving aerobic or facultative bacteria in addition to anaerobes, antimicrobial therapy must cover the key pathogens of all types. Some of the drugs discussed earlier have significant activity against certain aerobes as well, but ordinarily it is necessary to add another agent to cover the other flora.

In general, for therapy of serious anaerobic infections, antimicrobials should be given parenterally in the maximum approved dosages, taking into account the weight and renal and hepatic function of the patient. This is because penetration of drugs into abscesses, necrotic tissue, and poorly perfused tissue, all common in serious anaerobic infections, is less than optimal.

Relatively prolonged therapy is also an important consideration in anaerobic infections to avoid relapse; for example, lung abscess usually requires therapy for several weeks, empyema for 2 to 3 months, and actinomycosis for 6 to 12 months or longer. Duration of therapy must be individualized, taking into account the site, type, extent, and severity of the infection, the nature of the infecting organisms, whether or not the host is immunocompromised or in poor condition because of associated or underlying illness, the speed of response to treatment, and other such factors.

PORPHYROMONAS	SUTTERELLA WADSWORTHENSIS	F. NUCLEATUM	F. MORTIFERUM AND F. VARIUM	OTHER FUSOBACTERIUM	B. WADSWORTHIA
	Metronidazole	Ciprofloxacin	Clindamycin Tetracycline	Ceftazidime Moxalactam Ciprofloxacin Sparfloxacin Azithromycin	
Tetracycline	Clindamycin		Ciprofloxacin Sparfloxacin		
Fleroxacin Lomefloxacin		Fleroxacin Lomefloxacin Clarithromycin Erythromycin Roxithromycin	Fleroxacin Lomefloxacin Azithromycin Clarithromycin Erythromycin Roxithromycin	Fleroxacin Lomefloxacin Clarithromycin Erythromycin Roxythromycin	Amoxicillin Ampicillin Penicillin G

Suggested Reading

Duerden BI, Drasar BS, eds: *Anaerobes in human disease*, Chichester, UK, 1991, Wiley-Liss.

Finegold SM: Anaerobic infections in humans: an overview, *Anaerobe* 1:3, 1995.

Finegold SM: *Anaerobic bacteria in human disease*, New York, 1977, Academic Press.

Finegold SM, George WL, eds: *Anaerobic infections in humans*, San Diego, 1989, Academic Press.

Summanen P, et al: *Wadsworth anaerobic bacteriology manual*, ed 5, Belmont, CA, 1993, Star Publishing.

Willis AT: *Clostridia of wound infection*, London, 1969, Butterworths.

ANTHRAX AND OTHER *BACILLUS* SPECIES

Boris Velimirovic

Anthrax is primarily a disease of grazing domestic animals. It is an acute disease caused by the spore-forming, gram-positive, nonmotile, toxin-producing aerobic rod *Bacillus anthracis*. It is the oldest known zoonosis with worldwide distribution: rare and sporadic and almost disappearing in the United States and in central and northern Europe, moderately common in southern Europe and common in the former Soviet Union, in tropical and subtropical Africa, Asia, the Caribbean, and South America. The most affected countries are Turkey, Afghanistan, Iran, Pakistan, the Central Asian republics of the former Soviet Union, and sub-Saharan and South Africa. The incidence of human anthrax has decreased considerably in all countries since the introduction of an effective vaccine for use in animals. The frequency of infections in humans depends on the prevalence of the disease in livestock, which increases in years of drought.

■ EPIDEMIOLOGY

The ability to form spores permits the organism to survive environmental and disinfective measures that destroy most other bacteria. Public health problems largely arise from its long persistence in the soil (up to 90 years). In the Anglo-American biologic warfare experiments conducted in 1942 to 1943 on the uninhabited island of Gruinard off the western coast of Scotland, an estimated 4×10^{14} spores were exploded over the surface. Animal tests for more than 20 years demonstrated the persistence of virulent spores, eventually eliminated by disinfection of the area with a mixture of formaldehyde and sea water. Concern about the military use of anthrax during the 1991 Persian Gulf War resulted in vaccination of U.S. troops. It was estimated that 100 L of spores sprayed over a city could kill 3 million people. In August 1991, Iraq admitted to a United Nations inspection team that it had conducted research on the offensive use of *B. anthracis* before the Persian Gulf War, and in 1995, admitted to "weaponizing" anthrax.

Anthrax bacteria are easy to cultivate and mass produce, and about 30 countries have the capacity to do so. Accidents are also possible, such as the one that occurred in 1979 after an explosion in a Soviet biologic laboratory in former Sverdlovsk (now Ekaterinburg), which generated an aerosol causing at least 42 deaths from anthrax pneumonia. The largest recorded outbreak of cutaneous anthrax in humans occurred in Zimbabwe during the civil war in 1979 to 1980, affecting six of the eight provinces. More than 10,000 human cases and 1832 deaths were documented secondary to an unprecedented outbreak in cattle. It was alleged that this was a deliberately produced enzootic by aerial spread as part of the war efforts.

Infection of the skin comes about by direct occupational contact with contaminated goat hair, wool, hides, bone meal, and other similar products during processing, spinning, and weaving or by direct contact such as with infected carcasses, tissues, and meat.

Inhalation anthrax results from aspiration of *B. anthracis* or spores via small aerosolized *bacillus*-bearing particles. If they are less than 5 µm in size, the spores germinate in the alveoli and multiply. They can also be ingested and absorbed through intestinal mucosa. Vegetative forms multiply in the regional lymph nodes, producing toxin. If transported through oral mucosa, they can produce a cervical form. There is no evidence that milk from infected animals transmits the disease. Biting flies and other insects may perhaps be the mechanical vectors. Incubation is usually 48 hours but may be longer.

For epidemiologic purposes, the disease is divided into agricultural and industrial anthrax; the occupational history is important. At particular risk are veterinarians, veterinary assistants, herders, agricultural and ranch workers, slaughterhouse employees, tannery and textile industry workers, home craftsmen using imported yarn from endemic areas (24 cases in Switzerland in 1978 to 1981), and people handling bone-meal fertilizer. The statement that approximately 90% of human cases reported in recent years occurred in mill workers handling imported goat hair is perhaps valid for inhalation anthrax in a few western industrialized countries, but definitely not true for the world as a whole.

■ PATHOGENESIS

Anthrax bacilli proliferate at the site of entry and are numerous beneath the central necrotic area of the skin lesion. They are transported to the regional lymph nodes, producing a hemorrhagic lymphadenitis. If they penetrate the blood-stream, septicemia can cause metastatic lesions practically everywhere, with hemorrhagic edema and necrosis.

The virulence of the organism is variable, determined by at least two factors: an extracellular toxin and the capsular polypeptide. The number of organisms in the initial inoculum also plays a role. The toxin causes vascular permeability, edema and fluid loss, and oligemic shock, which is the mechanism of death. The toxin consists of at least three components—edema factor, protective antigen, and lethal factor—each of which is nontoxic but acts synergistically. Differing concentrations of individual toxins in any given strain of *B. anthracis* lead to varying pathogenicity and virulence. Systemic shock and death from anthrax primarily result from the effects of cytokines produced by macrophages stimulated by the lethal toxin.

■ CLINICAL PICTURE

Infection occurs in three distinct forms: cutaneous, pulmonary, and intestinal.

Cutaneous Infection
The most common form accounts for up to 98% of all cases. There are two types: dry and edematous. After an incubation period of 1 to 7 days, a small red papule develops at the entry points on the exposed parts of the skin—a minor injury, cut, or abrasion—or after active rubbing on the skin with the fingers, usually on the hand or other parts of the upper extremities, on the face (about half of all cases), lips, eyebrows, or neck, but also eyelids, feet, upper chest or back, breast, penis, and scrotum. This papule progresses within 12 to 48 hours to a fluid-filled blister. The fluid in the vesicle is initially clear, but soon it becomes dark and bluish black. The blister is surrounded by inflammation, extensive hard induration, edema in the adjacent deeper tissues, lymphadenitis, and lymphadenopathy. There is no carbuncle. Fever is mild, the lesion is not painful, double lesions occur. Satellite vesicles can develop near the initial lesion. The vesicle ruptures and develops into a pustule (*pustula maligna*); the tissue necrotizes and progresses to a lesion that is relatively painless, and then it becomes a dark or black eschar (*anthrax* is the Greek word for black) of about 1 to 3 cm in diameter or larger. This heals and the scab falls off, leaving a scar (Figure 1). The differential diagnosis includes plague and leishmaniasis in endemic areas.

In untreated cases, there may be hematogenous spread via regional lymph nodes, fever, and bacteremia, which may be fatal in 5% to 20% of cases. Localization on the head or neck has a more serious prognosis. Up to 80% of cases of cutaneous anthrax heal spontaneously without treatment.

Pulmonary Infection
Pulmonary (inhalation) anthrax is a rare disease; only two cases were reported between 1920 and 1990 in the United States. It is almost invariably fatal (Figure 2). The illness is biphasic; the initial phase lasts about 4 days and is manifested by a "flulike" illness with a nonproductive cough suggestive of mild bronchopneumonia, atypical pneumonia, influenza, psittacosis, tularemia, legionnaires' disease, *hantavirus* pulmonary syndrome, and pneumonic plague. Ra-

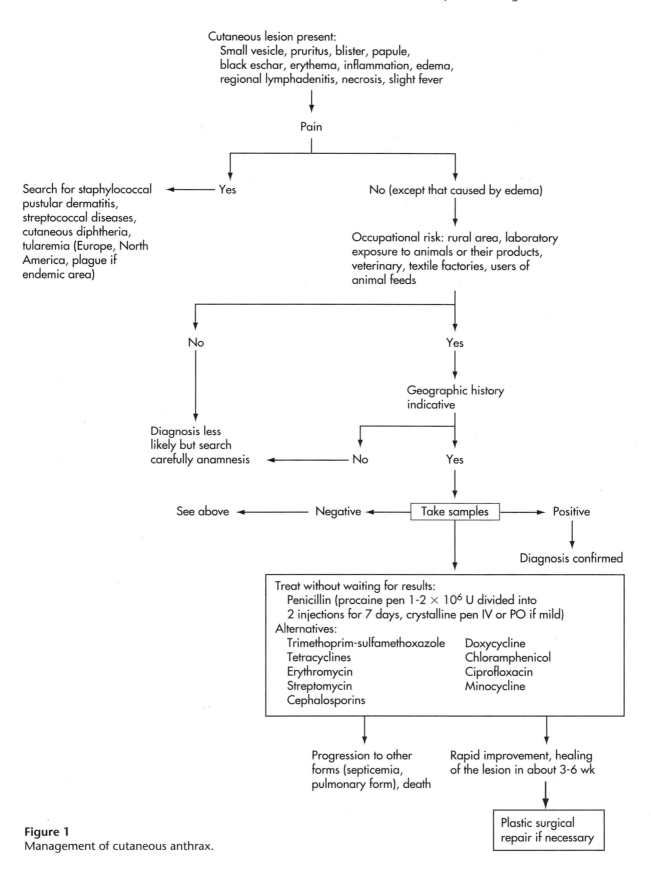

Figure 1
Management of cutaneous anthrax.

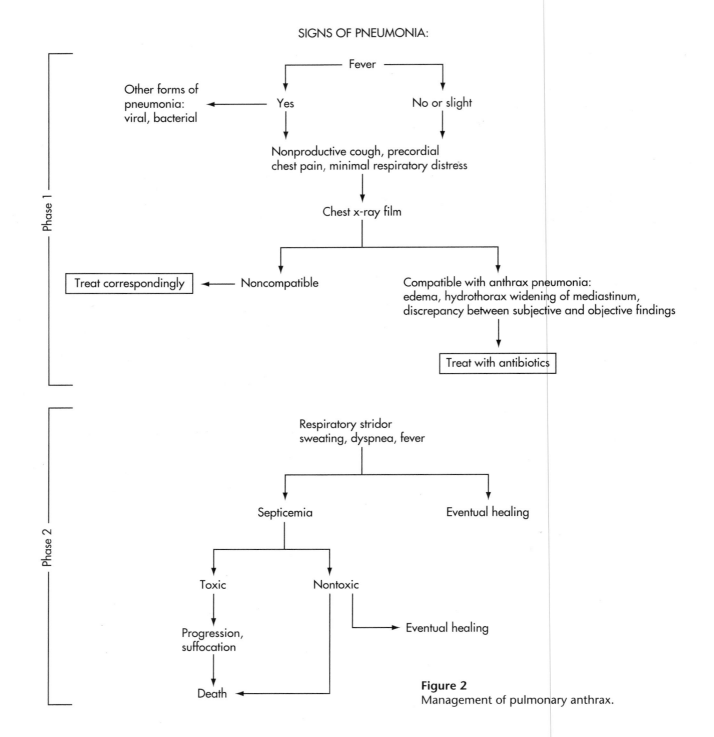

Figure 2
Management of pulmonary anthrax.

diographs may show mediastinal widening. The victim may die within 24 hours.

After several days and often after an apparent improvement from the primary phase (in which the patient is well oriented, alert, and unagitated), there is a sudden onset of rapidly progressive respiratory failure, acute dyspnea, circulatory collapse, cyanosis, stridor, signs of pleural effusion, and an elevated temperature. The patient usually dies of toxemia and suffocation within 24 hours of the onset of this second stage. Postmortem findings are of massive pulmonary edema, hemorrhagic mediastinitis, and hydrothorax. Not all persons who inhale the spores develop clinical disease. Subclinical infection, as assumed on the basis of serologic tests, may provide some protection against a new challenge. The pulmonary form of anthrax worries authorities most because of its potential for mass casualties.

Intestinal Infection

The intestinal form is difficult to diagnose. It appears 2 to 5 days after ingestion of meat contaminated with spores of *B. anthracis,* which penetrate the intestinal mucosa. The local ulcerative lesions, most often in the ileocecal region but also in the jejunum, are similar to those of the cutaneous form and are accompanied by nonspecific symptoms such as nausea, vomiting, dizziness, anorexia, fever, abdominal pain, splenomegaly, bloody diarrhea, and hemorrhagic ascites in the absence of liver damage. This may progress to shock and renal failure. About half the patients die. Local lesions, hemorrhagic spots in the serosa, and a typical small, soft, necrotic spleen are characteristic postmortem findings. A gastric form is extremely rare.

Other Clinical Forms

Meningeal anthrax follows cutaneous disease in up to 3% to 5% of cases; it rarely results from inhalation. The hemorrhagic meningitis produced is almost invariably fatal in 2 to 4 days, but successful treatment is documented. Renal, oropharyngeal, and ophthalmic forms have been described.

The incidence of milder or subclinical cases in cutaneous and pulmonary forms, and of chronic cases in the intestinal form, is unknown. The differential diagnosis of anthrax must consider staphylococcal pustular dermatitis, streptococcal lesions, cutaneous diphtheria and plague, any pneumonia in the respiratory form, and various enteric infections in the intestinal form. It is assumed that the clinical disease provides permanent immunity.

■ LABORATORY DIAGNOSIS

Diagnosis is made by visualization and culture of *B. anthracis* from pus, blood, exudates, or cerebrospinal fluid. *B. anthracis* measures 3 to 8 μm by 1 to 1.5 μm and is surrounded by a large capsule. It is strongly gram positive and non–acid fast. Methylene blue, Wright-Giemsa, and toluidine blue stains are commonly used to demonstrate anthrax bacilli in blood smears. Giemsa or Odd's stain is best to stain spores. In the gastrointestinal form, the organism can be demonstrated in vomitus or feces, and in the pulmonary form in sputum or hemoptysized specimens. Bacilli are usually not present in the bloodstream in large numbers except in septicemia just before death.

The bacillus can be identified by specific fluorescent antibody techniques in tissue sections. Examination of paired sera by indirect microhemagglutination or enzyme-linked immunosorbent assay (ELISA) may be helpful. Unfortunately, the diagnosis of inhalation and intestinal anthrax is usually made postmortem.

■ THERAPY

Treatment should be started on suspicion, without waiting for laboratory confirmation (see Figure 1). The drug of choice is procaine penicillin 1 to 2 million units daily divided into 2 intramuscular (IM) injections initially and continued as single daily doses thereafter for 7 days. However, in the cutaneous form, a shorter course may be equally effective. Benzyl penicillin, intravenous penicillin G, or crystalline penicillin may also be given. Complete sterilization of the wound is achieved in cutaneous anthrax within 24 hours. The edema resolves within about 5 days; it may increase in the first 24 to 48 hours because of the release of toxin from disintegrating bacilli.

In the pulmonary and septicemic forms, dosages from 10 to 40 million units of penicillin G per day have been recommended (see Figure 2). Other broad-spectrum antibiotics, such as tetracycline, doxycycline, erythromycin, chloramphenicol, streptomycin, cephalosporins, ciprofloxacin, and trimethoprim-sulfamethoxazole are effective in monkeys. In plague-endemic areas, streptomycin or tetracycline is recommended in cases of diagnostic doubt. In milder forms, oral penicillin can be given. Minocycline is recommended for treatment and urgent prophylaxis of infection caused by tetracycline-resistant *B. anthracis* strains.

■ PREVENTION

Prevention of cutaneous anthrax is possible by immunization of persons at high risk (e.g., veterinarians in endemic areas, workers in imported-wool processing plants and textile factories) with a cell-free vaccine prepared from a culture filtrate of a nonvirulent, nonencapsulated strain containing the protective antigen (PA) absorbed to aluminum hydroxide gel. The vaccine is given parenterally, three doses at 2-week intervals followed by three booster inoculations at 6-month intervals, and then annual booster inoculations. Little is known about the protective effect of vaccine in inhalation anthrax in humans. In experiments, rhesus monkeys survived exposure to a lethal dose only when vaccine and antibiotics (penicillin, ciprofloxacin, and doxycycline) were given simultaneously.

The human live vaccine has been licensed for use in certain endemic areas and reserved as an emergency method to be applied in a critical situation. In addition, scarification and subcutaneous administration and aerosol were used in the former USSR. In 1996, the State Research Institute of Applied Microbiology of Obolensk, Russia, claimed that it had developed a novel vaccine against anthrax in humans, supposed to have not only antitoxic but also antispore activity. The best measure to eliminate human anthrax is control in domestic animals by effective surveillance and the immunization of animals in endemic areas.

A licensed vaccine, currently given to American military personnel, is an aluminum hydroxide–adsorbed preparation (Michigan Biological Product Institute) derived from culture fluid supernatant taken from an attenuated strain. It raises strong humoral immunity specifically to lethal toxin. The vaccination series consists of six subcutaneous doses at 0, 2, and 4 weeks, then at 6, 12, and 18 months, followed by annual boosters. If a biologic warfare attack is threatened or may have occurred, prophylaxis of unimmunized persons with ciprofloxacin (500 mg orally twice a day), or doxycycline (100 mg orally twice a day) is recommended. Should an anthrax attack be confirmed, chemoprophylaxis should be continued for at least 4 weeks and until at least three doses of vaccine have been received by all those exposed.*

■ BACILLACEAE INFECTIONS

Non-*anthracis* bacilli are ubiquitous gram-positive, spore-forming organisms that were once believed to be nonpathogenic but are now recognized as causing a variety of infections, injuries, and skin abrasions from road contact in motor vehicle accidents.

Many ubiquitous saprophytic species of aerobic spore-forming bacilli are hard to classify or to distinguish from *B. anthracis* except on the basis of pathogenicity. The *Bacillus* species most commonly encountered are *B. cereus*, *B. subtilis*, and *B. licheniformis*. Bacilli more or less closely resembling the anthrax bacillus have been isolated from soil, water, meat, fish, bone meal, wool, dust, oil cake, and less often from animals and humans. These organisms have been termed *Bacillus pseudoanthracis* or *Bacillus anthracoides*. Other *Bacillus* species have occasionally been responsible for disseminated infections in immunocompromised hosts.

B. cereus is a gram-positive aerobic or facultatively anaerobic spore-forming rod. It is ubiquitous and is present in soil, dust, water, and on vegetation, food, and spices. It is part of the normal fecal flora. *B. cereus* food poisoning is a toxin-mediated disease, rather than infection. It causes a short-incubation emetic illness and a long-incubation diarrheal illness, both by production of enterotoxins. The emetic illness often results from eating poorly preserved or nonrefrigerated fried or boiled rice. The symptoms develop 1 to 6 hours after ingestion. Patients usually recover within 24 hours. The diarrheal syndrome is characterized by abdominal pain and watery stools. It has an incubation time of 10 to 12 hours. Other toxins may contribute to the pathogenicity of *B. cereus* in nongastrointestinal disease. Ten other *Bacillus* species isolated from clinical material other than feces or vomitus were commonly dismissed as saprophytes or opportunistic pathogen contaminants. They are presently recognized as an infrequent cause of serious systemic infection, transient bacteremia, and bronchopneumonia, particularly in neonates and drug addicts, the immunosuppressed, hemodialysis and postsurgical patients, and those with prosthetic implants such as ventricular shunts.

---

*For the purchase of large quantities of vaccine for use in humans in the United States, contact the Bureau of Disease Control and Laboratory Services, Michigan Department of Public Health, P.O. Box 30035, 3500 North Logan Street, Lansing, MI 48909. In Europe, contact the Pasteur Institute, 28 Rue du Docteur Roux, 75724 Paris, Cedex 15, France, telephone: 1-45.68.80.00. Regarding individual persons, contact the Biologic Drugs Division, Bureau of Laboratories, Centers for Disease Control and Prevention, Atlanta, Georgia 30333.

The most common severe infections are ocular, including endophthalmitis, panophthalmitis, and keratitis, usually with the characteristic corneal ring abscesses. Even with prompt surgical and antimicrobial treatment, enucleation of the eye and blindness can often result. Simultaneous therapy via more than one route may be required in ocular infection.

Septicemia, meningitis, endocarditis, necrotizing pneumonia, lung abscess, fasciitis, osteomyelitis, and surgical and traumatic wound infections are other manifestations of severe disease. *B. cereus* and most other nonanthrax *Bacillus* species are considered resistant to older penicillins and cephalosporins, including the third generation. They are usually susceptible to treatment with clindamycin, vancomycin, chloramphenicol, and erythromycin. They are also susceptible to aminoglycosides. Vancomycin is considered by some authors as the drug of choice for serious *Bacillus* infections. An addition of fosfomycin to the antibiotic regimen is reported to have resulted in complete cure in the cerebrospinal fluid when vancomycin alone failed. Many strains of *B. cereus* isolated from milk in Nairobi, Kenya in 1996 showed resistance to eight commonly used antimicrobial agents

In India, filarial lymphedema is complicated by frequent episodes of dermatolymphadenitis, which do not depend on the presence or absence of microfilariae. *B. cereus* and various cocci have been isolated by biopsies and from the blood. Antibiotic therapy is effective in prevention and treatment. *Bacillus* spores may survive treatment with common disinfectants (except 2% glutaraldehyde, soaking for 10 hours), and they may resist boiling.

Suggested Reading

Abramova FA, et al: *Pathology of inhalation anthrax in 42 cases from the Sverdlovsk outbreak, 1979* Proc Natl Acad Sci USA 90:2291, 1993.

Bastian L, Weber S, Regel G: *Bacillus cereus* pneumonia after thoracic trauma, *Anaestesiol Intensivmed Notfallmed Schmerztherap* 32:124, 1997.

Drobniewski FA: *Bacillus cereus* and related species, *Clin Microbiol Rev* 6:324, 1993.

Franz DR, et al: Clinical recognition and management of patients exposed to biological warfare agents, *JAMA,* 278:5, 1997.

Hanna PH: How anthrax kills, *Science,* 280:1671, 1998.

Koneman E, et al: *Diagnostic microbiology,* ed 5, Philadelphia, 1997, Lippincott-Raven.

Preston R: The bioweaponeers, *New Yorker,* 74:52, March 9, 1998.

Velimirovic B: Anthrax. In Standards Commission of the International Committee of the Office International des Epizooties: *Manual of recommended diagnostic techniques and requirements for biological products,* 15:1, 1989, Paris.

Velimirovic B: Anthrax in europe, *Rev Sci Tech Off Int Epiz* (Paris) 3:527, 1984.

Whitford HW: Anthrax. In Steele JH ed.: *Handbook series on zoonoses. Section A, bacterial, rickettsial, and mycotic diseases,* vol 1. Boca Raton, FL, 1979, CRC Press.

World Health Organization: *Health aspects of chemical and biological weapons.* Report of a WHO working group of consultants, Geneva, Switzerland, 1999, World Health Organization.

BARTONELLOSIS (CARRIÓN'S DISEASE)

Craig J. Hoesley
C. Glenn Cobbs

Bartonellosis is a bacterial disorder with a striking geographic distribution: the western slope of the Peruvian, Ecuadorian, and Colombian Andes 2000 to 8000 feet (725 to 2900 meters) above sea level. The causative microorganism, *Bartonella bacilliformis*, is a small, motile, gram-negative bacillus. Other members of the *Bartonella* genus causing human disease include *B. henselae* (cat-scratch disease, bacillary angiomatosis) and *B. quintana* (trench fever, bacillary angiomatosis). Bartonellosis, also known as *Carrión's disease*, is restricted to the Andes region of South America because its vector, a sandfly, *Lutzomyia (Phlebotomus) verrucarum*, is restricted to this area.

The clinical manifestations of this unique biphasic illness have been studied extensively. After inoculation by the bite of an infected sandfly, the bacteria enter the endothelial cells of blood vessels and replicate during the incubation period. Within 2 to 6 weeks after infection, the nonimmune host develops Oroya fever (erythrocytic invasive phase), which is characterized by anorexia, headache, malaise, and a potentially striking hemolytic anemia (Figure 1). Most commonly, only a few red blood cells are parasitized, and the disease is subclinical or mild without anemia. Less commonly severe disease may occur with up to 100% of erythrocytes parasitized resulting in profound hemolytic anemia and a high mortality. In addition to the anemia, leukopenia with decreased absolute CD4 cell counts produces transient immunosuppression. Lymphadenopathy and hepatomegaly occur, but splenomegaly is less common and, if present, may suggest some other disorder. This initial phase of infection ends with the sudden disappearance of bacteria from the erythrocytes. During the acute or convalescent stage of Oroya fever, secondary infections with *Salmonella, Mycobacterium tuberculosis,* amoebae, and malaria are possible and contribute significantly to the overall mortality of this disorder.

Individuals who survive the acute phase of infection may or may not develop the cutaneous stage of the disease. Within weeks to months after resolution of the acute phase, superficial and/or subcutaneous nodules evolve in crops on exposed skin. These skin lesions, known as *verruga peruana*, resemble Kaposi's sarcoma or bacillary angiomatosis. Verruga may persist for several months to 1 year and typically resolve spontaneously with little or no residua. Individuals who recover from either of the clinical forms of bartonellosis are immune; recurrent Oroya fever does not occur, and recurrent cutaneous manifestations are rare. In 1885, Daniel Carrión, a Peruvian medical student, proved that Oroya fever and verruga peruana were different manifestations of the same infectious agent. He inoculated himself with blood taken from a verruga of an infected patient and, approximately 3 weeks later, developed fever and severe hemolytic anemia that ultimately resulted in his death. In honor of these contributions, bartonellosis is also commonly termed *Carrión's disease.*

The diagnosis is suggested by the clinical picture and by the examination of the peripheral blood film. Bacilli may be seen within red blood cells, either singly or in pairs or clusters. The microorganism may be cultured on media containing 5% or more of rabbit, sheep, or horse blood in the presence of 5% CO_2 and an incubation temperature of 29° C. In addition, a variety of immunologic tests detect antibodies to *B. bacilliformis,* including an IgM fluorescence antibody test, an IgG fluorescence antibody test, an IgG enzyme-linked immunosorbent assay, and an indirect hemagglutination antibody test. Commercial assays are not

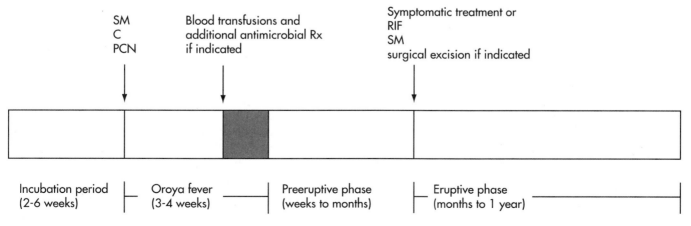

Figure 1
Bartonellosis (Carrións disease) Clinical course and treatment. *SM,* Streptomycin; *C,* chloramphenicol; *PCN,* penicillin; *RIF,* rifampin.

Table 1   Therapy of *Bartonella* Disease

OROYA FEVER PHASE

Agent of choice	Chloramphenicol
Alternative agents	Penicillins
	Streptomycin
	Erythromycin
	Quinolones
	Tetracycline

VERRUGA PHASE

Agent of choice	Rifampin
	Streptomycin
Alternative agents	Erythromycin and sulfonamides

available, and the sensitivity and specificity of these serologic tests are unknown.

In untreated patients, Oroya fever has a reported mortality of 40% to 85%, whereas mortality is reduced to less than 10% in patients treated with appropriate antimicrobial therapy. Many individuals may survive the acute illness only to succumb to opportunistic infections, such as *Salmonella*, tuberculosis, toxoplasmosis, and coccidioidomycosis.

BARTONELLA (ROCHALIMAEA) INFECTION

William A. Schwartzman

Over the past 5 years *Bartonella* (formerly *Rochalimaea*) species have been identified as agents of an expanding array of clinical syndromes. Clinical and histopathologic aspects of these infections differ in immunocompromised and immunocompetent patients, as do responses to antimicrobial therapy. This chapter presents the recognized clinical spectrum of *Bartonella* infections, methods of diagnosis, and antimicrobial therapy. The major clinical presentations are described in Table 1.

■ THERAPY

Table 1 lists therapeutic options for *Bartonella* disease. Chloramphenicol is the agent of choice for the acute Oroya fever phase, usually at 2 to 4 g/day for 7 days. Alternative agents that appear to be effective include penicillin, erythromycin, tetracycline, and fluoroquinolones. In the cutaneous verrugal phase, therapy with rifampin and streptomycin has been associated with rapid clearing of the skin lesions. A combination of erythromycin and sulfonamides has been effective in patients with refractory cutaneous lesions. Blood transfusions may be indicated as supportive therapy in patients experiencing massive parasitism and severe anemia during the Oroya fever phase of the disorder.

Prevention of infection requires control of the vector with insecticides and the use of insect repellant and bed netting by nonimmune individuals visiting endemic areas.

Suggested Reading

Alexander B: A review of bartonellosis in Equador and Columbia, *Am J Trop Med Hyg* 52:354, 1995.

Garcia-Caseres U, Garcia F: Bartonellosis. An immunodepressive disease and the life of Daniel Alcides Carrion, *Am J Clin Pathol* 95:S58, 1991.

Ihler G: *Bartonella bacilliformis:* dangerous pathogen slowly emerging from deep background, FEMS Microbiology Letters 144:1, 1996.

■ DISEASES CAUSED BY *BARTONELLA* SPECIES

Four *Bartonella* species are known to cause human disease: *B. quintana, B. henselae, B. elizabethae,* and *B. bacilliformis* (Table 2).

B. quintana was first identified as the agent of Quintan fever by Enrique da Rochalima during World War I. Also called trench fever, this relapsing febrile illness was transmitted by body lice to thousands of combatants, resulting in severe morbidity. It is characterized by fever and prostration lasting as long as 2 weeks, with occasional relapses. Patients may remain bacteremic with *B. quintana* for weeks after clinical resolution of trench fever. Although it was thought to be relatively rare after World War II, modern diagnostic techniques have uncovered several recent outbreaks of urban trench fever among chronic alcoholics, and several cases of culture-negative endocarditis caused by *B. quintana* have been described in this population. In addition, many cases of bacillary angiomatosis in immunocompromised patients result from infection with *B. quintana*, although most re-

Table 1   Clinical Presentations of *Bartonella* Infection

ALL SYNDROMES	IMMUNOCOMPETENT	IMMUNOCOMPROMISED (CELL-MEDIATED IMMUNITY)
Cat-scratch disease	Yes	*Bartonella*-related adenopathy
Bacillary angiomatosis	Rare	HIV+, malignancy, transplant
Parenchymal peliosis	Not reported	HIV+
Fever, bacteremia	Yes	HIV+, malignancy
Infective endocarditis	Yes	HIV+
Osteomyelitis	CSD*	Bacillary angiomatosis
Aseptic meningitis		HIV+
Retinitis/optic neuritis	CSD*	HIV+
Encephalopathy	CSD*	HIV+

HIV, Human immunodeficiency virus.
*Described in the context of cat-scratch disease (CSD).

Table 2   Diseases Caused by *Bartonella* Species

SPECIES	DISEASE	RESERVOIR	VECTOR
B. quintana	Trench fever	Unknown	Unknown
	Bacillary angiomatosis		
	Parenchymal peliosis		
	Infective endocarditis		
B. henselae	Cat-scratch fever	Domestic cat	Domestic cat (flea?)
	Fever, bacteremia		
	Bacillary angiomatosis		
	Parenchymal peliosis		
	Optic neuritis		
	Aseptic meninigitis		
	Recurrent pyogenic granuloma		
B. elizabethae	Infective endocarditis		
B. bacilliformis	Carrión's disease	Unknown	*Lutzomyia verrucarum*

ported cases appear to be caused by *B. henselae*. The reservoir for *B. quintana* has not been discovered.

B. henselae is the agent of cat-scratch disease. This entity was originally a clinical diagnosis based on four criteria: (1) history of cat scratch, (2) inoculation papule, (3) positive skin test with cat-scratch skin test antigen, and (4) demonstration of pleomorphic bacilli in tissue with Warthin-Starry silver stain. Today, the skin test antigen is not used, and the relatively nonspecific Warthin-Starry stain is supplemented by improved culture methods, polymerase chain reaction (PCR), and serologic methods. Most cases of cat-scratch disease occur in fall and winter in children and young adults with pet cats. Roughly 87% of patients have subacute or chronic regional lymphadenopathy, predominantly of the upper extremities, head, and neck. Lymph nodes may suppurate and cause great discomfort, which can be alleviated by aspiration. These cases usually resolve without antimicrobial therapy in 1 to 2 months. Some patients (10% to 13%) present with unusual or severe sequelae of cat-scratch disease (Table 3).

B. henselae, as well as *B. quintana,* causes bacillary angiomatosis and bacillary parenchymal peliosis, mainly in immunocompromised patients. The domestic cat is the main reservoir for this species, and as many as 47% of apparently healthy cats may be bacteremic with *B. henselae.* A recent study demonstrates *B. henselae* within the erythrocytes of

Table 3   Unusual Manifestations of Cat-Scratch Disease

Parinaud's oculoglandular syndrome
Prolonged fever and prostration
Osteomyelitis
Granulomatous hepatitis or splenitis
Optical neuritis
Encephalopathy with seizure or coma
Myelitis
Glomerulonephritis
Reactive arthritis

bacteremic cats. The cat's fleas as well as cat bites and scratches may play roles in human transmission.

B. elizabethae has been identified in one patient with infective endocarditis and in a dog with infective endocarditis. Its reservoir is unknown.

B. bacilliformis, which causes Carrión's disease, is found in the Andes Mountains at altitudes between 2000 and 8000 feet (725 to 2900 meters) above sea level. This infection may present as severe febrile illness accompanied by hemolysis and circulatory collapse, or encephalitis with cerebral vasculopathy and infarction. Patients who survive the acute phase may develop cutaneous or parenchymal vasculoproliferative lesions called verruga peruana, which are histologically similar to those seen in bacillary angiomatosis. *B. bacilliformis* is

Table 4   Treatment of *Bartonella* Infection

PRESENTATION	ANTIMICROBIAL	ROUTE	DURATION
Classic CSD	None		
Severe CSD	TMP-SMX	IV q6h by weight	
	Rifampin	PO	7-10 days, monitor response
	Gentamicin	IV	
	Ciprofloxacin	PO IV	
Bartonella endocarditis	Erythromycin		4-6 wk; standard indications for valve
	Doxycycline	IV 1 g q6h with rifampin 300 mg bid;	replacement
	Clarithromycin	consider gentamicin	
Barionella septicemia	Erythromycin	IV 1 g q6h with rifampin 300 mg bid	4 wk
	Doxycycline		
	Clarithromycin		
Bacillary angiomatosis,	Erythromycin	IV, then PO usually sufficient if able	4-5 wk
Parenchymal peliosis	Doxycycline	to take oral meds	
	Clarithromycin		
	Ciprofloxacin		
	(relapses reported)		
	Azithromycin		
Aseptic meningitis	Erythromycin	IV, then PO after clinical response	IV 7-14 days; total duration 4-6 wk
Retinopathy	Doxycycline		
Encephalopathy	Clarithromycin		
	Ciprofloxacin		
	Azithromycin		

CSD, Cat-scratch disease; *TMP-SMX*, trimethoprim-sulfamethoxazole.

discussed in more detail in the chapter *Bartonella bacilliformis (Carrión's Disease)*.

■ DIAGNOSIS

Bartonella species are best cultured from blood using fresh (14 days) 5% rabbit blood. Columbia or Brucella agar and lysis centrifugation tubes (Wampole) improve yield. Because these bacteria grow slowly, infected blood cultures may not trigger CO_2-based automated systems such as BACTEC. If *Bartonella* bacteremia is suspected, blood culture bottles should be held for 4 weeks and the medium stained with acridine orange and enhanced Gram stain. Fluid staining for gram-negative organisms should be subcultured on fresh rabbit blood agar at 35° C (95° F) in 5% CO_2 with high humidity and held for 4 weeks. Isolates may be identified by PCR, cellular fatty acid profiles, and indirect fluorescent assay (IFA) with specific murine or goat antisera. Isolation from tissue is best achieved by mincing and grinding tissue under sterile conditions and incubating with bovine pulmonary artery cell monolayers in 5% CO_2 in glutamate and pynavate supplemented M199 medium, then plating supernatants on fresh blood agar as previously described.

Bartonella may also be identified in tissue and body fluids by PCR amplification of characteristic genetic sequences (16S rDNA) from samples directly, then sequencing the product or performing restriction fragment length profiles. PCR-based diagnostic tests for *Bartonella* are commercially available.

Two serologic methods are available for diagnosis of *Bartonella* infections. Enzyme-linked immunosorbent assay (ELISA) and IFA both measure antibodies in body fluids, usually serum, plasma, or cerebrospinal fluid. The IFA available through the Centers for Disease Control and Prevention does not discriminate between specific IgG and IgM antibodies and does not distinguish among species of *Bartonella*. Whole-cell ELISA, which provides information on IgG and IgM *Bartonella* antibody levels, also has no proven efficacy in distinguishing *Bartonella* species. If using serologic methods to diagnose *Bartonella* infections, clinicians must observe both acute and convalescent antibody levels to derive useful information.

■ THERAPY

There are no data based on controlled trials of antimicrobials for *Bartonella* infections. However, a few empirically derived general principles of antimicrobial therapy for *Bartonella* infections are extremely helpful (Table 4).

Host Considerations

Immunocompetent patients with *Bartonella* infections do not generally demonstrate the dramatic and reliable response to antimicrobial therapy seen in immunocompromised patients. Therefore antimicrobial therapy for uncomplicated cat-scratch disease in a normal host is usually not warranted, and simple aspiration of a painful lymph node may be sufficient. Retrospective analysis of antimicrobial efficacy in one large database suggested that trimethoprim-sulfamethoxazole, rifampin, gentamicin, and ciprofloxacin reduced the length and severity of illness in patients with severe, febrile cat-scratch disease.

Immunocompetent patients with proven or suspected *Bartonella* endocarditis, fever, bacteremia, encephalopathy, ocular pathology, extranodal cat-scratch disease, or a long course characterized by fever and severe constitutional symptoms, all merit parenteral antimicrobial therapy. Long courses (4 to 6 weeks) are probably warranted in all bacteremic patients to prevent relapse.

Immunocompromised patients generally respond well to antimicrobial therapy, but must also be treated with 4- to 6-week courses to prevent relapse. Endocarditis and septicemia require parenteral therapy, but bacillary angiomatosis and parenchymal peliosis may respond well to oral therapy, depending on the severity of the illness.

Bartonella infections behave like those caused by intracellular agents. Lysis-centrifugation cultures enhance yield; bacteremias tend to relapse if not treated with prolonged courses; and the most successful antimicrobial regimens are those with good intracellular activity. Indeed, they appear within erythrocytes in cats, but there is as yet no well-defined intracellular habitat for these agents in humans. Erythromycin is the mainstay of treatment for *Bartonella* infections in immunocompromised patients. Doxycycline, clarithromycin, rifampin, azithromycin, and ciprofloxacin have reported efficacy in these patients in small uncontrolled observations. There are anecdotal reports of treatment failures with ciprofloxacin. Patients with severe septicemia or endocarditis may benefit from the addition of rifampin.

Suggested Reading

Adal KA, Cockerell CJ, Petri WA Jr: Cat scratch disease, bacillary angiomatosis and other infections due to *Rochalimaea*, *N Engl J Med* 330:1509, 1994.

Koehler JA, Glaser CA, Tappero JW: *Rochalimaea henselae* infection, a new zoonosis with the domestic cat as reservoir, *JAMA* 271:531, 1994.

Lucey D, et al: Relapsing illness due to *Rochalimaea henselae* in immunocompetent hosts: implication for therapy and new epidemiological associations, *Clin Infect Dis* 14:683, 1992.

Lyon LW: Neurologic manifestations of cat-scratch disease: report of a case and review of the literature, *Arch Neurol* 25:23, 1971.

Margileth AM: Antibiotic treatment for cat-scratch disease: clinical study of therapeutic outcome in 268 patients and a review of the literature, *Pediatr Infect Dis J* 11:474, 1992.

Schwartzman WA: *Rochalimaea* infections: an expanding spectrum. State of the art clinical article, *Clin Infect Dis* 15:893, 1992.

Welch DF, et al: *Rochalimaea henselae* sp. nov., a cause of septicemia, bacillary angiomatosis, and parenchymal bacillary peliosis, *J Clin Microbiol* 30:275, 1992.

BORDETELLA

Sarah S. Long

Bordetellae are non–carbohydrate-fermenting tiny gram-negative coccobacilli that grow aerobically on starch blood agar or completely synthetic media with nicotinamide for growth, amino acids for energy, and charcoal or cyclodextrin resin to absorb fatty acids and other inhibitory substances. *Bordetella pertussis* is the sole species that expresses the major virulence protein pertussis toxin and is the sole cause of epidemic pertussis and the usual cause of sporadic pertussis. *Bordetella parapertussis* is an occasional cause, and *Bordetella bronchiseptica*, a common animal pathogen causing kennel cough in dogs, snuffles in rabbits, and atrophic rhinitis in swine, has been the cause in individual case reports of upper and lower respiratory tract disease, endocarditis and septicemia, posttraumatic meningitis, and peritonitis, especially in immunodeficient adults exposed to pets. *Bordetella holmesii* is a recently described cause of individual cases of septicemia, endocarditis, and respiratory failure. Its natural habitat is unknown.

Neither natural infection nor immunization provides lifelong immunity to pertussis. The current practice of partial control of pertussis through immunization in the first 6 years of life, waning immunity 5 years after vaccination, and diminishing opportunity for natural boosting of immunity has led to broad susceptibility of adults to infection and outbreaks of disease in residential facilities for the elderly. Adults are the major reservoir for *B. pertussis*. Since 1990, the reported incidence of pertussis has increased in the United States, primarily because of an increase in incidence among persons age 10 years or older. In multiple studies of adolescents, university students and health care workers who have coughing illnesses lasting for more than 7 days, approximately 20% have pertussis. Fewer than one tenth of cases are accurately diagnosed or appropriately treated. Clues to pertussis are coughing for more than 1 week, paroxysmal cough, and cough with posttussive vomiting. Patients are usually afebrile and have few upper and no lower respiratory tract signs or symptoms and no myalgia or malaise. Adults describe a typical paroxysm as beginning with an aura of anxiety, followed by strangulating cough, feeling of suffocation, and then exhaustion. Whoop is uncommon, and patients are well between paroxysms. Laboratory evaluations are usually not helpful, and lymphocytosis is mild or absent.

Diagnosis can be confirmed easily in the escalating phase of illness by culture (more sensitive) or direct fluorescent antibody test (performed by experienced laboratory personnel) of specimen obtained by aspiration or swabbing of posterior nasopharynx. Regan-Lowe transport medium is nutritive for Bordetellae and inhibits normal flora; use is essential to maximize culture results. Regan-Lowe agar with cephalexin, 10 to 40 mg/L, or Stainer-Scholte medium with cyclodextrin is preferred for culture. Experience with polymerase chain reaction testing of direct specimens is promising. Serologic tests are confusing because of difficulty differentiating vaccine-induced from infection-induced antibody

Table 1 Evaluation of Therapies for Pertussis

THERAPEUTIC AGENTS	EFFICACY	RECOMMENDATION
Erythromycin	Effective in rendering noncontagious with or without amelioration of symptoms	Yes
Albuterol	Conflicting data No rigorous trial has shown benefit	No
Corticosteroids	No rigorous trial performed	No
Pertussis immunoglobulin	Hyperimmune IVIG product in clinical trials	No

IVIG, Intravenous immunoglobulin.

response, and they are not easily obtained. Adenoviruses, *Mycoplasma pneumoniae*, parainfluenza, influenza, and respiratory syncytial virus are only occasional causes of pertussis-like illnesses.

THERAPY

Therapies for pertussis are summarized in Table 1. An antimicrobial agent is always given when pertussis is suspected or confirmed for potential clinical benefit and to limit the spread of infection to others. Erythromycin, 40 to 50 mg/kg/day orally in four divided doses (maximum, 2 g/day) for 14 days, is standard treatment. Small studies of erythromycin ethylsuccinate 50 mg/kg/day divided into two doses or 60 mg/kg/day divided into three doses, and erythromycin estolate, 40 mg/kg/day divided into two doses, showed elimination of organisms in 98% of children. Shorter courses have been associated with bacteriologic and clinical relapse. In separate small studies, erythromycin estolate, 40 mg/kg/day (maximum dose, 1 g/day) in three divided doses for 7 days; clarithromycin, 10 mg/kg/day (maximum, 400 mg) divided into two doses for 7 days; and azithromycin, 10 mg/kg/day (maximum, 500 mg) once daily for 5 days, were bacteriologically effective. In vitro *B. pertussis* is exquisitely susceptible to erythromycin, quinolones, some newer macrolides, and third-generation cephalosporins. Rare isolates resistant to erythromycin have been reported. Ampicillin, rifampin, and trimethoprim-sulfamethoxazole have modest activity, but first- and second-generation cephalosporins do not. In clinical studies erythromycin is superior to amoxicillin for eradication of *B. pertussis* and is the only agent with proven efficacy. Activity of drug at site of colonization rather than intrinsic resistance is the limiting factor for pathogen eradication. *B. parapertussis* is less susceptible in vitro to all agents except erythromycin. *B. bronchiseptica* is susceptible in vitro to antipseudomonal penicillins, aminoglycosides, and quinolones but generally is not susceptible to cephalosporins. Clinical failure has occurred with agents effective in vitro. *B. holmesii* has in vitro susceptibilities similar to *B. bronchiseptica,* but isolates have been susceptible to third-generation cephalosporin.

Convalescence is protracted, with exacerbations of cough with subsequent respiratory illnesses; these are not caused by reinfection or reactivation of *B. pertussis*. Secondary sinusitis, otitis media, bronchitis, or pneumonia can complicate *B. pertussis* infection, which denudes ciliated epithelium and inhibits local phagocytic function. Pathogens of secondary infections are *Streptococcus pneumoniae, Staphylococcus aureus, Haemophilus influenzae,* and *Moraxella catarrhalis.*

CONTROL MEASURES

Erythromycin, 40 to 50 mg/kg/day orally in four divided doses (maximum, 2 g/day) for 14 days, should be given promptly to all household contacts and other close contacts regardless of age or history of immunization. Studies have repeatedly shown efficacy of chemoprophylaxis in maternal-neonatal exposure and in households, residential facilities, and communities, and have elucidated that the majority of contacts in household or residential facilities are or will become infected when a case of pertussis is recognized. Clarithromycin and azithromycin have potentially but unproven usefulness in those who do not tolerate erythromycin. Antimicrobial prophylaxis is not routinely recommended for exposed health care workers but has been found effective as part of multifaceted control measures in major outbreaks. Infected cases and contacts should be excluded from high-risk situations (e.g., school, health care facilities) until 5 days of appropriate treatment is completed.

Immunization is evaluated for close contacts younger than 7 years. Acellular pertussis (aP) containing vaccines are preferred. DTaP is given to children who are underimmunized (with further doses to complete recommended series), those who received a third dose 6 months or more before exposure, and those who received a fourth dose 3 years or more before exposure. Pertussis vaccine is not recommended for those 7 years of age or older. Acellular pertussis vaccines have been immunogenic and safe when used in adults to control outbreaks and in recent studies. In the future, recommendations may include postexposure vaccination and routine booster vaccinations throughout life.

Suggested Reading

American Academy of Pediatrics: Pertussis. In Peter G, ed: *2000 Red Book: report of the Committee on Infectious Diseases,* ed 25, Elk Grove Village, IL, 2000, American Academy of Pediatrics.

Centers for Disease Control and Prevention: Summary of notifiable diseases, United States, 1996, *MMWR* 45(S3), 1997.

Cherry JD: Epidemiologic, clinical and laboratory aspects of pertussis in adults, *Clin Infect Dis* 28(S2):S112, 1999.

Guris D, et al: Changing epidemiology of pertussis in the United States: increasing reported incidence among adolescents and adults, 1990-1996, *Clin Infect Dis* 28:1230, 1999.

Haiduven DJ, et al: Standardized management of patients and employees exposed to pertussis, *Infect Control Hosp Epidemiol* 19:861, 1998.

Hallander HA: Microbiological and serological diagnosis of pertussis, *Clin Infect Dis* 28 (S2):S99, 1999.

Long SS, Welkon CJ, Clark JL: Widespread silent transmission of pertussis in families: antibody correlates of infection and symptomatology, *J Infect Dis* 161:480, 1990.

Sprauer MA, et al: Prevention of secondary transmission of pertussis in households with early use of erythromycin, *Am J Dis Child* 146:177, 1992.

Weber DJ, Rutala WA: Pertussis: an underappreciated risk for nosocomial outbreaks, *Infect Control Hosp Epidemiol* 19:825, 1998.

MORAXELLA (BRANHAMELLA)

Michael J. Gehman
Abdolghader Molavi

■ *MORAXELLA CATARRHALIS*

Moraxella catarrhalis is a gram-negative diplococcus with kidney-shaped cells, morphologically indistinguishable from *Neisseria* species. Described originally as *Micrococcus catarrhalis,* this organism has undergone several changes of nomenclature in the past four decades. It was classified in the genus *Neisseria* (*Neisseria catarrhalis*) in 1920, reclassified as *Branhamella catarrhalis* in 1970, and then, on the basis of DNA homology, placed in the genus *Moraxella* in 1984. The taxonomic position of this organism remains uncertain, and the inclusion of both cocci (*Moraxella catarrhalis*) and rods (other *Moraxella* species) in the same genus is confusing. Both designations, *Moraxella catarrhalis* and *Branhamella catarrhalis,* are commonly used today, sometimes in the form of *Moraxella (Branhamella) catarrhalis.*

M. catarrhalis has been recovered exclusively from humans and is a normal inhabitant of the upper respiratory tract. It is isolated from nasopharyngeal cultures in 40% to 75% of healthy infants and children 1 to 2 years old. The proportion of children that are colonized with *M. catarrhalis* decreases with age. Approximately 1% to 5% of healthy middle-age adults are colonized by *M. catarrhalis.* Adults with chronic lung disease and the elderly have significantly higher rates of upper respiratory tract colonization. Several studies have demonstrated a strong seasonal variation, with substantially higher rates of colonization in winter months in both adults and children. Furthermore, there is a significant regional variation in the rates of colonization. The colonization is prompted by adherence of the organism to pharyngeal epithelial cells, which is mediated by host and/or bacterial factors.

■ CLINICAL SYNDROMES

For more than 80 years, *M. catarrhalis* was regarded as a nonpathogenic commensal of the upper respiratory tract. During the past two decades, it has been recognized as an important cause of lower respiratory tract infection in adults with chronic obstructive lung disease and the elderly, acute sinusitis in children, and acute otitis media in infants and children.

M. catarrhalis is a well-recognized cause of lower respiratory tract infection in adults, particularly in the setting of chronic obstructive pulmonary disease and other chronic lung diseases. Acute exacerbation of chronic bronchitis is the most common lower respiratory tract infection caused by this organism. It is characterized by cough, purulent sputum, shortness of breath, and occasionally low-grade fever. Pneumonia occurs predominantly in persons older than 50 years of age but can occur in younger individuals. It is usually mild to moderate in severity, and the chest radiograph shows either patchy or lobar alveolar infiltrates. Bacteremia is rare, and pleural effusion and empyema are uncommon. A presumptive diagnosis can be made from the sputum smear, which shows many polymorphonuclear leukocytes with intracellular and extracellular gram-negative diplococci, somewhat resembling the urethral discharge smear of a patient with gonorrhea. Because the organism is somewhat resistant to decolorization, this step of Gram staining requires special attention.

M. catarrhalis is also a well-recognized cause of lower respiratory tract infections in children, particularly those younger than 1 year of age and those with asthma. It can also cause a crouplike illness, manifested by fever and stridor, in young children.

M. catarrhalis lower respiratory tract infections occur predominantly in winter and early spring. This seasonal variation is similar to that seen for nasopharyngeal colonization, suggesting an association between colonization and lower respiratory tract infection.

M. catarrhalis is a common cause of acute otitis media in infants and children. It is isolated from the middle-ear fluids obtained by tympanocentesis in 15% to 20% of infants and children with acute otitis media, making it the third leading cause of this infection after *Streptococcus pneumoniae* and nontypable *Haemophilus influenzae.* The clinical manifestations of otitis media caused by *M. catarrhalis* are indistinguishable from those caused by other organisms. In a study of acute otitis media in adults, *M. catarrhalis* was isolated from 3% of the middle-ear aspirates.

M. catarrhalis is a common cause of acute sinusitis in children. It is isolated, alone or in combination with other bacteria, from the sinus aspirates of 15% to 20% of children with clinical and radiographic evidence of acute sinusitis and is only exceeded by *S. pneumoniae* and nontypable *H. influenzae* as a causative agent.

Outbreaks of nosocomial infection caused by *M. catarrhalis,* mostly involving the lower respiratory tract, have been reported in the past two decades. Most of these outbreaks have occurred in the respiratory care and neonatal intensive care units. Hand carriage has been implicated as a possible mode of spread.

Other infections caused by *M. catarrhalis* are uncommon. Bacteremia occurs in immunocompromised hosts (usually without an evident portal of entry), patients with chronic lung disease (commonly secondary to lower respiratory tract infection), and normal hosts. Other infections include meningitis (mainly in children), endocarditis, septic arthritis, osteomyelitis, laryngitis, ophthalmia neonatorum, keratitis, pericarditis, and peritonitis associated with continuous ambulatory peritoneal dialysis.

■ SUSCEPTIBILITY TO ANTIMICROBIAL AGENTS

Approximately 95% of *M. catarrhalis* isolates in the United States produce a beta-lactamase and are resistant to penicillin, ampicillin, and amoxicillin. The two beta-lactamases produced by this organism (BRO-1, BRO-2) are chromosomal in origin and hydrolyze penicillin, ampicillin, and extended-spectrum penicillins but are inhibited by clavulanate, sulbactam, and tazobactam. Beta-lactamase production in *M. catarrhalis* can be rapidly detected by nitrocefin, a chromogenic cephalosporin, which produces color in the presence of beta-lactamase. If the organism is beta-lactamase positive, it should be considered resistant to all penicillins (with the exception of beta-lactam/beta-lactamase inhibitor combinations) and the first-generation cephalosporins. Routine beta-lactamase testing of *M. catarrhalis* is not cost-effective because of the high incidence of beta-lactamase–positive strains.

M. catarrhalis is susceptible to amoxicillin-clavulanate, ampicillin-sulbactam, piperacillin-tazobactam, second-generation cephalosporins (including the oral agents cefuroxime, cefaclor, cefprozil, and loracarbef), third-generation cephalosporins (including the oral agents cefixime and cefpodoxime), aztreonam, and imipenem. It is also sensitive to macrolides (erythromycin, clarithromycin, and azithromy-cin), trimethoprim-sulfamethoxazone (TMP-SMX), quinolones, and tetracyclines. About 6.5% of strains exhibit in vitro resistance to TMP-SMX.

■ THERAPY

Because nearly all strains of *M. catarrhalis* are beta-lactamase positive, ampicillin or amoxicillin should not be used for the therapy of infections caused by this organism, unless the isolate is known to be beta-lactamase negative. For acute otitis media or sinusitis caused by *M. catarrhalis,* documented by tympanocentesis or sinus aspiration respectively, amoxicillin-clavulanate administered for 10 days (otitis media) or 2 weeks (sinusitis) is the drug of choice. If the isolate is known to be beta-lactamase negative, amoxicillin alone may be substituted for the prescribed duration. The second- and third-generation oral cephalosporins are effective alternatives. In patients with known allergy to penicillin, a macrolide (erythlomycin, clarithromycin, or azithromycin), TMP-SMX, or a quinolone may be used.

Acute exacerbations of chronic bronchitis caused by *M. catarrhalis* may be treated with amoxicillin-clavulanate, tetracyclines, TMP-SMX, an oral second-generation cephalosporin, clarithromycin, azithromycin, or a quinolone.

In more serious infections, such as pneumonia, parenteral antibiotics are generally preferred. The drug of choice for *M. catarrhalis* pneumonia is ampicillin-sulbactam; however, ceftriaxone could also be used. In patients with known penicillin allergy, any of the parenteral quinolones (ciprofloxacin or levofloxacin), parenteral macrolides, or TMP-SMX are effective.

Suggested Reading

Christensen JJ: *Moraxella (Branhamella) catarrhalis:* clinical, microbiological and immunological features in lower respiratory tract infections, *APMIS* 88(suppl):1, 1999.

Doern GV, et al: Prevalence of antimicrobial resistance among 723 outpatient clinical isolates of *Moraxella catarrhalis* in the United States in 1994 and 1995: results of a 30-center national surveillance study, *Antimicrob Agents Chemo* 40:2884, 1996.

Enright MC, McKenzie H: *Moraxella (Branhamella) catarrhalis*—clinical and molecular aspects of a rediscovered pathogen, *J Med Microbiol* 46:360, 1997.

McGregor K, et al: *Moraxella catarrhalis:* clinical significance, antimicrobial susceptibility and BRO beta-lactamases, *Eur J Clin Microbiol Infect Dis* 17:219, 1998.

Murphy TF: *Branhamella catarrhalis:* epidemiology, surface antigenic structure, and immune response, *Microbiol Rev* 60:267, 1996.

Thorsson B, Haraldsdottir V, Kristjansson M: *Moraxella catarrhalis* bacteremia. A report on 3 cases and a review of the literature, *Scand J Infect Dis* 30:105, 1998.

Verghese A, Berk SL: *Moraxella (Branhamella) catarrhalis, Infect Dis Clin North Am* 5:523, 1991.

BRUCELLOSIS

Carlos Carrillo
Eduardo Gotuzzo

Brucellosis is a zoonotic disease found in Latin America, Mediterranean countries (Spain, Italy, Greece), and Arabian countries (Iraq, Kuwait). According to the Centers for Disease Control and Prevention (CDC), the number of cases dropped from 6147 in 1947 to 104 in 1991 with modern bovine brucellosis eradication, mainly by pasteurization of milk or dairy products.

Most cases of brucellosis in the United States are related to occupational exposure to *Brucella abortus*. The affected are mainly men and occasionally laboratory and technical personnel. However, in Texas and Florida, the ingestion of unpasteurized dairy products is the common mechanism, and the pathogen responsible is *Brucella melitensis,* attacking men and women in equal proportion and sometimes children. *B. melitensis* produces a more severe clinical pattern and can even produce a chronic form. The attack rate is higher, especially in family outbreaks, with rare subclinical infections. *B. abortus* produces a mild disease with low attack rates (<10%) and more subclinical cases.

■ CLINICAL MANIFESTATIONS

Brucellosis is one of the most protean diseases because any system can be involved. We prefer to divide it into three forms.

Acute Brucellosis
Usually, there is high fever, mainly in the evening, with malaise, headache, perspiration, arthralgias, and myalgias. In most cases, constipation, back pain, and loss of weight (as much as 20 pounds in 2 months) are found. Generally, granulomatous hepatitis, hematologic disorders, and articular compromise (especially, peripheral arthritis and sacroiliitis) are seen.

In this form of the disease, any of the routine agglutination assays produce an appropriate diagnosis (immunofluorescence [IF], enzyme-linked immunosorbent assay [ELISA], counterimmunoelectrophoresis [CIE], and Bengal rose test) with high specificity and sensitivity. Rarely, false-positive results may be caused by *Francisella tularensis* and *Yersinia enterocolitica.* With the epidemic of cholera in Latin America, the cross-reaction between *Vibrio cholerae* and *Brucella* is significant, producing false-positive serology to *Brucella* in patients with cholera. Even vaccines against cholera produce false-positive reactions transiently.

The medium Ruiz-Castañeda with Carrillo's modification (addition of 0.025% sodium phosphate sulphonate [SPS] and 0.05% of cysteine) increased the yield of *Brucella.* In the acute form, two blood cultures are as efficient as one bone marrow culture.

Subacute Brucellosis (Figure 1)
Subacute form (undulant fever or Malta fever) is the typical and classic form described in endemic areas. There is intermittent low fever, often with articular compromise (peripheral arthritis, sacroiliitis and/or spondylitis), hematologic changes (e.g., pancytopenia, thrombocytopenia, hemolytic anemia), or hepatic damage (granulomatous hepatitis). Patients with incomplete treatment are also included in this form of brucellosis.

In this form of the disease, the 2-mercaptoethanol test detects IgG, and titer above 1:80 defines active infection. *Brucella* is isolated in 40% to 70% of serial blood cultures; the bone marrow culture (0.5 to 1 ml of aspirate from the iliac crest) permits isolation in 90% of these patients.

Chronic Brucellosis (Figure 2)
In the chronic form with more than 1 year of illness, there usually is an afebrile pattern with myalgia, fatigue, depression, arthralgias, and so on. The most important differential diagnosis is chronic fatigue syndrome.

Other localized forms are granulomatous or recurrent uveitis and spondylitis. Peripheral arthritis and sacroiliitis are rare.

This form of disease is produced mainly by *B. melitensis.* It is found mainly in adults older than 30 years of age, especially older than 50 years old, and is rare in children.

The routine serologic tests and blood cultures give a diagnosis only 10% to 20% of the time. We recommend Coombs' test specific for *Brucella* or blocking antibodies. The bone marrow in our experience produces a positive culture in 50% to 75% of patients.

■ THERAPY

The intracellular character of *Brucella* results in an important therapeutic challenge, especially in subacute and chronic forms. Antibiotics should have in vitro activity, but the intracellular concentration must be adequate.

Tetracyclines have shown excellent in vitro activity throughout the world. The MIC^{90} (minimum inhibitory concentration) was 2 µg/ml for tetracycline and 0.125 µg/ml for doxycycline in our surveillance in Peru. During the past 25 years, the antibiotic activity pattern of tetracycline against *B. melitensis* has not changed, which is remarkable because these are still our drugs of choice.

In addition, oxytetracycline and doxycycline showed that the minimal bactericidal concentration (MBC) was equal to MIC. All these features in conjunction with worldwide experience point to tetracyclines as the keystone of treatment.

The differences among tetracyclines are tolerance, dosage, and safety profile; however, the new ones have better tolerance and fewer side effects and can be used with meals without reducing efficacy. We prefer to use doxycycline or minocycline.

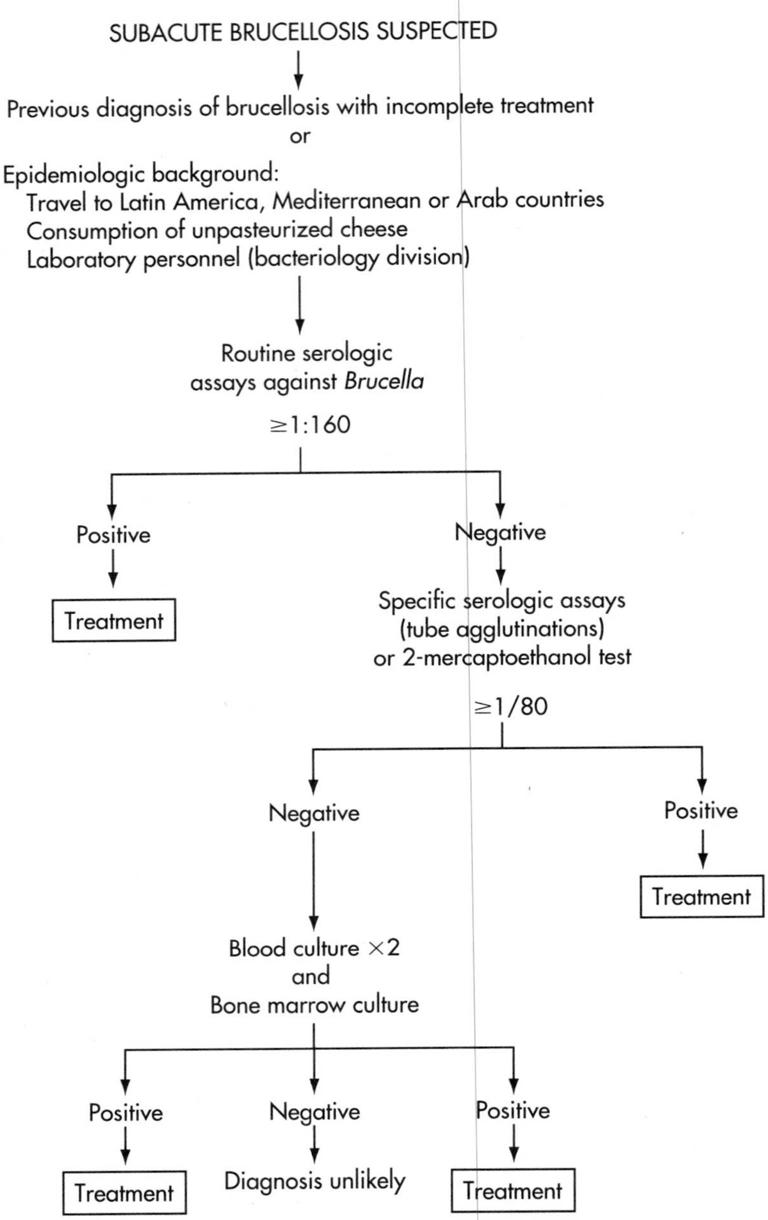

SUBACUTE BRUCELLOSIS SUSPECTED

↓

Previous diagnosis of brucellosis with incomplete treatment
or

Epidemiologic background:
    Travel to Latin America, Mediterranean or Arab countries
    Consumption of unpasteurized cheese
    Laboratory personnel (bacteriology division)

↓

Routine serologic
assays against *Brucella*

≥1:160

Positive   Negative

↓   ↓

[Treatment]   Specific serologic assays
                                            (tube agglutinations)
                                         or 2-mercaptoethanol test

                                                  ≥1/80

                  Negative   Positive

                     ↓   ↓

             Blood culture ×2   [Treatment]
                    and
            Bone marrow culture

       Positive   Negative   Positive

          ↓   ↓   ↓

   [Treatment]   Diagnosis unlikely   [Treatment]

Figure 1
Algorithm for the evaluation and treatment of subacute brucellosis.

The other important aspect is the need to combine antibiotics to reduce the rate of relapse. Most antibiotics can reduce the fever, but recurrence is high.

Rifampin has been introduced as a preferential agent because of its excellent in vitro activity and intracellular concentration. The possibility of rapid resistance was shown in our strains when 5 of 10 strains exposed in vitro to rifampin developed resistance by the seventh day.

The third effective group of drugs against *Brucella* is the aminoglycosides, with good in vitro activity and good clinical response. The largest study was done with streptomycin; however, gentamicin, netilmicin, and amikacin showed the same and even better results in open trials.

Comparative studies have been done of doxycycline plus rifampin versus doxycycline plus streptomycin (D-S). Both schedules had a high cure rate (more than 95%); however, D-S had a lower relapse rate.

The doxycycline levels in the plasma of patients treated with rifampin were significantly lower than those of patients treated with D-S. Patients who were rapid acetylators had lower levels because they had higher clearance rates. In addition, the half-life and the area under the curve were significantly lower in these patients. All these new data suggest that relapses may result from this interaction.

Adults

Our standard treatment for adult patients is oral doxycycline, 100 mg twice a day for 45 days, plus streptomycin, 1 g intramuscularly per day for 2 weeks (prolonging treatment with streptomycin for more than 2 weeks has not proved to be more effective); or doxycycline, 100 mg twice a day, plus rifampin, 600 mg once a day, both for 45 days. Only in a case of spondylitis, endocarditis, or brain abscess do we prolong treatment for 3 months.

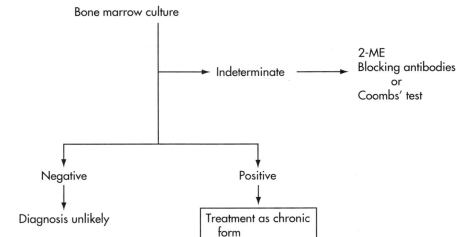

CHRONIC BRUCELLOSIS SUSPECTED

Chronic fatigue syndrome with epidemiologic background

Spondylitis with osteoblastic and osteoclastic lesions

Granulomatous uveitis or panuveitis

Depression with low-grade fever and arthralgias

Tube agglutination against brucella

Bone marrow culture

Indeterminate → 2-ME
Blocking antibodies
or
Coombs' test

Negative

Positive

Diagnosis unlikely

Treatment as chronic form

Figure 2
Algorithm for the evaluation and treatment of chronic brucellosis.

In chronic brucellosis we prefer to use standard treatment for 45 days and then 3 months of doxycycline only. Some experts recommend adding levamisole for this special form during 3 months.

Children
In children younger than 8 years of age, tetracyclines cannot be used. The combination of rifampin, 15 to 20 mg/kg once a day for 4 weeks, and aminoglycosides at standard dose for 5 to 10 days is highly effective in children.

The use of cotrimoxazole has also been recommended in children. Cotrimoxazole may be used 240 mg for 4 weeks plus rifampin 20 mg/kg once a day for 4 weeks. This schedule has a high level of tolerance and few adverse effects; however, the efficacy is not as acceptable as with other schedules. Some report excellent results of cotrimoxazole for 4 weeks plus gentamicin for 5 to 10 days.

Pregnancy and Brucellosis
Brucellosis during pregnancy is a special problem because the best drug should be avoided and the clinical course and fetal prognosis are poor.

In our experience with more than 70% women with brucellosis, early and adequate treatment showed excellent evolution of pregnancy, and the babies were normal. However, when antibiotic treatment is begun late, the prognosis is worse.

The best schedule is cotrimoxazole plus rifampin for 6 weeks. Folic acid supplements should be given.

Another option is aminoglycoside for 10 days plus rifampin or cotrimoxazole for 6 weeks.

Other Antibiotics
Some drugs, such as chloramphenicol, erythromycin, ampicillin, and cephalosporins, showed moderate in vitro activity, but the clinical experience is not as good as with the other drugs.

Recently, the fluoroquinolones showed better in vitro activity, and they have good intracellular penetration. However, some trials showed that norfloxacin and ciprofloxacin had less clinical efficacy. Only ofloxacin in one trial showed good efficacy.

Steroids
We recommend corticosteroids only for 3 to 6 weeks for uveitis and for 2 to 10 weeks for severe thrombocytopenic purpura. If there is no response, we maintain steroids for 2 to 4 months. After this time if the thrombocytopenia is still evident, we recommend splenectomy.

Suggested Reading
Ariza JF, et al: Treatment of human brucellosis with doxycycline plus rifampin or doxycycline plus streptomycin: a randomized double-blind study, *Ann Intern Med* 117:25, 1992.

Colmenero JD, et al: Possible implication of doxycycline-rifampin interaction for treatment of brucellosis, *Antimicrob Agent Chemother* 38:2798, 1994.

Gotuzzo E, Carrillo C: Brucella arthritis. In Espinoza L, Goldberg D, Arnett F, Alarcon G, eds: *Infections in the rheumatic diseases,* Orlando, FL, 1988, Grune & Stratton.

Monir Mad Kour M: *Brucellosis, Editorial,* Cambridge, UK, 1989, Butterworths.

Solera J, Martínez-Alfaro E, Saez L: Meta-análisis sobre la eficacia de la combinación de rifampicina y doxiciclina en el tratamiento de la brucelosis humana, *Med Clin (Barc)* 102:731, 1994.

Young EJ: Human brucellosis. *Rev Infect Dis* 15:821, 1983.

Zavala-Trujillo I, et al: Brucellosis, *Infect Dis Clin North Am* 8:225, 1994.

CAMPYLOBACTER

David W.K. Acheson

Campylobacter (Greek *campylo,* curved; *bacter;* rod) are motile, non–spore-forming gram-negative rods. They are a very common cause of gastrointestinal (GI) infection in humans in many parts of the world. *Campylobacter* organisms were first isolated in the early 1900s from aborted sheep fetuses. However, it was many years later and not until the 1970s that *Campylobacter* were isolated from stool. There are many members of the genus *Campylobacter;* the major enteric pathogen for humans is *C. jejuni,* although *C. coli, C. fetus, C. upsaliensis,* and *C. lari* are also pathogenic to humans. *C. jejuni* is associated with GI disease, and *C. fetus* usually causes systemic infection, often in debilitated patients. *Campylobacter* is microaerophilic, and although all will grow at 37° C (98.6° F), *C. jejuni* grows best at 42° C (107.6° F). A number of selective media are in use, including Skirrows, Butzler's, and Campy-BAP. Although several serotypes of *C. jejuni* have been reported, there are few data regarding the relative virulence of these different types, although some appear to be more closely associated with the development of Guillain-Barré syndrome (GBS) than others.

■ EPIDEMIOLOGY

Campylobacter is the most commonly diagnosed enteric bacterial infection in many parts of the United States and Europe. It is estimated that there are more than 2.5 million cases per year in the United States. It is especially common in children younger than 1 year of age and in young adults, and it occurs most often in the summer. *Campylobacter* species are found in fowl and many wild and domestic animals, and most human infections probably result from contamination of milk and other animal food sources, especially poultry. The organisms can also be transmitted by direct contact with infected animals and contaminated water, and cross-contamination between infected poultry and other foods is probably one of the most frequent modes of transmission. Small numbers of organisms may cause disease; as few as 800 have been shown to cause infection in volunteer studies, but the infecting dose is usually about 10^4. Although asymptomatic carriage of *Campylobacter* is thought to be uncommon in developed countries, in less developed nations carriage rates as high as 37% have been reported among children.

■ CLINICAL FEATURES

The incubation period for *C. jejuni* infection varies and is typically between 1 and 7 days, with most cases occurring 2 to 4 days after exposure. Very short incubation periods of less than 12 hours have been reported. *C. jejuni* illness typically presents with a prodrome of fever, headache, myalgia, and malaise for up to 24 hours before intestinal symptoms develop. The fever may be as high as 40° C (104° F), and the diarrhea varies from a few loose stools to copious watery discharge. Blood is often present in the stool but varies in amount. The illness usually lasts less than a week, but patients untreated with antibiotics often continue to excrete the organisms for several weeks. Bacteremia is rare in *C. jejuni* infections, although focal infections such as endocarditis, meningitis, septic abortion, acute cholecystitis, pancreatitis, and cystitis have all been documented. Postinfectious reactive arthritis may also occur, especially in HLA-B27–positive individuals. One of the most serious consequences of infection with *C. jejuni* is the development of GBS. This is an autoimmune disorder of the peripheral nervous system resulting in an ascending flaccid paralysis that carries a mortality rate of up to 5%. GBS is thought to be caused by molecular mimicry between polysaccharides on the outer surface of *C. jejuni* and gangliosides in the myelin sheaths of peripheral nerves.

In contrast to *C. jejuni, C. fetus* commonly produces systemic disease, often in vascular sites: endocarditis, pericarditis, and mycotic aneurysms of the abdominal aorta. Central nervous system infections such as meningoencephalitis also occur with *C. fetus,* as do other localized infections, including septic arthritis, spontaneous bacterial peritonitis, salpingitis, lung abscess, empyema, cellulitis, urinary tract infection, vertebral osteomyelitis, and cholecystitis. In patients with acquired immunodeficiency syndrome (AIDS), *Campylobacter* species other than *C. fetus* and *C. jejuni* may also cause bacteremia.

■ DIAGNOSIS

Campylobacter have a characteristic darting motility, and a presumptive diagnosis of *Campylobacter* infection may be made by examination of stool passed within 2 hours using direct darkfield or phase-contrast microscopy. Leukocytes and red cells are also often seen in stool samples, with 75% of patients having polymorphonuclear leukocytes in their stool. Confirmation of the diagnosis of *C. jejuni* infection is based on a positive stool or blood culture, although *Campylobacter* is fastidious and may die during transport to the laboratory. DNA probes, polymerase chain reaction, and serologic testing all have been used to confirm diagnosis but are not routinely available. Direct detection of *Campylobacter* antigens in stool using enzyme immunoassays is a new approach that is now commercially available. This method has the attraction of not requiring live organisms but has the detraction of not producing an isolate that will be available for antimicrobial sensitivity testing. *C. fetus* may be isolated from blood held in culture up to 14 days. The fastidious nature of the organisms means that failure to culture *Campylobacter* does not rule them out as the cause of significant clinical disease.

■ THERAPY

As with many diarrheal diseases, fluid replacement is the most important therapy in *Campylobacter* diarrhea. Oral rehydration is usually adequate, but patients with severe dehydration should be given volume replacement with intravenous solutions of electrolytes and water.

Most *Campylobacter* infections are mild and self-limited and do not result in a visit to a physician. These mild infections require no specific treatment. Treating patients later in the course of the disease (after several days of symptoms) will remove *Campylobacter* from the stool, but it is not likely to have a dramatic effect on the duration of symptoms. Treating early and empirically may reduce the length of time that a patient is symptomatic. Person-to-person spread generally is not considered a major concern with *Campylobacter,* so treating to prevent this is not generally recommended (except in the case of food handlers). However, there may be exceptions to this, for example, the reduction of spread in day-care settings. In general, antibiotics are recommended only for patients with severe infection, including those with significant fever or volume loss, frequent bloody diarrhea, prolonged or severe symptoms, and an immunocompromised status. Antibiotic therapy can have a dramatic positive effect on symptoms of *C. jejuni* infection, justifying a trial of therapy in severe or persistent illness.

C. jejuni is usually susceptible to many antimicrobial agents in vitro, including macrolides, tetracyclines, aminoglycosides, chloramphenicol, quinolones, and nitrofurans (Table 1). They are inherently resistant to trimethoprim and most cephalosporins except cefotaxime, ceftazidime, and cefpirone. Erythromycin has consistently been the drug most widely used in the treatment of *C. jejuni* because it is inexpensive, safe, and time tested. Erythromycin treatment will terminate gastrointestinal shedding of *Campylobacter*

Table 1 Recommended Antimicrobial Agents for *Campylobacter*

	DRUG	DOSAGE AND DURATION
Preferred	Erythromycin	Adults: 500 mg PO bid ×7 days Children: 30-50 mg/kg/day qid ×7 days
Alternative	Ciprofloxacin	Adults: 500 mg PO bid ×7 days
Other agents	Nitrofurans (furazolidone) Aminoglycosides Chloramphenicol	

within 24 to 72 hours, which should be kept in mind when treating infections in day-care or preschool settings to avoid spread of the disease. Resistance to erythromycin has been reported but is generally low in *C. jejuni*; it is higher in *C. coli.* Erythromycin stearate is resistant to acid and poorly absorbed, so it is the preparation of choice for treating *Campylobacter.* In children, erythromycin ethylsuccinate should be used. Of the other macrolides, clindamycin, azithromycin, and clarithromycin are all active but offer little advantage over erythromycin. Fluoroquinolones are generally very active against *Campylobacter,* and there was a period when it appeared that these would be the drugs of choice. However, there are increasing problems with fluoroquinolone resistance. In Sweden, quinolone resistance in clinical isolates of *C. jejuni* increased more than 20-fold in the early 1990s. There has also been a documented rise in the incidence of resistance to quinolones in other parts of Europe since 1992, with up to 57% of *C. jejuni* and 43% of *C. coli* isolates being resistant (determined by disk diffusion using naladixic acid and ciprofloxacin). Other studies from Spain have confirmed this trend, with 30% to 40% of *C. jejuni* strains being resistant to three fluoroquinolones. Similar trends of increasing fluoroquinolone resistance are occurring in the United States. Despite the initial enthusiasm for this group of drugs, they are expensive, they are not recommended for children in the United States, and the increasing resistance problems make them an unsuitable first choice of therapy. Extraintestinal infection with *C. jejuni* needs at least 10 days of treatment, and systemic infection with *C. fetus* warrants 2 to 3 weeks of therapy.

■ PROGNOSIS AND PREVENTION

Most patients recover totally following infection with *C. jejuni.* Complications such as reactive arthritis and GBS are unusual. Systemic *C. fetus* infections have a significant mortality, especially in patients with underlying disease such as diabetes mellitus or cirrhosis or who are immunocompromised. Transmission of *Campylobacter* infection can be reduced by careful food handling, with special attention to cross-contamination from poultry products. Proper cooking of food, pasteurization of milk, and protection of water supplies are all critical in preventing infection with *Campylobacter.*

Suggested Reading

Giesendorf BAJ, et al: Development of species-specific DNA probes for *Campylobacter jejuni, Campylobacter coli,* and *Campylobacter pylori* by polymerase chain reaction fingerprinting, *J Clin Microbiol* 31:1541, 1993.

Nachamkin I, Allos B, Ho T: *Campylobacter* species and Guillain-Barré syndrome, *Clin Microbiol Rev* 11:555, 1998.
Skirrow MB: *Campylobacter* enteritis: a "new" disease, *BMJ* 2:9, 1977.
Skirrow MB, Blaser MJ: *Campylobacter jejuni.* In Blaser MJ, et al, eds: *Infections of the gastrointestinal tract,* New York, 1995, Raven Press.

CLOSTRIDIA

Richard Quintiliani
Romelle Belmonte

The Clostridia include bacterial species that are responsible for generating some of the most potent toxins known to humans. They are obligate, anaerobic, spore-forming bacilli that live in soil and the intestinal tract of animals and man. Of the 83 clostridial strains, approximately 30 are clearly or potentially pathogenic. Distinctive types of infection have been associated with certain species of *Clostridium:* gastrointestinal illness with *C. perfringens* and *C. difficile;* neurologic syndromes with *C. botulinum* and *C. tetani;* focal suppurative infections, myonecrosis, and gas gangrene with *C. perfringens, C. novyi, C. septicum, C. histolyticum, C. bifermentans,* and *C. fallax;* and bacteremia with *C. perfringens, C. septicum,* and *C. tertium.*

■ GASTROINTESTINAL ILLNESS

Clostridium perfringens

One of the most common and dangerous causes of food poisoning in humans is caused by *C. perfringens.* Of the five strains of *C. perfringens* (A through E), type A causes most cases of foodborne illness and infectious diarrhea. The usual sources are meat and meat products. Diarrhea and crampy symptoms are believed to be caused by a protein toxin called *C. perfringens* enterotoxin. On rare occasions, type C causes foodborne infections that result in necrotizing enteritis. First reported in Germany between 1946 and 1949, it is now found only in the highlands of Papua New Guinea, where it is known as *pigbel* because of its association with pig feasts. It is believed that the disease results from deficiency or absence of intestinal proteolytic enzymes specific for the type C toxin, which is usually caused by nutritional factors or inhibitors in the diet or both. A vaccine has been developed against the beta toxin and was successful in preventing necrotizing enteritis in those at risk.

Laboratory Diagnosis

Criteria used to establish the diagnosis of *C. perfringens* food poisoning include (1) more than 10^5 *C. perfringens* organisms per gram of incriminated food; (2) median spore count of more than 10^6 per gram of stool from ill persons, and (3) isolation of the same serotype of *C. perfringens* from stool and suspected food. Molecular methods for detection of *C. perfringens* include enzyme immunoassay for detection of toxins as well as gene probe or PCR assays for detection of toxin gene.

Clinical Features and Therapy

After an incubation period of 8 to 12 hours, the patient develops diarrhea (90% of cases), midepigastric pain (80%), nausea (25%), fever (24%), and vomiting (9%). The disease is typically self-limited and resolves in less than 24 hours. Therapy is supportive, with fluid replacement playing a major role. Antibiotics and drugs that inhibit intestinal peristalsis are not indicated and may even prolong the illness.

Clostridium difficile

C. difficile, the agent that causes pseudomembranous colitis associated with antibiotic therapy, is discussed in the chapter *Antibiotic-Associated Diarrhea.*

■ BOTULISM

Botulism is a neuroparalytic illness caused by a neurotoxin produced from the anaerobic, spore-forming bacterium *C. botulinum.* The disease can be categorized as (1) foodborne, (2) wound, (3) infant, and rarely (4) adult infectious botulism. Since 1973, 24 cases of foodborne botulism, 3 cases of wound botulism, and 71 cases of infant botulism have been reported annually to the Centers for Disease Control and Prevention (CDC). The antigenically distinct toxins are designated A to G, with type A being the most common cause of foodborne botulism. On a weight basis, botulism toxins are the most potent poisons known. Purified botulinum toxin is used to treat various medical conditions such as strabismus, torticollis, blepharospasm, oromandibular dystonia, achalasia, and spasmodic dysphonia. On the other hand, botulinum toxin has been used in developing biologic agents by some countries as well as terrorist groups.

Foodborne Botulism

Foodborne botulism is caused by ingestion of preformed toxin in contaminated foods, with home-canned or prepared foods being the most often implicated vehicle. Botulism typically begins as neuromuscular blockade resulting in symmetric weakness, usually beginning 12 to 36 hours after ingestion of contaminated food. Patients are usually alert and afebrile. The most common complaints include weakness, lassitude, dizziness, diminished salivation, ileus, bladder distension, and constipation. Stabilization ensues, usually with complete recovery over days to months. Like tetanus, botulism does not result in long-term immunity.

Botulism is underdiagnosed because many clinicians are unfamiliar with the disease. Many cases are initially misdiagnosed as a cerebrovascular accident or other more common clinical entities such as Guillain-Barré syndrome or myasthenia gravis. Initial testing may include brain imaging, lumbar puncture, electromyography, or edrophonium chloride testing. The diagnosis of botulism is confirmed by (1) demonstration of botulinum toxin in serum by intraperitoneal injection into mice, (2) isolation of *C. botulinum* in stool, or (3) identification of toxin, the organism, or both in food.

Patients with botulism should be monitored initially in an intensive care unit (ICU) setting. The mainstay of treatment is supportive therapy with mechanical ventilation. If food exposure was recent, gastric lavage should be attempted. Cathartics and enemas are given to remove unabsorbed toxin from the colon. Cathartic agents containing magnesium should be avoided because of the theoretic concern that increased magnesium levels may enhance the action of botulinum toxin. The administration of antitoxin is the only specific pharmacologic treatment available. The CDC and the local health department should be informed for further investigation of suspected cases and to obtain antitoxin. The administration of trivalent equine antitoxin to humans by the intravenous route neutralizes toxin molecules not bound to nerve endings. A single vial (7500 IU of type A, 5500 IU of type B, and 8500 IU of type E antitoxin) per patient is now administered, and it is believed that no additional doses are necessary. Because the antitoxin is equine, patients should be tested for hypersensitivity. In the absence of infectious complications, antibiotic treatment has no value. Prophylactic immunization with a vaccine against botulism is protective; however, the vaccine is unlicensed, and the vaccination process should start months before exposure. Table 1 lists tests that are useful in the diagnosis of botulism.

Wound Botulism

First recognized in 1943, wound botulism usually results from severe trauma and open fractures contaminated by soil. Recently, intravenous drug abuse has been implicated. The clinical manifestations are similar to foodborne botulism except for the absence of gastrointestinal symptoms. The median incubation period is longer (7 days with a range of 4 to 14 days). Fever may be present because of wound infection.

Botulism antitoxin is administered as in foodborne botulism together with debridement of contaminated wounds. Anaerobic cultures of the wound should be obtained. Al-

Table 1   Useful Tests in Diagnosing Botulism

TEST	RESULT CONSISTENT WITH BOTULISM
INITIAL TEST	
Brain imagining (CT or MRI)	Normal
Lumbar puncture	Normal
Electromyography	Decreased amplitude of action potentials in involved muscle groups
Rapid repetitive electromyography (20-50 Hz)	Facilitation (increasing pattern of action potential amplitude)
Edrophonium chloride test	Negative
CONFIRMATORY TEST	
Mouse inoculation test for toxin (serum, stool, or food)	Positive
Stool culture for *Clostridium botulinum*	Positive
Identification of toxin or organism in food	Positive

Modified from Shapiro RL, Hatheway C, Swerdlow DL: *Ann Intern Med* 129:221, 1998.
CT, Computed tomography; *MRI,* magnetic resonance imaging.

though its efficacy has not been proved, intravenous penicillin, 10 to 20 million units per day, should be given.

Infant Botulism

First described in 1976, infant botulism is the most common cause of botulism in the United States. The disease most commonly occurs during the second month of life. The usual source of the organism is soil, but honey has been implicated in some cases. Supportive care remains the mainstay of treatment, with intubation or tube feeding sometimes becoming necessary. There is no evidence to support the use of antibiotics or botulinum antitoxin. It is believed that the antitoxin might result in lysis of intraintestinal organisms, thus liberating more neurotoxin into the gut. The safety and efficacy of human botulism immunoglobulin is being determined. This product is available in the United States solely for the treatment of infant botulism. For information on obtaining human botulism immunoglobulin, contact the California Department of Health Services at 510-540-2646 (24 hours).

◼ TETANUS

C. tetani is commonly found in soil all over the world. It is a strict anaerobe and often possesses terminal endospores that give the organism a drumstick appearance. About 1 million cases of tetanus occur annually worldwide, mostly in developing countries. About 50 to 100 cases of tetanus are reported each year in the United States, mostly in patients older than 60 years of age.

Two toxins are generated by *C. tetani*. Tetanospasmin is responsible for the clinical manifestations associated with tetanus. The role of tetanolysin in human tetanus is unclear.

Common portals of entry are wounds, burns, tympanic membrane perforation from otitis media, and skin ulcers. Infection of the umbilical stump can cause neonatal tetanus.

The incubation period is usually 7 to 21 days but ranges from 2 days to months. A shorter incubation period correlates with severe disease and frequent complications. The most common presenting complaints are trismus (lockjaw), generalized weakness, stiffness, cramping, difficulty swallowing, and difficulty in urination. Increasing muscle rigidity with reflex spasms ensues. Contraction of facial muscles results in a characteristic expression, risus sardonicus. These muscle spasms can result in hypoxia from laryngospasm or tonic contraction of respiratory muscles.

Local tetanus is manifested by fixed rigidity of muscles at or near the site of injury, probably resulting from partial immunity to tetanospasmin, but can progress to generalized tetanus. Cephalic tetanus is a rare manifestation of tetanus and usually results from otitis media or head wounds. It is manifested by dysfunction of one or more cranial nerves, usually the facial nerve and trismus. Neonatal tetanus presents as severe generalized disease within the first 2 weeks of life, usually the result of an infected umbilical stump. Children of nonimmunized mothers are at risk for developing neonatal tetanus. Infants show weakness and inability to suck, with tetanic spasms and rigidity developing later.

Diagnosis and Therapy

Diagnosis is based primarily on the history and clinical presentation. A complete immunization history should be obtained if possible. A serum antitoxin level of 0.01 IU/ml or higher or a history of immunization makes the diagnosis unlikely. Cerebrospinal fluid studies are generally within normal limits. Isolation of *C. tetani* from the wound does not prove the diagnosis because it can be part of normal skin flora. Differential diagnosis of tetanus includes meningitis, strychnine poisoning, severe hypocalcemia, subarachnoid hemorrhage, and oculogyric crisis secondary to strychnine poisoning. Management guidelines are outlined in Table 2. Guidelines for tetanus prophylaxis in wound management are provided in Table 3.

■ GAS GANGRENE

Clostridial gas gangrene or myonecrosis is usually a fulminant infection characterized by muscle necrosis and systemic toxicity. The most common organism isolated is *C. perfringens,* which accounts for 80% of cases. *C. novyi, C. septicum, C. histolyticum, C. fallax,* and *C. bifermentans* are sometimes implicated. Gas gangrene can occur in a variety of clinical settings and can be divided into posttraumatic or postoperative, or it may occur spontaneously, usually in patients with diabetes, peripheral vascular disease, or an underlying malignancy.

The incubation period averages about 4 days, with the patient initially presenting with severe, persistent pain at the site of the wound. Tachycardia, mental changes, hypertension, and renal failure can be seen in its acute phase. The skin is edematous, with gas sometimes noted on palpation, often along with hemorrhagic bullae. Approximately 15%

Table 2   Guidelines for Initial Management of Tetanus

1. Thorough history and physical examination, including immunization history and portal of entry.
2. Hospitalization in intensive care unit. Surroundings should be dark and quiet; avoid unnecessary manipulations.
3. Assess airway and ventilation; endotracheal intubation with neuromuscular blockage as needed. Severe laryngospasm may require tracheostomy.
4. Administer benzodiazepine (intravenous midazolam, 5 to 15 mg/hr, or intravenous diazepam, at 5-mg increments) to control muscle rigidity; taper slowly. The use of intrathecal baclofen or intravenous dantrolene has been reported to be effective in controlling muscle spasm.
5. Obtain baseline antitoxin levels and strychnine and dopamine antagonist assays.
6. Administer human tetanus immunoglobulin (HTIg) 500 U intramuscularly and give tetanus toxoid or diphtheria-pertussis-tetanus vaccine (0.5 ml IM), as indicated for age, at another site.
7. Initiate nutritional support.
8. Debride wound; administer penicillin, 1-10 million units per day, or metronidazole, 500 mg bid for 10 days.
9. For autonomic instability, consider labetalol or morphine.
10. Start prophylactic heparin.

Table 3   Tetanus Prophylaxis in Wound Management

HISTORY OF ADSORBED TETANUS TOXOID (DOSES)	CLEAN MINOR WOUNDS		ALL OTHER WOUNDS	
	Td*	TIG	Td*	TIG
Unknown or <3	Yes	No	Yes	Yes
>3	No†	No	No‡	No

Adapted from American Academy of Pediatrics: Tetanus. In Pickering LK (ed): *2000 Red Book: Report of the Committee on Infectious Diseases,* ed 25, Elk Grove Village, IL, 2000, American Academy of Pediatrics, p. 566.
Td, Adult-type tetanus and diphtheria toxoids; *TIG,* tetanus immunoglobulin.
*For patients 7 years of age or older. For patients younger than 7, diphtheria-pertussis-tetanus toxoid is preferred.
†Unless it is more than 10 years since previous dose.
‡Unless it is more than 5 years since previous dose.

have associated bacteremia. Gram stain of the wound discharge usually shows gram-positive or gram-variable rods with few or no white cells.

Immediate surgical debridement is the cornerstone of treatment. Intravenous penicillin, 24 million units divided every 4 to 6 hours per day with the use of intravenous clindamycin, 900 mg every 8 hours, to add synergy is a reasonable choice. Addition of an aminoglycoside or a third-generation cephalosporin (e.g., ceftriaxone, cefotaxime) should be used in mixed infections that include gram-negative organisms. Other antibiotics that can be used include metronidazole, chloramphenicol, tetracycline, and beta-lactam–beta-lactamase inhibitor combinations. The use of hyperbaric oxygen remains controversial.

CLOSTRIDIAL BACTEREMIA

Bacteremia caused by clostridial species can have a fulminant course. *C. perfringens* account for 60% of isolates. Many patients may have no symptoms attributable to the bacteremia and have been admitted to the hospital for another medical condition. These patients with so-called benign clostridial bacteremia do not require antibiotic therapy. Two-thirds are mostly from intraabdominal sources. The second most common *Clostridium* species isolated from blood is *C. septicum,* which is usually associated with underlying hematologic malignancy, colonic carcinoma, or cyclic neutropenia.

Virtually all *C. perfringens* species are susceptible to penicillin although some resistance to low levels of penicillin have been encountered. Metronidazole, clindamycin, and chloramphenicol are alternatives in a penicillin-allergic patient. *C. septicum* is extremely sensitive to penicillin as well as to other antibiotics. *C. tertium* is unusual in that it is resistant to beta-lactam antibiotics as well as to clindamycin and metronidazole. The organism is uniformly sensitive to vancomycin, trimethoprim-sulfamethoxazole, and ciprofloxacin.

Suggested Reading

Bodey GP, et al: Clostridial bacteremia in cancer patients, *Cancer* 67:1928, 1991.

Ernst ME, et al: Tetanus: pathophysiology and management, *Ann Pharmacother* 31:1507, 1997.

Shapiro RL, Hatheway C, Swerdlow DL: Botulism in the United States: a clinical and epidemiologic review, *Ann Intern Med* 129:221, 1998.

CAT-SCRATCH DISEASE

Andrew M. Margileth

Cat-scratch disease (CSD) a zoonotic bacterial infection, commonly presents as a chronic (usually ≥3 weeks) lymphadenitis in the cervical or axillary regions. It is usually benign and self-limiting. About 24,000 cases occur annually in the United States, resulting in more than 2000 hospitalizations. Contact with a cat, especially a kitten, or cat fleas are major risk factors for the disease. Rarely, CSD has been reported with dog contact only. CSD is caused by a fastidious gram-negative bacillus (*Bartonella henselae* or *clarridgeiae*) that has been cultured from skin, blood, and lymph nodes. The adenopathy (≥10 mm) is commonly regional and tender initially. In one third of our patients, multifocal adenitis occurred. Following cat contact (95%) or scratches (66%) before the adenopathy, the patient or parent often notes a primary inoculation skin papule or eye lesion. Adenopathy persists for several weeks to months, then gradually resolves spontaneously. However, 12% of patients have atypical manifestations, including the oculoglondular syndrome of Parinaud, neuroretinitis, encephalopathy, systemic disease, granulomatous hepatitis, thrombocytopenic purpura, osteomyelitis, thoracopulmonary disease, and rarely, a breast tumor or chest wall abscess. Clinical features observed in 1733 patients with CSD are noted (Table 1).

About 80% of patients are younger than 21 years of age. Systemic disease (severe malaise, weight loss, prolonged fevers, fatigue, encephalopathy) occurs in 2% to 3% of patients. Morbidity appears to be greater in adolescents and adults. Recently, reports of severe disseminated disease characterized by hepatic and/or splenic abscesses, neuroretinitis, pleuritis, and generalized lymphadenitis, with epithelioid angiomatosis and granulomatous osteomyelitis, have occurred in both immunocompetent and immunocompromised patients. Bacillary angiomatosis and bacillary peliosis (liver, spleen) are vascular proliferative manifestations of *Bartonella* infection *(B. henselae, B. quintana)* that occur predominately in human immunodeficiency virus (HIV)-infected patients involving skin, bone, brain, and lymph nodes.

A tuberculin test (PPD) should be performed to rule out tuberculosis. The diagnosis of CSD is based on clinical features and is confirmed with specific serologic studies. Performance of a *Bartonella* polymerase chain reaction (PCR) hybridization assay on lymph node and/or abscess aspirates or a biopsy specimen provide the highest diagnostic sensitivity. Less sensitive serologic tests for diagnosis are available from several commercial laboratories. Enzyme-linked immunoassay (EIA) to detect IgM *B. henselae* antibodies are only 71% sensitive in patients who fulfilled two or more criteria for CSD. The Centers for Disease Control and Prevention (CDC) perform a very sensitive (96%) immunofluorescent antibody assay (IFA) for *B. henselae* antibody. Cat-scratch skin-test antigens used since 1947 also are very sensitive (98%), with induration of 5 mm or more providing a diagnosis within 48 to 72 hours. However, serologic and CSD antigen skin tests are usually negative during the first week of illness. Diagnostic criteria are listed in Table 2.

THERAPY

General

Management consists primarily of careful observation over several (2 to 6) months, during which time spontaneous involution of the lymphadenopathy should occur. Extra bed

Table 1 Clinical Features in 1733 Patients with Cat-Scratch Disease, April 1975 through 1999

SYMPTOMS AND SIGNS	PERCENTAGE OF PATIENTS*	DURATION (DAYS)
Adenopathy	100.0†	14-730
Adenopathy only	50.0	14-730
Malaise/fatigue	29.4	1-21
Fever (38.3° to 41.2° C)	28.0	1-65
Anorexia, emesis	14.5	3-30
Headache	13.0	1-7
Splenomegaly	9.5	7-30
Sore throat	7.0	1-5
Exanthem	5.0	5-17
Conjunctivitis	3.3	1-20
Seizures/coma	2.7	1-5
Arthralgia	2.5‡	3-42‡
Blindness	2.0	30-200

*$N = 1733$.

†Three adults with systemic disease, neuroretinitis had no adenopathy.

‡Data from 1989 through 1999.

Table 2 Diagnosis of Cat-Scratch Disease

Lymphadenopathy (≥10 mm) present ≥3 weeks.*
1. Cat or flea contact with or without a scratch mark or a regional inoculation lesion (skin papule, eye granuloma, mucous membrane)
2. Laboratory: negative PPD or serology for other infectious causes of adenopathy; sterile pus aspirated from node, polymerase chain reaction assay positive; *Bartonella henselae* or *Afipia felis,* highest sensitivity; CT scan: liver/spleen abscesses
3. Positive enzyme-linked immunoassay or immunofluorescent antibody assay serology test >1:64 for *B. henselae* or *Bartonella clarridgeiae;* fourfold rise in titer between acute and convalescent specimens is definitive
4. Biopsy of node, skin, liver, bone, or eye granuloma showing granulomatous inflammation compatible with cat-scratch disease; positive Warthin-Starry silver stain

*Three of four criteria confirm the diagnosis; in an atypical case all four criteria may be needed.

rest may reduce extreme fatigue. Aspirin (65 mg/kg of body weight per day in six doses) or acetaminophen (60 mg/kg of body weight per day in six doses) is effective for the pain of tender adenitis. Application of warm, moist compresses to areas of lymph node swelling and to primary inoculation lesions for 1 to 2 hours, four to six times daily, results in less pain, more rapid involution, and occasionally, spontaneous drainage, especially from fluctuant lesions.

If suppuration occurs (15% of patients), incision and drainage should be avoided because chronic sinus tract discharge may occur and persist for several months. Needle aspiration relieves painful adenopathy and provides material for cultures or PCR tests. After one or two aspirates, the patient usually becomes symptom free within 24 to 48 hours. The technique for needle aspiration is as follows: after the area is washed with povidone-iodine cleanser, an 18- or 19-gauge needle is inserted through 1 to 2 cm of normal, unanesthetized skin at the base of the mass to avoid forming a chronic sinus tract in the event that a tuberculous lesion is present. Surgical excision of the nodes is usually not indicated unless one suspects a noninfectious etiology, such as a neoplasm.

Specific

A relatively healthy child, adolescent, or adult with typical CSD does not require antibiotic therapy. Recent literature suggests that each of the following five drugs has been found efficacious in over 60% of patients with systemic symptoms and/or severe lymphadenitis: azithromycin (Zithromax), 5 to 12 mg/kg/day once daily for 5 to 7 days, is 90% effective (maximum dose, 500 mg). Oral trimethoprim-sulfamethoxazole (TMP-SMX), 10 mg/kg of the trimethoprim component two or three times daily for 10 to 14 days, may result in prompt improvement. Rifampin, 10 to 20 mg/kg/day in two to three doses for 10 to 21 days, is 80% effective (maximum daily dose, 600 mg). In patients older than 12 years of age, ciprofloxacin, 20 to 30 mg/kg/24 hr in two divided doses for 10 to 14 or more days, may be very effective. In severely ill patients, gentamicin sulfate, 5 mg/kg/24 hr, given every 8 hours intramuscularly, was shown to be quite effective in selected patients (Table 3).

Other commonly used antibiotics are ineffective in patients with typical CSD. Paradoxically, CSD in patients with acquired immunodeficiency syndrome (AIDS) has responded dramatically to erythromycin, doxycycline, or antimycobacterial antibiotics used for several weeks to several months. Oral clarithromycin (Biaxin), 7.5 mg/kg in two doses (maximum daily dose, 1 g), is also effective therapy for immunocompromised patients.

Oral glucocorticoids cannot be routinely recommended despite anecdotal reports of several severely ill patients with systemic disease who responded to prednisone 2 mg/kg/24 hr for 5 to 7 days.

Prognosis

The prognosis is excellent. Lymphadenopathy usually regresses spontaneously in 2 to 6 months. One attack of CSD appears to confer lifelong immunity in children and adolescents. However, three adults have been reported with recurrence of lymphadenopathy 6 to 13 months after their initial diagnosis. Fatal complications have not been documented. Most patients with encephalitis and neuroretinitis have recovered completely during 6 to 12 months.

Prevention

The patient with CSD does not require isolation or quarantine; no evidence exists that the disease can spread directly from one person to another. Because the cats involved are invariably healthy, disposal is not recommended. Healthy kittens have been reported to have chronic bacteremia (*B. henselae* or *B. clarridgeiae*) lasting for several months to 2 years. Rigorous control of flea infestation in pets is essential for immunocompromised subjects. About 5% of other family members acquire the disease. Because 31% of American households (about 60 million) own cats and a larger number of households own cats worldwide, CSD is difficult to prevent. Preventive measures include declawing and regular nail clipping of young cats, keeping cats indoors, ensur-

Table 3 Antibiotic Therapy

ANTIBIOTIC*	ROUTE	DOSAGE	FREQUENCY	DURATION (DAYS)
Azithromycin (Zithromax)	PO	5-12 mg/kg (maximum, 500 mg/day)	Once daily	7-10
Ciprofloxacin	PO	20-30 mg/kg	q12h	≥10-21
Gentamicin	IM or IV	5 mg/kg	q8h	5-10
Rifampin	PO	10-20 mg/kg (maximum, 600 mg/day)	q8-12h	10-21
TMP-SMX	PO	10-20 mg/kg TMP 50-100 mg/kg SMX	q8-12h	≥10-14

TMP-SMX, Trimethoprim-sulfamethoxazole.
*A higher dose may be necessary if lymphadenopathy is over 5 cm or an abscess is present.

ing flea control, properly handling the litter box, washing hands after close contact with a cat or especially a kitten, and washing bites and scratches with soap and water.

Suggested Reading

Bass JW, Vincent JM, Person DA: The expanding spectrum of *Bartonella* infections. II. Cat-scratch disease, *Pediatr Infect Dis J* 16:163, 1997.

Boyer KM: Bartonella (cat scratch disease). In Feigin RD, Cherry JD, eds: *Textbook pediatric infectious disease*, ed 4, Philadelphia, 1998, WB Saunders.

Brouqui P, et al: Chronic *Bartonella quintana* bacteremia in homeless patients, *N Engl J Med* 340:184, 1999.

Kordick DL, Breitschwerdt EB: Persistent infection of pets within a household with three *Bartonella* species, *Emerg Infect Dis* 4:325, 1998.

Margileth AM, Baehrens DF: Chest wall abscess due to cat scratch disease (CSD) in an adult with antibodies to *Bartonella clarridgeiae*: case report and review of the thoracopulmonary manifestations of CSD, *Clin Infect Dis* 27:353, 1998.

CHLAMYDIA PNEUMONIAE (TWAR)

Lisa A. Jackson
J. Thomas Grayston

Chlamydia pneumoniae, also known as TWAR, is an important cause of both lower and upper respiratory tract infections worldwide. In the United States, it accounts for approximately 10% of cases of community-acquired pneumonia and 5% of cases of bronchitis in adults and is estimated to cause between 37,000 and 50,000 hospitalized pneumonia cases each year. Pneumonia and bronchitis are the most commonly recognized clinical manifestations of *C. pneumoniae* infection. Other reported syndromes include sinusitis, pharyngitis, otitis media, endocarditis, and myocarditis. Unlike many other respiratory pathogens, *C. pneumoniae* infection does not demonstrate seasonal variation.

Infection appears to be uncommon before age 5 years in industrialized countries but is increasingly common in older children, with a peak incidence of acute infection, as demonstrated by antibody conversion, among children 5 through 14 years of age. Many of these infections are asymptomatic. By age 20, approximately 50% of persons have detectable levels of antibody to the organism, and the seroprevalence increases to approximately 75% in the elderly. Because antibody titers decline with time, the persistently high seropositivity rates documented in the older age groups suggests that boosting of the antibody response by reinfection is common.

C. pneumoniae is rarely documented as a cause of acute lower respiratory tract infection in infants but is an important etiology of pneumonia among older children, especially in the outpatient setting. Up to 28% of cases of pneumonia among school-age children have been attributed to *C. pneumoniae*. Among adults, the highest rates of pneumonia caused by *C. pneumoniae* are among the elderly, and the organism is a significant cause of morbidity among nursing home residents.

As with the other bacterial causes of atypical pneumonia, the clinical manifestations of acute respiratory infection caused by *C. pneumoniae* are nonspecific. Upper respiratory symptoms, such as rhinitis, sore throat, or hoarseness, may be reported initially. These symptoms may then diminish over days to weeks, followed by the onset of cough, which is a predominant symptom in *C. pneumoniae* respiratory infections, thus at times producing a biphasic pattern of illness/symptoms. Although *C. pneumoniae* can cause severe infection, most cases are relatively mild and are associated with a low mortality rate.

The duration from onset of symptoms to presentation for medical evaluation tends to be longer for infections caused by *C. pneumoniae* than for those caused by other respiratory agents. Patients with *C. pneumoniae* infection are also less likely to give a history of fever or to have an elevated temperature documented on clinical presentation than patients with respiratory infection due to other agents. In addition to having a gradual onset, symptoms from *C. pneumoniae* respiratory infections may be prolonged, with cough and malaise persisting for several weeks or months despite appropriate antibiotic therapy.

A single, subsegmental, patchy infiltrate is the classic radiographic appearance associated with atypical pneumonias and is commonly seen with *C. pneumoniae* infection. However, this pattern is also common in cases of pneumonia caused by typical bacterial pathogens, including *S. pneumoniae*. In addition, other radiographic features, such as lobar or sublobar consolidation, interstitial infiltrates, bilateral involvement, pleural effusion, and hilar adenopathy may also be demonstrated with *C. pneumoniae* infection, although less often. Therefore the pattern of infiltrates on chest radiography is not a reliable indicator of the probable etiologic agent for cases of community-acquired pneumonia. As with other atypical pathogens, the white blood cell count is usually not elevated with *C. pneumoniae* infection, and other laboratory findings are nonspecific.

C. pneumoniae has also recently been associated with atherosclerotic cardiovascular disease by seroepidemiologic studies, detection of the organism in atherosclerotic plaque specimens, experimental in vitro cell culture studies, and animal model studies. Currently, several large, randomized controlled trials are being conducted to determine whether antibiotic treatment directed against *C. pneumoniae* can decrease the risk of cardiac events among persons with documented coronary artery disease.

■ LABORATORY DIAGNOSIS

Laboratory confirmation of infection is limited. Isolation of *C. pneumoniae*, an obligate intracellular parasite, is difficult and requires cell culture; furthermore, reliable serologic tests, which have limited commercial availability, optimally require paired sera with the convalescent serum obtained at least 3 weeks after onset. Of the available serologic tests, the microimmunofluorescence test is both sensitive and specific for *C. pneumoniae* infection. Acute infection is indicated by a fourfold rise in titer, an IgM titer of 16 or higher, or an IgG titer of 512 or higher. Preexisting antibody is indicated by IgG titer greater than 16 and less than 512.

A chlamydial complement fixation test is also available, which is genus specific but not species specific and therefore may be positive in persons with *C. psittaci* infection. Complement fixation antibodies are often absent in patients reinfected with *C. pneumoniae*, limiting the usefulness of the test among older patients.

Table 1   Oral Antibiotics Recommended for Treatment of *C. pneumoniae* Infections

ANTIBIOTIC	DOSAGE	DURATION
Erythromycin	500 mg qid*	2 wk
Tetracycline	500 mg qid	2 wk
Doxycycline	100 mg bid	2 wk
Azithromycin	500 mg on day 1; 250 mg/day on days 2-5	5 days
Clarithromycin	250 mg bid	1-2 wk

*Alternatively, 250 mg qid for 21 days may be used if the higher dosage is not tolerated.

Recently, the polymerase chain reaction has been used to identify *C. pneumoniae* to specific DNA in throat swabs and other clinical specimens. Although not yet commercially available, this technique holds promise for future use as a rapid diagnostic test.

■ THERAPY

Erythromycin, tetracycline, and doxycycline are active in vitro against *C. pneumoniae* and have traditionally been recommended as first-line therapy (Table 1). Newer macrolide-like antibiotics, such as azithromycin and clarithromycin, are also active in vitro, achieve high intracellular concentrations, and are better tolerated than erythromycin. The limited available data from clinical evaluations suggest that azithromycin and clarithromycin are at least as effective as erythromycin against *C. pneumoniae* respiratory infections and so may be considered as either first-line therapy or alternatives to the traditional agents in the treatment of suspected *C. pneumoniae* infections. Some quinolones, including levofloxacin, sparfloxacin, and grepafloxacin, also appear to be active in vitro and may be considered for therapy. The organism is not susceptible to penicillin, ampicillin, or sulfa drugs.

Clinical reports indicate that symptoms may persist or recur after conventional or longer courses of treatment with erythromycin, doxycycline, or tetracycline. Therefore, if these agents are used, a minimum of 10 to 14 days of treatment is recommended. If azithromycin or clarithromycin is used, the standard course of therapy indicated for treatment of respiratory infections is recommended. If symptoms persist despite treatment, a second course with a different antibiotic may be effective.

Suggested Reading

Grayston JT: Infections caused by *Chlamydia pneumoniae* strain TWAR, *Clin Infect Dis* 15:757, 1992.

Grayston JT: Does *Chlamydia pneumoniae* cause atherosclerosis and coronary artery disease? *Arch Surg* 134:934, 1999.

Kuo CC, Jackson LA, Campbell LA, Grayston JT: *Chlamydia pneumoniae* (TWAR), *Clin Microbiol Rev* 8:451, 1995.

Marston BJ, et al: Incidence of community-acquired pneumonia requiring hospitalization, *Arch Intern Med* 157:1709, 1997.

CHLAMYDIA PSITTACI (PSITTACOSIS)

Alfred E. Bacon III

One of three species of the genus *Chlamydia psittaci* was identified simultaneously by three investigators in 1930. Its association with human disease dates to reports as early as the late 1800s. *C. psittaci* has a wide range of host species, including birds, humans, and lower mammals. *Chlamydia pneumoniae*, on the other hand, is found only in humans, and *Chlamydia trachomatis* is found only in humans and mice.

The systemic illness associated with *C. psittaci* has been termed *psittacosis* because of its association with parrots and psittacine birds. Subsequently, many avian species have been found to harbor *C. psittaci* and to transmit the organism to humans, causing disease. The term *ornithosis* would be more appropriate; however, it is not traditional.

Not only is avian-to-human transmission of *C. psittaci* documented, but human-to-human transmission can also occur, particularly in outbreaks and clusters. These modes of transmission contribute to both epidemic and sporadic cases of psittacosis. Mammals (sheep, goats, cattle) can rarely transmit the organism to humans.

Individuals epidemiologically at risk for *C. psittaci* infection include those exposed to aviaries and abattoir and veterinary workers. Poultry breeders (particularly turkey farmers) are at significant risk, accounting for most outbreaks. A variable degree of illness exists in the birds infected with *C. psittaci*, ranging from asymptomatic to full-blown disease manifested by anorexia, dyspnea, and diarrhea. Birds may resolve the illness spontaneously, and a waxing and waning clinical course is not unusual. Therefore, a history of contact with birds is pertinent even if the bird is seemingly healthy.

■ CLINICAL SYNDROMES

C. psittaci is inhaled in aerosol form from the vector and travels to the alveoli. It disseminates to regional lymph nodes and the reticuloendothelial system. Multiple organ involvement is not uncommon, and the systemic nature of this disease cannot be overstated. The clinical syndrome classically presents as pneumonitis, although systemic infection in the absence of pneumonia has been described. Endocarditis, rash, panniculitis, and a pseudotyphoid presentation can occur. An association with reactive arthropathy and HLA-B27 seropositivity has been noted. Recently, a follicular conjunctivitis has been described caused by "nontrachoma" chlamydia, including *C. psittaci*.

The incubation period ranges from 5 to 21 days, and in up to 20% of patients, no history of exposure to a bird can be elicited. More than 80% of patients present with fever, cough, and sweats. Headache, sometimes a very prominent symptom, may separate it from other infectious diseases, particularly in the setting of pneumonitis. Nausea and vomiting are uncommon. Diarrhea is very common. All these phenomena represent the systemic nature of *C. psittaci* infection.

Physical findings commonly include pulmonary consolidation and an altered mental status. As with other intracellular pathogens, a temperature-pulse dissociation is often reported. Laboratory data are rarely unique to *C. psittaci* infection; however, hepatocellular damage is present in almost 50% of patients. An abnormal chest x-ray film is evident in 80% of infected individuals, almost uniformly a lobar infiltrate as opposed to a diffuse pattern.

■ DIAGNOSIS

The diagnosis of *C. psittaci* infection is based on serologic confirmation of exposure to the pathogen in the proper clinical setting. As with most atypical pneumonia cases, a thorough history looking for exposures, systemic symptoms, and atypical features is crucial. Culturing the organism is difficult and hazardous in the laboratory. Two serologic assays are readily available. A complement fixation antibody assay with a fourfold or greater change in titer between acute and convalescent phase sera confirms the diagnosis. A random titer greater than 1:32 with a compatible illness is presumptively diagnostic. The complement fixation assay, however, does cross-react with *C. trachomatis* and *C. pneumoniae*. More recently used is a serum microimmunofluorescence assay. This also requires evaluation of acute and convalescent serologic specimens. In the acute setting, when therapy is initiated, the diagnosis of *C. psittaci* infection truly rests on clinical grounds, with an exposure history and a compatible clinical presentation.

■ THERAPY

Table 1 outlines therapeutic options in *C. psittaci* infection. The therapy of choice for *C. psittaci* infections, both systemic and limited, is a tetracycline. Doxycycline, 100 mg orally twice a day, is the preferred agent. The systemic nature of the infection requires a prolonged course of therapy, and most authors suggest a course of at least 14 days and up to 21 days. In patients with endocarditis, a more prolonged course is necessary. Patients with *C. psittaci* endocarditis

Table 1 Therapeutic Options in *Chlamydia psittaci* Infections

ANTIMICROBIAL	DOSAGE
Doxycycline	100 mg bid, 14-21 days
Erythromycin	500 mg qid, 21 days
Azithromycin	1 g, then 500 mg qd, 10-14 days
Chloramphenicol	500 mg q6h, 14-21 days
Tetracycline HCl	500 mg qid, 14-21 days
Levofloxacin	500 mg qid, 14-21 days

rarely have survived without valve replacement in addition to doxycycline therapy.

Traditionally, erythromycin, 500 mg orally four times a day, is the second-line drug for *C. psittaci* pneumonia. Because relapses and failures in therapy have been reported, a 21-day course of therapy is indicated. Newer macrolide agents, particularly azithromycin, have been studied in chlamydia infections, specifically *C. psittaci*. Azithromycin appears both in vitro and in vivo to be an excellent alternative to doxyocycline. A 7-day course at 10 mg/kg of body weight has been effective in experimental models. This reflects the increased intracellular concentration of this agent as well as the prolonged half-life. There are fewer data to support the use of clarithromycin. This agent has been shown to be effective in the treatment of infections caused by other *Chlamydia* species.

In the treatment of conjunctivitis where *C. psittaci* is suspected, a 4- to 10-week course of either doxycycline or erythromycin is appropriate.

More traditional agents have also shown efficacy, including chloramphenicol, 500 mg four times a day for 14 days. Patients failing this regimen have done well with the addition of rifampin.

There are growing data on the use of quinolones in the management of *C. psittaci* infections. These agents have shown excellent activity against other *Chlamydia* species and ofloxacin, 200 mg orally twice a day, or levofloxacin, 500 mg orally daily, is not an unreasonable alternative in patients intolerant to the agents previously discussed.

Many reports in the literature demonstrate a prompt clinical response to doxycycline in patients infected with *C. psittaci*. A patient's failure to show symptomatic improvement within 48 hours should prompt a reevaluation of the diagnosis or a suspicion of deep-seated infection such as endocarditis.

Suggested Reading

Centers for Disease Control and Prevention: Compendium of measures to control *Chlamydia pscittai* infection among humans (psittacosis) and pet birds (avian chlamydia), *MMWR* 47(suppl): 1, 1998.

Leitman T, et al: Chronic follicular conjunctivitis associated with *Chlamydia psittaci* or *Chlamydia pneumoniae, Clin Infect Dis* 26:1335, 1998.

Niki Y, et al: In vitro and in vivo activities of azithromycin, a new azalide antibiotic, against *Chlamydia, Antimicrob Agents Chemother* 38:2296, 1994.

Schlossberg D: *Chlamydia psittaci* (psittacosis). In Mandel GL, Bennett JE, Dolin R, eds: *Mandell, Douglas and Bennett's principles and practice of infectious diseases,* ed 4, New York, 1995, Churchill Livingstone.

Schlossberg D, et al: An epidemic of avian and human psittacosis, *Arch Intern Med* 153:2594, 1993.

Yung AP, Grayston ML: Psittacosis: a review of 135 cases, *Med J Aust* 148:228, 1988.

CORYNEBACTERIA

Carlos H. Ramírez-Ronda
Carlos R. Ramírez-Ramírez

■ *CORYNEBACTERIUM DIPHTHERIAE* (DIPHTHERIA)

Diphtheria is an acute, infectious, preventable, and sometimes fatal disease caused by *Corynebacterium diphtheriae*. The infection is usually localized to the upper part of the respiratory tract and the skin; from here it gives rise to local and systemic signs. These signs are the result of a toxin produced by the microorganisms multiplying at the site of infection. The systemic complications particularly affect the heart and the peripheral nerves.

Cause

Diphtheria is distributed worldwide, with the highest incidence in temperate climates. It occurs predominantly under poor socioeconomic conditions, where crowding is common and where many persons are either not immunized or inadequately immunized.

The only significant reservoir of *C. diphtheriae* is the human host. The organism is transmitted directly from one person to another, and intimate contact is required. Transmission is usually by way of infected droplets of nasopharyngeal secretions. Infective skin exudate has been involved in human-to-human transmission. Transmission may also occur via animals, fomites, or milk.

Immunity depends on antitoxin in the host's blood. Antitoxin is formed by immunization or by clinical or subclinical infection, including skin infections. The Schick test consists of an intradermal injection of 0.1 ml of purified diphtheria toxin dissolved in buffered human serum albumin. This is injected into the volar surface of one arm, and 0.1 ml of purified diphtheria toxoid is used as a control in the other arm. The test can be used to assess the immune status of the subject. Reaction to toxin but not to toxoid indicates that the patient is immune and that levels of antitoxin exceed 0.03 U/ml. This test provides only an estimate of immunity, and the inability to perform it should not delay treatment of asymptomatic contacts of diphtheria. The Schick test is not to be used before adult immunization.

Clinical Features

Diphtheria may be symptomless or rapidly fatal. The incubation period varies from 1 to 7 days but is most commonly 2 to 4 days.

Anterior Nares Diphtheria
The infection is localized to the anterior nasal area and is manifested by unilateral or bilateral serous or serosanguineous discharge that erodes the adjacent skin, resulting in small crusted lesions. The membrane may be seen in the nose.

Tonsillar (Faucial) Diphtheria
Tonsillar diphtheria is the most common presentation and the most toxic form. The onset is usually sudden, with fever rarely exceeding 38° C (100.4° F), malaise, and mild sore throat. The pharynx is moderately infected, and a thick, whitish gray tonsillar exudate is often seen. The tonsillar and cervical lymph nodes are enlarged. The exudate may extend to other areas and result in nasopharyngeal diphtheria and massive cervical lymphadenopathy (bull neck appearance). The most common complaints are sore throat (85%), pain on swallowing (23%), nausea and vomiting (25%), and headache (18%).

Pharyngeal Diphtheria
Pharyngeal diphtheria is diagnosed when the membrane extends from the tonsillar area to the pharynx.

Laryngeal and Bronchial Diphtheria
Laryngeal and bronchial diphtheria involves the larynx. The voice becomes hoarse, and inspiratory and expiratory stridor may appear; dyspnea and cyanosis occur, and the accessory muscles of respiration are used. Tracheostomy or intubation is needed.

Cutaneous Diphtheria
Classically described as diphtheria in tropical areas, cutaneous diphtheria now is seen in nontropical areas as well. It takes the form of a chronic nonhealing ulcer, sometimes covered with a grayish membranous exudate. Another form is secondary infection of a preexisting wound. Finally, superinfection with *C. diphtheriae* may occur in a variety of primary skin lesions, such as impetigo, insect bites, ectyma, and eczema.

Complications of Diphtheria
Myocarditis
Although electrocardiographic (ECG) changes have been described in up to 25% of cases, overt clinical myocarditis is less common. The onset is insidious, occurring in the second or third week of the infection. The patient exhibits a weak, rising pulse; distant heart sounds; and profound weakness and lethargy. Overt signs of heart failure can occur. The most common ECG changes are flattening or inversion of T waves, bundle branch block or intraventricular block, and disorders of rhythm. Serial determination of serum glutamic oxaloacetic transaminase (SGOT) levels identifies most patients with myocarditis. The prognosis is poor, especially when heart block supervenes.

Peripheral Neuritis
The most common form of cranial nerve palsy is paralysis of the soft palate. There may be nasal regurgitation and/or nasal speech. This condition is usually mild, and recovery occurs within 2 weeks. Ciliary paralysis and oculomotor paralysis are the next most common forms. Peripheral neuritis affecting the limbs may appear during the fourth to eighth week. It is usually manifested by weakness of the dorsiflexors and decreased or absent deep-tendon reflexes. Diphtheritic polyneuritis has been described after cutaneous diphtheria.

Diagnosis
Diagnosis is made on clinical grounds and can be confirmed by laboratory tests (Figure 1). The clinical features of a fully developed diphtheritic membrane especially in the pharynx, are sufficiently characteristic to suggest diphtheria and for treatment to be started immediately.

Specific diagnosis of diphtheria depends completely on demonstration of the organism in stained smears and its recovery by culture. In experienced hands, methylene blue–stained preparations are positive in 75% to 85% of cases. The bacilli can be recovered by culture in Loeffler's medium within 8 to 12 hours if patients have not been receiving antimicrobial agents. The presence of beta-hemolytic streptococci does not rule out diphtheria because such streptococci are recovered in up to 20% to 30% of patients with diphtheria.

The differential diagnosis of tonsillar-pharyngeal diphtheria should include streptococcal pharyngitis, adenoviral exudative pharyngitis, infectious mononucleosis, and Vincent's angina, among others (Table 1).

Therapy
The best and most effective treatment of diphtheria is prevention by immunization with diphtheria toxoid. The most important aspect of treatment is to administer the antitoxin as soon as diphtheria is clinically suspected, without awaiting laboratory confirmation. The patient should be hospitalized, isolated, and kept in bed for 10 to 14 days (see Figure 1).

Use of Antitoxin
The antitoxin is equine and the minimal effective dose remains undefined; therefore dosage is based on empiric judgment. It is usually accepted that for patients with mild or moderate cases, including those with tonsillar and pharyngeal membrane, 50,000 U IM is enough (for a child, 30,000 U). In severe cases, such as with a more extensive membrane and/or thrombocytopenia, 60,000 to 120,000 U depending on severity is the recommended dose; critically ill patients should receive at least half of it by slow intravenous infusion.

Before administration of the antitoxin, any history of allergy or reactions to horse serum or horse dander must be determined. All patients must be tested for antitoxin sensitivity with dilute horse antitoxin in saline 1:10 and an eye test. This is followed by a scratch test with a 1:100 dilution; if negative in half an hour, the scratch test is followed by an intradermal test, 1:100 dilution. If all tests are negative, antitoxin can be given. The intravenous route is recommended. A slow intravenous infusion of 0.5 ml antitoxin in 10 ml saline is followed in half an hour by the balance of the dose in a dilution of 1:20 with saline, infused at a rate not to exceed 1 ml/min. Others give the antitoxin dose intramuscularly in mild to moderate cases only.

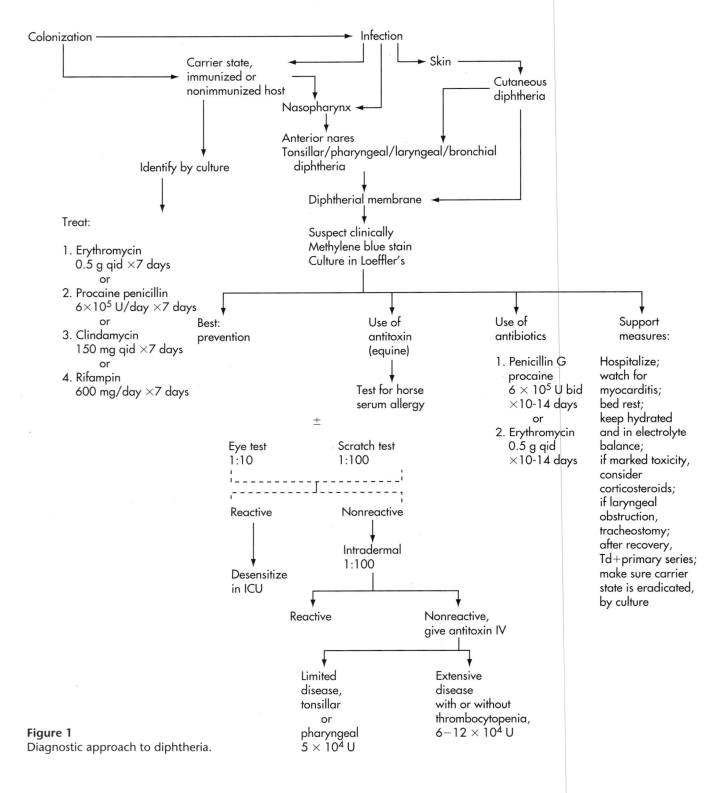

Figure 1
Diagnostic approach to diphtheria.

Table 1 Differential Diagnosis of Diphtheria	
AFFECTED AREA	**OTHER CONDITION**
Nose	Sinusitis, foreign body, snuffles of congenital syphilis, rhinitis
Fauces and pharynx	Streptococcal or adenoviral exudative pharyngitis, ulcerative pharyngitis (herpetic, coxsackie-viral), infectious mononucleosis, oral thrush, peritonsillar abscess, retropharyngeal abscess, Vincent's angina, lesions associated with agranulocytosis or leukemia
Larynx	Laryngotracheobronchitis, epiglottitis
Skin	Impetigo, pyogenic ulcers, herpes simplex infection

If the patient is sensitive to horse serum, desensitization should be carried out with care, preferably in an intensive care unit. Epinephrine, intubation equipment, and respiratory assistance should be available. The following doses of horse serum antitoxin should be injected at 15-minute intervals if no reaction occurs:

1. 0.05 ml of 1:20 dilution subcutaneously
2. 0.10 ml of 1:10 dilution subcutaneously
3. 0.3 ml of 1:10 dilution subcutaneously
4. 0.1 ml of undiluted antitoxin subcutaneously
5. 0.2 ml of undiluted antitoxin subcutaneously
6. 0.5 ml of undiluted antitoxin subcutaneously
7. Remaining estimated therapeutic dose intramuscularly

During all tests and upon injection of antitoxin, a syringe containing epinephrine 1:1000 dilution in saline should be at hand to be used immediately in a dose of 0.01 ml/kg subcutaneously or intramuscularly at any sign of anaphylaxis. A good precaution is to have open venous access with normal saline prior to the test. If needed, a similar amount of epinephrine diluted to a final concentration of 1:10,000 in saline may be given slowly intravenous and repeated in 5 to 15 minutes. Other information and instructions in the package insert accompanying the antitoxin should be observed.

Antibiotics

C. diphtheriae is susceptible to several antimicrobial agents. After cultures have been performed, antibiotics should be administered to prevent multiplication of the microorganism at the site of infection and to eliminate the carrier state. Penicillin G, the drug of choice, is usually given as procaine penicillin, 600,000 U intramuscularly (IM) every 12 hours for 10 to 14 days. Erythromycin, also very active against the diphtheria bacillus, is given at 2 g/day divided in four doses for the same period.

Supportive Measures

Complications such as dehydration, malnutrition, and congestive heart failure should be diagnosed promptly and properly treated. In cases of severe laryngeal involvement,

marked toxicity, or shock, corticosteroids (prednisone 3 to 5 mg/kg/day) have been advocated, but there are no hard data on their effectiveness. For laryngeal obstruction with respiratory stridor, a tracheotomy must be performed promptly.

Before the patient is discharged, specimens from throat and nose or suspected lesions should be cultured. At least two and preferably three consecutive negative cultures should be obtained.

After recovery, toxoid administration against tetanus and diphtheria (Td) should be administered to complete a primary immunization series if the patient has not been immunized.

Carriers

The chronic carrier state may occur despite immunity derived either from clinical diseases or from immunization. The carrier state occasionally persists in the absence of antecedent disease. Erythromycin, 0.5 g orally four times a day for 7 days in adults, is the treatment of choice for the carrier state. Alternative antibiotics are procaine penicillin G, 600,000 U IM daily for 14 days; clindamycin, 150 mg orally four times a day for 7 days; or rifampin, 600 mg/day orally for 7 days.

Epidemics

The approach to epidemic disease is as follows:

1. Identify all primary cases, hospitalize, and treat.
2. Use toxoid in all the population at risk.
3. Culture all contacts for diphtheria, and treat all persons with *C. diphtheriae* in throat, nose, or skin lesions with erythromycin for 7 days to eliminate carrier state.
4. Watch primary contacts closely during the first week of exposure and treat at first signs or symptoms. Alternatively, all susceptible primary contacts can be given 1500 to 3000 U of diphtheria antitoxin, administered as previously described, in addition to toxoid. This low-level dose will boost them while they are forming their antibody.

Prevention

Children who have had a complete course of primary immunization with diphtheria-tetanus-pertussis (DTP) vaccine may be given a booster injection on exposure to diphtheria. This is done in case of outbreaks but is not routine. Antibiotic prophylaxis is highly effective.

Household and other close contacts of a patient with diphtheria should be observed attentively for 7 days. They should receive either an intramuscular injection of 1.2 million units of benzathine penicillin or a 7-day course of erythromycin taken orally. Cultures should be performed before and after treatment. An injection of toxoid appropriate for age and immunization status can also be given. Susceptible close contacts who have had no (or only one) prior injections of toxoid should promptly be given 3000 to 10,000 units (depending on body size) of antitoxin, with the usual precautions being followed. When indicated, active immunization with toxoid should be continued to completion.

Routine immunization for diphtheria is discussed in the chapter *Immunizations*.

■ NONDIPHTHERITIC CORYNEBACTERIA

Nondiphtheritic corynebacteria were once considered comensals. They are present in the skin and often are recovered from blood cultures. The presence of the microorganism in the blood has been considered contaminant, but there are many instances in which nondiphtheritic corynebacteria are associated with bacteremias, sepsis, pneumonias, endocarditis, central nervous system infections, and intraocular infections, especially in immunocompromised patients and patients with vascular and central nervous system catheters and prosthetic devices. A common predisposing factor is neutropenia.

The diagnosis of infections with nondiphtheritic corynebacteria usually involves their recovery from blood or other sterile body fluid. Corynebacteria can be identified by conventional methods, but over the last few years, a new system, the Rapid CORYNE System, was found to be excellent and an alternative to conventional methods.

Clinically, there are no specific findings that suggest nondiphtheric corynebacteria, but their association with central lines, skin, and subcutaneous infections in immunocompromised patients leads the clinician to associate a given infection with a gram-positive rod. Table 2 lists the epidemiology and clinical features of selected nondiphtheric corynebacteria.

■ *CORYNEBACTERIUM* GROUP JK

Corynebacterium group JK is gram-positive coccobacillus or coccus resembling the streptococcus. Characteristically, it shows high-grade antibiotic resistance, being susceptible only to vancomycin in vitro and in vivo.

Clinical Features
Diseases associated with *Corynebacterium* group JK include soft-tissue infections, pneumonitis with or without cavitation, continuous ambulatory peritoneal dialysis–related peritonitis, neurosurgical shunt infections, skin rash, catheter-related epicardial abscess, and endocarditis. It should always be considered a possible cause of sepsis in the neutropenic patient and in patients with prosthetic devices in place.

Therapy
Despite their high antibiotic resistance, this corynebacteria remain susceptible to vancomycin. Total effective duration of treatment has not been established. Clinical response must be followed, usually treating for 4 to 6 weeks. Newer fluoroquinolones, mainly ciprofloxacin, have also shown good results. Infected prosthetic material often requires removal.

Corynebacterium minutissimum
Infection with *C. minutissimum* usually involves the skin, and the classical disease entity is erythrasma. Erythrasma is a skin infection characterized by brownish-reddish macules that itch and when exposed to a Wood's lamp fluoresce. The most frequent location is the intertriginous areas.

Bacteremia with *C. minutissimum* has been described in patients with leukemia in blast crisis. There are also reports of trichomycosis axillaris associated with this Corynebacteria.

Corynebacterium ulcerans
C. ulcerans, like *C. diphtheriae*, produces diphtheria toxin by lysogeny but without apparent clinical consequences. However, there are documented reports of *C. ulcerans* bacteremias with cardiac and central nervous system involvement as well as pneumonia.

Corynebacterium pseudotuberculosis
Infection with *C. pseudotuberculosis* is associated with exposure to farm animals or consumption of raw milk. Clinically, it presents as a suppurative granulomatous lymphadenitis most likely related to the dermonecrotic toxin it produces. This organism responds to long-term treatment with erythromycin or tetracycline.

Corynebacterium bovis
Most infections reported with *C. bovis* are associated with central nervous system processes. There have been cases of meningitis, epidural abscesses, and shunt infections.

Corynebacterium pseudodiphthericum
Sites of infection caused by *C. pseudodiphthericum* include heart valves, wounds, urinary tract, and lungs, with pneumonia and necrotizing tracheitis. The susceptibilities of this microorganism are varied, with both susceptibility and resistance to erythromycin, clindamycin, and penicillin. There is a case of response to penicillin intravenously (12 million units daily for 14 days).

Corynebacterium striatum
Persons with an underlying immunosuppressive process are usually victims of *C. striatum*. There are reports of pneumo-

Table 2 Epidemiology and Clinical Features of Selected Nondiphtheric Corynebacteria

CORYNEBACTERIUM	EPIDEMIOLOGY	CLINICAL FEATURES
C. group JK	Skin, systemic	Soft-tissue, pneumonias, shunt infections; skin rash; endocarditis
C. minutissium	Skin	Erythrasma, reddish-brown macular lesions, fluoresce under Wood's lamp
C. ulcerans	Skin, systemic	Cardiac and central nervous system involvement; diseases in horses and cattle
C. pseudotuberculosis	Skin exposure, farm animals, raw milk	Dermonecrotic toxin, suppurative granulomas, lymphadenitis, disease in farm animals
C. bovis	Shunts, skin	Meningitis, spinal epidural; abscess; ventriculoperitoneal or jugular shunts
C. pseudodiphtericum	Systemic	Pneumonia endocarditis, tracheitis, urinary tract
C. striatum	Immunosuppressed	Pneumonias, meningitis, abscesses, bacteremias

nias, pulmonary abscesses, meningitis, and bacteremias with *C. striatum.* Most patients have been treated with vancomycin.

Others

There have been reports of Corynebacterium CDC group A-4 associated with native valve endocarditis in immunocompetent patients as well as sepsis in immunocompromised hosts with infected Hickman catheters. *C. aquaticum,* an environmental organism of fresh water, has been associated with septicemia in a neutropenic patient with an indwelling central venous catheter who used untreated stored rainwater to shower. *C. afermentans* (CDC group ANF-1) was reported causing endocarditis in a prosthetic valve.

Therapy

Some corynebacteria are susceptible to erythromycin, sulfonamides, chloramphenicol, gentamicin, impinem, some of the newer fluoroquinolones, and vancomycin. For most serious and systemic infections, we prefer to use vancomycin at 1 g every 12 hours for at least 2 weeks in adults with normal renal function. In some patients, especially immu-

nocompromised patients, combination therapy can be used with vancomycin plus imipenem at 500 mg IV every 6 hours, vancomycin plus rifampin at 600 mg daily orally, or vancomycin plus ciprofloxacin at 750 mg orally every 12 hours for 2 to 4 weeks. Erythromycin at a dosage of 2 to 4 g in divided doses can be used as an alternative regimen. The optimal effective therapy for these infections has not been determined, but 8 weeks of treatment are often required. For unresponsive cases, surgical consultation is recommended.

Suggested Reading

Brown A: Other corynebacteria. In Mandell GL, Bennett JE, Dolin R, eds: *Mandell, Douglas and Bennett's principles and practice of infectious diseases,* ed 4, New York, 1995, Churchll Livingstone.
Halsey N: Corynebacteria. In Gorbach SL, Barlett JG , Blacklow NR, eds: *Infectious diseases,* Philadelphia, 1998, Saunders.
Koopman JS, Campbell J: The role of cutaneous diphtheria infections in a diphtheric epidemic, *J Infect Dis* 131:239, 1975.
Lipsky BA, et al: Infections caused by nondiptheria corynebactaria, *Rev Infect Dis* 4:1220, 1982.
MacGregor RR: *Corynebacterium diphtheriae.* In Mandell GL, Bennett JE, Dolin R, eds: *Mandell, Douglas and Bennett's principles and practice of infectious diseases,* ed 4, New York, 1995, Churchill Livingstone.

EHRLICHIOSIS

James G. Olson
Joseph E. McDade

Ehrlichiae are small, gram-negative, obligate intracellular bacteria. Several species are pathogenic for humans and produce a wide spectrum of clinical manifestations, ranging from relatively mild, flulike illnesses to multisystem, fatal infections. Ehrlichiae are transmitted to humans by the bite of infected ticks, which acquire ehrlichiae by feeding on infected mammals.

In the United States, the human ehrlichioses exist as two clinically similar illnesses caused by two different etiologic agents. *Ehrlichia chaffeensis* and an agent similar or identical to *E. phagocytophila.* Infections with the respective agents have been termed *human monocytic ehrlichiosis* (HME) and *human granulocytic ehrlichiosis* (HGE) because *E. chaffeensis* preferentially infects peripheral blood monocytes, whereas *E. phagocytophila* is found primarily in polymorphonuclear leukocytes. The two forms of ehrlichiosis can also be distinguished epidemiologically, as the occurrence of the respective illnesses mirrors the distribution of their different tick vectors. *E. chaffeensis* infections occur primarily in the southeastern and midwestern states, coincident with the

distribution of its principal vector, *Amblyomma americanum.* Most cases of *E. phagocytophila* infection have been reported in the northeastern states and upper Midwest (especially New York, Connecticut, Minnesota, and Wisconsin), coincident with the distribution of its primary vector *Ixodis scapularis. I. scapularis* also serves as the vector of *Borrelia burgdorferi,* the agent of Lyme disease, and a dual infection with both agents is possible. Infection with a third species of ehrlichiae, *E. ewingii,* has been reported in a small series of patients in Missouri, but it is not known whether this agent is a significant cause of human illness. Human ehrlichial infections have also been reported outside the United States (Table 1).

■ CLINICAL MANIFESTATIONS

Patients with ehrlichial infections generally seek treatment from a health care provider in their first week of illness. Unfortunately, early clinical signs and symptoms of ehrlichiosis are remarkably nonspecific and may mimic various other infectious and noninfectious conditions, including Rocky Mountain spotted fever (RMSF), murine typhus, influenza, measles, infectious mononucleosis, rubella, enteroviral infections, meningococcemia, leptospirosis, thrombotic thrombocytopenic purpura, idiopathic thrombocytopenic purpura, immune complex vasculitides, and other illnesses. Patients typically exhibit fever, headache, myalgias, and gastrointestinal symptoms. Rash is a relatively common (>60%) manifestation of ehrlichial infection in pediatric patients but is present in only about a third of adult patients

Table 1   Features of Ehrlichioses

ETIOLOGIC AGENT	DISEASE	PRINCIPAL VECTOR	CASE/FATALITY RATIO TREATED (UNTREATED)	ECOLOGY OF EXPOSURE AREAS	GEOGRAPHIC DISTRIBUTION
Ehrlichia chaffeensis	Human monocytic ehrlichiosis (HME)	*Amblyomma americanum*	<5% (unknown)	Grassy areas, forest edges, roadsides, hiking trails, stream banks, unmowed areas around homes (most common from May to September)	Southeastern and south-central United States (most common in Oklahoma, Missouri, Tennessee, Arkansas, Georgia); possibly Portugal, Mali, and Italy
The agent of human granulocytic ehrlichiosis (HGE) (closely related to or identical to *Ehrlichia phagocytophila*)	Human granulocytic ehrlichiosis (HGE)	*Ixodes scapularis*	<5% (unknown)	Grassy areas, forest edges, roadsides, hiking trails, stream banks, unmowed areas around homes (most common from May to September)	Northeastern coastal and upper midwestern United States (most common in New York, Wisconsin, Minnesota, Connecticut, Massachusetts); Europe (Slovenia and possibly Germany, Sweden, Switzerland, and United Kingdom), Bulgaria, Denmark

with HME and far less common among persons with HGE. When present, the rash may be variable and has been described as macular, papular, or both, and occasionally petechial or erythematous. Eschars, a prominent feature of several other rickettsioses, have not been reported for the ehrlichioses. Pulmonary manifestations of varying severity are noted in 30% to 55% of patients with ehrlichial infections. Central nervous system manifestations, including confusion, lethargy, photophobia, vertigo, ataxia, and seizures, occur in about 20% of patients. Hematologic and blood chemistry abnormalities, particularly leukopenia, thrombocytopenia, anemia, elevated levels of hepatic transaminases (especially aspartate aminotransferase), and hyponatremia, are often identified in persons with ehrlichioses and provide clues to the diagnosis. Leukopenia, especially absolute lymphopenia, is particularly common. Complications include adult respiratory distress syndrome, renal failure, neurologic disorders, and disseminated intravascular coagulation in 10% to 20% of patients. The case/fatality ratios for ehrlichiosis, reported in different patient series, vary considerably. Ratios approached 10% in early studies, when ehrlichiosis was a new disease that was not promptly recognized and treated. Certainly, HME and HGE can be life-threatening illnesses if untreated, but case/fatality ratios now appear to be less than 5% for both illnesses. Fatal outcomes have been reported most often among the elderly, the immunocompromised, or persons with other underlying illnesses.

■ DIAGNOSIS

At present, there are no routinely available laboratory tests that provide prompt diagnosis for acute ehrlichiosis. Suc-

cessful patient outcomes are guided by the clinical acumen of the evaluating health care provider and by therapeutic decisions based on a presumptive diagnosis developed from clinical suspicion and the epidemiologic setting. Relevant epidemiologic features to be recognized or elicited by physicians include the following:

1. *Exposures:* A history of a tick bite or exposure to ticks may be elicited by questioning patients about leisure and/or occupational outdoor activities (e.g., hunting, fishing, hiking, gardening, forestry) in the weeks preceding the illness. Exposures to ticks may also arise from contacts with certain animals (e.g., field rats or mice, deer, dogs) that may serve as reservoirs for ehrlichiae and as hosts for vector ticks.
2. *Geography:* Awareness of disease-endemic areas is invaluable and may sensitize physicians to subtle clues observed in patients with an acute febrile illness of otherwise unknown cause. In addition, ehrlichiosis may be acquired during travel to different states and other continents. The ehrlichioses are not restricted to rural settings; in fact, ehrlichial infections may occur more often in suburban than in rural habitats in certain areas of the United States.
3. *Seasonality:* The occurrence of ehrlichioses is directly related to the life cycles and natural histories of their tick vectors; approximately 90% of ehrlichial infections in the United States occur between April and September, coincident with peak vector activity and abundance.

Serologic assays remain the primary confirmatory method for ehrlichiosis. Depending on the patient and on the particular disease, however, diagnostic antibody titers to *E. chaffeensis* or *E. phagocytophila* may not appear until

14 days after the onset of symptoms. Indirect immunofluorescence assays are the most widely available tests for ehrlichioses and are offered through some commercial laboratories, state public health laboratories, and the Centers for Disease Control and Prevention (CDC). Paired (acute-phase and convalescent-phase) serum specimens are preferred for serologic testing to demonstrate a fourfold rise in antibody titer. Antibodies to *E. chaffeensis* may cross-react with *E. phagocytophila* and vice versa, thereby hindering identification of the specific etiologic agent. However, patients should receive the same therapy and supportive care regardless of the specific infectious agent. Availability of other diagnostic techniques, including polymerase chain reaction assays of acute-phase whole blood or tissues, immunohistochemistry of biopsied tissues, and direct isolation, is generally restricted to CDC laboratories, some state public health laboratories, or specialized research laboratories. The ehrlichioses are occasionally diagnosed by direct visualization of the distinctive intracytoplasmic aggregates of bacteria (known as *morulae*) in leukocytes in peripheral blood, bone marrow, or cerebrospinal fluid. However, this method lacks sensitivity because morulae are identified in fewer than 10% of patients with HME and fewer than 25% of patients with HGE.

■ TREATMENT

Most antimicrobials used as empiric therapies for bacterial infections in febrile patients (e.g., beta-lactams, macrolides, aminoglycosides, and sulfa-containing drugs) are characteristically ineffective in treating ehrlichiosis. (Suggested treatment regimens for ehrlichioses are described in Table 2.) Tetracyclines are bactericidal against ehrlichiae and are the drugs of choice for treating ehrlichial infections. Doxycycline (e.g., Vibramycin, Doryx, Monodox) is generally preferred over other tetracyclines because of its reduced phototoxicity, safety in patients with renal insufficiency, reduced deposition in teeth and bones, and longer plasma half-life (18 hours). Because tetracyclines may cause staining and hypoplasia of developing tooth enamel, routine use of tetracyclines in children younger than 8 years of age has been discouraged. However, because the degree of dental staining is dose and duration dependent (the threshold for cosmetically perceptible staining appears to be six or more multiple-day courses of therapy), the actual risk of discoloration appears minimal following a single short course of doxycycline. Thus the benefit of tetracycline use in children with potentially life-threatening rickettsial and ehrlichial infections far exceeds the risks, and doxycycline remains the antimicrobial of choice in pediatric patients of any age. Doxycycline is effectively administered orally in most cases. Intravenous therapy is given to hospitalized patients with vomiting, severe multisystem disease, or obtundation. Tetracyclines are contraindicated in pregnant women because of the risk of severe maternal hepatotoxicity and pancreatitis, as well as interference with normal development of teeth and long bones in the fetus.

Chloramphenicol (Chloromycetin) is occasionally used as an alternative therapy for other rickettsial diseases, but the efficacy of this drug in the treatment of ehrlichial infections is uncertain. Treatment failures have been described, and

Table 2	Antimicrobial Therapy of Ehrlichial Infections	
DRUG	**DOSAGE**	**ROUTE**
Doxycycline*		
Adults and children >45 kg	200 mg/day in two divided doses	PO or IV
Children <45 kg	3 mg/kg/day in two divided doses	PO or IV
Tetracycline		
Adults and children >8 years	25-50 mg/kg/day in four divided doses	PO
	10-20 mg/kg/day in four divided doses	IV
Chloramphenicol†		
Rifampin‡		

*Doxycycline is the antimicrobial of choice for all ehrlichial infections in adults and children but is contraindicated in pregnancy.
†Efficacy of chloramphenicol in the treatment of ehrlichiosis is uncertain. Oral formulation is unavailable in the United States.
‡Limited clinical data to suggest efficacy in pregnant patients with ehrlichiosis.

chloramphenicol is neither bacteriostic nor bactericidal against *Ehrlichia* species in vitro. Oral chloramphenicol has been unavailable in the United States since 1995. The only systemic formulation of chloramphenicol currently available is parenteral sodium succinate.

Rifampin (e.g., Rifadin, Rimactane) shows significant in vitro bactericidal activity against *E. chaffeensis* and *E. phagocytophila,* and anecdotal reports describe rapid clinical improvement in patients with HGE treated with rifampin in the second and third trimesters of pregnancy.

The efficacy of currently available quinolones against the ehrlichioses has not been evaluated by clinical trials. Ciprofloxacin is not active against *Ehrlichia* species in vitro and should not be used to treat these infections. In vitro studies also indicate that several newer quinolones possess bacteriostatic and/or bactericidal activities against ehrlichiae (e.g., trovafloxacin); however, these drugs have not been evaluated in patients with active disease.

Therapy with sulfa-containing antimicrobials is contraindicated, and evidence indicates that these drugs may increase the severity of several rickettsial infections, including RMSF, fleaborne typhus, and possibly ehrlichiosis.

Although no consensus exists regarding the optimal length of therapy for ehrlichiosis, the best guide appears to be the clinical response: clinicians should continue antibiotic coverage for at least 3 days following defervescence for a minimum total course of 5 days. In general, patients become afebrile within 24 to 48 hours after initiation of effective therapy, and the total duration of treatment is 5 to 10 days. Longer courses of doxycycline (10 to 21 days) may be warranted in select patients with HGE if coinfection with *Borrelia burgdorferi* is suspected.

Severely ill patients may develop marked hypotension, oliguria, and shock. Close hemodynamic and electrolyte monitoring, coupled with careful fluid replacement and pharmacologic blood pressure support, may be warranted. Marked anemia and thrombocytopenia can develop in some patients, thus requiring that close attention be paid to blood counts. Standard criteria for transfusion of red cells and platelets should be followed.

Prophylactic therapy in non-ill patients who have had recent tick bites is not warranted. Administration of doxycycline prior to the onset of symptoms may only delay the onset of clinical disease.

Suggested Reading

Bakken JS, et al: Clinical and laboratory characteristics of human granulocytic ehrlichiosis, *JAMA* 275:199, 1996.

Dumler JS, Bakken JS: Ehrlichial diseases of humans: emerging tick-borne infections, *Clin Infect Dis* 20:1002, 1995.
Fishbein DB, Dawson JE, Robinson LE: Human ehrlichiosis in the United States, 1985-1990, *Ann Intern Med* 120:736, 1994.
Nicholson WL, et al: An indirect immunofluorescence assay using a cell culture-derived antigen for detection of antibodies to the agent of human granulocytic ehrlichiosis, *J Clin Microbiol* 35:1510, 1997.

ENTEROBACTERIACEAE

Thomas Butler

The Enterobacteriaceae are a family of gram-negative bacteria that normally reside in the intestines of humans and other animals. Members of these genera are the leading causes of human infectious diseases affecting the urinary tract, intestine, lung, and nervous system, and of the production of localized inflammation in the form of abscesses and the generalized systemic illness known as sepsis, or systemic inflammatory response syndrome. These diverse infections are common causes of severe disease and death, and accordingly, they require prompt antimicrobial therapy and sometimes surgical intervention.

This chapter covers genera that are important causes of human illness (Table 1). Some genera in the Enterobacteriaceae family—*Salmonella, Shigella,* and *Yersinia*—are not included here because separately covered in other chapters.

■ CLINICAL PRESENTATION AND DIAGNOSIS

Most patients with infections caused by members of Enterobacteriaceae have fever, often with chills, sweating, headache, and malaise. Other symptoms are more variable, depending on the site of infection. Although all the pathogenic species of Enterobacteriaceae can cause infection at any bodily site, each species is associated preferentially with certain clinical presentations (see Table 1). The most common site is the urinary tract, which gives rise to increased urinary frequency, dysuria, suprapubic or back pain, and sometimes hematuria. Physical examination may reveal tenderness localized to the suprapubic or costovertebral regions over the kidneys or a generalized abdominal tenderness. The prostate gland may be enlarged or tender. Localization of infection in the urinary tract occurs in one or both kidneys (pyelonephritis), in the bladder (cystitis), or in the prostate (prostatitis), but precise localization by symptoms or signs

Table 1 Enterobacteriaceae	
PATHOGEN	**CLINICAL SYNDROMES**
Citrobacter diversus, C. freundii, C. amalonaticus	Nosocomial infections of urinary tract, lungs; neonatal meningitis, brain abscess
Edwardsiella tarda	Rare cause of gastroenteritis, abscess, meningitis; septicemia
Enterobacter cloacae, E. aerogenes, E. agglomerans	Nosocomial infections of lung, urinary tract, surgical wounds, burns; septicemia; diabetic ulcers
Escherichia coli	Most common cause of community acquired urinary tract infection, and urosepsis; common cause of gastroenteritis; nosocomial lung infection, septicemia; neonatal meningitis, abscess, peritonitis
Hafnia alvei	Rare cause of nosocomial infection
Klebsiella pneumoniae, K. ozaenae, K. rhinoscleromatis, K. oxytoca	Occasional cause of lung infection, empyema, urinary tract infection, sepsis; nosocomial infections of lung, urinary tract, surgical wounds, intravenous catheters, biliary tract, septicemia
Morganella morganii	Rare cause of nosocomial infections of urinary tract, lungs, septicemia
Proteus mirabilis, P. vulgaris, P. myxofaciens	Occasional cause of urinary tract infection, lung infection, sepsis; nosocomial infections of urinary tract, lungs, surgical wounds, septicemia
Providencia alcalifaciens, P. stuartii, P. rettgeri	Nosocomial infections of urinary tract, septicemia
Serratia marcescens, S. liquifaciens, S. rubidaea, S. odorifera	Nosocomial infection of lungs, urinary tract, surgical wounds, skin, septicemia; endocarditis, osteomyelitis in drug addicts

Excluding *Salmonella, Shigella,* and *Yersinia,* which are covered elsewhere.

of localized tenderness often cannot be accomplished by the examining physician. The diagnostic proof of urinary tract infection is urine showing microscopic pyuria and bacteriuria.

Another common infection caused by Enterobacteriaceae is sepsis. The symptoms include fever, chills, anorexia, vomiting, headache, diminished mental alertness, and prostration. There is often an antecedent or concomitant urinary infection, but the symptoms are more severe than in uncomplicated urinary infections, necessitating hospitalization and sometimes intensive care for intravenous fluids and monitoring of vital signs. Patients with sepsis show fever (temperature >38° C, or 100.4° F) or hypothermia (temperature <36° C, or 96.8° F), tachycardia, and tachypnea. The white blood cell count is usually above 12,000/ml^3 or may be below 4000/ml^3, and the percentage of band forms of polymorphonuclear leukocytes (PMLs) is often greater than 10. In some cases, the systolic blood pressure is below 90 mm/Hg. When the blood pressure remains low after an intravenous fluid bolus of at least 500 ml of normal saline, this is called *septic shock*. The diagnostic proof of sepsis is a positive blood culture. Sepsis is most likely to occur in immunocompromised patients, such as those with cancer receiving chemotherapy, patients receiving corticosteroids, patients with renal failure, and patients with cirrhosis. Mortality in severe sepsis or septic shock is about 50% and is highest in patients with underlying disease such as malignancy, cardiac disease, emphysema, cirrhosis, and renal failure.

Infections of the gastrointestinal tract with *Escherichia coli* may cause gastroenteritis with fever, vomiting, and diarrhea. Only strains of *E. coli* that are enterotoxigenic by virtue of carrying certain plasmids cause acute watery diarrhea. Persons are at increased risk for acquiring these infections when traveling in countries such as Mexico and Guatemala. The serotype of *E. coli* O157:H7 is enterohemorrhagic; it can cause bloody diarrhea after ingestion of incompletely cooked beef or foods contaminated with juices of infected beef. This infection can result in the serious complication of the hemolytic-uremic syndrome.

Less common clinical presentations of Enterobacteriaceae include pneumonia, abscesses, and meningitis. Nosocomial infections have increased in recent years and are likely to occur in patients who have already received antimicrobial treatment and have underlying malignancies, burns, diabetes mellitus, immunosuppression, or low birth weight in infancy. Community-acquired pneumonia caused by *Klebsiella pneumoniae* sometimes occurs in debilitated persons such as alcoholics. Patients who are placed on mechanical ventilators in intensive care units are at high risk for bacterial pneumonia; the most common causative organisms are *Pseudomonas aeruginosa* and Enterobacteriaceae including *K. pneumoniae, Enterobacter aerogenes,* and *Serratia marcescens*. The presentation of pneumonia includes cough productive of purulent yellow or green or blood-tinged sputum, dyspnea, and pleuritic pain. For hospitalized patients on mechanical ventilators, pneumonia is suspected when fever appears and suction of the endotracheal tube produces copious fluid with a yellow, green, or red coloration. The proof of pneumonia is radiographic infiltrates. Enterobacteriaceae as the cause of pneumonia is established

by a Gram stain of sputum or tracheal aspirate showing plentiful PML with a predominance of gram-negative bacilli. The culture of sputum is used to confirm the results of the Gram stain. Abscesses caused by Enterobacteriaceae manifest as abdominal pain, fever, diarrhea, ileus, intestinal perforation, or jaundice. The abscesses are localized in places such as in the liver, spleen, intestinal wall, peritoneum, or retroperitoneum. Most abscesses in these abdominal locations originate from the intestine, either by translocation of bacteria or by direct extension or perforation, and they frequently contain anaerobic bacteria (*Bacteroides* species, peptostreptococci, or *Clostridium* species) in addition to Enterobacteriaceae. Enterobacteriaceae rarely cause meningitis except for neonatal meningitis caused by *E. coli*. In adults, Enterobacteriaceae may cause meningitis in the elderly and sometimes after trauma or surgical procedures affecting the brain or spinal cord.

Spontaneous bacterial peritonitis may accompany preexisting ascites. The two most common causes of spontaneous bacterial peritonitis are *Streptococcus pneumoniae* and *E. coli*

Enterobacteriaceae may cause localized infections in other sites. These clinical presentations include septic arthritis, pericarditis, endocarditis, empyema, myositis, osteomyelitis and cholecystitis. When the common bile duct is occluded by a stone or tumor, Enterobacteriaceae may cause ascending cholangitis.

The diagnosis of these infections can be rapidly made by Gram stain of appropriate fluid. A Gram stain of uncentrifuged urine is advised. One or more gram-negative rod per oil immersion field suggests Enterobacteriaceae urinary tract infection. Likewise, Gram stain of sputum, spinal fluid, and other relevant fluids can provide diagnostic information on the day of the first examination.

Quantitative cultures of urine using a calibrated loop should be done in cases of suspected urinary tract infection. A clean-catch midstream collection is advised to reduce likelihood of contamination. In patients who are incontinent, uncooperative, or showing abnormal urinary retention, the bladder should be catheterized to obtain urine. Counts of a single bacterial species of at least 10^5/ml of voided urine suggest a significant infection; counts between 10^4 and 10^5 may represent a significant infection but should be repeated to confirm the infection. Bacterial counts less than 10^4 per milliliter of urine obtained by catheter or suprapubic aspiration should be considered significant because bladder urine is normally sterile. In a patient with an indwelling urinary catheter in place for more than 48 hours, a specimen for culture is preferably obtained after removal of the catheter to exclude bacterial colonization of the catheter lumen.

Blood should be cultured by venipuncture in patients with sepsis or fever with suspected infection at any of several sites. Standard techniques of skin cleansing should be followed to decrease likelihood of contamination. Blood should be obtained from at least two venipuncture sites to show reproducible results and to exclude contamination in the event that a possible contaminant is obtained from only one site. About 10 ml of blood should be obtained from each venipuncture, with 5 milliliters placed into each of two bottles, one for aerobic and one for anaerobic growth. The bottles should contain adequate broth volume to dilute the blood 10:1 to reduce concentrations of antibiotic and other growth-inhibiting substances in plasma. As the Enterobacteriaceae are both aerobic and facultatively anaerobic, they grow under both aerobic and anaerobic conditions. A positive blood culture for Enterobacteriaceae is useful not only for the diagnosis of sepsis, but also for determining which pathogen originating from a site such as the lung or wound—which sometimes show growth of multiple organisms—is the most significant pathogen, and hence has the highest priority for specific antimicrobial therapy.

■ THERAPY

Antimicrobial therapy should be guided by susceptibility testing. Most laboratories use disk diffusion in agar to report whether an organism shows susceptibility, resistance, or intermediate susceptibility to any specified drug. These designations are based on achievable serum concentrations of drug after administration of a usual dose. Urinary concentrations usually exceed these levels, but concentrations in other fluids, such as cerebrospinal fluid, may be considerably less.

The drugs listed in Table 2 are recommended as initial choices pending the results of culture and susceptibility testing. In the absence of Gram stain results, empiric therapies sometimes have to be started before any diagnostic information is available. After results of culture and antimicrobial susceptibilities are available, the therapy can often be changed to a narrower-spectrum drug that is preferably less toxic and less expensive than the initial therapy. For example, a patient with urosepsis caused by *E. coli* susceptible to ampicillin or cefazolin should be treated with one of these agents in place of the more nephrotoxic aminoglycoside or the more expensive third-generation cephalosporin, aztreonam, or imipenem. Multiply resistant Enterobacteriaceae are common, however, especially in nosocomial *Enterobacter* infection, with resistance mediated by inducible chromosomal beta-lactamase or plasmid-mediated beta-lactamases, which can confer resistance to third-generation cephalosporins.

Once the drug of choice has been determined, the duration of therapy must be decided. Three days of therapy is optimal for uncomplicated urinary infections in women. For complicated urinary infections with suspected sepsis or for urinary tract infections in men, courses of 7 to 14 days are appropriate to ensure cure and to prevent relapse. To

Table 2   Antimicrobial Drugs for Therapy of Infections Caused by Selected Species of Enterobacteriaceae

INFECTION	DRUG OF CHOICE	ALTERNATIVES
Escherichia coli		
Acute uncomplicated urinary tract infection in female patient	TMP-SMX orally	Amoxicillin-clavulanate, ampicillin, fluoroquinolone,[a] tetracycline[b]
Pyelonephritis, complicated urinary infection, urinary infection in male patient, sepsis	Third-generation cephalosporin[c] intravenously	Gentamicin,[d] ampicillin, ampicillin-sulbactam, amoxicillin, amoxicillin-clavulanate
Diarrhea caused by enterotoxigenic or enterohemorrhagic strains	TMP-SMX orally	Tetracycline,[b] fluoroquinolone[a]
Klebsiella pneumoniae	Third-generation cephalosporin[c] or gentamicin[d]	Cefazolin, cefoxitin, piperacillin,[e] imipenem,[f] aztreonam, TMP-SMX, fluoroquinolone,[a] tetracycline[b]
Enterobacter aerogenes	Imipenem[f] or cefepime plus	Third-generation cephalosporin,[c] ticarcillin,[g] piperacillin,[e] aztreonam, fluoroquinolone[a]
Enterobacter cloacae	gentamicin[c]	
Proteus mirabilis	Ampicillin	Gentamicin, cefazolin
Proteus vulgaris, Morganella morganii, Providencia spp.	Gentamicin,[d] third-generation cephalosporin[c]	Ticarcillin,[g] piperacillin,[e] imipenem,[f] aztreonam, TMP-SMX, fluoroquinolone[a]
Serratia marcescens	Third-generation cephalosporin[c]	Gentamicin,[d] imipenem,[f] aztreonam, fluoroquinolone,[a] ticarcillin,[g] piperacillin,[e] TMP-SMX
Citrobacter spp.	Imipenem[f]	Cefazolin, ticarcillin[g]
Hafnia alvei	Same as for *Enterobacter aerogenes*	
Edwardsiella tarda	Treatment not indicated for gastroenteritis	Tetracycline,[b] cefazolin, ampicillin
Gastroenteritis, bacteremia, abscess, meningitis	Gentamicin[d]	

TMP-SMX, Trimethoprim-sulfamethoxazole.

[a]Fluoroquinolone indicates choice of ciprofloxacin, norfloxacin, ofloxacin, enoxacin, lomefloxacin, levofloxacin, or sparfloxacin.

[b]Doxycycline may be substituted for tetracycline and is preferred sometimes for its twice daily dosing and greater ease of use in renal failure.

[c]Third-generation cephalosporins are cefotaxime, ceftriaxone, ceftazidime, ceftizoxime, and cefoperazone. Third-generation cephalosporins should be used with caution or avoided when *Enterobacter* infections are suspected or present because they induce beta-lactamase production, rendering these organisms multiresistant and causing an associated increase in mortality. The fourth-generation cephalosporin cefepime is more active against *Enterobacter* spp., including infections resistant to third-generation cephalosporins.

[d]Other aminoglycosides, including tobramycin, amikacin, and netilmicin, may be substituted for gentamicin.

[e]Mezlocillin may be substituted for piperacillin.

[f]Meropenem may be substituted for imipenem and has greater activity against some strains of Enterobacteriaceae.

[g]Carbenicillin may be substituted for ticarcillin. Both antibiotics have the same spectrum of activity, but the lower recommended doses of ticarcillin expose patients to lesser amounts of the sodium salt.

establish that a urinary tract infection has been effectively treated, a quantitative urine culture should be repeated after 3 days or more of therapy and should show no growth or fewer than 10^4 organisms/ml. For infection of soft tissue, including pneumonia, bronchitis, abscesses after drainage, meningitis, arthritis, and peritonitis, the duration of therapy should be about 7 to 14 days, individualized to the speed of resolution. Therapy may be continued until 2 to 4 days after fever and other signs of disease have disappeared. For patients with endocarditis or osteomyelitis, treatment is recommended to continue for about 6 weeks.

Oral administration of antimicrobials is the most convenient and least expensive for outpatients with most forms of infection that are not clinically severe. For uncomplicated urinary infection and soft-tissue infections of lung, skin, and intestine of mild to moderate degrees of severity, the oral route is preferred. For patients requiring hospitalization because of greater clinical severity, age older than 60 years, or underlying disease, the intravenous or intramuscular route is preferred to ensure adequate tissue concentrations of drug. After a few days of parenteral therapy and clinical improvement, most patients may be safely switched to oral therapy, usually in the outpatient setting. For patients with endocarditis or osteomyelitis, the full course of therapy is usually given parenterally because of the requirement of high blood concentrations of drug for about 6 weeks for cure.

Surgical drainage is an essential part of the therapy of localized infections caused by Enterobacteriaceae. Abscesses in common areas such as the liver and other intraabdominal or retroperitoneal sites, including perinephric, diverticular, and appendiceal sites, should be promptly drained in the operating room. Similarly, infected fluids such as accompany empyema and septic arthritis require drainage by insertion of a chest tube and by arthrotomy or aspiration, respectively.

Dosages of antimicrobial drugs vary with body weight and renal function. The usual dosages and other pharmacologic data are supplied in the chapter *Antimicrobial Agent Tables*. For gentamicin and other aminoglycosides, blood levels should be monitored periodically for adjustment of dosage. For gentamicin, tobramycin, and netilmicin, peak concentrations of 4 to 10 Mg/ml and trough concentrations less than 2 Mg/ml are advised. For amikacin, peak concentrations should be 15 to 30 µg/ml and trough less than 10 µg/ml.

Certain groups of patients with infections caused by Enterobacteriaceae have to be treated differently from others. Pregnant women should never receive tetracycline, doxycycline, chloramphenicol, ciprofloxacin, or any other fluoroquinolone because of their toxicity to bony development in the fetus. Trimethoprim-sulfamethoxazole (TMP-SMX) should be used with caution during pregnancy and is contraindicated at term. Tetracycline and doxycycline should be avoided in children younger than 10 years of age to avoid staining of teeth. Ciprofloxacin and other fluoroquinolones are not approved for use in children until age 18 years because they may affect cartilage development in growing bones.

The cost of antimicrobial therapies can be very great for the patient or insurer and should be minimized in a manner that does not compromise therapeutic efficacy. The cost of a course of treatment varies with the route of administration, whether a drug is off patent and available in generic form, the duration of treatment, and the practice of local pharmacies to buy large lots of drugs at discounted prices. In general, oral drugs are significantly less expensive than parenteral ones. Generic preparations of oral drugs are the least expensive. They include (see Table 2) TMP-SMX, ampicillin, amoxicillin, tetracycline, doxycycline, and cephalexin. Oral drugs that remain on patent and are more expensive include amoxicillin-clavulanate, the fluoroquinolones, cefaclor, cefpodoxime, cefuroxime-axetil, and cefixime. For intravenous therapies, the generic drugs that should be used when possible include ampicillin, cefazolin, gentamicin or tobramycin, and tetracycline. The remaining parenteral drugs, such as ampicillin-sulbactam, ticarcillin-clavulanate, piperacillin-tazobactam, imipenem, meropenem, aztreonam, third-generation cephalosporins, and cefepime remain the most expensive and should be used only when less expensive alternatives are unsatisfactory.

The management of severe sepsis or septic shock due to Enterobacteriaceae requires admission to an intensive care unit. Intravenous normal saline or lactated Ringer's solution to expand plasma volume is given in volumes of at least 500 ml to adults to ensure adequate intravascular fluid volume. Oxygen should be administered to obtain at least 90% saturation of hemoglobin. In severe cases, mechanical ventilation will be required to achieve adequate oxygenation. In cases of shock, vasopressors such as dopamine, epinephrine, and norepinephrine are needed to raise the blood pressure.

Suggested Reading

D'Agata E, et al: The molecular and clinical epidemiology of Enterobacteriaceae-producing extended-spectrum β-lactamase in a tertiary care hospital, *J Infect* 36:279, 1998.

Jacobson KL, et al: The relationship between antecedent antibiotic use and resistance to extended-spectrum cephalosporins in group I β-lactamase-producing organisms, *Clin Infect Dis* 21:1107, 1995.

Janda JM, Abbott SL: Infections associated with the genus *Edwardsiella*: the role of *Edwardsiella tarda* in human disease, *Clin Infect Dis* 17:742, 1993.

Jones RN: Important and emerging β-lactamase-mediated resistances in hospital-based pathogens: the amp C enzymes, *Diagn Microbiol Infect Dis* 31:461, 1998.

Mimoz O, et al: Cefepime and amikacin synergy in vitro and in vivo against a ceftazidime-resistant strain of *Enterobacter cloacae*, *J Antimicrob Chemother* 41:367, 1998.

Piddock LJV, et al: Prevalence and mechanism of resistance to "third-generation" cephalosporins in clinically relevant isolates of Enterobacteriaceae from 43 hospitals in the UK, 1990-1991, *J Antimicrob Chemother* 39:177, 1997.

Sanders WE, Sanders CC: *Enterobacter* spp.: pathogens poised to flourish at the turn of the century, *Clin Microbiol Rev* 10:220, 1997.

Sanders WE, Tenney JH, Kessler RE: Efficacy of cefepime in the treatment of infections due to multiply resistant *Enterobacter* species, *Clin Infect Dis* 23:454, 1996.

Shih C-C, et al: Bacteremia due to *Citrobacter* species: significance of primary intraabdominal infection, *Clin Infect Dis* 23:543, 1996.

ENTEROCOCCUS

Ronald N. Jones

In the past 15 years, the enterococci have emerged as major hospital-acquired (nosocomial) pathogens. They are now the third most common cause of nosocomial bloodstream infection and the second most common cause of nosocomial wound and urinary tract infection. The emergence of this genus may in part be related to patterns of general antimicrobial use in the hospital and in particular to widespread use of extended-spectrum cephalosporins, monobactams, fluoroquinolones, carbapenems, and aminoglycosides.

Cephalosporins are not potent or bactericidal against enterococci, and they may therefore result in a selective advantage for this genus. Enterococcus faecalis produce most human infections (70% to 95%), and Enterococcus faecium accounts for most (8% to 16%) of the remainder. Antimicrobial resistance is a particular problem among E. faecium isolates. Other species of interest are Enterococcus casseliflavus and Enterococcus gallinarum, not because of the frequency with which they are isolated (usually among top five), but because of the intrinsic low-level resistance to vancomycin (e.g., the vanC genotype and resultant resistant or intermediate phenotype).

In addition to the problems posed by the increasing frequency of enterococcal infection, the therapy of these infections has become very difficult as resistance to ampicillin, high-level resistance to aminoglycosides, and most recently glycopeptide (vancomycin and teicoplanin) resistance have narrowed the proven therapeutic options. In addition, the value (because of risk of failure) of trimethoprim-sulfamethoxazole (TMP-SMX) in therapy even for urinary tract infection has become controversial. All enterococci are intrinsically resistant to achievable in vivo levels of aminoglycosides; however, synergic killing may occur when aminoglycosides are combined with a cell wall–active agent such as a penicillin or a glycopeptide. Strains resistant to high levels of aminoglycoside (>500 µg/ml of gentamicin or >1,000 µg/ml of streptomycin) are not susceptible to the synergic codrug activity of the aminoglycosides. It is clinically significant that cross-resistance to the synergic activity of the aminoglycosides is incomplete between gentamicin (and the related compounds tobramycin, netilmicin, amikacin, kanamycin, and isepamicin) and streptomycin. Streptomycin may be used successfully in combination to treat some high-level gentamicin-resistant strains. The selection of the appropriate aminoglycoside codrug should be directed by validated in vitro susceptibility tests.

Resistance to vancomycin is more common with E. faecium isolates than with E. faecalis, but it may occur with either species. Reports in the USA in the late 1990s suggest that the overall vancomycin-resistant rate for enterococci is approaching 20% among blood stream infections, and higher resistance rates for some other drugs and species limit therapeutic choices (Table 1). Acquired vancomycin resistance is often associated with resistance to teicoplanin (Van A phenotype or vanA genotype) or may occur in the absence of cross-resistance to teicoplanin (Van B phenotype or vanB genotype), and this difference may be clinically significant in nations where teicoplanin is available. Intrinsic low-level resistance to both glycopeptides has been observed in E. casseliflavus and in E. gallinarum and is called the Van C phenotype that has a specific genotype.

For the clinician, the problems posed by the emergence of resistance have been exacerbated by the technical difficulties in reliable detection of these resistances. In vitro resistance to TMP-SMX as a result of the ability of the most prevalent enterococci to use thymidine or thymine in the susceptibility test medium has been addressed by the use of media free of or low in concentration for these antagonists. However, there are significant amounts of antagonists in the urine, and therefore the meaning of test results performed in these "improved" media is doubtful. Routine testing against ampicillin without testing for organism beta-lactamase production may result in false-susceptible results. However, beta-lactamase production is an exceedingly uncommon mechanism of resistance (<0.1%) among E. faecalis isolates. A number of problems with the detection of high-level aminoglycoside resistance using the most prevalent automated and commercial broth microdilution susceptibility test systems (Vitek, MicroScan) have been reported, although in some cases these now appear to have been resolved. Similarly, with vancomycin resistance both automated susceptibility test system and disk diffusion test interpretive criteria have required modifica-

Table 1   Susceptibility Rates of 2246 Enterococcal Strains Isolated from the SENTRY Antimicrobial Surveillance Program Hospital Patients in 1997 to 1999 (>30 Medical Centers in the United States)*

| | % SUSCEPTIBLE | | |
ANTIMICROBIAL AGENT	ALL ENTEROCOCCI (2246)	E. FAECALIS (1338)	E. FAECIUM (456)
Ampicillin	78	98	12
Gentamicin	71	74	59
Streptomycin	60	67	30
Vancomycin	85	97	46
Quinupristin-dalfopristin	25	2	92

*Data on file, University of Iowa College of Medicine (Iowa City, Iowa).

tion to enable consistent, accurate detection of resistant strains.

Empiric therapy of enterococcal infection is not satisfactory given the complexity of resistance patterns, and therefore, availability of prompt, reliable susceptibility test results is indispensable. At present, disk diffusion susceptibility testing, Etest (AB Blodisk, Solna, Sweden), Vitek System (personal experience), and the reference broth microdilution or agar dilution methods are reliable methods for detection of important enterococcal resistances.

■ ENTEROCOCCAL BLOODSTREAM INFECTION

Isolation of enterococci from the blood may occur with or without endocarditis. In community-acquired enterococcal bloodstream infection approximately one third of cases are associated with endocarditis, compared with fewer than 5% of nosocomial enterococcal bacteremias. These nosocomial infections are usually associated with urinary tract disease or instrumentation, intraabdominal infection, intravascular devices, neoplastic disease, and significant neutropenia.

Infective endocarditis, even when caused by more susceptible strains of enterococci, is more difficult to achieve cures for than endocarditis due to viridans streptococci. Only two thirds of patients will be cured if a penicillin is used alone. A combination of a cell wall–active agent (a penicillin or glycopeptide) with an aminoglycoside for 4 to 6 weeks is recommended. In general, ampicillin (two or four times as active) is used in preference to penicillin; however, the scientific basis for this pattern of use is less than compelling on potency issues alone. High-dose penicillins (ampicillin, 2 g every 4 hours, or penicillin G, 18 to 30 million U/day) are appropriate, combined with gentamicin, 1 mg/kg every 8 hours or the use of the less toxic pattern of once-daily dosing. However, limited clinical information supports the use of once-daily aminoglycosides in this clinical setting. Monitoring of aminoglycoside serum concentrations is essential to ensure adequate therapeutic levels and to minimize toxicity during the extended therapeutic course. (See also the chapter *Endocarditis of Natural and Prosthetic Valves: Treatment and Prophylaxis.*)

The choice of an aminoglycoside for combination therapy is between gentamicin and streptomycin. Gentamicin is generally preferred because synergic killing is more consistent, ototoxicity is less, and facilities to measure serum levels are more easily available. Enterococcal strains resistant to high levels of aminoglycoside in vitro are not susceptible to synergic killing with a penicillin or glycopeptide, and in such patients use of aminoglycosides constitutes exposure to potential toxicity for no apparent clinical benefit. Cross-resistance between gentamicin and streptomycin is not universal, and strains resistant to one should be tested against the other. Optimal therapy is not well defined for strains resistant to high levels of both aminoglycosides. Prolonged therapy with high dosages of a penicillin, possibly by continuous infusion, may be successful in some cases. Combination therapy with vancomycin and a penicillin has also been reported successful.

Enterococcal resistance to penicillin and vancomycin and

to high levels of aminoglycoside will be increasingly encountered in hospital practice and possibly in clinic patients. There is no established therapy for this group of organisms. Vancomycin-resistant enterococci of the Van B phenotype remain susceptible to teicoplanin, which is not available in the United States. Teicoplanin is not bactericidal alone, and combinations with an aminoglycoside appear appropriate for strains for which the combination will be synergistic. It is important that teicoplanin be used in adequate dose, particularly if used alone. Not less than 6 mg/kg twice on the first day and once daily thereafter is required for effective therapy of serious infection, and doses of 10 to 15 mg/kg have been used without serious toxicity. Monitoring for adequacy of trough levels (at least 20 µg/ml) is important where feasible, although facilities for such monitoring may not be available. Serum inhibitory and bactericidal titers may be as useful. Teicoplanin resistance has emerged on chemotherapy.

Therapy with teicoplanin is not an option for Van A strains, and this is the predominant pattern (60% to 70% g. strains) of vancomycin resistance in the United States. Various therapeutic approaches have been suggested, but none are widely accepted. Chloramphenicol and doxycycline have demonstrated a variable degree of activity (>50% to 90% susceptible by NCCLS criteria; Table 2) against the multidrug-resistant enterococci. Case reports indicate that these drugs used alone or with codrugs have been successful in a high percentage of cases, but each is only bacteriostatic. Combinations of both drugs are also not bactericidal. Even with eradication of enterococci from the bloodstream, mortality remains high (30% to 50%). Fluoroquinolones (ciprofloxacin, levofloxacin, gatifloxacin, and moxifloxacin) may have value for tested susceptible strains (see Table 2), although resistance may emerge rapidly when these drugs are used alone. Their action on susceptible strains can be bactericidal. Combinations of ampicillin and a fluoroquinolone have been found bactericidal for some strains. In vitro and animal studies support the use of a combination of novobiocin and a fluoroquinolone for some isolates, although in our experience the high degree of protein binding for novobiocin (>95%) significantly reduces its activity. Pristinomycins (quinupristin-dalfopristin or Synercid) are generally bacteriostatic agents available for use for therapy of *E. faecium* infection. These agents are not active against *E. faecalis* strains. A variety of other fluoroquinolones in development (see Table 2) are more active against enterococci than ciprofloxacin and may have expanded potential for future use. Evernimicin (formerly SCH27899), oxazolidinones (linezolid or U100766), and glycylcyclines are other highly effective investigational compounds of recent interest (see Table 2). However, most of these drugs demonstrate little bactericidal action against multidrug-resistant enterococci and their success awaits reports from Phase III clinical trials.

Therapy for enterococcal bloodstream infection in the absence of endocarditis follows the same general principles as for endocarditis except that bactericidal therapy may not be necessary. Bactericidal effect should be sought in the immunocompromised patient. Empiric therapy for such patients should be initiated with vancomycin, since patients likely to develop nosocomial enterococcal infection are also at risk for infection with methicillin-resistant

Table 2 In Vitro Susceptibility of Alternative Antimicrobial Agents for U.S. Enterococcal Isolates with Resistance to Glycopeptides (VRE Strains; 354 Isolates in 1999)

ANTIMICROBIAL AGENT	% BY CATEGORY		
	SUSCEPTIBLE	INTERMEDIATE	RESISTANT
FLUOROQUINOLONES			
Ciprofloxacin	3	2	95
Gatifloxacin	6	5	89
Levofloxacin	3	6	91
PRISTINOMYCINS			
Quinupristin-dalfopristin	82	6	12
EVERNINOMICINS			
Evernimicin (SCH27899)	100	0	0
GLYCYLCYCLINES			
GAR-936	100	0	0
OXAZOLIDONES			
Linezolid (U100766)	100	0	0
OTHERS			
Chloramphenicol	90	5	5
Doxycycline	53	20	27
Novobiocin	100	0	0
TMP-SMX	28	4	68
Clindamycin	0	0	100
Erythromycin	3	0	97
Imipenem	0	0	100

Modified from results of the SENTRY Antimicrobial Surveillance Program (University of Iowa College of Medicine, Iowa City, IA); Jones and Barrett (1995); Jones et al. (1996, 1997, 1999); and Pfaller et al. (1999).
TMP-SMX, Trimethoprim-sulfamethoxazole (1:19 ratio).

coagulase-negative staphylococci. As with all other pathogens, removal of potential foci of infection, such as an indwelling device, and drainage of an abscess, is essential for successful therapy.

■ THERAPY OF MODERATE INFECTION AND URINARY TRACT INFECTION

In the absence of immediate susceptibility test results, ampicillin is a reasonable option for therapy of moderate infections and particularly for urinary tract infection, given the high levels of ampicillin achieved in urine. Nitrofurantoin is also active against most enterococci and is useful in therapy of urinary tract infection.

Clearly, these approaches must be modified in the context of local epidemiology and emergence of resistant strains. In centers with very high incidence of infection with ampicillin-resistant enterococci, usually *E. faecium,* this may not be appropriate therapy. For infection with drug-resistant organisms, the options are similar to those discussed for bloodstream infection, except that synergic combinations are usually not necessary.

■ ENTEROCOCCAL CARRIAGE

There is no general acceptance that fecal carriage of multidrug-resistant enterococci is an indication for therapy; however, given the risk to the patient of subsequent disseminated infection, there is high epidemiologic interest in this issue. It seems reasonable to review the patient's

therapy with a view toward discontinuation of any nonessential antimicrobials that might confer a selective advantage for the enterococci. There have been reports of the successful use of oral bacitracin to eradicate fecal carriage of vancomycin- and ampicillin-resistant enterococci.

■ COMMENTS

Therapy of enterococcal infections is one of the most challenging areas in the contemporary treatment of infectious ndisease. Good laboratory support is essential to management of these infections in the most appropriate manner with minimal toxicity. Given the emerging inadequacies of our therapeutic armamentarium and the clear evidence that nosocomial spread of this pathogen can occur, an aggressive stance with respect to hospital environment surveillance and infection control are of critical importance. Also, more study will be required to develop new therapeutic agents and to focus our treatments on existing antimicrobial agents that produce acceptable enterococcus infection eradication.

Suggested Reading

French GL: Enterococci and vancomycin resistance, *Clin Infect Dis* 27 (suppl 1):S75, 1998.

Jarvis WR: Epidemiology, appropriateness, and cost of vancomycin use, *Clin Infect Dis* 26:1200, 1998.

Jones RN, Barrett MS: Antimicrobial activity of SCH 27899, oligosaccharide member of the everninomicin class with a wide Gram-positive spectrum. *J Clin Microbiol Infect* 1:35, 1995.

Jones RN, Johnson DM, Erwin ME: In vitro antimicrobial activities and spectra of U-100592 and U-100766, two novel fluorinated oxazolidinones. *Antimicrob Agents Chemother* 40:720, 1996.

Jones RN, Low DE, Pfaller, MA: Epidemiologic trends in nosocomial and community-acquired infections due to antibiotic-resistant Gram-positive bacteria: the role of streptogramins and other newer compounds, *Diagn Microbiol Infect Dis* 33:101, 1999.

Jones RN, et al, the SCOPE Hospital Study Group: Nosocomial enterococcal blood stream infections in the SCOPE Program: antimicrobial resistance, species occurrence, molecular testing results, and laboratory testing accuracy, *Diagn Microbiol Infect Dis* 29:95, 1997.

Landman D, Quale JM: Management of infections due to resistant enterococci: a review of therapeutic options, *J Antimicrob Chemother* 40:161, 1997.

Linden PK, et al: Differences in outcomes for patients with bacteria due to vancomycin-resistant *Enterococcus faecium* or vancomycin-susceptible *E. faecium, Clin Infect Dis* 22:663, 1996.

McDonald LC, et al: Vancomycin-resistant enterococci outside the health-care setting: prevalence, sources, and public health implications, *Emerg Infect Dis* 3:311, 1997.

Pfaller MA, et al, The SENTRY Participants Group: Survey of blood stream infections attributable to Gram-positive cocci: frequency of occurrence and antimicrobial susceptibility of isolates collected in 1997 in the United States, Canada, and Latin America from the SENTRY Antimicrobial Surveillance Program, *Diagn Microbiol Infect Dis* 33:283, 1999.

ERYSIPELOTHRIX

W. Lee Hand
Hoi Ho

*E*rysipelothrix rhusiopathiae, a pleomorphic, gram-positive bacillus, is the only species of the genus *Erysipelothrix*. This organism causes both a self-limited soft-tissue infection (erysipeloid) and serious systemic disease. *E. rhusiopathiae* is widespread in nature and infects many domestic animals. Swine are probably the major reservoir of *E. rhusiopathiae*. This microorganism is also found in sheep, cattle, horses, and dogs, as well as in fish and crabs. Human infection usually results from occupational exposure. Butchers, fishermen, abattoir workers, farmers, and veterinarians are at risk for *Erysipelothrix* infections.

The clinical spectrum of human infection includes localized cutaneous infection, diffuse cutaneous disease, and systemic bloodstream infection.

■ LOCALIZED CUTANEOUS INFECTION

Erysipeloid of Rosenbach, the localized cutaneous form of illness, is the most common human infection caused by *E. rhusiopathiae*. Fingers and/or hands (sites of exposure) are almost always involved in this soft-tissue infection. Mild pain may occur at the site of inoculation, followed by itching, throbbing pain, burning, and tingling. The characteristic skin lesion slowly progresses from a small red dot at the site of inoculation to a fully developed erysipeloid skin lesion, consisting of a well-defined purplish center with an elevated border. Patients often complain of joint stiffness and pain in the involved fingers, but swelling is minimal or absent. Small, hemorrhagic, vesicular lesions may be present at the site of inoculation. Pain may be disproportionate to the degree of apparent involvement. Local lymphangitis or adenitis develop in 30% of patients. However, systemic symptoms such as high fever or chills are uncommon, occurring in perhaps 6% of patients.

A provisional diagnosis is based on a history of contact with potentially contaminated materials or occupational exposure, plus compatible physical findings. Gram-stained smears and cultures of aspirated material from skin lesions are often negative because the organism is deep within the dermis.

Most of these infections are acquired from an aquatic environment. Other infections from aquatic sources are discussed in the chapter *Recreational Water Exposure.*

■ DIFFUSE CUTANEOUS DISEASE

Most erysipeloid skin lesions resolve even without specific treatment. However, erysipeoid occasionally will progress to the diffuse cutaneous form in untreated patients. Eating of contaminated meat has also been reported as a cause of this clinical entity. The characteristic purplish skin lesions expand with gradual clearing of the center. Bullous lesions may appear at the primary site or at distant locations. These patients often have systemic symptoms such as high fever, chills, and arthralgias. Blood cultures are invariably negative.

■ SYSTEMIC INFECTION (BACTEREMIA OR ENDOCARDITIS)

Bacteremic infection caused by *E. rhusiopathiae* is generally a primary infection and not the result of dissemination from localized cutaneous disease. Nevertheless, one third of patients with bloodstream infection have skin lesions suggestive of erysipeloid. Persistent bacteremia with *E. rhusiopathiae* has been reported after eating contaminated seafood. Cutaneous serpiginous lesions or multiple bullous lesions over the trunk and extremities may be seen. Most patients have fever for 2 to 3 weeks before presentation. Fever and chills may resolve spontaneously, but relapse is to be expected.

Table 1 Antibiotic Therapy for *Erysipelothrix Rhusiopathiae* Infection

TYPE OF *ERYSIPELOTHRIX* INFECTION	ANTIBIOTICS OF CHOICE		
	DRUG	DOSE AND ROUTE	DURATION
MILD			
Primary	Penicillin V	500 mg q6h PO	7 days
Alternatives	Ciprofloxacin (other fluoroquinolones may be used)	250 mg q12h PO	7 days
	Clindamycin	200 mg q8h PO	7 days
	Erythromycin (other macrolides may be used)	500 mg q6h PO	7 days
SEVERE (BACTEREMIC)			
Primary	Penicillin G	2-4 million units q4h IV	4 wk
Alternatives	Ceftriaxone	2 g q24h IV	4 wk
	Imipenem	500 mg q6h IV	4 wk
	Ciprofloxacin (other IV fluoroquinolones may be used)	400 mg q12h IV	4 wk

Patients with severe underlying heart disease or liver disease may present with a clinical picture resembling gram-negative sepsis. More than one third of patients with disseminated infection are alcoholics, and chronic liver disease is a major predisposing factor. Bacteremia has also been reported in immunocompromised individuals, who often are receiving corticosteroid and/or cytotoxic drug treatment for collagen-vascular disease or malignancy.

E. rhusiopathiae bacteremia is associated with a severe clinical course and is often complicated by endocarditis. *Erysipelothrix* endocarditis often results in extensive destruction of native cardiac valves, especially the aortic valve. Approximately one third of patients die because of this complication, and an additional one third require cardiac valvular replacement. Absence of typical findings of endocarditis on initial physical examination or echocardiography does not exclude this diagnosis in patients with positive blood cultures. Reported complications of endocarditis have included acute renal failure resulting from proliferative glomerulonephritis.

Earlier publications indicated that 90% of bacteremic infections were associated with endocarditis. This perceived high frequency may, at least in part, be a result of reporting bias because a number of bacteremic cases without endocarditis have been reported more recently.

The diagnosis of disseminated *E. rhusiopathiae* infection depends on identification of this organism in blood cultures. Commercial media are satisfactory for isolation from blood, and growth is usually detected in 2 or 3 days.

■ THERAPY

Erysipeloid may resolve spontaneously within 3 weeks, but treatment with an appropriate antibiotic hastens the healing process and prevents relapse. Local therapy with rest and heat is helpful for patients with painful, swollen lesions or arthritis. The involved hand or finger should be carried in a sling or splint. Surgical incision or debridement of the localized lesions is not necessary.

Penicillin and imipenem are the most active antibiotics against *Erysipelothrix* with in vitro testing. Penicillin is a time-tested, effective agent for treatment of all forms of *E. rhusiopathiae* infection. Other beta-lactam antibiotics are also active against the organism. Fluoroquinolones and clindamycin demonstrate good in vitro activity. Erythromycin, tetracyclines, and chloramphenicol have less predictable activity against *Erysipelothrix* and should not be used in the treatment of disseminated infection. *E. rhusiopathiae* is resistant to sulfonamides, trimethoprim-sulfamethoxazole, aminoglycosides, and vancomycin.

Antibiotic therapy should be based upon the clinical picture and results of blood cultures (Table 1). Oral antibiotic therapy is appropriate for localized cutaneous infection. Parenteral antibiotic treatment is indicated if patients have systemic infection or severe diffuse cutaneous disease. Penicillin G has been the historic drug of choice. Alternatives include ceftriaxone, imipenem, and fluoroquinolones. Patients with bacteremia or endocarditis should receive at least 4 weeks of intravenous antibiotic therapy.

Suggested Reading

Gorby GL, Peacock JE: *Erysipelothrix rhusiopathiae* endocarditis: microbiologic, epidemiologic, and clinical features of an occupational disease, *Rev Infect Dis* 10:317, 1988.

Klauder JV: Erysipeloid as an occupational disease, *JAMA* 111:1345, 1938.

Reboli AC, Farrar WE: *Erysipelothrix rhusiopathiae*: an occupational pathogen, *Clin Microbiol Rev* 2:354, 1989.

Soriano F, et al: In vitro susceptibilities of aerobic and facultative non-spore-forming gram-positive bacilli to HMR 3647 (RU66647) and 14 other antimicrobials, *Antimicrob Agents Chemother* 42:1028, 1998.

Venditti M, et al: Antimicrobial susceptibilities of *Erysipelothrix rhusiopathiae*, *Antimicrob Agents Chemother* 34:2038, 1990.

HACEK

Christopher H. Cabell
Daniel J. Sexton

The acronym *HACEK* describes a heterogeneous group of organisms that share two major characteristics. First, they are fastidious gram-negative rods that require forethought and special measures to culture in the microbiology laboratory. Second, they have a predilection to infect heart valves. The HACEK group includes *Haemophilus* species (except *H. influenzae*), *Actinobacillus actinomycetemcomitans*, *Cardiobacterium hominus*, *Eikenella corrodens*, and *Kingella* species. These organisms are infamous for their ability to cause endocarditis although, rarely, they cause a variety of other infections (Table 1). For example, human bites can result in cellulitis or abscess formation resulting from HACEK organisms, especially *Eikenella* species, and various *Haemophilus* species can cause epiglottitis or brain abscesses.

Members of the HACEK group are normal indigenous flora of the oral cavity. Systemic hematogenous spread may occur after dental manipulation or secondary to periodontal disease. Thereafter, individuals with underlying valvular heart disease are at risk of developing endocarditis. Antibiotic prophylaxis before dental manipulation does not ensure complete prevention against these fastidious organisms. However, the risk of endocarditis is very small after dental manipulation, even in patients with significant valvular disease. Millions of patients undergo dental procedures annually, yet the cases of infective endocarditis (IE) caused by HACEK group organisms are rare.

■ DIAGNOSIS

The key to the diagnosis of HACEK infections is suspicion by the treating physician. Without proper information, the microbiology laboratory may not take necessary steps to culture these organisms. Most laboratories routinely discard blood culture bottles after 7 days. Many members of the HACEK group may not be detectable in culture bottles after a week of incubation. To detect HACEK group organisms, blood cultures must be subcultured onto agar plates, which are incubated for an additional 2 to 3 weeks. HACEK organisms typically grow on 5% sheep blood and chocolate agar but not on MacConkey's agar. Because growth is often poor or absent in an unenhanced atmosphere, incubation in 5% to 10% carbon dioxide (CO_2) is recommended. After growth is observed, standard biochemical tests will identify individual HACEK species.

■ CLINICAL FEATURES

The clinical features of endocarditis caused by members of the HACEK group are identical to the clinical features of IE caused by more typical pathogens, with two exceptions. First, HACEK cases appear culture negative initially. Second, HACEK group infections are often complicated by large bulky vegetations.

■ THERAPY

There have been no large trials to evaluate the best therapy for IE caused by HACEK group organisms. Currently available information is in the form of small case series or individual case reports. In the past, ampicillin plus an aminoglycoside was the therapy of choice. This treatment was advocated because synergy between beta-lactams and aminoglycosides was demonstrated in vitro, but such synergy has not been conclusively proved in the clinical setting with HACEK infections. Moreover, a number of case reports have documented therapeutic failures of combined therapy with ampicillin and gentamicin in the treatment of *A. actinomycetemcomitans* and *Haemophilus* infections. In addition, a number of recent reports have described beta-lactamase production by numerous strains of HACEK group organisms. Because of their fastidious growth requirements, susceptibility testing is difficult. We and others believe that HACEK group organisms should be considered ampicillin resistant unless proved otherwise. In light of this, we do not advocate ampicillin as therapy for HACEK group organisms.

Most HACEK organisms, with the notable exceptions of *A. actinomycetemcomitans* and *E. corrodens,* are susceptible to first- and second-generation cephalosporins, and virtually all species are susceptible to third-generation cephalosporins. Therefore we believe the best therapy for IE caused by HACEK group bacteria is cefotaxime or ceftriaxone. We advocate using ceftriaxone, 2 g intravenously (IV) or intramuscularly (IM) once daily, because of its convenience and suitability for outpatient parenteral therapy (Table 2). The duration of therapy for native valve endocarditis should be at least 4 weeks; at least 6 weeks of therapy is recommended for prosthetic valve endocarditis.

HACEK group organisms are also susceptible in vitro to most fluoroquinolones, trimethoprim-sulfamethoxazole, and aztreonam. Thus one of these agents may be used in the beta-lactam–intolerant patient. There is a growing body of evidence to support the use of ciprofloxacin as outpatient therapy for HACEK endocarditis.

A number of investigators advocate empirical therapy with either ceftriaxone along with an aminoglycoside or ciprofloxacin until sensitivities return. A fluoroquinolone such as ciprofloxacin is the preferred alternative for patients who are allergic to a beta-lactam. Ciprofloxacin is an appropriate choice for the outpatient segment of therapy because of its high bioavailability after oral ingestion and excellent safety profile. However, because of the lack of published data about fluoroquinolone therapy for HACEK group bacterial infections, we prefer to use ceftriaxone as initial therapy. Despite the technical difficulties in obtaining in vitro susceptibility results, we advocate obtaining such results to confirm sensitivity to the agents being used or contemplated for use. Careful follow up of all patients undergoing treatment is also recommended, including periodic assessment of clinical and microbiologic response using careful examinations and follow-up blood cultures. Careful monitoring

Table 1   HACEK-Associated Infections

Haemophilus aphrophilus 　　　*haemolyticus* 　　　*parahaemolyticus* 　　　*parainfluenzae* 　　　*paraphrophilus* 　　　*segnis*	Brain abscess, endocarditis, endophthalmitis, epiglottitis, hepatic abscess, intraabdominal infection, meningitis, neonatal sepsis, necrotizing fasciitis, otitis media, pneumonia, sinusitis, septic arthritis, urinary tract infection
Actinobacillus actinomycetemcomitans	Brain abscess, cellulitis, empyema, endocarditis, endophthalmitis, osteomyelitis, periodontal infection, parotitis, pericarditis, pneumonia, synovitis, thyroid abscess, urinary tract infection
Cardiobacterium hominis	Endocarditis, meningitis
Eikenella corrodens	Abscessed tooth, Bartholin's gland abscess, brain abscess, cellulitis, conjunctivitis, dacryocystitis, empyema, endocarditis, endometritis, gingivitis, intraabdominal abscess, intravascular space infections, keratitis, liver abscess, mediastinitis, meningitis, mycotic aneurysm, otitis externa, parotitis, pericarditis, pneumonia, septic pulmonary emboli, subdural empyema, thyroid abscess, thyroiditis
Kingella dentrificens 　　　*indologenes* 　　　*kingae*	Abscess, endocarditis, epiglottitis, intervertebral diskitis, meningitis, oropharyngeal infections, osteomyelitis, septic arthritis

Table 2   Antibiotics Recommended for Serious Infections

	ANTIBIOTIC	DOSAGE AND ROUTE	LENGTH OF THERAPY
First choice	Ceftriaxone	2 g IV or IM qd	4-6 wk
Alternative	Ciprofloxacin	500 mg PO q12h	4-6 wk

for compliance is advised for all patients treated with oral therapy.

HACEK group organisms are usually susceptible to tetracycline and chloramphenicol; however, both of these agents are bacteriostatic and would be poor choices for endovascular infections. Most HACEK group members are resistant to metronidazole, vancomycin, erythromycin, and clindamycin.

■ PROGNOSIS

Patients with endocarditis caused by HACEK group organisms have a favorable prognosis. In general, there is a low complication and mortality rate, and most infections can be cured without surgical intervention. This is true in native valve as well as prosthetic valve endocarditis.

■ NONENDOCARDIAL INFECTIONS

Nonendocardial infections caused by HACEK group organisms are rare. Such infections are usually responsive to short courses of antibiotic therapy. Surgical drainage is indicated for abscesses. Some authorities have recommended that septic arthritis caused by *Kingella kingae* be treated with 3 to 4 weeks of parenteral therapy followed by an additional 3 weeks of antibiotics by mouth, but this recommendation is not based on controlled clinical data.

Suggested Reading

Babinchak TJ: Oral ciprofloxacin therapy for prosthetic valve endocarditis due to *Actinobacillus actinomycetemcomitans*, *CID* 21:1517, 1995.

Das M, et al: Infective endocarditis caused by HACEK microorganisms, *Ann Rev Med* 48:25, 1997.

Kaplan AH, et al: Infection due to *Actinobacillus actinomycetemcomitans*: 15 cases and review, *Rev Infect Dis* 11:46, 1989.

Wilson WR, et al: Antibiotic treatment of adults with infective endocarditis due to streptococci, enterococci, staphylococci, and HACEK microorganisms, *JAMA* 274:1706, 1995.

HELICOBACTER PYLORI

Zhannat Z. Nurgalieva
David Y. Graham

*H*elicobacter pylori infection is one of the most common chronic infections worldwide and is responsible for tremendous morbidity and mortality. The natural niche for the organism is the human stomach, where it causes destructive inflammation (e.g., gastritis). Before the discovery of *H. pylori,* gastritis was an important topic of research because it had been recognized that it was the basic pathology underlying gastric cancer and peptic ulcer disease. The ability to cultivate *H. pylori,* the proof that it caused gastritis and that gastritis healed following cure of the infection, together resulted in major changes in thinking about a number of important gastrointestinal diseases. *H. pylori* is now accepted as the major cause of gastric ulcer and duodenal ulcer disease, gastric cancer, and primary B-cell gastric lymphoma. Its role in nonulcer dyspepsia remains unclear.

■ THE BACTERIUM

Although they were unable to isolate the organism, in the 1970s Steer and colleagues brought attention to the fact that gastritis appeared to be strongly associated with a bacterium. In the early 1980s, Barry Marshall, working in the laboratory of Stewart Goodwin, was able to culture *H. pylori.* The hospital pathologist, Robin Warren, had noted that the gastric bacteria had morphology similar to *Campylobacter jejuni.* This observation provided the key to the cultivation of the organism as well as its initial classification as a *Campylobacter. H. pylori,* as the organism is now known, is a microaerophilic, gram-negative, spiral rod approximately 0.6×3.5 μ with unipolar flagella. The biochemical features that help identify it include the presence of urease, oxidase, and catalase.

■ EPIDEMIOLOGY

The primary reservoir for the infection is humans. The bulk of the data regarding transmission is consistent with person-to-person spread. The infection is usually acquired in childhood and clusters within families. Risk factors for *H. pylori* infection include birth in a developing country, low socioeconomic status, crowded living conditions, large family size, unsanitary living conditions, unclean food or water, presence of infants in the home, and exposure to gastric contents of infected individuals. *H. pylori* has been cultured from stools and gastric contents, suggesting that both fecal-oral and oral-oral are possible routes of transmission. In countries with unclean water supplies, there is also evidence for waterborne transmission.

Worldwide, the best correlates with a high prevalence of *H. pylori* infection are low socioeconomic status and unsanitary living conditions. Even in developed countries where the overall prevalence is low (e.g., approximately 35% in the United States), the infection is prevalent in some populations, for example, those with low socioeconomic status and immigrants from developing countries. The natural history of the infection in developed countries is to disappear, and in all age groups, the prevalence is falling. This decline in prevalence is possibly related to the widespread use of antibiotics.

■ GASTRITIS

After gaining access to the stomach, *H. pylori* begins to dictate its conditions. The eventual outcome of an infection is the result of the interactions between the host and the bacterium. *H. pylori* has a number of virulence factors responsible for colonization, including motility, the ability to withstand the acid environment of the stomach, and the ability to attach to the surface cells of the stomach. Flagellae allow the bacterium to burrow through the mucus to the mucosal surface, where it is protected from the acidic gastric fluid. Although *H. pylori* can attach to superficial gastric mucus cells and resist clearance from the stomach, small numbers can also be found within epithelial cells. It has been suggested that this intracellular location may serve as a sanctuary, allowing evasion of host defenses, and may be responsible for the failure of topical antibiotic therapy.

Attachment to the gastric mucosa is associated with local production of proinflammatory cytokines (e.g., interleukin [IL]-8), which is seen histologically as infiltration of the mucosa by polymorphonuclear leukocytes, ultimately leading to the characteristic histologic pattern of an acute inflammatory reaction superimposed on chronic inflammation with organized lymphoid follicles. *H. pylori* that contain a functional *cag* pathogenicity island (CPI) result in a greater inflammatory response than do those without this feature. These CPI-positive *H. pylori* are associated with increased risk of developing a symptomatic *H. pylori* disease such as peptic ulcer or gastric cancer. There is considerable interest in other putative virulence factors such as the vacuolating cytotoxin, VacA, but there are no consistent data to confirm that any of these other putative virulence factors have disease specificity. It is increasingly recognized that the host response to the infection and to the environment, rather than some feature of the organism, are the most important factors predicting outcome. For example, worldwide, CPI-positive *H. pylori* are the predominant type irrespective of whether the presentation is that of asymptomatic gastritis or a symptomatic *H. pylori* disease.

The outcome of an *H. pylori* infection can be related to the pattern of gastritis within the stomach. The stomach can be considered as having two regions, the acid-secreting corpus and the non–acid-secreting antrum and cardia. Whereas *H. pylori* colonize the entire surface of the stomach, the gastric corpus is relatively resistant to an *H. pylori*–mucosal interaction that results in significant inflammation. Overall, the data are consistent with acid secretion being the critical variable that "restricts" *H. pylori* inflammation to the antrum and cardia. *H. pylori*–induced inflammation of the gastric corpus leads to a reduction in acid secretion such that the greater the ability to secrete acid, the more likely that corpus inflammation is minimal. Events that reduce acid secretion, such as febrile illness in childhood, highly selective vagotomy, and use of potent antisecretory drugs, all are associated with an increase in corpus inflammation as well as expansion of inflammation from the antrum into the corpus. The typical pattern of gastritis associated with duodenal ulcer disease is antral predominant (or corpus sparing) gastritis, which reflects normal or increased acid secretion. This pattern of gastritis is associated with an increased risk of developing duodenal ulcer disease. Atrophic pangastritis with low to absent acid secretion is the phenotype associated with an increased risk of developing gastric cancer.

The key variables that predict which pattern of gastritis develops are the host and the environment (especially the diet). Putative virulence factors such as a CPI-positive *H. pylori* infection increase the risk of a symptomatic outcome but not which outcome. For example, in many countries, such as Japan, almost all *H. pylori* are CPI positive, and yet there has been a rapid decrease in pangastritis and gastric cancer and a concomitant increase in duodenal ulcer disease. This dramatic change is associated with changes in the sanitation, diet, and disease, without changes in the genetics of the hosts or in the characteristics of the strains of *H. pylori* that predominate.

■ IS THERE A PROTECTIVE ROLE FOR *H. PYLORI* IN RELATION TO GASTROESOPHAGEAL REFLUX DISEASE?

Gastroesophageal reflux disease (GERD) is common in Western countries but rare in countries where gastric cancer is common. As noted, the different patterns of gastritis portend different outcomes, with corpus gastritis being associated with reduced acid secretion. It is not surprising that there is this inverse relation because GERD, and its complications, such as Barrett's epithelium and adenocarcinoma of the distal esophagus, require acid to reflux in addition to an impairment of barrier function of the distal esophagus/lower esophageal sphincter. In countries where atrophic pangastritis is common, acid secretion is reduced to such an extent that the incidence of symptomatic GERD is low irrespective of the prevalence of patients with abnormal gastroesophageal barrier function. In these patients, *H. pylori* corpus gastritis is akin to lifetime antisecretory therapy.

The epidemiology of GERD is what one would predict. Both GERD and Barrett's esophagus are uncommon where *H. pylori* corpus gastritis is common. Elimination of *H. pylori* from such a population associated with treatment or through improvements in lifestyle, socioeconomic status, and sanitation results in an increase in acid secretion such that those with abnormal gastroesophageal barriers may develop symptomatic GERD. This epidemiology has been taken out of context to even suggest that *H. pylori* may have a protective role against GERD and adenocarcinoma of the distal esophagus/proximal stomach. This is clearly faulty

reasoning because using the best-case scenario (i.e., the highest incidence of Barrett's esophagus complicated by adenocarcinoma, and the least risk of typical *H. pylori*–associated gastric cancers) shows that the trade-off is that one new Barrett's cancer occurs whereas at least 50 gastric cancer deaths are prevented. Thus the concept of protection is based on a misinterpretation of epidemiology instead of an understanding of the pathophysiology. The recent recognition that long-term, high-level antisecretory therapy with H_2-receptor antagonists or proton pump inhibitors is associated with an acceleration of corpus gastritis in those with *H. pylori* infection suggests that it may be prudent to treat the infection in those with GERD in whom more than prn (as-needed) therapy is contemplated.

■ DIAGNOSIS OF *H. PYLORI* INFECTION

A number of tools are available to reliably diagnose *H. pylori* infection. Noninvasive methods include serologic tests, urea breath tests, and fecal antigen testing. Tests that require gastric biopsy include culture, rapid urease testing, and histology. The method of choice depends on availability, cost, and whether endoscopy is otherwise indicated. Because the diagnosis of an active *H. pylori* infection should be followed by therapy, the primary consideration for testing is the willingness to treat the infection.

The ^{13}C-urea breath test is the best test for both diagnosis and follow-up of therapy for an *H. pylori* infection. Serologic testing using laboratory ELISA testing or in-the-office rapid test is a less expensive alternative for patients with known or suspected peptic ulcer disease. Although serologic tests are excellent to diagnose *H. pylori* infection, antibody titers fall slowly and thus cannot be relied on to confirm cure or identify failure of therapy. Although "for research only" IgM and IgA antibody tests are widely available from commercial laboratories, they should be avoided because none are currently FDA approved and in our experience have such poor sensitivity as to be worthless for clinical decision making. A laboratory report with results of IgM or IgA antibodies should alert the physician to the fact that their laboratory may be using unapproved tests.

False-negative results are possible with all the tests that require the presence of live *H. pylori*, including culture, histology, rapid urease testing, and urea breath testing. Negative tests should be interpreted with caution if the patient has taken drugs that reduce the bacterial load such as antibiotics, bismuth, or proton pump inhibitors. In general, one should stop these drugs for 1 to 2 weeks before testing. H_2-receptor antagonists do not adversely affect any of these tests (although they apparently adversely affect the ^{14}C-urea breath test) and can be continued if needed to control symptoms.

Histology provides a permanent record and allows identification of the pattern and severity of gastritis. Prospective studies have consistently shown that hematoxylin and eosin (H&E) staining of gastric mucosal biopsies has poor sensitivity and specificity for active *H. pylori* infection. A special stain should be requested such as the Genta or El-Zimaity triple stains or the combination of H&E and the Diff-Quik stains.

■ TREATMENT OF *H. PYLORI* INFECTION

There is universal agreement that the presence of current or past peptic ulcer disease is an indication for testing based on the fact that cure of the infection will generally cure the disease. Other possible indications include the presence of peptic ulcer disease or gastric cancer in a first-degree relative because both are associated with markedly increased risks of developing symptomatic *H. pylori* disease. Probably the most common indication is suspected peptic ulcer disease (i.e., dyspepsia) because it is recognized that the population of patients with dyspepsia is enriched with patients with as-yet-undiagnosed peptic ulcer disease.

There are three steps in therapy: diagnosis, antimicrobial therapy, and confirmation of cure (Figure 1). No one should receive combination antibiotic therapy who does not have the infection because they can experience only side effects with no chance for benefit. The ideal combination therapy would be simple, effective, inexpensive, and without severe and serious side effects, as well as have a high rate of success. Such a combination is not available, but there are a number of effective regimens. Antimicrobial therapies have evolved from single antibiotics to combinations of three or four drugs. The antimicrobials that have proved useful are amoxicillin, tetracycline, metronidazole, clarithromycin, furazolidone, and bismuth (Table 1). Proton pump inhibitors also inhibit *H. pylori* growth in vivo and have proved valuable

adjuvants to therapy. All the antimicrobial drugs can be taken with meals without concern for possible interactions (e.g., bismuth and tetracycline).

The stomach is a hostile environment for antibiotics. In addition to the acidic conditions, the surface mucus and many surface cells are lost with each meal, gastric secretions dilute and wash out the antibiotics, and any intraluminal antibiotics are rapidly emptied from the stomach. It is unclear how much of the effect of the antibiotics is topical and how much systemic, but both probably are important. Effective combination therapy typically uses two antibiotics plus a bismuth (subsalicylate, citrate, or ranitidine bismuth citrate) or a proton pump inhibitor. Antisecretory therapy with a proton pump inhibitor or an H_2-receptor antagonist increases the pH of the stomach, thus making pH-sensitive antibiotics more effective as well as reducing the tendency of the stomach to wash out and dilute the antibiotics. Amoxicillin and clarithromycin are both pH sensitive, and effectiveness is improved by the addition of antisecretory therapy. Bismuth, metronidazole, furazolidone, and tetracycline are relatively pH dependent, although effectiveness is probably increased by addition of antisecretory drugs.

Drug combinations should be administered at least twice daily, and some therapies require administration three or four times a day. The optimum duration of therapy is unknown, but head-to-head comparisons have typically shown that 10 or 14 days is superior to 7 days (with 14 days

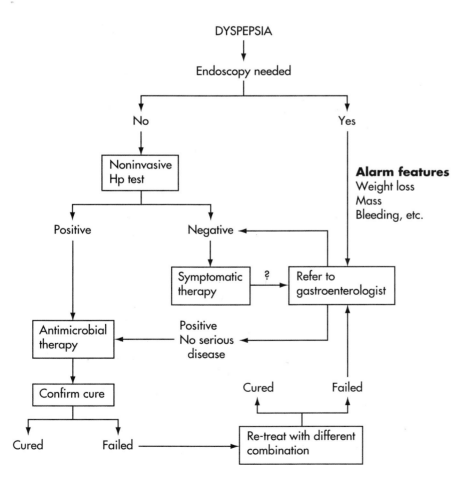

Figure 1
One approach to the evaluation of patients presenting with dyspepsia. It has become apparent that in the United States, where the incidence of gastric cancer is very low, noninvasive testing with serology, urea breath testing, or fecal antigen testing is sufficient and that endoscopy can be reserved for those with alarm symptoms. Referral to a gastroenterologist should be considered for those with alarm symptoms, those who have failure of symptoms to resolve after successful therapy, and those who fail one or more courses of therapy. The exception is those with clear-cut gastroesophageal reflux disease whose symptoms are not anticipated to resolve after successful cure of *H. pylori*. Those older than 50 with a long history of symptomatic gastroesophageal refux would be one group for whom referral should be considered to exclude Barrett's esophagus.

Table 1   Most Effective Combination Therapies for *Helicobacter pylori* Infection

TRIPLE THERAPIES FOR 14 DAYS[a], TWICE A DAY
- Proton pump inhibitor[b] + amoxicillin,[c] 1 g, + clarithromycin,[d] 500 mg, or metronidazole,[e] 500 mg
- Ranitidine bismuth citrate + amoxicillin,[c] 1 g, + clarithromycin,[d] 500 mg, or metronidazole[d] 500 mg

QUADRUPLE THERAPY FOR 14 DAYS
- Proton pump inhibitor once or twice a day + four-times-a-day bismuth (subsalicylate or citrate) two tablets and tetracycline[f] HCl,[e] 500 mg, + metronidazole, 500 mg three times a day

FURAZOLIDONE SALVAGE THERAPY FOR 14 DAYS
- Proton pump inhibitor once or twice a day + four-times-a-day bismuth (subsalicylate or citrate) two tablets and tetracycline[f] HCl, 500 mg, + furazolidone, 100 mg three times a day

[a]14 days of therapy appears best, although 10 days may be sufficient for these proton pump triple therapies.
[b]All proton pump inhibitors appear equal in this regard.
[c]Ampicillin cannot be substituted for amoxicillin.
[d]Azithromycin or erythromycin cannot be substituted.
[e]Tinidazole can be substituted.
[f]Doxycycline cannot be substituted.

usually being better than 10 days). We recommend a duration of at least 10 days, and we routinely prescribe a 14-day course of antimicrobial therapy. Large head-to-head comparisons of pump inhibitors have shown that twice-a-day administration is superior to once a day. The primary impediments to successful therapy are the presence of antibiotic-resistant *H. pylori*. Resistance has been described to all the commonly used antibiotics but is generally uncommon. Resistance to bismuth has not been described.

In general, resistance to one antibiotic in a combination therapy acts to functionally remove that antibiotic, and the results are what one would expect from the remaining antimicrobial agents. For example, in the case of clarithromycin resistance, the results with amoxicillin-clarithromycin-proton pump inhibitor combination therapy are what one would expect with the dual combination of amoxicillin and a proton pump inhibitor. The exception is metronidazole resistance, where increasing the dose may increase the cure rate despite the presence of metronidazole-resistant *H. pylori*. Thus multidose quadruple therapy consisting of bismuth, tetracycline, metronidazole, and a proton pump inhibitor is generally effective despite the presence of metronidazole resistance.

The choice of therapy should ideally depend on the results of antimicrobial susceptibility testing. This is generally not available. Studies are under way to provide regional data regarding antibiotic resistance. In general, resistance correlated with prior use of the antibiotic such that metronidazole resistance is high in immigrants from developing countries and in women who have been treated for vaginal infections. Clarithromycin resistance is highest in elderly patients with chronic lung disease who regularly receive macrolide antibiotics for respiratory complaints.

■ CONFIRMATION OF CURE

Therapy should be followed by confirmation of cure. The confirmatory test should be delayed until 4 to 6 weeks after the end of antimicrobial therapy to allow the bacteria, if present, an opportunity to repopulate the stomach. Drugs that inhibit *H. pylori*, such as proton pump inhibitors, should not be allowed for 1 week and probably 2 weeks before testing. The urea breath test is the ideal method for evaluating the outcome of therapy. An alternative approach would be to use the stool antigen test. If neither are available and endoscopy is the only option, it is prudent to reserve posttherapy testing for those at high risk of a bad outcome if therapy failed (e.g., after bleeding from an ulcer).

■ TREATMENT FAILURES

Because antibiotic susceptibility testing is generally unavailable, the operational approach has been to give a second course avoiding those antibiotics used the first time. For example, triple therapy with amoxicillin, clarithromycin, and a proton pump inhibitor might be followed by quadruple therapy with bismuth, tetracycline, metronidazole, and a proton pump inhibitor. There are no extensively studied salvage therapies for those who have failed several courses of therapy. We have found that quadruple therapy is generally effective despite metronidazole resistance. An alternative approach is to use furazolidone (100 mg three times daily) in place of metronidazole in quadruple therapy. This antimicrobial is monoamine oxidase (MAO) inhibitor and interacts with many foods and drugs, and it is prudent to read the package insert and give the patient a detailed list of foods and drugs to avoid.

Suggested Reading

Dixon MF, et al: Classification and grading of gastritis: the updated Sydney System. International Workshop on the Histopathology of Gastritis, Houston 1994, *Am J Surg Pathol* 20:1161, 1996.

El-Zimaity HM, et al: Histologic assessment of *Helicobacter pylori* status after therapy: comparison of Giemsa, Diff-Quik, and Genta stains, *Mod Pathol* 11:288, 1998.

Graham DY: Antibiotic resistance in *Helicobacter pylori*: implications for therapy, *Gastroenterology* 115:1272, 1998.

Graham DY: *Helicobacter pylori* infection in the pathogenesis of duodenal ulcer and gastric cancer: a model, *Gastroenterology* 113:1983, 1997.

Graham DY, Yamaoka Y: *H. pylori* and *cagA*: relationships with gastric cancer, duodenal ulcer, and reflux esophagitis and its complications, *Helicobacter.* 3:145, 1998.

Howden CW, Hunt RH. Guidelines for the management of *Helicobacter pylori* infection: ad hoc committee on Practice Parameters of the American College of Gastroenterology, *Am J Gastroenterol* 93:2330, 1998.

GONOCOCCUS— NEISSERIA GONORRHOEAE

John H. Powers
Michael F. Rein

Neisseria gonorrhoeae is the second most common sexually transmitted bacterial pathogen after *Chlamydia trachomatis*, resulting in an estimated 600,000 to 800,000 cases per year in the United States. Unchecked infection can result in sterility or ectopic pregnancy. The gonococcus causes disease by attaching to columnar or cuboidal epithelial cells. Pili and outer membrane proteins mediate attachment. The organism penetrates between and through the cells to submucosal areas, where it elicits a neutrophilic host response. Definitive diagnosis is based on isolation of the organism in culture or identification by one of the newer nonculture techniques, such as enzyme-linked immunosorbent assay (ELISA) or DNA probe.

Acute urethritis, presenting as some combination of urethral discharge and dysuria, is the primary manifestation of disease in men, although infected men may be asymptomatic carriers. Gram stain of a smear of urethral discharge may be used for presumptive diagnosis of gonococcal urethritis. Gram-negative diplococci in neutrophils are found in 90% of men with this disease, and the finding is 98% specific.

In women, the primary site of infection is the endocervix. Asymptomatic infection is more common in women than in men. Although the organism can be isolated from the urethra and periurethral (Skene's) and Bartholin's glands, these are rarely the sole site of infection. Gram stains of cervical smears from infected women are 97% specific for the disease when intracellular organisms are present. However, the sensitivity of the Gram stain is only 50% to 70% in this setting, which probably obviates the use of the Gram stain for presumptive diagnosis in women.

Anorectal gonorrhea occurs in up to 40% of women with endocervical disease and is also noted in homosexual men. Most patients with *N. gonorrhoeae* cultured from this site are asymptomatic, but acute proctitis may be present. Most patients with pharyngeal infection are also asymptomatic. Gonococcal conjunctivitis in adults produces a range of degrees of inflammation.

Disseminated gonococcal infection is uncommon overall, occurring in only 0.5% to 3% of infected patients. The predominant clinical presentation of disseminated infection is the arthritis-dermatitis syndrome, which usually manifests as asymmetric migratory polyarthritis, arthralgias, or tenosynovitis accompanied in 33% to 50% of cases by small painful papules or pustules on an erythematous base. Complement deficiency has been noted in up to 13% of patients with disseminated disease.

■ THERAPY

Uncomplicated anogenital infection with *N. gonorrhoeae* can be treated with a single dose of an appropriate medication. Treatment has been complicated by the emergence of resistance to various antimicrobials. The susceptibility of the gonococcus to penicillin has been severely compromised by the organism's acquisition of a plasmid that codes for the production of beta-lactamase, yielding the so-called penicillinase-producing strains of *N. gonorrhoeae* (PPNG). Chromosomally mediated resistance, which codes for alteration of the penicillin-binding proteins, has also resulted in decreasing sensitivity of the organism. The increased worldwide prevalence of these two mechanisms of resistance has resulted in the recommendation that penicillin no longer be used as an empirical treatment for gonococcal infections. Chromosomal and plasmid-mediated resistance to tetracyclines, now noted worldwide, has also precluded the use of tetracyclines in anti-gonococcal therapy. Up to half of isolates demonstrating chromosomal resistance to penicillin are also resistant to trimethoprim-sulfamethoxazole (TMP-SMX), and this drug should be avoided when alternatives are available. Clinical failures with quinolone antibiotics have been described since 1990. Failures with 500 mg of ciprofloxacin and 400 mg of ofloxacin have been reported in the United Kingdom, Australia, Canada, Hong Kong, and the United States. Strains with decreased susceptibility to quinolones have been divided into those with intermediate (minimum inhibitory concentration [MIC] of ≥ 0.125 µg/ml to 0.5 µg/ml for ciprofloxacin and ≥ 0.5 µg/ml to 1.0 µg/ml for ofloxacin) and high-level (MIC ≥ 1.0 µg/ml for ciprofloxacin and ≥ 2.0 µg/ml for ofloxacin) resistance. Intermediately resistant strains may still respond to standard, Centers for Disease Control and Prevention (CDC) recommended doses of quinolones, but smaller doses (e.g., 250 mg of ciprofloxacin) may result in therapeutic failure. The prevalence of strains with decreased susceptibility to quinolones increased dramatically in some geographic locations in the 1990s. In Hong Kong, the Philippines, and Thailand, 36%, 54%, and 22% of strains, respectively, have decreased susceptibilities to quinolones, with high-level resistant strains accounting for 10%, 12%, and 1%, respectively, of these. In a 1994 survey, 1.3% of U.S. strains had decreased susceptibilities, with 0.04% of these exhibiting high-level resistance. The mechanism of resistance to quinolones is usually mutation in the *gyrA* gene coding for the A subunit of DNA gyrase, also known as *topoisomerase II*. Mutation in the *parC* gene of topoisomerase IV appears to be associated with higher MICs than mutations in *gyrA* alone, and strains with MICs 2.0 µg/ml or greater are more likely to possess both mutations. Reduced permeability through the cytoplasmic membrane may also contribute to low-level quinolone resistance. Given the public health implications of the spread of the organism in the population and the potential for the further emergence of resistance to antimicrobials, regimens with less than 95% efficacy are considered unacceptable. The treatment of gonococcal disease is further complicated by frequent coinfection with *Chlamydia trachomatis* in genital infections, proctitis, and conjunctivitis.

Table 1   Oral Regimens for Treatment of Localized Gonococcal Infection, Including Urethritis, Cervicitis, Pharyngitis, and Proctitis

DRUG	REGIMEN (SINGLE DOSES)	CDC RECOMMEN-DATION	SAFETY IN PREGNANCY	SAFETY IN AGE <16 YR	EFFECTIVE IN PHARYNX	COMMENTS
Ciprofloxacin	500 mg	Yes	No	No	Yes	
Ofloxacin	400 mg	Yes	No	No	Possibly effective	300 mg bid for 7 days covers gonorrheal and chlamydial infection
Norfloxacin	800 mg	Alternative	No	No	No	Limted data
Enoxacin	400 mg	Alternative	No	No	Limited data	Resistance rapidly developing in some areas of Far East
Lomefloxacin	400 mg	Alternative	No	No	Limited data	Very limited experience
Cefixime	400 mg	Yes	Yes	Yes	Limited data but probably effective	
Cefpodoxime proxetil	200 mg	No	Yes	Yes	Probably not	Limited experience
Azithromycin	2 g	No	Yes	Yes	Very limited data	May cause gastro-intestinal upset at this dose; effective against chlamydial infection as well
Grepafloxacin	400 mg	No	No	No	No data	400 mg/day for 7 days; treats chlamydial NGU

Table 2   Parenteral Regimens for Treatment of Localized Gonococcal Infection, Including Urethritis, Cervicitis, Pharyngitis, and Proctitis

DRUG	REGIMEN (SINGLE DOSES)	CDC RECOMMEN-DATION	SAFETY IN PREGNANCY	SAFETY IN AGE <16 YR	EFFECTIVE IN PHARYNX	COMMENTS
Ceftriaxone	125 mg	Yes	Yes	Yes	Yes	
Ceftriaxone	250 mg	Formerly	Yes	Yes	Yes	Partial activity against coincident incubating syphilis
Ceftizoxime	500 mg	Alternative	Yes	Yes	Probably	
Cefotaxime	500 mg	Alternative	Yes	Yes	Probably	
Cefotetan	1 g	Alternative	Yes	Yes	Probably	
Spectinomycin	2 g	Alternative	Yes	Yes	No	

Oral Therapy (Table 1)

The fluoroquinolone class of antibiotics has demonstrated efficacy in all forms of uncomplicated anogenital gonococcal disease and can all be given as a single oral dose. These agents can be used in patients with immediate hypersensitivity reactions to beta-lactam antibiotics but are currently contraindicated in pregnant women and children because of the possibility of toxicity at the epiphyseal growth plate. Reduced susceptibility and outright resistance of *N. gonor-rhoeae* to quinolones is common enough in Asia that consideration should be given to alternative therapy in travelers returning from these regions. The newer quinolone, grepafloxacin, is indicated in the treatment of uncomplicated gonorrhea but does not seem to offer any particular advantage over other agents in this class. Trovafloxacin has been associated with rare cases of liver toxicity and is no longer indicated for uncomplicated disease. Given the similar mechanisms of resistance, it must be assumed that gono-

Table 3   Regimens for Treatment of Disseminated Gonococcal Infection

DRUG	REGIMEN	CDC RECOMMEN-DATION	SAFETY IN PREGNANCY	SAFETY IN AGE <16 YR	COMMENTS
Ceftriaxone	1 g IM or IV q24h	Yes	Yes	Yes	Use until clinical improvement, then complete 7-10 days of therapy with cefixime, 400 mg PO bid; ciprofloxacin, 500 mg PO bid; or ofloxacin, 400 mg PO bid; use cefixime for patients <17 yr of age.
Ceftizoxime	1 g IV q8h	Alternative	Yes	Yes	Use until clinical improvement, then complete 7-10 days of therapy with cefixime, 400 mg PO bid; ciprofloxacin, 500 mg PO bid; or ofloxacin, 400 mg PO bid; use cefixime for patients <17 yr of age.
Cefotaxime	1 g IV q8h	Alternative	Yes	Yes	Use until clinical improvement, then complete 7-10 days of therapy with cefixime, 400 mg PO bid; ciprofloxacin, 500 mg PO bid; or ofloxacin, 400 mg PO bid; use cefixime for patients <17 yr of age.
Spectinomycin	2 g IM bid	Alternative	Yes	Yes	Primarily for use in the setting of allergy to the beta-lactams; use until clinical improvement, then complete 7-10 days of therapy with ciprofloxacin, 500 mg PO bid, or ofloxacin, 400 mg PO bid.

cocci resistant to one quinolone are cross-resistant to other members of this class. Oral cephalosporins are also effective treatment. Cefixime and cefpodoxime have been studied, although clinical experience is greater with the former drug. Cefixime seems to have efficacy in the treatment of pharyngeal gonorrhea, but this regimen has been tested in only a few patients with this condition. There have been unacceptably high failure rates in pharyngeal gonorrhea with other oral cephalosporin regimens.

Parenteral Therapy

Third-generation cephalosporins such as ceftriaxone, cefotaxime, cefotetan, and ceftizoxime appear to have equal efficacy when given as a single intramuscular (IM) dose (Table 2). Clinical experience is greatest with ceftriaxone. This drug has the longest half-life and is injected in the smallest volume. A dose of 125 mg of ceftriaxone is effective, and this regimen is recommended by the CDC. Only the 250-mg dose of ceftriaxone has been studied in pregnant women. The smallest vial of ceftriaxone available for clinical use contains 250 mg, and unless more than one patient is to be treated, the use of the lower dose does not result in cost savings. Resistance to cefoxitin has developed in several areas, often in association with high-level tetracycline resistance. Cefoxitin should therefore no longer be used in the treatment of uncomplicated gonorrhea.

The aminocyclitol spectinomycin is an alternative for patients who are pregnant or for children who have a history of immediate hypersensitivity to beta-lactams. Resistance has been noted in Korea, and the drug does not reach adequate concentrations in saliva, rendering it ineffective in the treatment of pharyngeal disease. Parenteral aminoglycosides, especially gentamicin, have been included in inpatient regimens for the treatment of pelvic inflammatory disease.

Nonstandard Therapy

The monobactam aztreonam and the carbapenems imipenem-cilastatin and meropenem are uniformly effective against *N. gonorrhoeae* but are costly and available only in intravenous form. These drugs are never primary therapy for gonorrhea. Penicillins formulated with a beta-lactamase inhibitor (i.e., amoxicillin-clavulanate, ampicillin-sulbactam, ticarcillin-clavulanate, and piperacillin-tazobactam) are costly, and although they are effective against PPNG strains, they may not be effective against chromosomally mediated resistance.

The dose of the macrolide azithromycin required to eradicate the gonococcus (2 g orally) is twice that used in the single-dose treatment of nongonococcal urethritis. This high dosage often causes gastrointestinal upset and is far more expensive than alternative regimens.

Extragenital Disease

A single dose of ceftriaxone, 125 mg IM in children or 1 g IM in adults, cures gonococcal conjunctivitis, but long-term follow-up is lacking, and 7 to 10 days of a parenteral drug may be the safest alternative. Although saline flushing of the conjunctiva has been used, topical antibiotics have no proved additional benefit.

No prospective studies on the treatment of disseminated gonococcal infection have been performed since 1976; hence, recommendations are empirical because the worldwide spread of resistant gonococci occurred after that time. The gonococcal arthritis-dermatitis syndrome should be treated with ceftriaxone. Regimens using other third-generation cephalosporins should be equally effective. If frank septic arthritis is not present, the patient can be switched to oral cefixime or ciprofloxacin or an equivalent dose of another oral cephalosporin or quinolone to complete 7 to 10 days of therapy. The actual optimal duration of therapy is unknown. Spectinomycin is an alternative for pregnant women, children, and those who are allergic to beta-lactams. Gonococcal endocarditis should be treated with 4 weeks of an appropriate parenteral regimen, preferably ceftriaxone or another third-generation cephalosporin. Meningitis should be treated for 10 to 14 days. Penicillin therapy may still be used if the isolate in question is found to be susceptible to the drug, with an MIC of 2 μg/ml or less.

Any regimen used to treat genital infections, conjunctivitis, or proctitis must include treatment for possible coinfection with *C. trachomatis* (Table 3). Dual therapy may also slow the emergence of resistance if the gonococcal isolate is also susceptible to the antichlamydial agent. It is also important to treat sexual contacts of patients with gonorrhea to prevent spread in the population as well as reinfection of the patient. Given the emergence of gonococcal resistance to virtually all classes of antimicrobials, it is important to obtain appropriate cultures and susceptibility testing on all those patients who do not improve on therapy, once reinfection and nonadherence to medication have been ruled out.

Suggested Reading

Centers for Disease Control and Prevention: 1998 guidelines for treatment of sexually transmitted diseases, *MMWR* 47(RR-1):1, 1998.

Fox KK, et al: Antimicrobial resistance in *Neisseria gonorrhoeae* in the United States, 1988-1994: the emergence of decreased susceptibility to the fluoroquinolones, *J Infect Dis* 175:1396, 1997.

Handsfield HH, Weisner PJ, Holmes KK: Treatment of the gonococcal arthritis-dermatitis syndrome, *Ann Intern Med* 107:692, 1976.

Knapp JS, et al: Fluoroquinolone resistance in *Neisseria gonorrhoeae*, *Emerg Infect Dis* 3:33, 1997.

Lind I: Antimicrobial resistance in *Neisseria gonorrhoeae*, *Clin Infect Dis* 24(suppl):S93, 1997.

Rein MF: Gonorrhea, *Curr Opin Infect Dis* 4:12, 1991.

HAEMOPHILUS

Feng-Yee Chang
Victor L. Yu

Members of the genus *Haemophilus* are gram-negative bacteria that constitute part of the normal flora of the respiratory tract of humans and many animal species. The *Haemophilus* species, *H. influenzae*, *H. parainfluenzae*, *H. aphrophilus*, *H. paraphrophilus*, *H. aegyptius*, and *H. ducreyi*, are well-documented human pathogens, and *H. haemolyticus*, *H. segnis*, and *H. parahaemolyticus* have been implicated infrequently.

H. influenzae is indigenous to humans only. *H. influenzae* in cultures obtained from the upper (but not from the lower) respiratory tract is a normal finding because up to 80% of persons are carriers. Although most people are colonized with unencapsulated strains, 3% to 5% of individuals are colonized with encapsulated strains, most commonly serotype b. The type b capsule is a major virulence factor, and type b strains cause 95% of systemic *H. influenzae* infections in children.

Two clinical patterns of *H. influenzae* disease are seen: the most serious is invasive infection such as meningitis, septic arthritis, epiglottitis, and cellulitis; bacteremia is common. Invasive infections are usually caused by type b strains and are seen in young children during the winter. The second presentation is less serious but occurs more frequently as a result of contiguous spread of *H. influenzae* within the respiratory tract, leading to otitis media, sinusitis, conjunctivitis, or pneumonia. These infections are usually caused by unencapsulated strains.

Haemophilus species other than *H. influenzae* cause a variety of diseases, including respiratory tract infection, endocarditis, septicemia, meningitis, brain abscess, and soft-tissue infections. *H. ducreyi* is the causative agent of chancroid. *H. influenzae aegyptius* causes Brazilian purpuric fever, which arises as conjunctivitis in young children and then progresses to sepsis with purpura.

The correct diagnosis of *Haemophilus* infections relies on isolation of the organism or detection of capsular antigen. Nasopharyngeal culture for *H. influenzae* is not helpful because of the high carriage rate among healthy persons. Cultures of blood, cerebrospinal fluid (CSF), and other normally sterile fluids (e.g., from joints or pleural, subdural, or pericardial spaces) are diagnostic. Cultures in cases of epiglottitis are generally positive but should be taken only when the airway can be protected. Needle aspiration of the middle ear (tympanocentesis), maxillary sinus, an area of cellulitis, or lung may occasionally yield the organism. Specimens should also be Gram-stained. The morphology of *Haemophilus* is variable, appearing as coccobacilli or filamentous rods. Pleomorphic character, small size, and inconsistent uptake of dyes often render identification by stains difficult. In about 70% of cases of meningitis, small coccobacillary organisms are visible on CSF. Detection of capsular antigen in serum, CSF, or concentrated urine using immunoelectrophoresis, latex agglutination, or enzyme-linked immunosorbent assay (ELISA) may be diagnostic and can be found in up to 90% of culture-proved cases of meningitis. It may be especially useful in patients who have received empirical antibiotic therapy because even if the culture is rendered negative by antibiotics, antigen remains detectable in infected pleural fluid, pericardial fluid, joint fluid, or CSF.

■ ANTIBIOTIC THERAPY

Meningitis and epiglottitis caused by *H. influenzae* type b can be rapidly fatal. For many years, ampicillin and chloramphenicol were the mainstays of therapy. However, increasing resistance to both ampicillin and chloramphenicol has necessitated major changes in antibiotic therapy. Third-generation cephalosporins are extremely active against *H. influenzae*, with achievable CSF concentrations one hundred to several thousand times greater than the minimal inhibitory concentration (MIC), and are the preferred antibiotics for meningitis treatment. The use of cefotaxime or ceftriaxone treatment of meningitis may result in fewer neurologic sequelae than chloramphenicol therapy and is at least as effective as the combination of chloramphenicol and ampicillin. Meropenem may also be used as an alternative. The usual duration of therapy is 7 to 10 days, depending on clinical response. Repeat lumbar puncture for CSF culture to validate cure is usually unnecessary in patients who have a clinical response.

Use of corticosteroid therapy to reduce cerebral edema and other complications has been controversial. However, one study has suggested that deafness was decreased by dexamethasone.

Treatment of serious infection caused by nontypable *H. influenzae*, such as meningitis, lower respiratory tract infections, tubal abscess, and neonatal sepsis, requires systemic antibiotics. Cephalosporins, including second-generation (cefuroxime) and third-generation agents, are most commonly used. Chloramphenicol is also effective, but blood concentrations must be monitored in premature infants. Sinusitis and otitis media caused by nontypable *H. influenzae* can usually be treated with oral amoxicillin. If ampicillin resistance is common in the geographic area, then amoxicillin-clavulanate, trimethoprim-sulfamethoxazole (TMP-SMX), an oral second-generation cephalosporin, or azithromycin is effective (Tables 1 and 2).

H. influenzae is often implicated with other respiratory pathogens in chronic bronchitis. Antibiotic therapy for excerbations of chronic bronchitis is commonly used in adult patients with chronic obstructive pulmonary disease, although efficacy is uncertain. Worsening cough with increasing purulence of sputum is the primary indication. The most inexpensive oral agents, including TMP-SMX, doxycline, and amoxicillin, are recommended. Amoxicillin-clavulanate, oral cephalosporins, azithromycin, and fluoroquinolones are alternatives. Third-generation parenteral cephalosporins are used for severe and life-threatening pneumonia. Duration is 7 to 10 days. Some authorities

Table 1 Treatment for *Haemophilus* Infection

ORGANISMS	DISEASES	PREFERRED ANTIBIOTICS	ALTERNATIVES
H. influenzae *H. parainfluenzae* *H. aphrophilus* *H. paraphrophilus*	Serious infection cellulitis pneumonia	Ceftriaxone, ceftioxime, cefotaxime	Ampicillin (if beta-lactamase negative)
	Meningitis	Ceftriaxone/ceftotaxime	Ampicillin (if beta-lactamase negative) or chloramphenicol
	Otitis, sinusitis	Amoxicillin (if beta-lactamase negative), amoxicillin-clavulanate, or cefuroxime	TMX-SMX, cefaclor, cefixime, loracarbef, cefprozil, cefpodoxime, or azithromycin
	Exacerbations of chronic bronchitis	TMP-SMX or doxycycline	Amoxicillin (if beta-lactamase negative) or amoxicillin-clavulanate, cefaclor, cefixime, azithromycin, or clarithromycin
H. parainfluenzae, *H. aphrophilus,* *H. paraphrophilus*	Endocarditis	Ampicillin (if beta-lactamase negative) with gentamicin	Ceftriaxone
H. ducreyi	Chancroid	Ceftriaxone, azithromycin, or erythromycin	Amoxicillin-clavulanate or TMP-SMX

TMP-SMX, Trimethoprim-sulfamethoxazole.

Table 2 Recommended Dosages of Antibiotic Therapy in *Haemophilus* Infection

	CHILDREN	ADULTS	
DRUG	**DOSE, INTERVAL**	**DOSE, INTERVAL**	**DAILY DOSE FOR SERIOUS INFECTION**
Amoxicillin	13.3 mg/kg q8h PO	0.25-0.5 g q8h PO	1.5 g
Ampicillin	25 mg/kg q6h PO	0.5-1 g q6h PO	4 g
	25-(100)* mg/kg q6h IV/IM	1-2 g q4-6h IV/IM	8-(12)* g
Amoxicillin-clavulanate	13.3 mg/kg q8h PO	0.25-0.5 g q8h PO	1.5 g
Cefaclor	6.6-13.3 mg/kg q8h PO	0.25-0.5 g q8h PO	1.5 g
Cefixime	8 mg/kg/day q12-24h PO	0.4 g/day q12-24h PO	0.4 g
Cefpodoxime	5 mg/kg q12h	0.2-0.4 g q12h	0.4-0.8 g
Cefuroxime axetil	0.125-0.5 g q12h PO	0.125-0.5 g q12h PO	0.5-1 g
Cefuroxime	50-240 mg/kg/day q6-8h IV/IM	0.75-1.5 g q8h IV/IM	4.5 g
Cefprozil	15 mg/kg q12h	0.25-0.5 g q12h	0.5-1 g
Loracarbef	7.5-15 mg/kg q12h	0.2-0.4 g q12h	0.4-0.8 g
Cefotaxime	50-(200)* mg/kg/day q4-6h IV/IM	1-2 g q4-12h IV/IM	6-(12)* g
Ceftizoxime	50 mg/kg q6-8h IV/IM	1-4 q8-12h IV/IM	6-(12)* g
Ceftriaxone	50-100 mg/kg/day q12-24h IV/IM	1-2 q12-24h IV/IM	2-(4)* g
Chloramphenicol	12.5-(25)* mg/kg q6h IV/IM	12.5-(25)* mg/kg q6h IV/IM	4 g*
Erythromycin	12.5 mg/kg q6h PO	0.25-5 g q6h PO	2 g
	3.75-12.5 mg/kg q6h IV/IM	0.25-1 q6h IV	4 g
Azithromycin	Not available	0.25-0.5 g q24h	0.5 g
Clarithromycin	7.5 mg/kg q12h PO	0.25-0.5 g q12h PO	0.5-1 g
Doxycycline†	2.2 mg/kg q12-24h PO/IV/IM	0.1 g q12-24h PO/IV/IM	0.2 g
Ciprofloxacin	Not recommended	0.25-0.75 g q12h PO	1.5 g
		0.2-0.4 g q12h IV	0.8g
Ofloxacin	Not recommended	0.2-0.4 g q12h PO/IV (infuse over 60 min)	0.8 g
TMP-SMX	4-5 mg/kg q6-12h (as TMP) PO	160 mg q12h (as TMP) PO	320 mg (as TMP) PO
	4-5 mg/kg q6-12h (as TMP) IV	4-5 mg/kg q6-12h (as TMP) IV	1.2 g TMP, 6 g SMX IV
Meropenem	40 mg/kg q8h	1.0 g q8h IV	3 g
Gentamicin	2.5 mg/kg q8h IV/IM	1-1.7 mg/kg q8h IV/IM	3-5 mg/kg

*For meningitis or life-threatening infections.
†Use in children older than 7 years.
TMP-SMX, Trimethoprim-sulfamethoxazole.

recommend sputum culture before initiation of therapy, but we do not, because culture results do not necessarily correlate with clinical response.

■ PREVENTION

Four vaccines are licensed for active immunization against invasive type b infections. Conjugate vaccines are administered at the same time as diphtheria-pertussis-tetanus and polio immunizations as part of the routine program of childhood immunizations. The inclusion of conjugate type b vaccine in the routine immunization schedule has resulted in a dramatic decline in invasive type b disease in children in the United States. Chemoprophylaxis for those with close contact to patients with *H. influenzae* meningitis, such as day-care or household contact, is indicated. The drug of choice is oral rifampin, 20 mg/kg (maximum 600 mg), in a single daily dose for 4 days.

Individuals with immunodeficiencies, especially those with primary deficiency of antibody synthesis, have increased susceptibility to infection with *H. influenzae,* particularly nontypable strains. They may benefit from passive infusion of immunoglobulin preparations administered either intramuscularly or intravenously.

Suggested Reading

deGroot R, et al: Antibiotic resistance in *Haemophilus influenzae:* mechanisms, clinical importance and consequences for therapy, *Eur J Pediatr* 150:543, 1991.

Herbert MA, Moxon RE: *Haemophilus influenzae.* In Yu VL, Merigan TC Jr, Barriere SL, eds: *Antimicrobial therapy and vaccines,* Baltimore, 1999, Williams & Wilkins.

Isada CM: Antibiotics for chronic bronchitis with exacerbations, *Semin Resp Infect* 8:243, 1993.

Moxon ER: *Haemophilus influenzae:* In Mandell G, Bennett JE, Dolin R, eds: *Principles and practice of infectious diseases,* ed 4, New York, 1995, Churchill Livingstone.

LEGIONELLOSIS

Lütfiye Mülazimoglu
Victor L. Yu

Legionellae are gram-negative, aerobic, uncapsulated bacilli. They are nutritionally fastidious and require special laboratory growth media for growth. More than 40 different *Legionella* species have been identified. *Legionella pneumophila* is responsible for 85% of human infections, followed by *Legionella micdadei* (the Pittsburgh pneumonia agent), and *L. bozemanii, L. dumoffii, L. longbeachae,* and *L. feeleii. L. pneumophila* contains 14 serogroups, but serogroup 1 is the predominant pathogen.

The source of the organism is usually the water distribution system. The mode of transmission is aspiration, aerosolization, or instillation of water contaminated with *Legionella* into the respiratory tract. Cooling towers have been implicated in some reports, but their actual role in disseminating the organism has been questioned. Air conditioning systems have never been rigorously implicated in cases of Legionnaires' disease.

Legionnaires' disease is pneumonia caused by *Legionella pneumophila* and is the predominant manifestation of *Legionella* infection. The disease presents with a broad spectrum of illness, ranging from a mild cough and low-grade fever to stupor, respiratory failure, and multiorgan failure.

Cigarette smoking; chronic lung disease; immunosuppression, especially with corticosteroids; and transplant surgery are major risk factors.

■ CLINICAL MANIFESTATIONS

The clinical presentation is that of an acute pneumonia. Early in the illness, patients have nonspecific symptoms, including malaise, myalgias, and anorexia. Fever is virtually always present, and 20% of patients have temperatures in excess of 40° C (104° F). Cough occurs in 80% of patients and can be mild and only slightly productive. In 10% of cases, hemoptysis occurs. Chest pain, pleuritic or nonpleuritic, is prominent for 10% of patients and, when coupled with hemoptysis, may be mistaken for pulmonary embolization. Watery diarrhea, nausea, vomiting, and abdominal pain are seen in 25% to 40% of cases. Headache and mental status changes are the most common neurologic symptoms.

The chest radiograph cannot distinguish Legionnaires' disease from other pneumonias. The initial finding on chest radiograph is usually a unilateral alveolar infiltrate, which can progress to the other lobes with consolidation. Diffuse interstitial infiltrates are seen in 25% of patients. Circumscribed peripheral opacities may be seen in immunosuppressed patients receiving corticosteroids; these opacities tend to expand and cavitate. Pleural effusion is seen in one third of patients. Progression of infiltrates on chest radiographs despite appropriate antibiotic therapy is common; radiologic improvement lags behind clinical improvement, and radiographic abnormalities may persist for up to 4 months.

Although there are a few clinical clues suggestive of Legionnaires' disease (Table 1), the presentation is nonspe-

Table 1   Clinical Signs Suggestive of Legionnaires' Disease

High fever, often over 40° C (104° F)
Diarrhea
Hyponatremia (serum sodium 131 mmol/L)
Gram stain of respiratory specimen with numerous neutrophils but no organism
Failure to respond to beta-lactam agents or aminoglycosides

Table 2   Antibiotic Dosages for *Legionella* Infection

ANTIMICROBIAL AGENT	DOSAGE*
Azithromycin[†]	500 mg PO or IV q24h
Clarithromycin	500 mg PO or IV q12h
Roxithromycin	300 mg PO q12h
Erythromycin	1000 mg IV q6h
	500 mg PO q6h
Levofloxacin[†]	500 mg PO or IV q24h
Ciprofloxacin	400 mg IV q12h
	750 mg PO q12h
Doxycycline[†]	100 mg PO or IV q12h
Minocycline[†]	100 mg PO or IV q12h
Tetracycline	500 mg PO or IV q6h
Trimethoprim-sulfamethoxazole	160/800 mg IV q8h
	160/800 mg PO q12h
Rifampin	300-600 mg PO or IV q12h

*Dosages are based on clinical experience, not on controlled trials.
[†]We recommend doubling the first dose.

cific and specialized laboratory tests are necessary for definitive diagnosis.

Extrapulmonary *Legionella* infections are rare, but the clinical manifestations are often dramatic. *Legionellae* have been implicated in cases of sinusitis, cellulitis, pancreatitis, peritonitis, and pyelonephritis in immunosuppressed patients. The most common extrapulmonary site is the heart. Myocarditis, pericarditis, postcardiotomy syndrome, and prosthetic-valve endocarditis have been reported. *Legionella* wound infections are caused by exposure of existing wounds to water contaminated with *Legionella*.

Pontiac fever is an acute, self-limiting, flulike illness. Pneumonia does not occur. The predominant symptoms are malaise, myalgias, fever, chills, and headache. Complete recovery is the rule even without any specific therapy.

■ LABORATORY FINDINGS

Patients often have moderate leucocytosis. Hyponatremia (serum sodium concentration <131 mmol/L) occurs significantly more often in Legionnaires' disease than in other pneumonias.

The definitive method for the diagnosis of legionellosis is culture of the organism. Sputum from patients suspected of having legionellosis should be cultured (regardless of the quality of specimen) on special culture media: buffered charcoal yeast extract agar with inhibitors. Macroscopically visible colonies are seen in 3 to 5 days.

Although the organisms are gram-negative bacilli, they are not usually visible on Gram stain of sputum. Direct fluorescent antibody staining is rapid and highly specific. Sensitivity is 30% to 70%, but a large number of microorganisms are required for visualization.

Serologic tests are useful primarily for epidemiologic studies because acute and convalescent sera are required. The diagnosis is based on a fourfold rise in the antibody titer to 1:128 or greater. A single titer of 1:128 or more in a patient with pneumonia is suggestive.

Detection of *Legionella*-soluble antigens in urine is a rapid and highly sensitive test but is available only for *L. pneumophila* serogroup 1. However, this serogroup causes the large majority of *Legionella* cases. Antigen in urine is detectable 3 days after the onset of clinical disease. It is often easier to obtain a urine sample than respiratory tract specimens, and unlike culture, the test result remains positive for weeks despite specific antibiotic therapy.

Polymerase chain reaction–based assays applied to clinical specimens are specific but not more sensitive than culture.

■ ANTIBIOTIC THERAPY (Table 2)

The new macrolides, especially azithromycin, have displaced erythromycin as the antibiotic of choice. The new macrolides have more potent intracellular activity within alveolar macrophages and leukocytes, and higher lung tissue and respiratory secretion concentrations. Furthermore, the new macrolides have improved pharmacokinetic properties, which allow once- or twice-daily dosing and produce significantly fewer adverse effects than erythromycin.

Parenteral therapy is preferred initially because the gastrointestinal manifestations of Legionnaires' disease may interfere with absorption. When objective clinical response is documented (usually defervescence in 3 to 5 days), oral therapy can then be used. Total duration of therapy is 10 to 14 days. Azithromycin need be given only 7 to 10 days. A 21-day course has been recommended for immunosuppressed patients. For patients with acquired immunodeficiency syndrome (AIDS), we recommend continuing oral maintenance antimicrobial agent therapy until the infiltrates on chest radiograph resolve; close follow up for recurrence is necessary.

For nosocomial pneumonias and nursing home pneumonias in which *Legionella* is considered a potential pathogen, the quinolones—especially ciprofloxacin and levofloxacin—are ideal antibiotics because the quinolones cover gram-negative bacilli, which are common pathogens in the hospital or nursing home settings.

For transplant recipients in whom *Legionella* is a potential pathogen, a quinolone is recommended, especially ciprofloxacin or levofloxacin. The macrolides, except azithromycin, interact with the immunosuppressive agents cyclosporin and tacrolimus used in transplantation.

For patients with prosthetic valve endocarditis we would administer a combination of a quinolone or azithromycin with rifampin for 3 months if the infected valve is replaced and for 6 months if the infected valve is not removed. For patients with extrapulmonary disease, we recommend a quinolone or a new macrolide (azithromycin, clarithromycin, roxithromycin) for 14 to 21 days; combination with rifampin might be considered in severely ill patients.

Mortality rates vary from 0% to 11% for appropriately treated immunocompetent patients in the community setting and reach 40% for appropriately treated immunosuppressed patients. The mortality rates increase to 30% and 80% with inappropriate therapy, respectively, for both groups.

■ PREVENTION

Hospital-acquired legionellosis can be prevented by disinfection of the hospital water distribution system. Two methods are reliable and cost-effective. The superheat and flush method requires heating the water such that the distal outlet temperature is 70° to 80° C (158° to 176° F) and rinsing the outlets for at least 30 minutes. It has the advantage of halting an outbreak, but efficacy is only short term (months). Copper-silver ionization units are effective in the long term (Tarn-Pure). Hyperchlorination has been abandoned because of marginal efficacy, high cost, damage to the piping system by corrosion, and production of carcinogenic byproducts in water.

Suggested Reading

Edelstein PH: Antimicrobial chemotherapy for Legionnaires' disease, *Clin Infect Dis* 16:741, 1993.

Stout JE, Yu VL: Legionellosis, *N Engl J Med* 337:682, 1997.

Vergis EN, Yu VL: Legionella species. In Yu VL, Merigan T Jr, Barriere SL, eds: *Antimicrobial therapy and vaccines,* Baltimore, 1999, Williams & Wilkins.

LEPROSY

J.B. Stricker
Clay J. Cockerell

■ EPIDEMIOLOGY

Leprosy is an ancient disease that has been the cause of great morbidity and mortality for centuries. Despite the cause of the condition now being known, the disease is still feared and misunderstood by laypersons in the modern era. The causative agent, *Mycobacterium leprae,* multiplies very slowly in the host and is an obligate intracellular parasite. It grows best at 33° C (91.4° F), which accounts for its predilection for cooler parts of the body such as the skin, testis, anterior segment of eye, mucous membranes of nasal passages, and ear lobes and extremities. The phenolic glycolipid in the capsule is, in part, related to the pathogenesis and causes foamy histiocytes to accumulate in tissue. Leprosy is relatively difficult to transmit, and most individuals are only minimally susceptible to it. Those who acquire it initially develop a single lesion that often heals spontaneously. In some patients, however, the initial lesion does not resolve, and if treatment is not initiated, there is strong likelihood that the disease will progress to a more advanced stage.

Leprosy is endemic in a number of regions, especially the tropics and subtropics, including south and southeast Asia, Mexico and Central America, Africa, China, the Middle East, India, southern Europe, and the southern United States. However, isolated pockets of disease are found in many parts of the world, and as a consequence of international travel, affected individuals may be encountered in any location. Worldwide, 10 to 12 million people are infected. In the United States, infected patients may be found in any state, but most are in California, Hawaii, Florida, Texas, and Louisiana. In the United States, approximately 85% of cases are seen in immigrants, although it is endemic in southeastern Louisiana and in south-central Texas.

The exact mechanism of transmission is unclear, although it is thought to be spread by aerosolized particles landing on and passing through nasal mucosa. Organisms may occasionally enter the body through broken skin, but such cases are rare and poorly documented. Armadillos are known to harbor *M. leprae,* and a number of cases have been traced to exposure to these animals, although direct transmission of the organism to humans has not been definitively demonstrated.

■ PATHOPHYSIOLOGY

The clinical disorder recognized as leprosy develops as a consequence of both the host's immune reaction to *M. leprae* as well as from direct effects of bacillary spread and multiplication. Those susceptible to infection demonstrate an impaired cell-mediated immune response to the organism. This is thought to result from a genetic predisposition because cases cluster in families, and there is a high concordance rate in identical twins. Furthermore, preliminary studies have linked susceptibility to leprosy with the NRAMP-1 gene, which controls innate immunity to mycobacterial infections in mice. The microorganism has a tropism for nerves that become damaged as a consequence of immune reactions to intraneural bacilli as as well physical effects induced by proliferation of bacilli within nerves. As a consequence, many of the clinical manifestations are caused by peripheral nerve damage with loss of motor and sensory function leading to ulcers, contractures, and loss of tissue substance. Other tissues, such as the skin, may harbor innumerable organisms in some forms of the disease, and deforming cutaneous nodules may develop. Immune reactions to organisms in skin lead to severe forms of vasculitis with extensive cutaneous necrosis.

CLASSIFICATION AND CLINICAL PRESENTATION

There may be a number of different presentations in patients with leprosy, depending on the level of immunity and the duration of the disease. Individuals with the early indeterminate form present with one or more scaly hypopigmented anesthetic macules of the skin appearing initially on the face, although the limbs, trunk, or buttocks may be involved. If untreated, this may progress to any form of the disease. Others present only with sensorimotor neuropathy with enlargement of the peripheral nerves without skin lesions. Nerves affected most commonly include the ulnar and median nerves, often resulting in a claw hand deformity; the common peroneal nerve, leading to foot drop; the posterior tibial nerve, which results in claw toes and plantar insensitivity; and the facial, radial cutaneous, and great auricular nerves. Other areas of the body, such as the nasopharynx, eyes, and testicles, may also be involved.

Classically, patients present with symptoms that can range from one pole (tuberculoid) to another (lepromatous) or anywhere in between (borderline tuberculoid, borderline, or borderline lepromatous). Tuberculoid leprosy is the form with a small number of asymmetric skin lesions that are hypopigmented, have sharp borders, and are associated with anesthesia. Commonly, cutaneous nerves are enlarged and few bacilli are present on biopsy (paucibacillary form). Lepromatous leprosy presents as widely distributed symmetric skin lesions that can manifest as macules, papules, plaques, or nodules, which are red to brown. Often, it can also present as diffuse thickening of the skin with loss of underlying adnexa. Biopsy shows many bacilli (multibacillary form). Borderline cases may present anywhere between these two extremes.

A number of different schemes have been developed to clinically classify patients so that treatment can be tailored appropriately. The World Health Organization (WHO) classification is the most commonly used system, although the Ridley-Jopling classification was the first to be developed and is based on clinical signs and symptoms. The WHO classification is based on the number of skin lesions and number of bacilli present in smears. Patients with five or fewer skin lesions without evidence of bacilli on skin smears are considered paucibacillary, whereas those with six or more skin lesions with or without bacilli on skin smears are considered to be multibacillary. The clinical forms in the Ridley-Jopling classification referred to as indeterminate, tuberculoid, and borderline tuberculoid correlate with paucibacillary disease, whereas those with borderline, borderline lepromatous, and polar lepromatous forms have multibacillary disease.

Leprosy in reaction refers to clinical disease produced when there is a change in the host's immune response to *M. leprae*. There are two forms of reactional leprosy. Type I reactions are induced by cell-mediated immunity and are referred to as *upgrading* and *downgrading* reactions. Upgrading reactions are characteristically seen in patients with borderline lepromatous disease who undergo a shift toward more tuberculoid (paucibacillary) forms. These may develop after induction of therapy. Downgrading reactions occur with transformation from a tuberculoid to a more lepromatous (multibacillary) form and often develop in the absence of treatment. Both may appear similar clinically and are manifest by erythema and edema of existing skin lesions associated with painful neuropathy and ulceration. Type II reactions are immune complex–mediated and include erythema nodosum leprosum (ENL) and Lucio's phenomenon. Both of these are manifestations of immune complex–mediated vasculitis that lead to prominent inflammation and often ulceration with acute damage to nerves. Patients present with fever, multiple erythematous tender nodules, and varying degrees of neuritis, edema, arthralgias, leukocytosis, iridocyclitis, pretibial periostitis, orchitis, and nephritis.

DIAGNOSIS

The diagnosis of leprosy must be considered in anyone with a history of travel to indigenous areas with unusual skin lesions or a sensorimotor neuropathy. The diagnostic evaluation includes a thorough physical examination, especially a detailed neurologic examination in the search for tender and enlarged nerves as well as motor and sensory testing and skin smears. Smears are made by making small slits in skin lesions, smearing exudate on a slide, and staining for acid-fast bacilli. Other modalities, such as the lepromin skin test, polymerase chain reaction for *M. leprae,* and measurement of phenolic glycolipid-1 (PGL-1) antibody, may be useful in selected circumstances, but clinical assessment remains paramount. At present, *M. leprae* has not been cultured but will proliferate in the nine-banded armadillo as well as in nude mice and a few other other animals.

TREATMENT

Treatment depends on whether the individual has paucibacillary or multibacillary disease. Virtually all patients are treated with a regimen of multiple drugs as recommended by the WHO (Table 1). Dapsone and clofazimine are weakly bactericidal when used alone, although they are mycobactericidal and kill more than 99% of bacilli when used in combination. Rifampin is highly bactericidal alone, although its use alone is not recommended because antibiotic resistance may develop. Minocycline, ofloxacin, and clarithromycin have also shown effectiveness. Administration of antibiotics renders the patient noninfectious in a matter of weeks.

Paucibacillary patients receive a supervised dose of rifampin, 600 mg orally once per month for 3 months, and a daily unsupervised dose of dapsone, 100 mg orally for 6 months. At the end of 6 months, therapy is discontinued. Multibacillary patients receive a supervised dose of rifampin, 600 mg orally once monthly, a 300-mg dose of clofazimine, and an unsupervised daily dose of dapsone, 100 mg orally, and a 50-mg daily oral dose of clofazimine for 12 months. In patients with high bacillary indices (at least 10 bacilli per oil immersion field), 24 months of therapy is recommended, which is a significant improvement from prior regimens, which were lifelong. Relapses should be treated in the same manner as the initial disease, providing

Table 1 World Health Organization Recommended Drug Therapy

	PAUCIBACILLARY	MULTIBACILLARY
Monthly, supervised	600 mg rifampin	600 mg rifampin *and* 300 mg clofazimine
Daily, unsupervised	100 mg dapsone	100 mg dapsone *and* 50 mg clofazimine
Duration of therapy	6 mo	12 mo
Follow-up	2 yr	5 yr

Table 2 Recommended Treatment of Reversal Reactions

	TYPE I REACTION	ERYTHEMA NODOSUM LEPROSUM
Mild	Symptomatic	NSAIDs, symptomatic
Severe	40-60 mg prednisolone	40-60 mg prednisolone *or* 300 mg clofazimine (chronic) *or* 300-400 mg thalidomide
Duration	Slowly taper as tolerated	Slowly taper prednisolone as tolerated Taper clofazimine to 100 mg in 12 months Taper thalidomide as tolerated to 100 mg, discontinue as soon as indicated

NSAIDs, Nonsteroidal antiinflammatory drugs.
Note: All patients should receive prednisolone in the presence of neuritis.

there is no drug resistance. A single oral-dose regimen of three drugs consisting of 600 mg rifampicin, 400 mg ofloxacin, and 100 mg of minocycline (ROM) has demonstrated similar bactericidal activity and relapse rates in paucibacillary patients, although it was less effective in producing clinical improvement. Studies are ongoing to discover shorter, simpler, and more effective regimens.

All patients are evaluated monthly or more frequently, depending on complications for at least 2 years for paucibacillary patients and at least 5 years for multibacillary patients. Most programs continue inspections for 5 to 10 years in all patients. Relapse rates are approximately 1% in both paucibacillary and multibacillary patients. The WHO recommends that all patients be instructed to recognize the signs and symptoms of recurrent disease as well as adverse reactions to medications. It may take up to 5 years for bacilli to be completely cleared in patients with multibacillary disease. Although many of the neurologic problems may be permanent, skin lesions usually disappear within 1 year of treatment and reappearance of skin lesions is highly suggestive of relapse.

Major drug side effects are relatively uncommon with present regimens. Clofazimine may cause gastrointestinal symptoms and a purplish skin discoloration, which clear with discontinuation of the drug. Dapsone often causes mild anemia, although severe anemia may result in patients with glucose-6-phosphate dehydrogenase deficiency, so all patients should be tested for this enzyme before initiation of therapy. Other side effects include agranulocytosis, cutaneous eruptions, peripheral neuropathy, gastrointestinal distress, and nephrotic syndrome. It is of interest that, when given in combination with rifampicin, dapsone is cleared from the plasma 7 to 10 times more quickly, although this has been shown to affect clearance of bacilli. Rifampicin, in the doses advocated by the WHO, rarely causes adverse effects but may cause discoloration of the urine, stool, and other body fluids. Pregnant women have safely taken dapsone and clofazimine, but experience with rifampicin is limited.

■ TREATMENT OF REVERSAL REACTIONS

Early diagnosis and prompt treatment of reversal reactions is of great importance to prevent many of the deforming complications of leprosy (Table 2). Up to 25% of patients

will develop a reversal reaction, usually during therapy. Mild reactions can be treated symptomatically; however, severe type I reactions with neuritis or silent neuropathy require prompt initiation of systemic glucocorticoid therapy, starting at a minimum dose of 40 to 60 mg of prednisolone, tapering once the reaction is controlled. In patients with nerve damage from reactional leprosy for 3 to 6 months, the response to therapy is less than 67%. When present for longer than 6 months, the response to therapy is even poorer. Mild to moderate ENL can be treated with nonsteroidal antiinflammatory drugs (NSAIDs) and other symptomatic modalities. Severe ENL or the presence of neuritis requires prednisolone (as prescribed in type I reactions). Clofazimine is useful for chronic reactions, and its use has been credited with the overall decrease of ENL in leprosy. Patients are given 300 mg/day orally until lesions begin resolving, following which the dose is tapered slowly to 100 mg over 12 months. Thalidomide, 300 to 400 mg orally, will supress ENL within 48 hours and is considered the drug of choice by many leprologists. Its high teratogenic potential has prevented its widespread use, although it is now available. Patients receiving thalidomide should have the dose tapered to 100 mg after a therapeutic response is noted, and if possible, the drug should be discontinued. Side effects of thalidomide include somnolence and peripheral neuropathy, the latter of which can be permanent and may be difficult to distinguish from neuropathic changes of leprosy. Ophthalmologic complications associated with Hansen's disease, such as iridocyclitis and lagophthalmos, should be managed by an ophthalmologist if possible.

Suggested Reading

Jacobson RR, Krahenbuhl JL: Leprosy, *Lancet* 353:655, 1999.
Physicians Desk Reference, ed 53, Montvale, NJ, 1999, Medical Economics Data Production.
Whitty CJM, Lockwood DNJ: Leprosy—new perspectives on an old disease, *J Infect* 38:2, 1999.
WHO Study Group: *Chemotherapy of leprosy* (WHO tech rep ser no 847), Geneva, 1994, World Health Organization.

MENINGOCOCCUS AND MISCELLANEOUS NEISSERIAE

Charles Davis
Edmund C. Tramont

■ MENINGOCOCCAL INFECTION

Meningococcal infection, first recognized nearly two centuries ago as epidemic cerebrospinal fever, occurs worldwide as epidemic, endemic, and sporadic cases. Worldwide, most cases are caused by serogroups A to C, whereas in the United States, serogroups B and C predominate (see the following). Humans are the only natural reservoir for the bacteria. Transmission of the organism occurs from person to person by direct contact with contaminated respiratory secretions or airborne droplets with subsequent colonization of the nasopharynx. Nasopharyngeal carriage approximates 5% to 15% in nonepidemic periods but may approach 50% to 95% during epidemics, especially serogroup A epidemics. The carriage rate is also increased when there is crowding, such as in military barracks, dormitories, prisons, and sporting events. The oropharyngeal and nasopharyngeal carriage may persist for several weeks to several months. Sexual transmission of meningococci in women and homosexual men may result in anogenital carriage. Most cases of disease (e.g., bacteremia, menigitis) occur in children between 6 months and 5 years of age. With rare exceptions, most invasive meningococci are encapsulated. Invasive disease occurs almost exclusively in persons who lack specific antimeningococcal antibody to the colonizing strain of organism. Individuals with complement component deficiencies are at increased risk for developing invasive meningococcal infections because their serum loses the ability of complement-mediated lysis of the bacteria. Hence, complement deficiency should be considered in persons with recurrent episodes of invasive meningococcal infection. Asplenic patients are also at increased risk for acquiring invasive meningococcal disease. On rare occasions, persons may develop serum IgA antibodies that block the bactericidal action of IgG and IgM antibodies.

Clinical Features

The clinical consequences of meningococcal infection are the result of meningococcal endotoxin release and subsequent activation of the procoagulation, anticoagulation, fibrinolysis, complement, and kallikrein-kinin cascades together with the release of inflammatory mediators. The clinical manifestation of meningococcal infection varies from a mild transient bacteremia to fulminate meningococcemia and/or meningitis and death. Most commonly, *Neisseria meningitidis* acquisition results in asymptomatic colonization of the nasopharynx. The mildest form of invasive disease is manifested by a transient bacteremia. Symptoms begin insidiously with fever, malaise, and symptoms of an upper respiratory tract infection. A few petechial skin lesions may appear, but neither signs nor symptoms of sepsis or meningitis develops. Symptoms usually resolve spontaneously within 24 to 48 hours. Acute meningococcemia, which often follows several days of upper respiratory tract symptoms, is heralded by fever, chills, malaise, weakness, headache, myalgias, and nausea and/or vomiting. Skin manifestations, especially a petechial rash, raises the index of suspicion for meningococcal infection. They usually appear in crops on the ankles, wrists, axilla, trunk, and mucous membranes, while the palms, soles, neck, and face are usually spared. The rash may also be urticarial, maculopapular, ecchymotic, or gangrenous. However, the rash may not develop (Table 1).

Fulminate meningococcemia, also called *Waterhouse-Friderichsen syndrome* or *purpura fulminans,* complicates acute meningococcemia in 5% to 15% of cases and is associated with the rash progressing into massive skin and mucosal hemorrhage, disseminated intravascular coagulopathy (DIC), and vascular collapse and is associated with a high mortality, sometimes within hours. Death, usually

Table 1   Differential Diagnosis of Rash and Meningitis
Neisseria meningitidis
Haemophilus influenzae b
Streptococcus pneumoniae
Rickettsiae, especially Rocky Mountain spotted fever
Viruses, especially echovirus and coxsackievirus
INFECTIONS THAT MAY BE ASSOCIATED WITH PETECHIAL RASHES
Bacterial
N. meningitidis
H. influenzae type b
N. gonorrhea
S. pneumoniae
S. pyogenes
E. coli
Klebsiella species
Pseudomonas species
Streptobacillus moniliformis (rat-bite fever)
Viral
Enteroviruses
Rubella
Atypical measles
Epstein-Barr virus
Cytomegalovirus, congenital
Colorado tick fever
Arboviruses
Rickettsial
Rickettsia rickettsii (RMSF)
Rickettsia prowazekii (epidemic typhus)
Spirochetes
Leptospirosis
Parasites
Plasmodium falciparum
Endocarditis
Disseminated intravascular coagulopathy associated with septicemia

associated with adrenal hemorrhage, may occur despite appropriate therapy.

Meningitis may occur with or without any manifestations of meningococcemia. Clinically, meningococcal meningitis resembles an acute meningitis of any cause, presenting with fever, headache, altered sensorium, and nuchal rigidity.

On rare occasions, a chronic meningococcemia develops. This is characterized by intermittent febrile episodes, lasting 2 to 10 days, accompanied by a variety of skin lesions (macular, maculopapular, petechiae, ecchymotic, or pustular), arthralgias or arthritis, myalgias, and splenomegaly. The infection may last for months and can be fatal, but it usually resolves spontaneously.

Occasionally, meningococcemia may produce oropharyngitis, sinusitis, pneumonia, conjunctivitis, endophthalmitis, proctitis, urethritis, cervicitis, immune-mediated arthritis, endocarditis, myocarditis, pericarditis, and pelvic inflammatory disease (PID). Except in advanced cases, the response to appropriate antibiotic treatment is usually dramatic.

Culture and Laboratory Findings

N. meningitidis is an aerobic, oxidase-positive, gram-negative diplococcus that grows best at 35° to 37° C (95° to 98.6° F) in a moist environment of 5% to 7% carbon dioxide. Oxidative metabolism of glucose and maltose but not sucrose, lactose, or fructose is the major means for differentiating *N. meningitidis* from other *Neisseria* species. The organism is surrounded by a polysaccharide capsule that provides the basis for serogrouping. The meningococcus has been classified as serogroups A, B, C, D, 29E; I, J, K, L, W-135, X, Y, Z and nontypable (indicates organism is uncapsulated). Serogroups A, B, C, W-135, and Y are responsible for most cases of invasive disease. With rare exceptions, invasive meningococci are encapsulated, attesting to the virulence conveyed by the polysaccharide capsule, whereas meningococci colonizing mucous membranes often are not encapsulated.

When possible, specimens should be cultured for *N. meningitidis* before antibiotics are instituted. For culture of a normally sterile site, such as blood or cerebrospinal fluid (CSF), nonselective agar is preferred. A selective antibiotic-containing medium, such as Thayer-Martin, Martin-Lewis, or New York City culture media, is necessary when the culture specimen is obtained from a nonsterile site such as the oropharynx or urethra. If petechial or hemorrhagic lesions are present, meningococci may be demonstrated in up to 70% of cases on Gram staining, fluorescent staining, acridine orange staining or even methylene blue staining of tissue fluid extracted from these lesions. Organisms may also be demonstrated in the buffy coat of peripheral blood.

In patients with meningitis, the CSF is generally cloudy with a leukocytosis consisting predominantly of polymorphonuclear neutrophils associated with hypoglycorrhachia. The Gram stain of the CSF is positive in about 75% of cases. The CSF and blood are the most common sources of positive cultures. Rapid identification of *N. meningitidis* capsular polysaccharide in CSF, serum, and urine by latex particle agglutination (LPA) is also available, but its sensitivity in the CSF is no better than that of a Gram stain. The LPA test is most useful to establish the diagnosis in patients who have received prior antibiotics. As with any laboratory test, a negative LPA does not rule out the diagnosis. Specificity may be hampered by the potential cross reactivity of the group B test antiserum with the K1 antigen of *Escherichia coli*.

Therapy

Penicillin G remains the drug of choice for all forms of meningococcal disease. Penicillin G therapy should be administered intravenously (IV), at least initially. Adults should receive 300,000 U/kg IV daily divided every 4 hours. Infants should receive 250,000 U/kg/day IV in divided doses every 4 hours.

However, initial antimicrobial therapy is often empirically based on the clinical presentation, which may be indistinguishable from other bacterial infections such as *Streptococcus pneumoniae, Staphylococcus aureus,* or other gram-negative organisms. Thus, without a specific diagnosis, initial empirical therapy should be with broad-spectrum cephalosporin antibiotics such as cefuroxime, ceftriaxone, cefotaxime, and ceftazidime or ampicillin plus an aminoglycoside, either gentamicin, netilmycin, or amikacin. However, the existence of ampicillin-resistant strains of meningococcus is well documented. Chloramphenicol is primarily of historical importance; however, it remains an effective substitute in patients allergic to penicillin, even though high-level resistance has begun to emerge in Asia and in Europe; the dosage is 100 mg/kg/day in divided doses every 6 hours up to 4 g/day. Even though sulfonamides have been used with success in the past, they should not be used empirically because of unpredictable susceptibility of the organism (Table 2).

Seven to ten days of therapy is sufficient to sterilize the patient, with the antibiotic being given intravenously for at least the first 4 days. Supportive care is extremely important. Potential complications such as volume depletion, acidosis, hypoxemia, and adrenal insufficiency should be anticipated and managed appropriately. Long-term sequelae include hearing loss, other cranial palsies, and mental retardation. Steroid therapy is indicated when acute adrenal insufficiency is a possibility, especially when the patient has progressed into the Waterhouse-Friderichsen syndrome. Dexamethasone, 0.15 mg/kg every 6 hours in infants and 8 to 12 mg every 12 hours in children and adults, is recommended. Some clinicians also use short-term steroids (3 days) in patients with meningitis (personally recommended by us). The management of DIC may also be necessary, but the use of heparin in such cases remains controversial. Immunoglobulin therapy with high titers of antibody to core antigen and/or to tumor necrosis factor have been of little benefit.

Prevention

Most cases of *N. meningitidis* are sporadic. However, person-to-person transmission has been a source of "household" outbreaks (close contacts). *N. meningitidis* is harbored in the nasopharynx of patients and asymptomatic carriers. The organism is spread through direct contact, especially respiratory droplets. The risk of contracting a symptomatic *N. meningitidis* infection is approximately 4 cases per 1000 among persons who have had "close contact" with a known carrier or patient with a virulent strain. This risk of developing invasive disease is greatly minimized by chemoprophy-

Table 2   Treatment of Meningococcal Meningitis

ANTIBIOTIC	INTRAVENOUS DOSAGE*	COMMENT
Penicillin G	Adults: 300,000 U/kg/day divided q4h Children: 250,000 U/kg/day divided q4h	Remains drug of choice; exceeds usual MIC with meningeal inflammation; relatively resistant strains reported
Ampicillin	Adults: 12 g qd divided q4h Children: 50-75 mg/kg q6h	As effective as penicillin; exceeds MIC with meningeal inflammation
Ceftriaxone	Adults: 1g q12h Children: 80-150 mg/kg/day divided q12h or qd	Good CNS penetration; exceeds usual MIC
Cefotaxime	Adults: 8-12g/day divided q4h Children: 200 mg/kg/day divided q6-8h	Exceeds usual MIC with meningeal inflammation
Ceftazidime	Adults: 1-2 g q8-12h Children: 125-150 mg/kg/day divided q8h	Exceeds usual MIC with meningeal inflammation
Chloramphenicol	Adults: 25 mg/kg q6h (maximum 4g/day) Children: 25 mg/kg q6h	Concentrates in CSF; because of potential to cause irreversible aplastic anemia (1:10,000 to 1:40,000) it is rarely used in United States but is used more frequently in emerging countries
Ciprofloxacin	Adults: 400-600 mg q12h Children: 10-15 mg/kg q12h	Appropriate spectrum and pharmacokinetics; few studies in children

MIC, Minimal inhibitory concentration; *CNS*, central nervous system; *CSF*, cerebrospinal fluid.
*In all instances treatment should extend 7 to 10 days.

Table 3   Considered Close Contacts of an Index Case

All household members
Day-care workers
Preschool workers
Classmates (daycare and preschool)
Health care workers with contact with oral and/or respiratory secretions
Workers and classmates in boarding schools
Workers and classmates if two or more cases occur in a 6-month period
The index case, if treated with penicillin or chloramphenicol
Living in a common military barrack

---

laxis: administering prophylactic antibiotics to individuals who have had "close contact" to an index case. Defining a "close contact" is problematic; however, the Centers for Disease Control and Prevention (CDC) has defined a *close contact* as "those residing with the index case or spending four or more hours with the index case for 5 of 7 days before the onset of illness" (Table 3). Those at increased risk for infection include all household members and day-care or preschool workers and classmates of the diagnosed patient. Health care workers are considered to be at risk only if they have intimate contact with the patient's secretions, such as providing mouth-to-mouth resuscitation before the patient being started on appropriate antibiotic therapy. The incubation period is 2 to 10 days. Thus prophylaxis should be considered for those who have had close contact with the untreated index case during the incubation period.

Rifampin remains the drug of choice for chemoprophylaxis. Rifampin, 600 mg PO every 12 hours for four doses for adults or 10 mg/kg every 12 hours for four doses for children, eradicates meningococci for 75% to 98% of carriers. However, rifampin-resistant meningococcus have emerged, even during chemoprophylaxis. Alternatives that have been shown to be effective include ceftriaxone, ciprofloxacin, ofloxacin, azithromycin, minocycline, and spectinomycin. A single intramuscular injection of ceftriaxone, 250 mg in adults and 125 mg in children, is 97% effective in eradicating the carrier state; however, the cost, availability, and route of administration limit worldwide use. Ciprofloxacin, 500 mg as a single dose, has an efficacy rate of 89% to 97%; however, its use is contraindicated in pregnant females, and it is not licensed for use in children younger than 18 years of age. However, studies including children younger than 12 years of age have found the drug to be highly efficacious and without any untoward sequelae. A single dose of ofloxacin, 400 mg, was found to be 97% effective in eradicating carriage; however, it has the same limitations as ciprofloxacin. A single 500-mg dose of azithromycin had a 93% efficacy rate at eradicating meningococcal carriage. Minocycline is effective, given at a dosage of 100 mg twice a day for 5 days, but an unacceptable incidence of vestibular side effects precludes its routine use. Spectinomycin (Spiramycin) is the primary prophylactic agent in many European countries, given at a dosage of 500 mg orally four times a day for 5 days to adults and 10 mg/kg orally four times a day for 5 days in children. Unfortunately, sulfonamide resistance is too highly prevalent and should be used only if the isolate from the index case is known to be sensitive. One must be aware that chemoprophylaxis with penicillin prevents invasive disease but does not predictably eradicate the carrier state and therefore transmission (Table 4).

Immunity to invasive meningococcal disease is correlated directly with bactericidal antibody to the capsular polysaccharide except for serogroup B. Hence group-specific meningococcal polysaccharide vaccines have been developed. Vaccine immunoprophylaxis is recommended for high-risk groups, such as persons with terminal complement compo-

Table 4 Antibiotics Used for Chemoprophylaxis of *Neisseria meningitidis*

ANTIBIOTIC COMMENT	EFFICACY AT ERADICATING NASOPHARYNGEAL CARRIAGE	DOSAGE
RIFAMPIN Drug of choice Safety in pregnancy not demonstrated Body fluid discoloration May render birth control pills ineffective	75%-98%	Adults: 600 mg PO q12h ×4 doses Children ≥1 mo: 10mg/kg PO q12h ×4 doses Children <1 mo: 5mg/kg PO q12h ×4 doses
CEFTRIAXONE Can be given to young children and pregnant women	92%-97%	Adults: 250 mg IM ×1 dose Children <15: 125 mg IM ×1 dose
CIPROFLOXACIN Safety in pregnancy not established Not licensed in children under 18 years	89%-97%	Adults: 500 mg PO ×1 dose
OFLOXACIN Same as for ciprofloxacin	97%	Adults: 400 mg PO ×1 dose Children: 200 mg PO ×1 dose
SPIRAMYCIN	90%-95%	Adults: 500 mg PO qid ×5 days Children: 10mg/kg PO qid ×5 days
MINOCYCLINE Proved effective but vestibular toxicity Not to be used in pregnant or lactating women	90%-95%	Adults: 100 mg PO q12h ×5 days Children: 1 mg/kg PO q12h ×5 days
SULFADIAZINE Excellent CNS penetration Cannot be given to persons with G6PD deficiency Resistance limits its usefulness[*]	95%	Adults: 1g PO q8h ×3 days Children: 1g PO q12h ×3 days
AZITHROMYCIN	93%	Adults: 500 mg PO ×1 dose

CNS, Central nervous system; *G6PD,* glucose-6 phosphate dehydrogenase.
[*]Sulfadiazine sensitive = ≤0.1 mg/100 ml.

nent deficiencies, those who have anatomic or functional asplenia, military trainees, and college or boarding school first-year students 15 to 20 years of age. Immunization may benefit travelers to areas in which *N. meningitidis* is hyperendemic (Nepal, New Delhi, sub-Saharan Africa, the "meningitis belt" from Senegal in the west to Ethiopia in the east), particularly if their stay is prolonged.

Licensed meningococcal vaccine consists of a mixture of purified high-molecular-weight capsular polysaccharides from serogroups A, C, Y, and W-135. This tetravalent vaccine has virtually eliminated meningococcal disease caused by these serogroups in U.S. military recruits. There is as yet no vaccine to prevent group B disease. The duration of immunity induced is not precisely known but it is estimated to be at least 2 to 3 years. In a 3-year study, efficacy declined from greater than 90% to less than 10% in children younger than 4 years of age at the time of vaccination, whereas for those who were 4 years of age or older at the time of vaccination, the efficacy was 67% 3 years later. Licensed meningococcal vaccine is poorly immunogenic in children younger than 2 years of age; therefore only chemoprophylaxis can be relied on for the prevention of secondary cases of meningococcal disease in this age group. Revaccination should be considered for persons at high risk for infection, such as those remaining in or traveling to areas where the disease is epidemic and in children at high risk who were first vaccinated when they were younger than 4 years of age.

Natural immunity develops in most individuals by age 5 years as a consequence of asymptomatic nasophayngeal or gastrointestinal carriage of other cross-reacting microbial species.

■ INFECTIONS WITH OTHER *NEISSERIA* SPECIES

The nonpathogenic *Neisseria* species include *N. lactamica, N. sicca, N. subflava, N. mucosa, N. flavescens, N. cinerea, N. kochii, N. elongata,* and *N. polysaccharea* are usually commensulates of the oropharynx and nasopharynx. Infections caused by these organisms are extremely rare, occurring primarily in immunosuppressed hosts, especially those who are hypogammaglobulinemic or have defective antibody production (i.e., chronic lymphocytic leukemia). The relative lack of virulence of these organisms is attributed to the lack of encapsulation, and hence they have no predilection to resist bacterial lysis by nonspecific components of the blood or to invade the meninges. Thus they are easily controlled by normal innate host defense mechanisms.

Because these organisms normally reside in the oropharynx, local extension of infection is most commonly to the ear, sinuses, and lung. Conjunctivitis, meningitis, endophthalmitis, endocarditis, and urethritis have also been reported, attesting to the common tissue tropism that these sites share with the oropharynx. These nonpathogenic *Neisseria* are easily treated with penicillin, cephalosporin, or quinolone antibiotics.

Suggested Reading

Centers for Disease Control and Prevention: Control and prevention of meningococcal disease: recommendations of the advisory committee on immunization practices (ACIP), *MMWR* 46:1, 1997.

deKleijn ED, et al: Pathophysiology of meningococcal sepsis in children, *Eur J Pediatr* 157:869, 1998.

Derkx B, et al: Randomized, placebo-controlled trial of HA-1A, a human monoclonal antibody to endotoxin, in children with meningococcal septic shock, *Clin Inf Dis* 28:770, 1999.

Jones GR, et al: Lack of immunity in university students before an outbreak of Serogroup C meningococcal infection, *J Infect Dis* 181:1172, 2000.

LISTERIA

Bennett Lorber

The bacterium *Listeria monocytogenes* is an uncommon cause of illness in the general population. However, in some groups, including neonates, pregnant women, the elderly, immunosuppressed transplant recipients, and others with impaired cell-mediated immunity, it is an important cause of life-threatening meningoencephalitis and bacteremia. Ingestion of large numbers of listeriae in contaminated food may produce fever and diarrhea in healthy persons.

L. monocytogenes is an important cause of zoonoses, especially in herd animals. It is widespread in nature, being found commonly in soil, decaying vegetation, and as part of the fecal flora of many mammals. The organism has been isolated from the stool of approximately 5% of healthy adults with higher rates of recovery reported from household contacts of patients. Many foods are contaminated with *L. monocytogenes*, and recovery rates of 15% to 70% or more are common from raw vegetables, raw milk, fish, poultry, and meats, including fresh or processed chicken and beef available at supermarkets or deli counters. Ingestion of *L. monocytogenes* must be an exceedingly common occurrence.

There are 1000 to 2000 cases of invasive disease (bacteremia or meningitis) per year in the United States, with 250 to 450 deaths. The highest infection rates are seen in infants younger than 1 month of age and adults older than 60 years. Pregnant women account for 27% of all cases and 60% of cases in the 15- to 40-year age group. Almost 70% of nonperinatal infections occur in those with hematologic malignancy, acquired immunodeficiency syndrome (AIDS), or organ transplantation or those receiving corticosteroid therapy; but seemingly normal persons may develop invasive disease, particularly those older than 60.

Foodborne outbreaks of invasive human listerial infection have been documented with vehicles including coleslaw, milk, soft cheeses, and ready-to-eat pork products. Food appears to be an important source of sporadic listeriosis also, as illustrated by recent Centers for Disease Control and Prevention (CDC) studies in which cases were more likely than controls to have eaten soft cheeses or deli counter meats, and 32% of sporadic cases could be attributed to these foods. Alkalinization of the stomach by antacids, H_2 blockers, or ulcer surgery may promote infection. Evidence from cases related to specific ingestions points to incubation periods ranging from 11 to 47 days with a mean of 31 days.

In the intestine, *L. monocytogenes* crosses the mucosal barrier, perhaps aided by active endocytosis of organisms by endothelial cells. Once in the bloodstream, hematogenous dissemination may occur to any site; *L. monocytogenes* has a particular predilection for the central nervous system (CNS) and the placenta.

Except for vertical transmission from mother to fetus and rare instances of cross-contamination in the delivery suite or newborn nursery, human-to-human infection has not been documented.

■ CLINICAL SYNDROMES

Infection in Pregnancy

During gestation, there is a mild impairment of cell-mediated immunity, and pregnant women are prone to develop listerial bacteremia. CNS infection, the most commonly recognized form of listeriosis in other groups, is extremely rare during pregnancy in the absence of other risk factors. Bacteremia usually occurs in the third trimester and is manifested clinically as an acute febrile illness, often accompanied by myalagias, arthralgias, headache, and backache. Of perinatal infections, 22% result in stillbirth or neonatal death; premature labor is common. Untreated bacteremia is generally self-limited, although, if there is a complicating amnionitis, fever in the mother may persist until the fetus is spontaneously or therapeutically aborted. Early diagnosis and antimicrobial treatment can result in the birth of a healthy infant.

Neonatal Infection

When in utero infection occurs, it may precipitate spontaneous abortion and the fetus may be stillborn or die within hours of a disseminated form of listerial infection known as *granulomatosis infantiseptica*, which is characterized by widespread microabscesses and granulomas. In this entity, abundant bacteria are often visible on Gram stain of meconium.

More commonly, neonatal infection manifests like group B streptococcal disease in one of two forms: (1) an early-onset sepsis syndrome usually associated with prematurity and probably acquired in utero, and (2) a late-onset meningitis occurring about 2 weeks postpartum in term babies most likely infected by organisms present in the maternal vagina at parturition.

Bacteremia

In recent clinical series, bacteremia without an evident focus has been the most common manifestation of listeriosis in compromised hosts; meningitis is second in frequency. Clinical manifestations are similar to those seen with other etiologies of bacteremia and typically include fever and myalgias; a prodromal illness with diarrhea and nausea may occur. Because immunocompromised patients are more likely than healthy persons to have blood cultured during febrile illnesses, transient bacteremia in otherwise healthy persons may go undetected.

Central Nervous System Infection

The organisms that most commonly cause bacterial meningitis (*Streptococcus pneumoniae, Neisseria meningitidis, Haemophilus influenzae*) rarely cause parenchymal brain infections such as cerebritis and brain abscess. In contrast, *L. monocytogenes* has tropism for the brain itself (particularly the brainstem) as well as for the meninges. Many patients with listerial meningitis have altered consciousness, seizures, and/or movement disorders and truly have a meningoencephalitis.

Meningitis

As reported by the CDC in 1990, *L. monocytogenes* was the fifth most common cause of bacterial meningitis behind *H. influenzae, S. pneumoniae, N. meningitidis,* and group B streptococcus, but it had the highest mortality at 22%. In 1995, 5 years after the introduction of *H. influenzae* conjugate vaccines, *H. influenzae* had become less common than *L. monocytogenes,* which accounted for 20% of cases in neonates and 20% in persons older than 60 years of age. Worldwide *L. monocytogenes* is one of the three major causes of neonatal meningitis, is second only to pneumococcus as a cause of bacterial meningitis in adults older than 50, and is the most common cause of bacterial meningitis in patients with lymphomas, organ transplant recipients, or those receiving corticosteroid immunosuppression for any reason.

Clinically, meningitis caused by *L. monocytogenes* is usually similar to that caused by more common etiologies; features particular to listerial meningitis are summarized in Table 1.

Brainstem Encephalitis (Rhombencephalitis)

In contrast to other listerial CNS infections, brainstem encephalitis is an uncommon form of listerial encephalitis that usually occurs in healthy adults. The typical clinical picture is one of a biphasic illness with a prodrome of fever, headache, nausea, and vomiting lasting about 4 days followed by the abrupt onset of asymmetric cranial nerve

Table 1 Clinical Features Particular to Listerial Meningitis as Compared with More Common Bacterial Etiologies

Presentation usually acute but may be subacute and may mimic tuberculous meningitis

Nuchal rigidity less common (not present in 15%-20% of adult cases)

Movement disorders (ataxia, tremors, myoclonus) are more common (15%-20%)

Seizures are more common (≥25%)

Fluctuating mental status is common

Blood cultures are more likely positive (75%)

Cerebrospinal fluid:
  Gram stain is negative in most (organisms seen in approximately 40%)
  Cerebrospinal fluid glucose is not low in most (normal >60%)
  Mononuclear cell predominance is present in about one third of cases

deficits, cerebellar signs, and hemiparesis and/or hemisensory deficits. Nuchal rigidity is present in about one half; cerebrospinal (CSF) findings are only mildly abnormal, with a positive CSF culture in about 40%; and almost two thirds are bacteremic. Magnetic resonance imaging (MRI) is superior to computed tomography (CT) for demonstrating rhombencephalitis.

Brain Abscess

Macroscopic brain abscesses account for about 10% of CNS listerial infections. Bacteremia is almost always present, and concomitant meningitis with isolation of *L. monocytogenes* from the CSF is found in 25%; both of these features are rare in other forms of bacterial brain abscess. About one half of cases occur in known risk groups for listerial infections. Abscesses located in the thalamus, pons, and medulla are common; these sites are exceedingly rare when abscesses are caused by other bacteria.

Endocarditis

Listerial endocarditis accounts for about 7.5% of adult listerial infections, produces both native valve and prosthetic valve disease, and has a high rate of septic complications and a mortality of 48%. Listerial endocarditis, but not bacteremia per se, may be an indicator of underlying gastrointestinal tract pathology, including cancer.

Localized Infection

There are rare reports of focal infections involving skin, conjunctivae, bones, joints, and visceral organs. There is nothing clinically unique about these localized infections.

Gastroenteritis and Fever

Two recent outbreaks have provided convincing evidence that *L. monocytogenes,* when ingested in large quantities, can cause fever and diarrhea. One outbreak followed ingestion of contaminated chocolate milk and the other, contaminated corn salad. Fever, diarrhea, chills, and headache were the major symptoms. The incubation period averaged 20 hours, and the diarrheal illness lasted about 2 days. *L. monocytogenes* should be considered as a possible etiology of foodborne outbreaks of febrile gastroenteritis when routine stool cultures fail to identify a pathogen.

DIAGNOSIS

Listeriosis should be given strong consideration as part of the differential diagnosis in any of the following clinical settings:

- Neonatal sepsis or meningitis
- Meningitis or parenchymal brain infection in patients with hematologic malignancies, AIDS, organ transplantation, or corticosteroid immunosuppression
- Meningitis or parenchymal brain infection in adults older than 50 years of age
- Simultaneous infection of meninges and brain parenchyma
- Subcortical brain abscess
- Fever during pregnancy, particularly in the third trimester
- Blood, CSF, or other normally sterile specimen reported to have "diphtheroids" on Gram stain or culture
- Foodborne outbreak of febrile gastroenteritis when routine cultures fail to identify a pathogen

In clinical specimens, the organisms may be Gram variable and look like diphtheroids, cocci, or diplococci. Laboratory misidentification as diphtheroids, streptococci, or enterococci is not uncommon, and the isolation of a "diphtheroid" from blood or CSF always should alert one to the possibility that the organism is really *L. monocytogenes*. Antibodies to listerial-specific antigens have not proved useful for the diagnosis of invasive disease but may be helpful in identifying those with noninvasive disease (asymptomatic infection, gastroenteritis) during foodborne outbreaks. As mentioned, MRI is superior to CT for demonstrating parenchymal brain involvement, especially in the brainstem.

TREATMENT

There have been no controlled trials to establish a drug of choice or duration of therapy for listerial infection. Our guidelines appear in Table 2. Ampicillin is generally considered the preferred agent. Based on synergy demonstrated both in vitro and in animal models, most authorities suggest adding gentamicin to ampicillin for treatment of bacteremia in patients with severely impaired T-cell function and in all cases of CNS infection and endocarditis. In one uncontrolled study, the combination of trimethoprim-sulfamethoxazole (TMP-SMX) plus ampicillin was associated with a lower failure rate and fewer neurologic sequelae than ampicillin combined with an aminoglycoside.

For patients intolerant of penicillins, TMP-SMX as a single agent is thought to be the best alternative. Chloramphenicol, previously regarded as the agent of choice for penicillin-allergic patients, should not be used because of unacceptable failure and relapse rates.

Reports have documented the utility of erythromycin and tetracycline in isolated cases, but these agents are unreliable and should be avoided. Quinolones either do not have good in vitro activity or lack clinical data to support use. No currently available cephalosporin should be used; they have limited activity, and meningitis has developed in patients while receiving cephalosporins. Both imipenem and meropenem have been used successfully; because imipenem may produce seizures, meropenem is preferred.

Vancomycin has been used with success in a few penicillin-allergic patients, but others have developed listerial meningitis while receiving the drug. Rifampin is quite active in vitro and is known to penetrate into phagocytic cells; however, clinical experience is minimal, and in animal models, the addition of rifampin to ampicillin was not more effective than ampicillin alone.

Patients with CNS infection or endocarditis and a history of allergy to *both* penicillins and sulfonamides should be desensitized and treated with ampicillin rather than choosing another agent. A single initial dose of vancomycin could be given while performing desensitization.

Meningitis dosages should be used for all patients even in the absence of CNS or CSF abnormalities because of the high affinity of this organism for the CNS. Patients with meningitis should be treated for at least 3 weeks; bacteremic patients without CSF abnormalities can be treated for 2 weeks.

Patients with rhombencephalitis or brain abscess should be treated for at least 6 weeks and followed with serial MRI

Table 2 Intravenous Therapy of Listerial Infection				
SYNDROME	**ANTIBIOTIC***	**DOSAGE (PER DAY)**	**INTERVAL**	**MINIMUM DURATION**
Meningitis	Ampicillin plus Gentamicin	200 mg/kg 5 mg/kg	q4h q8h	3 wk
Brain abscess or rhombencephalitis	Ampicillin plus Gentamicin	200 mg/kg 5 mg/kg	q4h q8h	6 wk
Endocarditis	Ampicillin plus Gentamicin	200 mg/kg 5 mg/kg	q6h q8h	6 wk
Bacteremia	Ampicillin	200 mg/kg	q6h	2 wk

*Penicillin-allergic patients without endocarditis can be treated with trimethoprim-sulfamethoxazole alone, using 15 mg/kg of trimethoprim daily at 6- to 8-hour intervals. Patients with endocarditis should be desensitized to ampicillin and treated as above.

studies or CT scans. Endocarditis should be treated for 4 to 6 weeks.

Iron is a virulence factor for *L. monocytogenes*, and clinically, iron overload states are risk factors for listerial infection. Therefore, in patients with iron deficiency, it seems prudent to withhold iron replacement until treatment is completed.

Corticosteroids appear to be important adjunctive agents in treating the most common forms of bacterial meningitis. Their role in the treatment of listerial CNS infection is unknown, but they should probably be avoided because impairment of cellular immunity from corticosteroid therapy is a major risk factor for the development of listeriosis.

Suggested Reading

Cherubin CE, et al: Epidemiological spectrum and current treatment of listeriosis, *Rev Infect Dis* 13:1108, 1991.

Dalton CB, et al: An outbreak of gastroenteritis and fever due to *Listeria monocytogenes* in milk, *N Engl J Med* 336:100, 1997.

Farber JM, Peterkin PI: *Listeria monocytogenes*, a food-borne pathogen, *Microbiol Rev* 55:476, 1991.

Gellin BG, Broome CV: Listeriosis, *JAMA* 261:1313, 1989.

Hof H, Nichterlein T, Kretschmar M: Management of listeriosis, *Clin Microbiol Rev* 10:345, 1997.

Khayr WF, Cherubin CE, Bleck TP: Listeriosis: review of a protean disease, *Infect Dis Clin Pract* 1:291, 1992.

Lorber B: Listeriosis. State-of-the-art clinical article, *Clin Infect Dis* 24:1, 1997.

Nieman RE, Lorber B: Listeriosis in adults: a changing pattern. Report of eight cases and review of the literature, 1968-1978, *Rev Infect Dis* 2:207, 1980.

Schuchat A, Swaminathan B, Broome CV: Epidemiology of human listeriosis, *Clin Microbiol Rev* 4:169, 1991.

NOCARDIA

Lisa Haglund
George S. Deepe, Jr.

*N*ocardia species are soilborne bacteria that are aerobic and slow growing. In culture, they may require 2 to 4 weeks before colonies appear. Nocardia are gram-positive and weakly acid-fast filaments, 0.5 to 1.0 μ in diameter, that branch at right angles. Four nocardial species are pathogenic for humans: the *N. asteroides* group (which includes *N. nova* and *N. farcinica*), *N. brasiliensis*, *N. otitidiscaviarum* (*N. caviae*), and *N. transvalensis*.

Nocardiosis is typically a suppurative infection with multiple abscesses. It is rarely granulomatous and not fibrotic. Acquisition of infection is by the respiratory tract or by traumatic inoculation. Although *Nocardia* are ubiquitous, they rarely colonize the human respiratory tract. Accordingly, treatment should be initiated when *Nocardia* are repeatedly isolated from pulmonary specimens, particularly from an immunocompromised host. Antimicrobial therapy (alone or in combination with surgical drainage) is recommended, and the duration of therapy must be prolonged to prevent relapse.

Of patients with systemic nocardiosis, 50% to 75% possess underlying risk factors. Predisposing conditions are listed in Table 1. As the number of solid organ and bone marrow transplants increases, the incidence of nocardiosis has risen, particularly in those patients surviving more than 1 year after transplant. Nocardiosis remains an uncommon opportunistic complication of human immunodeficiency virus (HIV) infection. One explanation is that the prophylactic use of trimethoprim-sulfamethoxazole (TMP-SMX), pyrimethamine, or dapsone for *Pneumocystis carinii* prevents nocardiosis. However, this is not the case because the infection has developed in patients receiving these drugs.

■ PATHOGENESIS OF SYSTEMIC NOCARDIOSIS

Neutrophils inhibit the growth of *Nocardia*, but organisms are not killed until cell-mediated immunity is activated. If cellular immunity is impaired, the organism causes indolent abscesses and then slowly spreads to distant sites such as the brain or cerebrospinal fluid. Illness is usually subacute to chronic but may be fulminant in an immunocompromised host. Weight loss, anorexia, and fatigue are common in systemic nocardiosis.

Table 1 Risk Factors for Systemic Nocardiosis			
Chronic pulmonary disease	Solid organ transplantation	Systemic lupus erythematosus	Renal failure
Alcoholism	Bone marrow transplantation	Systemic vasculitis	Whipple's disease
Cirrhosis	Chronic corticosteroid use	Ulcerative colitis	Hypogammaglobulinemia
Lymphoreticular malignancy	Cushing's syndrome	Sarcoidosis	Human immunodeficiency virus infection

■ MYCETOMA, CUTANEOUS NOCARDIOSIS, TRAUMATIC NOCARDIOSIS

Nocardial species can cause mycetoma, which typically manifests as a swollen area with sinuses draining purulent material. Unlike other causes of mycetoma (botryomycosis and *Actinomyces israelii*), nocardial mycetoma may present without grain formation. Primary cutaneous nocardiosis manifests as nontender, red, irregularly shaped, raised lesions. Occasionally, these form sinuses and drain purulent material. Regional lymphadenopathy is occasionally observed. Nocardia arthritis usually presents as a monarthritis, commonly involving the knee. Disease is often inoculated through a puncture wound. Other inoculation nocardial infections described include postoperative wound infections (including mediastinitis after cardiac transplantation) and osteomyelitis.

■ PULMONARY NOCARDIOSIS

Pulmonary disease is apparent in 65% to 85% of systemic nocardial infections. The roentgenographic features include infiltrates that may cavitate, sometimes accompanied by empyema or pericarditis. There is no specific radiographic appearance; thus a high degree of suspicion must be maintained to make the diagnosis. Sputum cultures may be overgrown with other organisms before nocardia colonies appear. Therefore it may be helpful to notify the microbiology laboratory to hold cultures for *Nocardia*.

■ NOCARDIA MENINGITIS AND BRAIN ABSCESS

Central nervous system (CNS) nocardiosis is detected in 20% to 40% of systemic nocardial infections. Two thirds have clinical findings such as fever, headache, stiff neck, or altered mental status. Hypoglycorrhachia is found in two thirds of patients. Mildly elevated cerebrospinal fluid protein and a neutrophilic pleocytosis of approximately 1000 white blood cells are usually found. Nocardial brain abscess can be a complication of nocardial meningitis or can present in the absence of meningitis. Although meningitis without underlying brain abscess has been described, this is unusual and an underlying abscess should always be suspected. Because of the high incidence of CNS infection, an imaging study of the brain should be performed if any personality or neurologic changes are found during workup of systemic nocardiosis.

■ THERAPY OF NOCARDIOSIS: SULFONAMIDE THERAPY

Sulfonamides are currently the first-line agents for nocardiosis, and sulfadiazine, 6 to 8 g/day given intravenously (IV) or orally (PO), is a typical adult regimen. TMP-SMX is an alternative first-line treatment for nocardiosis, although it has never been shown to be superior to a sulfonamide alone. Table 2 summarizes typical dosages and durations of therapy for sulfonamide therapy of nocardiosis.

Sulfadiazine became a commonly used agent by 1940. As a short-acting sulfonamide with rapid absorption and prompt urinary excretion, it had to be given in large dosages for therapeutic effect. Unfortunately, with its low urinary solubility, there is a high incidence of crystalluria.

TMP-SMX is a well-absorbed combination agent with a long plasma half-life of 11 and 9 hours for TMP and SMX, respectively. It is available orally as single- or double-strength tablets (80 mg TMP plus 400 mg SMX, and 160 mg TMP plus 800 mg SMX, respectively) and as a liquid suspension containing 40 mg TMP plus 200 mg SMX per 5 ml. It is also available IV (5 ml = 80 mg TMP plus 400 mg SMX).

The most common side effects of TMP-SMX are upper gastrointestinal symptoms and skin rashes (3% to 4% each). Leukopenia, thrombocytopenia, and megaloblastic changes can develop rarely. Adverse effects of sulfonamide therapy include acute renal failure as a result of tubular damage from sulfa crystalluria. This effect may be prevented by adequate hydration and by alkalinizing the urine. Hepatitis, intrahepatic cholestasis, pancreatitis, and aseptic meningitis have been reported with TMP-SMX. Serious adverse reactions are rare and include anaphylaxis and Stevens-Johnson syndrome, and hematologic effects include thrombocytopenia, leukopenia, and hemolytic anemia.

TMP-SMX and other sulfonamides should not be given to patients with a demonstrated deficiency of folic acid or glucose-6-phosphate dehydrogenase. In HIV-infected patients, there is an increased incidence of adverse reactions to TMP-SMX, including reversible hyperkalemia, and a severe hypersensitivity reaction with fever, hypotension, and multiorgan involvement on rechallenge with the drug 2 to 3 weeks after previous course of therapy.

■ OTHER AGENTS WITH ANTINOCARDIAL ACTIVITY

Susceptibility studies of *Nocardia* are technically difficult and are not standardized. Thus they are most reliable from an experienced laboratory. Speciation can also guide antimicrobial therapy because different species vary in in vitro susceptibilities (Table 3). The parenteral agents with greatest in vitro activity include imipenem-cilastatin (500 mg IV every 6 hours), amikacin (5 mg/kg IV every 8 hours), cefotaxime (2 g IV every 8 hours), or ceftriaxone (2 g IV every 12 hours) (Table 4). In vitro susceptibility does not uniformly correlate with clinical outcome in humans. With susceptible organisms, these agents have been as efficacious as sulfonamides in animal models; in fact, they may be more rapidly bactericidal than sulfonamides. So far, no large human case series has been published establishing clinical superiority of these alternative parenteral regimens to sulfonamide therapy, but case reports suggest these may be useful second-line therapy. In CNS nocardiosis, it is worthwhile to recall that seizures are a potential side effect of imipenem-cilastatin therapy.

Tetracyclines manifest excellent activity against nocardial species. Minocycline has the best in vitro activity among the tetracyclines and is given 300 mg orally twice daily for 3 to 6 months (see Table 4). Its drawbacks include poor cerebrospinal fluid penetration and side effects of vertigo, making it unsuitable for CNS nocardial disease. Although quinolones

Table 2   Sulfonamide Dosage and Duration of Therapy for Treatment of Nocardia

TYPE OF NOCARDIOSIS	DOSAGE (DIVIDED BID-QID)	DURATION	COMMENTS
Cutaneous	5-10 mg/kg/day TMP-SMX	6-12 wk	Longer for extensive disease or bony involvement as seen in mycetoma
Pulmonary	10 mg/kg/day TMP-SMX	3-6 mo	
Central nervous system	15 mg/kg/day TMP-SMX 50-100 mg/kg/day sulfadiazine	6 mo	6 mo minimum duration for immuno-compromised host

*TMP-SMX dosage based on mg/kg of the trimethoprim (TMP) component.

Table 3   Therapies for Nocardiosis Based on Species

NOCARDIA SPECIES	MAY BE SUSCEPTIBLE TO:	MAY BE RESISTANT TO:
N. asteroides and N. transvalensis	Sulfonamides, imipenem-cilastatin, or minocycline	—
N. brasiliensis	Amoxicillin-clavulanic acid	—
N. nova	Erythromycin or ampicillin	—
N. farcinica	Check susceptibilities	Third-generation cephalosporins or aminoglycosides (except amikacin)
N. otitidiscaviarum (N. caviae)	Check susceptibilities	Sulfonamides, imipenem-cilastatin

Table 4   Other Regimens for Treatment of *Nocardia*

DRUG	DOSAGE	DURATION	COMMENT
Minocycline	300 mg PO bid	3 to 6 mo	Useful for prolonged disease; poor central nervous system penetration
Imipenem-cilastatin	500 mg IV q6h	Until oral agent can be given	Dosage must be adjusted for renal failure
Ceftriaxone	2 g IV q12h	Until oral agent can be given	
Cefotaxime	2 g IV q8h	Until oral agent can be given	
Amikacin	5 mg/kg IV q8h	Until oral agent can be given	Nephrotoxic; dosage must be adjusted for renal failure

show some in vitro activity, MIC-90s for most nocardial species are higher than achievable serum concentrations, and few patients with systemic nocardiosis have received quinolones therapeutically.

Suggested Reading

Bross JE, Gordon G: Nocardial meningitis: case reports and review, *Rev Infect Dis* 13:160, 1991.

Palmer DL, Harvey RL, and Wheeler JK: Diagnostic and therapeutic considerations in *Nocardia asteroides* infections, *Medicine* 53:391, 1974.

Smego RA Jr, Moeller MB, Gallis HA: Trimethoprim-sulfamethoxazole therapy for nocardia infections, *Arch Intern Med* 143:711, 1983.

Uttamchandani RB, et al: Nocardiosis in 30 patients with advanced human immunodeficiency virus infection: clinical features and outcome, *Clin Infect Dis* 18:348, 1994.

Wallace RJ Jr, et al: Antimicrobial susceptibility patterns of *Nocardia asteroides*, *Antimicrob Agents Chemother* 32:1776, 1998.

PASTEURELLA MULTOCIDA

David S. Stephens
Molly E. Eaton

*P*asteurella multocida ("killer of many species") is a gram-negative, pleomorphic coccobacillus best known for its association with infections due to animal bites. However, this organism can cause many human infections, some of which can be life-threatening.

P. multocida is found worldwide. It commonly colonizes the upper respiratory tract of many animals, most notably cats (70% to 90%), but also dogs (50% to 66%), pigs, rats, opossums, birds, reindeer, cattle, buffalo, monkeys, wolves, Tasmanian devils, and camels. It causes a number of diseases in animals, including pneumonia in sheep and goats, hemorrhagic septicemia (shipping fever) in cattle, fowl cholera in birds, and snuffles in rabbits. Human infection is usually related to animal exposure. Direct inoculation by a bite or scratch is the most common mode of transmission of *P. multocida* to humans. Inoculation can also occur by nontraumatic animal contact, as when a wound is licked by an animal. The second mode of transmission is by colonization of the human respiratory tract occurring with exposure to animals such as nuzzling or grooming of pets. The organism has been cultured from the respiratory tract of healthy veterinary workers and animal handlers as well as from ill patients. Infection also occasionally occurs with no history of animal contact.

Identification of *P. multocida* in the microbiology laboratory can sometimes be a problem. On Gram stain, *Pasteurella* can resemble *Haemophilus* species, *Neisseria* species, or other gram-negative bacilli. However, differential growth on selective media and the results of biochemical tests should allow proper identification.

■ CLINICAL PRESENTATION

Infections caused by *P. multocida* can be divided into three groups: bite wound infections, infections of the respiratory tract, and invasive infection.

■ BITE WOUND INFECTION

Bite wounds account for 60% to 86% of *P. multocida* infections. *P. multocida* is found as a pathogen in 75% of infected cat bites and in up to 50% of infected dog bites. Most of the bite wounds grow multiple organisms. Infection with *P. multocida* is characterized by extremely rapid onset. Local pain and inflammation often occur within 4 to 6 hours of the injury and almost always within 24 hours. Purulent drainage is present in 40% and lymphangitis in 20%, but fever and systemic symptoms are usually absent. Abscesses can develop. Rapid inflammatory reaction with no fever should prompt the clinician to suspect *P. multocida* in a bite wound infection.

Bite wound infections with *P. multocida* can lead to serious sequelae, even with aggressive and appropriate antibiotic and surgical management. Tendon sheath infection (tenosynovitis) is a common complication. Osteomyelitis often results from cat bites, probably because the deep punctures may penetrate the periosteum. Poor functional outcome is common with these infections, especially when they involve the extremities. In patients with risk factors for invasive infections as discussed subsequently, an apparently insignificant and uninfected wound may be associated with serious sequelae weeks later.

■ RESPIRATORY TRACT INFECTION

Respiratory tract infection is a second, but much less common, type of infection seen with *P. multocida*. The organism may cause bronchitis, pneumonia, empyema, sinusitis, epiglottitis, and otitis media. Patients almost always have some underlying respiratory illness, such as chronic obstructive pulmonary disease, bronchiectasis, chronic sinusitis, or pulmonary neoplasm. These patients may do well once appropriate antibiotic therapy is instituted, but the outcome is closely related to the severity of the underlying illness.

■ INVASIVE OR DISSEMINATED INFECTION

Rarely, invasive or disseminated infection occurs with *P. multocida*. These infections spread hematogenously from wounds or from pulmonary colonization. Invasive infections generally occur in the very old, in the very young, during pregnancy, in patients with liver disease, or in other conditions of immune compromise. They may occur long after animal contact, but usually there is some history of exposure.

Septic arthritis, unlike osteomyelitis, is more common from hematogenous spread than direct inoculation. Often, the affected joint is proximal to but not contiguous with an inoculation site. The joints most commonly involved are prosthetic joints and those already affected by arthritides.

Meningitis caused by *P. multocida* is reported in several series; 50% of patients are less than a year old, and 30% are older than 60 years of age. Patients present with the classic symptoms of meningitis. Cerebrospinal fluid examination usually shows a neutrophilic pleocytosis and low glucose. The organism can be seen on Gram stain in 50% to 80% percent but is usually mistaken for *Haemophilus influenzae* or *Neisseria meningitidis*. Once appropriate antibiotics are started, the prognosis depends on the patient's underlying condition.

Bacteremia is documented in 20% to 30% of invasive infections with a known source and also occurs with no apparent focus. Liver dysfunction, solid tumors, and leukemias are risk factors for bacteremia. The fatality rate is as high as 30% to 35% in patients with cirrhosis and bacteremia.

Peritonitis may occur in patients with liver disease. In some cases, it may be related to endoscopic procedures that transfer the organism from the upper respiratory tract to the gastrointestinal tract with deranged mucosal integrity (e.g., bleeding varices). It has also been reported in several patients on peritoneal dialysis whose cats bit or licked the dialysis tubing. Other serious infections caused by *P. multocida* include endocarditis, pyelonephritis, subdural empyema, mycotic aneurysm, vascular graft infection, endophthalmitis, appendiceal abscess, liver abscess, chorioamnionitis, neonatal sepsis, and chronic ulceration of the penis.

■ THERAPY

Antibiotics

In general, the antibiotic of choice for treatment of *P. multocida* infections is penicillin. Human infection with *P. multocida* resistant to penicillin is rarely reported, but 20% to 30% of bovine and porcine species are resistant. Therefore antibiotic susceptibility testing should be performed. Ampicillin and the other penicillin derivatives are also effective, but the semisynthetic penicillins such as oxacillin and nafcillin have variable efficacy. Third-generation cephalosporins and most second-generation cephalosporins are very effective, but the first-generation cephalosporins and cefaclor are not reliable, especially in oral doses. *P. multocida* is uniformly sensitive to tetracycline and chloramphenicol. Many strains are resistant to erythromycin, especially at levels achievable with oral dosing. Most strains are only moderately sensitive to aminoglycosides and are universally resistant to clindamycin and vancomycin. Fluoroquinolones, azithromycin, clarithromycin, and trimethoprim-sulfamethoxazole (TMP-SMX) have good in vitro activity. Clinical experience with these agents is limited, but they are options for patients with allergies to penicillin and cephalosporins who cannot take tetracycline. Tables 1 and 2 show appropriate antibiotics and doses.

Prophylactic Antibiotic Therapy for Bite Wounds

The value of "prophylactic" antibiotic therapy is unclear. The decision to prescribe antibiotics at the time of injury depends on the risk of infection, which can be assessed by the criteria in Table 3. Additional specific risk factors for *P. multocida* are listed in Table 4. In general, if a wound shows no sign of infection after 24 hours, *P. multocida* infection is unlikely to develop. However, for individuals with underlying risk factors and bites at risk for *P. multocida* infection, prophylaxis is reasonable even if they present late. For further discussion of the management of bite wounds, see the chapter *Human and Animal Bites*.

Treatment of Infected Wounds

Infected wounds should have deep cultures performed before the initiation of therapy. Surgical evaluation should be performed as necessary, especially when joints or extremities are involved or when there is extensive tissue damage. If infection with intense local inflammation develops within 24 hours, *P. multocida* should be strongly suspected. Because

Table 1   Antibiotic Susceptibilities of *Pasteurella multocida*

USUALLY SUSCEPTIBLE	VARIABLE	USUALLY RESISTANT
Penicillin and derivatives	Semisynthetic penicillins	Vancomycin
Ampicillin (± sulbactam)	Oxacillin	Clindamycin
Amoxicillin (± clavulanate)	Dicloxacillin	Erythromycin (oral)
Ticarcillin (± clavulanate)	Cloxacillin	
Piperacillin (± tazobactam)	Nafcillin	
Second- and third-generation cephalosporins*	Cefaclor	
Cefuroxime	First-generation cephalosporins	
Cefotetan	Cephalexin	
Cefoxitin	Cefazolin	
Cefixime†	Cephradine	
Cefprozil†	Cefadroxil	
Loracarbel†	Erythromycin (IV)	
Cefpodoxime†	Aminoglycocides	
Ceftriaxone	Gentamicin	
Ceftizoxime	Tobramycin	
Cefotaxime	Amikacin	
Ceftazidime		
Ciprofloxacin†		
Trimethoprim-sulfamethoxazole†		
Aztreonam		
Imipenem		
Tetracycline		
Doxycycline		
Chloramphenicol		

*Cefaclor, an oral second-generation cephalosporin, is often not effective.
†There are few clinical data on the use of these agents but by in vitro testing they should be effective.

Table 2 Doses of the Most Efficacious Agents for Treatment of *Pasteurella multocida*

AGENT	ORAL	PARENTERAL
Penicillin V	500-750 mg q6h	
Penicillin G		10 million to 20 million units/day divided q4h
Amoxicillin (± clavulanate)	250-500 mg q6h	
Ampicillin	250-500 mg q6h	1-2g q4-6h
Ampicillin-sulbactam		1.5-3 g q6h
Ticarcillin-clavulanate		3.1 g q4-8h
Piperacillin		3-4 g q4-6h
Cefuroxime	250-500 g q12h	750 mg-1.5 g q8h
Cefoxitin		1-2 g q4-8h
Cefotaxime		1-2 g q4-8h
Ceftriaxone		1-2 g q24h
Ciprofloxacin	500-750 mg q12h	400 mg q12h
TMP-SMX	160 mg TMP (1 DS tab) bid	10 mg/kg/day TMP divided q6-12h
Aztreonam		500 mg-2 g q6-12h
Imipenem		500 mg-1 g q6-8h
Tetracycline	250-500 mg q6h	500 mg-1 g q12h
Doxycycline	100-200 mg q12h	100-200 mg q12h
Chloramphenicol	12.5-25 mg/kg q6h	12.5-25 mg/kg q6h

TMP-SMX, Trimethoprim-sulfamethoxazole; DS, double strength.

Table 3 Risk Factors for Wound Infection

	HIGH	LOW
Type of wound	Puncture Crush injury Foreign material introduced	Laceration No contamination
Species of animal	Cat, pig, bovine	Dog, rodent
Delay before presentation	>8 hr	<6 hr >48-72 hr, no infection yet
Management before presentation	Poor cleaning	Good cleaning
Site of wound	Extremity, especially hand	Trunk, buttocks, head, minor facial wounds
Patient characteristics	>55 yr or <1 yr of age Immune compromise Liver disease	No underlying disease

Table 4 Risk Factors for *Pasteurella multocida* Infection

WOUND	PATIENT
Deep puncture	<1 yr or >55 yr of age
Feline, porcine	Liver disease, especially cirrhosis
Deep feline scratch	Solid tumors, leukemias
	Immune modulating medications
	Chronic respiratory disease
	Collagen-vascular disease
	Pregnancy
	Artificial heart valve
	History of cranial trauma or surgery

the rate of serious sequelae is high, the clinician should have a low threshold for admission and surgical consultation. If infection develops only after 24 to 48 hours, gram-positive organisms are more likely to be the cause, and therapy should be directed toward *Staphylococcus, Streptococcus* species, and anaerobes. However, if the patient has underlying risk factors for *P. multocida* infection, coverage for that organism should be included in the regimen. Table 1 shows the antibiotics of choice for *P. multocida*. Uncomplicated cellulitis should be treated for 7 to 10 days, but more complicated wound infections may require longer treatment. The same antibiotics are appropriate for therapy at the time of the bite; however, if no infection develops, the duration of therapy should be only 3 to 5 days.

Therapy for Other *P. multocida* Infections

The most important factor in successful treatment of other *P. multocida* infections is suspicion of the organism. A history of animal contact should always be obtained and the patient examined carefully for signs of even minor trauma. Gram stains of wounds or purulent collections are positive in up to 50% of cases. If *P. multocida* infection is a possibility, therapy should be initiated with a penicillin or a third-generation cephalosporin. Tetracycline, fluoroquinolones, and TMP-SMX are alternatives if beta-lactam allergy is present. In the case of meningitis in the patient allergic to cephalosporins, chloramphenicol can be used. Once antibiotic susceptibilities have been ascertained, therapy can be narrowed. As with other suppurative infections, purulent collections should be drained. The optimal duration of treatment for respiratory and invasive infections has not been defined, but it is usually similar to that of other bacterial infections of the same site and should be guided by clinical response.

Suggested Reading

Goldstein EJC: Bite wounds and infection, *Clin Infect Dis* 14:633, 1992.

Kumar A, Devlin HR, Vellend H: *Pasteurella multocida* meningitis in an adult: case report and review of the literature, *Rev Infect Dis* 12:440, 1990.

McDonough JJ, Stern PJ, Alexander JW: Management of animal and human bites and resulting human infections, *Curr Clin Top Infect Dis* 8:11, 1987.

Raffi F, et al: *Pasteurella multocida* bacteremia: report of 13 cases over 12 years and review of the literature, *Scand J Infect Dis* 19:385, 1987.

Talan DA, et al: Bacteriologic analysis of infected dog and cat bites, *N Engl J Med* 340:85, 1999.

Weber DJ, Hansen AR: Infections resulting from animal bites, *Infect Dis Clin North Am* 5:663, 1991.

Weber DJ, et al: *Pasteurella multocida* infections: report of 34 cases and review of the literature, *Medicine* 63:133, 1984.

PNEUMOCOCCUS

Maurice A. Mufson

Infections caused by *Streptococcus pneumoniae* (the pneumococcus) hold major importance today because of (1) continuing high rates of occurrence, especially among infants and very young children and elderly adults; (2) persistently high case fatality rates, especially in invasive infections; (3) rapidly evolving penicillin-resistant (PRSP) and multidrug-resistant (MDRP) isolates of the pneumococcus during the last 2 decades; (4) the availability and use of an effective polyvalent polysaccharide vaccine; and (5) the development of conjugated pneumococcal vaccines for use in infants and children. Pneumococcal pneumonia ranks first among community-acquired pneumonias; pneumococcal meningitis ranks second among bacterial meningitides; and pneumococcal otitis media predominates among cases of otitis in infants and children.

The dilemma physicians face in the treatment of pneumococcal illnesses encompasses two aspects: (1) rapid identification of pneumococcus as the pathogen, especially for invasive disease, and (2) selection of an appropriate initial antibiotic regimen that covers susceptible, PRSP, and MDRP isolates before culture results become known. Usually pneumococcal pneumonia can be suspected only on the basis of clinical and epidemiologic findings. A Gram stain of sputum adds a modest degree of confidence in establishing the diagnosis. Lacking definitive laboratory evidence of invasive pneumococcal infection, namely a positive blood culture, the treatment of community-acquired pneumococcal pneumonia (or any community-acquired pneumonia) can be approached by initiating empiric antibiotic therapy according to the guidelines of the American Thoracic Society (ATS) and Infectious Diseases Society of America (IDSA). These guidelines provide a framework for promptly selecting an appropriate antibiotic regimen in advance of the results of blood cultures and antibiotic sensitivity tests.

By contrast, a diagnosis of pneumococcal meningitis can be confirmed during the initial examination of the patient by a Gram stain of cerebrospinal fluid. Other available techniques for testing cerebrospinal fluid include the capsular swelling technique with polyvalent pneumococcal capsular antiserum (omniserum from the Danish Statens Serum Institut in Copenhagen) and immunoelectrophoresis. Antibiotics specific for the treatment of pneumococcal meningitis can be administered from the outset. However, the possibility that a PRSP or MDRP isolate caused the meningitis should influence the physician's choices of antibiotics (see the following).

No means exist for determining whether a serious pneumococcal infection is caused by PRSP or MDRP at the time a treatment decision must be made. When PRSP or MDRP causes infection, prompt and appropriate antibiotic treatment remains crucial to a successful outcome. Knowledge of the epidemiologic patterns of PRSP and MDRP in a community can assist in judging the likelihood of a resistant infection. During the 1990s, the occurrence of PRSP and MDRP increased substantially throughout many communities in the United States. PRSP and MDRP infections pose a major threat to the effective treatment of pneumococcal infections, especially isolates that exhibit high resistance to penicillin. Pneumococcal isolates highly resistant to penicillin usually show resistance to several other antibiotics, which further limits treatment options.

The issues of treatment of PRSP and MDRP also signal the importance of preventing serious pneumococcal infection in high-risk persons. The current polyvalent vaccine composed of 23 capsular polysaccharides induces anticapsular antibody sufficient to provide a protective efficacy rate of about 75% in immunocompetent persons. Widely used, pneumococcal vaccine can protect high-risk persons. Infants and children younger than 2 years of age respond poorly to the vaccine. They respond well to conjugate vaccines consisting of a protein carrier and pneumococcal capsular polysaccharides specific for this age group. Conjugate vaccine induces high levels of anticapsular antibody in infants and children; one such vaccine became licensed recently for use in children 2 years and younger.

■ INFECTIONS CAUSED BY PNEUMOCOCCUS

Pneumonia

Pneumococcal pneumonia, the most common infection caused by pneumococcus and the most common community-acquired pneumonia, is accompanied by bacteremia in about one fifth of cases. Bacteremic infections need to be treated promptly and aggressively. The incidence of bacteremic pneumococcal pneumonia is highest in children younger than 4 years of age and adults 60 years of age and older. In children younger than 4 years of age, the incidence of bacteremic pneumococcal pneumonia is about 45 to 60 cases per 100,000 population, and in adults 60 years of age and older, it ranges from 27 to 76 cases per 100,000 population. The case fatality rate in bacteremic pneumococcal pneumonia among adults older than 50 years of age varies between 15% and 25%, depending on the population at risk; it increases with each decade. Nonbacteremic pneumococcal pneumonia holds little risk of death; it carries a case fatality rate of less than 4%. Blood cultures must be done to assess the invasive nature of the infection; a single set of cultures obtained before the start of antibiotic treatment is adequate to isolate the organism.

When a definitive diagnosis of pneumococcal pneumonia can be made by diagnostic tests, including recognition of the pneumococcus in Gram smear of expectorated sputum or isolation of the organism from the blood or pleural fluid, the physician can select appropriate antibiotic treatment (Table 1). The first-line recommendation for adults infected with a penicillin-susceptible isolate and a mild or moderate pneumonia, for example in a young adult, that can be treated on an ambulatory basis, is amoxicillin-clavulanate, 875 mg orally twice daily for 7 to 10 days. Adults, especially elderly adults, with more severe pneumonia requiring hospitalization, need to be treated with penicillin G, 2 million U every 4 hours intravenously (IV), plus a macrolide, such as erythromycin, 500 mg orally twice daily. However, until the organism can be tested for antibiotic sensitivity, the physician must gauge the likelihood that a PRSP or MDRP isolate caused the infection and choose an antibiotic regimen accordingly (see Table 1). Importantly, invasive pneumococcal pneumonia caused by intermediate PRSP isolates can be successively treated with penicillin G, 2 million U every 2 hours, or amoxicillin-clavulanate, 875 mg orally twice daily or ceftriaxone or cefotaxime. Although infections with highly penicillin-resistant isolates might respond to very high dosages of penicillin G, the prudent approach dictates treatment with antibiotics other than penicillin. In these cases, the clinician should treat with ceftriaxone, 1 to 2 g every 24 hours IV/IM, or cefotaxime, 1 to 2 g every 6 hours IV/IM, plus either a newer macrolide, such as

Table 1   Recommendations for the Treatment of Proved Pneumococcal Pneumonia When a Culture Is Positive

SENSITIVITY TEST RESULTS	SEVERITY OF PNEUMONIA	ANTIBIOTIC CHOICE	RECOMMENDED TREATMENT SCHEDULE	ALL ANTIBIOTIC OPTIONS
Susceptible	Ambulatory treatment (less severe, younger person)	First-line	Amoxicillin-clavulanate, 875 mg bid ×7-10 days orally	Penicillin orally or amoxicillin-clavulanate
		Second-line	Erythromycin, 250 mg q6h orally ×7-10 days, or clarithromycin, 500 bid orally ×7-14 days	Macrolide, such as erythromycin or clarithromycin or an oral fluoroquinolone, such as levofloxacin or sparfloxacin
	In-hospital treatment (more severe, older adult, >60 yr)	First-line	Penicillin, 2 million U q4h IV ×7-10 days, *plus* erythromycin, 500 mg bid orally or IV	Penicillin G or amoxicillin-clavulanate *plus* erythromycin or a newer macrolide
		Second-line	Levofloxacin, 500 mg q24h IV	Other newer oral fluoroquinolone, such as sparfloxacin
PRSP/MDRP	Ambulatory treatment (less severe younger person)	First-line	Clarithromycin, 500 mg bid orally ×7-14 days	Newer macrolide, such as azithromycin or clarithromycin or a second-generation oral cephalosporin
		Second-line	Levofloxacin, 500 mg daily orally ×7-10 days	Newer oral fluoroquinolone, such as levofloxacin or sparfloxacin
	In-hospital treatment (more severe, older adult >60 yr)	First-line	Ceftriaxone, 1-2 g q24h IV, *plus* clarithromycin, 500 mg bid orally	Third-generation cephalosporin, such as ceftriaxone or cefotaxime, *plus* newer macrolide, such as azithromycin or clarithromycin
		Second-line	Ceftriaxone, 1-2 g q24h IV, *plus* levofloxacin, 500 mg q24h IV	Third-generation cephalosporin, such as ceftriaxone or cefotaxime, *plus* a newer fluoroquinolone, such as levofloxacin or sparfloxacin

PRSP, Penicillin-resistant *Streptococcus pneumoniae; MDRP,* multidrug-resistant pneumonia.

clarithromycin, 500 mg orally twice daily, or azithromycin, 500 mg IV daily, or a fluoroquinolone such as levofloxacin, 500 mg daily IV or orally.

When culture results are not available, the treatment of a presumed pneumococcal pneumonia follows the guidelines for the empiric treatment of community-acquired pneumonia (Table 2). Usually, the person at highest risk of adverse outcome and presumed invasive infection should be treated with two antibiotics, namely a third-generation cephalosporin and a macrolide. Several regimens can be used; for example, ceftriaxone, 1 to 2 g every 24 hours IV, or cefotaxime, 1 to 2 g every 6 hours IV, plus azithromycin, 500 mg daily IV (and changed to orally after a few days), or erythromycin, 500 mg every 6 hours orally or IV, or clarithromycin, 500 mg orally twice daily for 7 to 10 days (see Table 2). As the patient improves, cephalosporin antibiotics administered IV can be changed to an appropriate oral cephalosporin, such as cefuroxime-axetil.

Meningitis

Pneumococcal meningitis, the second most common bacterial meningitis, occurs mainly in older adults; in adults older than 50 years of age, the incidence is about 1 to 3.5 cases per 100,000 population. It is fatal in about 10% to 60% of cases, depending on the adult population studied. The highest case fatality rates occur in persons older than 50 years of age. Among children, the case fatality rate is low, 6% to 15%, but substantially higher than the case fatality rate in bacteremic pneumococcal pneumonia.

Meningitis needs to be recognized immediately and treated quickly and appropriately. Confirmation of pneumococcal meningitis can be done in almost all cases by recognition of the typical morphology of *Streptococcus pneumoniae* on a Gram smear of cerebrospinal fluid. Lacking a positive Gram smear, another rapid diagnostic test, such as immunoelectrophoresis, may be used.

Children and adults infected with a penicillin-susceptible isolate should be treated with penicillin, 4 million U every 24 hours IV. When a PRSP/MDRP infection is suspected or proved in children, the treatment includes a third-generation cephalosporin, such as ceftriaxone, 200 m/kg/day IV, plus vancomycin, 15 mg/kg/day every 6 hours IV (and dexamethasone, 0.4 mg/kg every 12 hours for 2 days). Among adults with a suspected or proved PRSP or MDRP meningitis, the treatment includes a third-generation cephalosporin, such as ceftriaxone, 2 g every 12 hours IV, plus vancomycin, 15 mg/kg daily (Table 3). Vancomycin should be used only when a PRSP or MDRP infection is suspected or proved; indiscriminate use of vancomycin can encourage the emergence of resistant isolates. If dexamethasone is added to the treatment regimen of an adult, rifampin, 600 mg daily IV or orally, should be given in lieu of vancomycin.

Otitis Media

Streptococcus pneumoniae ranks among the top three common pathogens of acute otitis media (AOM) in children (with *Haemophilus influenzae* and *Moraxella catarrhalis*). PRSP and MDRP also represent an increasing problem in the treatment of otitis media. In children with a penicillin-susceptible pneumococcal AOM, amoxicillin, 80

Table 2 Recommendations for the Treatment of Presumed Pneumococcal Pneumonia on a Empiric Basis before Diagnostic Tests or Culture Results Become Positive

SENSITIVITY TEST RESULTS	SEVERITY OF PNEUMONIA	ANTIBIOTIC CHOICE	RECOMMENDED TREATMENT SCHEDULE	RECOMMENDED ANTIBIOTIC OPTIONS
Susceptible or PRSP/MDRP	Ambulatory treatment (less severe, younger person)	First-line	Azithromycin, 500 mg day 1; days 2-5, 250 mg orally; or clarithromycin, 500 bid orally ×7-14 days	Newer macrolide, such as azithromycin or clarithromycin
		Second-line	Levofloxacin, 500 mg daily orally ×7-10 days	Newer macrolide, such as azithromycin or clarithromycin or a second-generation oral cephalosporin or newer oral fluoroquinolone, such as levofloxacin or sparfloxacin
	In-hospital treatment (more severe, older adult, >60 yr)	First-line	Ceftriaxone, 1-2 g q24h IV, *plus* clarithromycin, 500 mg bid orally, or azithromycin, 500 mg daily IV	Third-generation cephalosporin, such as ceftriaxone or cefotaxime or a cephalosporin with antipseudomonal activity, such as ceftazidime *plus* a newer macrolide, such as azithromycin or clarithromycin
		Second-line	Ceftriaxone, 1-2 g q24h IV, *plus* levofloxacin, 500 mg q24h IV	Third-generation cephalosporin, such as ceftriaxone or cefotaxime or a cephalosporin with antipseudomonal activity, such as ceftazidime *plus* newer oral fluoroquinolone, such as levofloxacin or sparfloxacin

PRSP, Penicillin-resistant *Streptococcus pneumoniae; MDRP,* multidrug-resistant *Streptococcus pneumoniae.*

Table 3　Recommendations for the Treatment of Pneumococcal Meningitis

SENSITIVITY TEST RESULTS	AGE GROUP	ANTIBIOTIC CHOICE	RECOMMENDED TREATMENT SCHEDULE	RECOMMENDED ANTIBIOTIC OPTIONS
Susceptible	Child	First-line	Penicillin G, 4 million U q4h IV	Penicillin G
	Child	Second-line*	Vancomycin, 15 mg/kg/day, and rifampin, 600 mg daily IV or orally	Vancomycin and rifampin; or chloramphenicol
	Adult	First-line	Penicillin G, 4 million U q4h IV	Penicillin G
	Adult	Second-line*	Vancomycin, 15 mg/kg/day, and rifampin, 600 mg daily IV or orally	Vancomycin and rifampin
PRSP/MDRP	Child	First-line	Ceftriaxone, 200 mg/kg/day IV, *plus* vancomycin, 15 mg/kg/day q6h IV (and dexamethasone, 0.4 mg/kg q12h ×2 days)	Third-generation cephalosporin, such as ceftriaxone or cefotaxime *plus* vancomycin (and dexamethasone)
	Adult	First-line	Ceftriaxone, 2 g q12h IV, *plus* vancomycin, 15 mg/kg/day (or rifampin, 600 mg daily IV or orally if dexamethasone given)	Third-generation cephalosporin, such as ceftriaxone or cefotaxime, *plus* vancomycin (or rifampin, if dexamethasone given)

PRSP, Penicillin-resistant *Streptococcus pneumoniae*; MDRP, multidrug-resistant *Streptococcus pneumoniae*.
*This treatment schedule for penicillin-allergic persons.

mg/kg/day, remains first-line therapy; other treatment regimens (especially for children who fail amoxicillin) include amoxicillin-clavulanate, 45 mg/kg/day; oral cefuroxime-axetil; or IM ceftriaxone, 50 mg daily. When PRSP or MDRP are suspected, the clinician should treat with amoxicillin-clavulanate or IM ceftriaxone.

In adults, AOM can be treated with amoxicillin-clavulanate, erythromycin, one of the newer macrolides, or sulfamethoxazole-trimethoprim. When PRSP or MDRP are likely, a macrolide should be used.

Pneumococcal Polysaccharide Vaccine

The currently licensed 23-valent pneumococcal polysaccharide received approval for general use in 1983 for administration to persons at high risk of serious pneumococcal infection. Safe and cost-effective, pneumococcal vaccine should be offered to all persons age 65 years and older, persons resident in nursing homes or other chronic care facilities, all immunocompetent persons age 2 years and older with underlying disease (e.g., heart and lung diseases, renal disease, and diabetes mellitus) that place them at increased risk of serious pneumococcal pneumonia, and all immunocompromised persons, including those with functional and anatomic asplenia, lymphoma, leukemia, and human immunodeficiency disease (HIV). The 23 vaccine types account for about 90% of invasive disease in the United States. Repeat doses of vaccine are recommended for persons 65 years of age and older who received the first dose of vaccine before 65 years of age and at least 5 years earlier, persons who received only the 14-valent vaccine, and those undergoing chronic renal hemodialysis. Antibody wanes in time in all adults, and second doses of vaccine provide satisfactory booster responses. A repeat dose of vaccine about 7 years after the first dose of 23-valent vaccine should be considered for elderly patients at high risk for serious pneumococcal disease.

Immunocompetent children age 2 years and younger fail to develop adequate antibody responses to the 23-valent vaccine. They should be immunized with a protein-conjugated pneumococcal vaccine specific for this age group.

Suggested Reading

Bartlett JG, et al: Community-acquired pneumonia in adults: guidelines for management, *Clin Infect Dis* 26:811, 1998.

Mufson MA, Stanek RJ: Bacteremic pneumococcal pneumonia in one American city: a twenty-year longitudinal study, 1978-1997, *Am J Med* 107:34S, 1999.

Niederman MS, et al: Guidelines for the initial management of adults with community-acquired pneumonia: diagnosis, assessment of severity, and initial antimicrobial therapy, *Am Rev Respir Dis* 148:1418, 1993.

Stanek RJ, Mufson MA: A 20-year epidemiological study of pneumococcal meningitis, *Clin Infect Dis* 28:1265, 1999.

PSEUDOMONAS

Barbara Menzies
David W. Gregory

Infections with *Pseudomonas* species cause substantial morbidity and mortality and are difficult to treat. *Pseudomonas aeruginosa,* an aerobic, gram-negative rod and the fifth most frequently isolated nosocomial pathogen, commonly causes pneumonia, bacteremia, urinary tract infections, and surgical wound infections (Table 1). Two related species, *Stenotrophomonas maltophila* and *Burkholderia cepacia,* are briefly discussed here.

■ EPIDEMIOLOGY

The epidemiology of *P. aeruginosa* infections reflects its predilection for moist environments. In hospitals, *P. aeruginosa* has been isolated from respiratory devices, disinfectants, distilled and tap water, and sinks. *P. aeruginosa* can readily colonize the upper respiratory tract of mechanically ventilated patients, burn wounds, and the gastrointestinal tract of patients receiving chemotherapy or broad-spectrum antibiotics. Colonization usually precedes tissue invasion.

■ ANTIMICROBIAL THERAPY

Although several antipseudomonal antibiotics exist (Table 2), intrinsic or acquired drug resistance and bacterial persistence at sites of infection complicate management and eradication. Beta-lactam antibiotics active against *P. aeruginosa* include the extended-spectrum penicillins, some third-generation cephalosporins, the carbapenems, and the monobactam aztreonam. Newer agents such as meropenem and cefepime may be useful in treating multidrug-resistant strains. Initial selection of an agent should be guided by the site of infection, the patient's allergic history, and the institutional antibiogram, if known. Subsequent modification may be based on the susceptibility profile of the isolate.

The aminoglycosides gentamicin, tobramycin, and amikacin have excellent in vitro activity against *P. aeruginosa.* The concentration-dependent bactericidal activity and the postantibiotic effect of aminoglycosides provide the rationale for single daily dosing (i.e., high dosages of aminoglycoside at extended intervals). Renal function and serum aminoglycoside levels should be monitored.

The quinolones have become increasingly important, given their excellent activity against *P. aeruginosa* and other bacteria, excellent tissue penetration, good oral bioavailability, and safety profile. Ciprofloxacin is still the most active quinolone against *P. aeruginosa,* although others such as trovafloxacin, sparfloxacin, and levofloxacin have moderately good activity.

Table 1   Risk Factors for *P. aeruginosa* Infections

TYPE OF INFECTION	SETTING
Bacteremia	Neutropenia, pulmonary or urinary tract focus, burn wound
Pneumonia	Mechanical ventilation, neutropenia, cystic fibrosis
Endocarditis	Intravenous drug abuse, prosthetic heart valve
Meningitis, brain abscess	Hematogenous or contiguous spread, neurosurgery, penetrating head trauma
Urinary tract infection	Bladder instrumentation
Osteomyelitis, septic arthritis	Contiguous or hematogenous spread, intravenous drug use (e.g., sternoclavicular joint)
Osteochondritis	Puncture wounds of the feet
Malignant external otitis	Advanced age, diabetes
Green nail syndrome	Wet skin, water immersion

Table 2   Antimicrobial Agents for *P. aeruginosa**

BETA-LACTAMS	QUINOLONES
Piperacillin, 3-4 g IV q4-6h, with tazobactam, 3.375 g IV q6h	Ciprofloxacin, 200-400 mg IV q12h, or 500-750 mg PO q12h
Ticarcillin, 3 g IV q3-6h, with clavulanate 3.1 g IV q4-6h	Levofloxacin, 250-500 mg IV/ PO qd
Mezlocillin, 3 g IV q4h	Trovafloxacin, 200-300 mg IV qd, or 100-200 mg PO qd
Ceftazidime, 1-2 g IV q8h	**AMINOGLYCOSIDES†‡**
Cefoperazone, 2-4 g IV q6h	Gentamicin, 3-5 mg/kg/day IV in 3 divided doses
Cefepime, 1-2 g IV q12h	Tobramycin, 3-5 mg/kg/day IV in 3 divided doses
Aztreonam, 1-2 g IV q8h	Amikacin, 15 mg/kg/day IV in 2 divided doses
Imipenem, 0.5 -1 g IV q6h	
Meropenem, 0.5-1 g IV q6h	

*Suggested dosing in adult patients with normal renal and hepatic function.
†Suggested loading doses for traditional dosing: gentamicin and tobramycin, 2 mg/kg; amikacin, 7.5 mg/kg.
‡Once-daily administration has been shown to be efficacious, less nephrotoxic, and less ototoxic. Initial dosing for gentamicin and tobramycin, 5 mg/kg; for amikacin, 15 mg/kg.

Combination therapy with a beta-lactam and an aminoglycoside agent is recommended for most serious infections. In vitro synergy between the two agents and postponement of antibiotic resistance form the basis of the practice. Synergy between quinolones and other classes of antimicrobials has not been observed in vitro.

■ INFECTIONS CAUSED BY *P. AERUGINOSA*

Respiratory Infections

P. aeruginosa pneumonia may follow colonization of patients in the setting of mechanical ventilation, antibiotic administration, neutropenia, acquired immunodeficiency syndrome, and chronic pulmonary disease, particularly in patients with cystic fibrosis (Table 3). Lower respiratory tract

Table 3   Management of *P. aeruginosa* Infections

INFECTION	ANTIBIOTICS	ADJUNCTIVE
Bacteremia	AP beta-lactam + AG or Q	Identify source
Pneumonia	AP beta-lactam + AG or Q	Pulmonary toilet
Endocarditis	Ticarcillin + tobramycin (8 mg/kg/day)	Valvulectomy for persistent bacteremia
Meningitis	Ceftazidime + AG	Intrathecal AG
Urinary tract	Monotherapy (e.g., AP beta-lactam ± AG or Q)	Remove urinary catheter if possible
Malignant external otitis	AP beta-lactam + AG or Q	Surgery may be necessary
Osteomyelitis	AP beta-lactam + AG or Q	Surgical debridement

AP, Antipseudomonal; *AG,* aminoglycoside; *Q,* quinolone.

infection may be distinguished from airway colonization by an increase in quantity and purulence of respiratory secretions. Clinical manifestations may be fulminant with fever, chills, dyspnea, productive cough, and systemic toxicity. Diffuse bronchopneumonia with nodular infiltrates is commonly seen on chest radiograph. Pneumonia may be accompanied by bacteremia, particularly in neutropenic patients. Empiric antimicrobial treatment in the neutropenic patient with fever and lung infiltrate should include coverage for *P. aeruginosa.* Conventional antimicrobial therapy for *P. aeruginosa* pneumonia includes an antipseudomonal beta-lactam combined with an aminoglycoside or a quinolone.

Patients with cystic fibrosis are prone to chronic lower respiratory infections with mucoid strains of *P. aeruginosa.* These infections usually persist for a lifetime, with frequent acute exacerbations manifested by decreased exercise tolerance, increased cough and sputum, and weight loss. Therapy consists of a semisynthetic penicillin such as ticarcillin or piperacillin and an aminoglycoside. These patients may require large doses because of altered pharmacokinetics. Aggressive physiotherapy, nutrition, and hydration are essential.

Bacteremia

Bacteremia may complicate *P. aeruginosa* infections at other sites. Predisposing factors include neutropenia, hematologic malignancy, organ transplantation, vascular and urinary tract catherization, and antibiotic use. The lower respiratory tract is the most common source of *Pseudomonas* bacteremia, followed by skin, soft tissues, and the urinary tract.

No distinct clinical characteristics differentiate *P. aeruginosa* bacteremia from other gram-negative bacteremias. Most patients have fever, tachycardia, and tachypnea. Many have signs of systemic toxicity, with hypotension, shock, disseminated intravascular coagulopathy, and altered mental status. Skin manifestations include papules, bullae, and rarely, ecthyma gangrenosum (Figure 1), a focal skin lesion characterized by hemorrhage, necrosis, and vascular invasion by bacteria. Prompt initiation of combination antimicrobial therapy is crucial because there is high mortality. Therapy should continue for 2 to 3 weeks in seriously ill patients. An aggressive search for the source of the bacteremia is important.

Infective Endocarditis

Endocarditis caused by *P. aeruginosa* occurs primarily in the setting of intravenous drug use and less commonly with prosthetic heart valves. Intravenous drug users acquire this organism from nonsterile diluents such as tap water or nonsterile paraphernalia. Fever and bacteremia are invariably present. Tricuspid valve infection, which is typical, commonly presents with signs of septic pulmonary embolism. If treatment is early and aggressive with effective antibiotics, cure may be achieved without surgery. Tricuspid valvulectomy may be necessary in the event of bacteriologic failure or recurrence. Involvement of the aortic and mitral valves may manifest as a severe acute illness with sepsis and large arterial emboli necessitating early surgical valve replacement in addition to antimicrobial treatment. Combination therapy with a beta-lactam agent and an aminoglycoside in high doses (e.g., tobramycin 8 mg/kg/day) is recommended. Antibiotic therapy should be continued for at least 6 weeks.

Urinary Tract Infections

P. aeruginosa is the third most common nosocomial urinary pathogen. These infections are most commonly associated with indwelling urinary catheters. Bacteremia, a common complication, may lead to metastatic infection (e.g., vertebral osteomyelitis). Symptomatic urinary tract infections should be treated by removing the catheter when possible and by administering an antibiotic. Monotherapy with a beta-lactam antipseudomonal agent or a quinolone suffices unless there is complicating bacteremia or upper tract infection. Oral quinolones may be used successfully even in complicated urinary tract infections. A 7- to 10-day course of treatment is adequate for uncomplicated cases. Longer courses, at least 2 to 3 weeks, are necessary for pyelonephritis, renal abscess, or complicating bacteremia. Asymptomatic bacteriuria need not always require treatment. Eradication of the bacteriuria is often impossible if the patient has an anatomic abnormality or a foreign body, and antibiotics in this setting may only select a more resistant organism.

Meningitis

P. aeruginosa is a rare cause of meningitis and brain abscess. Infection may occur by (1) extension from a contiguous structure such as mastoid or sinuses, (2) direct inoculation from penetrating trauma or neurosurgical procedures, or (3) metastatic spread from a distant site. Ceftazidime is the antimicrobial of choice because of its excellent in vitro activity and its ability to penetrate cerebrospinal fluid (CSF). Aztreonam and the carbapenems have good in vitro activity, but experience with these agents is limited. Addition of an aminoglycoside may be justified on the basis of possibly

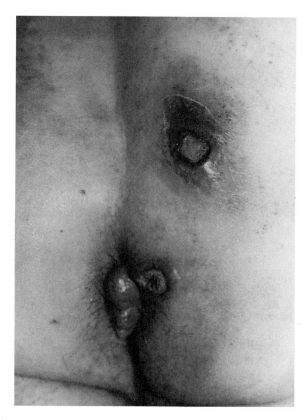

Figure 1
Ecthyma gangrenosum in patient with *Pseudomonas* bacteremia.

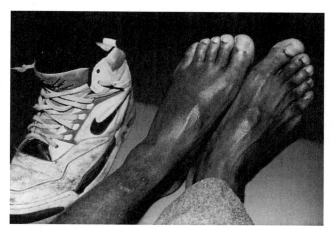

Figure 2
Acute pseudomonas osteochondritis with cellulitis following nail puncture wound of sole. Note swelling of left foot.

conferring synergy and preventing emergence of drug resistance. Because of poor penetration of aminoglycosides into CSF, intrathecal or intraventricular doses may be required. There are anecdotal reports of successful therapy with parenteral ciprofloxacin, but quinolones should be used only when other drugs have failed or when organisms are resistant to beta-lactam agents. Cure of *Pseudomonas* central nervous system infections may require surgical drainage of brain abscesses, debridement of infected tissues, and removal of prosthetic materials. A minimum of 2 weeks and as many as 6 weeks of antimicrobial therapy may be necessary.

Bone and Joint Infections

P. aeruginosa causes osteomyelitis and septic arthritis as a result of hematogenous dissemination or contiguous spread. Vertebral osteomyelitis usually occurs in elderly patients with urinary tract infections associated with bladder instrumentation and in intravenous drug users. Neck or back pain with paraspinal tenderness is a common presentation. Computed tomography (CT) and magnetic resonance imaging (MRI) are sensitive diagnostic means of defining the extent of disease. The pathogen can be isolated by needle aspiration or biopsy under fluoroscopic or CT guidance. Occasionally, surgical exploration for biopsy, culture, and decompression is necessary. Removal of prosthetic materials is usually necessary. Combination antibiotic therapy with an antipseudomonal beta-lactam and either an aminoglycoside or quinolone should be used for a minimum of 4 to 6 weeks.

Monotherapy has been used successfully, but treatment failures have occurred.

Contiguous osteomyelitis arises from direct extension of infected overlying skin and soft tissues or penetrating trauma. *P. aeruginosa* may be implicated in this setting in patients with infected diabetic foot ulcers. Vascular insufficiency and the polymicrobial nature of this infection may complicate management. The goal of therapy is to achieve effective levels of antimicrobials in bone and soft tissues. Prolonged antimicrobial treatment (up to 6 weeks) including a beta-lactam antipseudomonal agent and an aminoglycoside has been the current standard, but quinolones either used alone or in combination with a beta-lactam have proved efficacy in open trials.

Osteochondritis of the foot involving bone and fibrocartilaginous joints is seen following puncture wounds through the soles of footwear colonized by *P. aeruginosa* (Figure 2). Treatment consists of surgical debridement combined with an antimicrobial agent such as ceftazidime or ciprofloxacin for a minimum of 4 weeks.

Ear Infections

External otitis media is most commonly caused by *P. aeruginosa* and is usually associated with immersion (swimmer's ear). Patients complain of pain and pruritus; examination reveals edema, exudate, and erythema of the pinna and external canal. This infection is treated with topical agents such as antibiotic drops (polymixin, neomycin, and hydrocortisone) or dilute acetic acid.

A more invasive and necrotizing process involving the bone and soft tissues of the external auditory canal and with potential to extend to the temporal bone and base of the skull is referred to as *malignant external otitis* (Figure 3). This principally affects elderly persons with diabetes mellitus. Otalgia and purulent drainage from the external canal are present. Neurologic complications such as cranial nerve palsies may become manifest. CT or MRI is useful to delineate the extent of bone and soft-tissue destruction and monitor treatment. Because debridement may be necessary, surgical consultation is advised. Combination antimicrobial

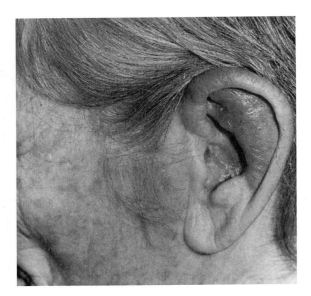

Figure 3
Invasive external otitis in elderly diabetic patient.

treatment is recommended for a minimum of 4 weeks. The course of treatment should be extended to 6 to 8 weeks for more extensive disease.

Skin Infections

Exposure to contaminated whirlpools, hot tubs, and swimming pools may produce *P. aeruginosa* folliculitis, a diffuse red maculopapular or vesicopustular rash (Figure 4). The eruption is self-limited and does not require specific antimicrobial treatment.

Burn wounds may become colonized and subsequently infected with *P. aeruginosa*. Bloodstream invasion may thus occur, resulting in septicemia. Systemic antibiotic combinations should be administered. A topical agent such as mafenide acetate or silver sulfadiazine should be used to reduce burn wound colonization. Avoidance of hydrotherapy also reduces the risk of pseudomonas infections in burn patients.

Persons with a history of submersion of the hands may develop greenish discoloration of the nail plates and *Pseudomonas* nail bed infection. This condition has been called *green nail syndrome* (Figure 5). Treatment requires elimination of the exposure; orally administered ciprofloxacin is a useful adjunct.

■ INFECTIONS CAUSED BY RELATED SPECIES

Stenotrophomonas (formerly *Xanthomonas*) *maltophilia* is a nosocomial, gram-negative pathogen that may cause bacteremia, pneumonia, and wound infection. *S. maltophilia* nosocomial pneumonia is associated with mechanical ventilation, tracheostomy, use of nebulizers, and previous exposure to broad-spectrum antibiotics. Patients usually have preexisting lung conditions such as chronic obstructive pulmonary disease. Isolation of *S. maltophilia* from the respiratory tract in ventilator-associated pneumonia is an

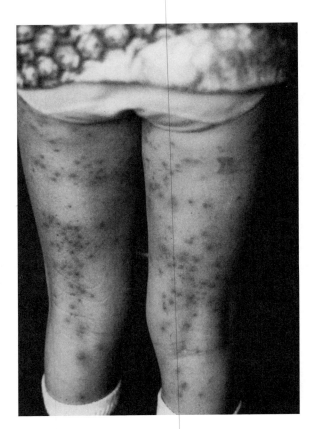

Figure 4
Red papular rash of *Pseudomonas* folliculitis.

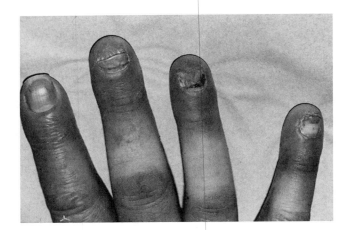

Figure 5
Nail of digits discolored by green pigment of *Pseudomonas aeruginosa*.

important predictor of mortality. Management of *S. maltophilia* pneumonia and other infections are often difficult because the organism is usually resistant to most antipseudomonal beta-lactams, carbapenems, and aminoglycosides. Trimethoprim-sulfamethoxazole (TMP-SMX) has been regarded as the antibiotic of choice for therapy. Ceftazidime, ticarcillin-clavulanate, and the quinolones have variable activity among strains. Combination therapy with TMP-SMX and a beta-lactam such as ticarcillin-clavulanate or ceftazidime (if susceptibility is documented) has been proposed based on in vitro synergy and anecdotal reports of clinical efficacy.

Burkholderia (formerly *Pseudomonas*) *cepacia* is an opportunistic pathogen that may colonize the respiratory tract of a patient with cystic fibrosis and lead to persistent disease with progressive respiratory failure. Therapy is thwarted by antibiotic resistance to many beta-lactam agents and aminoglycosides. Susceptibility to quinolone agents is variable. TMP-SMX, the carbapenems (imipenem and meropenem), and chloramphenicol may have activity.

Suggested Reading

Baltch Al, Smith RP, eds: *Pseudomonas aeruginosa: infections and treatment,* New York, 1994, Dekker.

Denton M, Kerr KG: Microbiological and clinical aspects of infection associated with *Stenotrophomonas maltophilia,* Clin Micro Rev 11:57, 1998.

Hill M, et al: Antibiotic therapy for *Pseudomonas aeruginosa* bacteremia: outcome correlations in a prospective study of 200 patients, *Am J Med* 87:540, 1989.

Korvick JA, Victor Yu: Antimicrobial agent therapy for *Pseudomonas aeruginosa*: minireview, *Antimicrob Agents Chemother* 35:2167, 1991.

RAT-BITE FEVERS

Neil S. Lipman

For 2300 years, illness associated with rat bites has been recognized in India, which is believed to be the country of origin for the disease. The first recorded description of rat-bite fever was in lectures by a physician at Yale in the early nineteenth century. It was not until 1902 that Japanese workers describing the clinical entity in a European journal coined the term *Rattenbisskrankeit,* or rat-bite fever. Rat-bite fever comprises two clinically similar but distinct bacterial diseases caused by two unrelated agents, *Streptobacillus moniliformis* and *Spirillum minus.* The organisms are distributed worldwide, with *S. moniliformis* more common in the United States and *S. minus* more common in the Far East.

Rat-bite fevers are most often associated with the bite of laboratory or wild rats but may follow contact with rat-contaminated materials. A number of recently reported cases were not associated with rat bites or contact, although all patients had a history of occupational exposure to rat-infested areas. Disease caused by these agents has also followed contact with a variety of other species, including mice, gerbils, guinea pigs, squirrels, dogs, cats, ferrets, turkeys, and weasels. Estimates are that upward of 14,000 rat bites occur annually in the United States, most of them to individuals of low socioeconomic status in cities. Diagnosis is rare, likely resulting from a low incidence of disease despite substantial potential exposure, a low index of suspicion of attending physicians, the routine postexposure use of effective antimicrobials, and the difficulty of isolating the organism in the laboratory. More than 50% of the reported cases in the United States are associated with children younger than 12 years of age. Rat-bite fever also is an occupational disease of laboratory workers; it is the most commonly reported zoonosis associated with laboratory rats.

The rat is the natural reservoir and primary host of both *S. moniliformis* and *S. minus,* neither of which is routinely associated with natural disease in the rat. Nasopharyngeal commensals, the organisms may be found in other tissues, including the urine and blood. Surveys of wild rats report carrier rates up to 50%. Estimates of infection rates in laboratory rats during the first half of the twentieth century were similar to those reported for wild populations, but modern production techniques and maintenance, in concert with frequent monitoring of commercial suppliers, have reduced this rate dramatically. Because of the difficulty in isolating the organism and the lack of a reliable serologic test, the actual carrier rate in laboratory rats is unknown. Although disease in humans has occasionally been associated with other species, these species are not believed to be commensal carriers.

■ PRESENTATION

Rat-bite fevers are acute, systemic illnesses with relapsing fever. Streptobacillary rat-bite fever, streptobacillary fever, or streptobacillosis follows infection with *S. moniliformis.* Haverhill fever and epidemic arthritic erythema are diseases caused by streptobacillosis acquired through ingestion of contaminated water, raw milk, or food. Sodoku, which derives from the Japanese word for rat *(so)* and poison *(doku),* spirillary rat-bite fever, and spirillosis are diseases resulting from *S. minus* infection. Although similar, these diseases can be differentiated clinically (Table 1). Streptobacillary rat-bite fever has a shorter incubation period than the spirillary form and is often accompanied by rash and arthralgia. Haverhill fever is more commonly associated with vomiting, diarrhea, and sore throat. An indurating chancre develops at the site of inoculation and accompanies clinical signs in the spirillary form. Dual infections, albeit extremely rare, may occur. Most cases of streptobacillary disease spontaneously resolve within 2 weeks. If the patient goes untreated, arthritis, endocarditis, myocarditis, pericarditis, hepatitis, pancreatitis, prostatitis, pneumonia, nephritis,

Table 1   Clinical Features of Rat-Bite Fevers

CLINICAL FEATURES	STREPTOBACILLARY FORM	SPIRILLARY FORM
Incubation period	2-10 days	7-21 days
Fever	+++	+++
Chills	+++	+++
Myalgia	+++	+++
Rash	++	++
	Morbilliform/petechial	Maculopapular
Lymphadenitis	+	++
Arthralgia, Arthritis	++	−
Indurated bite wound	−	+++
Recurrent fever/constitutional signs (untreated)	Irregular periodicity	Regular periodicity

meningitis, abscessation, septicemia, and chorioamnionitis may result; of untreated cases, 13% are fatal. The clinical course of disease in infants may be particularly rapid and fatal.

S. moniliformis is a fastidious, facultatively anaerobic, highly pleomorphic, asporogenous, gram-negative rod measuring less than 1 × 1 to 5 μm long. Curved and looping, nonbranching filaments as long as 150 μm may be formed. Characteristic bulbous swellings may be observed in older cultures. The bacterium has two phases, the bacillary and the cell wall–deficient L-phase. Spontaneous conversion from one form to another, which alters the organism's sensitivity to antimicrobial agents, may be responsible for clinical relapses and resistance to therapy. The incubation period of streptobacillary rat-bite fever is 2 to 10 days; however, onset usually occurs within 3 days of exposure. Clinical signs develop despite rapid healing of the bite wound, presumably as a result of bacteremia and septicemia. Illness of sudden onset is characterized by remittent chills, fever, headache, and myalgia. A morbilliform or petechial rash develops in 75% of patients, often within days of onset, on either the lateral or extensor surfaces of the extremities and occasionally involving the palms and soles. Occasionally, the rash may be generalized. Simultaneous with rash development, approximately 50% of patients have severe arthralgia or frank arthritis of at least one, but often more than one, large joint. Untreated, the course is biphasic, with fever and symptoms diminishing 2 to 5 days after onset and recurring several days later. Relapsing fever with return of constitutional symptoms of 1 to 6 days duration are not uncommon. *S. moniliformis*, identified by fatty acid profile, has also been associated with abscesses of the genital tract from three women.

In the United States, the spirillary form is considerably less common than streptobacillary disease and is rarely associated with infection acquired from laboratory rats. *S. minus* is a gram-negative aerobic, motile, rigid spiral bacterium. It is 0.2 to 0.5 × 3 to 5 μm long and has two to six wide angular windings and pointed ends with one flagellum at each pole. Illness follows an incubation period, usually 7 to 21 days but sometimes as short as 2 days or as long as months. There is initial healing of the bite wound. Subsequently, an indurated chancre or eschar develops at the wound site and is accompanied by a regional lymphadenitis and lymphangitis, fever, rigors, myalgia, and in about 50% of the cases, an erythematous maculopapular rash originat-

ing from the wound. Arthritis is uncommon. Untreated, fevers and other symptoms resolve but then recur regularly.

■ DIAGNOSIS

Diagnosis is suggested by rat bite and clinical presentation. Patients may present without a history of rat bite or after a prolonged disease course. Definitive diagnosis depends on isolation of the organism. A high index of suspicion in the laboratory is often necessary because these organisms are extremely difficult to isolate. *S. minus* cannot be grown on any artificial medium. It may be demonstrated in darkfield microscopy in wet mounts of blood, exudate from the bite wound, cutaneous lesions, and lymph nodes. Isolation requires intraperitoneal inoculation of infected materials into guinea pigs or mice followed by darkfield examination of the animal's blood or peritoneal exudate 1 to 3 weeks later.

S. moniliformis is difficult to identify in most hospital laboratories because of its fastidious growth requirements and slow growth. The organism may be demonstrated by Giemsa stain in blood, synovial fluid, or other body fluids; samples should be mixed with 2.5% sodium citrate to prevent clotting before examination. Blood and joint fluid should be cultured in media enriched with 15% blood, 20% horse or calf serum, or 10% to 30% ascitic fluid. Media used successfully include blood agar bases, chocolate agar, Schaedler agar, thioglycollate broth, meat-infusion broth, and tryptose-based media. Nalidixic acid can be added to the media to prevent overgrowth by gram-negative bacteria. Brain-heart infusion cysteine broth supplemented with Panmede, a papain digest of ox liver, has been recently advocated. The medium should not contain sodium polyanethol sulfonate (SPS), an anticoagulant and bacterial growth promoter used in blood culture media because it inhibits the growth of the organism. Inoculated media are incubated at 35° C (95° F) in humidified 7% to 8% carbon dioxide atmosphere. Characteristic "puffballs" appear after 2 to 6 days in broth; on agar, 1- to 2-mm round, gray, smooth, glistening colonies are observed. L-forms produce colonies with a typical fried-egg appearance. Identification is made by biochemical profile. The API ZYM system and fatty acid profiles may be valuable in rapid identification. The slide agglutination test used to evaluate a patient's serum for the presence of specific streptobacillus agglutinins is no longer available.

Differential diagnosis of rat-bite fevers can be broad to include septic arthritides such as Lyme disease, gonococcal arthritis, and brucellosis and noninfectious inflammatory polyarthropathies such as rheumatoid arthritis. Presentation with fever and rash mimics systemic lupus erythematosus, viral exanthems, rickettsial infections, secondary syphilis, and drug reactions. A biologic false positive for syphilis occurs in up to 25% of patients with streptobacillary disease and in up to 50% of cases with the spirillary form.

■ THERAPY

Both streptobacillary and spirillary forms of rat-bite fever respond well to appropriate antimicrobial therapy. *S. minus* is more sensitive to therapy. Penicillin is the drug of choice for both organisms, and a dramatic response to therapy may be expected. Dosage of 400,000 to 600,000 U/day for at least 7 days is recommended for uncomplicated forms of the disease. The dosage should be raised to 1.2 million U/day until antimicrobial sensitivity is determined if an adequate response is not observed. Endocarditis, if present, should be treated parenterally with 15 to 20 million U/day for 4 to 6 weeks. Tetracycline and streptomycin are effective alternatives in penicillin-allergic patients. Amoxicillin-clavulanate, second- and third-generation cephalosporins, chloramphenicol, clindamycin, erythromycin, and vancomycin have been used successfully. Treatment failures have been re-ported with erythromycin. Prophylactic administration of penicillin may be considered following a rat bite although the risk of nascent infection is low. However, prophylaxis should be a high consideration in infants because of the possibility of rapid progression and severe outcomes.

Suggested Reading

Cole JS, Stoll RW, Bulger RJ: Rat-bite fever: report of three cases, *Ann Intern Med* 71:979, 1969.

Edwards R, Fitch RG: Characterization and antibiotic susceptibilities of *Streptobacillus moniliformis*, *J Med Microbiol* 21:39, 1986.

Holroyd KJ, Reiner AP, Dick JD: *Streptobacillus moniliformis* polyarthritis mimicking rheumatoid arthritis: an urban case of rat-bite fever, *Am J Med* 85:711, 1988.

Pins MR, et al: Isolation of presumptive *Streptobacillus moniliformis* from abscesses associated with the female genital tract, *Clin Infect Dis* 22:471, 1996.

Rogosa M: *Streptobacillus moniliformis* and *Spirillum minus*. In Lennette EH, Balows A, Hausler WJ, editors: *Manual of clinical microbiology*, ed 4, Washington, DC, 1985, American Society for Microbiology.

Roughgarden JW: Antimicrobial therapy of ratbite fever, *Arch Intern Med* 116:39, 1965.

Sens MA, et al: Fatal *Streptobacillus moniliformis* infection in a two-month old infant, *Am J Clin Pathol* 91:612, 1989.

Will LA: Rat-bite fever. In Beran G, ed: *Handbook of zoonoses*, ed 2, Boca Raton, FL, 1994, CRC Press.

Wullenweber M: *Stretobacillus moniliformis*—a zoonotic pathogen. Taxonomic considerations, host species, diagnosis, geographical distribution, *Lab Anim* 29:1, 1995.

SALMONELLA

Bruce S. Ribner

The salmonellae are gram-negative, non–spore-forming; facultatively anaerobic bacteria in the family Enterobacteriaceae. More than 2300 different serotypes of *Salmonella* have been identified.

Salmonellae are widely distributed in nature. They are generally found in the gastrointestinal (GI) tracts of the hosts with which they are associated. Some salmonellae, such as *S. typhi* and *S. paratyphi,* are found to colonize only the human GI tract. Other *Salmonella* species, such as *S. typhimurium,* have a wide range of hosts, including humans. Finally, some organisms, such as *S. dublin* and *S. arizona,* are rarely found in the GI tracts of humans. The specificity and range of the different serotypes helps determine the epidemiology of infections caused by these bacteria.

Infections caused by the salmonellae are grouped into three major syndromes: gastroenteritis, typhoid or enteric fever, and localized infections outside of the GI tract. Although there is considerable overlap between these syndromes, their epidemiology and clinical presentations are distinct enough to make discussion by syndrome useful.

■ GASTROENTERITIS

Gastroenteritis accounts for most *Salmonella* infections in humans. The incidence of *Salmonella* gastroenteritis in the United States has doubled over the past three decades. Much of this increase has been attributed to the widespread contamination of chickens and eggs as the industry became increasingly centralized. Most cases of *Salmonella* gastroenteritis are traced to the ingestion of inadequately cooked poultry or eggs, either directly or through consumption of such foods as Caesar salad, sauces containing raw eggs, and inadequately cooked stuffing contaminated by salmonellae from raw poultry. Beef, milk, and rarely, fruits and vegetables have also been responsible for salmonellae infections. Pet reptiles such as turtles and lizards, and baby ducklings and chicks often have asymptomatic colonization of the GI tract. Young children who play with these animals often forget to wash their hands before eating, resulting in *Salmonella* gastroenteritis. Individuals at greatest risk for acquiring disease are neonates, those with achlorhydria or who are taking antacids, transplant recipients, individuals with lymphoma, and patients with acquired immunodeficiency syndrome.

Salmonella gastroenteritis has an incubation period of 12 to 72 hours. The typical illness is accompanied by fever, nausea, vomiting, abdominal cramping, and watery diarrhea; it lasts 4 to 7 days. The stool usually contains neutrophils, but dysentery, with gross blood and pus in the stool, is uncommon. Patients with *Salmonella* gastroenteritis occasionally have headaches and myalgias. Bacteremia, seen in approximately 5% of patients, is most common in those with underlying diseases. Bacteremia tends to occur early during the course of the illness. *Salmonella* gastroenteritis is typically a mild disease; it rarely leads to severe dehydration and cardiovascular collapse. Severe forms are most likely to be seen in infants, debilitated patients, or patients with immunologic impairment.

Approximately 50% of newborns with *Salmonella* gastroenteritis have GI carriage of the organism for more than 6 months. This rate decreases as age increases. Fewer than 10% of adults remain colonized at 3 months. The administration of antibiotics during the early phase of illness may actually increase the likelihood of carriage.

■ TYPHOID OR ENTERIC FEVER

Typhoid fever is caused by salmonellae such as *S. typhi* and *S. paratyphi*, which are almost exclusively associated with humans. Transmission is by ingestion of food or water contaminated by other humans. In contrast to *Salmonella* gastroenteritis, the incidence of typhoid fever in developed countries has decreased markedly over the past few decades as sanitation and the quality of the water supply have improved. Most typhoid fever in the United States is acquired during foreign travel. A high percentage of infections acquired in the United States result from the ingestion of food prepared by chronic carriers, many of whom picked up the organism in another country.

Typhoid fever has an incubation period of 3 to 60 days, depending on the size of the inoculum and the host's health. Typhoid fever manifests as fever, abdominal pain, hepatosplenomegaly, headache, and myalgia. Diarrhea is rare after the first few days. Although classic typhoid fever is characterized by a temperature-pulse dissociation with bradycardia in the face of a high fever, this phenomenon is uncommon. Rose spots, which are faint, maculopapular, salmon-colored blanching lesions found predominantly on the trunk, are seen in approximately one third of patients. Biopsy of these lesions often yields the infecting organism.

Some 90% of patients with typhoid fever have bacteremia during the first week of illness. This percentage decreases as the illness progresses. Positive stool cultures do not appear before the second week of illness, and the rate increases until by the third week 75% of patients have positive stool cultures. The white cell blood count is usually low in relation to the degree of illness. Occasionally, an absolute leukopenia is seen.

The patient with untreated typhoid fever will have 4 to 8 weeks of sustained fever. Mortality of untreated disease is estimated to be 15% worldwide but only 1% in the United States. Mortality is highest in the immunocompromised, especially those with hemoglobinopathies, malaria, schistosomiasis, and infection with human immunodeficiency virus (HIV). The major complication of untreated disease is hemorrhage from intestinal perforation secondary to ulceration and necrosis of the Peyer's patches in the ileum. Such hemorrhage may be seen during the third or fourth week of illness when the patient actually seems to be improving. Other complications include pericarditis, orchitis, splenic and hepatic abscesses, cholangitis, meningitis, and pneumonia. Of untreated patients, 10% relapse.

Enteric fever occasionally can be mimicked by infection with non-*Salmonella* pathogens (e.g., *Yersinia*, *Campylobacter*, *Pseudomonas*, and Epstein-Barr virus).

■ LOCALIZED INFECTIONS OUTSIDE OF THE GASTROINTESTINAL TRACT

On rare occasions, *Salmonella* infection may present as a localized infection at a site other than the GI tract. This is most likely in patients with underlying diseases. Thus sustained bacteremia with *S. choleraesuis* or *S. dublin* suggests seeding of an atherosclerotic plaque or infection of the clot within a preexisting aneurysm, especially if the patient is elderly. If infection is localized to the abdominal aorta, surgery is generally necessary because medical management alone is associated with high mortality. Rarely, sustained bacteremia may represent endocarditis with valve ring or septal abscess.

Localized disease may also present as a hepatic or splenic abscess, especially if the patient has biliary tract stones, cirrhosis, or cholangitis. Although one fourth of patients with typhoid fever may have positive urine cultures with *Salmonella*, actual infection of the urinary tract is rare in the absence of nephrolithiasis, renal schistosomiasis, or renal tuberculosis.

Salmonellae are the second most common cause of gram-negative meningitis in neonates. They are also a common cause of osteomyelitis in children with hemoglobinopathies.

Approximately 2% of individuals who have *Salmonella* gastroenteritis will develop Reiter's syndrome. This occurs within 2 weeks of the onset of diarrhea and is associated with human leukocyte antigen (HLA)-B27.

■ CHRONIC CARRIAGE

Because *Salmonella* is excreted in the stool of a high percentage of those recovering from acute *Salmonella* infection for many months, the chronic carrier state is not considered to occur unless the organism persists in the stool for more than 1 year. This occurs in approximately 1% to 4% of those with *S. typhi* infection and less than 1% of those infected with other serotypes. Biliary tract carriage is most likely to occur in the elderly and those with cholelithiasis. Urinary tract carriage is most likely in those with schistosomiasis and nephrolithiasis. Many chronic carriers have no clear history of a preceding acute *Salmonella* infection.

■ DIAGNOSIS

Serum antibodies against salmonellae are long-lived, and measuring them is rarely useful for the diagnosis of acute disease. The diagnosis of acute disease is based on culture of stool, blood, urine, or other body fluids.

■ THERAPY

General Considerations

Widespread resistance to chloramphenicol, ampicillin, and trimethoprim-sulfamethoxazole (TMP-SMX) now exists among the salmonellae, especially in the Indian subcontinent, Middle East, and Southeast Asia. In developed countries, an increase in 4-fluoroquinolone resistance has recently been observed, possibly due to the addition of quinolones to animal feeds. As a result, ciprofloxacin and ceftriaxone have become the agents of choice for initial treatment of *Salmonella* infection if susceptibility data are not available (Table 1). Because ciprofloxacin is not recommended for children or pregnant women, most authorities recommend that the initial treatment of severe *Salmonella* infections in children and pregnant women be with ceftriaxone until antibiotic susceptibilities are available. Therapy may be switched to ampicillin-amoxicillin or TMP-SMX once the organism is known to be susceptible. Although the response to chloramphenicol is equivalent to that of the other agents, chloramphenicol is rarely used because of concern over its side effect of aplastic anemia. Ofloxacin and the other 4-fluoroquinolones are generally thought to be as effective as ciprofloxacin, but there is more experience with ciprofloxacin.

Gastroenteritis

The treatment of *Salmonella* gastroenteritis is fluid and electrolyte replacement. Antibiotics should not be routinely administered because they have little effect on clinical outcome and increase the relapse rate and the likelihood of chronic carriage. Antibiotics are recommended only for individuals who are immunocompromised and at particular risk for bacteremia and metastatic spread. Such patients include neonates, those older than 50 years of age with atherosclerotic disease or intravascular prostheses, those infected with HIV, transplant patients, and individuals with hemoglobinopathies.

Typhoid Fever

Treatment of adults with typhoid fever consists of ciprofloxacin or ceftriaxone. In children and pregnant women, severe disease should be treated with ceftriaxone. The patient may be switched to oral TMP-SMX or amoxicillin as his or her condition improves and antibiotic susceptibility data become available. Most authorities recommend a short course of dexamethasone for severe disease with altered mental status or shock.

Localized Infection

Localized infection should initially be treated with ciprofloxacin or ceftriaxone until antibiotic susceptibility data are available. Surgical intervention to drain an abscess or for resection of an infected intravascular lesion is often essential.

Chronic Carriage

Chronic carriage has been eradicated by administration of 6 weeks of amoxicillin plus probenecid or TMP-SMX plus

Table 1 Therapy of Salmonella Infections	
SYNDROME	**SUGGESTED THERAPY**
GASTROENTERITIS	
Normal host	None
Immunocompromised adult	Ciprofloxacin, 500 mg PO bid for 3 to 5 days or Ceftriaxone, 2 g IV qd for 3 days
Neonate or immunocompromised child	Ceftriaxone, 80 mg/kg up to 2 g IV qd for 3 days; may switch to PO amoxicillin or TMP-SMX once stable and susceptibility data available
TYPHOID FEVER	
Adult	Ciprofloxacin, 500 mg PO bid for 10 days or Ceftriaxone, 2 g IV qd for 5 days
Children, pregnant women	Ceftriaxone, 80 mg/kg up to 2 g IV qd for 5 days; may switch to PO amoxicillin or TMP-SMX once stable and susceptibility data available
All patients with typhoid fever should receive dexamethasone, 3 mg/kg IV once, followed by 1 mg/kg IV q6h for 7 doses.	
CHRONIC CARRIER	
Adult	Ciprofloxacin, 500 mg PO bid for 4 wk
Child, pregnant women	Amoxicillin, 30 mg/kg up to 2 g PO q8h for 6 wk plus Probenecid, 30 mg/kg/day

TMP-SMX, Trimethoprim-sulfamethoxazole.

rifampin, but recent studies suggest that 4 weeks of cipro-floxacin are more effective than either of these regimens. Although success rates are lower in the face of cholelithiasis, it is still appropriate to attempt eradication of carriage with antimicrobials. If initial medical therapy is not successful, surgical correction of anatomic abnormalities such as chole-lithiasis should be attempted.

Suggested Reading

Centers for Disease Control and Prevention: *Addressing emerging infectious disease threats: a prevention strategy for the United States,* Atlanta, GA, 1994, US Department of Health and Human Services, Public Health Service.

Hedberg CW, MacDonald KL, Osterholm MT: Changing epidemiology of food-borne disease, *Clin Infect Dis* 18:671, 1994.

Keusch GT: Salmonellosis. In *Harrison's principles of internal medicine,* ed 14, New York, 1997, McGraw-Hill.

Miller SI, Pegues DA: *Salmonella* species (including Salmonella typhi). In Mandell GL, Bennett JE, Dolin R, eds: *Mandell, Douglas, and Bennett's principles and practice of infectious diseases,* ed 5, New York, 2000, Churchill Livingstone.

STAPHYLOCOCCUS

Carol A. Kauffman

Suzanne F. Bradley

Treatment of staphylococcal infection depends on the site involved, the severity of infection, and the antibiotic suscep-tibility pattern of the organism causing the infection. Al-though most serious staphylococcal infections are caused by coagulase-positive staphylococci *(Staphylococcus aureus),* in-fections caused by coagulase-negative staphylococci (e.g., *Staphylococcus epidermidis*) are increasing and may also be life-threatening. *S. aureus* is a highly invasive pathogen, able to spread hematogenously to many organs and leading to metastatic foci of infection. Coagulase-negative staphylo-cocci generally require the presence of prosthetic material to gain a foothold and cause infection.

■ SUSCEPTIBILITY TO ANTIBIOTICS

Staphylococci have a propensity to develop resistance to an-tibiotics relatively quickly. Virtually all staphylococci should be considered resistant to penicillins that are susceptible to penicillinase (e.g., amoxicillin, ampicillin, piperacillin, me-zlocillin, ticarcillin). However, the addition of clavulanic acid, sulbactam, or tazobactam to several of the aforemen-tioned penicillins renders them resistant to penicillinase and thus useful for treating staphylococcal infections. Examples are amoxicillin-clavulanic acid (Augmentin), ampicillin-sulbactam (Unasyn), pipercillin-tazobactam (Zosyn), and ticarcillin-clavulanic acid (Timentin).

Cephalosporins are useful for the treatment of staphylo-coccal infections. First-generation cephalosporins (cefazo-lin, cephalexin) are the most active, followed by second-generation agents (cefuroxime, cefotetan, cefoxitin). Third-generation (ceftriaxone, cefotaxime) and fourth-generation (cefipime) cephalosporins have less activity. Only first-generation cephalosporins should be used for serious staph-ylococcal infections.

Since the 1970s, both *S. aureus* and coagulase-negative staphylococci have become increasingly resistant to penicillinase-resistant penicillins (nafcillin, methicillin, oxa-cillin) and the penicillins that are combined with sulbactam, tazobactam, and clavulanic acid. These methicillin-resistant *S. aureus* (MRSA) and methicillin-resistant *S. epidermidis* (MRSE) are common in hospitals throughout the United States, Europe, and Australia, and in some medical centers, they account for as many as 50% of all *S. aureus* isolates causing nosocomial infections. These organisms are usually resistant to other classes of antibiotics (cephalosporins, macrolides, clindamycin), and vancomycin is often the only effective treatment for serious infections.

Although it may be tempting to treat both methicillin-susceptible *S. aureus* (MSSA) and MRSA infections with vancomycin, this practice should be discouraged. MSSA infections clear more slowly when treated with vancomycin than with a beta-lactam antibiotic. Also, overuse of vanco-mycin has contributed to the increase in vancomycin-resistant enterococci (VRE), and recently vancomycin-resistant MRSA have also been isolated from patients on long-term vancomycin treatment. Thus organisms that are identified as MSSA should be treated with a penicillinase-resistant beta-lactam antibiotic; vancomycin should be used only if the infecting organism is MRSA.

The situation with coagulase-negative staphylococci is more difficult because the assays used by most laboratories to determine methicillin resistance are not as well estab-lished for coagulase-negative staphylococci as for *S. aureus.* Thus some authorities recommend the use of vancomycin for serious coagulase-negative staphylococcal infections de-spite susceptibility patterns suggesting methicillin suscepti-bility. A new diagnostic test that detects the presence of the *mec*A gene that encodes for methicillin resistance is used in some laboratories for both *S. aureus* and coagulase-negative staphylococci; however, it is not yet clear if this test, which is costly and labor intensive, is more accurate for determining methicillin resistance.

For patients allergic to beta-lactam antibiotics, other antimicrobial agents for staphylococcal infections include (depending on susceptibility results) trimethoprim-sulfamethoxazole (TMP-SMX); quinolones, such as levofloxacin or ciprofloxacin; clindamycin; erythromycin; and vancomycin. With the exception of vancomycin, the use of these antistaphylococcal agents generally should be restricted to the treatment of localized, uncomplicated infections. Organisms that are resistant to erythromycin but susceptible to clindamycin should not be treated with clindamycin because cross-resistance to this antibiotic is almost always induced within several days.

■ INFECTION CONTROL ISSUES

Because of the difficulty in treating MRSA infections and the propensity for *S. aureus* to spread among patients from the hands of health care workers, guidelines for the control of MRSA within acute-care hospitals have been issued. Patients who have MRSA isolated should be placed in a private room in Contact Precautions, ensuring that health care workers wear gloves for general care of the patient, don gowns when performing tasks likely to result in contamination of clothing by secretions, and assiduously wash their hands before and after patient care. Special care should be taken with wounds from which MRSA has been isolated and with sputum in a patient with pneumonia due to MRSA.

Decolonization of patients who are infected or colonized with MRSA is generally not carried out, in part, because the effect is transient and recolonization the rule. However, it has been known for some time that colonization of nares and skin before a surgical procedure is associated with an increased risk of postoperative staphylococcal wound infection. Recent data suggest that transient decolonization of the nares by application of mupirocin ointment can decrease the risk of postoperative wound infection. However, the drug is not approved for this indication, and treatment of all patients preoperatively is discouraged because resistance to mupirocin has been shown to develop rapidly in hospitals in which treatment is widespread. Many authorities advocate using this drug only for efforts designed to disrupt transmission during outbreaks.

■ INFECTIONS CAUSED BY *S. AUREUS*

Skin and Soft-Tissue Infections

The most common infections caused by *S. aureus* are skin and soft-tissue infections. Folliculitis, furuncles, abscesses, and wound infections are common and can often be treated with oral antibiotics. Beta-lactam antibiotics (penicillinase-resistant penicillins and first-generation cephalosporins) are the most effective drugs for treating these infections (Table 1). In addition to antibiotic therapy, incision and drainage of abscesses is crucial to early resolution of infection.

Cellulitis is commonly caused by *S. aureus* and may be difficult to differentiate from that caused by beta-hemolytic streptococci. Initial treatment of cellulitis should always include drugs effective against both *S. aureus* and beta-hemolytic streptococci. Therefore penicillinase-resistant penicillins or first-generation cephalosporins are used until the organism is identified and antimicrobial susceptibilities are reported. Many patients require intravenous administration of antibiotics until the acute illness has improved, and then therapy can be switched to oral agents. Initial therapy with nafcillin or cefazolin, followed by dicloxacillin or cephalexin, is preferred.

Osteoarticular Infections

S. aureus is the leading cause of osteoarticular infections. These infections are difficult to treat and often require long-term therapy with intravenous antibiotics. Most difficult to treat are those patients who have prosthetic joints or hardware in place. Nafcillin or vancomycin should be used until antibiotic susceptibilities are available. In the case of septic arthritis, drainage of infected synovial fluid is essential to preserve joint function and eradicate infection. Intravenous therapy should continue for at least 3 to 4 weeks. For treatment of osteomyelitis, intravenous antibiotics should be given for a minimum of 6 weeks. Patients with vertebral osteomyelitis, paraspinous abscess, and/or epidural abscess often require treatment beyond 6 weeks to prevent relapse. This usually can be accomplished by giving an appropriate oral agent following the course of intravenous antibiotics.

Pulmonary Infections

Staphylococcal pneumonia is now mostly seen in elderly patients with underlying illnesses. Abscesses and empyema commonly complicate staphylococcal pneumonia. Treatment should be with nafcillin or vancomycin, based on the organism's susceptibilities, and should continue for 2 to 4 weeks depending on the patient's response. Drainage of loculated fluid in the pleural space is essential for resolution of infection.

Bacteremia

Bacteremia may reflect a transient event, often associated with a removable focus, most often an intravascular catheter, or it may be the first indication of deep-seated visceral infection, including endocarditis. If a catheter is the presumed source of the infection and it has been promptly removed, the length of therapy can be guided by the presence or absence of a vegetation by echocardiography. The patient can be treated with nafcillin or cefazolin for MSSA or vancomycin for MRSA bacteremia. All patients with *S. aureus* bacteremia should have, in addition to routine clinical assessment for visceral foci of infection, diagnostic tests that include transesophageal echocardiography to help define whether endocarditis is present. If there is no clinical, laboratory, or echocardiographic evidence for endocarditis or other visceral infection, then treatment for a total of 2 weeks is appropriate. For patients in whom deep-seated infections are documented and for those in whom the clinical suspicion of endocarditis is high, longer courses of therapy (4 to 6 weeks) are required. Under no circumstances should patients simply have the catheter removed without antibiotic treatment because of the propensity of *S. aureus* to seed to multiple organs, including brain, spleen, kidney, joints, and bones.

Table 1   Treatment of Noncardiac Infections Caused by *Staphylococcus aureus*

INFECTION	FIRST-LINE DRUGS*	SECOND-LINE DRUGS*†	COMMENTS
Folliculitis, furunculosis, minor abscesses and wound infections	Dicloxacillin, 250 mg, or cephalexin, 250 mg q6h PO for 7-10 days	Clindamycin, 300 mg, or erythromycin, 250 mg q6h PO for 7-10 days	Usually community acquired, rarely caused by MRSA
Cellulitis	Nafcillin, 1 g q4h, or cefazolin, 1 g q8h IV for 10-14 days	Vancomycin, 1 g q12h IV for 10-14 days	Usually community acquired, rarely caused by MRSA; after patient afebrile and nontoxic, switch to oral cephalexin or dicloxacillin
Major abscesses and wound infections			
MSSA	Nafcillin, 2 g q4h, or cefazolin, 2 g q8h IV for 2 wk	Vancomycin, 1 g q12h IV for 2 wk	Drainage of abscesses important
MRSA	Vancomycin, 1 g q12h for 2 wk		
Osteomyelitis			
MSSA	Nafcillin, 2 g q4h, or cefazolin, 2 g q8h, IV for 6 wk	Vancomycin, 1 g q12h IV for 6 wk	Vertebral osteomyelitis, with or without paraspinous or epidural abscess, often requires longer duration of therapy
MRSA	Vancomycin, 1 g q12h IV for 6 wk		
Septic arthritis			
MSSA	Nafcillin, 2 g q4h, or cefazolin, 2 g q8h IV for 3-4 wk	Vancomycin, 1 g q12h IV for 3-4 wk	Repeated needle aspiration, arthroscopic drainage, or operative drainage of joint fluid essential to resolution of infection
MRSA	Vancomycin, 1 g q12h IV for 3-4 wk		
Pneumonia			
MSSA	Nafcillin, 2 g q4h IV for 2-4 wk	Vancomycin, 1g q12h IV for 2-4 wk	Empyema, when present, must be drained
MRSA	Vancomycin, 1 g q12h IV for 2-4 wk		
Bacteremia			
MSSA	Nafcillin, 2 g q4h IV (see text for discussion regarding length of therapy)	Vancomycin, 1 g q12h IV (see text for discussion regarding length of therapy)	Length of therapy depends on source of bacteremia and whether visceral foci of infection, including endocarditis are present; careful diagnostic workup and clinical assessment of the patient is essential
MRSA	Vancomycin, 1 g q12h IV (see text for discussion regarding length of therapy)		

MRSA, Methicillin-resistant *Staphylococcus aureus*; *MSSA,* methicillin-susceptible *Staphylococcus aureus.*
*Usual adult dosages. Dosages of cefazolin and vancomycin depend on renal function. Vancomycin levels should be checked to ensure proper dosing.
†Second-line drugs used mostly for patients allergic or intolerant to beta-lactam antibiotics.

Endocarditis

The most serious staphylococcal infection is endocarditis. Patients with left-sided cardiac lesions often have metastatic abscesses in spleen, brain, kidney, and myocardium, and the mortality rate varies from 25% to 70%, depending on the host and the extent of infection. Transesophageal echocardiography has become an important tool for both diagnostic and therapeutic reasons. The patient must be monitored closely for symptoms and signs of septic complications that require surgical intervention. Right-sided endocarditis is most commonly found in intravenous drug users. In that population, the mortality rate is significantly lower, and shorter courses of therapy may be indicated.

For details of specific antibiotic regimens for endocarditis, see the chapter *Endocarditis of Natural and Prosthetic Valves.*

Toxic Shock Syndrome

Under certain conditions, such as those brought about by the use of tampons during menstruation and the packing of surgical wounds, *S. aureus* elaborates toxins that lead to multiorgan system disease in the absence of bacteremia. Treatment of shock and the removal of tampons or surgical packing are the primary goals of therapy. Antistaphylococcal therapy is secondary, initiated primarily to eradicate the carriage of toxin-producing *S. aureus* strains (see the chapter *Staphylococcal and Streptococcal Toxic Shock and Kawasaki Syndromes*).

■ INFECTIONS CAUSED BY COAGULASE-NEGATIVE STAPHYLOCOCCI

Infections caused by coagulase-negative staphylococci are often hospital-acquired and are usually associated with prosthetic devices. Because coagulase-negative staphylococci are often resistant to many antibiotics, the most consistently reliable antibiotic for initial therapy is vancomycin. Recent data note the benefit of using rifampin as an adjunctive agent in the treatment of infected prosthetic devices. The recommended treatment regimen for prosthetic valve endocarditis is vancomycin or nafcillin combined with rifampin for 6 weeks and gentamicin for 2 weeks (see the chapter *Endocarditis of Natural and Prosthetic Valves*). For prosthetic joint infections, vancomycin or nafcillin, with rifampin, for 6 weeks is recommended. Antimicrobial therapy alone often fails in patients with prosthetic device infections, necessitating the removal of the device for cure. Infected intravenous devices that are easily removed, such as central venous catheters, peripherally inserted central catheters (PICC lines), and midline catheters should be removed and 7 to 10 days of antimicrobial therapy given. For those intravenous devices that are more difficult to remove, such as Hickman or Groshong catheters and subcutaneous ports, a 2-week trial of vancomycin or nafcillin with or without rifampin may be adequate. However, if relapse occurs in this setting or if tunnel infection or septic phlebitis is present, the catheter or port should be removed (see the chapter *Intravascular Catheter–Related Infection*).

Suggested Reading

Fowler VG Jr, et al: Outcome of *Staphylococcus aureus* bacteremia according to compliance with recommendations of infectious diseases specialists: experience with 244 patients, *Clin Infect Dis* 27:478, 1998.

Jernigan JA, Farr BM: Short-course therapy of catheter-related *Staphylococcus aureus* bacteremia: a meta-analysis, *Ann Intern Med* 119:304, 1993.

Lowy FD: *Staphylococcus aureus* infections, *N Engl J Med* 339:520, 1998.

Raad I, Alrahwan A, Rolston K: *Staphylococcus epidermidis:* emerging resistance and need for alternative agents, *Clin Infect Dis* 26:1182, 1998.

Raad II, Sabbagh MF: Optimal duration of therapy for catheter-related *Staphylococcus aureus* bacteremia: a study of 55 cases and review, *Clin Infect Dis* 14:75, 1992.

STREPTOCOCCUS GROUPS A, B, C, D, AND G

Dennis L. Stevens
J. Anthony Mebane
Karl Madaras-Kelly

■ CLASSIFICATION

More than 50 years ago, Lancefield divided streptococci into groups based on carbohydrates present in the cell wall and designated the groups A through H and K through T. In addition, streptococci may be classified by their characteristics on culture on sheep blood agar. Beta-hemolytic streptococci produce zones of clear hemolysis around each colony; alpha-hemolytic streptococci (*Strepococcus viridans*) produce a green discoloration characteristic of incomplete hemolysis; absence of hemolysis is characteristic of gamma streptococci.

■ GROUP A

Pharyngitis

The sole member of Lancefield group A is *Streptococcus pyogenes.* This organism produces a variety of suppurative infections. All group A streptococcal infections have their highest incidence in children younger than age 10. About 5% to 20% of the population harbor group A streptococcus in their pharynx, and some are colonized on their skin. Group A streptococcus is ubiquitous in the environment, but with rare exceptions is exclusively found in or on the human host. Streptococcal pharyngitis, the most common infection caused by this organism, is characterized by the onset of sore throat, fever, painful swallowing, and chilliness. These symptoms combined with submandibular adenopathy, pharyngeal erythema, and exudates correlate with positive throat cultures in 85% to 90% of cases. Sore throat without fever or any of the other signs and symptoms has a low predictive value for pharyngitis caused by group A streptococcus. Rapid strep tests correlate with positive cultures in 68% to 99% of cases, but results depend greatly on the individual performing the test as well as the bacterial colony count. Colony counts greater than 100 per plate correlated with positive rapid strep tests in 95% of patients, and counts less than 100 per plate correlated with positive rapid strep tests for only 68% of patients.

Therapy

Penicillin remains the drug of choice for group A streptococcal pharyngitis and tonsillitis (Table 1). In the past, the purpose of treatment of streptococcal pharyngitis was largely to prevent postinfectious immunologic sequelae. However, because some patients with pharyngitis have subsequently developed streptococcal toxic shock syndrome with or without necrotizing fasciitis, it seems prudent to diagnose and treat streptococcal pharyngitis aggressively in an attempt to prevent this complication as well. Antibiotic treatment of streptococcal pharyngitis reduces pharyngeal pain and fever by approximately 24 hours in children.

Penicillin treatment within 10 days of the onset of pharyngitis is extremely effective in the prevention of rheumatic fever, although it is unclear whether it prevents poststreptococcal glomerulonephritis. Penicillin fails to eradicate group A streptococcus from the pharynx in 5% to 25% of patients with pharyngitis or tonsillitis, although penicillin resistance has never been documented. The most likely explanation for such failure, particularly in patients with tonsillitis, is the inactivation of penicillin by beta-lactamases produced by cocolonizing organisms such as *Staphylococcus aureus*, *Haemophilus influenzae*, *Moraxella catarrhalis*, and *Bacteroides fragilis*. A second course of penicillin fails in more than 50%

Table 1 Streptococcal Infections

ORGANISM	LANCEFIELD GROUP	TYPE OF INFECTION	THERAPY
Streptococcus pyogenes	A	Pharyngitis and impetigo	Benzathine penicillin IM, 1.2 million units for adults; 600,000 U for children <60 lb
			Penicillin G or V, PO 400,000 U qid for 10 days for adults; 200,000 U qid for children <60 lb
			Erythromycin ethyl succinate, PO 40 mg/kg/day
		Recurrent streptococcal pharyngitis, tonsillitis	Same as above or ampicillin + clavulanic acid, PO 20-40 mg/kg/day
			Oral cephalosporin
			Clindamycin, PO 10 mg/kg/day in 4 doses
		Cellulitis and erysipelas	Nafcillin, IV 8-12 g/day for 7-10 days
			Penicillin G or V, PO 200,000 U qid for 10 days
			Dicloxacillin, PO 500 mg qid for 10 days for adults
		Necrotizing fasciitis, myositis, and streptococcal toxic shock syndrome	Clindamycin, IV 900 mg q8h in adults and penicillin, IV 4 million U q4h for adults
		Prophylaxis of rheumatic fever	Benzathine penicillin, IM 1.2 million U q28 days
			Penicillin G, PO 200,000 U bid for children <60 lb
			Sulfadiazine, 1 g/day for patients >27 kg; 500 mg/day for patients <27 kg
			Erythromycin, PO 250 mg bid
Streptococcus agalactiae	B	Neonatal sepsis	Penicillin, IV 100,000-150,000 U/kg/day in 2-3 divided doses for infants <7 days of age
			Penicillin, IV 200,000-250,000 U/kg/day in 4 divided doses for infants >7 days of age
			Ampicillin, IV 100 mg/kg/day in 2-3 divided doses for infants <7 days of age
			Ampicillin, IV 150-200 mg/kg/day in 4 divided doses for infants >7 days of age
		Postpartum sepsis	Ampicillin, IV 8-12 g in 4-6 divided doses or penicillin 12-24 million U/day for adults
		Septic arthritis	Penicillin or ampicillin as for neonatal sepsis or postpartum sepsis above
		Soft-tissue infection Osteomyelitis	Penicillin or ampicillin as for postpartum sepsis above
Streptococcus equi	C	Bacteremia Cellulitis Pharyngitis	Penicillin as for streptococcal toxic shock syndrome above
*Enterococcus faecalis**	D	Endocarditis Bacteremia Urinary tract infection Gastrointestinal abscess	Ampicillin + gentamicin
Streptococcus bovis	D	Bacteremia Abscesses	Penicillin as for *Streptococcus equi* above
Streptococcus canis	G	Bacteremia Cellulitis Pharyngitis	Penicillin as for *Streptococcus equi* above

*See the chapter *Enterococcus* for more details.

of patients and treatment with dicloxacillin, a cephalosporin, Augmentin, erythromycin, or clindamycin will subsequently cure 90% to 95% of patients. Preparations containing procaine penicillin G plus benzathine penicillin are no more effective than benzathine alone but are less painful on injection. Ceftriaxone is under study for this indication. Resistance to erythromycin is about 5% in the United States, but in 1970, it reached a prevalence of 70% in Japan during a period of extensive erythromycin use in that country. In Finland and Sweden, emergence of erythromycin resistance has also paralleled erythromycin use.

Prophylactic treatment for populations at risk (e.g., schools, military) is indicated during epidemics of streptococcal pharyngitis when rheumatic fever is prevalent. The incidence of rheumatic fever has declined in developed nations but flourishes in Third World countries. Antistreptococcal prophylaxis should be continuous in individuals with a history of rheumatic fever. Benzathine penicillin given intramuscularly once each month has the greatest efficacy, although oral agents such as phenoxymethyl penicillin are also effective. In recent years, the U.S. military has demonstrated that such prophylaxis, particularly benzathine penicillin, prevents epidemics of streptococcal infections among young soldiers living in crowded conditions. Routine follow-up culture to verify eradication is not recommended except in patients with a history of rheumatic fever. Following appropriate treatment for symptomatic pharyngitis, treatment is not needed for continued positive cultures unless symptoms recur.

Scarlet Fever

Severe cases of scarlet fever were prevalent in the United States, western Europe, and Scandanavia during the nineteenth century, and mortality rates of 25% to 35% were not uncommon. In contrast, scarlet fever today is rare and, when it occurs, is very mild. The primary site of infection is usually the pharynx, although surgical site infections have also been described. Classically, a diffuse, erythematous rash with sandpaper consistency appears 2 days after the onset of pharyngitis. Circumoral pallor and "strawberry" tongue are common findings, and desquamation occurs approximately 6 to 10 days later. The cause of the rash is uncertain, although most agree that extracellular toxins, likely the pyrogenic exotoxins formerly called "scarlatina toxins," are responsible. Treatment of the underlying infection with penicillin (see section on pharyngitis) and general supportive measures are indicated. Specifically, severe hyperpyrexia (fevers to 107° to 110° F [41.7° to 43.3° C]) have been described, and antipyretics may be necessary to prevent febrile seizures.

Pyoderma (Impetigo Contagiosa)

Impetigo is a superficial vesiculopustular skin infection. Although *Staphylococcus aureus* is the most common organism isolated, group A streptococcus is likely the most significant pathogen. Impetigo is most common in patients with poor hygiene or malnutrition. Colonization of the unbroken skin occurs first; then minor abrasions, insect bites, and so on initiate intradermal inoculation. Single or multiple thick, crusted, golden-yellow lesions develop within 10 to 14 days.

Penicillin orally or parenterally, or bacitracin or mupirocin topically, is effective treatment and will reduce transmission of streptococci to susceptible individuals. None of these treatments, including penicillin, prevents poststreptococcal glomerulonephritis.

Erysipelas

Erysipelas occurs most commonly in the elderly and very young. It is caused almost exclusively by group A streptococcus and is characterized by an abrupt onset of fiery red localized swelling on the face or extremities. Distinctive features are well-defined margins, particularly along the nasolabial fold, scarlet or salmon red rash, rapid progression, and intense pain. Flaccid bullae may develop during the second to third day of illness, and desquamation of the involved skin occurs 5 to 10 days into the illness. In contrast, the rash of scarlet fever is generalized, has a diffuse pink or red hue that blanches on pressure and has a sandpaper consistency. The organism is present in the lesion, although it is difficult to culture. Treatment with penicillin, a cephalosporin, or nafcillin is effective. Swelling may progress despite treatment, although fever, pain, and the intense redness usually diminish with 24 hours of treatment.

Cellulitis

Streptococcus pyogenes (group A streptococcus) is the most common cause of cellulitis, and although group A is the most common, beta-hemolytic streptococci of groups B, C, and G also cause cellulitis in specific clinical settings. Patients with chronic venous stasis or lymphedema are predisposed to recurrent cellulitis caused by groups A, C, and G streptococci. Cellulitis in diabetic and elderly patients, particularly those with peripheral vascular disease, may also be caused by group B streptococci. Clinical clues to the category of cellulitis such as dog bite (*Capnocytophaga*), cat bite (*Pasteurella multocida*), human bite (mouth anareobes and *Eikinella corrodens*), freshwater injury (*Aeromonas hydrophila*), seawater (*Vibrio vulnificus*), and furuncles (*S. aureus*) are extremely important. Definitive diagnosis in the absence of such factors rests on aspiration of the leading edge of the cellulitic lesion. At best, a bacterial cause is established in only 15% of cases. Cellulitis caused by groups A, B, C, and G streptococcus responds to penicillin, nafcillin, erythromycin, clindamycin, and a variety of cephalosporins. Ceftriaxone, cefpodoxime proxetil, and cefuroxime axetil have the greatest in vitro activity, and all have FDA-approved indications for the treatment of streptococcal cellulitis. Although most quinolones have efficacy in the treatment of cellulitis, older quinolones such as ciprofloxacin should be avoided because of their poor in vitro activity against streptococci. Newer quinolones may be considered as second-line therapy.

Invasive Group A

In the past 10 years, there has been an increase in the number of severe group A streptococcal soft-tissue infections and bacteremia, associated with shock and death in 30% to 70% of cases. Shock and organ failure early in the course of infection define streptococcal toxic shock syndrome, and the inciting infection may be necrotizing fasciitis, myositis, pneumonia, peritonitis, septic arthritis, uterine infection, and others. Predisposing factors include varicella virus infections, penetrating or blunt trauma, and nonsteroidal antiinflammatory agents.

Therapy

When large numbers of streptococci accumulate, more organisms are in the stationary phase and are less affected by beta-lactam antibiotics (the Eagle phenomenon). The decreased expression of critical penicillin-binding proteins in such slow-growing bacteria presumably explains the lack of efficacy of penicillin. In vitro, clindamycin—but not penicillin—prevents synthesis of toxins. Interestingly, in experimental necrotizing fasciitis and myositis, clindamycin has markedly better efficacy than penicillin. Thus some authorities recommend treatment with both penicillin and clindamycin (and debridement when appropriate). Uncontrolled observations suggest that intravenous immunoglobulin may be helpful as well.

■ GROUP B

Streptococcus agalactiae (the only species in Lancefields' group B) colonize the vagina, gastrointestinal tract, and occasionally the upper respiratory tract of normal humans. Group B streptococci are the most common cause of neonatal pneumonia, sepsis, and meningitis in the United States and Western Europe, with an incidence of 1.8 to 3.2 cases per 1000 live births. Preterm infants born to mothers who are colonized with group B streptococci in the third trimester and have premature rupture of the membranes are at highest risk for early-onset pneumonia and sepsis. The mean time of onset is 20 hours, and symptoms are respiratory distress, apnea, and fever or hypothermia. Ascent of the streptococcus from the vagina to the amniotic cavity causes amnionitis. Infants may aspirate streptococci either from the birth canal during parturition or from amniotic fluid in utero. Radiographic evidence of pneumonia and/or hyaline membrane disease is present in 40% of cases. Type III strains account for most cases of group B streptococcal meningitis.

Late-onset neonatal sepsis occurs 7 to 90 days postpartum. Symptoms are fever, poor feeding, lethargy, and irritability. Bacteremia is common, and meningitis occurs in 80% of cases.

The standards of modern day prenatal care include swab culture of the lower vagina and anorectum for these organisms at 35 to 37 weeks' pregnancy. Women presenting in labor without such cultures can be screened with a rapid antigen-detecting kit, although the false-negative rate may be 10% to 30%. Both passive immunization with intravenous immunoglobulin and active immunization with multivalent polysaccharide vaccine show promise and in the future may become the best approach to prevention of neonatal sepsis as well as postpartum infection in the mother.

Adults with group B infections include postpartum women and patients with peripheral vascular disease, diabetes, or malignancy. Soft-tissue infection, septic arthritis, and osteomyelitis are the most common presentations.

Therapy

Penicillin is the treatment of choice, although in practice many neonates are empirically treated with ampicillin, 100 to 200 mg/kg/day, plus gentamicin. Once the diagnosis is established, penicillin or ampicillin should be given (Table 1). Adults should receive 12 million to 24 million units of penicillin per day for bacteremia, soft-tissue infection, or osteomyelitis; the dosage should be 8 to 12 g of ampicillin or 24 million units per day of penicillin for meningitis. Vancomycin or a first-generation cephalosporin is the alternative for patients allergic to penicillin. Intrapartum administration of ampicillin to women colonized with group B streptococcus who had premature labor or prolonged rupture of the membranes prevents group B neonatal sepsis. Infants should continue to receive ampicillin for 36 hours postpartum.

■ GROUPS C AND G

Groups C and G, which may be isolated from the throats of both humans and dogs, produce streptolysin O and resemble group A in colony morphology and spectrum of clinical disease. Before rapid identification tests were developed, many infections caused by groups C and G, such as pharyngitis, cellulitis, skin and wound infections, endocarditis, meningitis, osteomyelitis, and arthritis, were mistakenly attributed to group A. Rheumatic fever following group C or G streptococcal infection has not been described. These strains also cause recurrent cellulitis at the saphenous vein donor site in patients who have undergone coronary artery bypass surgery. Both organisms are susceptible to penicillin, erythromycin, vancomycin, and clindamycin.

■ GROUP D

Group D consists of gram-positive, facultatively anaerobic bacteria that are usually nonhemolytic but may demonstrate alpha- or beta-hemolysis. *Streptococcus faecalis,* renamed *Enterococcus faecalis,* was previously classified as group D because it hydrolyzes bile esculin and possesses the group D antigen. *Streptococcus bovis* is also a cause of subacute bacterial endocarditis and bacteremia often in patients with underlying gastrointestinal malignancy. Enterococci are commonly isolated from stool, urine, and sites of intraabdominal and lower-extremity infection. Enterococci cause subacute bacterial endocarditis and have become an important cause of nosocomial infection, not because of increased virulence, but because of antibiotic resistance. First, person-to-person transfer of multidrug-resistant enterococci is a major concern to hospital epidemiologists. Second, superinfections and spontaneous bacteremia from endogenous sites of enterococcal colonization are described in patients receiving quinolone or moxalactam antibiotics. Last, conjugational transfer of plasmids and transposons between enterococci in the face of intense antibiotic pressure within the hospital milieu have created multidrug-resistant strains, including some with vancomycin and teicoplanin resistance.

Therapy

Serious infections with enterococci, such as endocarditis or bacteremia, require a synergistic combination of antimicrobials, that is, ampicillin or vancomycin together with an aminoglycoside (see also the chapter *Enterococcus*). Unlike enterococci, *S. bovis* remains highly sensitive to penicillin.

Suggested Reading

American Academy of Pediatrics: *Report of the committee on infectious diseases* 1991, Elk Grove Village, IL, 1991, American Academy of Pediatrics.

Baker CJ, Edwards MS: Group B streptococcal infections. In Remington JS, Klein JO, eds: *Infectious diseases of the fetus and newborn infant,* ed 3, Philadelphia, 1991, Saunders.

Bisno AL: Group A streptococcal infections and acute rheumatic fever, *N Engl J Med* 325:783, 1991.

Pfaller MA, et al: Nosocomial streptococcal bloodstream infections in the SCOPE program: species and occurrence of resistance. The SCOPE hospital study group, *Diagn Microbiol Infec Dis* 29:259, 1997.

Stevens DL: Invasive group A streptococcus infections, *Clin Infect Dis* 14:2, 1992.

Stevens DL, et al: Severe group A streptococcal infections associated with a toxic shock like syndrome and scarlet fever toxin A, *N Engl J Med* 321:1, 1989.

VIRIDANS STREPTOCOCCI

Chatrchai Watanakunakorn

Viridans streptococci are a heterogeneous group of microorganisms that produce alpha (partial) hemolysis when cultivated on sheep blood agar. They are normal inhabitants of the mouth, oropharynx, and upper intestinal tract. They are present in throat cultures of healthy individuals, and clinical microbiology laboratories report the results as normal throat flora. When isolated from other clinical specimens, they are often reported as alpha-hemolytic streptococci. Some laboratories speciate these organisms if they are isolated from blood cultures or from a usually sterile area. Table 1 lists the most common species of viridans streptococci isolated from blood cultures.

◼ INFECTIONS

Viridans streptococci are important causes of infective endocarditis. In addition, bacteremia, septicemia, normal flora mixed aerobic-anaerobic pulmonary infections, and primary brain abscess are important infections caused by viridans streptococci.

Infective Endocarditis

Viridans streptococci are the bacteria that typically cause subacute bacterial endocarditis (SBE). This may occur in patients with certain underlying heart conditions and poor dental hygiene, or following oral upper respiratory tract procedures without antibiotic prophylaxis. The clinical course is usually indolent. (See the chapter *Endocarditis of Natural and Prosthetic Valves.*)

Bacteremia and Septicemia

Transient bacteremia due to viridans streptococci may occur in daily life, especially in individuals with poor dental hygiene or periodontal disease. This may be subclinical or associated with a mild transient febrile illness, especially in healthy individuals. However, viridans streptococcal septicemia, either monomicrobial or polymicrobial, can be associated with significant mortality. A toxic shock syndrome characterized by hypotension, rash with palmar desquamation, acute renal failure, adult respiratory distress syndrome, and occasionally death, has been described with viridans streptococcal septicemia in patients with malignant diseases. Predisposing factors include chemotherapy-induced oral mucositis, leukopenia, prophylactic administration of trimethoprim-sulfamethoxazole or quinolone, and use of antacids or histamine type 2 (H_2) antagonists.

Normal Flora Mixed Aerobic-Anaerobic Pulmonary Infections

Pulmonary infections due to mixed aerobic and anaerobic microorganisms are the result of aspiration of oropharyngeal contents. Predisposing conditions include periodontal disease, gingivitis, depressed cough and gag reflexes, dysphagia from esophageal disease, depressed consciousness, seizures, and ethanol abuse. These patients may have pneumonia in the dependent segments, and that may lead to necrosis with abscess formation and/or empyema. Foul odor of sputum and/or empyema fluid suggests this diagnosis. The purulent sputum contains numerous pus cells and cultures reported as normal flora. Empyema fluid may grow alpha-hemolytic streptococci. Sputum specimens are not suitable

---

Table 1 Most Common Species of Viridans Streptococci Isolated from Blood Cultures (in Descending Order of Frequency)

S. sanguis
S. mitis
S. salivarius
S. intermedius
S. uberis
S. mutans
S. constellatus
S. (Gemella) morbillorum

Table 2 Antibiotic Treatment of Viridans Streptococcal Endocarditis (See Also the Chapter *Endocarditis of Natural and Prosthetic Valves: Treatment and Prophylaxis*)

Any of the following regimens
1. Penicillin G, 12 million to 18 million units per day in 4 divided doses, plus gentamicin, 1 mg/kg IV q8h for 2 weeks.
2. Penicillin G, 12 million to 18 million units IV per day in 4 divided doses for 4 weeks.
3. Ceftriaxone, 2 g IV or IM daily for 4 weeks.
4. Ceftriaxone, 2 g IV or IM, plus gentamicin, 3 mg/kg once daily for 2 weeks.
5. Vancomycin, 15 mg/kg not to exceed 1 g IV q12h for 4 weeks.

Regimen 5 should be used in patients with history of immediate-type penicillin allergy.
For prosthetic valve endocarditis, use penicillin or vancomycin as above for 6 weeks with gentamicin for at least 2 weeks.

Table 3 Treatment Regimens

VIRIDANS STREPTOCOCCAL SEPTICEMIA
Treat for 2 weeks with any of the following regimens
1. Penicillin G, 10 million units IV per day in 4 divided doses
2. Ampicillin, 1-2 g IV q6h
3. Cefazolin, 1 g IV q8h
4. Clindamycin, 300 mg IV or PO q8h

NORMAL FLORA AEROBIC-ANAEROBIC PULMONARY INFECTION
Clindamycin, 900 mg IV q8h for 2-3 weeks, then 300 mg PO q8h for 2-3 weeks

PRIMARY BRAIN ABSCESS
Treat for at least 6 weeks with either of the following regimens
1. Metronidazole, 500 mg IV or PO q6h, plus penicillin G, 4 million units IV q4h.
2. Metronidazole, 500 mg IV or PO q6h, plus cefotaxime, 2 g IV q4-6h

for anaerobic culture, but proper anaerobic culture of empyema fluid should yield anaerobes. Chest tube drainage is needed for treatment of empyema.

Primary Brain Abscess

Viridans streptococci with or without anaerobes are important causes of primary brain abscess of unknown source. Headache of increasing severity in a seemingly healthy individual is a common presenting symptom, often without fever or neurologic deficit. There may be papilledema. Lumbar puncture is contraindicated. Computed tomography with intravenous contrast materials is the diagnostic method of choice. The abscess will manifest as ring-enhancing lesions, either single or multiple. Definitive diagnosis is by aspiration of the abscess by craniotomy or a stereotactic needle. Small abscesses can be successfully treated with antibiotic alone without open drainage. Large abscesses should be drained surgically.

■ THERAPY

With few exceptions, viridans streptococci are susceptible to penicillin and other beta-lactam antibiotics. Most strains are also susceptible to erythromycin and clindamycin, although there may be 5% to 10% resistance.

Table 2 lists recommended antibiotic treatment regimens for viridans streptococcal endocarditis. Table 3 lists recommended antibiotic regimens for the treatment of septicemia, normal flora mixed aerobic-anaerobic pulmonary infections, and primary brain abscess.

Suggested Reading

Elting LS, Bodey GP, Keefe BH: Septicemia and shock due to viridans streptococci: a case-control study of predisposing factors, *Clin Infect Dis* 14:1201-1207, 1992.

Gudiol F, et al. Clindamycin vs penicillin for anaerobic lung infections: High rate of penicillin failures associated with penicillin-resistant *Bacteroides melaninogenicus*, *Arch Intern Med* 150:2525-2529, 1990.

Sexton DJ, et al: Ceftriaxone once daily for four weeks compared with ceftriaxone plus gentamicin once daily for two weeks for treatment of endocarditis due to penicillin-susceptible streptococci, *Clin Infect Dis* 27:1470-1474, 1998.

Seydoux C, Francioli P: Bacterial brain abscess: factors influencing mortality and sequelae, *Clin Infect Dis* 15:394-401, 1992.

Watanakunakorn C, Pantelakis J: Alpha-hemolytic streptococcal bacteremia: A review of 203 episodes during 1980-1991, *Scand J Infect Dis* 25:403-408, 1994.

Wilson WR, et al: Antibiotic treatment of adults with infective endocarditis due to streptococci, enterococci, staphylococci, and HACEK organisms, *JAMA* 274:1706-1713, 1995.

POSTSTREPTOCOCCAL IMMUNOLOGIC COMPLICATIONS

Barbara W. Stechenberg

Infections caused by group A beta-hemolytic *Streptococcus* (*Streptococcus pyogenes*) are unusual in that they have been associated with nonsuppurative complications, acute rheumatic fever (ARF), and acute glomerulonephritis. These distinct clinical entities are not related to toxic effects of the organism and follow the infections by an interval during which immunologic mechanisms are triggered. Table 1 compares some features of two clinical syndromes. This chapter describes clinical manifestations and treatment for these sequelae.

■ ACUTE RHEUMATIC FEVER

ARF is a multisystem collagen-vascular disease that follows untreated or undetected group A streptococcal pharyngitis in 1% to 3% of persons. It is seen most commonly in children ages 5 to 17 and is associated with a genetic predisposition. There also appear to be strains of *S. pyogenes* more likely to be implicated in this condition (see Table 1).

The diagnosis of ARF is made clinically and is based on the modified Jones criteria (Table 2). The presence of two major or one major and at least two minor criteria suggests the diagnosis. Recent infection with *S. pyogenes* also must be suggested by either isolation of the organism from the throat or serologic evidence in the form of elevation of antistreptolysin-O, antihyaluronidase, or antideoxyribonuclease B titers. The exception to this rule is chorea, which becomes manifest 2 to 6 months after infection, by which time evidence of a recent streptococcal infection may be lacking.

The most common clinical manifestations of ARF are carditis and arthritis. The former usually presents as a significant murmur, most commonly mitral insufficiency. Both myocarditis and pericarditis may accompany this valvulitis. It is the only manifestation that may result in residual disease. The arthritis is a migratory polyarthritis that generally involves the medium-size joints (elbows, wrists, ankles, and knees). In adults, the clinical presentation may be purely migratory and not necessarily additive. Pain is often striking. Another characteristic finding is the dramatic response of the arthritis to salicylate therapy. Chorea known as *Sydenham chorea* or *St. Vitus dance*, usually occurs as an isolated, often subtle, neurologic disorder with behavioral aspects. Erythema marginatum and subcutaneous nodules are rarely seen. The strongest diagnoses of ARF are based on carditis or chorea. The weakest is based on arthritis as a single major manifestation with two minor criteria.

Table 1 Comparison of Acute Rheumatic Fever (ARF) and Acute Poststreptococcal Glomerulonephritis (AGN)

FEATURE	ARF	AGN
Prior infection	Pharyngitis	Pharyngitis or pyoderma
M-types	1, 3, 5, 6, 18	Pharynx: 1, 2, 3, 4, 12, 15, Skin: 4, 9, 52, 55, 59, 60, 61
Latency	2-4 wk	Throat: 10 days Skin: 3 wk
Recurrences	Common	Rare
Antibiotic prophylaxis	Useful	Not useful
Sequelae	Common (heart)	Rare

Table 2 Modified Duckett Jones Criteria for Acute Rheumatic Fever*

MAJOR CRITERIA	MINOR CRITERIA
Carditis	Previous rheumatic fever
Arthritis	Clinical
Chorea	Fever
Erythema marginatum	Arthralgia
Subcutaneous nodules	Laboratory
	Prolonged PR interval
	Elevated acute-phase reactants: erythrocyte sedimentation rate, C-reactive protein, white blood cell count

*Requirements: (1) evidence of antecedent group A streptococcal infection and (2) two major criteria or one major and at least two minor criteria.

Prevention

Primary prevention of ARF requires the proper diagnosis and treatment of *S. pyogenes* pharyngitis. The accepted standard of care is the performance of a throat culture or rapid streptococcal antigen detection test. If the latter is negative, a throat culture should be done because of the variable sensitivity of that test. Treatment of streptococcal pharyngitis should be undertaken, generally with oral phenoxymethyl penicillin (penicillin V) at 250 to 500 mg, two or three times a day for 10 days; if compliance is an issue, benzathine penicillin G, 1.2 million units intramuscularly (IM) (if >60 lbs, 27 kg; or 600,000 U if <27 kg), is acceptable. For patients allergic to penicillin, erythromycin, 50 mg/kg/day (maximum, 1 g/day) in three or four divided doses for 10 days, is the antibiotic of choice. Prompt treatment should prevent most cases of ARF after symptomatic pharyngitis. Initiation of therapy up to 8 days after infection begins is probably beneficial.

Therapy

Treatment of ARF involves three important areas: eradication of *S. pyogenes*, treatment of the acute manifestations, and prevention of both recurrences and infective endocarditis in those with residual carditis. The first is accomplished with the regimens for primary prevention. These regimens should be used even if the throat culture is negative at the time of diagnosis of ARF. The mainstay of treatment of ARF is salicylates, both for arthritis and mild to moderate carditis. A dosage of 70 to 80 mg/kg/day should be initiated to produce a therapeutic blood level of 20 to 25 mg/dl. This is continued for at least 2 weeks, until acute inflammation has subsided, and then weaned gradually over the next 2 to 4 weeks. Patients with arthritis should be repeatedly evaluated for carditis during the initial 2 weeks. Persons with severe carditis and/or congestive heart failure should be treated with steroids, usually prednisone at 2 mg/kg/day acutely for at least 2 weeks, with a gradual withdrawal over 4 to 6 weeks, with the introduction of salicylates to prevent rebound. Supportive care of carditis is important; digitalization should be done slowly starting with one quarter of the usual initial dose.

Sydenham chorea is usually self-limited over several weeks. If symptoms are debilitating, phenobarbital may be started at 15 to 30 mg every 6 to 8 hours. Haloperidol is an alternative. Bed rest must be used judiciously; it is more important in patients with acute carditis and chorea. It is used during the acute phase and then liberalized on an individual basis.

Secondary Prevention

Secondary prevention of infection with *S. pyogenes* is based on the fact that persons with ARF have at least 10% to 30% chance of recurrence of ARF when reinfected with this organism. Because of concerns about compliance, benzathine penicillin G, 1.2 million units IM every 4 weeks, is recommended, particularly in the first 5 years after clinical presentation, and in persons with carditis. In areas of high prevalence of ARF, this regimen should be given every 3 weeks. Oral penicillin, 250 mg twice a day, is an acceptable alternative. Patients allergic to penicillin are treated with sulfadiazine, 500 mg twice a day. Erythromycin, 250 mg twice daily, should be reserved for persons allergic to both penicillin and sulfa. The duration of secondary prevention is controversial; many believe it should be lifelong, but there is evidence for discontinuing at age 21 or after 5 years (whichever is longer). Persons with residual carditis should be educated about the importance of oral hygiene. They should receive antibiotics for prophylaxis against infective endocarditis. (See the chapter *Endocarditis of Natural and Prosthetic Valves: Treatment and Prophylaxis.*)

■ ACUTE POSTSTREPTOCOCCAL GLOMERULONEPHRITIS

Poststreptococcal acute glomerulonephritis (AGN) is an inflammatory disorder of the glomeruli. It occurs when soluble IgG immune complexes are deposited at the glomerular basement membrane, causing complement activation and release of cytokines. This leads to infiltration of inflammatory cells. The streptococcal antigen involved has not been completely elucidated. It can follow either throat or skin infection with *S. pyogenes*. Table 1 list the major strains associated with AGN and designated nephritogenic; the incidence of AGN has decreased remarkably in the last 20 years, perhaps with a decrease in these M-types. AGN has rarely been associated with infection with group C streptococci.

The epidemiology of AGN reflects that of streptococcal pharyngitis (age 5 to 15 years; winter to spring) and pyoderma (younger age; summer months). Prompt therapy does not prevent AGN. The incubation period is about 10 days with pharyngeal strains and about 3 weeks following pyoderma.

Clinical manifestations include edema (85%), gross hematuria (25%), and hypertension (60% to 80%). A consequence of volume overload, the hypertension may lead to encephalopathic changes in a small number of patients. Symptoms referable to the cardiovascular system (cardiomegaly, congestive heart failure, pulmonary edema) are sometimes present. Fever is uncommon. Some patients have a mixed acute nephritis/nephrotic syndrome with ascites and anasarca. AGN is typically self-limited, with spontaneous diuresis and improvement in hypertension within 1 week. In fact, up to 50% have been asymptomatic during outbreaks. In children, fewer than 2% of cases are complicated by acute renal failure. This number may be higher in adults. Progression to chronic renal failure is also very unlikely.

Freshly voided urine typically demonstrates mild proteinuria, red and white blood cells, and red and white blood cell casts. Gross hematuria (usually brown) disappears rapidly, although microscopic hematuria persists for months as does the proteinuria. Striking hypocomplementemia is seen in 90% of patients, primarily C3 and CH50 with a normal C4. Diagnosis is supported by the latter finding in association with evidence of preceding *S. pyogenes* infection. Following pharyngeal infection, antistreptolysin-O elevations are common. However, it is less useful following skin infections, after which anti-DNAase B or antihyaluronidase are more likely to be high. Attempts to culture the organism also should be undertaken.

Therapy

Therapy is supportive. Antibiotics should be given to eradicate any streptococcal carriage. However, no data have demonstrated that this therapy either prevents AGN or alters its natural history. As noted for ARF, penicillin is the agent of choice. Either benzathine penicillin G, 1.2 million units IM, or phenoxymethyl penicillin (Pen-V), 250 to 500 mg two to three times a day orally, are appropriate. Erythromycin, 250 mg four times a day, is an alternative for individuals allergic to penicillin. Oral therapy should be continued for 10 days. Patients with obvious edema, hypertension, or azotemia may require hospitalization, although most patients respond to careful restriction of fluid and salt intake. Diuretic therapy is usually successful in controlling hypertension. Prognosis is generally excellent. Relapses are rare.

There is no need for antibiotic prophylaxis to prevent future attacks because repeated episodes are rare.

Suggested Reading

Berrios X, et al: Discontinuing rheumatic fever prophylaxis in selected adolescents and young adults, *Ann Intern Med* 118:401, 1993.
Bisno AL: Group A streptococcal infections and acute rheumatic fever, *N Engl J Med* 325:783, 1991.

Popovic-Polovic M, et al: Medium and long-term prognosis of patients with acute post-streptococcal glomerulonephritis, *Nephron* 58:393, 1991.

Special Writing Group of the Committee on Rheumatic Fever, Endocarditis and Kawasaki disease: Guidelines for the diagnosis of acute rheumatic fever, *JAMA* 268:2069, 1992.

Tejani A, Ingulli E: Post-streptococcal glomerulonephritis, *Nephron* 55:1, 1990.

Veasy GL, Hill HR: Immunologic and clinical correlations in rheumatic fever and rheumatic heart disease, *Pediatr Infect Dis J* 16:400, 1997.

SHIGELLA

David W. K. Acheson

Shigella belongs to the family Enterobacteriaceae and closely resembles *Escherichia coli* at the genetic level. Four species of *Shigella*—*S. dysenteriae, S. flexneri, S. boydii,* and *S. sonnei*—are differentiated by group-specific polysaccharide antigens of lipopolysaccharide, designated A, B, C, and D, respectively. *S. dysenteriae* consists of 10 antigenic types, of which type 1 produces a potent cytotoxin known as Shiga toxin. *S. flexneri* is divided into 6 types and 14 subtypes, and *S. boydii* into 18 serologic types. Although there is only one *S. sonnei* serotype, there are at least 20 colicin types. Shigellae are biochemically very similar, and differentiation among species is based primarily on serologic methods using group and type-specific antisera.

■ EPIDEMIOLOGY

Shigellosis occurs throughout the world with varying species distribution. *S. dysenteriae* and *S. flexneri* are the predominant species in developing countries, whereas *S. sonnei* is the major isolate in developed countries, accounting for more than three quarters of the isolates in the United States. *S. flexneri* is being seen more frequently in the United States in homosexual men and is thought to be transmitted sexually in this group. *S. boydii* is uncommon except in the Indian subcontinent. Fecal-oral transmission is the typical way for these bacteria to spread. They will colonize only in humans and some nonhuman primates, so typically the route of spread is human-to-human via contaminated food (often salads) or water, and the disease is often associated with poor personal hygiene. One of the most striking features of shigellosis is the exceedingly small inoculum of organisms required to cause disease. As few as 10 to 100 *S. dysenteriae* have been shown to cause dysentery in adults. The other species may require 1000 to 10,000 bacteria, but this is still a small enough dose to be readily transmitted by fecal contamination of hands, water supply, or food.

■ CLINICAL FEATURES

Shigellosis characteristically begins with constitutional symptoms, including fever, fatigue, anorexia, and malaise. Watery diarrhea usually develops and may become bloody and progress to dysentery within a few hours or days. The latter classically consists of a small amount of blood and mucus but may be grossly purulent. Progression to clinical dysentery is uncommon in *S. sonnei* infection, occurs more often in *S. boydii* infection, is common in *S. flexneri,* and occurs in most patients when *S. dysenteriae* is the cause. Although fluid loss is usually not a major problem in shigellosis (usually no more than 30 ml/kg/day), hyponatremia can be severe because of inappropriate secretion of antidiuretic hormone, especially in infants infected with *S. dysenteriae* type 1 or *S. flexneri.*

Shigellosis may cause both local and systemic complications. Intestinal obstruction and toxic megacolon during shigellosis are uncommon in the United States but occur regularly in developing countries and are associated with high mortality. *Shigella* bacteremia is considered to be uncommon; however, when routinely looked for, it is not rare and has been documented in 4% of a series of patients in Bangladesh. Bacteremic patients were more likely to die, and mortality in *Shigella* sepsis was 21% compared with 10% in the absence of bacteremia. Systemic complications are especially frequent during infection with *S. dysenteriae,* including toxic megacolon and leukemoid reactions with leukocyte counts in excess of 50,000 per deciliter. Hemolytic uremic syndrome (HUS) and neurologic complications, especially seizures, may occur. HUS is associated with the Shiga toxins produced by *S. dysenteriae* and may result in significant morbidity and mortality. Other complications include reactive arthritis, especially after infection with *S. flexneri.* The pathogenesis of shigellosis is highly complex, involving multiple genes in both chromosomal and plasmid locations. Several reviews have been published on this topic. (See the suggested readings at the end of this chapter.)

■ DIAGNOSIS

Shigellosis may be diagnosed clinically, microbiologically, or serologically. Patients with the classical picture of dysentery, with frequent small-volume bloody stools, abdominal cramps, tenesmus, and large numbers of leukocytes in the stool, especially if febrile, can be given a presumptive diagnosis of shigellosis. Studies in Bangladesh indicate that 85% of patients with shigellosis had more than 50 leukocytes per high-power field. This level is higher than usual in other enteric infections. *Shigella* are especially fastidious and rapidly die off if stool samples are not properly handled. The best way to isolate *Shigella* is to obtain stool as opposed to rectal swabs, rapidly inoculate specimens onto selective culture plates, and quickly incubate them at 37° C (98.6° F). To optimize isolation, a variety of media such as MacConkey, deoxycholate, and eosinmethylene blue, and highly selective media such as Hektoen-enteric, salmonella-shigella, and xylose-lysinedeoxycholate should be used. Detection of antibodies to *Shigella* lipopolysaccharide is an alternative but is generally used for epidemiologic studies and not for routine diagnosis in the clinical microbiology laboratory. Molecular techniques, including DNA probes and polymerase chain reaction techniques, have also been described for the detection of *Shigella* but are not routinely used except in research.

■ THERAPY

Diarrhea from *Shigella* is generally not severely dehydrating; however, replacement of lost fluids and electrolytes is the most important therapy and can often be done orally. Most infections in developed countries are caused by *S. sonnei* and are self-limiting within a few days. In more severe infections, usually those caused by *S. flexneri* or *S. dysenteriae*, hyponatremia with serum sodium below 120 mmol/L may be a significant problem requiring infusion of 3% hypertonic saline 12 ml/kg over 2 hours to raise the serum sodium by around 10 mmol/L. This therapy must be combined with restricted access to drinking water. Hypoglycemia, also a common problem in children with shigellosis in developing countries, may require intravenous replacement therapy. One way to do this is rapid infusion of glucose 1 g/kg body weight over 5 to 10 minutes, and then a continuous infusion of glucose, 50 g/L, until the infection is under control. Shigellosis involves major catabolic stress, and nutritional replacement is an important part of therapy.

Specific therapy in shigellosis requires the administration of antimicrobial agents that shorten the illness and reduce the mortality. Many *Shigella* carry resistance for streptomycin, tetracycline, and chloramphenicol; more are now resistant to ampicillin and depending on locale, a varying proportion are also resistant to trimethoprim-sulfamethoxazole (TMP-SMX). Globally, there are increasing problems with resistance in *Shigella*. In a study from Turkey published in 1998, of 289 *Shigella* strains isolated from children, 75% of the isolates were *S. sonnei* and 24.8% were *S. flexneri*. 79% of the isolates were resistant to streptomycin, 56% to tetracycline, 55.7% to TMP-SMX, 27.7% to ampicillin, and 19.7% to chloramphenicol. None of the isolates was resistant to ciprofloxacin, naladixic acid, cephalothin, ampicillin-sulbactam, and ceftriaxone. The authors concluded that TMP-SMX should not be used empirically in the treatment of shigellosis. In a second study undertaken between 1996 and 1997 at Kasturba Medical College Hospital, Manipal, five strains of *S. flexneri* and one strain of *S. dysenteriae* (out of a total of 29 isolates found during the study period) were found to show resistance to naladixic acid and the newer fluoroquinolones (ciprofloxacin, norfloxacin, and ofloxacin). Since 1983 in England and Wales, the incidence of resistance to ampicillin in *S. dysenteriae*, *S. flexneri*, and *S. boydii* infections has increased from 42% to 65%, and the incidence of resistance to trimethoprim from 6% to 64%. For *S. sonnei*, almost 50% of isolates were resistant to ampicillin or trimethoprim and 15% were resistant to both antimicrobials. However, it is important to remember that many of these infections were likely imported from other countries. The conclusion in the United Kingdom was that if it is necessary to commence treatment before the results of laboratory-based sensitivity tests are available, the best options would be to use naladixic acid for children and a fluoroquinolone antibiotic for adults. However, quinolone-resistant *S. flexneri* 2a was reported in Japan in 1998, so even this strategy is not without potential problems. In the United States and other developed countries, it is possible to use an oral or parenteral third-generation cephalosporin or, in the case of adults, a fluoroquinolone (Table 1). Therapy should be maintained for 5 days. In the United States, the fluoroquinolones are not currently approved for use in those younger than 17 years of age because of a concern that they will

Table 1 Antimicrobial Therapy for Shigellosis			
	DOSAGE		
DRUG	**CHILDREN**	**ADULTS**	**COMMENTS**
FIRST-LINE AGENTS			
Ciprofloxacin	Not recommended in United States	500 mg bid	Little resistance to date
Other 4-quinolones	Not recommended in United States	Variable	
Naladixic acid	55 mg/kg/day	1 g qid	Not licensed in the United States
Ampicillin	100 mg/kg/day	500 mg qid	Increasing resistance
Trimethoprim-sulfamethoxazole	10/50 mg/kg/day bid	1 DS tablet bid	Increasing resistance
SECOND-LINE AGENTS			
Amdinocillin	80 mg/kg/day	400 mg qid*	Resistance rare
Cefixime	8 mg/kg/day	400 mg/day*	
Ceftriaxone	50 mg/kg/day	1-2 g/day*	

DS, Double strength.
*Use not routine in adults.

damage cartilage. Currently, there is so much flux in the resistance patterns that the recommendation is to obtain cultures and sensitivity before commencing a patient on an antibiotic. This will allow the physician to alter therapy if needed when culture results are available. The guidelines in Table 1 are general and will not be valid in all parts of the world because of these changing resistance patterns.

Suggested Reading
Acheson DWK, Donohue-Rolfe A, Keusch GT: The family of Shiga and Shiga-like toxins. In Alouf JE, Freer JH, eds: *Sourcebook of bacterial protein toxins,* New York, 1991, Academic Press.

Acheson DWK, Keusch GT: *Shigella* and enteroinvasive *Escherichia coli*. In Blaser MJ, et al, eds: *Infections of the gastrointestinal tract,* New York, 1995, Raven Press.
Aysev AD, Guriz H: Drug resistance of *Shigella* strains isolated in Ankara, Turkey, 1993-1996, *Scand J Infect Dis* 30:351, 1998.
Cheasty T, et al: Increasing incidence of antibiotic resistance in Shigellas from humans in England and Wales: recommendations for therapy, *Microb Drug Res* 4:57, 1998.

TULAREMIA

Richard B. Hornick

Francisella tularensis is an unusual gram-negative, rod-shaped bacteria that causes the disease tularemia. *F. tularensis* is unusual because of its virulence, the geographic distribution of the few known varieties, and the organism's unique preference for residing inside macrophages. Tularemia is acquired in most patients through contact with infected tissues of cottontail or jackrabbits or from bites of dogs, cats, snakes, and other animals that have become contaminated from biting or eating infected rabbits. Human infections can be induced by ticks, mosquitoes, and deer flies that have fed on an infected animal.

Tularemia has an American heritage. McCoy studied a plaguelike disease in ground squirrels in 1911 in Tulare County, California. Dr. Edward Francis subsequently selected the name tularemia (1921) for the disease because his investigations demonstrated that a bacteremia must occur and because of the first demonstration of infected animals in Tulare County. The organism was subsequently named *Francisella tularensis* to honor the extensive studies of Dr. Francis. Further studies have identified infection in more than 100 wild and domestic animals and the ectoparasites and biting insects that feed on them.

One of the two major strains is unique in the United States. Type A—biovar tularensis—is found often in cottontail rabbits. It is highly virulent, (cottontails die within a week); very few organisms (50) infected subcutaneously or aerosolized and inhaled as small particles (5 μ) by volunteers will induce disease. Type B strains (biovar palaeattica) are found in Europe and Asian countries, as well as in North America. This strain is less virulent in that mortality and morbidity are less in infected persons than that induced by type A. Volunteers were infected with doses 1000 times greater than with type A. Type B is found in rodents, woodchucks, and contaminated water. It does not kill cottontail rabbits.

■ TYPES OF INFECTIONS

There are four types of disease, each related to the route of infection: ulceroglandular, pneumonitis, typhoidal, and oculoglandular. In nature the mechanisms of transmission are through minute cuts or pores in the skin, producing an ulcer; the organisms are often acquired when skinning or eviscerating an infected animal. In this process of eviscerating, large numbers of organisms can be aerosolized from the organs, especially the liver. Small numbers of these may reach the lower levels of the lung and cause pneumonitis. Ticks may deposit the organisms on the skin adjacent to the site of their bite. The organism will then be transmitted into the skin when the wound is scratched or rubbed.

The incubation period for the ulceroglandular form of tularemia is 2 to 6 days. Patients usually present with an ulceration of a finger, often around the edge of the nail bed. Regional draining lymph nodes enlarge and may become fluctuant if antibiotic therapy has not been administered. These nodes will heal without being drained when appropriate antibiotic therapy is given. Some nodes, when incised, resolve very slowly despite antibiotic therapy.

The incubation period for the most serious form of tularemia, pneumonitis, is 4 to 6 days. The affected areas of the lung may be difficult to interpret on chest radiographs. The pattern of several rounded opacities suggests tularemia. However, few patients demonstrate this radiographic picture. Various radiographic findings may be present, including lobar pneumonia, pleural effusions, abscess, mediastinal adenopathy, and tracheal compression. Oculoglandular tularemia presents with small yellowish granulomatous lesions on the palpebral conjunctivae. The preauricular lymph nodes enlarge and are tender. Untreated, the cornea may be perforated by the infectious process. Contaminated fingers rubbing an eye can initiate the infection. Spread from ulceroglandular disease can also induce pneumonitis.

Typhoidal tularemia occurs when the ingested organisms spread throughout the body from the oropharynx. Cervical lymph nodes are enlarged, and mesenteric nodes may also be involved and cause abdominal pain. Very large numbers of *F. tularensis* are required. The gastrointestinal tract appears to be resistant to infection or disease.

■ DIAGNOSIS

Each of these clinical presentations is difficult to diagnose, especially in patients remote from endemic areas. Historical facts regarding recent exposures to animals, ticks, and deer flies, among others, provide a significant assist and will direct therapeutic options. Fever and chills are common with each form of disease. The ulcer may have a black base, similar to that caused by *B. anthracis*. Very little pus is present in the ulcer.

Patients with pneumonia are quite ill, with chills, fever, substernal burning, and nonproductive cough. Headache, myalgia, photophobia, malaise, and extreme fatigue are common but not distinctive. Cervical lymph nodes may be enlarged and these, plus the substernal burning in a patient with a sudden onset of pneumonitis and the history of direct or indirect animal exposure, should raise concerns about tularemia.

Laboratory findings are not helpful; the leukocyte count will be normal if no abscess is present, despite the obvious pneumonitis or ulceroglandular disease. Blood, sputum, and other culture specimens can be obtained, but the laboratory must be alerted to the possibility of tularemia. Laboratory personnel have become infected from laboratory accidents. Appropriate class 4 facilities are needed to prevent spread to humans or laboratory animals.

Serologic studies are the safest method to make a diagnosis. However, the agglutinating antibodies do not appear for 7 to 10 days and peak at 3 to 4 weeks. Paired specimens of serum obtained 2 weeks apart with a fourfold rise in titer is confirmatory. A single specimen with a titer of 1:160 or greater without any prior known exposure to *F. tularensis* is diagnostic. Polymerase chain reaction (PCR) is a quick method but available only in experimental laboratories.

Skin Tests
Although the skin test is a reliable diagnostic tool (the test can be positive in the first week of disease), the antigen is not readily available. The Centers for Disease Control and Prevention (CDC) in Atlanta may be able to provide the test solution.

■ TREATMENT

Streptomycin therapy changed tularemia from a deadly disease to one that was readily controlled. It is very effective. Patients should receive 1 g every 12 hours for 10 days. Prompt defervesence will occur. Appropriate dosage adjustments are needed when renal insufficiency is present. Gentamicin also is effective, 5 mg/kg/day with normal renal function. Tetracycline and chloramphenicol are effective but are second choices to the aminoglycosides; they are not bactericidal, and responses are slower with relapses possible. The fluoroquinolone group is effective in experimental animals and in in vitro tests. They have not been fully evaluated in patients. No antibiotic-resistant strains have been isolated from patients with tularemia.

Mortality from pneumonia caused by type A is less than 1% to 2% if treatment is instituted promptly. Without appropriate therapy, mortality approaches 50%. Type B pneumonitis is milder.

Ulceroglandular disease caused by type A has a 5% mortality if untreated; type B ulceroglandular infection is indolent and self-limited without antibiotic therapy.

Isolation of patients is unnecessary; no evidence of person-to-person spread has been documented.

An effective live attenuated vaccine is available for those with occupations that expose them to infected animals or ectoparasites. It is available from the U.S. Army Medical Research Institute of Infectious Diseases, Fort Detrick, Maryland, 21702.

Suggested Reading
Fulop M, Leslie D, Titball R: A rapid, highly sensitive method for the detection of *Francisella tularensis* in clinical samples using the polymerase chain reaction, *Am J Trop Med Hyg* 54:364, 1996.
Gill V, Cunha BA: Tularemia pneumonia, *Semin Resp Infect* 12:61, 1997.
Jacobs RF: Tularemia, *Advan Ped Infect Dis* 12:55, 1996.
Steinmann TL, et al: Oculoglandular tularemia, *Arch Ophthalmol.* 117:131, 1999.
Waag DM, et al: Immunogenicity of a new lot of *Francisella tularensis* vaccine strain in human volunteers, *FEMS Immuno Med Microbiol* 13:205, 1996.

TUBERCULOSIS

Asim K. Dutt
William W. Stead

In the United States, the epidemiology of tuberculosis (TB) is changing rapidly. Infection by human immunodeficiency virus (HIV) and the increase in homelessness, poverty, and drug abuse are major factors in this change. TB occurs most commonly among ethnic minorities, African-Americans, and Hispanics 25 to 44 years of age. Immigrants from developing countries with a high prevalence of TB and drug resistance have contracted almost one third of the new cases in this country in the past several years. Drug-resistant disease is a major concern.

■ DIAGNOSIS

When pulmonary TB is suspected, three spontaneously produced sputum specimens should be examined by microscopy and culture. If necessary, sputum production may be induced by inhalation of aerosol of warm saline (Figure 1). Methods such as early-morning gastric lavage and laryngeal swab on suction are less productive. When suspicion of TB is high and microscopy is negative on at least three specimens, a bronchial washing or transbronchial biopsy through a fiberoptic bronchoscope or postbronchoscopy sputum may be productive. In an unconscious patient, tracheal aspiration or transthoracic needle aspiration of the lung may be needed to obtain a specimen. On rare occasions diagnosis must be made by open lung biopsy.

Positive sputum microscopy suggests TB, but the only positive identification of *Mycobacterium tuberculosis* is by culture or DNA probe to distinguish it from less virulent mycobacteria. Drug susceptibility testing should be performed.

For the diagnosis of extrapulmonary TB secretions and/or biopsy, material must be obtained from the site (see Figure 1). In the case of tuberculous meningitis it may be necessary to initiate therapy empirically because the disease may become irreversible before the diagnosis can be made.

■ THERAPY

Principles of Chemotherapy

Table 1 lists drugs, dosages, and major side effects. Several first-line bactericidal drugs are commonly combined initially because they reduce the bacterial population rapidly without the risk of resistance. Second-line drugs are most useful when resistance to two or more first-line drugs is found or they cannot be used because of life-threatening side effects or intolerance (Figure 2).

The bactericidal drugs in suitable combinations actually kill actively multiplying extracellular bacilli in TB lesions. Rapid elimination of these bacilli renders the sputum bacteriologically negative, leading to cure. No bactericidal drug should be used alone to treat active TB because this inevitably leads to resistance to that drug. When initial therapy fails at this stage, the sputum bacteriology does not become negative, as shown by persistence of positive sputum smears beyond 3 months. Failure of therapy usually results from emergence of drug-resistant organisms, most often due to poor compliance, prescription of an inadequate regimen, or inadequate dosage of individual drugs.

In the continuation phase of therapy, the drugs slowly eliminate small populations of intermittently metabolizing persisters in the closed caseous lesion or within macrophages. Incomplete therapy may lead to relapse after discontinuation of treatment, often with drug-sensitive organisms.

Drug-Resistant Organisms

The inclusion of a number of drugs in a regimen should be based on the awareness of the circumstances under which drug-resistant bacilli are likely to be present (Table 2).

At the minimum, a four-drug regimen should be initiated when drug resistance is likely, until susceptibility results are available. The number of drugs in the initial regimen may have to be increased to five to seven if the organisms are resistant to three or more drugs and HIV infection is present, as often occurs in large cities in the United States and in many developing countries.

Drug Regimens

Any of several drug regimens with variable durations may be selected according to the local conditions.

Nine-Month Regimen

Since the mid 1970s, Arkansas Department of Health physicians have treated patients with isoniazid (INH) and rifampin (RIF) in a combination capsule (Rifamate) for 9 months. The therapy may be administered daily or, as in most cases, twice weekly. The Arkansas regimen consists of INH-RIF two capsules daily for 1 month followed by two INH-RIF capsules and two 300-mg INH tablets twice weekly for another 8 months. Several thousand patients have been treated, and the success rate is greater than 95%. Development of drug resistance has not been a problem because the patient cannot take a single drug alone, and side effects are minimal. The cost of medication is quite reasonable.

The main objection to a two-drug regimen is possible presence of drug-resistant bacilli during initial therapy. In Arkansas, the incidence of initial or primary resistance is less than 3%. Morever, patients with risk factors (see Table 2) are excluded from this regimen. However, the regimen should never be prescribed in large cities, in places with high prevalence of primary drug resistance, or in certain areas of the United States such as the Mexican border and areas in which Southeast Asians have settled.

We still find this regimen useful in the initial treatment of elderly persons in whom the disease is generally caused by recrudescence of an infection acquired many years ago, when drug resistance was not a problem. Moreover, the twice-weekly schedule is easily supervised when needed, either by health care personnel or by relatives or friends.

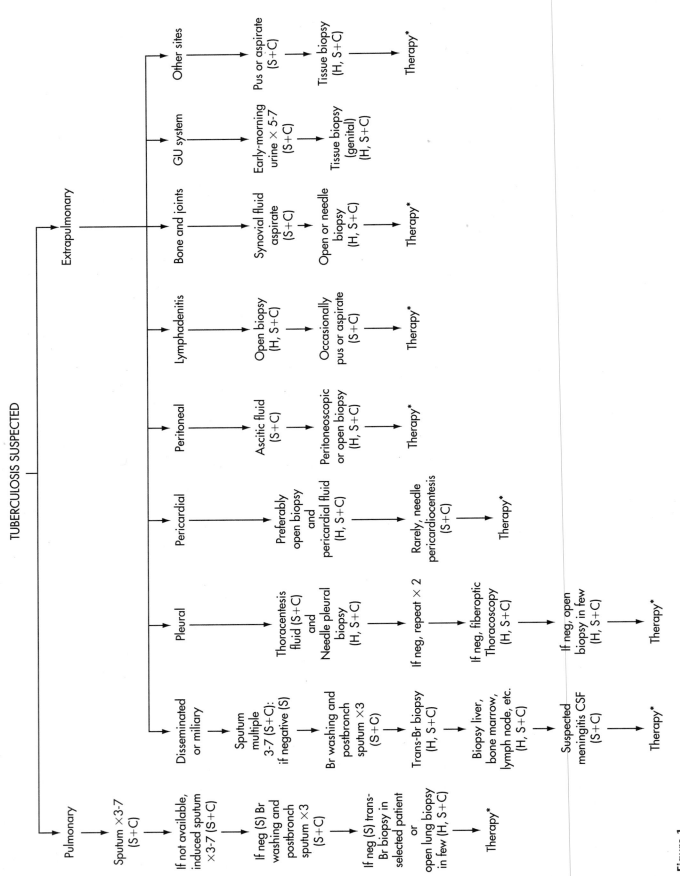

Figure 1

Diagnosis of suspected TB. *S,* Smear; *C,* culture for mycobacteria; *H,* histology; *Br,* bronchial; *Bronch,* bronchoscopy; *CSF,* cerebrospinal fluid; *Bx,* biopsy; *neg,* negative; *GU,* genitourinary.

*Therapy started in suspected cases, awaiting culture results and/or clinical response.

Table 1 Antituberculosis Drugs

DRUG	DAILY DOSAGE	TWICE-WEEKLY DOSAGE	SIDE EFFECTS	MODE OF ACTION
FIRST-LINE DRUGS				
Streptomycin, other aminoglycosides	10-15 mg/kg (usually 0.5-1 g) 5 days/wk	20-25 mg/kg (usually 1-1.5 g) IM	Cranial nerve VIII damage (vestibular and auditory), nephrotoxicity, allergic fever, rash	Active against rapidly multiplying bacilli in neutral or slightly alkaline extracellular medium
Capreomycin	Same as aminoglycosides	Same as aminoglycosides	Same as aminoglycosides	Same as aminoglycosides
Isoniazid	5 mg/kg (usually 300 mg) PO or IM	15 mg/kg (usually 900 mg) PO	Peripheral neuritis, hepatotoxicity, allergic fever and rash, lupus erythematosus phenomenon	Acts strongly on rapidly dividing extracellular bacilli; acts weakly on slowly multiplying intracellular bacilli
Rifampin	10 mg/kg (usually 450-600 mg) PO	10 mg/kg (usually 450-600 mg) PO	Hepatotoxicity, nausea, vomiting, allergic fever and rash, flulike syndrome, petechiae with thrombocytopenia or acute renal failure during intermittent therapy	Acts on both rapidly and slowly multiplying extracellular and intracellular bacilli, particularly on slowly multiplying persisters
Rifamate (INH 150 mg + RIF 300 mg)	2 capsules daily PO	2 capsules + 2 tablets of INH (300 mg)	Same as for INH and RIF	Same as INH and RIF
Rifater (INH 50 mg + RIF 120 mg + PZA 300 mg)	5-6 capsules daily PO	May be used	Same as for INH, RIF, and PZA	Same as INH, RIF, and PZA
Rifabutin (RBT)	150-300 mg PO	150-300 mg PO	Same as RIF, uveitis, arthralgia, leukopenia	Same as RIF
Rifapentene (RPT)	150 mg once weekly PO	Not used	Same as RIF and RBT Not used in HIV-infected persons	Same as RIF Long half-life
Pyrazinamide	25-30 mg/kg (usually 2.5 g) PO	45-50 mg/kg (usually 3-3.5 mg) PO	Hyperuricemia, hepatotoxicity, allergic fever and rash	Active in acid pH medium on intracellular bacilli
Ethambutol	15-25 mg/kg (usually 800-1600 mg) PO	50 mg/kg PO	Optic neuritis, skin rash, hyperuricemia	Weakly active against both extracellular and intracellular bacilli to inhibit the development of resistant bacilli
SECOND-LINE DRUGS				
Ethionamide	10-15 mg/kg (usually 500-750 mg) in divided doses PO	Not used	Nausea, vomiting, anorexia, allergic fever and rash, hepatotoxicity, neurotoxicity	Same as ethambutol
Cycloserine	15-20 mg/kg (usually 0.75-1 g) in divided doses with 200 mg pyridoxine PO	Not used	Personality changes, psychosis, convulsions, rash	Same as ethambutol
Paraminosalicylic acid	150 mg/kg (usually 12 g) in divided doses PO	Not used	Nausea, vomiting, diarrhea, hepatotoxicity, allergic rash and fever	Weak action on extracellular bacilli; inhibits development of drug-resistant organisms
Thiocetazone*	150 mg PO	Not used	Allergic rash and fever, Stevens-Johnson syndrome, blood disorders, nausea, vomiting	Same as paraminosalicylic acid
Clofazimine (antileprosy)	100 mg tid PO	Not used	Pigmentation of skin, abdominal pain	Active against *Mycobacterium intracellulare*
NEWER AGENTS				
Ofloxacin	400 mg q12h	Not used	Gastrointestinal: diarrhea, nausea, abdominal pain, anorexia; central nervous system: dizziness, restlessness, nightmares, ataxia, seizures	Rapidly multiplying bacilli at neutral or alkaline pH
Ciprofloxacin	750 mg q12h	Not used	Same as ofloxacin	Same as ofloxacin
Azithromycin	500 mg/day, up to 30 days	Not used	Diarrhea, nausea, abdominal pain, elevation of liver enzymes	Rapidly multiplying bacilli in macrophages against *M. intracellulare*
Clarithromycin	1 g q12h	Not used	Same as azithromycin	Same as azithromycin

*Not available in the United States.

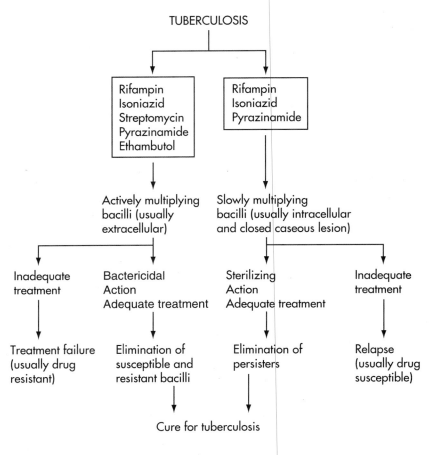

Figure 2
Principles of chemotherapy of tuberculosis.

Table 2 Conditions and Patients with Increased Risk of Drug-Resistant Tuberculosis (TB)

History of treatment with anti-TB drugs, including preventive therapy

Patients from areas with high prevalence of initial or primary drug resistance (>4%) (e.g., urban population in the northeastern United States, Florida, California, U.S.-Mexican border)

Foreign-born persons from areas with high prevalence of drug-resistant TB (e.g., Southeast Asia, Mexico, South America, Africa)

Contacts of persons with drug-resistant disease

Disease in persons who are homeless, drug abusers, and HIV infected

Persons with positive sputum smears and cultures after 3 mo of chemotherapy

Six-Month Regimen

The addition of pyrazinamide (PZA), 25 to 30 mg/kg, to the INH, 300 mg, and RIF, 600 mg daily, for the initial 2 months, followed by INH, 300 mg, and RIF, 600 mg daily, or INH, 900 mg, and RIF, 600 mg twice weekly for another 4 months (a total of 6 months), has proved highly successful. The Centers for Disease Control and Prevention (CDC) American Thoracic Society guidelines recommend this regimen if the prevalence of primary drug resistance is less than 4% (Table 3, option 1).

The three-drug regimen reduces the duration of therapy to 6 months. Addition of PZA accelerates reduction of the bacterial population and adds little to the toxicity of the regimen, although its cost is greater. The addition of a third drug, PZA, ensures against failure in the event of initial resistance to either INH or RIF. In clinical studies, 6 months of therapy with these drugs has been less effective in RIF-resistant cases than in INH-resistant cases.

Six-Month Therapy When Resistance is Suspected

When drug resistance is suspected or likely, at least four-drug therapy consisting of INH 300 mg, RIF 600 mg, PZA 25 to 35 mg/kg, and streptomycin (SM) 0.5 to 1 g IM 5 days a week or ethambutol (EMB) 25 mg/kg should be administered initially (option 1, Table 3). After drug susceptibility results are available, usually 2 months, the regimen is modified accordingly. If the organisms are found to be susceptible to both drugs, therapy is completed with INH-RIF daily or twice weekly for another 4 months. In cases of INH resistance, therapy may consist of RIF, PZA, and EMB for another 6 to 7 months. INH should be included in the regimen because of its action on persisters, which generally remain INH sensitive. In RIF-resistant cases, other bactericidal drugs should be continued for at least 10 to 12 months to prevent relapse.

Treatment of Multidrug-Resistant Disease

Where the prevalence of multidrug resistance (MDR) and HIV infection are very high, it is necessary to initiate a five-

Table 3 Regimens for the Initial Treatment of TB

| TB WITHOUT HIV INFECTION | | | TB WITH HIV INFECTION |
OPTION 1	OPTION 2	OPTION 3	
INH, RIF, PZA (if initial INH resistance is <4%) daily for 8 weeks, followed by INH and RIF daily or twice weekly for 16 wk Add EMB or SM if resistance is (>4%)	INH, RIF, PZA EMB, or SM daily for 2 wk, then twice weekly for 6 wk (DOT), subsequently INH and RIF twice weekly for 16 wk (DOT)	INH, RIF, PZA, EMB, or SM 3 times a week for 6 mo (DOT)	Option 1, 2, or 3 for a total of 9 mo, at least 6 mo beyond culture conversion
Total treatment 6 mo (at least 3 mo past culture conversion)	Total treatment 6 mo	Total treatment 6 mo	Total treatment 6-9 mo

From Centers for Disease Control and Prevention: Initial therapy for tuberculosis in the era of multidrug resistance: Recommendations of the Advisory Council for the Elimination of Tuberculosis, *MMWR* 42 (RR-7):1-8, 1993.
INH, Isoniazid; *RIF,* rifampin; *PZA,* pyrazinamide; *EMB,* ethambutol; *SM,* streptomycin; *DOT,* directly observed therapy.

to seven-drug regimen, including second-line drugs. This is applicable to large urban populations such as New York City, Miami, parts of New Jersey, and San Francisco, as well as persons from developing countries.

In the treatment of MDR disease, that is, resistance to INH and RIF, some basic principles must be followed: (1) A single drug must not be added to a failing regimen. (2) At least three new drugs the patient has not yet taken should replace the existing drug regimen until the susceptibility results are available. (3) The total duration of therapy must be prolonged to 24 months or more. (4) The regimen should include an injectable drug for at least 4 months after the culture is converted to negative. (5) Directly observed therapy (DOT) should be used to ensure compliance, because it is the patient's last chance at a cure.

Most drugs used for MDR disease are second-line drugs (see Table 1)—ethionamide, cycloserine, paraaminosalicylic acid (PAS), capreomycin, and kanamycin. Newer drugs, fluoroquinolones (ciprofloxacin and ofloxacin), and amikacin are available but unproven. Finally, clofazimine and thiocetazone (not available in the United States) may be used but also are unproven. These second-line drugs are often rather toxic, and close monitoring is necessary. Monthly bacteriologic studies are necessary to monitor response to treatment.

Because of high failure and relapse rates in MDR TB, surgical resection of the major diseased area of the lung is again becoming necessary after reasonable medical treatment has been given to reduce the bacterial load.

Preventive therapy for recent contacts with MDR TB is controversial. However, two possible regimens are PZA plus EMB and PZA plus ciprofloxacin or oxafloxacin for 12 to 24 months, during which periodic clinical, bacteriologic, and radiologic monitoring must be maintained.

Treatment Regimens for HIV-Infected Persons

Current 6 month treatment in the United States consisting of INH, RIF, PZA, and EMB or SM daily for 2 months followed by INH and RIF daily or twice weekly for another 4 months is not adequate in HIV-infected patients. The CDC recommends that therapy for patients with HIV infection be prolonged to 9 months or for at least 6 months following conversion of sputum cultures to negative (Table 3). Treatment-limiting side effects are frequent in HIV infected patients, and they require innovative measures. Intermittent regimens (two or three doses a week) are generally well tolerated in such situations.

The protease inhibitors and nonnucleoside reverse transcriptase inhibitors (NNRTIs) have considerable interactions with rifamycins (RIF, rifabutin [RFB], and rifapentene [RPT]) as a result of induction or inhibition of hepatic cytochrome CYP450 enzyme system. Out of these rifamycins, RFB has substantially less activity as an inducer.

For HIV-infected persons who are receiving therapy with protease inhibitors or NNRTIs, RIF is replaced with RFB 300 mg daily. The twice-weekly dosage remains the same. However, if the patient is taking indinavir, nelfinavir, or amprenavir, the daily dose of RFB is decreased to 150 mg, but twice-weekly dosage remains unchanged to 300 mg. Also, if the patient is taking efavirenz, the daily or twice-weekly dosage of RFB is increased from 300 to 450 mg.

The dosage of protease inhibitors or NNRTIs may be increased 20% to 25% when used with rifabutin (RFB). However, periodic check with HIV RNA level is necessary to assess decreased antiretroviral drug activity. Concurrent use of rifabutin (RFB) is avoided with ritonavir and delavirdine.

Smear-Negative Tuberculosis

Positive sputum smears indicate a large bacterial population and advanced disease, while negative smears generally suggest less advanced disease. We have treated a large number of patients having three initial specimens with negative smears but one or two positive cultures with INH and RIF for 6 months. Relapses are no more common than in smear-positive cases treated for 9 months. Occasionally a patient who is smear-negative is also culture negative, but is treated for TB on the basis of clinical and x-ray findings. Regimens for such patients have included 4 months of INH plus RIF. Another suggested regimen for smear-negative TB is INH, RIF, PZA, and EMB for 4 months.

Extrapulmonary Tuberculosis

The bacterial load in extrapulmonary TB usually is much smaller than in cavitary pulmonary TB. Thus 6- to 9-month regimens (see Table 3) are adequate for treatment of extrapulmonary TB. Figure 1 indicates the steps in the diagnosis of pulmonary and extrapulmonary TB. We have successfully treated many patients with extrapulmonary TB with INH and RIF, but the increasing incidence of drug resistance necessitates additional drugs. It is generally recommended that the duration of therapy be prolonged in TB spondylitis (Pott's disease).

Directly Observed Therapy

DOT is the best method to ensure compliance, avoid selective ingestion of medication by the patient, and minimize the risk of developing resistant disease. World Health Organization (WHO) strongly recommends that all tuberculosis medication should be given under a directly observed treatment program. The supervision required for DOT is difficult for physicians in managed care and is best turned over to the local public health unit.

The fact that most of the 6-month regimens may be given intermittently two or three times per week has led to the development of some innovative regimens. The Denver regimen consists of DOT administration of daily INH, RIF, PZA, and SM or EMB for 2 weeks, followed by twice-weekly doses for 6 weeks and then twice-weekly administration of INH or RIF for another 16 weeks. Another DOT regimen is INH, RIF, PZA, and EMB or SM three times a week for 6 months (see Table 3, options 2 and 3).

Therapy in Special Situations
Pregnancy

Treatment with INH, RIF, and EMB is safe in pregnancy. SM should not be used because of toxicity to eighth nerve of the fetus. Experience with PZA is limited in pregnancy, and at present it should be avoided if possible.

Renal Failure

INH and RIF dosage need not be altered in renal failure because these drugs are excreted by the liver. Renal dialysis patients should receive the drugs after dialysis. EMB dosage must be reduced to 8 to 10 mg/kg in advanced renal failure. SM and aminoglycosides should be avoided in these patients, and the level should be monitored if they must be used in very unusual circumstances. PZA dosage should be reduced to 15 to 20 mg/kg.

Liver Disease

Alcoholic liver disease does not preclude use of antituberculosis drugs. However, monitoring for side effects must be careful and regular. In overt liver failure, the therapy should consist of INH and EMB until liver function returns to normal. At that time, RIF and/or PZA may be added to the regimen.

Combined Preparations

In the United States, two commercial preparations of combination drugs are available. It is advantageous to use combination preparations because they preclude the taking of only one bactericidal drug, which encourages drug resistance. Rifamate is a combination capsule of INH 150 mg and RIF 300 mg, and two capsules are the recommended daily dose. Another preparation, Rifater, contains INH 50 mg, RIF 120 mg, and PZA 300 mg in each tablet; the recommended dose is five tablets daily. We strongly recommend the use of combination preparations for therapy as a safeguard against development of drug resistance, particularly for patients not on DOT.

Corticosteroid Therapy

Corticosteroids are not routinely used in the treatment of TB. Prednisone, 20 to 30 mg/day, may improve the general sense of well-being, reduce fever, increase appetite, and improve nutrition of markedly toxic or severely debilitated patients. The drug should be tapered off gradually after 4 to 8 weeks. In disseminated TB associated with hypoxemia and respiratory failure, prednisone, 40 to 60 mg a day, may improve oxygenation. Steroids have been successfully used in AIDS patients with TB, but they may promote opportunistic infections. Most authorities believe that complicated tuberculous meningitis should be treated with prednisone, 60 to 80 mg/day, slowly tapered after 8 to 12 weeks. Some advise corticosteroid therapy for all cases of tuberculous pericarditis to prevent constrictive pericarditis.

■ MONITORING AND FOLLOW-UP OF PATIENTS

Intense bacteriologic monitoring is necessary during therapy of pulmonary TB. We recommend that three to five specimens of bronchial secretions (sputum) be examined initially by smear and culture, followed by drug susceptibility testing. During therapy, at least one specimen of sputum should be examined every 2 weeks until conversion to negative occurs. This permits early detection of noncompliance and impending failure. After completion of treatment, to detect early relapse, one specimen every 3 months three times should be examined before discharging the patient from the clinic.

Monitoring for side effects should be done monthly after explaining to the patient the symptoms of side effects for which to be alert (e.g., nausea, vomiting, anorexia, dark urine, jaundice). Blood should be collected for baseline complete blood count, renal, and hepatic function tests. We do not recommend routine monthly blood studies. Rather, the patients are advised to discontinue medication when symptomatic, and to report for repeat hepatic function studies at that time. The drugs are then adjusted to the laboratory findings. For EMB, vision and color studies are performed monthly, and for SM, monthly examination for balance and hearing loss.

Serum concentrations of the drugs should be checked in patients who fail to respond to adequate therapy, such as remaining bacteriologically positive beyond 3 months or more after good chemotherapy. In some patients, absorption from the gut may be deficient. This may occur particularly with rifampin. Based on the levels, the dosage of the drugs may be adjusted to achieve therapeutic levels. This may prevent failure of therapy and development of drug resistance. Laboratories equipped to determine serum levels of the drugs are available at National Jewish Hospital, Denver, Colorado, or at University of Alabama, Birmingham, Alabama.

■ PROPHYLAXIS

For prophylaxis, see the chapter *Nonsurgical Antimicrobial Prophylaxis.*

Suggested Reading

Centers for Disease Control and Prevention: Initial therapy for tuberculosis in the era of multidrug resistance: Recommendations of the Advisory Council for the Elimination of Tuberculosis, *MMWR* 42(RR-7):1, 1993.

Centers for Disease Control and Prevention: Prevention and treatment of tuberculosis among patients infected with human immunodeficiency virus: principles of therapy and revised recommendation, *MMWR* 47(RR-20):1, 1998.

Dutt AK, Moers D, Stead WW: Short course chemotherapy for extrapulmonary tuberculosis, *Ann Intern Med* 104:771, 1986.

Dutt AK, Stead WW: Medical perspective: present chemotherapy for tuberculosis, *J Infect Dis* 146:698, 1982.

Goble M, et al: Treatment of 171 patients with pulmonary tuberculosis resistant to isoniazid and rifampin, *N Engl J Med* 328:527, 1993.

Iseman MD: Treatment of multidrug-resistant tuberculosis, *N Engl J Med* 329:784, 1993.

Weiss SE, et al: The effect of directly observed therapy on the rates of drug resistance and relapse in tuberculosis, *N Engl J Med* 330:1179, 1994.

NONTUBERCULOUS MYCOBACTERIA

Dina B. KiaNoury
Henry Yeager, Jr.

The nontuberculous mycobacteria (NTM) are rather ubiquitous in our environment. The common NTM species include *Mycobacterium avium complex* (MAC), *M. kansasii*, and the rapidly growing mycobacteria (RGM) species, which includes *M. chelonae*, *M. fortuitum*, and *M. abscessus*. The less common mycobacterium species include, among others, *M. scrofulaceum*, *M. marinum*, *M. ulcerans*, *M. haemophilum*, and *M. szulgai*. Infection is thought to occur from environmental exposure to the NTM. The portals of entry for infection with these species are thought to be the gastrointestinal and respiratory tracts, and via direct inoculation of the skin and soft tissues. No human-to-human transmission is thought to occur.

The most common isolated manifestation of NTM infection in immunocompetent patients is chronic pulmonary disease. The most common patients with this form of infection are typically older white male adults. Most will have underlying lung disease, such as bronchiectasis, cystic fibrosis, previous pulmonary tuberculosis, and chronic obstructive pulmonary disease. A second group that is being seen with greater frequency is elderly white females with no known predisposing factors. The disease is commonly in the lingula or right middle lobe. Symptoms are usually insidious and may vary to include weakness, night sweats, weight loss, chronic productive cough, dyspnea, and hemoptysis.

Lymphadenitis is the most common disease manifestation of NTM infection in children. *M. tuberculosis* accounts for only about 10% of all mycobacterial lymphadenitis cases in children, but approximately 90% of those in adults.

Infection usually occurs in children ages 1 to 5 years. Symptoms are most often minimal, with low-grade fevers and unilateral involvement of the submandibular, submaxillary, preauricular, and cervical lymph nodes. Nearly all of the NTM have been found to cause infections of the skin, soft tissues, and joints, but the most common are secondary to *M. fortuitum*, *M. abscessus*, *M. marinum*, *M. chelonae*, and *M. kansasii*. Inoculation usually results after surgery or local trauma, such as stepping on a nail, has occurred.

Dissemination in immunocompromised patients has been reported for several of the NTM species. Although most commonly seen in patients infected with the human immunodeficiency virus (HIV), it has also been reported to occur in other immunosuppressed states.

■ *MYCOBACTERIUM AVIUM* COMPLEX (MAC)

M. avium and *M. intracellulare* have been commonly referred to as *MAC*. These have been found in soil, water, and in dairy products. In the southeastern United States, MAC is the most common of the NTM to cause pulmonary disease. MAC infection has been the most common bacterial infection among patients infected with HIV. MAC infections are increasingly common in elderly white females without evidence of preexisting lung disease. Disease can be localized to an organ (e.g., cervical lymphadenitis in children, of which MAC is the most common cause) or disseminated.

■ MAC INFECTION IN HIV

Dissemination may occur in up to 20% to 40% of patients with HIV in the absence of chemoprophylaxis. Risk factors for dissemination include a CD4 count of less than 100 cells/μl, average of 25 to 30 cells/μl, and anemia (hemoglobin <8 g/dl). Symptoms can include fever, weight loss, night sweats, abdominal pain, diarrhea, and anemia with or without an elevated alkaline phosphatase. Diagnosis is made by at least one positive blood culture or alternatively with a positive bone marrow, liver, or lymph node biopsy culture. The predictive value of a stool culture is low.

In adults with acquired immunodeficiency syndrome (AIDS) who have a CD4 count of less than 50, prophylaxis with one of the following regimens is recommended (Table 1): rifabutin, 300 mg/day, clarithromycin, 500 mg twice daily; azithromycin, 1200 mg once a week; or azithromycin once a week plus rifabutin, 300 mg/day. It is important to exclude active infection with MAC or MTB before initiating MAC prophylaxis. This is done by performing a chest radiograph and a tuberculin skin test, and if any systemic signs of infection, such as fever, night sweats, or weight loss are present, at least one blood culture for MAC.

In disseminated disease, treatment should include clar-

Table 1   Treatment of Nontuberculous Mycobacterial Infections

NTM SPECIES	DISEASE	TREATMENT	COMMENTS
MAC (*M. avium* and *M. intracellulare*)	Disseminated	Clarithromycin, 500 mg bid, or azithromycin, 250-500 mg qd, plus ethambutol, 15 mg/kg/day ± rifabutin	Continue treatment for life. Prophylaxis is recommended for adults with AIDS who have a CD4 count <50.
	Pulmonary disease in non-HIV	Clarithromycin, 500 mg bid, or azithromycin, 250-500 mg, plus rifampin, 600 mg qd, or rifabutin, 300 mg qd, plus ethambutol, 25 mg/kg/day for 2 mo and then 15 mg/kg/day ± streptomycin for the first 2 months; for patients older than 70 or of low weight, consider a modified regimen	Treat for at least 1 yr after cultures become negative.
M. kansasii	Pulmonary and extrapulmonary	Isoniazid, 300 mg/day, plus rifampin, 600 mg/day, plus ethambutol, 25 mg/kg/day for 2 months followed by 15 mg/kg	Treat for at least 1 yr after cultures become negative. Rifampin should be replaced with either clarithromycin or rifabutin in HIV-positive patients using protease inhibitors.
Rapidly growing mycobacteria (RGM) (*M. fortuitum, M. chelonae, M. abscessus*)	Soft-tissue infections, localized		Do sensitivities to clarithromycin, ciprofloxacin, doxycycline, amikacin, tobramycin, imipenem.
	Mild	Oral meds only	Remove foreign body or catheter.
	Extensive	IV meds for 2-4 wk, followed by oral meds; total 3-6 mo	
	Soft-tissue infections, disseminated	*M. chelonae,* 1× daily tobramycin + clarithromycin 2-4 wk, then clarithromycin only for total of 6 mo	
		M. abscessus—same as *M. chelonae,* except use amikacin instead of tobramycin	
	Chronic pulmonary infection		
	M. abscessus	Cefoxitin + amikacin IV 2-4 wk, then suppressive therapy with macrolide	About 80% of all RGM lung infections.
	M. fortuitum	Multiple oral meds for 6 mo, with or without 2-4 wk IV treatment at first	About 20% of all RGM lung infections.
M. scrofulaceum	Lymphadenitis	Excisional biopsy Clarithromycin-containing regimen	Excision yields an approximately 95% cure. Incision and drainage or percutaneous biopsy is contraindicated.
M. marinum	Skin and soft-tissue infections	Surgical debridement, cryosurgery, or electrodessication	Superficial skin lesions may resolve without treatment.
		For somewhat extensive infections: minocycline or doxycycline, 100 mg bid, or trimethoprim-sulfamethoxazole, 160/800 mg bid	A response to treatment may not be seen for up to 3 wk. Treat for at least 3 mo.
		For more extensive infections: rifampin, 600 mg/day, plus ethambutol, 15 mg/kg/day	
M. ulcerans	Skin infections	Surgical excision for widespread skin involvement ± rifampin and sulfamethoxazole	
M. haemophilum	Skin infections	Depends on in vitro susceptibility testing	Duration of therapy depends on clinical response.

HIV, Human immunodeficiency virus.

ithromycin, 500 mg twice daily or daily azithromycin, 250 to 500 mg, plus ethambutol 15 mg/kg and should be continued for life. A third drug (e.g., rifabutin, 300 mg/day) may be added to the regimen. Some success has been shown with the use of interferon gamma in cases of refractory disseminated infection in patients with non-HIV familial mycobacteriosis.

■ MAC INFECTION IN THE IMMUNOCOMPETENT PATIENT

In non-AIDS patients the predominant infection is in the lungs, and diagnosis requires repeated isolation of MAC in two or more sputum samples with a consistent radiographic picture of active lung disease. The typical chest radiograph in patients, male or female, with preexisting lung disease will reveal bilateral or unilateral upper lobe predominant, fibronodular disease, with or without cavitation. This is similar to the findings of MTB infection. However, cavity walls may be thinner, and there are far fewer cases with pleural effusion than with MTB.

The pattern may be different in older patients, mostly white women, without preexisting lung disease, with scattered nodular infiltrates of the bilateral lower lobes associated with pleural thickening and bronchiectasis. The lingula and right middle lobe appear to be most frequently involved. This has been commonly referred to as the *Lady Windermere syndrome*. Pulmonary MAC disease may also present as a solitary nodule. Skeletal abnormalities such as pectus excavatum and scoliosis have been associated with an increased risk for MAC infection.

In non-HIV patients, the daily treatment regimen for pulmonary disease secondary to MAC infection should include clarithromycin, 500 mg twice daily, or azithromycin, 250 mg, plus rifampin, 600 mg or rifabutin, 300 mg, plus ethambutol, 25 mg/kg for 2 months and then 15 mg/kg. Treatment should be continued until cultures are negative for at least 1 year. Streptomycin may be added to the above regimen two to three times per week for additional coverage during the first 8 weeks. Treatment of MAC pulmonary disease is difficult secondary to frequent medication intolerance. Although no controlled trials have been performed, lobectomy for localized disease that has not responded to medical therapy has been performed with some success.

■ *MYCOBACTERIUM KANSASII*

M. kansasii is the second most common NTM to cause pulmonary disease in the United States. The organism is most prevalent in the midwest and southwest. Only occasionally will dissemination occur. HIV patients infected with this organism typically have an average CD4 count of less than 200 cells/μl. The course after infection with *M. kansasii* can be an indolent or rapidly progressive one. When isolated from respiratory culture *M. kansasii* is considered to be an invasive pathogen. Radiographic findings will typically show diffuse reticulonodular infiltrates with an upper lobe predominance.

The treatment regimen for extrapulmonary as well as pulmonary disease is the same and should include 18 months of isoniazid, 300 mg/day, plus rifampin, 600 mg/day, plus ethambutol, 25 mg/kg/day for the first 2 months, then 15 mg/kg/day. Therapy should continue for a minimum of 12 months after cultures become negative. In HIV-positive patients taking protease inhibitors, rifampin should be replaced with either clarithromycin or rifabutin.

■ RAPIDLY GROWING MYCOBACTERIA

The rapidly growing mycobacteria (RGM) include *M. chelonae, M. fortuitum,* and *M. abscessus*. These have been isolated from the soil and natural water supplies and primarily cause cutaneous disease. Most cases are sporadic and community acquired. Nosocomial outbreaks associated with wound infections and case clustering have been reported in patients who have undergone cardiac surgery, line placement, continuous ambulatory peritoneal dialysis catheters, total hip replacement, pacemaker insertion, and breast augmentation.

Patients who develop pulmonary disease from infection with the RGM have been observed to have similar characteristics to the elderly white females without underlying lung disease who get MAC lung infection. This is most often as *M. abscessus,* less for *M. fortuitum*. The course can be slow and progressive. Chest radiographs most commonly reveal a diffuse, reticulonodular, or mixed alveolar-interstitial pattern. Cavitation is uncommon.

The treatment of choice for the soft tissue infections caused by the RGM is surgical debridement and antibiotics. For pulmonary or other deep organ infection therapy is usually with antibiotics alone. The RGM are usually resistant to the standard antimycobacterial drugs and therefore susceptibility testing should be done with other antibiotics to which they may be responsive, such as amikacin, clarithromycin, erythromycin, sulfamethoxazole, doxycycline, cefoxitin, and ciprofloxacin. At least six months of daily therapy with amikacin, 10 to 15 mg/kg, plus cefoxitin, 200 mg, should be given for serious infections with *M. fortuitum,* or 3 months of the same for serious *M. chelonae* infection. For milder *M. fortuitum* infection, sulfamethoxazole, 3 g/day, or doxycycline, 200 mg/day, can be used if the organism is sensitive. For milder *M. chelonae* infections, erythromycin, 2 g/day, can be used if in vitro sensitivities permit.

M. abscessus, formerly a subspecies of *M. chelonae,* can cause pulmonary as well as cutaneous disease. In fact, it is the most common rapid grower to cause pulmonary disease. As is true for *M. fortuitum* and *M. chelonae,* drug resistance is a serious problem resulting in high relapse rates. The organism will often show in vitro susceptibility to only intravenous antibiotics. Eradication of *M. abscessus* from sputum is difficult, and persistent presence of the organism is associated with chronic progressive lung disease. Although not curative, some improvement has been reported after 2 to 6 weeks of therapy with amikacin and cefoxitin. Usually this is followed by oral suppressive therapy with a macroslide *M. fortuitum*. Pulmonary disease can often be treated successfully with two oral antibiotics to which the bacteria are sensitive.

■ *MYCOBACTERIUM SCROFULACEUM*

M. scrofulaceum is an occasional pathogen and is the second most common cause of NTM lymphadenitis in children. Diagnosis is by pathologic demonstration of lymph nodes with granulomatous inflammation, with or without the presence of AFB, and cultures positive for *M. scrofulaceum*. Percutaneous biopsy or incision and drainage is not recommended, as fistula formation with chronic drainage may occur. Excisional biopsy is the definitive treatment and results in an approximately 95% cure rate. If response is poor or disease is extensive, then treatment with a clarithromycin-containing regimen should be considered. If MTB cannot be excluded because of the age of the child (i.e., older than 5 years), a positive PPD skin test, or bilateral cervical lymph node involvement, treatment with isoniazid, rifampin, and ethambutol should be instituted pending culture results.

■ *MYCOBACTERIUM MARINUM*

M. marinum infection infects the skin and soft tissues and is commonly acquired after exposure to stagnant water, such as in fish tanks. Known as "swimming pool granuloma" or "fish tank granuloma," lesions are usually solitary and ascending, resembling sporotrichosis. They present as slow-growing, nodular verrucous or ulcerating lesions of the extremities. Diagnosis is made by biopsy and culture.

Superficial skin lesions may resolve spontaneously, but deeper infections and bone involvement require therapy. For small, superficial lesions surgical debridement, cryosurgery, or electrodessication may be all that is required. Treatment in adults can include clarithromycin, 500 mg twice daily, minocycline or doxycycline at a dosage of 100 mg twice daily, trimethoprim-sulfamethoxazole at 160 to 800 mg twice daily, or rifampin, 600 mg/day plus ethambutol at a dosage of 15 mg/kg/day. For mild to moderate disease, minocycline, doxycycline, or trimethoprim-sulfamethoxazole can be used. For more extensive disease, rifampin and ethambutol are recommended. A response to treatment may not be seen for up to 3 weeks, and therapy should continue for at least 3 months. Recurrences are common and may respond to the reinstitution of therapy.

■ *MYCOBACTERIUM ULCERANS*

M. ulcerans is mainly a disease of the tropics and only a few cases have been reported in the United States. Patients develop skin lesions, usually of the extremities, after exposure. Lesions appear as erythematous nodules with peripheral expansion, central necrosis and undermining. Diagnosis is made by biopsy which shows necrosis with a neutrophil predominant infiltrate which is histologically different when compared to the other NTM, which have pathologic findings similar to MTB.

As is the case with *M. marinum*, surgical excision for widespread skin involvement is recommended. The role of drugs, especially rifampin and trimethoprim-sulfamethoxazole, is controversial.

■ *MYCOBACTERIUM HAEMOPHILUM*

M. haemophilum predominantly infects the skin, causing multiple cutaneous ulcerating lesions of the extremities, usually over joints. The organism has also been isolated from sputum, bone and synovial fluid. Dissemination can occur in patients with AIDS or other immunocompromised states. Infection has also been reported in renal transplant and bone marrow transplant patients. Diagnosis can be difficult because of specific growth requirements required by this organism when compared with other NTM.

Although no studies have compared the efficacy and duration of therapy of the various drugs for *M. haemophilum*, in vitro susceptibility testing suggests that this organism is sensitive to ciprofloxacin, cycloserine, rifabutin, and kanamycin. It appears to be less sensitive to the standard antimycobacterial regimens. The duration of therapy should depend on the clinical response.

■ *MYCOBACTERIUM SZULGAI*

M. szulgai can cause skin, joint, lymphatic, pulmonary and disseminated disease. If isolated, this organism should be considered a pathogen. Treatment with rifampin and higher than usual doses of isoniazid, streptomycin, and ethambutol has been successful.

Suggested Reading

Griffith DE, Girard WM, Wallace RJ Jr: Clinical features of pulmonary disease caused by rapidly growing mycobacteria, *Am Rev Respir Dis* 147:1271, 1993.

Patz EF, Jr, Swensen SJ, Erasmus J: Pulmonary manifestations of nontuberculous mycobacterium, *Radiol Clin North Am* 33:719, 1995.

Wallace RJ, et al: Diagnosis and treatment of disease caused by nontuberculous mycobacteria (ATS statement), *Am J Respir Crit Care Med* 156:SI, 1997.

VIBRIOS

Duc J. Vugia

Vibrios are motile, rod-shaped, facultative-anaerobic, gram-negative bacteria that can cause gastroenteritis, wound infection, and septicemia in humans. They are naturally found in marine, estuarine, and brackish waters in the United States and in other parts of the world. In the United States, they are recovered from the environment most commonly in summer and fall, when the water is warm. Vibrios have also been isolated from a variety of fish and shellfish, including oysters, clams, mussels, crabs, and shrimp. Human cases of illness associated with *Vibrio* infection occur mostly in summer and fall and usually follow ingestion of raw or undercooked shellfish, particularly oysters, or exposure of a wound to fish, shellfish, or seawater. In countries with endemic or epidemic cholera, infection with *V. cholerae* may occur after ingestion of any contaminated food or water; in the United States cholera is endemic along the Gulf Coast.

Analysis of 5S ribosomal ribonucleic acid sequence revealed 34 *Vibrio* species, 12 of which have been isolated from human clinical specimens. The major clinical presentations associated with infection with these 12 species are shown in Table 1.

Rarely, vibrios have also been recovered from bone, cerebrospinal fluid, ear, gallbladder, sputum, and urine.

■ GASTROENTERITIS AND CHOLERA

Clinical Presentation

Gastroenteritis is the most common clinical presentation of infection with most pathogenic vibrios. The disease ranges in severity from mild, self-limited diarrhea to frank, life-threatening cholera.

Cholera is a profuse, watery diarrhea mediated via an enterotoxin produced by epidemic strains of *V. cholerae* O1 and O139 and by some non-O1 strains. After attachment of toxigenic vibrios to intestinal epithelial cells, the cholera toxin, consisting of one A (activation) unit and five B (binding) units, is generated. It stimulates intracellular cyclic adenosine monophosphate (cAMP), resulting in a secretory diarrhea. Other symptoms include nausea, vomiting, abdominal cramps, and muscle cramps of extremities; fever is typically not seen because the disease is toxin-mediated and there is no invasion of the intestinal epithelium. Illness develops 4 hours to 5 days after ingestion of the bacteria and can rapidly lead to severe dehydration, electrolyte imbalance, acidosis, and death. Cholera usually lasts less than 7 days even without antibiotic therapy.

Gastroenteritis caused by vibrios other than *V. cholerae* O1 and O139 may also be mediated via an enterotoxin, but the diarrhea is normally not so severe. However, bloody stool, low-grade fever, and elevated white blood cell count may be noted along with nausea, vomiting, and abdominal cramps. The median incubation period is 1 day, ranging from 4 hours to 5 days, and the duration of illness is typically less than 7 days, ranging from 1 to 15 days.

Therapy

For cholera, prompt fluid volume and electrolyte replacement with an appropriate intravenous or oral solution is critical. If the patient has severe dehydration (loss of at least 10% of body weight) or cannot drink, intravenous fluid replacement with Ringer's lactate is recommended. Other intravenous solutions do not contain similar proportions of necessary electrolytes and are therefore not optimal. If the patient can drink, a solution containing adequate electrolyte replacement is recommended, such as those prepared with the oral rehydration salts endorsed by the World Health Organization or commercially available Rehydralyte.

Treatment of cholera with antimicrobials will decrease shedding of vibrios and duration of illness. Multidrug-resistant strains of *V. cholerae* O1 have emerged in Africa and in Asia in recent years; antibiotic susceptibility testing should be performed on isolates from cholera patients. In adults, if infection was acquired in Asia or Africa, ciprofloxacin, either 500 mg orally twice daily for 3 days or 1 g orally in a single dose, is the antimicrobial treatment of choice. For cholera acquired in the Americas, where tetracycline resistance is not yet a problem, doxycycline, 100 mg orally twice daily for 3 days, or tetracycline, 500 mg orally four times daily for 3 days, is still effective. For tetracycline-resistant cholera in children, there is concern for possible arthropathy with using quinolones, but that risk is probably low for a short course such as with ciprofloxacin 30 mg/kg up to a maximum of 1 g divided into two oral doses daily for 3 days. An alternative is erythromycin 30 to 50 mg/kg up to a maximum of 2 g divided into four doses daily for 3 days.

For severe or prolonged gastroenteritis due to other vibrios, fluid and electrolyte replacement along with tetracycline or doxycycline treatment is in order. However, mild or moderate gastroenteritis is usually self-limited and may not need therapy other than oral rehydration.

■ EXTRAINTESTINAL INFECTIONS

Clinical Presentations

For extraintestinal sites, wound infection and septicemia are the most common clinical presentations. Wound infection with vibrios occurs after exposure of a break in skin to seawater or after a skin injury from handling fish or shellfish. Wound infection may be mild and self-limited or severe and invasive. Septicemia, which may be primary following ingestion or secondary (e.g., following wound infection), indicates severe disease.

Among vibrios causing extraintestinal infections, *V. vulnificus* often causes two important clinical syndromes: primary septicemia and wound infections. Primary septicemia occurs predominantly in adults with liver disease, including cirrhosis and hemochromatosis, with alcoholism, with other chronic underlying diseases, including renal failure and diabetes, or with immune suppression, including cancer and

Table 1   Association of *Vibrio* with Major Clinical Presentations

SPECIES	CLINICAL PRESENTATIONS		
	GASTROENTERITIS	WOUND INFECTION	SEPTICEMIA
V. cholerae			
O1	++	+	+
O139	++		+
Other non-O1	++	+	+
V. alginolyticus	+	++	+
V. carchariae		+	
V. cincinnatiensis			+
V. damsela		+	+
V. fluvialis	++	+	+
V. furnisii	+		
V. hollisae	++	+	+
V. mimicus	++	+	+
V. metschnikovii	+	+	+
V. parahaemolyticus	++	+	+
V. vulnificus	+	++	++

++, Common; +, rare.

HIV infection. In these susceptible persons, septicemia usually follows ingestion of raw shellfish, typically oysters. Between 7 and 48 hours after eating shellfish containing *V. vulnificus,* infected patients present with fever, chills, nausea, vomiting, abdominal pain, diarrhea, mental status changes, suggestive skin lesions (including bullae, cellulitis, and ecchymoses), and often hypotension or shock. Mortality for patients with *V. vulnificus* primary septicemia is greater than 50%, and it increases greatly with hypotension within 12 hours of hospitalization and when appropriate antibiotic therapy is delayed beyond 72 hours after onset of illness.

V. vulnificus wound infection, on the other hand, results from injury to the skin from handling fish or shellfish or exposure of a fresh wound to seawater. Any healthy person may acquire this infection, but persons with the underlying diseases listed previously are at higher risk for secondary septicemia and death. Infected persons develop inflammation of the wound, fever, and chills 4 hours to 4 days after exposure. Wound infections range from mild cellulitis to severe necrotizing fasciitis and myositis requiring extensive debridement or amputation. Secondary disseminated skin lesions such as bullae may be caused by secondary septicemia.

Therapy

For invasive diseases of *Vibrio,* particularly *V. vulnificus,* prompt treatment with early antibiotic administration, appropriate wound management, and supportive care are crucial. Tetracycline, 500 mg four times daily, the antimicrobial treatment of choice, should be started empirically, intravenously in severe cases, pending laboratory confirmation. The duration of treatment should be individualized to the presentation and clinical course but should probably be considered for at least 10 to 14 days. Alternatives include quinolones and chloramphenicol, to which vibrios are also susceptible. Necrotic tissue should be surgically debrided.

■ LABORATORY DIAGNOSIS

For a patient with a gastrointestinal or cholera-like illness thought to be caused by *Vibrio,* physicians should specify culture for vibrios when ordering stool cultures. Ideally, specimens should be collected before treatment with antimicrobials. Vibrios are isolated by direct inoculation of stool onto a selective medium, such as thiosulfate-citrate-bile-salts-sucrose (TCBS) agar.

Selective media are not necessary for extraintestinal infections because common media used to culture blood and wounds contain at least 0.5% sodium chloride, which is adequate to grow halophilic (salt-loving) vibrios.

For cholera patients already treated with antimicrobials and whose stool culture was either negative or not processed for vibrios, *V. cholerae* vibriocidal or antitoxin antibodies can be detected by serologic assays.

■ PREVENTION

Most *Vibrio* gastroenteritis, cholera, and primary septicemia caused by *V. vulnificus* can be prevented. For travelers, prevention of cholera should include recognizing that cholera exists in the country being visited and taking appropriate precautions with all foods and drinks. In general, well-cooked foods and hot or carbonated drinks are safe. The currently available parenteral vaccine is not recommended because it is only 50% effective and the duration of protection lasts only 3 to 6 months. More effective oral vaccines are commercially available recently but only outside the country. In the United States, *Vibrio* gastroenteritis can be prevented by avoiding consumption of raw or undercooked shellfish. Patients with underlying liver and other chronic diseases or with immunosuppression, which put them at increased risk of *V. vulnificus* septicemia, should avoid raw oysters and other raw shellfish.

Wound infections are probably not preventable because vibrios exist naturally in certain waters and on a variety of fish and shellfish. Nonetheless, an exposure history in a patient with an infected wound should raise clinical suspicion and consideration of treatment for possible infection with a *Vibrio*.

Suggested Reading

Hlady WG, Klontz KC: The epidemiology of *Vibrio* infections in Florida, 1981-1993, *J Infect Dis* 173:1176, 1996.

Hoge CW, et al: Epidemiology and spectrum of *Vibrio* infections in a Chesapeake Bay community, *J Infect Dis* 160:985, 1989.

Janda JM, et al: Current perspectives on the epidemiology and pathogenesis of clinically significant *Vibrio* spp, *Clin Microbiol Rev* 1:245, 1988.

Mahon BE, et al: Reported cholera in the United States, 1992-1994. A reflection of global changes in cholera epidemiology, *JAMA* 276:307, 1996.

YERSINIA

Royce H. Johnson

*Y*ersinia genus includes several species. The most important for human disease are *Y. enterocolitica, Y. pseudotuberculosis,* and *Y. pseudotuberculosis* subspecies *pestis*. More commonly *Y. pseudotuberculosis* subspecies *pestis* is listed as *Y. pestis*. *Y. pseudotuberculosis* and *Y. pestis* are clearly closely related species by analysis of the genome. However, *Y. enterocolitica* and *Y. pseudotuberculosis* produce clinically similar disease and both are quite distinct from that produced by subspecies *Y. pestis;* hence, in this chapter the older terminology *Y. pestis* will be used, and *Y. enterocolitica* and *Y. pseudotuberculosis* discussed separately.

■ YERSINIA PESTIS

In 1894, Alexander Yersin identified the cause of bubonic plague, a disease known since antiquity. In the United States, *Y. pestis* is a zoonosis, with human infection an incidental event. Domestic dogs and cats can also play a role in the transmission of the disease. Most cases occur in New Mexico, Arizona, and California.

Y. pestis usually results from the bite of an infected flea. Less commonly, the ingestion of contaminated meat may result in infection. Inhalation of infected aerosols results in a primary pneumonic disease. Ninety percent of infected individuals present with lymphadenitis or bubonic disease. Incubation is typically 2 to 6 days. Inguinal and femoral nodes are most frequently involved; cervical and axillary lymph node inflammation is less frequent. Disease without lymphadenitis may present as septicemia without localizing findings and represents a substantial problem in differential diagnosis. A careful epidemiologic history is essential in the diagnostic evaluation of patients. Less common sites of infection include the eye, skin, and meninges.

Specimens and cultures from patients with suspected *Y. pestis* must be handled with extreme caution. Smear and culture of lymph node aspirate, sputum, cerebrospinal fluid, buffy coat, or blood should be undertaken as directed by the clinical presentation. A gram stain or the preferred Wayson's stain should be prepared. *Y. pestis* has the classic bipolar safety pin morphology on direct smear. *Y. pestis* is easily propagated on normal laboratory media aerobically or anaerobically. Identification can be undertaken with any of a number of systems appropriate for gram-negative organisms. Difficulty with an exact identification sometimes occurs. All suspected specimens should be referred to an appropriate Public Health Reference Laboratory for confirmation whether identification is clear or not.

Therapy

Therapy of the most common early bubonic manifestation of *Y. pestis* infection is uncomplicated and highly effective (Table 1). Treatment of more severe cases with pneumonia, meningitis, sepsis, and shock often meet with little success. The mortality of untreated cases is greater than 50%. Early treatment can reduce mortality to approximately 5%. Many antimicrobial regimens have been recommended; however, none has been subjected to a controlled trial. Streptomycin has been used since 1948 with great success, although this drug may not be readily available in the United States, necessitating the use of alternative regimens. When streptomycin is available it should be used at a dosage of 15 mg/kg/day every 12 hours. Intramuscular (IM) treatment is recommended, but intravenous (IV) therapy can be used if required by the clinical circumstances. A 10-day course of streptomycin is recommended. Appropriate monitoring for renal, vestibular, and auditory toxicity is required. Doxycycline, 100 mg orally (PO) every 12 hours for 10 days, also has demonstrable efficacy. Tetracyclines are not appropriate for children younger than 8 years of age or for pregnant women. In children, pregnant females, and patients with meningitis, IV and PO chloramphenicol can be used as an alternative. Initial doses of 1 g (25 mg/kg) followed by 500 mg (15 mg/kg) every 6 hours can be used for a total

Table 1 Therapy of *Yersinia pestis*

PREFERRED ANTIBIOTIC	CLASSIFICATION FOR USE
Streptomycin, 15 mg/kg/day q12h IM (or IV if necessary)	If immediate availability is a problem, call direct to Pfizer Pharmaceuticals
Tetracycline HCl, 500 mg-1 g PO q6h	IV not available, not for use during pregnancy or in children <8
Doxycycline, 100 mg PO or IV q12h	Not for use during pregnancy or in children <8
Chloramphenicol, 1 g (25 mg/kg) IV or PO q6h with dosage reduction as patient stabilizes to 500 mg (15 mg/kg) q6h	Predominately for patients with meningitis and children in whom tetracycline is not indicated

Table 2 Therapy of *Yersinia enterocolitica*

PREFERRED AGENTS FOR SERIOUS ILLNESS	AGENTS LIKELY TO BE EFFECTIVE	AGENTS NOT LIKELY TO BE EFFECTIVE
Fluoroquinolones Ceftriaxone	Doxycycline Trimethoprim-sulfamethoxazole Aminoglycosides Aztreonam Imipenem Chloramphenicol*	Penicillin Ampicillin Amoxicillin-clavunulate First-generation cephalosporins

*Not recommended in usual circumstances.

course of 10 days. Trimethoprim-sulfamethoxazole, other aminoglycosides, and third-generation cephalosporins are likely to be effective. Recently, some question has been raised regarding the efficacy of ciprofloxacin and other fluoroquinolones. No evaluable data exist regarding this issue. There has also been a disturbing case report of drug-resistant *Y. pestis* in an isolate from Madagascar. Resistance to ampicillin, chloramphenicol, kanamycin, streptomycin, sulfonamides, and tetracyclines were found. This appeared to be based on a plasmid derived from enteric organisms.

■ *YERSINIA ENTEROCOLITICA* AND *YERSINIA PSEUDOTUBERCULOSIS*

Y. enterocolitica is an increasingly well-recognized pathogen with protean manifestations. *Y. pseudotuberculosis,* a much rarer pathogen, causes gastrointestinal illness and rarely sepsis. *Y. enterocolitica* is widely distributed in nature and also has been identified in food, particularly pork, contaminated milk, and untreated water. Only certain serotypes of *Y. enterocolitica* typically produce gastrointestinal disease. The O:3 serogroup is most commonly responsible for disease in the United States. This serogroup can be distinguished by its failure to ferment D-xylose.

Unlike many enteric pathogens, *Y. enterocolitica* is found most often in cool climates. The disease is reported most commonly from Northern Europe, Japan, Canada, and the United States. The incubation period is 1 to 14 days, typically at the shorter end of this spectrum.

Individuals with iron overload or receiving treatment with desferrioxamine are at increased risk, as are individuals who are immunocompromised. Alkalinization of the stomach may also create an increased risk of infection.

The most common presentations of *Y. enterocolitica* are enteritis or enterocolitis. Children are the most frequently affected. The most typical illness is suggestive of shigellosis, with diarrhea (occasionally bloody), fever, abdominal pain, and vomiting. *Y. enterocolitica* may manifest as mesenteric lymphadenitis and present with abdominal pain that mimics appendicitis. The distinction from true appendicitis can often be made by careful ultrasound or computed tomography (CT) evaluation. *Y. enterocolitica* can also cause suppurative infections: pharyngitis with or without cervical lymphadenitis, hepatic abscess, and pulmonary, genitourinary, and musculoskeletal infections. Bacteremia, endocarditis, pericarditis, and myocarditis have all been reported. Rare cutaneous infections have also been described.

Yersinia enterocolitica has also been shown to precipitate disease through immunopathologic mechanisms. Erythema nodosum, anterior uveitis, and reactive arthritis have all been reported.

Yersinia enterocolitica grows on usual laboratory media, but very slowly. It is often overgrown by rapidly growing fecal flora in gastrointestinal specimens. Selective media or cold enrichment may enhance recovery when this pathogen is suspected.

Therapy

Antimicrobial therapy has not been shown to alter the course or outcome of *Y. enterocolitica* infection of the gastrointestinal tract or typical mesenteric lymphadenitis. However, current practice (Table 2) is to treat such patients when disease is recognized. Nongastrointestinal bacteremic or localized infections should clearly be treated.

Because of beta-lactamase activity that is specific for different serotypes and biotypes, resistance to older beta-lactam antibiotics is common. Penicillin, ampicillin, and first-generation cephalosporins are ineffective. Amoxicillin-clavulanate also appears to be ineffective because of a cephalosporinase activity that is not inhibited by clavulanate. Antipseudomonal penicillins and second-generation cephalosporins are not sufficiently active to be recommended on a routine basis. Only limited clinical information on aztreonam and imipenem-cilastatin is available; in vitro susceptibility testing suggests that these agents are active. Third-generation cephalosporins, especially ceftriaxone, have in vitro and clinical data to suggest significant utility, though there have been clinical failures. Similarly, aminoglycosides, chloramphenicol, trimethoprim-sulfamethoxazole, and doxycycline may be useful. Doxycycline may be particularly useful in less critically-ill patients. Probably the best information on in vitro sensitivity, animal models, and anecdotal human experience is for fluoroquinolones. These data suggest that these agents may be the drugs of choice for severe *Y. enterocolitica* infection.

Duration of treatment shown to be effective has varied between 2 to 6 weeks. Initial therapy is most typically begun with an intravenous drug in severely ill individuals, with completion of therapy on an oral basis.

Yersinia pseudotuberculosis rarely requires therapy when presenting as mesenteric adenitis or gastrointestinal disease. Patients with sepsis may be treated with streptomycin or doxycycline; ampicillin can also be used.

Suggested Reading

Abe J, et al: Clinical role for a superantigen in *Yersinia pseudotuberculosis* infection, *J Clin Invest* 99:1823, 1997.

Butler T: *Yersinia* infections: centennial of the discovery of the plague bacillus, *Clin Infect Dis* 19:655, 1994.

Gage KL, Dennis DT, Tsai TF: Prevention of plague: recommendations of the Advisory Committee on Immunization Practices, *MMWB* 45(RR-14), 1996.

Galimand M, et al: Multidrug resistance in *Yersinia pestis* mediated by a transferable plasmid, *N Engl J Med* 10:677, 1997.

Giamarellou H, et al: *Yersinia entercolitica* endocarditis: case report and literature review, *Euro J Clin Microbiol Infect Dis* 14:126, 1995.

Heijden I, et al: *Yersinia enterocolitica*: a cause of chronic polyarthritis, *Clin Infect Dis* 25:831, 1997.

Hoogkamp-Korstanje JAA, Stolk-Engelaar VMM: *Yersinia enterocolitica* infection in children, *Pediatr Infect Dis J* 14:771, 1995.

Jelloul L, et al: Mesenteric adenitis caused by *Yersinia pseudotuberculosis* presenting as an abdominal mass, *Euro Journal Pediatric Surg* 7:180, 1997.

Stolk-Engelaar VMM, Hoogkamp-Korstanje JAA: Clinical presentation and diagnosis of gastrointestinal infections by *Yersinia enterocolitica* in 261 Dutch patients, *Scand J Infect Dis* 28:571, 1996.

Verhaegen J, et al: Surveillance of human *Yersinia enterocolitica* infections in Belgium: 1967-1966, *Clin Infect Dis* 27:59, 1998.

MISCELLANEOUS GRAM-POSITIVE ORGANISMS

Roberto Baun Corales
Steven K. Schmitt

■ *PEDIOCOCCUS* SPECIES

Pediococci are gram-positive cocci that grow in pairs and tetrads. Normal inhabitants of the gastrointestinal tract, they are used extensively in industry to ferment cheese and other dairy products, soy products, and alcoholic beverages. Eight species of *Pediococci* are recognized, but only the closely related *P. acidilactici* and *P. pentosaceus* have been identified as human pathogens. In recent years, these organisms have been increasingly recognized as a cause of bacteremia and pneumonitis in the immunocompromised host. These organisms have also been isolated from intraabdominal infections such as peritonitis and hepatic abscesses. Risk factors for *Pediococcus* infections include prior antibiotic therapy, abdominal surgery, and gastric feeding.

Diagnosis is made by isolation and identification of the organism from cultures of blood or other body fluids. As one of the lactic acid bacteria associated with foods, *Pediococcus* species may be difficult to distinguish from enterococci and *Leuconostoc* species. Approximately 95% of clinical isolates will cross-react with group D streptococcal antisera. Tests that aid in distinguishing pediococci from other organisms include a negative pyrrolidonylarylamidase (PYRase) test and the absence of gas production from glucose. With newer application of molecular genetic techniques to determine relatedness of food-associated lactic acid bacteria, reorganization of the genus with novel morphologic or phenotypic differentiation of *Leuconostoc* species from *Pediococcus* species is being studied.

Pediococci are intrinsically highly resistant to vancomycin and other glycopeptides. Most strains are moderately susceptible to penicillin and ampicillin. Minimum inhibitory concentrations (MICs) are variable for cephalosporins. Imipenem appears active against all isolates, as does gentamicin. Resistance to erythromycin, clindamycin, tetracycline, tobramycin, and amikacin has been described. If a serious *Pediococcus* infection is suspected (e.g., on the basis of the characteristic tetrad morphology on Gram stain), intravenous penicillin at a dosage of 12 million or more units daily or imipenem may be used as empiric therapy. Susceptibility testing, preferably by MIC rather than disk diffusion, should be performed to determine appropriate therapy (Table 1).

■ *LEUCONOSTOC* SPECIES

Leuconostoc species are gram-positive coccobacilli that recently have been increasingly recognized as human pathogens. These organisms are normally found in dairy products and vegetable matter and are used in the production of wine, dairy products, and dextrans. *Leuconostoc* species are not usually considered part of the normal human flora, but they have been isolated from the feces, vagina, and gastric fluid, primarily in hospitalized patients. Antibiotic therapy, particularly with vancomycin, to which leuconostocs are intrinsically resistant, may contribute to gastrointestinal colonization with these organisms.

Leuconostoc species may cause bacteremia in otherwise healthy neonates. Recent reports of other infections produced by these organisms include endocarditis caused by

Table 1   Recommended Drug of Choice for the Miscellaneous Gram-Positive Organisms

ORGANISM	ANTIBIOTIC (Ab) (ALTERNATIVE Ab)	ROUTE	DOSAGE	DURATION
Pediococcus	Penicillin G Imipenem (Cephalosporins)	IV	12 million U	(10-14 days)*
Leuconostoc	Penicillin G Ampicillin (Clindamycin) (Erythromycin)	IV	≥12 million U	(10-14 days)* 4 to 6 wk for endocarditis
Lactobacillus	Penicillin G Penicillin G gentamicin (Clindamycin) (Erythromycin)	IV IV IV	12 million U daily 20-24 million U daily for endocarditis 1.0 mg/kg q8h	(10-14 days)* 6 wk
Oerskovia	Penicillin G, TMP-SMX (Vancomycin)	IV	(Moderate to high dosage)*	4-6 wk for endocarditis
Rothia	Penicillin G, (Vancomycin) (Cephalosporins) (Fluoroquinilones)	IV	20 million U daily for endocarditis	6 wk
Arcanobacteria	Erythromycin Penicillin V Penicillin G ± aminoglycosides (Clindamycin) (Tetracycline)	PO/IV PO IV	40 mg/kg (four divided doses) 250-500 mg qid 2 million U q4h (for endocarditis)	10 days Until clinical response 4-6 wk

Rhodococcus	Vancomycin (V)
	V + imipenem or
	  rifampin (AIDS)
	Erythromycin
	  + rifampin
	(Sulfonamides)
	(Chloramphenicol)
		IV
		IV
		PO
		IV/PO
		PO
			1 g q12h
			500 mg q6h
			600 mg/day
			500 mg-1 g qid
			600 mg/day
				2 wk
				
				2-4 wk

*Suggested by some authorities.

Leuconostoc mesenteroides; empyema, and bacteremia caused by *Leuconostoc cremoris* in a burn patient; after liver transplantation; and from a thrombotized central venous catheter. Serious infections such as bacteremia and pneumonia almost always occur in immunocompromised patients, although a case of meningitis in a previously healthy teenager has been described. At least four *Leuconostoc* species (including *L. mesenteroides, L. paramesenteroides, L. cremoris,* and *L. citreum*) may cause human infections. Risk factors for *Leuconostoc* infection include lengthy hospitalization, intravascular catheters, prior antibiotic therapy, prematurity, short gut syndrome, and serious underlying disease.

Diagnosis is based on identification of the organism from cultures of blood or other sterile body fluids. On Gram stain the organisms appear as pairs or chains of slightly elongated gram-positive cocci that may appear rodlike. They may be difficult to distinguish from viridans streptococci, enterococci, lactobacilli, or pediococci. Helpful tests include the production of gas from glucose; a negative catalase, oxidase, and PYRase test; and the absence of arginine hydrolysis.

Leuconostoc isolates, like pediococci, are uniformly resistant to vancomycin and other glycopeptides. Most strains are susceptible to penicillin, clindamycin, and gentamicin. Susceptibility to the cephalosporins, quinolones, and trimethoprim-sulfamethoxazole (TMP-SMX) is variable. Penicillin, the drug of choice, should be given at relatively high dosages (≥12 million units daily). In the case of penicillin allergy or resistance, therapy should be based on results of susceptibility testing. Appropriate therapy may also include removal of potentially infected devices such as indwelling intravascular catheters.

■ *LACTOBACILLUS* SPECIES

Lactobacillus species are gram-positive rods that normally inhabit the human mouth, vagina, and gastrointestinal tract. More than 50 species of lactobacilli are recognized, many of which are used in the production of cheese, yogurt, pickles, and fermented beverages. Lactobacilli are widely considered to have low pathogenicity, and recent attention has focused on their possible roles as probiotic bacteria promoting beneficial health effects, as vehicles for oral immunization, and as part of treatment policies called *ecoimmunonutrition.* Nevertheless, they have been reported to cause many infections, including bacteremia, endocarditis, intraabdominal and hepatic abscesses, meningitis, and pneumonia. Risk factors for serious infections caused by *Lactobacillus* species include underlying immunocompromised state (including human immunodeficiency virus [HIV] disease) and gastrointestinal surgery. Prior antibiotic therapy, particularly with vancomycin (to which most lactobacilli are resistant), has also been identified as a clinical risk factor. In patients with *Lactobacillus* bacteremia and endocarditis, a recent review identified cancer, recent surgery, and diabetes mellitus as underlying risk factors. In this series, *Lactobacillus* bacteremia was a marker for serious and rapidly fatal underlying illness. Additional history of dental infection or manipulation is common.

Diagnosis is based on identification of the organism from sterile body fluids. Lactobacilli are gram-positive rods, but they may appear coccoid if grown on solid media. Cultures grown in broth are more reliable for assessing morphology. Some *Lactobacillus* isolates may be difficult to distinguish from *Leuconostoc* species and streptococci. The combination of tests for gas production from glucose, arginine hydrolysis, PYRase, and carbohydrate fermentations should allow proper identification.

Intravenous penicillin (≥12 million units daily) is generally the drug of choice for serious infections. Endocarditis should be treated with penicillin 20 million to 24 million units daily plus gentamicin for 6 weeks. Lactobacilli are usually resistant to glycopeptides such as vancomycin. Susceptibility to cephalosporins and quinolones is variable, and most isolates are resistant to tetracycline and TMP-SMX. Most strains are susceptible in vitro to clindamycin, a possible alternative therapy in penicillin-allergic patients, but few clinical data are available. In the patient allergic to beta-lactams who has endocarditis, penicillin desensitization should be considered.

■ *OERSKOVIA* SPECIES

Oerskovia species are yellow, gram-positive, non–acid-fast organisms with extensively branched filaments. They were first described by Orskov in 1938 as "motile *Nocardia*." Their usual habitat is soil, although they have also been isolated from decaying plant materials and grass cuttings. Two *Oerskovia* species have been recognized: *O. turbata* and *O. xanthineolytica*. Both are rare causes of opportunistic infection in humans, but should be considered as potential pathogens in the setting of indwelling devices. Reported infections caused by *Oerskovia* species include native and prosthetic valve endocarditis, peritonitis, central venous catheter infections, bacteremia in immunocompromised hosts (including patients with acquired immunodeficiency syndrome [AIDS]), prosthetic joint infection, keratitis, and endophthalmitis due to a penetrating eye injury. Several reported cases have been associated with exposure to soil and bacterial contamination of hydrophilic contact lens solutions.

The diagnosis of *Oerskovia* infections rests on laboratory identification from clinical specimens. Gram stain may reveal pleomorphic gram-positive rods. Culture reveals yellow colonies that are catalase positive when grown aerobically. They may be distinguished from other *Nocardia*-like organisms in that they are facultatively anaerobic and do not produce aerial mycelia. Identification is based on carbohydrate fermentation testing.

Successful treatment of *Oerskovia* infections generally requires removal of the contaminated foreign body in addition to appropriate antibiotic therapy. Antibiotics to which clinical isolates of *Oerskovia* have been reported to be susceptible include penicillin, vancomycin, TMP-SMX, cephalothin, and amikacin. Intermediate susceptibility or resistance has been described for ampicillin, ciprofloxacin, doxycycline, erythromycin, gentamicin, clindamycin, and the third-generation cephalosporins. Therapy should be based on susceptibility testing of the isolate. However, if Gram stain or initial culture results suggest *Oerskovia* infection, parenteral penicillin or TMP-SMX therapy should be begun while awaiting results of susceptibility testing.

■ *ROTHIA* SPECIES

Rothia dentocariosa is a small gram-positive pleomorphic rod. These organisms, common components of the normal oral microflora, were first isolated from carious dentine. The first description of human disease due to *Rothia* species was not reported until 1975, when the organism was recovered from a periappendiceal abscess. More recently, a number of case reports have described *Rothia* species as causing native and prosthetic valve endocarditis, aortic root abscess, and pneumonia. The patient often has a history of recent dental infection or dental manipulation; however, a recent report includes identification in throat cultures of healthy individuals. Complications, including mycotic aneurysm, cerebral abscess, and perivalvular abscess, are common. *Rothia* species may also cause bacteremia without endocarditis (particularly in immunocompromised patients), pneumonia, peritonitis, and infections of the head and neck. *Rothia dentocariosa* was recently isolated in lymph nodes of patients with cat-scratch disease (CSD), suggesting that it (along with other gram-positive rods) may have a role, together with *Bartonella henselae*, in the pathogenesis of CSD.

Diagnosis of *Rothia* infections depends on identification of the organism from the cultures of blood or other body fluids. *Rothia* species are catalase positive, nonmotile, urease negative and indole negative. The organisms may appear branched, resembling *Actinomyces* or *Nocardia* species. They are distinguished from these genera by carbohydrate fermentation testing.

Penicillin is the drug of choice for treatment of infections due to this organism. Because rare isolates may be resistant to penicillin, susceptibility testing should be performed. For endocarditis due to penicillin-susceptible strains, intravenous penicillin at dosages of 20 million units per day for 6 weeks is recommended. In the case of penicillin resistance or drug allergy, vancomycin, netilmicin, or teicoplanin therapy may be effective. *Rothia* species may also be susceptible in vitro to ciprofloxacin, rifampin, cephalosporins, and gentamicin. Resistance to amikacin, kanamcin, ciprofloxacin, and TMP-SMX has been described. Dental evaluation should also be considered in patients with infections due to *Rothia* species because carious or infected teeth may be a source of recurrent infection.

■ *ARCANOBACTERIUM* SPECIES

Arcanobacterium haemolyticum (formerly known as *Corynebacterium haemolyticum*) are facultatively anaerobic gram-positive to gram-variable pleomorphic rods (slender at first, sometimes clubbed, or in angular arrangements), nonmotile and nonsporulating. They are considered commensals of human nasopharynx and skin and are transmitted person-to-person by the droplet route. *Arcanobacterium* species have been recognized as causes of pharyngitis and cervical lymphadenopathy (indistinguishable from the pharyngitis caused by *S. pyogenes*) with additional symptoms of fever, pruritius, nonproductive cough, scarlatiniform skin rash with mild desquamation, and occasional formation of peritonsillar abscesses. Cutaneous infections, including ulcers, wound infection, cellulitis, and paronychia, are marked in some cases by the elaboration of lipid hydrolyzing enzyme (sphingomyelinase D), producing dermonecrosis. Sepsis syndrome has been seen, with intravenous drug abuse and diabetes identified as risk factors. Central nervous system (CNS) infections (brain abscess, cerebritis, meningitis), endocarditis, osteomyelitis, otitis media, sphenoidal sinusitis, empyema, and cavitary pneumonia have also been described.

Diagnosis is made by isolation and identification of the organism from cultures of blood, pharynx, skin lesions, or other clinical specimens (e.g., CNS abscess, cerebrospinal fluid [CSF], aortic valve, bone). On Loeffler's medium, the morphology closely resembles *Corynebacterium diphtheriae*. Tests that aid in diagnosis include fermentation of dextrose, lactose, and maltose but not mannitol or xylose. Colonies appear circular, discoid, opaque, and whitish, with a rough surface and friable consistency, a uniform feature at 48 hours of a black opaque dot at the center of each colony, and hemolysis at 24 to 48 hours incubation. Because *Archanobacterium* species may present as part of polymicrobic infections with typical respiratory pathogens, they are often overlooked. Diagnosis often occurs only after repeated isolation.

Most isolates of *A. haemolyticum* are susceptible to erythromycin, gentamicin, clindamycin, and cephalosporins. They are resistant to sulfonamides and nalidixic acid in vitro. The drug of choice is erythromycin, 40 mg/kg PO or IV in four divided doses per day (2 g maximum). Although there have been reports of treatment failure with penicillin attributed to tolerance and failure to penetrate the intracellular location of the pathogen, penicillins with or without aminoglycosides are also widely used antibiotics, in most cases with success.

■ *RHODOCOCCUS* SPECIES

Rhodococcus equi (formerly known as *Corynebacterium equi*), readily found in soil contaminated with stool of horses and other animals, are nonfastidious, strict aerobic gram-positive bacteria displaying rod-to-coccus pleomorphism, with fragmenting and occasionally palisading forms. *Rhodococcus* are well-documented veterinary pathogens, causing granulomatous pneumonia in foals. They have been recognized as opportunistic pathogens found in immunocompromised patients, including transplant patients and HIV-infected persons. Documented clinical presentations include slowly progressive granulomatous pneumonia, with lobar infiltrates progressing to cavitating lesions on chest radiograph; abscesses of the central nervous system, pelvis, and subcutaneous tissue; and lymphadenitis. Vertebral osteomyelitis and pulmonary malakoplakia have also been reported. Mortality exceeds 50% among AIDS patients with documented *R. equi* pneumonia, which is associated with a high rate of relapse despite adequate treatment.

R. equi forms salmon pink colonies on blood agar from clinical specimens after 2 to 3 days of incubation. Colonies can be mucoid and coalescing; growth on Lowenstein-Jensen medium allows earlier detection of pigment. Synergistic hemolysis (resembling the CAMP test), displayed by cross-streaking on sheep blood agar with any of a number of other bacteria, including *A. haemolyticum*, *Staphylococcus aureus*, and *Corynebacterium pseudotuberculosis* has been helpful in the diagnosis. In addition, *Rhodococcus* isolates are nonreactive to catalase and urease and exhibit acid-fast staining. Some diagnostic laboratories use a commercial kit (API CORYNE strip, bioMerieux-Vitek, Hazelwood, MO) for identification.

Most strains are susceptible to inhibition by glycopeptide antibiotics, rifampin, and macrolides. Resistance to beta-lactam antibiotics (except carbapenems) has been reported. The high relapse rate and attributable mortality rate, especially among AIDS patients, makes it difficult to recommend a standard treatment protocol. Repeat cultures are warranted during treatment to discover acquired resistance. A combination of at least two antibiotics parenterally (including a glycopeptide and rifampin) followed by oral maintenance therapy is recommended. Surgical lung resection has been used with some success, sometimes in combination with antimicrobial therapy. Antimicrobial prophylaxis may prove of benefit in AIDS patients.

Suggested Reading

Cornish N, Washington JA: Rhodococcus equi infections: clinical features and laboratory diagnosis (review), *Curr Clin Top Infect Dis* 19:198, 1999.

Dhodapkar KM, Henry NK: *Leuconostoc* bacteremia in an infant with short-gut syndrome: case report and literature review (review), *Mayo Clin Proc* 71:1171, 1996.

Ferraz V, McCarthy K, Smith D, Koornhof HJ: *Rothia dentocariosa* endocarditis and aortic root abscess, *J Infect* 37:292, 1998.

Handwerger S, et al: Infection due to *Leuconostoc* species: six cases and review, *Rev Infect Dis* 12:602, 1990.

Husni RN, et al: *Lactobacillus* bacteremia and endocarditis: review of 45 cases, *Clin Infect Dis* 25:1048, 1997.

Linder R: *Rhodococcus equi* and *Arcanobacterium haemolyticum*: two "coryneform" bacteria increasingly recognized as agents of human infection, *Emerg Infect Dis* 3:145, 1997.

Maguire JD, McCarthy MC, Decker CF: *Oerskovia xanthineolytica* bacteremia in an immunocompromised host: case report and review, *Clin Infect Dis* 22:554, 1996.

Mastro TD, et al: Vancomycin-resistant *Pediococcus acidilactici*: nine cases of bacteremia, *J Infect Dis* 161:956, 1990.

Waagner DC: *Arcanobacterium haemolyticum*: biology of the organism and disease in man, *Ped Infect Dis J* 10:933, 1991.

MISCELLANEOUS GRAM-NEGATIVE ORGANISMS

Judith L. Nerad
Sampath Kumar

Most gram-negative infections are caused by organisms in the Enterobacteriaceae or Pseudomonadaceae families; however, a few are caused by a heterogeneous group of gram-negative organisms. The clinical presentation varies widely, affecting different types of hosts and requiring a variety of antibiotics for therapy (Table 1). Varied predisposing environmental and host factors are outlined in Table 2).

■ *ACINETOBACTER*

Acinetobacter is a member of the family Neisseraceae, with perhaps 17 genospecies and 2 commonly recognized clinical species, *A. johnsonii* (formerly *A. calcoaceticus var. Iwoffi*) and A. *baumanni-A. calcoaceticus* complex (formerly *A. calcoaceticus anitratus*). They are usually seen as gram-negative coccobacilli and thus are easily confused with *Neisseria* or *Haemophilus*. They differ from Enterobacteriaceae in that they cannot grow anaerobically or reduce nitrates. They are distinguished from *Neisseria* and *Moraxella* in their reaction to the oxidase test. Virulence factors include a polysaccharide capsule that may prevent phagocytosis, fimbriae that potentiate adherence to epithelial cells, and a lipopolysaccharide known to be biologically active.

Acinetobacter is widely distributed in the environment, found in food, soil, water, and sewage. Typically, moist environments, including hospital equipment such as ventilator tubing, resuscitation bags, humidifiers, sinks, mist tents, dialysis baths, angiography catheters, pressure transducers, and plasma protein solutions, contain these organisms. They are found on the skin of many animal species and humans usually as commensal organisms. They are found in normal oral flora, the genitourinary tract, and the gastrointestinal tract.

Most infections are nosocomial, occurring in severely debilitated patients who have been exposed to antibiotics, surgery, or instrumentation. *Acinetobacter* infections have been reported from all organ systems, causing septicemia, endocarditis, meningitis, pneumonia, urinary tract infections, wound infections, abscesses, peritonitis, osteomyelitis, and eye infections. The most common sites are the respiratory and urinary tracts. The mortality can be as high as 36%. Community-acquired pneumonia has been reported infrequently, usually associated with underlying pulmonary disease, alcohol abuse, or non-Hodgkins lymphoma.

Acinetobacter is commonly multidrug resistant, and isolated pathogens must be evaluated as to specific sensitivity patterns within each hospital. Most strains are sensitive to imipenem-cilastatin, ceftazidime, cefotaxime, amikacin, trimethoprim-sulfamethoxazole (TMP-SMX), and minocycline. The quinolones are quite effective against *Acinetobacter*. Most strains are resistant to penicillin, ampicillin, first- and second-generation cephalosporins, gentamicin, chloramphenicol, and nalidixic acid. They are variably resistant to tetracycline, tobramycin, kanamycin, ureidopenicillin, and aztreonam. *A. baumanni* resistant to the carbapenems and amikacin have been more frequently reported. Ampicillin-sulbactam, and sulbactam alone, have been used with good success in these cases. Antibacterial resistance is greater among *anitratus* than *Iwoffi* species.

■ *ACHROMOBACTER*

Achromobacter is widely distributed in nature, including soil and water. It may be part of the normal flora of the lower gastrointestinal tract. It has been found as a contaminant in disinfectants, diagnostic tracer solutions, intravenous computed tomography contrast solutions, hemodialysis solutions, ventilators, humidifiers, and pressure transducers.

Table 1   Antimicrobial Therapy of Miscellaneous Gram-Negative Bacilli

ORGANISM	FIRST-LINE THERAPY	ALTERNATIVE THERAPY
Acinetobacter	Imipenem-cilastatin, ceftazidime, cefotaxime, amikacin, ciprofloxacin	TMP-SMX, minocycline, ureidopenicillins, aztreonam
Achromobacter	Imipenem-cilastatin, TMP-SMX	Quinolones, ceftazidime, piperacillin, ticarcillin
Alcaligenes	TMP-SMX, chloramphenicol	Ticarcillin-clavulanate, third-generation cephalosporins
Capnocytophaga DF-1	Clindamycin	Erythromycin, ciprofloxacin, third-generation cephalosporins
Capnocytophaga canimorsus	Penicillin	Erythromycin, ciprofloxacin, clindamycin, third-generation cephalosporins, TMP-SMX
Chromobacterium	Chloramphenicol, gentamicin, tetracycline	TMP-SMX
Flavimonas/ Chrysseomonas	Ciprofloxacin	Ureidopenicillins, third-generation cephalosporins, carbapenems, aminoglycosides
Chryseobacterium (Flavobacterium)	Clindamycin, rifampin, ciprofloxacin, TMP-SMX	Erythromycin, vancomycin, chloramphenicol

TMP-SMX, Trimethoprim-sulfamethoxazole.

Table 2   Environmental and Host Factors Predisposing to Infections with Miscellaneous Gram-Negative Bacilli

ORGANISM	ENVIRONMENTAL FACTORS	HOST FACTORS	INFECTION
Acinetobacter	Ventilator tubing, resuscitation bags, humidifiers, sinks, mist tents, dialysis bags, angiography and IV catheters, pressure transducers, plasma protein solutions	Severely debilitated, recent surgery, instrumentation	Septicemia, endocarditis, meningitis, pneumonia, UTI, wound infections, abscesses, peritonitis, osteomyelitis, eye infections
Achromobacter	Contaminant in disinfectants, diagnostic tracers solution, IV CT contrast, hemodialysis solutions, ventilators, humidifiers, pressure transducers	Severely debilitated, recent neurosurgery	Community-acquired bacteremia, meningitis, chronic otitis media, hospital-acquired meningitis, bacteremia, ventriculitis, endocarditis, endophthalmitis, corneal ulcers, pharyngitis, pneumonia, wound infections, peritonitis, UTI, abscesses
Alcaligenes	Dairy products, rotten eggs, hospital equipment	Severely debilitated	Septicemia, native and prosthetic valve endocarditis, meningitis, meibomianitis, chronic purulent otitis, pyelonephritis, hepatitis, appendicitis, diarrhea
Capnocytophaga	Normal oral, gastrointestinal, respiratory, and vaginal flora of humans *C. canimorsus* in canine oral flora	Severely immunocompromised, children with malignancies, neutropenia, mucositis, asplenia, alcohol abuse	Bacteremia, septicemia, keratitis, conjunctivitis, endophthalmitis, corneal ulcer, endocarditis, pericardial abscess, mediastinitis, lung and subphrenic abscess, empyema, peritonitis, abdominal abscess, septic arthritis, lymphadenitis, juvenile periodontitis
Chromobacterium	Enters through the skin or ingestion of contaminated food or water	Neutrophil defects (e.g., chronic granulomatous disease)	Local cellulitis, lymphadenitis, septicemia, osteomyelitis, arthritis, meningitis, ocular infections, and pneumonia
Chryseobacterium *(Flavobacterium)*	Soil, water, use of contaminated fluids in the hospital, nebulizers, flush solutions, pressure transducers, contaminated disinfectants and anesthetics, ice machines, peritoneal dialysis solutions	Neonates, premature infants, adult immunocompromised patients	Neonates: meningitis, hydrocephalus Adults: endocarditis, pneumonia, peritonitis, keratitis, wound infection, meningitis
Flavimonas/ *Chryseomonas*	Soil, water, flushing solutions	Patients with indwelling foreign material, malignancies, immunosuppressive therapy, postsurgical state, history IVDU, chronic renal failure, bone marrow transplant, cirrhosis	Septicemia, bacteremia, subdural empyema, pneumonia, peritonitis, biliary tract infection, abscesses, wound infection, empyema, line infections, prosthetic joint infections

UTI, Urinarty tract infection; *CT,* computed tomography; *IVDU,* intravenous drug use.

Achromobacter has been commonly reported as a causative agent in a variety of nosocomial and community-acquired infections. Community-acquired infections include bacteremia, meningitis, and chronic otitis media. Nosocomial outbreaks have also been reported, including meningitis and ventriculitis after neurosurgical manipulation, bacteremia, endocarditis, otitis, endophthalmitis, corneal ulcer, pharyngitis, pneumonia, wound infections, peritonitis, urinary tract infections, and abscesses. Mortality can approach 52% in patients with bacteremia.

Clinical isolates should be tested for sensitivity to antibiotics. Imipenem-cilastatin is the most consistently effective agent in vitro against *Achromobacter*. Piperacillin, carbenicillin, ticarcillin-clavulanic acid, and ceftazidime can also be effective. For severe infections, more than one drug may be necessary; however, synergistic combination therapy has not been established. Most strains are resistant to penicillin, ampicillin, first- and second-generation cephalosporins, and aminoglycosides. TMP-SMX, chloramphenicol, tetracycline, and quinolones exhibit variable activity.

■ *ALCALIGENES*

Alcaligenes consist of gram-negative rods or cocci that are motile with pertrichous flagella and are generally obligate aerobes. They are found in soil and water as well as on normal human skin and in gastrointestinal tract flora. Dairy products and rotten eggs have been sources of *Alcaligenes*. These organisms have also been isolated from hospital equipment.

Clinically important infections are found in severely debilitated patients. *Alcaligenes faecalis* isolation from the urine is often considered to be a contaminant. *Alcaligenes* isolated from the blood of patients with septicemia is thought to be associated with contaminated hospital equipment; however, blood isolates have also been obtained from patients without clinical evidence of sepsis. Clinical presentations include native and prosthetic valve endocarditis, meningitis, chronic purulent otitis, meibomianitis, pyelonephritis, hepatitis, appendicitis, and diarrhea. Often *Alcaligenes* is isolated with other flora as part of mixed infections.

Alcaligenes is generally susceptible to TMP-SMX and chloramphenicol. Sensitivity to beta-lactams and aminoglycosides is variable. On the basis of in vitro studies, third-generation cephalosporins or the addition of clavulanic acid to amoxicillin or ticarcillin may be more consistently effective, especially against *A. faecalis*. Greater resistance is seen in hospitals. Sensitivity to quinolones is variable.

■ *CAPNOCYTOPHAGA*

Capnocytophaga encompasses a group of capnophilic, microaerophilic gram-negative rods. The organisms are long, thin, and often fusiform, and they display gliding motility on agar media. Special selective media and carbon dioxide are required for optimal growth. There are few clinically relevant species of *Capnocytophaga*; *C. ochracea, C. sputigena,* and *C. gingivalis* were formerly identified as *Bacteriodes ochraceus* (Centers for Disease Control and Prevention dysgonic fermenter-1, or DF-1). These species are oxidase, catalase, and indole negative. *C. canimorsus,* formerly DF-2, and *C. cynodegmi,* formerly DF-2-like organism, have recently been established as *Capnocytophaga* species. These species are oxidase and catalase positive and indole negative, and they reduce nitrates.

C. ochracea, C. sputigena, and *C. gingivalis* are part of the normal flora of humans isolated from the vagina, gastrointestinal tract, and respiratory tract. Most clinically important infections are juvenile periodontitis or systemic disease in an immunocompromised patient. Immunocompromised patients with *Capnocytophaga* infection tend to be children with malignancies, be neutropenic, or have oral lesions (mucositis or ulceration). These patients usually have bacteremia and septicemia. In immunocompetent patients, *Capnocytophaga* commonly is a component of a polymicrobial infection of the respiratory tract or a contaminated wound. It has also been reported to cause keratitis, conjunctivitis, endophthalmitis, corneal ulcer, endocarditis, pericardial abscess, mediastinitis, lung and subphrenic abscesses, empyema, septic arthritis, cervical and inguinal lymphadenitis, sinusitis, thyroiditis, osteomyelitis, peritonitis, abdominal abscess, chorioamnionitis, and congenital bacteremia.

Capnocytophaga species are typically sensitive to clindamycin, erythromycin, tetracycline, chloramphenicol, quinolones, and imipenem-cilastatin. Susceptibilities are variable for penicillin, expanded-spectrum cephalosporins, and

metronidazole. In general, these organisms are resistant to aztreonam, aminoglycosides, vancomycin, trimethoprim, and polymyxin B. Beta-lactamase production has been reported in 2.5% to 32% of isolates. Clindamycin is thought to be the most active drug in vitro. It has been recommended that for immunocompromised patients, antibiotics should be given for 10 to 14 days after documenting negative blood cultures. For immunocompetent patients, the duration of therapy should be dictated by the site and extent of infection and should be given in conjunction with adequate surgical drainage.

C. canimorsus and *C. cynodegmi* are normal oral flora of dogs and cats. Of the two species, *C. canimorsus* has caused more infections, with a wide spectrum of illness ranging from mild to fulminant. More than 75% of cases report exposure to a dog, either through ownership or a bite. The most common clinical manifestations are septicemia and bacteremia, but *C. canimorsus* has been reported to cause meningitis, endocarditis, pneumonia, empyema, corneal ulcer, septic arthritis, cellulitis, and wound infections after a dog bite or cat scratch. Predisposing factors to infection are asplenia, alcohol abuse, and immunosuppression (steroids or hematologic malignancies). In predisposed persons, particularly asplenic patients, the infection tends to be fulminant, with shock, disseminated intravascular coagulation, gangrene, renal failure, and death.

The diagnosis is established by blood cultures, which turn positive within 1 to 14 days. In asplenic patients, the organism may be demonstrated in a Gram stain of the buffy coat. In one alcoholic patient, the organisms were seen on a peripheral blood smear.

C. canimorsus is reportedly susceptible to penicillins, imipenem, erythromycin, vancomycin, clindamycin, third-generation cephalosporins, chloramphenicol, rifampin, doxycycline, and quinolones but resistant to aztreonam. Susceptibility to aminoglycosides may depend on the method used. Penicillin is considered the drug of choice for these infections and for infections associated with dog bites.

■ *CHROMOBACTERIUM*

Chromobacterium violaceum is the only known pathogenic member of this genus and the only violet pathogenic bacterium. It is a slightly curved rod, facultatively anaerobic, that produces a water-insoluble violet tryptophan metabolite when grown aerobically. The organism grows within 24 hours on conventional media containing tryptophan. It is motile, with both polar and lateral flagellae that are antigenically distinct. Humans with neutrophil defects (e.g., chronic granulomatous disease) may be particularly susceptible to infections with this organism.

Chromobacterium is generally found in the environment (soil, fresh water, and food). It grows optimally at 20° to 37° C (68° to 98.6° F); hence, most infections have been documented in tropical or subtropical climates. It is a rare infection, thought to enter the body through the skin, although ingestion of contaminated food or water may play a role. The clinical presentation is usually manifest by local cellulitis and regional or diffuse lymphadenitis, then hematologic dissemination. Septicemia and multiorgan system failures then occur. Mortality is 60% to 70%, depending on the host and accuracy of diagnosis. Other presentations have included fever, skin lesions, abdominal pain, osteomyelitis, arthritis, meningitis, ocular infections, and pneumonia.

C. violaceum is generally very susceptible to chloramphenicol, gentamicin, and tetracycline. It is uniformly resistant to cephalosporins and generally resistant to most penicillins. It has variable sensitivity to some of the carboxypenicillins and ureidopenicillins. TMP-SMX has been used successfully as outpatient therapy after prolonged intravenous therapy with other agents.

■ CHRYSEOBACTERIUM (FLAVOBACTERIUM)

Chryseobacterium (Flavobacteria) are long, thin, slightly curved, occasionally filamentous, nonmotile gram-negative rods. They are common inhabitants of soil and water. *C. meningosepticum* is the species most commonly isolated, but *C. odoratum, C. balustinum,* and other *Flavobacterium* species have also been implicated in human disease.

Chryseobacteria are uncommon pathogens in adults, and rarely cause infections in children beyond the newborn period. In neonates, infection presents as sepsis and meningitis. Premature infants and those who are small for their gestational age seem to be at particular risk. The development of meningitis may be insidious. The prognosis is extremely poor, with mortality greater than 60%. Half of the survivors develop significant neurologic complications, including hydrocephalus. Meningitis has also been reported in adult immunocompromised patients. Other clinical presentations include endocarditis, pneumonia, peritonitis, keratitis, and wound infections. Most of the described cases are nosocomial infections associated with the use of contaminated fluids in the hospital (nebulizers, flush solutions for arterial catheters, pressure transducers, ice machines, contaminated disinfectants, contaminated anesthetics, peritoneal dialysis).

Antimicrobial susceptibilities vary with the method used; dilution methods are more reliable than agar disk diffusion methods. Most chryseobacteria produce beta-lactamases and are resistant to beta-lactam drugs, including aztreonam, ticarcillin, and the carbapenems. Most are resistant to aminoglycosides. Minocycline, doxycycline, clindamycin, TMP-SMX, and rifampin are active in vitro against most strains. Other drugs that have been used alone or in combination include erythromycin, chloramphenicol, ciprofloxacin, and vancomycin. Erythromycin and rifampin have both been given concurrently intravenously and intrathecally with some success. Development of resistance on therapy has been demonstrated with erythromycin, rifampin, ciprofloxacin, and TMP-SMX. This should be considered in cases of persistence of organisms in the cerebrospinal fluid (CSF).

Antimicrobial therapy should be continued for at least 2 weeks after sterilization of the CSF. Recovery is the rule in immunocompetent older patients infected with contaminated materials; however, the prognosis is poor in immunocompromised patients.

■ FLAVIMONAS/CHRYSEOMONAS

Flavimonas oryzihabitans and *Chryseomonas luteola* are motile aerobic gram-negative rods with a distinct yellow-orange pigment. After 48 hours of incubation, colonies are typically rough or wrinkled. They are nonfermentative, oxidase-negative, and catalase-positive, and they grow on MacConkey agar. They are found in water, soil, and other damp environments. Eighty-four percent of the reported cases have been associated with the presence of a foreign material, including intravascular catheters, dialysis catheters, or artificial grafts. Other associated host factors include malignancy, immunosuppressive therapy, postsurgical state, chronic renal failure, previous antibiotic therapy, intravenous drug use, long-term steroid use, liver cirrhosis, and bone marrow transplant.

The infections caused by these organisms include septicemia, bacteremia, line infections, pneumonia, prosthetic joint infections, subdural empyema, peritonitis, biliary tract infections, surgical wound infections, abscesses, and empyema.

According to the literature, both organisms are resistant to first- and second-generation cephalosporins and most isolates are resistant to ampicillin and tetracycline. They are sensitive to the ureidopenicillins, third-generation cephalosporins, carbapenems, aminoglycosides, and quinolones. There is a difference in susceptibility to cotrimoxazole: *C. luteola* is resistant and *F. oryzihabitans* is sensitive. Clinically, most patients have been treated with ciprofloxacin with a favorable outcome. The number of cases of infection is increasing because of increasing awareness of clinicians and the laboratory. The presence of foreign material, such as a central venous catheter or a joint prosthesis, may predispose patients to infections with these organisms.

Suggested Reading

Go ES, et al: Clinical and molecular epidemiology of *Acinetobacter* infections sensitive only to polymyxin B and sulbactam, *Lancet* 344:1329, 1994.

Nerad JL, Seville MT, Snydman DR: Miscellaneous gram negative bacilli: *Acinetobacter, Cardiobacterium, Actinobacillus, Chromobacterium, Capnocytophage,* and others. In Gorbach SL, Bartlett JG, Blacklow NR, eds: *Infectious diseases,* ed 2, Philadelphia, 1998, WB Saunders.

Rahav G, et al: Infections with *Chryseomonas luteola* (CDC Group Ve-1) and *Flavimonas oryzihabitans* (CDC Group Ve-2), *Medicine* (Baltimore) 74:83, 1995.

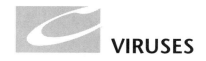

VIRUSES

EPSTEIN-BARR VIRUS AND OTHER CAUSES OF THE INFECTIOUS MONONUCLEOSIS SYNDROME

Jeffery L. Meier

Epstein-Barr virus (EBV) infects nearly all persons in the world at some time. The virus persists indefinitely in their B lymphocytes and is shed intermittently from salivary tissue into oral secretions. Transmission of EBV occurs when susceptible individuals come in close oral contact with infectious saliva. Casual contact is generally insufficient to transmit infection, and spread of EBV among susceptible household contacts is infrequent. Occasionally, the virus is transmitted by blood products or donor tissues. About 95% of all persons will have acquired EBV by the end of their third decade of life. Persons living with low standards of hygiene, such as occurs in developing countries or areas of low socioeconomic standing, often acquire EBV in childhood, and nearly everyone becomes infected by adulthood. In contrast, persons adhering to a high standard of hygiene will often have EBV infection delayed until adolescence or early adulthood, when sexual intimacy becomes a factor in transmission.

■ INFECTIOUS MONONUCLEOSIS

Presentation

Most EBV infections do not generate illness. When EBV does induce disease, the spectrum of illness is varied (Table 1). Infectious mononucleosis (IM) is the paradigmatic illness associated with EBV infection. The IM syndrome is largely the product of an exuberant immunologic response to a newly acquired EBV infection, and in healthy persons IM does not arise from EBV reactivation. This illness commonly occurs among adolescents and young adults (15 to 25 years) and seldom appears in persons of other ages. This is because most infants and children do not overtly exhibit findings of acute infection and most older adults are no longer susceptible to EBV, although they do retain the capacity to develop IM.

The diagnosis of IM is based on a characteristic clinical and laboratory presentation (Table 2). A primary EBV infection (IM) is exceedingly likely in persons presenting with the following: classic clinical triad of fever, pharyngitis, and cervical lymphadenopathy; absolute peripheral lymphocytosis; atypical lymphocytosis that is greater than 10% of the differential; and heterophile antibodies. As these criteria are relaxed, the probability of EBV causing the mononucleosis-like (mono) syndrome decreases accordingly. Conversely, the absence of any of these criteria does not rule out EBV. For example, as many as 5% to 10% of EBV mono episodes will remain heterophile negative. In addition, some of the classic features of IM may not be evident until later in the illness. Atypical lymphocytosis, for instance, may not be impressive until the second week of illness. Infants, young children, the elderly, and immunosuppressed persons are most likely to exhibit an atypical EBV mono syndrome.

Malaise and fatigue are often prominent symptoms of IM, and their resolution is generally more gradual than other symptoms. In exceptional cases, these symptoms may wax and wane for months, but they do not indicate continuing EBV activity. Mild retroorbital headache is also common in IM but short-lived. Prominent abdominal discomfort is unusual and should raise a concern of splenic rupture, as splenomegaly occurs in one half of IM cases. Fever is typically in the range of 38° to 39.5° C (100° to 103.1° F) and subsides in 1 to 2 weeks, although it may occasionally persist up to 4 weeks. Concomitant sweats and chills also occur. Fever above 40° C (104° F), which is rare, may signal a superimposed bacterial infection (e.g., bacterial pharyngitis or peritonsillar abscess). Exudative tonsillopharyngitis

Table 1   EBV-Related Illness
ACUTE
Infectious mononucleosis (IM)
Atypical presentations or complications of IM
CHRONIC
Chronic IM (extremely rare)
Oral hairy leukoplakia
LYMPHOPROLIFERATIVE DISORDERS
Consequence of congenital or acquired immunosuppression
X-linked (Duncan's syndrome)
OTHER DISORDERS
African Burkitt's lymphoma
Nasopharyngeal carcinoma
Smooth muscle cell tumors
AIDS lymphoma (especially of brain)
Some thymomas

EBV, Epstein-Barr virus; *AIDS,* acquired immunodeficiency syndrome.

Table 2 Clinical and Laboratory Findings in Uncomplicated Infectious Mononucleosis

	COMMON	OCCASIONAL	INFREQUENT
Symptoms	Sore throat, malaise, fatigue, headache, sweats	Anorexia, myalgia, chills, nausea	Cough, arthralgias, abdominal discomfort
Signs	Lymphadenopathy, fever, pharyngitis, splenomegaly	Hepatomegaly, palatal petechiae, periorbital edema	Rash, jaundice
Labs	>50% mononuclear cells >10% atypical lymphocytes Heterophile antibodies Mild LFT increase Mild thrombocytopenia Cold agglutinins	Mild neutropenia Antinuclear antibodies Rheumatoid factor	Bilirubinemia >3 mg/100 ml Hematuria Pyuria Proteinuria

Common, Present in more than 50%; *occasional,* present in 10% to 50%; *infrequent,* present in fewer than 10%; *LFT,* liver function test.

occurs in one third of uncomplicated IM cases; this usually resolves in the first 2 weeks of illness. Petechiae located on the uvula and at the junction of soft and hard palates suggest EBV but may be seen in other viral infections such as rubella. Symmetric posterior cervical lymphadenopathy is a common distinguishing mark of IM. Anterior cervical lymph node enlargement is common as well. Lymphadenopathy may take several weeks to resolve; rarely, it persists for months. Hepatitis, which is usually mild, is present in about 90% of IM episodes. Clinical jaundice is uncommon, as is an elevation of transaminases above 500 IU/L. Rash is distinctively unusual in the absence of antibiotics and, if present, often takes the form of a faint morbilliform eruption.

Elderly persons with an acute EBV illness are less likely to have pharyngitis, lymphadenopathy, and splenomegaly. In such episodes, a prolonged febrile course or jaundice occurs with greater frequency. Atypical lymphocytosis may be delayed and of lesser magnitude. Infants and young children with EBV mono are more likely to be heterophile negative and have coryza, exudative pharyngitis, rash, and hepatosplenomegaly.

Complications

Most episodes of IM are uneventful. However, any one of a wide range of complications may occur (Table 3). These complications may at times either greatly overshadow or develop in the absence of typical IM features. Most complications of IM resolve without sequelae, but rare fatalities do occur, largely as the result of encephalitis, splenic rupture, hepatitic failure, myocarditis, or bacterial infection related to neutropenia. Airway obstruction can arise from excessive hyperplasia of lymphoid tissue (i.e., tonsillar tissue) in Waldeyer's ring. Enlarged spleens are susceptible to traumatic rupture; spontaneous rupture is rare. Autoantibodies that may form during IM can cause critical hemolytic anemia, thrombocytopenia, or neutropenia.

IM may evolve into a life-threatening lymphoproliferative disorder in persons with profound acquired or congenital cellular immunodeficiency. In a rare inherited disease, the X-linked lymphoproliferative disorder, young males develop a fulminant mononucleosis after acquiring EBV. Many die of hemorrhage and infection; survivors have aplastic anemia, dysgammaglobulinemia, and lymphoma. EBV can also rarely provoke chronic IM, in which manifestations of

Table 3 Complications of Infectious Mononucleosis

Neurologic
  Encephalitis, meningitis, Guillain-Barré syndrome, Bell's palsy, optic neuritis, psychosis, transverse myelitis, Reye's syndrome
Splenic
  Traumatic rupture of enlarged spleen; rarely spontaneous rupture
Respiratory
  Upper airway obstruction from hypertrophy of lymphoid tissue, interstitial pneumonitis
Hematologic
  Autoimmune hemolytic anemia, critical thrombocytopenia, agranulocytosis, aplastic anemia, hemophagocytic syndrome
Hepatic
  Fulminant hepatitis, hepatic necrosis
Cardiac
  Myocarditis, pericarditis
Immunologic
  Anergy, lymphoproliferative syndromes, hypogammaglobulinemia
Dermatologic
  Cold-mediated urticaria, leukocytoclastic vasculitis, ampicillin-associated rash, erythema multiforme, erythema nodosum

persistent illness may include interstitial pneumonitis, massive lymphadenopathy, hepatosplenomegaly, marrow failure, dysgammaglobulinemia, Guillain-Barré syndrome, and uveitis. The diagnosis is substantiated by showing a high amount of EBV in tissues; EBV-specific antibodies also reach very high titers. Although a tiny proportion of persons with chronic fatigue syndrome develop this illness in association with a well-documented episode of primary EBV infection, there is no evidence that ongoing EBV activity is responsible for the syndrome.

Serology

Heterophile antibodies are a fairly specific marker of primary EBV infection because their appearance outside of this setting is rare. A heterophile response is occasionally seen in illnesses such as viral hepatitis, primary human immunodeficiency virus (HIV) infection, and lymphoma. Rapid latex

Table 4 Differential Diagnosis of Mononucleosis-Like Syndrome

VARIABLES	EBV	CMV	TOXOPLASMA	HIV	BACTERIAL PHARYNGITIS*	RUBELLA	HAV, HBV, HCV
Fever	++	++	+	++	++	+	++
Sore throat	++	+	+	++	++ abrupt	+/− coryza	−
Exudative pharyngitis	+	+/−	−	+/− aphthous ulcers	+	−	−
Anterior cervical LN	++	+	++	++	++	+	+/−
Posterior cervical LN	++	+	++	++	+/− mild	++	+/−
Rash	+/− but common with ampicillin	+	+/−	++	+/− scarlatiniform	++	+/−
Hepatitis	++	++	+	+	−	+/−	++
Jaundice	+/−	−	−	−	−	−	++
Splenomegaly	++	+	+/−	+/−	−	+/−	+
Atypical lymphs	++	++	+ <10% of cells	+/− <10% of cells	−	+/− <10% of cells	+ <10% of cells
Heterophile antibodies	++ absent in 5%-10%	−	−	−	−	−	−

++, Present in >50% of cases; +, present in 10%-50% of cases; +/−, present in 10% of cases; −, absent or rare; *EBV*, Epstein-Barr virus; *CMV*, cytomegalovirus; *HIV*, human immunodeficiency virus; *HAV*, hepatitis A virus; *HBV*, hepatitis B virus; *HCV*, hepatitis C virus; *LN*, lymphadenopathy; *Lymphs*, peripheral lymphocytes.
*Primarily beta-hemolytic streptococci; consider diphtheria, *Arcanobacterium hemolyticum*, *Neisseria gonorrhoeae*, mycoplasma, and Vincent's angina.

slide tests can reliably detect heterophile antibodies. These rapid tests have supplanted the traditional tests, such as the Paul-Bunnell-Davidsohn test, which define heterophile antibodies as those that react with epitopes on the surface of certain animal erythrocytes (e.g., causing sheep erythrocyte agglutination) but do not react with guinea pig kidney cells. These antibodies do not recognize EBV antigens, and their titers do not correlate with severity of illness. The antibodies resolve in 3 to 6 months and do not reappear.

EBV-specific serologies are useful to ascertain the role of EBV in illness not fulfilling the criteria of classic IM. Antiviral capsid antigen (anti-VCA) antibodies are demonstrable in virtually all acute episodes of IM. Anti-VCA IgM evolves quickly during primary EBV infection, is usually detectable when patients first present, and may linger for weeks to months. A comparison of paired acute and convalescent anti-VCA IgG titers is not usually helpful in the diagnosis of primary infection because the titer is often already near its peak when patients present with IM. This antibody titer falls slowly and persists lifelong, ranging from 1:40 to 1:2,560, as determined by the immunofluorescence assay (IFA). Antibodies to EBV early antigens (anti-EA) of the diffuse and restricted types develop in most IM cases and wane with time. The persistence of these antibodies in low titers is of no clinical significance. Antibodies to EBV nuclear antigens (anti-EBNA) are not detected in acute IM when assayed by the IFA technique but do appear in convalescence and persist for life.

Caution should be used when interpreting EBV-specific antibody titers. Comparison of results acquired at different times or in different places may be misleading. Furthermore, the newer immunoassays (e.g., enzyme-linked assays) in use are not directly comparable to the original IFA assay.

■ OTHER CAUSES OF MONO SYNDROME

Primary infections with cytomegalovirus (CMV), toxoplasma, HIV, rubella, and viral hepatitis (e.g., hepatitis A, B, and C), as well as bacterial pharyngitis, are often contemplated as other possible causes of mono syndrome, particularly when heterophile antibodies are absent. Although each of these other causes of mono syndrome may exhibit distinguishable clinical and general laboratory features (Table 4), the definitive diagnosis usually relies on the outcome of specific laboratory tests (Table 5). EBV should also be kept in the differential diagnosis of heterophile-negative mono syndrome.

Streptococcal pharyngitis may be distinguished from IM on the basis of its abrupt onset and lack of any associated posterior cervical lymphadenopathy, hepatosplenomegaly, and atypical lymphocytosis. Toxoplasmosis, which is an uncommon cause of mono syndrome, does not produce exudative pharyngitis or a peripheral atypical lymphocytosis that exceeds 10% of the differential. Rubella may present with fever and lymphadenopathy, but the rash, coryza, arthralgias, and minimal atypical lymphocytosis distinguish it from IM. The diagnosis of viral hepatitis is suggested by prominent hepatitic involvement in the absence of pharyngitis or marked lymphadenopathy.

CMV and HIV account for the majority of heterophile-negative mono episodes. CMV mono may closely resemble

Table 5 Diagnostic Studies in Mononucleosis-Like Syndrome

VARIABLES	EBV	CMV	TOXOPLASMA	HIV	BACTERIAL PHARYGITIS*	RUBELLA	HAV, HBV, HCV
Acute Antibody† Response	+ Heterophile + IgM VCA +/– anti-EA (IFA) – anti-EBNA (IFA)	+ IgM CMV	+ IgM toxo	– HIV EIA	None	+ IgM rubella	+ IgM HAV, + IgM HBc, none for HCV
Convalescent Antibody† Response	+/– Fourfold increase IgG VCA +/– anti-EA (IFA) + anti-EBNA (IFA)	+ Fourfold increase IgG CMV	+ IgG toxo seroconversion (several test-types available)	+ HIV EIA and confirmatory Western blot	+ Elevated or rising ASO or anti-DNase B	+ Fourfold increase IgG rubella	+ IgG HAV, + or – anti-HBs + IgG-HBc, + HCV EIA (confirmatory RIBA)
Nucleic Acid or Antigen Detection	None	+/– CMV pp65 or DNA detection in blood leukocytes	None	+/– p24 Ag + HIV RNA PCR	+ Rapid Strept test	None	+ HBs Ag + HCV RNA PCR
Culture	Impractical	+ Urine (+ saliva, +/– blood)	Impractical	Available, but insensitive and expensive	+ Throat swab, blood agar	Impractical	None

+, Typically present; +/–, sometimes present; –, usually absent; *EBV*, Epstein-Barr virus; *CMV*, cytomegalovirus; *HIV*, human immunodeficiency virus; *HAV*, hepatitis A virus; *HBV*, hepatitis B virus; *HCV*, hepatitis C virus; *VCA*, EBV viral capsid antigens; *EA*, EBV early antigens; *IFA*, immunofluorescence assay; *EBNA*, EBV nuclear antigens; *EIA*, enzyme-linked immunoassay; *HBc*, HBV capsid antigens; *HBs*, HBV surface antigen; *RIBA*, recombinant immunoblot assay; *pp65*, CMV tegument protein; *p24*, HIV core protein; *PCR*, polymerase chain reaction.

*Applies primarily to group A streptococcus; special media required to culture *C. diphtheriae, N. gonorrhoeae,* and *A. haemolyticum.*

†IgM and heterophile status determined with acute serum. Paired acute and convalescent sera should be analyzed simultaneously to accurately determine change in antibody titer.

IM because both often produce fever, mild hepatitis, and marked atypical lymphocytosis. However, cervical lymphadenopathy and pharyngitis tends to be milder in CMV mono. In the normal host, presence of anti-CMV IgM in serum, viremia, or viral antigen or DNA in peripheral blood leukocytes supports the diagnosis of acute CMV infection. Absence of culturable CMV in urine makes the diagnosis unlikely. Acute HIV infection is commonly accompanied by a mono syndrome. In acute retroviral syndrome, unlike IM, a rash is common, exudative pharyngitis is infrequent, tonsillar hypertrophy is minimal, and oral or genital ulcers are distinctive. A transient peripheral lymphopenia is followed 2 to 3 weeks later by lymphocytosis in which a small proportion of cells may be reactive. Detection of plasma HIV RNA or p24 antigen, in conjunction with a negative or indeterminate HIV serology, substantiates the diagnosis of acute retroviral syndrome.

■ MANAGEMENT

Epstein-Barr Virus

The management of primary EBV infection (Table 6) rarely demands more than general supportive care, which includes adequate rest, hydration, antipyretics, and analgesics. Complications of IM may require additional supportive measures (e.g., maintenance of airway during obstructive tonsillar enlargement or encephalitis, transfusions for severe hemolytic anemia or thrombocytopenia, splenectomy for splenic rupture). Activity should be restricted in proportion to the degree of symptoms and any splenomegaly. Most students can return to school in less than 2 to 3 weeks. Persons with acute IM are advised to avoid contact sports for 1 month or until absence of splenomegaly is verified. This recommendation derives from two observations. First, episodes of traumatic splenic rupture involve enlarged spleens and occur within the first month of illness. This rupture can occur in the early convalescent phase, as well as the acute symptomatic phase of the illness. Second, ultrasonography can detect significant splenomegaly that is often not appreciated on physical examination. This too resolves in 1 month. For the athlete with resolving IM who wants to participate in contact sports during the first month of illness, ultrasonography can be used to exclude nonpalpable splenomegaly.

The viral exudative tonsillopharyngitis that accompanies IM commonly leads to a search for beta-hemolytic streptococci. Anywhere from 3% to 30% of throat cultures obtained randomly during IM will grow group A streptococci, reflecting differences in the age of patients and in prevalence of streptococcal carriage in the community. Although streptococcal infection and colonization are clinically indistinguishable in persons with EBV pharyngitis, as many as 30% of individuals harboring this bacterium will eventually show serologic evidence of infection. For this reason, treatment for 10 days with penicillin or erythromycin is advised, particularly to prevent poststreptococcal sequelae. Ampicillin should not be used because it causes rash in more than 85% of cases; amoxicillin also appears to cause rash frequently. The empiric use of antibiotics in uncomplicated IM is inadvisable; studies have shown lack of benefit of such an approach.

Table 6 Management of Acute Infectious Mononucleosis

UNCOMPLICATED CASES
Supportive care: hydration, rest, antipyretic, analgesic (e.g., aspirin, acetominophen, or nonsteroidal antiinflammatory agent)
Activity restriction: restrict in proportion to degree of symptoms and splenomegaly; avoid contact sports for 1 mo or until absence of splenomegaly verified
If throat culture contains beta-hemolytic streptococci, treat with 10 days of penicillin or erythromycin
Avoid ampicillin- and amoxicillin-containing regimens
Glucocorticoid use is inadvisable

COMPLICATED CASES
Additional supportive care: maintenance of airway during obstruction or encephalitis; splenectomy for splenic rupture; transfusions for critical anemia or thrombocytopenia
Glucocorticoids are useful in selected situations*: impending airway obstruction from tonsillar enlargement; persistent severe illness; autoimmune hemolytic anemia or thrombocytopenia; aplastic anemia; considered in encephalitis, myocarditis, or pericarditis

*15- to 20-mg dose equivalent of prednisone four times per day for 2 to 3 days, then tapered over 1 to 2 wk.

Antiviral agents such as acyclovir, ganciclovir, and foscarnet can inhibit EBV replication during lytic (productive) infection but do not affect amplification of latent virus, which occurs when EBV-infected B cells proliferate. Both parenteral and high-dose oral acyclovir can effectively inhibit oropharyngeal shedding of EBV in uncomplicated IM, but neither route of therapy is clinically beneficial, and the proportion of circulating B cells containing EBV is not consistently reduced. There is also no compelling evidence that acyclovir is clinically beneficial in complications of IM, although it can repress viral replication while glucocorticoid is administered. Oral hairy leukoplakia is the only illness caused by EBV in which antiviral agents such as acyclovir (800 mg PO 5 times a day) are clearly efficacious. It is doubtful whether acyclovir offers any salutary effect in posttransplant lymphoproliferative disorders. Acyclovir appears to have been beneficial in some cases of chronic IM.

The routine use of a glucocorticoid (steroid) as therapy for uncomplicated IM is inadvisable. Although steroid therapy may modestly reduce the duration of fever and tonsillopharyngeal symptoms of uncomplicated IM, there are rare reports of encephalitis and myocarditis developing in association with its use. There are also theoretic concerns that steroids may adversely alter long-term immunity or number of cells latently infected by the virus. Steroids have not been shown to produce significant or reproducible effects on lymphadenopathy or hepatosplenic involvement. Given the unimpressive evidence of the overall benefit of steroids, experts have advised against their use in uncomplicated IM.

Steroids do have a role in the management of certain complications of IM (Table 6). Such therapy may quickly ameliorate impending airway obstruction from tonsillar enlargement. In exceptional situations of persistent severe infectious mononucleosis (i.e., fever, prostration, weight loss), a short course of steroids is worth consideration. Steroids may also reduce the severity of autoimmune thrombocytopenia and hemolytic anemia. Aplastic anemia may respond to this therapy as well. Steroid therapy can be considered in the intractable or desperate cases of encephalitis, myocarditis, and pericarditis. When required, steroid therapy is initiated with 15 to 20 mg of predisone-equivalent given orally (or intravenously) four times per day for 2 to 3 days, and then tapered over a period of 1 to 2 weeks.

Therapy of Other Causes of Mono Syndrome

The mono syndrome associated with either CMV, toxoplasma, HIV, rubella, or the hepatitis viruses is usually self-limited and, like IM, is primarily managed with supportive care. However, HIV, pregnancy, and underlying cellular immunosuppression are circumstances in which additional therapeutic measures may be required. For instance, specific antimicrobial therapy is warranted in persons with profound cellular immune deficiency who develop CMV mono or acute toxoplasmosis (see the chapters *Cytomegalovirus, Toxoplasmosis* and *AIDS: Therapy for Opportunistic Infections*). Because primary CMV, toxoplasma, and rubella infections in pregnancy pose a risk to the fetus of developing the TORCH syndrome, an obstetrician with expertise in this area should be consulted. Primary toxoplasmosis of pregnancy necessitates antimicrobial therapy (see the chapter *Toxoplasmosis*). Antiretroviral therapy given during pregnancy can substantially reduce perinatal HIV transmission, but its use requires knowledge of the attendant toxicities and risks (see the chapter *Pregnancy and the Puerperium: Infectious Risks*). Immediate antiretroviral therapy should be considered in persons with acute HIV infection, as current evidence suggests a benefit (see the chapter *HIV infection: Antiretroviral Therapy*).

Suggested Reading

Chervenick PA: Infectious mononucleosis: the classic clinical syndrome. In Schlossberg D, ed: *Infectious mononucleosis*, ed 2, New York, 1989, Springer-Verlag.

Schooley RT: Epstein-barr virus (infectious mononucleosis). In Mandell GL, Bennett JE, Dolin R, eds: *Mandell, Douglas, and Bennett's principles and practices of infectious diseases*, ed 5, New York, 2000, Churchill Livingstone.

Straus SE, et al: Epstein-Barr virus infections: biology, pathogenesis, and management, *Ann Intern Med* 188:45, 1993.

HERPES SIMPLEX VIRUSES

David W. Kimberlin
Richard J. Whitley

■ THE VIRUS

Herpesviruses are generally defined as large enveloped virions with an icosapentahedral nucleocapsid consisting invariably of 162 capsomeres arranged around a double-stranded DNA core. The two antigenically distinct types of herpes simplex virus (HSV) are HSV-1 and HSV-2. Considerable homology exists between the HSV-1 and HSV-2 genomes, with most of the polypeptides specified by one viral type being antigenically related to polypeptides of the other viral type. Although this results in considerable cross-reactivity between the HSV-1 and HSV-2 glycoproteins (g), unique antigenic determinants exist for each virus (e.g., gG-1 and gG-2). Surrounding the viral genome and nucleocapsid is a tightly adherent membrane known as the *tegument*. A lipid envelope containing the viral glycoproteins loosely surrounds the tegument.

■ PATHOLOGY AND PATHOGENESIS

Cutaneous HSV infection causes ballooning of infected epithelial cells, with nuclear degeneration and loss of intact cellular membranes. Infected epithelial cells either lyse or fuse to form multinucleated giant cells. With cell lysis, clear fluid containing large quantities of virus, cellular debris, and inflammatory cells accumulates between the epidermal and dermal layers. Multinucleated giant cells are usually present at the base of the vesicle. An intense inflammatory response extends from the base of the vesicle into the dermis. As the lesions heal, vesicular fluid becomes purulent as more inflammatory cells are recruited to the site of infection. Scab formation then follows. Scarring is uncommon.

When infection involves mucous membranes, shallow ulcers are more common than vesicles because of rapid rupture of the very thin cornified epithelium present at mucosal sites. Nevertheless, the histopathologic findings of mucosal lesions are similar to those of skin lesions.

■ EPIDEMIOLOGY

HSV-1 is found most commonly in the oropharynx, although any organ system can be involved. Factors that influence the frequency of primary HSV-1 infection include geographic location, socioeconomic status, and age. Throughout childhood and adolescence, African-Americans maintain approximately twice the prevalence of HSV-1 antibodies as Anglo children, with 40% of African-American children being seropositive for HSV-1 by 5 years of age. By the age of 60 years, however, both African-Americans and Caucasians have a similarly high prevalence of HSV-1 antibody (up to 90%).

Recurrences of herpes labialis have been associated with physical or emotional stress, fever, exposure to ultraviolet light, tissue damage, and immune suppression. As with primary infections, recurrent disease may occur in the absence of clinical symptoms. At any given time, 1% of normal children and 1% to 5% of normal adults asymptomatically excrete HSV-1.

HSV-2 causes 75% to 80% of the cases of genital HSV infections in the United States. As would be expected, antibodies to this virus are rarely found before the onset of sexual activity. Among adolescents and adults, factors that correlate with seroprevalence for HSV-2 include sex (higher for women than for men), race (higher for African-Americans than for Caucasians), marital status (higher for persons previously married than for single or married persons), and income level (higher probability for those persons earning lesser amounts of money).

The propensity for recurrence of genital HSV infection depends on a variety of factors, including sex (more common in men), viral type (more common with HSV-2), and the presence and titer of neutralizing antibodies (more common in the presence of high neutralizing antibody titers). Overall, 60% to 90% of patients with primary genital HSV-2 infection will experience clinically apparent recurrence of infection.

■ CLINICAL MANIFESTATIONS

Oropharyngeal HSV Infection

Primary oropharyngeal infection with HSV-1 occurs most commonly in young children between 1 and 3 years of age. It is usually asymptomatic. The incubation period ranges from 2 to 12 days, with an average of 4 days. Symptomatic disease is characterized by fever to 104° F, oral lesions, sore throat, fetor oris, anorexia, cervical adenopathy, and mucosal edema. Oral lesions initially are vesicular but rapidly rupture, leaving 1- to 3-mm shallow gray-white ulcers on erythematous bases. These lesions are distributed on the hard palate, the anterior portion of the tongue, along the gingiva, and around the lips (Figure 1). In addition, the lesions may extend down the chin and neck due to drooling. Total duration of illness is 10 to 21 days.

Primary infection in young adults has been associated with pharyngitis and often a mononucleosis-like syndrome. In such patients, ulcerative lesions on erythematous bases frequently are apparent on the tonsils.

Primary gingivostomatitis results in viral shedding in oral secretions for an average of 7 to 10 days. Virus can be isolated from the saliva of asymptomatic children and adults as well. Virus is also shed in the stool.

Recurrent orolabial HSV lesions are often preceded by a prodrome of pain, burning, tingling, or itching. These symptoms generally last for less than 6 hours, followed within 24 to 48 hours by the appearance of painful vesicles,

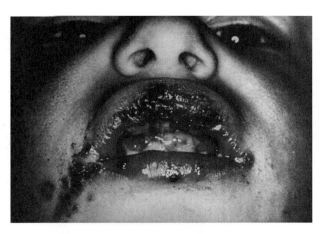

Figure 1
Herpes simplex gingivostomatitis. *(From Whitley RJ, Gnann JW: The epidemiology and clinical manifestations of herpes simplex virus infections. In Roizman B, Whitley RJ, Lopez C, eds: The human herpesviruses, New York, 1993, Raven Press.)*

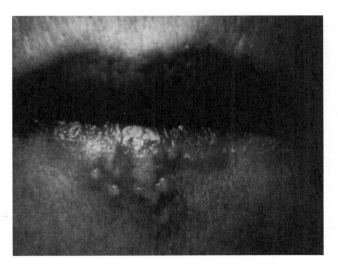

Figure 2
Recurrent herpes simplex labialis. *(From Whitley RJ, Gnann JW: The epidemiology and clinical manifestations of herpes simplex virus infections. In Roizman B, Whitley RJ, Lopez C, eds: The human herpesviruses, New York, 1993, Raven Press.)*

typically at the vermillion border of the lip (Figure 2). Lesions usually crust within 3 to 4 days, and healing is complete within 8 to 10 days. Recurrences occur only rarely in the mouth or on the skin of the face of immunocompetent patients.

Genital HSV Infection

Genital HSV-2 disease is usually acquired by sexual contact with an infected partner. The incubation period of primary disease ranges from 2 to 12 days. Lesions persist for an average of 21 days. In 70% of patients, primary infections are associated with fever, malaise, myalgias, inguinal adenopathy, and other signs and symptoms of systemic illness.

Complications include extragenital lesions, aseptic meningitis, and sacral autonomic nervous system dysfunction with associated urinary retention. Women tend to experience more severe primary infections and are more likely to develop complications.

In males, primary genital HSV infection usually manifests as a cluster of vesicular lesions on erythematous bases on the glans or shaft of the penis (Figure 3). In females, primary genital HSV lesions usually involve the vulva bilaterally (Figure 4). Concomitant HSV cervicitis occurs in 90% of women with primary HSV-2 infection of the external genitalia. In women, the lesions rapidly ulcerate and become covered with a gray-white exudate. Such lesions may be exquisitely painful.

Recurrent genital HSV-2 infection can be either symptomatic or asymptomatic. A prodrome of itching, burning, tingling, or tenderness may be noted several hours before a recurrence. The duration of disease is shorter during recurrent infection (7 to 10 days), and fewer lesions are present. In men, lesions usually appear on the glans, or shaft, of the penis. In women, lesions occur most commonly on the labia minora, labia majora, and perineum. Cervical excretion of HSV occurs in 10% of women with recurrent genital lesions. Systemic symptoms are uncommon in recurrent genital HSV disease.

Other Primary HSV Skin Infections

Alteration in the barrier properties of skin, as occurs in atopic dermatitis, can result in localized HSV skin infection (eczema herpeticum). Most cases resolve over a 7- to 9-day period without specific therapy. Localized cutaneous HSV infection after trauma is known as herpes gladitorium (wrestler's herpes or traumatic herpes).

Herpes simplex virus infection of the digits results in herpetic whitlow. Such lesions may be the result of autoinoculation, as in the case of infants, or exogenous exposure, as occurs among medical and dental personnel.

Ocular HSV Infection

Herpetic infection of the eye usually presents as either a blepharitis or a follicular conjunctivitis. As disease progresses, branching dendritic lesions develop. Symptoms include severe photophobia, tearing, chemosis, blurred vision, and preauricular lymphadenopathy. An ophthalmologist should always be involved in the care of such patients.

Central Nervous System HSV Infection

Central nervous system (CNS) signs and symptoms of HSV disease can begin suddenly or can follow a 1- to 7-day period

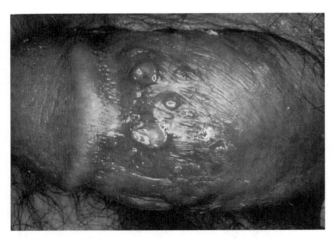

Figure 3
Primary genital HSV infection in men. *(From Whitley RJ, Gnann JW: The epidemiology and clinical manifestations of herpes simplex virus infections. In Roizman B, Whitley RJ, Lopez C, eds: The human herpesviruses, New York, 1993, Raven Press.)*

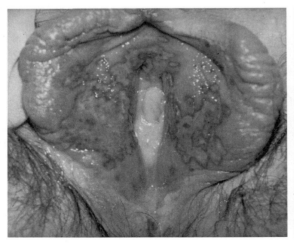
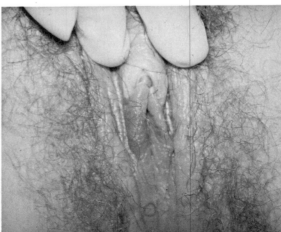

Figure 4
Genital HSV infection in women. *(From Whitley RJ, Gnann JW: The epidemiology and clinical manifestations of herpes simplex virus infections. In Roizman B, Whitley RJ, Lopez C, eds: The human herpesviruses, New York, 1993, Raven Press.)*

of nonspecific influenza-like symptoms. Prominent CNS features include headache, fever, behavioral disturbances, speech disorders, altered consciousness, and focal neurologic findings such as focal seizures.

Neonatal HSV Infections

Neonatal HSV infection can be classified as (1) disease localized to the skin, eye, and/or mouth (SEM); (2) encephalitis, with or without SEM involvement; and (3) disseminated infection that involves multiple organs, including the central nervous system, lung, gastrointestinal tract, liver, adrenals, skin, eye, and/or mouth. Infants with HSV disease are divided roughly evenly among these three categories. Infants with disseminated and SEM disease usually present for medical attention within the first 2 weeks of life, whereas infants with disease localized to the CNS usually present between the second and third weeks of life. Presenting signs and symptoms can include any combination of irritability, seizures (both focal and generalized), lethargy, tremors, poor feeding, temperature instability, bulging fontanelle, respiratory distress, jaundice, disseminated intravascular coagulopathy, shock, and cutaneous vesicles. It is important to note that more than 20% of infants with disseminated disease and 30% to 40% of infants with encephalitis will never have skin vesicles during the course of illness.

Herpes Simplex Virus in the Immunocompromised Host

Patients compromised by immunosuppressive therapy, underlying disease, or malnutrition are at increased risk for severe HSV infection. Disseminated disease may occur with widespread dermal, mucosal, and visceral involvement. Alternatively, disease may remain localized but persist for much longer periods of time than would be seen in immunocompetent hosts.

■ DIAGNOSIS

Serologic diagnosis of HSV infection currently is not of great clinical value, largely because commercially available serologic assays cannot distinguish between HSV-1 and HSV-2, although type-specific assays are pending Food and Drug Administration (FDA) approval. Isolation of HSV by culture remains the definitive diagnostic method of determining HSV disease outside of the central nervous system. If skin lesions are present, a scraping of the vesicles should be transferred in appropriate viral transport media on ice to a diagnostic virology laboratory. Other sites from which virus may be isolated include the cerebrospinal fluid (CSF), urine, throat, nasopharynx, conjunctivae, and duodenum. The presence of intranuclear inclusions and multinucleated giant cells on a Tzanck prep are indicative of, but not diagnostic for, HSV infection.

In HSV encephalitis, CSF findings are variable but often include a moderate pleocytosis with a predominance of mononuclear cells, elevated protein level, and normal or slightly decreased glucose. The electroencephalogram (EEG) generally localizes spike and slow wave activity to the temporal lobe, even when obtained very early in the disease course. Computed tomography (CT) of the brain may initially be normal or reveal only edema, but as the disease progresses can demonstrate temporal lobe involvement as well. Detection of HSV DNA in the CSF by polymerase chain reaction (PCR) has become the diagnostic method of choice; however, it must be performed only by a reliable laboratory.

■ TREATMENT

Herpes Labialis

Topical acyclovir is not efficacious in the treatment of orolabial herpes lesions. Orally administered acyclovir at a dosage of 400 mg five times daily for 5 days reduces the duration of pain and time to the loss of crusts by about one-third, but only if treatment is started during the prodromal or erythematous stages of recurrent infection. Thus oral acyclovir has a slight clinical benefit only if initiated very early after recurrence and cannot be recommended as routine treatment for herpes labialis in immunocompetent patients. There are no data to support the use of long-term suppressive treatment with acyclovir for the prevention of herpes labialis. Recently, denavir was licensed for the treatment of labial herpes in adults. Therapy results in approximately a 20% reduction in disease duration.

Genital Herpes

Acyclovir administered topically, orally, and intravenously is effective in the treatment of primary genital herpes in the normal host, decreasing the duration of symptoms, viral shedding, and time to healing of lesions (Table 1). However, neither systemic nor topical treatment of primary HSV lesions reduces the frequency or severity of recurrences. Episodic administration of oral or topical acyclovir for the treatment of recurrent genital HSV lesions provides only a modest benefit, with duration of lesions being shortened at most by 1 to 2 days. However, daily administration of oral acyclovir can effectively suppress recurrences of genital herpes in 60% to 90% of patients. Treatment should be interrupted every 12 months to reassess the need for continued suppression.

Both valaciclovir and famciclovir are now licensed for the treatment and suppression of recurrent herpes. There is a pharmacokinetic advantage with these medications. Valaciclovir is administered at 500 mg once daily. Famciclovir is administered at 250 mg three times daily.

Mucocutaneous HSV Infections in Immunocompromised Patients

In immunocompromised patients, topical, oral, and intravenous acyclovir all diminish the duration of viral shedding, as well as substantially improve time to cessation of pain and to total healing of HSV lesions. In addition, prophylactic administration of oral or intravenous acyclovir to such patients significantly reduces the incidence of symptomatic HSV infection (see Table 1). Valaciclovir and famciclovir also can be used in these populations.

Herpes Simplex Keratoconjunctivitis

Idoxuridine (Stoxil), trifluridine (Viroptic), and vidarabine ophthalmic drops all are effective and licensed for treatment of HSV keratitis. Trifluridine is the most efficacious and the

Table 1   Antiviral Therapy in Herpes Simplex Virus (HSV) Infections

TYPE OF INFECTION	DRUG	ROUTE AND DOSAGE[a]	COMMENTS
Genital HSV			
Initial episode	Acyclovir	200 mg PO 5 times/day ×10 days	Preferred route in normal host
		5 mg/kg IV q8h ×5 days	Reserved for severe cases
	Valaciclovir	1 g PO bid ×5-10 days	
	Famciclovir	250 mg PO tid ×5-10 days	
Recurrent episode			
	Acyclovir	200 mg PO 5 times/day ×5 days	
	Valaciclovir	500 mg PO bid ×5-7 days	
	Famciclovir	250 mg PO tid ×5-7 days	Titrate dosage as required
Suppresion			
	Acyclovir	400 mg PO bid	
	Valaciclovir	500 mg PO bid or 1 g day	
	Famciclovir	250 mg PO tid	
Mucocutaneous HSV in Immunocompromised patient	Acyclovir	200-400 mg PO 5 times/day ×10 days	
		5 mg/kg IV q8h ×7-10 days[b]	
	Valaciclovir	500 mg bid PO	
	Famciclovir	500 mg tid PO	
HSV encephalitis	Acyclovir	10 mg/kg IV q8h ×10-14 days[c]	
Neonatal HSV	Acyclovir[d]	20 mg/kg IV q8h ×14-21 days	
Herpetic conjunctivitis	Trifluridine	1 drop q2h while awake ×7-14 days	Alternative: vidarabine ointment

Adapted from Whitley R, Gnann J: *N Engl J Med* 327:782, 1992.
[a]The dosages are for adults with normal renal function unless otherwise noted.
[b]A dosage of 250 mg/m^2 should be given to children <12 years of age.
[c]A dosage of 500 mg/m^2 should be given to children <12 years of age.
[d]Acyclovir is not approved by the FDA for this indication.

easiest to administer, and as such is the drug of choice for HSV ocular disease (see Table 1).

Herpes Simplex Encephalitis

In patients with HSV encephalitis, acyclovir administration greatly reduces mortality and has a modest impact of morbidity. Dosage and length of therapy are shown in Table 1. Outcome is more favorable when therapy is instituted early in the disease course.

Neonatal HSV Infections

Although not licensed for this indication, acyclovir is the drug of choice in the treatment of neonatal HSV infection (see Table 1). Therapy is most efficacious if instituted early in the course of illness. Because of the exceptional safety profile of acyclovir, an intravenous dosage of 60 mg/kg/day

divided every 8 hours should be given. Duration of therapy is 14 to 21 days.

Infants with ocular involvement caused by HSV should receive topical antiviral medication in addition to parenteral therapy. Trifluridine is the treatment of choice for ocular HSV infection in the neonate (see Table 1).

Suggested Reading

Douglas JM, et al: Double-blind study of oral acyclovir for suppression of recurrences of genital herpes simplex virus infection, *N Engl J Med* 310:1551, 1984.

Whitley R, Gnann J: Acyclovir: a decade later, *N Engl J Med* 327:782, 1992.

Whitley RJ, et al: Herpes simplex encephalitis: vidarabine therapy and diagnostic problems, *N Engl J Med* 304:313, 1981.

Whitley RJ, et al: Changing presentation of neonatal herpes simplex virus infection, *J Infect Dis* 158:109, 1988.

VARICELLA-ZOSTER VIRUS

John A. Zaia

Varicella-zoster virus (VZV) is one of the eight known herpesviruses of humans and the cause of chickenpox (varicella) and shingles (zoster). Chickenpox, the exanthem caused by primary infection with VZV, usually occurs in children. Shingles, the clinical syndrome of segmental exanthem and pain caused by reactivation of latent VZV infection, usually occurs many years after the primary infection. In the immunodeficient person, both primary and reactivated VZV infection can lead to severe generalized virus dissemination, the life-threatening form of VZV infection. The availability of antiviral agents for management of VZV infection has raised the importance of recognizing this infection in high-risk groups. Before the VZV vaccine, approximately 3.7 million cases of chickenpox occurred each year, 83% in children younger than age 9 years. There are 300,000 cases of herpes zoster in the United States per year, and the incidence is constant for each age group through midadulthood. Thereafter, the incidence of zoster increases with age; persons age 80 and older have a 1 : 100 chance per year of developing shingles.

■ CLINICAL PRESENTATION

Chickenpox

In healthy children, VZV infection manifests as a vesicular exanthem often associated with prodromal malaise, pharyngitis, rhinitis, and abdominal pain. At the median, the rash appears 15 days after VZV exposure; the range is 10 to 21 days. The vesicular eruption emerges in successive crops over the first 3 to 4 days of illness, usually with concomitant exanthem. Each skin vesicle appears on an erythematous base, resulting in the descriptive image of a dew drop on a rose petal. This stage of infection may be missed because of rupture of the vesicle, which then undergoes inflammatory changes and crusting. The exanthem usually begins on the head and quickly progresses to the trunk, arms, and finally the legs. It is common to see all stages of the exanthem, including macules, vesicles, papules, and crusts, in the same region of the skin, and this should be looked for in the examination of the patient. Fever can be expected for the first 3 to 4 days of the exanthem, and much of the morbidity is associated with the extent of the cutaneous rash. In addition, primary VZV infection invades the mucosal surfaces of respiratory, alimentary, and genitourinary systems, and the patient with chickenpox can have severe laryngitis, laryngotracheobronchitis, vaginitis, urethritis, pancreatitis, and enteritis. Severe abdominal pain or back pain is a hallmark of progressive VZV infection in the immunocompromised individual.

The rate of complications is highest in persons younger than 1 year of age and older than 15 years of age. The complications that lead to hospitalization in VZV infection consist of bacterial superinfection of skin, dehydration, pneumonia, encephalitis, and hepatitis. Bacterial skin infections and bacterial pneumonias occur in the youngest groups, and before the antibiotic era, severe bacterial infections, including osteomyelitis, were fairly common in association with chickenpox. Encephalitis occurs in approximately 1 : 11,000 cases in the age group 5 to 14 years. Reye's syndrome, once a concern in VZV infection, has become uncommon because of the recommendation against aspirin use. With the availability of antiviral agents and of varicella-zoster immunoglobulin (VZIg), VZV-associated mortality has decreased to fewer than 100 deaths per year in the United States.

Shingles

Shingles occurs when VZV infection reactivates in cranial or spinal nerve ganglia and then spreads to the cutaneous nerves. The clinical presentation and major complications of this disease derive from the neural origin of the virus infection. The most common area of involvement is the trunk, presumably because this is the area of greatest primary infection, followed by cranial dermatomes and then by cervical and lumbar dermatomes. Thus, shingles presents with pain and with a vesicular eruption in a unilateral cutaneous distribution. Pain without rash, called *zoster sine herpete*, can be the only symptom of this disease. The pain of herpes zoster that persists after the healing of skin lesions is termed *postherpetic neuralgia*. This problem increases in frequency with age and is a major problem in patients older than 50. Virus reactivation in the spinal or cranial nerve ganglia causes intense inflammation with hemorrhagic necrosis of nerve cells, eventual destruction of portions of the ganglion, poliomyelitis of posterior spinal columns, and leptomeningitis. This intense inflammation results in nerve dysfunction manifested clinically by meningitis and myelitis, with or without paresis at sites of involved nerves. Thus, there may be weakness or paralysis of limbs, of facial muscles, and of muscles within abdominal viscera. In addition, intense inflammation of the cutaneous site of infection results in scarring of the involved epidermis. This is a particular concern when the cornea or other ophthalmic structures are involved.

■ DIAGNOSIS

The history and physical examination remain the primary methods for diagnosing chickenpox and shingles. In chickenpox, the clinician should look for lesions in all stages of development, including macules, vesicles, pustules, and crusted lesions. The rash of chickenpox can be mistaken for a diverse array of entities, such as rashes caused by herpes simplex virus, Coxsackie and other enteroviruses, mycoplasma, streptococcal impetigo, rickettsialpox, insect bites, and delayed-type hypersensitivity reactions such as poison ivy. In certain individuals, especially those at high risk for complications of VZV infection, specific diagnosis can be pursued by laboratory methods. The most rapid and accurate method is the direct immunofluorescent stain of a skin scraping for VZV antigen using a commercially available kit. The Tzanck prep, a method to demonstrate multinucleated giant cells in skin scrapings stained with Wright-Giemsa, has been superseded by this fluorescent antigen detection assay when the latter technique is available. Conventional methods of culture of VZV or serology for VZV antibody can also be used to confirm the diagnosis, but these are rarely necessary.

■ DETECTION OF SUSCEPTIBILITY TO VZV

The simplest method of reliably ruling out susceptibility to chickenpox is to obtain a history of chickenpox or of having cared for children with it. A positive history from adults has a 97% to 99% correlation with serologic confirmation. A negative history from an adult fails to conform to a negative serologic status in 72% to 93% of cases. Therefore serologic tests are necessary to determine whether a person with a negative history has been infected with VZV. Commercial assays, fluorescent or enzyme-linked immunoassays, and a rapid latex agglutination assay are very reliable except in persons who have received blood products and thereby acquired passive antibody.

■ THERAPY

Chickenpox
Overall Assessment
The goal in management is to treat the symptoms of primary VZV infection and to prevent complications if possible. A flowchart describing an approach is shown in Figure 1. The three stages of management are (1) establishing the likelihood of the diagnosis, (2) determining whether antiviral therapy is indicated, and (3) ruling out secondary bacterial infection, other complications, and failure of antiviral treatment. In children, chickenpox usually requires minimal medical attention, but if there is an atypical course or severe skin involvement, the patient should have a physical examination to assess the level of hydration, the need for temperature control, the baseline mental status, and other physical findings that suggest complications.

Symptomatic Therapy
Itching is the major symptom of chickenpox, and pruritic management is important. Warm baths containing baking soda (⅓ cup per bathtub) or emulsified oatmeal (Aveno) can temporarily relieve itching. This can be combined with the oral administration of either diphenhydramine (Benadryl), 1.25 mg/kg by mouth every 6 hours, or hydroxyzine (Atarax, Vistaril), 0.5 mg/kg by mouth every 6 hours. In older children, cold pramoxine HCl 1% lotion with calamine 8% (Caladryl) can be used, but this should be avoided in infants because of the risk of excessive surface exposure and absorption of drug or vehicle (alcohol 2.2%). Fever should be controlled with acetaminophen, and salicylates should not be used because administration of salicylates to children with chickenpox increases the risk of subsequent Reye's syndrome. For severe dysuria, a cold compress on the genital area during urination will ease the pain and minimize the likelihood of a functional bladder obstruction.

Antiviral Therapy
Acyclovir (Zovirax) is the only agent approved in the United States for the treatment of chickenpox. It is indicated for treatment of chickenpox in certain normal persons, for disseminated VZV infection in immunosuppressed persons, and for treatment of shingles (later section). Oral acyclovir should be used in otherwise healthy persons with chickenpox who are at risk for moderate to severe disease, such as those older than 12 years, those with chronic cutaneous or pulmonary disorders, those receiving chronic salicylate therapy, and persons receiving short or intermittent courses of corticosteroids or aerosolized corticosteroids (Table 1). The American Academy of Pediatrics (AAP) does not recommend that otherwise normal children under age 12 receive oral acyclovir for chickenpox. However, studies have shown that treatment of chickenpox within 24 hours of the onset of rash reduces the duration and magnitude of fever and the number and duration of skin lesions. Therefore some experts recommend using oral acyclovir in secondary household cases because disease is usually more severe in these children. The data are insufficient regarding the safety and efficacy of acyclovir therapy for infants younger than 12 months, and it is not recommended.

All adults with chickenpox should receive oral acyclovir, and those with rapidly progressive infection should be treated with intravenous acyclovir. All immunosuppressed persons with chickenpox should be treated with intravenous acyclovir because there is inadequate experience with the oral formulation. However, as noted by the AAP, some experts have used oral acyclovir in highly selected immunocompromised persons who are at relatively low risk for developing complications and in whom follow-up is ensured. Case-by-case evaluation of risks versus benefits is necessary, but for many groups, the risk of disseminating infection is sufficiently high and unpredictable to recommend intravenous treatment in nearly all cases. Acyclovir should not be used by exposed persons in an attempt to prevent chickenpox. It should be considered for the pregnant patient at risk for serious complications of varicella, but oral acyclovir is not recommended for routine use by the pregnant woman with uncomplicated chickenpox because the risks and benefits to the fetus and mother are mostly unknown. VZIg is licensed for use in high-risk individuals at the time of exposure to VZV infection but is not recommended for treatment of chickenpox.

Bacterial Infections
Pyoderma is the most commonly observed bacterial complication of varicella. It can be minimized by attention to good hygiene, including daily bathing with bacteriostatic soap, trimming of children's fingernails to minimize excoriation of itchy skin, and early recognition of superinfection. Streptococcal and staphylococcal bacterial infections can be associated with bacteremia and subsequent osteomyelitis, with scarlet fever, and with bacterial synergetic gangrene. Therefore aggressive management of bacterial infection is warranted.

Respiratory Tract Infection
In addition to the occasional laryngitis and laryngotracheobronchitis that can occur during chickenpox, bacterial superinfection can affect the lower respiratory tract, producing

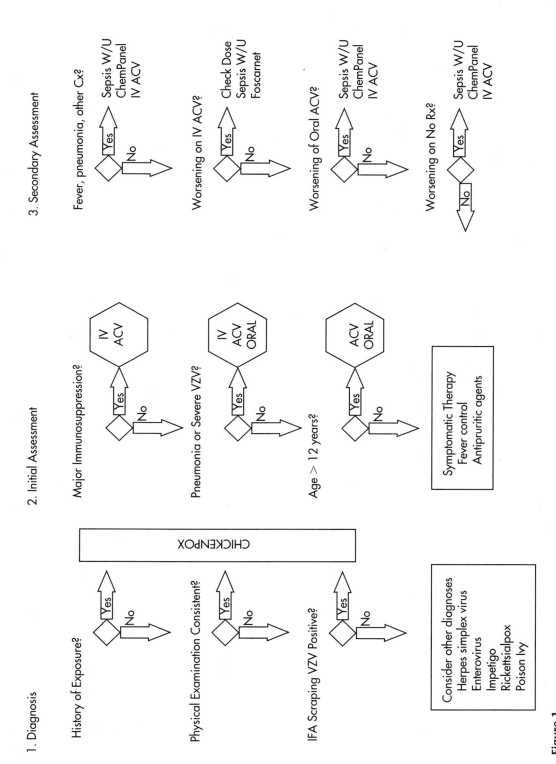

Figure 1
Algorithm for the management of chickenpox. *IV,* Intravenous; *ACV,* acyclovir; *Cx,* complications; *W/U,* workup; *IFA,* immunofluorescent antibody.

Table 1   Antiviral Treatment of Varicella-Zoster Virus (VZV) Infection[a]

AGENT	INDICATION	CREATININE CLEARANCE (ml/min/1.73 M²)	DOSE	DOSING INTERVAL	DURATION (DAYS)
Oral acyclovir	Chickenpox >age 12 yr	>25	20 mg/kg up to 800 mg	4 times/day	5 days
		10-25	Same	q8h	5 days
		0-10[b]	Same	q12h	5 days
	Shingles	>25	20 mg/kg up to 800 mg	5 times/day	5-7 days
		10-25	Same	q8h	5-7 days
		0-10[b]	Same	q12h	7 days
IV acyclovir	Life-threatening VZV infection	>50	500 mg/M² or 10 mg/kg[c,d]	q8h	7 days
		25-50	Same	q12h	7 days
		10-25	Same	q24h	7 days
		0-10[b]	250 mg/M²	q24h	7 days
Famciclovir	Shingles >18 years of age	>60	500 mg	q8h	7 days
		40-59	500 mg	q12h	7 days
		20-39	500 mg	q24h	7 days
Valacyclovir	Shingles >18 years of age	>50	1000 mg	q8h	7 days
		29-49	1000 mg	q12h	7 days
		10-29	1000 mg	q24h	7 days
		<10	500 mg	q24h	7 days
Foscarnet	Acyclovir-resistant VZV[e]	>100[f]	60 mg/kg	q8h	7-10 days

[a]See package insert for recommended dose adjustment of all drugs.
[b]An additional dose is recommended after each hemodialysis treatment.
[c]To minimize renal toxicity, an adequate urine output is required. This can be ensured if the acyclovir is infused at a concentration of approximately 4 mg/ml over 1 hour and the same volume of fluid is given over the next hour.
[d]Use ideal body weight for height to calculate dose in obese person: M^2, square meter of body surface area.
[e]Foscarnet is recommended by experts for treatment of life-threatening acyclovir-resistant VZV infection, but this is not an FDA-approved indication for foscarnet use. Appropriate informed consent should be obtained before such use.
[f]Foscarnet is nephrotoxic, and the dosage should be based on creatinine clearance. Guidelines for dosage adjustment are listed in the package information.

pneumonia and bronchitis. Pneumonia is most often caused by the usual respiratory pathogens, including *Streptococcus pneumoniae, Haemophilus influenzae,* and *Staphylococcus aureus.* Viral pneumonia is more likely to be a problem in older persons with chickenpox.

Gastrointestinal Complications

When death occurs during VZV infection, the gastrointestinal tract is invariably involved. Specific attention must be given to bleeding, particularly in the immunosuppressed person. Vomiting is not a usual part of the clinical course of this infection, and it should alert the physician to look for abdominal or central nervous system (CNS) complications. Also, surgical emergencies such as appendicitis and intussusception can occur during varicella. Mild hepatitis is seen in a majority of children with chickenpox, usually as a result of asymptomatic elevation of hepatic enzymes for which no treatment is necessary. However, elevation of serum or urinary amylase indicates pancreatitis, which may require supportive treatment. As noted, the concomitant use of aspirin in the child with chickenpox has been associated with an increased incidence of Reye's syndrome. Although this is rare today, Reye's syndrome and other metabolic diseases must be excluded in any child with varicella in whom there are vomiting and changes in mental status.

Encephalitis

Cerebral complications may be either cerebral or cerebellar abnormalities; the latter is a more benign disease. Cerebellar ataxia, the most common syndrome associated with varicella encephalitis, is generally a benign entity thought to be caused by postinfectious demyelination. There is no evidence that acyclovir treatment is necessary in postchickenpox cerebellitis, but it is prudent to include antiviral therapy in any cerebral presentation of VZV infection, especially if it may be associated with continued viral replication such as in AIDS or other immunosuppression.

Bleeding Disorders

Bleeding disorders during chickenpox are due to disseminated intravascular coagulation, vasculitis, or idiopathic thrombocytopenic purpura (ITP), which can occur during active infection or convalescence. It responds to conventional treatment for ITP.

Immunosuppressed Patients

Acyclovir is the only indicated drug for the treatment of VZV infections in the immunosuppressed patient, whether disseminated chickenpox, disseminated shingles, or localized shingles. Three other commercial antiviral drugs, valaciclovir (Valtrex), famciclovir (Famvir), and foscarnet (Foscavir) have activity against VZV. Valaciclovir and famciclovir are indicated only for the treatment of shingles in the immunocompetent person. Focarnet is used for the management of acyclovir-resistant VZV infection. Vidarabine has been used for acyclovir-resistant VZV infection, but usually only as an alternative to foscarnet.

Shingles
Overall Assessment

The major complication of shingles is postherpetic pain. For this reason, effective analgesic medication must be a principal part of treatment, and the initial assessment should be directed to a determination of general medical status and tolerance for narcotic-based therapy. In addition, there is increasing evidence that early antiviral therapy can lessen late neuralgia, and therefore, institution of specific anti-VZV agents is important in certain patients.

Symptomatic Therapy

A hallmark of shingles is intense inflammation, and the cutaneous site of disease can take weeks to heal. During the initial healing phase, the patient or caretaker should be instructed to have daily soaks with salt solutions and dressing changes to minimize bacterial infection and speed healing. If the eye is involved, an ophthalmologist should be consulted for use of topical antiinflammatory or antiviral medication and for long-term evaluation. Management of pain will vary from patient to patient, but it usually begins with acetaminophen-codeine combinations and increases to more potent analgesia if indicated. In severe postherpetic neuralgia, if there is no response to conventional pain management, tricyclic antidepressant medications such as amitriptyline (Elavil) can be tried, although this is not an indicated use. Local nerve block should be used in refractory pain. Topical pain medications are not recommended because the source of pain stimulation is central.

Use of corticosteroids in the acute phase of disease remains controversial, but a recent controlled study indicated no effect of steroids combined with acyclovir compared with acyclovir alone on postherpetic pain. However, steroids plus acyclovir produced earlier healing and less pain in the initial 2 weeks of shingles. There were more side effects with steroid use, and therefore the routine use of steroids for shingles cannot be recommended. It is possible that early treatment with antivirals alone can significantly reduce late postherpetic pain, and at present this must be the focus of initial therapy.

Antiviral Therapy

Acyclovir, valacyclovir, and famciclovir are approved in the United States for the treatment of shingles in otherwise normal persons (see Table 1). Acyclovir is the agent of choice for immunocompromised persons and is the only intravenous agent available for treatment of shingles. Valaciclovir and famciclovir are oral prodrugs of acyclovir and penciclovir, respectively. Safety and efficacy in children younger than 18 years have not been established for these agents. Also, because of the potential for tumorigenicity in rats, penciclovir should not be given to nursing mothers unless nursing is discontinued. Treatment should be given to those older than 50 because this population is at greatest risk for postherpetic neuralgia, and the decision to treat adults younger than

Table 2 Groups at Risk for Complications of Varicella-Zoster Virus (VZV) Infection*

Susceptible persons on immunosuppressive therapy†
Persons with congenital cellular immunodeficiency
Persons with an acquired immunodeficiency, including AIDS
Persons >20 years of age
Newborn infants exposed to onset of maternal varicella <5 days before or 2 to 7 days after birth
Premature infants weighing <1 kg‡

*Susceptible (antibody negative) persons exposed to VZV by indoor face-to-face contact with an infected person less than 2 days before or anytime during vesiculopustular stage of chickenpox are at highest risk and should receive varicella-zoster immunoglobulin.
†All cytoreductive chemotherapy and radiotherapy is considered immunosuppressive. The immunosuppressive dose of prednisone equivalent can vary in individual cases but is in the range of 1 to 2 mg/kg/day.
‡The risk of complications of VZV infection in this group, which is poorly defined, is based on the likelihood of protective maternal antibody versus gestational age at birth.

50 years of age with antiviral agents should be made on individual assessment. The advantages of prodrugs are the improved absorption and the convenient dosing intervals.

Exposure to VZV

The spread of infectious VZV from a person with chickenpox is by air droplets from nasopharyngeal secretions, which usually requires face-to-face exposure indoors but can also be via air currents to susceptible individuals without direct contact. The period of respiratory infectivity is generally considered to begin 48 hours before the onset of exanthem and to continue for 4 days after onset. In addition, the vesicular fluid can spread the virus by direct contact, so infectivity by contact with skin lesions is possible until they are crusted. Shingles can also spread by direct contact or by exposure to airborne infectious material. The incubation period for chickenpox after exposure to shingles is the same as for exposure to chickenpox—15 days, range 10 to 21 days. The clinical varicella attack rate in susceptible children on household exposure to chickenpox is approximately 90% and is 25% on exposure to household shingles.

Immunocompromised Host Exposed to VZV

Until the VZV vaccine became available in the United States, the only protection from VZV infection was passive immunization at the time of exposure. Families and school personnel must continue to be aware of exposure to VZV in high-risk persons so that VZIG can be administered within 96 hours. Any susceptible person at risk for complications of VZV (Table 2) should receive passive immunization if exposure was adequate to communicate disease and occurred within approximately 4 days. Adequacy of exposure is defined as indoor face-to-face exposure for 1 hour with a person during the infectious phase. VZIG should not be used in any person with a history of chickenpox except persons who have undergone bone marrow transplantation. Immunosuppressive therapy should be stopped during the incubation period, although this precaution is waived if the underlying disease requires continued treatment, such as initial therapy for acute leukemia.

Adults Exposed to VZV

More than 90% of adults have had VZV, and although reinfection occurs after exposure to chickenpox, these persons do not usually develop disease, although some cutaneous lesions can occur. Susceptible adults are at risk for life-threatening chickenpox, and they are the source of unexpected epidemics. One adult population known to have a high rate of susceptibility to chickenpox is immigrants from subtropical climates. Serologic tests of susceptibility should be considered in any such immigrants working in a health care setting. The decision to use VZIG in susceptible healthy adults following close exposure to VZV should be made on an individual basis, taking into consideration the person's health, the type of exposure, and the likelihood of previous chickenpox.

Nosocomial VZV

Control of nosocomial infections requires three actions: (1) routine continuous surveillance of VZV susceptibility among hospital staff, with VZV vaccination as indicated; (2) adequate isolation of contagious VZV infections; and (3) rapid evaluation of and response to exposure. Hospitals that care for immunodeficient children should screen staff at the time of employment for susceptibility. This can be done efficiently by performing antibody tests on those who have a negative or unknown history of chickenpox. Susceptible employees should be excluded from care of patients with VZV infection. Exposed susceptible health care workers should be furloughed from the tenth day after initial exposure until 21 days after the last exposure. If the VZV exposure is from a patient, he or she should be discharged if possible. If not, the patient should be placed in isolation designed to prevent spread of infection by both air and direct contact. Optimally, this consists of a private room with negative air pressure relative to the corridor, with gown, mask, and glove precaution guidelines posted on the door and restricted entry for susceptible persons. Isolation should remain in effect until skin lesions are crusted. After control of the source of infection, quick assessment of three types of information should be obtained: (1) the nature of the exposure and whether it is likely to result in secondary infections, (2) which of the exposed patients or staff are susceptible, and (3) which patients are at risk for complications. Thus, the initial step is to define the hospital areas in which a definitive VZV exposure occurred and then to focus on which patients in these areas are at risk for infection. Once susceptibility or positive history of varicella is determined and serologic evaluation of those with ambiguous or negative history is done, all susceptible patients who are exposed should be discharged if possible. Those remaining in the hospital should be placed in respiratory isolation between days 8 and 21 after exposure, or for 8 to 28 days for those receiving VZIG. Those remaining in the hospital without exposure should be placed in a cohort that protects them from exposures.

Management of the Pregnant Woman

A syndrome of congenital varicella consisting of low birth weight, cutaneous scarring, limb hypoplasia, microcephaly, and other brain and eye abnormalities can occur in the baby of a pregnant woman who has chickenpox but not shingles. Teratogenic damage results only from first- and second-trimester infection, and clinically apparent disease occurs only in approximately 2% of infants born after maternal varicella in early pregnancy. For this reason, experts advise that maternal chickenpox is not a medical indication for abortion. There is no reliable diagnostic method, including amniocentesis and ultrasound, for determining teratogenic intrauterine infection. It is recommended that after exposure in pregnancy, susceptibility should be determined and the susceptible person should be given VZIG.

Varicella Vaccine

A live, attenuated VZV vaccine (Varivax) was approved in the United States in 1995 and is recommended for all healthy, chickenpox-negative persons older than 12 months of age. In addition to normal children, it is particularly recommended for eligible health care and day-care workers, college students, prisoners, military recruits, nonpregnant women of childbearing age, and international travelers. After a single dose in children younger than age 12 years and two doses 1 month apart in older persons, protection from chickenpox can be expected in more than 94% of immunized persons. The vaccine is not recommended for infants younger than 1 year of age, for immunosuppressed persons, for those receiving salicylate therapy, for pregnant women, or for those allergic to components of the vaccine, including neomycin, gelatin, and monosodium glutamate.

Suggested Reading

Cohen JI, et al: Recent advances in varicella-zoster virus infection, *Ann Intern Med* 130:922, 1999.

Enders G, et al: Consequences of varicella and herpes zoster in pregnancy: prospective study of 1739 cases, *Lancet* 343:1548, 1994.

Snoeck R, Andrei G, De Clercq E: Current pharmacological approaches to the therapy of varicella zoster virus infections: a guide to treatment, *Drugs* 57:187, 1999.

Wood MJ, et al: A randomized trial of acyclovir for 7 days or 21 days with and without prednisolone for treatment of acute herpes zoster, *N Engl J Med* 330:896, 1994.

Zaia JA, Grose C: Varicella and herpes zoster. In Gorbach SL, Bartlett JG, Blacklow NR, eds: *Infectious diseases*, ed 2, Philadelphia, 1998, Saunders.

CYTOMEGALOVIRUS

Jeffery L. Meier

Nearly half of persons in the United States are infected with cytomegalovirus (CMV), although prevalence of infection ranges widely according to age, socioeconomic status, sexual habits, and race. The initial infection is followed by lifelong persistence of virus in fluctuating states of latency and reactivation. CMV-related illness is generally limited to persons with impaired or immature cellular immune systems, but a mononucleosis-like syndrome may indicate a primary CMV infection of healthy persons. An estimated 7000 infants per year in the United States have serious sequelae or die as a result of congenital CMV infection. Symptomatic congenital infections are most often a consequence of primary CMV infection during gestation. In immunocompromised persons, both primary and reactivation CMV infections can produce serious disease, although their relative likelihood of doing so varies greatly according to the particular type of patient afflicted. Such infections are themselves immunosuppressive, predisposing to other opportunistic infections and possibly accelerating HIV progression.

CMV establishes latency in monocytes and their precursors. Either primary or reactivation infection can yield asymptomatic viral shedding, which is augmented by immunosuppression. CMV is shed into saliva, breast milk, semen, cervical secretions, and urine. Infants and young children often shed CMV into urine, and sometimes into saliva, for several weeks to months after an asymptomatic primary infection. Hence, close contact with children, sexual contact, breast-feeding, and receiving donor blood or an organ are risks for CMV transmission.

■ DIAGNOSIS

The diagnosis of CMV-related disease in immunocompromised persons often relies on demonstration of characteristic cytomegalic inclusions in affected tissue. However, such an approach is not feasible or necessary in all patients. For instance, a person with advanced acquired immunodeficiency disease (AIDS) who has the typical retinal abnormalities of CMV retinitis does not require additional diagnostic studies. The positive and negative predictive values of qualitative CMV culture-, DNA-, or antigen-based assays for diagnosing CMV disease range widely according to clinical circumstances. For example, CMV growth from a blood buffy coat obtained from a febrile transplant recipient is highly predictive of CMV disease, whereas this finding has low predictive value in the febrile patient with AIDS. Recent modifications of DNA- and antigen-based assays to quantitate CMV amount in blood components or urine have greatly improved positive and negative predictive values for diagnosing CMV disease or determining risk of

disease. Although such tests are considered investigational and are not standardized, they will likely have important future roles in prevention and treatment of CMV disease. Assessment of CMV antibody levels in immunocompromised persons is seldom helpful in the diagnosis of CMV disease, except for determining serostatus. Interpretation of CMV-specific IgM antibody values is confounded by high rates of false-positive and false-negative findings in these patients. The laboratory diagnosis of CMV mononucleosis in the normal host is discussed in the chapter *Epstein-Barr Virus and Other Causes of the Infectious Mononucleosis Syndrome.*

■ MANAGEMENT

Two nucleoside analogs (ganciclovir and cidofovir), one pyrophosphate analog (foscarnet), and one antisense oligonucleotide (fomivirsen) are approved by the Food and Drug Administration (FDA) for the treatment of CMV infection. Each of these agents has been shown to delay progression of CMV retinitis in persons with AIDS. Ganciclovir and foscarnet are also effective treatments of CMV disease involving other organs or immunocompromised persons. Ganciclovir, acyclovir, valaciclovir, and CMV immunoglobulin variably prevent CMV disease in solid organ transplant recipients. Ganciclovir, and possibly CMV immunoglobulin, attenuates or prevents CMV disease in bone marrow transplant recipients. Oral ganciclovir may prevent or delay the first episode of CMV retinitis in persons having AIDS and fewer than 50 CD4 lymphocytes/μl, but its association with better vision or longer survival has not been demonstrated. The characteristics of these anti-CMV agents and specific recommendations for their use are provided in Table 1.

Ganciclovir

The action of ganciclovir, a guanosine analog, depends on its initial phosphorylation by the viral phosphotransferase UL97. Cellular enzymes further convert ganciclovir monophosphate to a triphosphate molecule. Ganciclovir triphosphate inhibits the viral DNA polymerase and is incorporated into replicating DNA to terminate chain elongation. The median effective inhibitory dose (ED_{50}) of ganciclovir for susceptible clinical CMV isolates is equal to or less than 6 μM. The standard intravenous dosing schedule (5 mg/kg every 12 hours) provides a peak serum ganciclovir level (peak and trough of 32.8 μM and 0.2 μM, respectively) that greatly exceeds the ED_{50} value of susceptible CMV strains. The intracellular half-life of 16.5 hours for the active metabolite of ganciclovir also contributes to the efficacy of this dosing schedule. Ganciclovir concentrations in vitreous and cerebrospinal fluid (CSF) are somewhat lower and more variable than that of serum, which accounts for some treatment failures of disease involving the retina or central nervous system. The 4.5-mg intraocular sustained-release device provides more favorable intravitreal ganciclovir concentrations. The bioavailability of oral ganciclovir is only 6% to 9%. Nonetheless, oral ganciclovir given 3 to 4.5 g/day in divided doses produces inhibitory concentrations in serum that are sufficient to prevent CMV disease in some patients. Ganciclovir is eliminated by the kidneys, requiring dosage adjustments according to creatinine clearance.

Table 1 CMV Prophylaxis and Treatment Regimens

AGENT	INDICATIONS	DOSING REGIMEN	TOXICITIES	MONITORING	COMMENTS
INTRAVENOUS					
Ganciclovir	Treatment of visceral or disseminated disease	Standard: 5 mg/kg q12h × 14-21 days Maintenance: 5 mg/kg/day	Catheter-related complications, neutropenia, thrombocytopenia, anemia	Standard dose: CBC and Cr biweekly Lower dose: CBC qwk, Cr q1-3wk	If ANC 500-1000, add filgrastim If ANC <500 or platelets <25 K, hold ganciclovir Increased toxicity of AZT or imipenem, increased level of ddl
	Prophylaxis or preemptive therapy in solid organ or bone marrow transplant recipients	5 mg/kg qd or bid; duration varies depending on risk for CMV disease			May cause infertility and may be teratogenic or embryotoxic Adjust dosage for reduced renal function
Foscarnet	Treatment of visceral or disseminated disease	Standard: 90 mg/kg q12h × 14-21 days Maintenance: 90-120 mg/kg/day	Catheter-related complications, nephrotoxicity, paresthesias, cation chelation, genital ulcerations, nausea	Standard dose: CBC, Cr, cations (K+, Mg++, Ca++), and phosphate 2-3× qwk Maintenance dose: Cr and electrolytes qwk CBC q2wk	If Cr >2.8, hold foscarnet until Cr ≤2.1 mg/dl Adjust dosage for reduced renal function Hydration reduces renal toxicity
Cidofovir	Treatment of retinitis	Standard: 5 mg/kg/wk × 2 Maintenance: 5 mg/kg q2wk	Nephrotoxicity, neutropenia, uveitis, ocular hypotony, probenecid rash Probenecid contraindicated in persons with severe sulfa allergy	Standard dose: Cr and UA every dose Maintenance dose: Same plus intraocular pressure qmo	1-2 L saline hydration, with 1 L given before cidofovir infusion; probenecid (4 g) given 3 hr before and 8 hr after cidofovir infusion Do not use if Cr >1.5 mg/dl CrCl ≤55 ml/min, ≥2+ proteinuria or receiving other nephrotoxic agents
INTRAOCULAR					
Fomivirsen	Treatment of retinitis, if refractory or intolerant to other therapies	Induction: 330 mg intravitreal injection every other week × 2 Maintenance: 150-330 mg intravitreal injection qmo	Uveitis, increased intraocular pressure	Ophthalmologic follow-up, with intraocular pressure	Do not use in patients recently (2-4 wk) treated with cidofovir Topical steroids useful for management of uveitis

Drug	Indication	Dosage	Adverse effects	Monitoring	Comments
Ganciclovir implant	Treatment of retinitis	Surgical: Intraocular implantation via pars plana of (4.5 mg) implant; replacement q6-8mo. Concomitant systemic therapy: see oral ganciclovir maintenance dosing	Transient blurred vision, retinal detachment, hemorrhage, infection	Ophthalmologic follow-up	Concomitant systemic therapy reduces risk of CMV disease in contralateral eye and other organs. Implant releases 1 μg/h of ganciclovir
ORAL Ganciclovir	Maintenance therapy of CMV retinitis. Prophylaxis in solid organ and bone marrow transplant recipients and AIDS patients	1-1.5 g tid, with food. 1 g tid, with food	Neutropenia	CBC and Cr q2wk	
Acyclovir	Prophylaxis in renal transplant recipients	800 mg qid			Acyclovir prophylaxis has been applied to other types of transplant recipients but is less effective than ganciclovir. Acyclovir is ineffective for CMV prophylaxis in persons with AIDS
Valaciclovir	Prophylaxis in solid organ transplant recipients	2 g qid	Hallucinations, confusion		Valaciclovir (8 g/day) is not recommended for CMV prophylaxis in persons with AIDS because of potential adverse events
CMV IMMUNOGLOBULIN CMV immunoglobulin intravenous (CytoGam)	Treatment of CMV pneumonitis in bone marrow transplant recipients. Prophylaxis in solid organ or bone marrow transplant recipients	400 mg/kg days 1, 2, and 7; 200 mg/kg day 14 plus IV ganciclovir (see IV ganciclovir); 50-150 mg/kg q2-4wk (various dosing regimens have been used)	Fever, myalgia, arthralgia, nausea, wheezing, hypotension, aseptic meningitis	Vital signs before, during, and after infusion	Derived from pooled adult human plasma containing high titers for antibody for CMV. Increase infusion rate as tolerated, 15-60 mg/kg/hr

CBC, Complete blood count; Cr, serum creatinine; ANC, absolute neutrophil count; AZT, zidovudine; CMV, cytomegalovirus; UA, urine analysis; AIDS, acquired immunodeficiency syndrome.

Resistance to ganciclovir can emerge during its extended use in persons with AIDS but seldom develops in transplant recipients. The AIDS Clinical Trials Group has designated CMV isolates as intermediate resistant with ED_{50} values greater than 6 μM but less than 12 μM and resistant with ED_{50} values equal to or greater than 12 μM. Resistance mostly results from mutations in the viral phosphotransferase and is less commonly due to mutations in the viral DNA polymerase. CMV isolates exhibiting high-level resistance (ED_{50} values $\geq$30 μM) often have mutations in both viral enzymes and are also likely to be resistant to cidofovir. Alternative treatments of ganciclovir-resistant virus include foscarnet, cidofovir, or fomivirsen, with the caveat that cidofovir and fomivirsen are only useful for CMV retinitis.

Clinical toxicity of ganciclovir includes granulocytopenia, thrombocytopenia, and anemia. A rise in creatinine was observed in bone marrow transplant recipients. Granulocytopenia can often be abrogated by colony-stimulating factors. In animal studies, ganciclovir was teratogenic and carcinogenic and caused infertility. Ganciclovir given intravenously poses a risk for catheter-related sepsis, whereas the intraocular implant may be complicated by endophthalmitis (0.3%). In persons with CMV retinitis, retinal detachments occur in nearly 15% of eyes containing implants placed by skilled ophthalmologists but also occur in a similar proportion of eyes treated with parenteral ganciclovir alone.

Ganciclovir has proved effective in the treatment of several forms of CMV disease and also in the prevention of initial or recurrent disease. The recommended dosing schedules and indications for use are provided in Table 1. Ganciclovir is typically used for treatment of CMV disease involving the retina, gastrointestinal tract, lung, or nervous system. In bone marrow transplant patients with CMV pneumonia, the combination treatment of intravenous ganciclovir and high-titer CMV immunoglobulin is believed to improve survival. Although ganciclovir implant is substantially better than systemic therapy in delaying progression of CMV retinitis in persons with AIDS, it should be used in conjunction with oral ganciclovir to reduce the incidence of new CMV disease. Ganciclovir has also been used to treat severe CMV disease in normal hosts, but its risk:benefit ratio must be carefully weighed because of potential bone marrow and gonadal toxicities. The use of ganciclovir to treat symptomatic congenital CMV infection is under study.

Foscarnet

Foscarnet (phosphonoformic acid) directly inhibits viral DNA polymerase activity. The drug is cleared by the kidneys, so dosage adjustment according to creatinine clearance is required. The major toxicity is renal impairment, which may be reduced by hydration. Mineral and electrolyte abnormalities, such as hypocalcemia, hyperphosphatemia, hypophosphatemia, hypokalemia, and hypomagnesemia, are common. Although managable, these abnormalities can precipitate seizures. Chelation of ionized calcium by foscarnet may result in numbness, tingling, and paresthesias, which may be prevented by slowing the infusion rate. Particular caution is advised when using the drug in persons with underlying cardiac or seizure disorders. Other notable adverse events include anemia, granulocytopenia, genital ulcers, and catheter-related sepsis. Foscarnet should not be used in persons receiving amphotericin B, aminoglycosides, intravenous pentamidine, or other nephrotoxic agents.

Intravenous foscarnet and intravenous ganciclovir are equivalent in efficacy for treatment of CMV retinitis and gastrointestinal disease. Foscarnet has some activity against human immunodeficiency virus (HIV) as well, which may partly explain its association with lower mortality compared with ganciclovir for initial treatment of CMV retinitis in persons with AIDS. Foscarnet also appears effective in treatment of other forms of CMV disease, including neurologic or pulmonary disease. One study found the combination of ganciclovir and foscarnet to be more effective than either drug alone in the treatment of relapsing CMV retinitis. Intravitreal administration of foscarnet has been used when other therapeutic options for CMV retinitis have been exhausted.

Cidofovir

The phosphorylation of cidofovir by cellular enzymes renders it active for inhibition of the viral DNA polymerase and termination of DNA chain elongation. The active metabolite has a long intracellular half-life (17 to 65 hours), which may partly account for the drug's prolonged anti-CMV effect. Cidofovir is a nephrotoxic drug that is contraindicated in persons who have preexisting renal insufficiency (Cr >1.5 mg/dl, CrCl ≤55 ml/min, or ≥2+ proteinuria) or are receiving other nephrotoxic agents. To minimize its nephrotoxicity, intravenous prehydration and administration of probenecid is necessary. Notably, probenecid is contraindicated in those persons with history of a severe sulfa allergy. Neutropenia, ocular hypotony, and metabolic acidosis (Fanconi's syndrome) are other potential toxicities of the drug. In animal studies, cidofovir was gonadotoxic, embryotoxic, and carcinogenic.

Intravenous cidofovir is efficacious in delaying progression of untreated CMV retinitis in persons with AIDS. Relapsing retinitis may also respond to cidofovir, although patients treated extensively with ganciclovir or foscarnet are more likely to fail cidofovir therapy. Unfortunately, treatment-limiting toxicity is common. Cidofovir has not been shown to be efficacious in treating CMV disease of other organs. Unlike ganciclovir and foscarnet, it is poorly effective in reducing CMV viremia in patients with AIDS.

Fomivirsen

Fomivirsen is a phosphorothioate antisense oligonucleotide that inhibits CMV replication by binding to and inactivating an essential viral messenger RNA (IE2). The mechanism of action of fomivirsen does not directly involve the viral phosphotransferase or DNA polymerase. Therefore this drug is active against CMV strains that are resistant to ganciclovir, foscarnet, and/or cidofovir. Fomivirsen is given only by intravitreal injection to provide local therapy of CMV retinitis and does not provide treatment of systemic CMV disease. Uveitis is a common complication of fomivirsen that can be alleviated with topical corticosteroid. Cidofovir may exacerbate uveitis and should not be used with fomivirsen. Increased intraocular pressure is also a common toxicity but is usually transient. Current use of fomivirsen is limited to treatment of CMV retinitis in persons with AIDS who are intolerant to or have failed other treatments.

Cytomegalovirus Immunoglobulin

Intravenous cytomegalovirus immunoglobulin (CMVIG) is human immunoglobulin that is fourfold to eightfold enriched in anti-CMV antibody titer compared with standard preparations of intravenous immunoglobulin. CMVIG is used for passive immunoprophylaxis to prevent or attenuate CMV disease in selected solid organ transplant recipients. It appears to be most beneficial in those patients at high risk of primary CMV infection. The role of CMVIG prophylaxis in bone marrow transplantation is controversial, but it may reduce the incidence of interstitial pneumonia among CMV-seropositive patients. CMVIG's use for preventing CMV

disease in solid and bone marrow transplant recipients has been largely supplanted by antiviral agents with superior efficacy and reduced cost. CMVIG remains useful in combination with intravenous ganciclovir to treat CMV pneumonia in bone marrow transplant recipients.

Suggested Reading

Crumpacker CS: Ganciclovir, *N Engl J Med* 335:721, 1996.

Goodrich JM, Boeckh M, Bowden R: Strategies for the prevention of cytomegalovirus disease after marrow transplantation, *Clin Infect Dis* 19:287, 1994.

Jacobson MA: Treatment of cytomegalovirus retinitis in patients with the acquired immunodeficiency syndrome, *N Engl J Med* 337:105, 1997.

Patel R, et al: Cytomegalovirus prophylaxis in solid organ transplant recipients, *Transplantation* 61:1279, 1996.

HUMAN HERPESVIRUSES 6, 7, AND 8

Ruth M. Greenblatt
Malcolm John

Human herpesviruses (HHV) 6, 7, and 8 are among the most recently identified human herpesviruses. All three are DNA viruses enclosed in a capsid and cause lytic and latent infection of lymphocytes and other cell types. Latent infection has been implicated in the etiology of several malignancies, although clear evidence of induction of malignancy exists only for HHV-8 at this time. Reactivation of latent infection occurs intermittently, with replication of virus in various tissues and secretions. HHV-6, -7, and -8 constitute a diverse group in terms of their biology and pathogenesis and the diseases they produce. Clinical presentation ranges from asymptomatic infection or mild illnesses, such as exanthem subitum in the case of HHV-6, all the way to life-threatening disease in the immune compromised host, such as Kaposi's sarcoma (KS) in the case of HHV-8. Selected clinical and virologic characteristics are summarized in Table 1, and limited antiviral treatment information is presented in Table 2.

■ HUMAN HERPESVIRUS 6

HHV-6 is a member of the Betaherpesvirinae group, of which cytomegalovirus (CMV) was the previously recognized human pathogen, and is placed in the genus *Roseolovi-*

rus. HHV-6 consists of two related variants, HHV-6A and HHV-6B, that cannot be distinguished by serologic tests but have distinctive molecular, cell culture, and clinical features. Both variants primarily infect CD4-positive T cells. Less is known about HHV-6A, which is not known to produce disease but has been isolated from acquired immunodeficiency syndrome (AIDS) patients and other immunocompromised individuals. HHV-6B is a cause of exanthem subitum (roseola infantum or sixth disease) and infections in immunocompromised hosts.

Shedding and Tissue Tropism

HHV-6B is shed in saliva, which is an important vehicle of transmission (perhaps most often from mother to child). The virus is not found in breast milk. After primary infection, viral replication occurs in salivary glands and recurs during periodic episodes of reactivation and shedding, which decrease in frequency over time. Virus can also be detected in peripheral blood mononuclear cells, and HHV-6 is capable of infecting natural killer cells, macrophages, epithelial cells, neurons, and a variety of other cell types. Both HHV-6 variants are highly neurotropic, perhaps indicating a central nervous system (CNS) site of latency. Viral DNA sequences can be detected in tissue and appear to be integrated at specific chromosomal locations.

Infection in Immunocompetent Hosts

Infection with both viruses is very common, approaching 100% of adults in the United States. After the attrition of maternal antibody, primary infection occurs most often during the first 2 years of life, generally between 6 and 12 months of age. Fever is generally present, can reach 40° C (104° F), and lasts 3 to 5 days. In 30% to 60% of children, fever is followed by a maculopapular rash that begins on the trunk. The rash can be confused for a medication allergy if antibiotics were administered during the febrile stage. Interestingly, about 60% of primary HHV-6 infections in Japan are diagnosed as exanthem subitum, whereas the diagnosis

Table 1 Clinical Features of Human Herpesviruses (HHV) 6, 7, and 8

VIRUS	AGE OF FIRST INFECTION	SITES OF SHEDDING	CLINICAL FEATURES OF PRIMARY INFECTION	CLINICAL FEATURES OF INFECTION IN COMPROMISED HOSTS
HHV-6A	Most before 2 yr	Serum, CSF	Not known	? pneumonitis, ? disseminated infections
HHV-6B	Most before 2 yr, perinatal transmission is possible	Saliva, cervical secretions, stool, serum	Pityriasis rosea, exanthem subitum, fever, uncommonly seizures, respiratory and GI symptoms	Pneumonitis, hepatitis, encephalitis, allograft rejection, suppression of bone marrow engraftment, retinitis, hemophagocytosis, dissemination, rash
HHV-7	Early childhood	Saliva, breast milk	Less common cause of exanthem subitum and other exanthems	Unknown
HHV-8	Most commonly after puberty, occasionally in childhood	Saliva, semen	None to febrile illness of infancy	Kaposi's sarcoma, multicentric Castleman's disease, body cavity–based lymphoma

CSF, Cerebrospinal fluid; *GI,* gastrointestinal.

Table 2 Summary of in Vivo and in Vitro Information Regarding Antiviral Treatment of Human Herpesviruses (HHV) 6, 7, and 8

VIRUS	TREATMENT INDICATION	DRUG	COMMENTS
HHV-6A	No clear indication, possible treatment of documented invasive disease in AIDS	Foscarnet possibly a first choice, ganciclovir, cidofovir	No proved efficacy in clinical trials, CMV dosing presumed to be required
HHV-6B	Treatment of documented (direct detection of virus) bone marrow, lung, brain infection in transplant recipient	Ganciclovir, foscarnet, cidofovir	No proved efficacy in clinical trials, CMV dosing presumed to be required
HHV-7	None known	None known	
HHV-8	KS, MCD in AIDS patient	1. HAART regimen	Potent antiretroviral combination treatment
		2. Cidofovir, or ganciclovir, or foscarnet	CMV dosing, duration not known
	KS in solid organ transplant recipient	1. Withdraw as much immunosuppressive therapy as possible	Proved efficacy
		2. Ganciclovir or foscarnet	Presumed CMV dosing, no clinical data, theoretic efficacy at best

AIDS, Acquired immunodeficiency syndrome; *CMV,* cytomegalovirus; *KS,* Kaposi's sarcoma; *MCD,* multicentric Castleman's disease; *HAART,* highly active antiretroviral therapy.

is made in only 9% to 40% of children in the United States. Other findings can include an enanthem on the soft palate and uvula, eyelid edema, and cervical adenopathy. Less commonly reported are otitis media, diarrhea, cough, or febrile convulsions. However, it is estimated that HHV-6 may account for 20% to 25% of all emergency room visits for children 6 to 12 months of age. Some studies have suggested that 13% to 33% of all febrile seizures in children less than 2 years of age may be caused by HHV-6. Rarely reported is severe illness evidenced by a mononucleosis-like syndrome, hepatitis, hemophagocytosis, thrombocytopenia, encephalitis, and/or fatal dissemination. As in many other viral illnesses, the severe complications are more common in adults with primary infection. HHV-6 has been implicated,

in theory, as an etiologic agent of multiple sclerosis and chronic fatigue syndrome. Detection of HHV-6 in these conditions may indicate etiology or reactivation triggered by local inflammation. HHV-6 has also been mentioned as having a possible etiologic role in several leukemias and lymphomas.

Infection in Immunocompromised Hosts

In immunocompromised hosts, such as bone marrow and solid organ transplant recipients, serious complications can occur. These include pneumonitis, encephalitis, and hepatitis, and may result in rejection of the allograft. Fever and skin rash are often reported. Most infections occur 2 to 4 weeks after transplantation. Active HHV-6 infections may occur concurrently with CMV or HHV-7, making distinction of the clinical manifestations caused by each virus difficult. Both variants of HHV-6 can be identified in compromised hosts, but again show distinctive patterns of tissue involvement. HHV-6B was predominantly identified in the brain, lungs, and peripheral blood leukocytes. HHV-6A was predominant in cerebrospinal fluid and serum and in patients with AIDS. Both variants can be detected in the lung of bone marrow transplant recipients with pneumonitis. HHV-6 also produces chronic infection in human immunodeficiency virus (HIV)-infected persons, with manifestations that include encephalitis, pneumonitis, and retinitis. HHV-6 can also suppress production of key inflammatory mediators and lymphocyte proliferative responses, producing defects in cell-mediated immunity. Like some other herpesviruses, HHV-6 increases susceptibility of CD4 cells to HIV and may facilitate HIV-disease progression. As is the case for CMV, combination antiretroviral therapy appears to have reduced the incidence of serious HHV-6 infections in AIDS.

Detection of Infection

The very high prevalence of infection and the course of intermittent reactivation must temper interpretation of diagnostic tests for HHV-6. Detection of virus does not necessarily indicate disease. Diagnosis of HHV-6 can be done both serologically and by viral detection. Viral culture of peripheral blood mononuclear cells is the gold standard for viral detection and can be accomplished using standard cell culture or shell vial techniques. Detection of HHV-6 DNA in either cellular or acellular specimens using polymerase chain reaction (PCR) is also suggestive of active HHV-6 replication and is positive in children with exanthem subitum and a variety of immunocompromised individuals. Immunohistochemistry tests can detect cells with active infection in biopsy or cytologic specimens. Serologic tests include indirect immunofluorescence assay (IFA), anticomplement immunofluorescence assay, competitive radioimmune assay, neutralization, and enzyme immunoassays (EIA). The EIA tests are more easily quantified and are less subjective. Primary infection can be demonstrated serologically by seroconversion of IgG from negative to positive in children and adults or the presence of IgM in children. The presence of IgM in adults may indicate either primary infection or reactivation from latency. A fourfold increase in serum IgG by IFA or a 16-fold increase by EIA suggests recent infection. In classic exanthem subitum, etiologic diagnosis is seldom necessary. In more complex cases, culture or PCR testing of blood, cerebrospinal fluid (CSF), and other body fluids have been used clinically.

Treatment

Information regarding the susceptibility of HHV-6 to antiviral agents is limited and based on in vitro testing. These preliminary studies suggest that HHV-6B is best inhibited by foscarnet and ganciclovir rather than acyclovir; a susceptibility pattern similar to that of CMV. HHV-6A has demonstrated consistent inhibition by foscarnet and variable inhibition by ganciclovir. Cidofovir and dexamethasone appear to have activity against both variants of HHV-6. Treatment is recommended for virologically confirmed infection in the

setting of posttransplant bone marrow suppression, encephalitis, or pneumonitis. Again analogous to CMV, bone marrow transplant recipients who receive high-dose acyclovir, despite lack of efficacy in vitro, appear to have fewer HHV-6 infections than patients who do not receive this treatment (see also the chapter *Classic Viral Exanthems*).

■ HUMAN HERPESVIRUS 7

HHV-7 is similar in morphology and genome sequence to HHV-6, the viruses resembling each other more than CMV. The virus is also a member of the Betaherpesvirinae group, genus *Roseolovirus* (along with HHV-6), and infects CD4-positive T lymphocytes. Primary infection occurs during childhood but may occur later than in HHV-6. Cross-reactivity between HHV-6 and HHV-7 in some assay systems may have complicated early studies of the viruses, and HHV-6 and HHV-7 may reactivate each other. Infection is common; serum antibodies can be identified in more than 85% of adults. Salivary shedding occurs even more often than in the case of HHV-6 (can be found in saliva from 75% of adults), and exposure to oral secretions is likely the major mode of transmission. The virus can be detected in breast milk, cervical tissue, and peripheral blood lymphocytes.

HHV-7 appears to be a cause of exanthem subitum but less commonly than HHV-6B. Other febrile illnesses of childhood have been reported in association with development of serum antibodies. HHV-7 has also been isolated from the peripheral blood mononuclear cells of patients with chronic fatigue syndrome, but the significance of this is not clear. The strongest evidence exists for a causative role of HHV-7 in pityriasis rosea. HHV-7 DNA has been found in the body fluids of patients with acute pityriasis rosea but not from those of healthy individuals or those with other illnesses. It is speculated that pityriasis rosea may be a manifestation of late primary infection with HHV-7 or more likely a result of reactivation given the epidemiology of serologic reactivity to human herpesvirus 7. HHV-7 infection results in downregulation of CD4 expression on lymphocytes, and thus could potentially influence the rate of lymphocyte infection with HIV. T cells that respond to HHV-6 antigens may also respond to HHV-7, perhaps providing some level of partial immunity. There is currently no published information on the treatment of apparent HHV-7 infections or information regarding sensitivity to antivirals.

■ HUMAN HERPESVIRUS 8

HHV-8 is a member of the Gammaherpesvirinae group, of which Epstein-Barr virus was the only previously recognized human pathogen. Relatively little is known about primary HHV-8 infection. In central Africa, a region in which KS was common before the HIV epidemic, HHV-8 infection appears to be a relatively common cause of the first febrile illness in infants and may be associated with respiratory symptoms in some cases. In these areas, an increasing incidence of HHV-8 infection occurs with age; prevalence of

Table 3 Clinical Characteristics of Conditions Associated with Human Herpesvirus 8 Infection

CONDITION	SETTING	CLINICAL CHARACTERISTICS
Classic KS	A rare condition seen among elderly men of Mediterranean or Ashkenazi Jewish descent; no known environmental etiologic precipitator	Often involves lower extremities, slowly progressive, primarily cutaneous, often not cause of death
Endemic KS	A relatively common cause of cancer (or a cancer-like condition) in children and adults residing in central Africa; no known environmental etiologic precipitator	Variable from mild (like classic) to locally aggressive disease
Iatrogenic KS	Seen in solid organ transplant recipients and other recipients of medication-induced immunologic suppression	Aggressive condition that often improves or resolves with withdrawal of immunosuppressive therapy and may recur with reinstitution
AIDS KS	AIDS-defining illness in HIV-infected patients, most often homosexual men (in developed countries); one of the most common HIV-associated malignancies, the incidence is falling	Often aggressive condition that progressively includes meta-static mucosal or cutaneous foci (often the mouth, face, and genitalia), and then may extend to lymphatic, pulmonary, and GI tract disease; often responds to potent anti-retroviral combination therapy
Multicentric Castleman's disease	HHV-8 DNA present in virtually all HIV-associated cases, approximately half of cases in HIV-uninfected persons	Associated with fever
Body cavity–based lymphoma	Most common in AIDS patients, most cases reported in men, but occurs in women; has been reported in recipients of solid organ transplants	Aggressive lymphoma not typically presents with ascites or pleural effusion

KS, Kaposi's sarcoma; *AIDS,* acquired immunodeficiency syndrome; *HIV,* human immunodeficiency virus; *GI,* gastrointestinal.

infection reaches 39% in early and 48% by late adolescence. In immunocompromised hosts, primary HHV-8 infection may be associated with transient development of KS and related conditions, or perhaps an increased risk of progressive KS. HHV-8 infection of peripheral blood mononuclear cells (PBMCs) appears to precede the onset of KS, at least in some patients.

Kaposi's Sarcoma, Multicentric Castleman's Disease, and Body Cavity–Based Lymphoma

Moritz Kaposi first described classic KS in 1872 as a rare skin tumor seen primarily in elderly men of Mediterranean or Ashkenazi Jewish origin. The clinical characteristics of conditions associated with HHV-8 infection are summarized in Table 3. Because several types of cells (many of which are inflammatory) are present in KS lesions, and not of a single clone or specific pattern of cytogenetic mutations as seen in most cancers, some researchers question whether KS is a true malignancy. The endemic, or African, form of KS was recognized in the early part of the twentieth century and is confined to equatorial areas where, until the AIDS era, it accounted for up to 10% of all malignancies. The iatrogenic form primarily occurs in solid organ transplant recipients and tends to be an aggressive illness with rapid dissemination, unless immunosuppressive therapies are discontinued. AIDS KS has a variable course, which can range from isolated skin lesions to more aggressive disease with rapid dissemination.

In a 1990 study, the risk of KS was at least 20,000 times greater among AIDS patients than the general population and 300 times greater among AIDS patients than other immunosuppressed groups. AIDS KS is most prevalent among men who have sex with men, regardless of intrave-

nous drug use. Overall, epidemiologic evidence supports the notion that AIDS KS is caused by a sexually transmissible agent. Early KS lesions appear as faint red-violet or brown macules that can be mistaken for more benign skin conditions. Lymphedema is common and can occur out of proportion to the extent of skin and lymphatic involvement, perhaps because of the release of inflammatory mediators.

HHV-8 DNA sequences have been identified in two other conditions that are associated with immunologic compromise. Multicentric Castleman's disease (MCD) is a rare condition characterized by angiofollicular hyperplasia associated with fever, adenopathy, and splenomegaly. It occurs most commonly, but not exclusively, in AIDS patients with KS. HHV-8 DNA sequences have been detected in mononuclear cells and lesional tissue from MCD patients.

Body cavity–based lymphomas (BCBLs) are true malignancies that have unique pathologic and clinical characteristics compared with other lymphomas: cases in men predominate, disease localizes to a body cavity, progression occurs rapidly, and morphology bridges large-cell immunoblastic and anaplastic types. HHV-8 DNA has been detected in BCBL in HIV-infected and uninfected persons but not in other lymphomas.

HHV-8 genes have been found to code for viral products that resemble cellular cytokines and other regulators of local immune response and tissue growth. These findings may provide insight into the mechanism by which the virus promotes development of KS, BCBLs, and MCD. Elevated blood levels of some of these viral inflammatory products are known to precede the onset of KS. HIV proteins may augment this inflammatory process, explaining the synergistic effect dual HIV/HHV-8 infection appears to have on the development of KS.

Detection of Infection

Standardized methods for detection of HHV-8 infections have not yet been established. Indirect IFAs and EIAs have been developed for the detection of antibodies to lytic and latent HHV-8 antigens. Antibody assays have ranged from 80% to 98% sensitivity in KS patients (when compared with PCR).

Epidemiology and Modes of Transmission

HHV-8 antibodies are highly prevalent among patients with KS and in homosexual men. The prevalence of serologic reactivity is also relatively high among in areas where KS was endemic before the AIDS epidemic. The prevalence of HHV-8 infections in various populations is summarized in Table 4. As is true of many herpes simplex virus infections and other sexually transmitted diseases (STDs), prevalence rates tend to increase with age and incidence peaks during years of greatest sexual activity.

If HHV-8 is sexually transmitted, it should be present in genital, oral, or gastrointestinal secretions. Most studies show that the detection of HHV-8 DNA in semen and genital tissues is limited to the high-risk populations of homosexual men, residents of central Africa, and persons with KS. HHV-8 DNA sequences have also been identified in saliva and oral tissues of patients with KS and in HIV-infected patients without KS. These studies indicate that HHV-8 is present in the oropharynx and could be transmitted via saliva contact in a manner analogous to Epstein-Barr virus. Curiously, HHV-8 has a far lower prevalence rate and later age of infection than is seen with HHV-6, HHV-7, and Epstein-Barr virus, infections in which saliva is more clearly a key vehicle for transmission.

Transmission via Allografts and Blood Products

KS is a relatively common cancer among solid organ transplant recipients and it is associated with HHV-8 infection. BCBL has also been reported in allograft recipients. HHV-8 can be transmitted via renal allografts, and screening of donated tissue has been recommended. Although KS can occur among patients who were infected with HHV-8 before receiving an allograft, it is unclear if the risk is greatest among persons who were HHV-8 infected or uninfected before transplantation. Because HHV-8 can be identified in blood from healthy donors, parenteral transmission of the pathogen is possible but does not appear to occur commonly.

Treatment

At present, treatment of HHV-8 infection itself is not recommended, even in HIV-infected persons and allograft recipients. Traditional treatment for KS, MCD, and BCBL includes reduction or elimination of any immunosuppressive treatment, chemotherapy, and/or radiation therapy. The clinical course of AIDS KS has improved greatly in the years since the introduction of protease inhibitor-containing antiretroviral regimens. Other antiviral agents have demonstrated efficacy in inhibiting HHV-8 itself. The recent finding from in vitro studies that ganciclovir, cidofovir, and foscarnet effectively inhibit HHV-8 DNA synthesis may lead to new treatment regimens that specifically target HHV-8. Parenteral administration of cidofovir, foscarnet, ganciclovir, and α-interferon have been reported to induce response or remission in patients with AIDS KS, often in conjunction with antiretroviral therapy and/or chemotherapy. Foscarnet has been used successfully to treat MCD. Foscarnet or ganciclovir may be effective in preventing KS among HIV-infected men, although this approach has been largely displaced by antiretroviral therapies. Dosage of the antiviral therapies is based on anticytomegalovirus therapy, specific dosing recommendations for HHV-8 are not available.

Table 4   Estimated Prevalence of Human Herpesvirus 8 Infection in Various Populations

POPULATION	% PREVALENCE
Homosexual men in industrialized countries	21-67*
Injection drug users in industrialized countries	5-50*
Heterosexual patients without HIV infection	<1-64*
U.S. women with HIV infection	4-15*

HIV, Human immunodeficiency virus.
*Prevalence rates depend on type of diagnostic test and are higher with lytic antigen and enzyme immunoassay types of tests.

Suggested Reading

Campadelli-Fiume G, Mirandola P, Menotti L: Human herpesvirus 6: an emerging pathogen, *Emerg Infect Dis* 5:353, 1999.

Dockrell DH, Smith TF, Paya CV: Human herpesvirus 6, *Mayo Clin Proc* 74:163, 1999.

Drago F, Rebora A: The new herpesviruses: emerging pathogens of dermatological interest, *Arch Dermatol* 135:71, 1999.

Greenblatt R: Kaposi's sarcoma and human herpesvirus-8, *Infect Dis Clin North Am* 12:63, 1998.

Kimberlin DW: Human herpesviruses 6 and 7: identification of newly recognized viral pathogens and their association with human disease, *Pediatr Infect Dis J* 17:59, 1998.

Lebbe C, et al: Clinical and biological impact of antiretroviral therapy with protease inhibitors on HIV-related Kaposi's sarcoma, *AIDS* 12:F45, 1998.

Levy J: Three new human herpesvirus (HHV6, 7, and 8), *Lancet* 349:558, 1997.

Oksenhendler E, et al: Transient angiolymphoid hyperplasia and Kaposi's sarcoma after primary infection with human herpesvirus 8 in a patient with human immunodeficiency virus infection, *N Engl J Med* 338:1585, 1998.

Regamey N, et al: Transmission of human herpesvirus 8 infection from renal-transplant donors to recipients, *N Engl J Med* 339:1358, 1998.

INFLUENZA

Neil Fishman
Harvey M. Friedman

Influenza is an important epidemic viral infection that has caused significant morbidity and mortality throughout history. The first worldwide pandemic was documented in 1580, and 31 pandemics have been described since then. The most severe occurred in 1918-1919, when 21 million deaths were recorded worldwide, including 549,000 in the United States. The last pandemic was in 1977, but milder epidemics continue to occur every 1 to 3 years. The Centers for Disease Control and Prevention (CDC) documented 10,000 to 40,000 excess deaths in the United States during each of the 19 epidemics from 1957 through 1986. The major causes of death are pneumonia and exacerbation of chronic cardiopulmonary conditions; of those who die, 80% to 90% are 65 years of age or older.

■ INFLUENZA VIRAL STRUCTURE AND PATHOPHYSIOLOGY

Influenza viruses are medium-size enveloped RNA viruses belonging to the family Orthomyxoviridae. Three genera, influenza virus types A, B, and C, have been described. Influenza A and B viruses are important causes of human disease, whereas influenza C virus causes only sporadic upper respiratory infections.

The morphologic characteristics of all influenza virus types are similar. The envelope is composed of a lipid bilayer, with a layer of matrix protein on the inner surface and spikelike surface projections of glycoproteins on the outer surface. These glycoproteins have either hemagglutinin or neuraminidase activity and are responsible for the attachment of the virus to human cells, for the release of virus from infected cells, and for the stimulation of the host immune response. Hemagglutinins initiate the infectious process by binding to surface receptors on respiratory epithelial cells; after proteolytic cleavage, the hemagglutinins fuse with the host cell membrane. The neuraminidase cleaves sialic acid that is present on the host cell surface and promotes release of viral particles from infected cells. Within the envelope are eight segmented pieces of nucleocapsid composed of a nucleoprotein and segmented single-stranded RNA.

■ EPIDEMIOLOGY

One of the most remarkable features of influenza virus is the frequency of changes in antigenicity. Antigenic variation is annual with influenza A virus but less common with influenza B virus. Therefore immunity to the influenza viruses is partial and temporary; this phenomenon explains why influenza remains a major epidemic disease of humans. Two types of antigenic variation have been described, principally involving the two external glycoproteins of the virus, hemagglutinin and neuraminidase. The more dramatic but less common alteration, antigenic shift, results from genetic reassortments. Shifts that produce immunologically novel strains of the influenza A virus herald the larger epidemics and worldwide pandemics; they tend to occur sporadically. Between World War I and the last pandemic in 1977, antigenic shifts occurred approximately every 10 to 15 years. The second and more common change, antigenic drift, is produced by a single point mutation in the hemagglutinin or neuraminidase genes that results in a change of just one or two amino acids. Antigenic shift is seen only with influenza A virus. Although antigenic drift affects both influenza A and B viruses, changes in the latter occur less frequently. Three subtypes of hemagglutinin, H1 (variants H0, H1, Hsw1), H2, and H3, and two subtypes of neuraminidase, N1 and N2, are recognized among influenza A viruses. Only a few strains of either virus tend to dominate during each annual influenza season.

Most human infections are acquired through human-to-human transmission of small-particle aerosols. Localized epidemics begin rather abruptly, usually in children, reach a sharp peak in 2 to 3 weeks, and last 5 to 6 weeks; attack rates during such outbreaks can approach 10% to 40%. Although influenza is virtually always active somewhere in the world, infection is most common during the winter. The peak influenza season extends from December through April in the Northern Hemisphere. Influenza season is defined by viral isolation, and an epidemic is defined by a rise in pneumonia and influenza deaths above the epidemic threshold in the CDC's 121-city mortality surveillance system. Although influenza affects all segments of the population, severe infections and major complications are most common in patients who are young, elderly, or debilitated.

In May 1997, a 3-year-old boy in Hong Kong contracted an acute, influenza-like illness and died 12 days later from complications consistent with Reye's syndrome. A virus was isolated from a tracheal aspirate and identified locally as influenza type A but did not react to antisera to recent isolates of human and swine subtypes. Further serologic and molecular characterization identified this as an H5N1 virus that was closely related to an isolate that was responsible for severe outbreaks of disease on three rural chicken farms in Hong Kong from late March to early May 1997. The death rate for the total of 6800 chickens on these farms exceeded 70%. This was the first documented isolation of an influenza A virus of this subtype from humans.

Although the case in May was considered an isolated incident with little or no person-to-person transmission, surveillance was increased. Seventeen new cases of human illness caused by the H5 virus were identified between November and late December 1997, five of which were fatal. Including the fatal index case in May, the case fatality rates were 18% in children and 57% in adults older than 17 years. An epidemiologic study found that all patients had been near live chickens in market places prior to the onset of illness, suggesting direct transmission from chickens rather than person-to-person spread. It is postulated that a nonpathogenic H5N1 influenza spread from migrating shorebirds to ducks by fecal contamination of water. The virus subsequently was transmitted to chickens, established infection in the live bird markets, and became highly pathogenic. On December 28, 1997, veterinary authorities began to slaughter all 1.6 million chickens present in wholesale facilities or vendors within Hong Kong, and importation from neighboring areas was stopped. No further human cases caused by avian influenza virus were detected until March 1999, when an H9N2 virus was isolated from two children. However, no additional cases have been reported at this time.

■ CLINICAL MANIFESTATIONS

Uncomplicated Influenza

Classic influenza is characterized by abrupt onset of symptoms after an incubation period of 1 to 2 days. Many patients can pinpoint the hour of onset. Systemic signs and symptoms predominate initially. They include fever, chills or rigors, headaches, myalgias, malaise, and anorexia. Myalgias and headache are the most troublesome symptoms, with severity related to the height of the febrile response. Severe pain of the intraocular muscles often can be elicited on lateral gaze. Myalgias in the calf muscles may be particularly prominent in children. The systemic symptoms usually persist for approximately 1 week. Respiratory symptoms such as dry cough and nasal discharge, also present at the onset of illness, begin to dominate the clinical presentation as fever resolves. Cough, the most common and troublesome of these later complaints, can take 2 weeks or more to resolve completely.

Complications of Influenza

The complications of influenza, which can be classified as pulmonary and nonpulmonary, result either from progression of the viral process itself or from secondary bacterial infections. Two manifestations of pneumonia associated with influenza, primary influenza viral pneumonia and secondary bacterial pneumonia, are well recognized (Table 1). Extrapulmonary complications of influenza occur less often and are most prevalent during larger, more severe outbreaks. These include myositis (more common with influenza B infection), myocarditis, pericarditis, transverse myelitis, encephalitis, and Guillain-Barré syndrome. A toxic shock–like syndrome has occurred in previously healthy children and adults during recent outbreaks of influenza A or B; this has been attributed to the effects of the viral infection on the colonization and replication characteristics of toxin-producing staphylococcus. Reye's syndrome has also been described in children treated with aspirin during influenza outbreaks.

■ DIAGNOSIS

Isolation of virus and detection of viral antigen in respiratory secretions offer the greatest utility for diagnosis in the setting of acute illness. Serologic tests such as hemagglutinin inhibition antibody titers that compare acute and convalescent sera are sensitive and specific but do not yield data in time to affect clinical decisions. In clinical practice, however, the diagnosis is usually established on epidemiologic grounds. A clinical presentation with fever, headache, myalgias, and cough is usually sufficient to diagnose influenza during a winter outbreak. Studies have documented the accuracy of clinical diagnosis during an influenza outbreak to be 60% to 85%.

Table 1 Pulmonary Complications of Influenza

FEATURE	PRIMARY VIRAL PNEUMONIA	SECONDARY BACTERIAL PNEUMONIA
Setting	Cardiovascular disease Pregnancy Young adults (in large outbreaks)	Age >65 years Chronic pulmonary, cardiac, or metabolic disease
History	Rapid progression after typical onset	Biphasic illness, with worsening after clinical improvement
Physical examination	Diffuse crackles	Consolidation
Sputum culture	Normal oral flora	*Streptococcus pneumoniae* *Staphylococcus aureus* *Haemophilus influenzae*
Isolation of influenza virus	Yes	No
Chest radiograph	Diffuse bilateral interstitial disease	Consolidation
Response to antibiotics	No	Yes
Mortality	Variable, high during some pandemics	Variable, generally low

■ THERAPY (TABLE 2)

Amantadine and rimantadine are approved in the United States for the treatment of influenza A. Amantadine has been shown to reduce the duration of signs and symptoms of clinical influenza by approximately 50% if therapy is instituted within 48 hours of onset. It also accelerates the resolution of small-airway dysfunction. However, amantadine causes several minor reversible central nervous system (CNS) toxicities, including insomnia, dizziness, nervousness, and difficulty concentrating. In addition, amantadine use is associated with an increased incidence of seizures in individuals with known seizure disorders. Rimantadine is structurally related to amantadine and appears to be of equal efficacy in the treatment of uncomplicated influenza. It may offer some advantages over amantadine in the management of elderly patients because CNS side effects occur less frequently (amantadine, 14%; rimantadine, 6%; placebo, 4%).

Table 2 Recommended Dosage for Amantadine and Rimantidine

ANTIVIRAL AGENT	1-9 YEARS	10-13 YEARS	14-64 YEARS	≥65 YEARS
Amantadine*				
Treatment†	5 mg/kg/day up to 150 mg in two divided doses	100 mg twice daily‡	100 mg twice daily	≤100 mg/day
Prophylaxis	5 mg/kg/day up to 150 mg in two divided doses	100 mg twice daily‡	100 mg twice daily	≤100 mg/day
Rimantadine§				
Treatmemt†	NA‖	NA‖	100 mg twice daily	100 or 200 mg/day¶
Prophylaxis	5 mg/kg/day up to 150 mg in two divided doses	100 mg twice daily‡	100 mg twice daily	100 or 200 mg/day¶

Adapted from recommendations of the Advisory Committee on Immunization Practices, Centers for Disease Control and Prevention, 1995.
*The drug package insert should be consulted for dosage recommendations for administering amantadine to persons with a creatinine clearance of 50 ml/min or less.
†Treatment should be instituted within 48 hours of the onset of symptoms and continued for 7 days.
‡Children 10 years of age or older who weigh under 40 kg should be administered amantadine or rimantadine 5 mg/kg/day.
§A reduction in dose to 100 mg/day of rimantadine is recommended for persons who have severe hepatic dysfunction or those with a creatinine clearance ≤10 ml/min. Other persons with less severe hepatic or renal dysfunction taking more than 100 mg/day of rimantadine should be observed closely, and the dosage should be reduced or the drug discontinued, if necessary.
‖NA, Not applicable (not approved for this indication).
¶Elderly nursing home residents should be administered only 100 mg/day of rimantadine. A reduction in dose to 100 mg/day should be considered for all persons 65 years of age or over if they have side effects when taking 200 mg/day.

There are several important pharmacokinetic differences between amantadine and rimantadine. Amantadine is excreted unchanged in the urine; therefore renal clearance is reduced substantially both in persons with renal insufficiency and in the elderly. In contrast, rimantadine undergoes extensive hepatic metabolism; less than 15% of the drug is excreted unchanged in the urine. Both drugs require adjustment of dosage in the setting of renal insufficiency, but rimantadine may be a safer choice in this setting. On the other hand, the clearance of rimantadine is decreased by 50% in patients with hepatic dysfunction; therefore amantadine may be a better agent for patients with underlying liver disease. Finally, rimantadine is more expensive than amantadine, with the average wholesale prices being $0.17 per 100 mg and $1.90 per 100 mg, respectively. Dosing guidelines are listed in Table 2. Amantadine and rimantadine are active only against influenza A; therefore because influenza A and B often cocirculate, treatment may not be effective in any given season. Resistance to both drugs emerges rapidly and has been described in influenza A isolates from treated patients. The isolation of resistant virus is not associated with a change in severity or duration of illness, but it does temper the enthusiasm of many clinicians for treating influenza with either drug.

Two new drugs, zanamivir (Relenza) and oseltamivir (Tamiflu), are available for treatment of influenza infection. Both drugs belong to a new class of antiviral compounds called neuraminidase inhibitors. Neuraminidase is a viral enzyme that cleaves sialic acid residues promoting the release of influenza virus from infected cells. The antiviral drugs inhibit neuraminidase activity and alter virus release. Zanamivir has poor oral bioavailability and is formulated as a dry powder for oral inhalation using a disk inhaler. Zanamivir at a dosage of 10 mg twice daily for 5 days given within 48 hours of onset of symptoms reduced the duration of influenza symptoms by 1 day. When given within 30 hours of onset of symptoms, zanamivir reduced the duration of illness by 3 days. Oseltamivir is the ethyl ester prodrug of the active compound and is well absorbed orally. When started within 40 hours of onset of symptoms, oseltamivir at a dosage of 75 mg twice daily reduced duration of symptoms by 1.3 days. In vitro, the drugs are active against both influenza A and B strains. In vivo, the drugs appear to be active against both strains, although the number of influenza B infections treated to date is small. Adverse effects are uncommon with both drugs. Resistance can develop while the patient is receiving therapy, although this is also uncommon. Treatment may reduce respiratory complications requiring use of antibiotics, although information remains limited on this issue.

■ PREVENTION

Vaccine

Inactivated virus vaccines are the mainstay of the prevention of influenza. Efficacy has ranged between 67% and 92%. Because influenza viruses undergo frequent antigenic alterations, a new vaccine containing antigens expected to predominate in the winter epidemic is prepared each year. In general, vaccines have contained both an A and a B virus. Two subtypes of influenza A have circulated in recent years; both have been included in the vaccine because the predominant strain cannot be predicted reliably. Influenza vaccination has been shown to reduce hospital admissions for influenza and pneumonia by 32% to 39%, and to decrease mortality from these conditions by 43% to 65%. Recommendations for the use of influenza vaccine are listed in Table 3. The only contraindication to vaccination is hypersensitivity to hens' eggs, in which the vaccine virus is grown. Adults with acute febrile illnesses usually should not be vaccinated until their symptoms have abated. However,

Table 3 Recommended Recipients of Influenza Vaccine
GROUPS AT INCREASED RISK FOR INFLUENZA-RELATED COMPLICATIONS
Persons ≥65 years of age
Residents of nursing homes and other chronic-care facilities that house persons of any age with chronic medical conditions
Adults and children with chronic disorders of the pulmonary or cardiovascular systems, including asthma
Adults and children who have required regular medical follow-up or hospitalization during the preceding year because of chronic metabolic diseases, including diabetes mellitus, renal dysfunction, hemoglobinopathies, or immunosuppression
Children 6 months to 18 years of age who are receiving long-term aspirin therapy and therefore might be at risk for developing Reye's syndrome after influenza
GROUPS THAT CAN TRANSMIT INFLUENZA TO PERSONS AT HIGH RISK
Physicians, nurses, and other personnel in both hospital and outpatient settings
Employees of nursing homes and chronic care facilities who have contact with patients or residents
Providers of home care to persons at high risk (e.g., visiting nurses and volunteer workers)
Household members (including children) of persons in high-risk groups
Anyone who wishes to avoid influenza

Adapted from recommendations of the Advisory Committee on Immunization Practices, Centers for Disease Control and Prevention, 1995.

minor illnesses with or without fever are not a contraindication. The optimal time for organized vaccination campaigns for persons in high-risk groups is usually mid-October through mid-November.

The vaccine should not be administered simultaneously with cytotoxic chemotherapy; the efficacy drops by 50% in this setting.

Influenza vaccine has produced protective antibody titers in vaccinated human immunodeficiency virus (HIV)-infected persons with high CD4+ T-lymphocyte cell counts, but there has not been a consistent antibody response in individuals with advanced HIV disease (HIV-1 RNA levels >100,000 copies/ml) and low CD4 counts (<200/ml). A second dose of vaccine does not improve the immune response in this latter group. Increases in plasma HIV-1 RNA levels after influenza vaccination appear to be transient and return to steady-state levels in 2 to 4 weeks; this is most likely to occur in those who develop an immune response to the vaccine. Deterioration of CD4 cell counts and progression of clinical HIV disease have not been reported in vaccinated persons. Because influenza can result in serious illness and complications and because influenza vaccination may result in the production of protective antibody titers, the Advisory Committee for Immunization Practices of the CDC concluded that vaccination will benefit many HIV-infected patients. However, some authorities recommend

that patients be on effective antiretroviral regimens with evidence of control of viral replication at the time of vaccination.

Influenza-associated excess mortality among pregnant women has not been documented except during the pandemics of 1918-1919 and 1957-1958. However, additional case reports and limited studies suggest that women in the third trimester of pregnancy and early puerperium, including women without underlying risk factors, may be at increased risk for serious complications from influenza. Therefore, because the influenza vaccine has been proved safe at any stage of pregnancy, vaccination is recommended for women who would be in the third trimester of pregnancy or early puerperium during the influenza season and for those who are otherwise at increased risk for influenza.

Chemoprophylaxis

Amantadine and rimantadine are approved for use as prophylactic agents against influenza. Their level of efficacy is about 50% to 80%, and protection may be additive to that of the vaccine. These drugs should be considered for prophylaxis for selected individuals for 5 to 7 weeks during an outbreak of influenza A virus but not influenza B, particularly for high-risk individuals who have not been vaccinated. In such situations either drug may be administered for just 2 weeks if vaccine is given simultaneously. Chemoprophylaxis may also be used to supplement protection offered by the vaccine in patients who may be expected to have a poor antibody response (see Table 2).

Zanamivir and oseltamivir are effective in preventing influenza infections. When given to healthy adult volunteers, zanamivir at a dosage of 10 mg/day was 67% effective in preventing laboratory confirmed cases of influenza A or B infections over a 4-week period. Over a 6-week period, oseltamivir at 75 mg/day was noted to reduce laboratory documented cases by 74%. These compounds has not been compared with each other or with amantadine and rimantadine for efficacy in prevention of influenza; however, potential advantages of the new compounds is that resistance appears less likely to develop and the drugs are active against influenza A and B strains. As of late 1999, these drugs had not been approved by the Food and Drug Administration (FDA) for prevention of influenza, although they were approved for treatment.

Suggested Reading

Betts, RF: Influenza virus. In Mandell GL, Bennett JE, Dolin R, eds: *Mandell, Douglas and Bennett's principles and practices of infectious diseases,* ed 4, New York, 1995, Churchill Livingstone.

Cox NJ, Hughes JM: New options for the prevention of influenza, *N Engl J Med* 341:1387, 1999.

Dolin R, et al: A controlled trial of amantadine and rimantadine in the prophylaxis of influenza A infection, *N Engl J Med* 307:580, 1982.

Douglas RG: Drug therapy: prophylaxis and treatment of influenza, *N Engl J Med* 322:443, 1990.

Recommendations and Reports: Prevention and control of influenza: recommendations of the advisory committee on immunization practices, *MMWR* 48(RR-4), 1999.

ACUTE AND CHRONIC PARVOVIRUS INFECTION

Neal S. Young

B19 parvovirus is the only member of the Parvoviridae family known to cause diseases in humans. Parvoviruses are small viruses with unenveloped icosahedral capsids that contain a single-stranded DNA genome. These physical properties contribute to viral resistance to heat, solvents, and extreme chemical conditions. Because of their limited genome, parvoviral propagation depends on infection of mitotically active cells. In the taxonomy of the parvovirus family, B19 and closely related simian parvoviruses constitute the *Erythrovirus* genus, separated from autonomous animal parvoviruses, dependoviruses, (which require coinfection with a second virus for propagation in cell culture) and insect parvoviruses called densoviruses.

B19 parvovirus has extreme tropism for human erythroid progenitor cells, which are responsible for the generation of circulating erythrocytes. In tissue culture, B19 has been propagated only in bone marrow, fetal liver, peripheral blood, and rather inefficiently in a few leukemic cell lines of megakaryocytoblastoid character. B19 replication in patients has been detected only in blood and marrow. Specificity for erythroid cells follows from the cellular receptor for the virus, globoside or P antigen, a tetrohexoseceramide present on erythroid cells, megakaryocytes, endothelial cells, and some placental cell types, as well as fetal liver and heart. Parvovirus infection is terminated by host production of neutralizing antibodies. Failure to produce neutralizing antibodies can result in persistent infection. Little is known of the cellular immune response.

■ B19 DISEASES

Serologic studies have shown that about half of the adult population have antibodies to B19 parvovirus; although most infection occurs during childhood, the seropositivity rate continues to rise with age. Probably the majority of infections are asymptomatic. Reliable diagnostic assays only recently have become widely available, and the full spectrum of B19 parvovirus infection has not been defined. The presence of immunoglobulin G (IgG) to virus only signifies past infection. IgM or virus DNA detected by direct hybridization testing indicates recent infection. The interpretation of a positive DNA study obtained by gene amplification (polymerase chain reaction) study is more problematic, as individuals may not clear small amounts of virus for many months after an acute infection.

Fifth Disease

This common childhood exanthem is caused by acute parvovirus infection. The slapped-cheek rash and the evanes-

cent maculopapular eruption over the trunk and proximal extremities are typical. Children may be febrile but usually have few symptoms. Meningitis and encephalitis have been reported as very rare complications. The blood of children with fifth disease contains IgM antibody to B19 but little if any virus; because the syndrome is due to immune complex formation between virus and antibodies, affected individuals are not considered infectious. Reassurance and antipyretics as needed are sufficient for this self-limited illness.

In adults, acute parvovirus infection may be more serious. Adults have more rheumatic complaints than children, and there may be frank joint inflammation or a pattern of distribution and chronicity mimicking rheumatoid arthritis; occasionally rheumatoid factor will be present. However, in most cases, symptoms resolve within a few days or weeks, and parvovirus is not a cause of rheumatoid arthritis. The basis of chronic joint complaints in some patients is not understood, but symptoms can be addressed with conventional antiinflammatory drug therapy.

Transient Aplastic Crisis and Other Hematologic Syndromes

Transient aplastic crisis is caused by parvovirus infection in patients with hemolytic anemia, compensated hemolysis (as in many cases of hereditary spherocytosis), or increased demand for red cell production (iron deficiency, acute hemorrhage). B19 probably briefly interrupts erythropoiesis in most persons infected, but without consequence because of the long survival of circulating red blood cells. Transient aplastic crisis is manifested by anemia, reticulocytopenia, and red cell aplasia in the marrow. There may be moderate thrombocytopenia and neutropenia in addition to the severe anemia, especially in patients with functioning spleens. The syndrome may be accompanied by marrow necrosis and may be fatal, especially in young children. As the anemia is self-limited, transfusion is adequate therapy. Specific antibody production terminates the episode and prevents recurrence.

Hemophagocytic syndrome, defined as acute pancytopenia with a characteristic marrow morphology showing reticuloendothelial cells ingesting hematopoietic cells, especially erythrocytes, typically follows herpesvirus infections, but well-characterized cases have been reported after B19 parvovirus as well. However, B19 parvovirus is not a common cause of classic aplastic anemia.

Hydrops Fetalis and Congenital Infection

Parvovirus infection of the pregnant woman may be transmitted to the fetus. Midtrimester events have been best characterized; first trimester infection may result in abortion, and third trimester infection has not been associated with adverse outcomes. Infection of the fetus is predominantly in the liver, the site of red cell production; the heart may also be affected (fetal myocardial cells express P antigen). Untreated, the infant develops severe anemia and heart failure leading to the massive edema of hydrops and death at birth or shortly afterward. In utero blood transfusions have apparently been successful in a few instances; however, fetal infection need not result in mortality or morbidity. As ultrasound diagnosis may not be definitive, a conservative recommendation is to document progressive hydrops on serial testing before intervention.

Congenital parvovirus infection after transfusion treatment of hydrops can produce chronic anemia from birth. Only a few infants have been described: in all, virus was localized to the marrow and did not circulate, and gene amplification was required to detect the low levels of B19 DNA. The pathology of the marrow was erythroid hypoplasia (Diamond-Blackfan anemia) or erythroid dysplasia resembling congenital dyserythropoietic states. There may be associated immunodeficiency; one infant died of overwhelming bacterial infection from a catheter source. Transfusions can maintain the hemoglobin, but immunoglobulin therapy has not been effective.

Persistent Infection

In the absence of an appropriate immune response, B19 infection can become chronic. Persistent infection has been observed in congenital immunodeficiency (Nezelof syndrome), acquired immunodeficiency syndrome (AIDS) secondary to human immunodeficiency virus (HIV) 1 infection, and during therapy with cytotoxic or immunosuppressive drugs. The deficit in the immune response may be subtle; B19 infection may be the only evidence of a congenital syndrome and the first sign of AIDS. Clinically, the patients have typical pure red cell aplasia with severe anemia, absent reticulocytes in the blood, and a paucity of red cell precursors in the marrow. Scattered giant pronormoblasts, the mark of B19 infection, may signal the diagnosis, which is established by DNA hybridization studies of serum.

Persistent infection results from inability to mount an effective humoral immune response, measured either as neutralizing antibodies in functional tissue culture experiments or by immunoblot binding of viral capsid proteins. Most AIDS patients lack any antibodies to B19; some congenital cases may have circulating IgM to B19 suggestive of a class-switch abnormality. Fortunately, commercial immunoglobulin preparations are a good source of effective antibodies to parvovirus. Administration of IgG IV 0.4 g/kg/day for 5 to 10 days terminates infection (Figure 1). The reticulocyte count dramatically increases after the first week, the marrow shows healthy normoblastic erythroid proliferation, and the hemoglobin rises to a level appropriate for the patient. Treatment can be curative, and the virus may no longer be detectable in some patients who have congenital immunodeficiency or whose immunosuppressive therapy is discontinued. In contrast, AIDS patients have intense chronic parvoviremia, and IgG treatment appears to reduce but not eliminate the virus (Figure 2). Although relapse after some months is common, recurrent anemia responds to a second course of IgG. Monthly maintenance injections of IgG have been used in a few patients.

■ OTHER POSSIBLE ASSOCIATIONS

B19 parvovirus' association with other clinical syndromes is less secure. Apparent links to childhood neutropenia, idiopathic thrombocytopenic purpura, vasculitis, and juvenile rheumatoid arthritis have not been reproducible. A major technical problem has been the use of gene amplification methods, which not only are susceptible to false positive

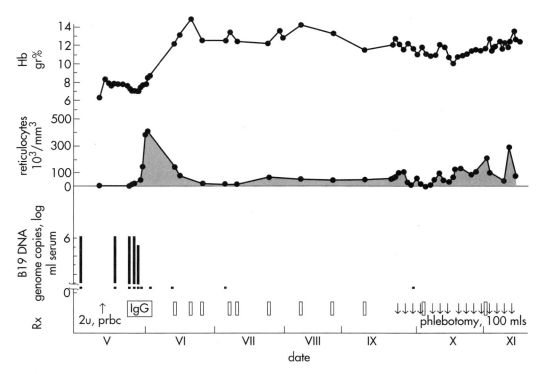

Figure 1

Clinical course of a patient with congenital immunodeficiency syndrome and persistent parvovirus infection treated with commercial immunoglobulin. The patient is apparently cured of the viral infection and pure red cell aplasia.

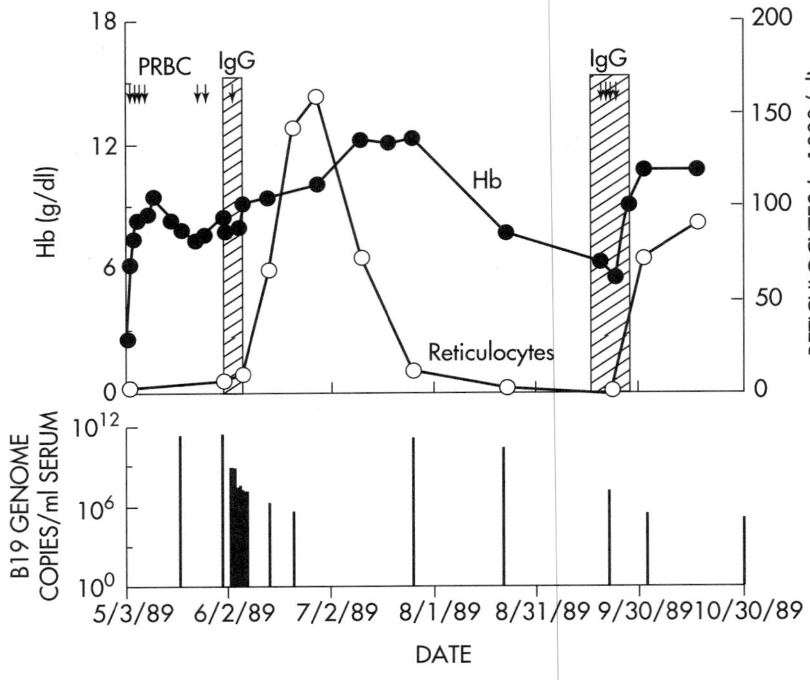

Figure 2
IgG treatment of B19 persistence in AIDS, illustrating recurrence predicted by molecular studies and the effectiveness of repeated treatment.

results but also are positive in a high proportion of normal individuals: viral DNA has been found in almost half of knee joints biopsied for trauma and in 20% of normal bone marrows using this sensitive method. Polymerase chain reaction–derived data that are reported without other clinical or serologic evidence of recent infection should be especially suspect. Nevertheless, B19 parvovirus may be linked to some types of hepatitis. In addition, paroxysmal cold hemoglobinuria, a severe childhood hemolytic anemia that usually follows on a viral illness, is a good candidate as a B19 parvovirus syndrome because of the presence of the pathogenic Donath-Landsteiner antibody, directed against erythrocyte P antigen, the virus' cellular receptor. Fetal and childhood myocarditis might also follow parvovirus infection, because the P antigen receptor is present on maturing heart cells.

■ VACCINE DEVELOPMENT

Effective vaccines to prevent parvovirus infection in animals have been produced by tissue culture modification of virus. For B19, which resists conventional cell culture, recombi-

nant empty capsids have been produced in a baculovirus system by expression of a portion of the parvovirus genome; they contain no viral DNA. Capsids enriched for the highly immunogenic VP1 protein elicit strong neutralizing antibody responses in test animals. Recombinant capsids are now in phase I toxicity trials in normal volunteers.

Suggested Reading

Frickhofen N, et al: Persistent parvovirus infection in patients infected with human immunodeficiency virus type 1 (HIV-1): a treatable cause of anemia in AIDS, *Ann Intern Med* 113:926, 1990.

Kurtzman G, et al: The immune response to B19 parvovirus infection and an antibody defect in persistent viral infection, *J Clin Invest* 84:1114, 1989.

Kurtzman JG, et al: Pure red cell aplasia of 10 years' duration due to B19 parvovirus infection and its cure with immunoglobulin infusion, et al: 321:519, 1989.

Serjeant GR, et al: Human parvovirus infection in homozygous sickle cell disease, *Lancet* 341:1237, 1993.

Sokal EM, et al: Acute parvovirus B19 infection associated with fulminant hepatitis of favourable prognosis in young children, *Lancet* 352:1739, 1998.

Young NS: Parvoviruses. In Fields BM, Knipe DM, eds: *Virology*, ed 3, New York, 1995, Raven Press.

PAPILLOMAVIRUS

Lawrence J. Eron

Human papillomaviruses (HPV) cause squamous epithelial tumors in the genital area and elsewhere on the body. Genital HPV infection, a sexually transmitted disease, is highly prevalent, infecting as many as 20% or more of the sexually active adult population, resulting in 1 million new cases each year in the United States. Approximately 75% of the sexual partners of persons with genital HPV infection also show evidence of infection, and given the extraordinarily high prevalence, it is no longer thought to be useful to routinely screen partners for infection.

There are more than 60 different DNA types of HPV, which are distinguished on the basis of hybridization. The genital HPV types fall into two groups, which produce two basically different diseases. In people infected with HPV types 6 and 11, exophytic condylomata (genital warts), having a cauliflowerlike appearance, develop on the external genitalia. This may be associated with low-grade dysplasia of the vulva, vagina, and cervix, termed *squamous intraepithelial lesions* (SIL) grade I. However, most infections are clinically inapparent (Figure 1). HPV types 16, 18, and 31 produce disease that is often subclinical (so-called flat warts) that can become more obvious when acetic acid is applied to the surface of the skin. These infections may result in moderately (SIL grade II) or highly (SIL grade III) dysplastic lesions evolving in many cases to carcinomas.

HPV may also infect the perianal region and the distal rectum above the dentate line. In human immunodeficiency virus (HIV)-infected individuals, small, innocent-appearing ulcers may be observed. A biopsy must be performed on these to evaluate for the development of squamous cell carcinomas of the rectum. HIV infection also increases the likelihood that dysplastic lesions of the cervix may become invasive carcinomas. Conversely, recurrent or refractory genital warts may be markers for concomitant infection by HIV, and it is important to test for HIV in patients with HPV infection, as with any other sexually transmitted disease.

■ CYTOTOXIC THERAPY

When HPV causes external genital warts, it may be viewed as only a minor cosmetic problem, but it is at the very least a public health problem. When HPV infects the cervix, it may be a premalignant condition ultimately evolving into carcinoma of the cervix. Treatments may be able to extirpate clinically evident disease without eliminating the underlying HPV infection. Moreover, eliminating a wart or dysplastic tissue may or may not decrease infectivity because the virus can be shed asymptomatically from apparently normal tissue adjacent to the treated area.

Further complicating the issue of treatment is the fact that most studies report a natural regression rate of about 20% for untreated or placebo-treated warts. On the other hand, pregnancy, diabetes, HIV, organ transplantation, and other immunosuppression may lead to more persistent disease with larger numbers of warts that resist any and all therapeutic interventions.

Over the last few years, new guidelines governing treatment of HPV infection have emerged. They suggest (1) clinicians should become familiar with and prescribe one patient-applied treatment (e.g., podophyllotoxin or imiquimod), and one provider-applied treatment (e.g., trichloroaectic acid [TCA] or cryotherapy) (Table 1); (2) the cure must not be worse than the disease; and (3) subclinical disease in the absence of dysplasia should not be treated.

Therapeutic methods may be categorized as cytotoxic, cytodestructive, or immune. Topical cytotoxic therapies are the most popular for external condylomata involving the penis, scrotum, and labia. Podophyllotoxin (Condylox), the active ingredient in podophyllin (which is no longer produced), is one of two therapies licensed for self-application by patients. It is applied to external warts twice daily for 3 days per week and may be repeated weekly for up to 5 weeks. It may cause local irritation and discomfort. Efficacy rates of 60% are achievable (Table 2). Recurrence rates are generally in excess of 33%.

A topical formulation of TCA or bichloroacetic acid (BCA) 50% to 85%, applied twice daily 3 days per week, can be used on pregnant women, unlike podophyllotoxin. When applied to external warts or vaginal warts, it produces a white slough that peels away in a few days and can be reapplied weekly. The efficacy rate is comparable to that of podophyllotoxin. As with podophyllotoxin, it is not as effective on highly keratinized squamous epithelium (the penile shaft, scrotum, and labia majora) as on wet areas (the prepuce of the penis and the labia minora).

In addition to external and vaginal warts, 5-fluorouracil (Effudex) can be applied to cervical areas, although it is not licensed for this indication. Although it is effective, it can also be intensely irritating when applied more often than once or twice weekly. It has been used as a cytotoxic adjuvant to laser therapy of the vagina and cervix, as well as for urethral warts. As with all cytotoxic therapies, significant relapse rates of 25% have been reported. 5-Fluorouracil with the vasoconstrictor epinephrine in a collagen gel implant, has been used via intralesional injection. Although intuitively this form of treatment would allow more focusing of therapy, modest clearance rates of 65%, with recurrence rates of 30% to 45%, are similar to what has been reported with the regular Effudex formulation.

Cidofovir, an acyclic nucleoside analog with broad-spectrum antiviral activity against DNA viruses, has been used in a topical formulation to treat external genital warts. Clearance rates up to 33% have been reported.

■ CYTODESTRUCTIVE THERAPY

Various procedures for the physical ablation of HPV-infected areas have been used. The most common approaches are surgical excision or cryotherapy applied to the

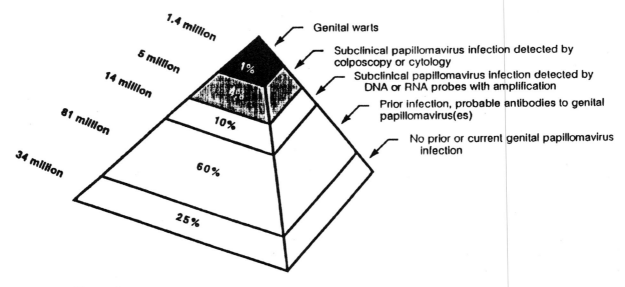

Figure 1
Estimated prevalence of genital human papillomavirus infection among men and women 15 to 49 years of age in the United States in 1994. (*Reprinted from Koutsky L:* Am J Med *102:3, 1997.*)

Table 1 Therapy of Choice for Genital Warts

LESIONS	CERVIX	URETHRAL	ALL OTHER SITES
Few, small	Cryotherapy Electro-cautery	5-FU	TCA Podophyllo-toxin Cryotherapy
Extensive	Laser	Laser	Cytodestruc-tive thera-pies
Recalcitrant or recurrent	Laser and interferon	Laser and inferferon	Interferon and cytodestruc-tive thera-pies

5-FU, 5-Fluorouracil; *TCA*, trichloroacetic acid.

Table 2 Clearance and Recurrence Rates in the Therapy of Genital Warts

TREATMENT	CLEARANCE RATE (%)	RECURRENCE RATE (%)
Podophyllin	40	50
Podophyllotoxin	60	33
Trichloroacetic acid	70	25
5-FU		
Urethra	90	10
Elsewhere	60	25
Cidofovir	33	—
Cryotherapy	80	25
Electrocoagulation	90	25
Laser	>90	10
Interferon	70	25
Imiquimod	56	15

5-FU, 5-Fluorouracil.

involved area by a nitrous oxide probe or by liquid nitrogen via two 1-minute freeze-thaw cycles. The latter method is the least painful cytodestructive therapy and does not require local anesthesia. It is more efficacious than the chemical therapies, generally achieving cure rates in the 80% range when used weekly for 3 to 6 weeks. As with chemical therapies, recurrences occur about 25% of the time.

Electrocoagulation of genital warts and loop electrical excisional procedure (LEEP) of dysplastic tissue of the cervix are somewhat more effective (80%) than cryotherapy but require local injection of lidocaine for anesthesia. Scarring may also result, and the use of an exhaust containment apparatus is recommended to capture the smoke plume, which may contain infectious HPV DNA. Disease recurs up to 25% of the time.

Laser ablation is the treatment of choice for cervical lesions. It offers precise control of depth of tissue destruction, unlike electrocoagulation and cryotherapy. However, as with electrocoagulation, it requires local or sometimes general anesthesia and is more expensive than any other treatment. Here, too, the smoke plume must be contained. Efficacy rates of 90% have been reported.

■ IMMUNE THERAPIES

Although exophytic warts or subclinical disease may be eradicated after treatment, adjacent normal tissue may still harbor silent infection by HPV. This reservoir probably is responsible for recurrences and possibly for asymptomatic transmission of HPV after treatment.

Immunotherapies offer the possibility of decreasing recurrence rates by enhancing host response, specifically cell-mediated immunity. By increasing helper CD4 and cytotoxic CD8 lymphocyte activity, they may be useful in patients whose disease fails to respond to cytotoxic and cytodestructive measures.

Because of their antiviral and immune-stimulating properties, in addition to their antiproliferative effects, interferons have been proposed to eradicate the viral reservoir. Interferon is effective when administered intralesionally, either 1 million units per wart, three times weekly (recombinant interferon-α2b, Intron-A, or α2a, Roferon) or when administered twice weekly (natural interferon-α, Alferon). Interferon-β (fibroblast interferon) has also been shown to be effective, but trials of immune interferon-γ have not shown consistent efficacy. All interferons have influenza-like side effects (myalgias, fever, and malaise), but these can be ameliorated by limiting doses to 5 million units per visit, by concomitant administration of acetaminophen, and by treatment late in the day so that the side effects, which appear 6 hours later, occur at bedtime.

Local subcutaneous injection of interferon in the anterior thigh (regional administration) has been proposed to have a greater effect than an intramuscular injection into the deltoid muscle (systemic administration). However, in both cases, effects on genital HPV have been minimal at best, in distinct contrast to effects on hepatitis B and C viruses when interferon is administered systemically.

Imiquimod 5% cream (Aldara) is a potent inducer of interferon and other cytokines. When topically applied thrice weekly for 8 weeks, clearance rates of 56% are achievable in women but not in men, in whom clearance rates are much lower. Recurrences occur in 13% to 19% of cases. The main advantage of imiquimod is that it is one of two patient-applied therapies, the other being podophyllotoxin.

Interferon therapy may best be reserved for refractory or recurrent warts. It may become a standard adjuvant to cytodestructive therapies to decrease the likelihood of relapse. As it has been shown to decrease the latent viral burden in tissue adjacent to clinically evident lesions that are treated, it may have a role in the control of transmission of HPV.

■ HPV VACCINES

HPV infection is potentially amenable to vaccination. Although there are many different genital HPV types, the viral genome is highly conserved. Moreover, HPV uses cellular enzymes to replicate and thus is not prone to mutation, in contrast to HIV, for example. Indeed, animal models suggest that both therapeutic and prophylactic applications for vaccine use are possible in humans.

The HPV genome consists of just eight genes, two of which are for coat proteins (L1 and L2). Neutralizing antibodies in animal models (canine HPV) seem to be sufficient to protect against viral challenge. Although it may be difficult to achieve high-titer neutralizing antibodies at mucosal surfaces, cytotoxic CD8 lymphocytes may eliminate nascently HPV-infected cells undergoing productive infection. Trials using a vaccine prepared from an HPV type 6 fusion protein between the products of the E7 and L2 gene are under way to determine whether genital warts can be made to regress more effectively with fewer recurrences than occur with cytotoxic and cytodestructive therapies.

Therapeutic vaccines have also been investigated in animal models with respect to cancer therapy, using HPV oncogene products E6 and E7. These vaccines can protect animals from challenge with tumors expressing E6 and E7 by serving as tumor-rejecting antigens using MHC-restricted cytotoxic CD8 lymphocyte responses. A recombinant vaccinia virus expressing E6 and E7 antigens from HPV 16 and 18 has been shown to be safe and immunogenic in humans. Thus the possibility of vaccinating women with preinvasive but high-grade SILs (or with low grade SILs or asymptomatic infection to potentially decrease infectivity by decreasing viral burden) may be more effective than in patients with cervical cancers, where a downregulation of MHC molecules may induce an immune tolerant state, precluding a robust immune response.

Suggested Reading

Beutner KR, et al: Genital warts and their treatment, *Clin Infect Dis* 28(suppl 1):S37, 1999.

Eron LJ: Human papillomaviruses and anogenital disease. In Gorbach SL, Bartlett JG, Blacklow NR, eds: *Infectious diseases*, Philadelphia, 1999, Saunders.

Galloway DA: Is vaccination against human papillomavirus a possibility? *Lancet* 351:22, 1998.

Krause SJ, Stone KM: Management of genital infection by HPV, *Rev Infect Dis* 12:S620, 1990.

DENGUE AND RELATED SYNDROMES

Niranjan Kanesa-thasan
Charles H. Hoke, Jr.

■ DENGUE

Dengue virus, a mosquito-transmitted flavivirus, is the most common arbovirus infection of man. Any of four dengue virus serotypes (1, 2, 3, and 4) may cause illness. Infection confers long-lasting protection against reinfection with the same serotype but not against other serotypes. Hence, repeated dengue virus infections are possible if an individual is exposed to several serotypes. Infection with dengue virus may result in dengue fever or the more severe forms of disease known as dengue hemorrhagic fever (DHF) and dengue shock syndrome (DSS).

Classical dengue, or breakbone fever, is typically a self-limited, nonfatal acute viral illness in adults. An incubation period of 3 to 8 days precedes the sudden onset of fever to 39° to 41° C (100.4° to 102.2° F), frontal headache, muscle ache, and retroorbital pain. Prominent malaise and arthralgias may be accompanied by altered taste perception, nausea, and vomiting. Minor hemorrhagic manifestations such as petechiae are common, but occasionally significant bleeding results from gastrointestinal ulcers. There is a characteristic transient depression of circulating neutrophil, lymphocyte, and platelet counts. Generally dengue fever resolves uneventfully, with defervescence in 7 days or less.

Occasionally, persons infected with dengue virus develop DHF at or near the time of defervescence, when systemic capillary leakage results in hemoconcentration (more than 20% rise in hematocrit) and thrombocytopenia (100,000/mm³). Manifestations of DHF include a positive tourniquet test, ascites, pleural effusion, and spontaneous bleeding. Coagulopathies are present in most affected individuals. DHF may rapidly progress to DSS, with rapid or feeble pulse, narrow pulse pressure (<20 mm Hg), hypotension, and clammy extremities. DSS typically occurs on day 4 or 5 of illness. The World Health Organization's clinical grading scheme for DHF based on severity may be helpful in classification and management of patients (Table 1). In this scheme, DSS is classified as grade III or IV DHF.

The risk of DHF is highest in individuals who were previously infected with another dengue serotype. DHF most often affects children in endemic areas, where several serotypes may cocirculate. However, adults may be at risk for DHF if a dengue serotype is introduced to the area after another serotype was widespread.

Diagnosis

Diagnosis is confirmed by isolation of virus and/or demonstration of dengue-specific IgM antibody in the serum. A fourfold rise in dengue hemagglutination-inhibiting antibody titer also provides evidence of infection. Serologic tests may be complicated by cross-reactive antibodies to another flavivirus, such as Japanese encephalitis virus or yellow fever virus. Virus is best isolated from serum collected from febrile patients, and dengue-specific antibody is detected in specimens obtained after defervescence. Hence, specimens should be acquired when possible during the febrile period and again after defervescence. Sera for virus isolation should be stored at −70° C (−94° F) and shipped on dry ice to a state health or Centers for Disease Control and Prevention laboratory; if such handling is not possible, storage and shipment at 4° C (39.2° F) is preferable to other procedures. Reverse transcriptase polymerase chain reaction has been used to detect circulating viral genome but has not been adapted for routine clinical use.

Clinicians should suspect dengue fever in travelers with acute febrile syndromes within 2 weeks of return from tropical countries. Malaria is clinically indistinguishable from dengue and should be ruled out, as it may be fatal without treatment. Other causes of acute fever and exanthem, such as measles, rubella, typhoid, and meningococcal disease, should be considered in the differential diagnosis. The hemorrhagic fever viruses (e.g., Ebola and Junin) and other exotic viruses with similar initial clinical presentations must be kept in mind if a patient with suspected DHF has a history of travel to a tropical or remote location (see the chapter *Viral Hemorrhagic Fevers*).

Therapy

Management of suspected dengue is complicated because diagnostic confirmation of infection is usually not available at the time of treatment. Furthermore, it is impossible to identify individuals at risk for severe dengue at the time of presentation. Treatment of uncomplicated dengue fever is supportive. Relief of symptoms may be achieved with nonsteroidal antiinflammatory agents; aspirin is best avoided because of the risks of bleeding and of Reye syndrome. All individuals suspected of having dengue should be monitored daily for sudden onset of restlessness, confusion, or lethargy. Examination should focus particularly on evaluation for pulse or blood pressure (BP) changes, cool extremities, thrombocytopenia, or elevated hematocrit. Hospital admission is required for individuals who demonstrate shock, evidence of bleeding, hemoconcentration, narrowed pulse pressure or hypotension, oliguria, significant prostration, or clinical deterioration, or concern that the individual cannot be adequately monitored at home. All cases of suspected or confirmed dengue should be reported to the state health department.

Treatment of severe dengue requires close monitoring and support of circulatory and hematologic status. These simple measures decrease mortality to less than 1%. The phenomena of DHF are reversible, and recovery is often rapid after appropriate supportive therapy. Hence, judicious use of fluid resuscitation and monitoring of vital signs (pulse, BP) and urine output are required to avoid both hypovolemia in initial stages of disease and fluid overload in the recovery phase. Frequent determinations of hematocrit and platelet counts aid monitoring of plasma repletion through resolution of hemoconcentration and thrombocy-

Table 1 Treatment and Classification of Dengue and Dengue Hemorrhagic Fever

GRADE	SYMPTOMS	SIGNS	TREATMENT
Dengue fever	Headache Retroorbital pain Myalgia	Fever (39°-40° C [100.4°-102.2° F]) Rash (blanching, erythematous)	Treat symptoms. 　Use antiinflammatory agents 　　(not aspirin). Monitor clinical status daily. Determine Hct and platelet count.
DHF grade I	Same as above	Hemoconcentration (>20% rise in Hct) Thrombocytopenia (<100,000/mm³) Positive tourniquet test	Same as above, plus: Monitor vital signs q2h, then q6h. Determine Hct, platelet count Provide oral hydration.
DHF grade II	Same as above	Hemoconcentration and thrombocytopenia Spontaneous bleeding	Same as above, plus: Type and cross-match. Determine PT and PTT.
DHF grade III	Restlessness Confusion Lethargy	Hemoconcentration and thrombocytopenia Rapid weak pulse Narrowed pulse pressure (<20 mm Hg) Hypotension Cold clammy skin	Same as above plus: Administer isotonic intravenous fluids 　(rapid 20 ml/kg bolus). Obtain electrolytes; ALT/AST. Monitor vital signs more frequently 　(≤q30min). Follow urine output.
DHF grade IV	Depressed sensorium Stupor	Hemoconcentration and thrombocytopenia Undetectable pulse and blood pressure	Same as above, plus: Administer intravenous colloid or 　plasma 10-20 ml/kg. Provide critical care support as needed.

Adapted from Technical Advisory Committee: *Dengue hemorrhagic fever: diagnosis, treatment, and control,* ed 2, Geneva, 1997, World Health Organization.

Hct, Hematocrit; *PT,* prothrombin time; *PTT,* partial thromboplastin time; *ALT,* alanine aminotransferase; *AST,* aspartate aminotransferase.

topenia. In addition, a rapid drop in hematocrit after fluid replenishment without improvement in vital signs may suggest onset of spontaneous bleeding. If bleeding is present, it is advisable to obtain blood for type and cross-match. Determination of the prothrombin and partial thromboplastin times may indicate degree of the coagulopathies associated with DHF. Disseminated intravascular coagulation is distinctly uncommon, and heparin should not be used for treatment.

Treatment of DSS requires aggressive use of isotonic (Ringer's lactate or physiologic saline, 20 mg/kg IV bolus) and colloid fluids (plasma or dextran compound 10 to 20 mg/kg IV as needed). In cases of profound shock, critical care support including ventilation may be required. Intravenous steroids do not decrease mortality in DSS. Ribavirin did not prevent dengue virus replication in animal trials, and its use in DHF or DSS is unjustified.

Prevention

Cases of dengue infection are increasing with the unchecked spread of the primary mosquito vectors, *Aedes aegypti* and *Aedes albopictus* (the tiger mosquito). Both species are well adapted to man and widely dispersed in cities throughout the world, including the United States. The vectors are daytime feeders and feed repeatedly indoors. Travelers in dengue-endemic areas should avoid mosquitoes during the day if possible, particularly at dawn and dusk. Use of insect repellents is strongly recommended.

■ DENGUELIKE ILLNESSES

Other mosquito-borne viruses may also cause epidemics of self-limited denguelike illnesses characterized by abrupt onset of fever, malaise, myalgias, arthralgias, headache, and rash. These arboviruses include the alphaviruses (chikungunya, O'nyong-nyong, Ross River, Mayaro, and Sindbis viruses) and flaviviruses (e.g., West Nile virus). Individual arboviruses may be more closely associated with particular manifestations (e.g., arthritis in chikungunya and Ross River virus infections, lymphadenopathy in West Nile virus fever). However, specific diagnosis of acute arboviral fevers on clinical grounds alone is impossible. Serologic or virologic diagnosis requires specialized research or public health laboratory support. Treatment is usually directed to relief of symptoms with antiinflammatory agents and fluids. Prevention comprises use of insect repellents and avoidance of mosquitoes.

Suggested Reading

Innis BL: Dengue and dengue hemorrhagic fever. In Porterfield J, Tyrrell D, eds: *Handbook of infectious diseases,* vol 3, Exotic viral infections, London, 1996, Chapman & Hall.

Rigau-Perez JG, et al: Dengue and dengue hemorrhagic fever, *Lancet* 352:971, 1998.

Suh KN, Kozarsky PE, Keystone JS: Evaluation of fever in the returned traveler, *Med Clin North Am* 83:997, 1999.

Technical Advisory Committee: Dengue hemorrhagic fever: diagnosis, treatment, prevention, and control, ed 2, Geneva, 1997, World Health Organization.

VIRAL HEMORRHAGIC FEVERS

Lucy E. Wilson
Michele Barry

Viral hemorrhagic fevers (VHFs) are viral illnesses characterized by a syndrome of fever, hemorrhage, and multisystem organ dysfunction, often leading to deaths in epidemic settings. With increasing international travel, the potential danger of transmission and importation of nonendemic VHFs has been the focus of intense media attention and public concern. This concern has evoked extensive guidelines for treatment and management of suspected VHF in the United States, which are summarized in this chapter. The epidemiology, clinical features, diagnostic evaluation, and treatment are delineated for the VHF syndromes likely to cause disease in humans (except for dengue fever and hantavirus, which are discussed in separate chapters). Clinical management of VHF in a community setting and the necessary biosafety precautions are reviewed in this chapter.

VHF syndromes associated with human disease are caused by RNA viruses classified in four distinct families: Arenaviridae, Bunyaviridae, Filoviridae, and Flaviviridae (Table 1). These agents share many common features:

1. Most are caused by infectious agents that are arthropodborne (mosquitoes, ticks); however, person-to-person transmission may occur with five viruses through direct contact with blood or secretions (i.e., Lassa, Marburg, Congo-Crimean, Ebola, and Sabiá). Animal excreta has also been implicated in transmission.
2. Asymptomatic animal reservoirs of viruses are generally rodents (i.e., hantavirus, Lassa, Guanarito, Junin, and Machupo) although monkeys and primates may perpetuate disease through a sylvatic cycle (i.e., yellow fever and dengue). Many viruses have not had reservoirs identified (i.e., Ebola, Marburg, and Sabiá).
3. Clinical manifestations of VHF are associated with a short incubation period; usually less than 21 days. Clinical pathology has common themes: capillary leak, thrombocytopenia, leukopenia, disseminated intravascular coagulation (DIC), and hepatocellular destruction are often described. Early vascular dysregulation with hypotension, flushing, and injected conjunctivae is commonly followed by hemorrhage, shock, and multiorgan dysfunction. Milder, undifferentiated febrile illnesses and subclinical infections with asymptomatic seroconversion and potential immunity have also been described for all of the VHF viruses (Table 2).
4. Diagnosis of VHF depends on the demonstration of the infecting virus in an acute serum sample by antigen-detection enzyme-linked immunosorbent as-

say (ELISA), or reverse transcription and subsequent polymerase chain reaction (RT-PCR). IgM antibodies can also be helpful in making a diagnosis in early convalescence by IgM capture ELISA technique. Classical histopathology in autopsy specimens may unfortunately be the first clue (Table 3).

5. Supportive therapy is the mainstay of management of most VHFs, better accomplished in countries with sophisticated technologic support that is often lacking in endemic developing countries. Antiviral therapy with ribavirin is recommended for all Arenaviridae and Bunyaviridae infections (with the exception of hantavirus pulmonary syndrome). Unfortunately, ribavirin is often difficult and expensive to obtain in an endemic setting.
6. Control measures generally involve meticulous hospital infection control efforts, strict isolation for certain agents, concurrent disinfection, and contact and source reporting to public health authorities. Some of the VHF viruses are preventable by vaccines (see Table 3).

■ SPECIFIC VHFS CAUSING DISEASE IN HUMANS

Yellow Fever
Epidemiology
Yellow fever virus is a member of Flaviviridae genus (*flavi* means "yellow") and is found in the tropical Americas and sub-Saharan Africa. Official reports from endemic areas involve about 3000 cases per year, but recent epidemics in Nigeria, Kenya, and the Amazon area have raised the annual incidence and caused a reemergence of disease. Urbanization of populations near forested areas has recently caused urban yellow fever, a cycle involving only mosquitoes and infected humans.

Clinical Features
Yellow fever carries a case-fatality rate of about 20%. It exists in two transmission cycles: a sylvatic or jungle cycle that involves mosquitoes and nonhuman primates, mostly monkeys, and an urban cycle. The urban cycle involves mosquitoes and infected humans. *Aedes aegypti* is the usual mosquito vector, but several other species have been implicated, including *Amblyomma* ticks.

After a person is bitten by a mosquito infected with yellow fever virus, the usual incubation period is 3 to 6 days. Most infected individuals suffer only mild illness with fever and malaise. About 15% develop a serious illness manifested by three phases. The first is an acute phase of fever, headache, myalgia, nausea, and vomiting; few physical specific signs are apparent at this stage, except for Faget's sign, a relative bradycardia with fever. The second phase is a period of "remission" in which the fever remits for 1 to 2 days. During the third phase, a "period of intoxication," fever recurs, accompanied by jaundice and hemorrhagic manifestations. "Black vomit" refers to the massive hemetemesis that can occur; 50% mortality can often be related to the liver failure, myocarditis, encephalopathy, and acute renal failure that occurs during this phase.

Table 1 Epidemiology of Viral Hemorrhagic Fevers

FAMILY	GENUS	VIRUS	HUMAN DISEASE	TRANSMISSION ROUTES	RESERVOIR	INCUBATION PERIOD (DAYS)	ENDEMIC AREAS
Arenaviridae	*Arenavirus*	Guanarito	Venezuelan HF	Rodent to human, via direct contact and by aerosolization of body fluids	Wild rodent	7-16	Venezuela
		Junin	Argentine HF	Same as above	Wild rodent	7-16	Argentina
		Machupo	Bolivian HF	Same as above	Wild rodent *Calomys callosus*	7-16	Northern Bolivia
		Sabia	Brazilian HF	Same as above, laboratory acquired	? Rodent	7-16	Brazil
		Lassa	Lassa fever	Same as above	*Mastomys natalensis* rodent	5-21	West Africa
Bunyaviridae	*Phlebovirus*	Rift Valley fever	Rift Valley fever	Mosquitoborne, contact with livestock, nosocomial spread	Wild and domestic mammals	2-5	Sub-Saharan Africa
	Nairovirus	Crimean-Congo HF	Crimean-Congo HF	*Hyalomma* tickborne, contact with infected animals, nosocomial spread	Hares, domestic animals birds, ticks	3-12	East Europe, Africa, Middle East, China
	Hantavirus	Hantaan	Hemorrhagic fever with renal syndrome (HFRS)	Rodent to human. Direct contact versus aerosolization of rodent body fluids	Wild rodents	9-35	Worldwide, especially in Asia (endemic in China), Europe
	Hantavirus	Puumala	HFRS	See above	See above	9-35	Europe
	Hantavirus	Seoul	HFRS	See above	See above	9-35	? Worldwide
	Hantavirus	Sin Nombre, New York-1, Bayou, Rio Mamore, Laguna Negra, and others	Hantavirus pulmonary syndrome	See above	See above	7-28	Americas
Filoviridae	*Filovirus*	Ebola	Ebola HF	Unknown	Person to person, monkey to human, nosocomial	3-16	Western sub-Saharan Africa, Philippines
		Marburg	Marburg HF	Unknown	See above	3-16	Western sub-Saharan Africa
Flaviviridae		Dengue (types 1-4)	Dengue HF	*Aedes aegypti* and *Aedes albopictus* Mosquitoborne	Monkeys, humans	3-15	Worldwide; hemorrhagic syndromes occur in Southeast Asia and Caribbean
		Kyasanur Forest disese	Kyasanur Forest disease	*Ixodid* tickborne	Monkeys, rodents, shrews	3-8	Kamataka State, India, Pakistan
		Omsk hemorrhagic fever	Omsk hemorrhagic fever	*Ixodid* tickborne, muskrats	Muskrat to human	3-8	Siberia
		Yellow fever	Yellow fever	Mosquitoborne (*Aedes aegypti*) *Amblyomma* ticks (rare)	Monkeys, humans	3-6	South America, West and East Africa

HF, Hemorrhagic fever.

Table 2   Clinical Features of Viral Hemorrhagic Fevers

VIRUS	EARLY CLINICAL FEATURES	ADVANCED CLINICAL FEATURES
ARENAVIRIDAE		
Junin Guanarito Machupo Sabia	Insidious onset of headache, fever, arthralgia, myalgia, anorexia, nausea, vomiting, constipation, photophobia, and pain in retroorbital, epigastric, and lumbar areas Ill appearing, with erythema of head and torso, occasionally with petechiae Moderate-to-severe leukopenia and thrombocytopenia Proteinuria and microscopic hematuria	Epistaxis, hematemesis, acute neurologic disease, pulmonary edema, intractable shock Neurologic disease (50%): tremors, delirium, oculogyrus, strabismus, dysarthria, intention tremor Superimposed bacterial and fungal infections
Lassa	Insidious onset of symptoms: fever, headache, sore throat, cough, abdominal pain, arthralgias, and low back pain Conjunctivitis and pharyngitis are common Acute phase lasts 1-4 wk	Hemorrhage, usually gastrointestinal, in up to 20% of cases Relative bradycardia, pleural/pericardial effusions, pneumonitis, encephalopathy, facial edema, shock Deafness in 30% during convalescence, often reversible
BUNYAVIRIDAE		
Rift Valley fever	Mild viral illness can occur with recovery and immunity Acute onset of fever, headache, back pain, myalgias, nausea, epigastric pain	Severe hemorrhage (epistaxis and gastrointestinal), icterus, hepatic necrosis, anuria, disseminated intravascular coagulation (DIC), and shock Retinal vasculitis and encephalitis may occur, but these patients do not develop hemorrhage
Crimean-Congo HF	Acute onset of fever, severe headache, chills, arthralgias, vomiting, prostration, myalgias in lower back and limbs; palatal petechiae and pharyngitis Thrombocytopenia, leukocytosis, and icterus	Most severe hemorrhage of all viral hemorrhagic fevers Hemorrhage on days 4-5 include epistaxis, gum bleeding, oozing, and gastrointestinal hemorrhage Large ecchymoses occur Fatality associated with pulmonary edema, hypovolemic shock, and DIC
Hantavirus with renal syndrome	*Five phases:* febrile, hypotensive, oliguric, diuretic, and convalescent phase *Febrile phase:* high fever, dizziness, frontal headache, ocular symptoms, severe abdominal and back pain, severe diarrhea *Diagnostic triad:* facial flushing, periorbital edema, and palatal/axillary petechiae Thrombocytopenia for first 10 days Most patients recover	*Hypotensive phase:* after 3-5 days, lasts 1-2 days Hemorrhage, shock and DIC may occur during the first three phases, usually occurring from day 3-6 *Oliguric phase:* overlaps with hypotensive phase and occurs 24 hr after shock; proteinuria, dialysis Profound central nervous system changes can occur Recovery involves the diuretic phase (tenth day of illness) and the prolonged convalescent phase
FILOVIRIDAE		
Ebola Marburg	*First week* Initial phase: fever, headache, conjunctivitis, myalgia, arthralgia, asthenia, vomiting, abdominal pain, nonbloody diarrhea, maculopapular rash with desquamation Marburg with enanthema Ebola with sore throat, "ghostlike" facies, encephalopathy	*Remission phase:* for 24-48 hr occurs before second phase *Second week: late phase:* normothermia, obtundation, delirium, convulsions, shock, tachypnea, hemorrhage, hepatitis, oliguria/anuria *Convalescent* patients can develop ocular diseases, orchitis, arthralgias, and alopecia
FLAVIVIRIDAE		
Dengue	Sudden onset of fever, severe headache, retroorbital pain, myalgias, low back pain: breakbone fever, rash After 5 days, diffuse morbilliform rash appears with puritus and desquamation; fever resolves Fever returns after 48 hours Hemorrhage can occur at any time during febrile phase	In setting of thrombocytopenia and hemoconcentration, WHO classification of severity criteria (grades 1-4): 1. Fever, systemic symptoms, positive tourniquet sign 2. Above and spontaneous bleeding 3. Above and circulatory failure and central nervous system changes 4. Above and profound hypotension/shock (also called *dengue shock syndrome*)
Yellow fever	5%-20% of all infected develop jaundice and clinical syndrome *Early phase:* viremia with fever, chills, severe headache, low back pain, myalgias, nausea, malaise, relative bradycardia (Faget's sign), conjunctival injection, coated tongue with red edges *Remission phase:* usually lasts 2-3 d	*Intoxication phase:* fever, jaundice, albuminuria, oliguria, hemorrhage (especially gastrointestinal), delirium, stupor, acidosis, shock; gastrointestinal hemorrhage ("black vomit"); thrombocytopenia, DIC, leukopenia, increased direct bilirubin, hepatitis, elevated creatinine, hypoglycemia, and encephalopathy

HF, Hemorrhagic fever; *WHO,* World Health Organization.

Diagnosis

Laboratory findings include leukopenia, thrombocytopenia, and abnormal coagulation parameters. Leukocytosis can evolve, as can elevated transaminases, hyperbilirubinemia, and hypoglycemia, all indicating incipient liver failure. Nephrotic range proteinuria and renal failure can occur. Yellow fever infection can be detected early in serum or blood using IgM-antibody capture ELISA or PCR; IgM-specific ELISA appears by the end of the first week. A fourfold or greater rise in titer in serum plaque neutralizing antibody, complement fixation, or hemagglutination inhibition antibodies is also diagnostic but requires paired acute and convalescent sera. Cell culture can detect virus in acute serum. Pathologic examination of liver with viral isolation provides a postmortem diagnosis; antemortem liver biopsy is usually contraindicated because of risk of bleeding diatheses.

Treatment and Prevention

No effective antiviral agent is available. All treatment is supportive. Index patients should be protected from mosquito bites for 5 days after illness to avoid spread. Blood and needle precautions should be instituted by health care attendants.

The best preventive measure against yellow fever infection is the live attenuated 17D vaccine. A single subcutaneous injection is immunogenic in 99% of recipients and probably offers lifelong duration of immunity, but 10-year boosting is suggested if travel to an endemic area is anticipated. Immunization during pregnancy should be postponed unless absolutely necessary, although it poses only a small risk to the fetus. On hypothetical grounds of dissemination, patients with symptomatic human immunodeficiency virus (HIV) infection or acquired immunodeficiency syndrome (AIDS) should not receive the live vaccine. Infants younger than 9 to 12 months of age should not receive the vaccine because vaccine-strain encephalitis has been described.

Lassa Fever
Epidemiology

Lassa fever virus is a member of the Arenaviridae genus and is endemic as well as epidemic in West Africa. RNA virus was first recognized in 1969, after a Nigerian outbreak among missionary nurses. It is estimated that there are 400,000 hospital admissions yearly for Lassa fever in West Africa, with 5000 of these admissions resulting in death.

Clinical Features

The vector for Lassa fever is the bush rodent *Mastomys natalensis*. Humans are infected when they come into contact with excreta or aerosolized body fluids from infected mice, via contact with an infected human, or from nosocomial transmission. Human-to-human infection is unlikely to be transmitted from inhalation of respiratory droplets, but rather from direct contact with human bodily fluid.

After an incubation period of 5 to 21 days, the acute phase of Lassa fever usually lasts between 1 and 4 weeks. In contrast to other hemorrhagic fevers, its onset is characteristically insidious, featuring fever, severe sore throat and headache, back pain, and abdominal pain. Severity of illness can vary, leading to an underestimation of the incidence of the disease and overestimation of the lethality of the disease.

The late phase of disease involves its hemorrhagic manifestations. In particular, the hemorrhagic manifestations are gastrointestinal, with death occurring from hypovolemic shock secondary to hemorrhage. Other late-stage features are relative bradycardia, pleural/pericardial effusions, pneumonitis, encephalopathy, facial edema, and endothelial and platelet dysfunction. DIC, however, does not occur.

The mortality rate of clinically apparent Lassa fever is estimated at 15%. A mortality rate of 80% is associated with an elevated aspartate aminotransferase (AST) (>150 IU/L) and high levels of viremia (>10^3 TCID$_{50}$/ml). Also, there is an increased mortality rate with pregnancy.

Diagnosis

Several clinical and serologic diagnostic modalities exist. First, clinical suspicion is paramount. One study reported good specificity (89%) and predictive value (80%) for diagnosing Lassa fever in patients who presented in an epidemic setting with the clinical triad of pharyngitis, retrosternal pain, and proteinuria.

Lassa fever can be serologically diagnosed in several ways. First, using acute serum via the ELISA test can be diagnostic of either IgG or IgM antibodies. Second, detection of a fourfold or greater rise in IgG serum titer, using paired acute and convalescent titers can be diagnostic. Third, antigen can be detected by RT-PCR of acute serum. However, there are geographic differences in primers. Finally, diagnosis by isolation of virus in cell culture is possible if the patient is acutely ill. Autopsy findings display focal necrosis of the spleen, liver, and adrenals.

Treatment

McCormick and others reported that patients treated with intravenous or oral ribavirin within the first 6 days of fever had a statistically significant decrease in mortality rate; ribavirin was also more effective than administering convalescent plasma. Laboratory markers that support ribavirin therapy include elevation of the AST greater than 150 and high levels of viremia. Ribavirin is recommended for all phases of the disease, including postexposure prophylaxis. If it is available, intravenous ribavirin should be chosen over oral ribavirin for severely ill patients. Prophylactic oral ribavirin is recommended for all close contacts who are not pregnant. For dosing recommendations, see Table 4.

Prevention

Prevention includes strict isolation and precautions at biosafety level 4 and prompt notification of local and national public health authorities. Control of rodents and proper storage of food may control rodent-to-human transmission. Prophylaxis of close or high-risk contacts with oral ribavirin should be considered (see Table 5 for definition of high-risk and close contact). There is no commercially available vaccine.

■ FILOVIRIDAE

Ebola and Marburg Viruses

Ebola and Marburg viruses are the two members of the Filoviridae genus. Both are enveloped, single-stranded RNA viruses. These two viruses can be genetically, serologically, and biochemically distinguished. Whereas Marburg is a

Table 3 Diagnosis and Treatment of Viral Hemorrhagic Fevers

VIRUS	DIAGNOSIS	ISOLATION/PRECAUTIONS	VACCINE AVAILABLE†	RIBAVIRIN?	OTHER THERAPY
ARENAVIRIDAE					
Guanarito	*Culture:* isolation of virus from body fluids via DFA method on cell culture	Strict isolation BSL-4	No	Yes	Supportive
Junin	*Serologic* *Antibodies:* IgM or IgG detection via ELISA and IFA methods; detection of a fourfold rise in IgG antibody titer (≥1:16) *Antigen:* RT-PCR of acute serum	Strict isolation BSL-4	Live attenuated (U.S. Army availability)	Yes Active in vitro	Convalescent phase plasma associated with decreased mortality rate if used within the first days of illness; associated increase in reversible late phase neurologic syndrome
Machupo		Strict isolation BSL-4	No	Yes Two case reports of successful outcome	Supportive
Sabia		Strict isolation BSL-4	No	Yes One case report of successful outcome	Supportive
Lassa		Strict isolation BSL-4	In development	Yes Treated with IV/PO within first 6 days of symptoms had statistically significant impact on mortality rate	Supportive
BUNYAVIRIDAE					
Rift Valley fever	*Culture:* virus isolation from blood or liver via cell culture or mouse inoculation *Antibodies:* IFA testing of acute serum after first 3-4 days of illness	Blood and body fluid precautions BSL-4 BSL-3 if vaccinated	Experimental inactivated vaccine (U.S. Army availability)	Yes Effective in nonhuman primates and mice	Supportive
Crimean-Congo HF	*Culture:* virus isolated by cell culture or mouse inoculation *Antibodies:* CF, HI, ELISA, neutralization, and IF methods; acute and convalescent serum *Antigens:* RT-PCR	Blood and body fluid precautions BSL-4	Yes Efficacy (available in Bulgaria)	Yes In vitro susceptibility Three cases of severe CCHF were treated successfully with ribavirin	No clear evidence for convalescent immune plasma

Organism	Diagnosis	Isolation/BSL	Vaccine	Antiviral	Treatment
Hantaan Puumala Seoul	*Cell culture* *Antibodies:* anti-Hantaan specific IgM antibodies in serum with ELISA or IFA; plaque reduction neutralization assay, acute and convalescent serum titers	None BSL-3	Yes ? Efficacy (available in Asia)	Yes Statistically significant improvement in outcome and reduction in mortality	Supportive; uncontrolled trial with reaferon had potential merit
Sin Nombre	*Antibodies:* IgM or IgG paired serum titers by ELISA, Western blot *Antigen:* detected in tissue by immunohistochemistry and RT-PCR		No	Sensitive in vitro No controlled trials in humans	Supportive, especially respiratory
FILOVIRIDAE Ebola Marburg	Electron microscopy of serum *Culture:* isolation from most body tissues at autopsy *Antibodies:* IFA at 8-10 days; titer >1:256; ELISA at 4-7 days; paired serum titers *Antigen:* RT-PCR for Ebola	Strict isolation BSL-4	No No	No No	Supportive
FLAVIVIRIDAE Dengue	Immunohistochemical staining of peripheral blood mononuclear cells *Serology* *Antibodies:* IgG or IgM via ELISA, HI, neutralization test or CF *Antigen:* isolated by immunoassay or PCR of blood	Blood precautions BSL-2	Experimental live attenuated vaccine against all four serotypes	No Ineffective in rodents	Supportive
Yellow fever	*Culture:* isolation of virus from acute serum in cell culture *Serology* *Antibodies:* IgG or IgM detection by ELISA, HI, neutralization test (5-7 days), or CF (7-14 days) Paired acute and convalescent sera *Antigen:* PCR of viral antigen acute serum	Blood and body fluid precautions BSL-3 Netting and isolation of index case during first 5 days of viremia	Yes Live attenuated Avoid with egg allergy, infants, and pregnant women <6 months pregnant	No	Supportive

DFA, Direct fluorescent antibody; *ELISA,* enzyme-linked immunosorbent assay; *IFA,* indirect fluorescent antibody; *RT-PCR,* reverse transcriptase polymerase chain reaction; *BSL,* biosafety level; *HF,* hemorrhagic fever; *CF,* complement fixation; *HI,* hemaqqlutination inhibition; *CCHF,* Crimean-Congo hemorrhagic fever.

Table 4 Ribavirin Therapy for Viral Hemorrhagic Fever

TREATMENT
30 mg/kg IV loading dose, then 16 mg/kg IV q6h for 4 days, then 8 mg/kg IV q8h for 6 days (total treatment time, 10 days)
PROPHYLAXIS
500 mg PO q6h for 7 days

Table 5 Isolation Management of a Potential Viral Hemorrhagic Fever

1. Isolate using universal precautions.
2. A negative-pressure room should be arranged, preferably with an anteroom for removing protective barriers and storing supplies.
3. All nonessential staff and visitors should be restricted.
4. Gloves and gowns should be worn by all persons entering room.
5. Face shields, surgical masks, and eye protection should be worn by persons coming within 3 feet of patient.
6. If a suspected viral hemorrhagic fever patient has a prominent cough, vomiting, diarrhea, or hemorrhage, personal protective respirators are recommended (high-efficiency particulate air respirators).
7. Chemical toilets should be used and all effluents disinfected with bleach before disposal into a municipal sewer system for up to 6 wk of convalescence or until patient is virologically negative.
8. Soiled linens should be double-bagged and either incinerated or autoclaved. Hot water cycle with bleach can be used if no sorting occurs.

---

fairly homogeneous virus, Ebola can be grouped into at least four different subtypes.

Marburg

Epidemiology. Marburg virus was first described in 1967, in commercial laboratory workers in Marburg, Germany, presenting with VHFs. Thirty-one cases were documented in this outbreak. Infected green monkeys imported from Uganda for research purposes were the identified carriers. Isolated cases have subsequently been reported in South Africa, Zimbabwe, and Kenya. No reservoir has been identified.

Ebola

Epidemiology. Ebola virus is a member of the Filoviridae genus and has been described in Western sub-Saharan Africa and from imported monkeys from the Philippines. Ebola was first described in 1976, when two outbreaks coincided in southern Sudan and northern Zaire. Ebola is the name of a small river in northwestern Zaire. Another outbreak occurred in Kikwit, Zaire, in 1995, and various cases have sporadically been reported. Ebola is subdivided into four genetically distinct subtypes: Zaire (EBO-Z), Sudan (EBO-S), Reston (EBO-R), and more recently, Ivory Coast (EBO-CI).

Characteristics of Marburg and Ebola Viruses

For both Marburg and Ebola viruses, the natural reservoir is unknown, although zoonotic transmission is postulated.

The original Marburg outbreak in Marburg, Germany, was associated with ill green monkeys (*Cercopithecus aethiops*) imported from Uganda. Likewise, the Reston, Virginia Ebola outbreak was linked to infected symptomatic cynomolgus monkeys (*Macaca fascicularis*) imported from the Philippines, but as in all other cases, no uninfected animal reservoir was identified.

Human-to-human transmission via intimate contact is documented in each disease. Nosocomial transmission is clearly documented via infected body fluids. Generally, transmission has occurred between close contacts, by sexual transmission, and from contaminated needles and syringes, not by casual contact. Airborne transmission was postulated to occur in the monkey-to-human Reston Ebola outbreak, but this mode of transmission has never been documented in human-to-human cases and is not thought to play an important role in transmission of Ebola. Primate-to-primate transmission is also described. All outbreaks have been self-limiting because of the institution of isolation precautions.

Clinical Features

The incubation period for Marburg and Ebola viruses is estimated at 3 to 16 days. Marburg virus carries a mortality rate of 23%, whereas Ebola virus has a wider range of mortality rate of 53% to 88%, varying by Ebola strain and available health resources.

The clinical features of Marburg and Ebola hemorrhagic fevers exhibit a biphasic illness pattern, punctuated by a remissionlike period. The initial phase is characterized by asthenia/weakness, the later phase by hemorrhage.

The first week of illness (the initial phase) is characterized by the acute onset of fever, headache, myalgias, and arthralgias. Next, patients experience conjunctivitis, vomiting, and nonbloody diarrhea with abdominal pain. A maculopapular rash with resultant desquamation occurs in approximately half of patients, usually by the fifth day of illness. In addition, on the fifth day of illness, patients start to develop signs of petechiae and hemorrhage.

Patients with Marburg virus tend to develop enanthema with mucosal erythema and eruption. Ebola cases show no enanthema, but patients complain of an intensely dry, sore throat with odynophagia, and also may complain of chest pain. Severely ill Ebola patients often exhibit profound lethargy and prostration, with deep-set eyes and an expressionless face, described as "ghostlike."

The remission phase of filovirus infection lasts for 24 to 48 hours before the second phase of morbidity. The late phase of disease, during the second week of illness, exhibits normothermia, tachypnea, shock, oliguria, and hemorrhage. Hepatitis with elevated transaminases occurs in both diseases. In Ebola patients, encephalopathy is common. Encephalopathic symptoms include irritability, confusion, obtundation, delirium, and convulsions. Hemorrhage has been reported in 45% to 78% of cases. Pregnant patients who contract Ebola experience fetal loss.

Death, usually occurring in the second week of illness, has been associated with mucosal bleeding, oozing from puncture sites, anuria, hiccups, tachypnea, and encephalopathy. Convalescence is often prolonged, lasting weeks, and can include orchitis, ocular diseases, arthralgias, and alopecia. Filovirus can be detected in semen up to 3 months after illness, and relapse of Marburg virus has been reported after 3 months of convalescence.

Diagnosis

Laboratory features include thrombocytopenia and early lymphopenia followed by a neutrophilic leukemoid response. Transaminitis (AST greater than alanine aminotransferase [ALT]), icterus, markedly elevated lactate dehydrogenase (LDH), and increased amylase are all prominent. Urinalysis reveals hematuria and proteinuria.

Several laboratory methods can be used to detect the Marburg and Ebola viruses. Both viruses can be isolated from the serum by electron microscopy. An indirect fluorescent antibody (IFA) test is used for the identification of both Marburg and Ebola virus and becomes positive around day 8 to 10. Serum IFA titers greater than 1:256 are generally considered positive. However, the IFA technique is considered imperfect because the specificity is low. Ebola antigen and antibody is also be rapidly detected by the more sensitive and specific technique of ELISA. Antibodies to Ebola are detectable in the first 4 to 7 days of illness, with large increases in titers during the second and third weeks of illness. IgM capture ELISA tests are usually positive early in convalescence and can be coupled with rising IgG antibody titers. RT-PCR can be used to detect low concentrations of Ebola viral RNA. At autopsy, Marburg and Ebola virus can be isolated from serum, blood, urine, pharyngeal swabs, semen, liver, and lymphoid tissue. Virus is detectable in semen for up to 3 months after recovery from infection and thus may be sexually transmissible.

Treatment

Because there is no known therapy for either viral hemorrhagic fever, supportive care is offered. Several trials have shown there is no efficacy for the use of interferon-α, convalescent plasma, or ribavirin.

Prevention

If Ebola or Marburg hemorrhagic fever is suspected, strict isolation of the index case is essential. Barrier precautions with gowns, gloves, and masks are required. Biosafety level 4 precautions are to be implemented, and local and national health authorities should be contacted immediately. All nonhuman primates suspected of disease should be quarantined.

Crimean-Congo Hemorrhagic Fever
Epidemiology

Crimean-Congo hemorrhagic fever (CCHF) is caused by the single-stranded RNA *Nairovirus* of the Bunyaviridae genus. CCHF has been identified in Africa, the Middle East, the Balkans, Russia, and Western China. It was first recognized in 1944 in Crimea as a hemorrhagic febrile illness.

The vectors are the *ixodid* ticks in the Hyalomma genus. Transmission is thought to occur between humans and from the blood, aerosols, or fomites from slaughtered cattle and sheep. Tick bites and direct handling or crushing of ticks is another route of transmission. Nosocomial infections via blood have been well documented. Community epidemics in endemic areas are postulated to occur via aerosol spread.

Subclinical or asymptomatic infections are thought to occur in endemic areas.

Clinical Features

CCHF is generally an acute and self-limiting disease, except in the event of an epidemic. Onset of disease is acute. After an incubation period of generally 3 to 6 days (but up to 12 days, especially in nosocomial cases), patients experience fever, severe headache, chills, arthralgias, vomiting, and prostration. Myalgias are concentrated in the lower back and limb area. The soft palate often develops a fine petechial rash, and the pharynx can be hyperemic. Facial flushing, conjunctivitis, bradycardia, and diarrhea may occur. Encephalopathy and pulmonary symptoms are less common, but the liver is often affected.

Mortality is reported to increase in epidemics, rising from 15% up to 70%. The most severe cases are reported in Asia, with lower mortality rates reported in Europe and Africa. Clinically, CCHF has the most severe bleeding and ecchymoses of all the hemorrhagic fevers. On day 4 to 5 of illness, severe hemorrhage occurs in up to 25% of patients. Hemorrhagic manifestations include gum bleeding and epistaxis, followed by gastrointestinal hemorrhage. Ecchymoses are often large and pressure-linked. Hematuria, proteinuria, azotemia, and liver involvement are associated with poor prognosis. Fatalities are associated with the development of pulmonary edema, hypovolemic shock, and DIC. Immunity develops after infection and is thought to persist indefinitely.

Diagnosis

Laboratory values feature thrombocytopenia, hemorrhage, leukopenia, and icterus. The laboratory diagnosis of Crimean-Congo viral infection can be achieved via several methods. Virus or antibodies should be detectable within 7 to 20 days after the onset of clinical symptoms. In addition, virus isolation from the serum of severely ill cases is usually positive in cell culture. Antibodies can be detected by complement fixation, hemagglutination-inhibition, ELISA, neutralization, and immunofluorescence techniques. Acute and convalescent serum can be used to identify virus-specific antibodies. RT-PCR can be performed on serum of acutely ill patients.

Treatment

Therapy for CCHF consists of rapid clinical diagnosis followed by the implementation of supportive therapy. Convalescent immune plasma therapy is not associated with improved outcome in patients with CCHF. In vitro, Crimean-Congo virus is susceptible to ribavirin. No formal clinical studies of ribavirin therapy for CCHF exist; however, three patients with documented severe CCHF were treated successfully with oral ribavirin. Thus treatment of suspected CCHF with ribavirin is recommended. Extrapolating from studies of the treatment of Lassa fever with ribavirin, intravenous ribavirin is the preferred route of administration for the treatment of CCHF.

Prevention

Prevention of CCHF entails the avoidance of exposure to tick bites. The slaughter of acutely viremic livestock may increase the risk of disease transmission. In appropriate

Table 6 Handling Laboratory Specimens

1. All laboratory testing should be minimized to reduce exposure risk.
2. Specimens should be placed in durable, leakproof containers and double-bagged and hand-carried directly to the laboratory by person collecting sample.
3. All specimen handling should be done under a class 2 laminar flow hood, and centrifugation should be performed in covered buckets with O-ring seals following appropriate biosafety level.
4. Decreasing viral concentration by using Triton X-100 (polyethylene glycol p-tert-octylphenyl ether); treatment with 10 μ of 10% Triton X-100/1 ml of serum for 1 hr dramatically reduces titer of viruses, although 100% efficacy cannot be assumed. Most laboratory testing can be performed after disinfection.
5. Routine automated analyzers should be disinfected after use (1:100 dilution household bleach, ¼ cup to 1 gallon water).
6. Virus isolation or cultivation must be done at BSL-4 facility if a BSL-4 virus is suspected (see Table 10).

Table 7 Suggested Equipment and Supplies for Anteroom Adjoining Patient's Room

Prescribed medications (analgesics, antipyretics, antibiotics)	Containers with solution for throat swabs and urine specimens
Resuscitation equipment	Labels
Material for physical examination	Marker pens
Portable x-ray machine	Plastic airtight bags (various sizes)
Electrocardiogram machine	Plastic trash bags
Intravenous equipment and supplies	Disinfectant solutions (see text)
Tourniquets	Chemical toilet
Dry gauze	Urinals
Alcohol swabs	Nursing supplies
Needles (various sizes)	Disposable linen, towels, pajamas, and so on
Syringes (various sizes)	Toilet articles
Plastic container for disposal of needles and other sharp equipment	Gowns, masks, surgical gloves, shoe covers, and protective eye wear for staff
Tubes for hematologic and Biochemical investigations	Housekeeping materials (absorbent towels for spills, and so on)
Blood-culture bottles	

From Centers for Disease Control and Prevention: *MMWR* 37(S-3):16, 1988.

areas, cattle dipping (to reduce the number of infected vectors) may decrease transmission rates to humans. Barrier nursing is essential in the clinical setting. Biosafety level 4 is required for the handling of laboratory specimens and infectious material. Prompt notification of local and national public health authorities is required. A formalin-inactivated vaccine has been used regionally in high-risk groups but is of limited efficacy.

Approach to a Suspected Case of VHF in a Community Setting

When travel or occupational history and physical signs suggest a VHF, such as exposure to an endemic area within 3 weeks, and fever, pharyngitis, conjunctivitis, skin rash predate rapid hemorrhage and shock, four immediate steps should immediately occur:

1. Isolate the patient with barrier nursing precautions. (Tables 5, 6, and 7).
2. Notify local and state health departments and the CDC—phone: 404-639-1115; 404-639-1511, or 404-639-2888 (after hours and weekends).
3. Determine the biosafety level to be achieved for the virus suspected (Table 8).
4. Begin surveillance of all contacts of index case since illness (Table 9).

Identifying an exposure to arthropods, rodents, or a tick bite and reviewing local virus transmission within geographic areas with a CDC epidemiology intelligence service officer will help distinguish VHF viruses from malaria, typhoid, shigella, leptospirosis, or rickettsial disease; all short-incubation diseases in the differential of imported fevers with multiorgan dysfunction. Epidemiologic studies of VHF in humans indicate that infection is not readily transmitted from person to person by the airborne route except in end-stage disease (i.e., a Lassa fever patient with extensive pulmonary involvement). Severe vomiting and

hemorrhagic shock may expose persons to massive secretions and aerosol exposure. VHF infection has not been reported to be transmitted during the incubation period before fever occurs.

Isolation should be in a single room with an adjoining anteroom serving as its only entrance. Ideally, a patient's room should be at negative pressure from the anteroom. The anteroom should contain supplies for routine care (see Table 7) as well as gloves, masks, and shoe covers. Patients should have a chemical toilet with all secretions, excretions, and other body fluids treated with disinfectant solution. All material leaving the room, including linen and pajamas, should be double-bagged in airtight bags. Outside bags should be sponged with disinfectant. Disposable items such as dressings and catheters should be placed in rigid containers of disinfectant solution, then sponged and incinerated.

Collecting and Handling Laboratory Specimens (see Table 6)

All hospital workers drawing blood or collecting secretions should ideally be responsible for double-bagging specimens, disinfecting exterior bagging with bleach, and hand-carrying specimens to the laboratory. Laboratory handling of a VHF specimen, disinfecting blood before handling, and disinfecting machinery after use is described in Table 6.

Treatment Regimens

Ribavirin has been used with some success for most Bunyaviridae and Arenaviridae infections (see Table 4 for dosage). Intravenous treatment can result in a mild hemolysis and transient LFT abnormalities. All VHF patients ideally should be aggressively supported in an intensive care setting.

Table 8   Major Viral Hemorrhagic Fevers (VHFs)

FAMILY/GENUS	DISEASE	LABORATORY BIOSAFETY LEVEL	INTER-HUMAN TRANSMISSIBILITY
ARENAVIRIDAE			
Lassa virus	Lassa fever	BSL-4	Person-to-person Rare nosocomial
Junin, Machupo, Guanarito and Sabia viruses	Various South American HFs	BSL-4	Rare nosocomial Rare interhuman
BUNYAVIRIDAE			
Phlebovirus	Rift Valley fever	BSL-3*/BSL-4	None
Nairovirus	Crimean-Congo HF	BSL-4	Occasional nosocomial
Hantavirus	HF with renal syndrome	BSL-3†	None
	Hantavirus pulmonary syndrome	BSL-3†	None
FILOVIRIDAE	Marburg and Ebola HF	BSL-4	5%-25% in unprotected patient care and household setting
FLAVIVIRIDAE	Yellow fever	BSL-3*	None
	Dengue HF/dengue shock syndrome	BSL-2	None

BSL, Biosafety level; *HF*, hemorrhagic fever.
*Laboratory workers must be protected by vaccine. In the case of Rift Valley fever virus, vaccinated workers use BSL-3 precautions within the laboratory, but additional precautions are required to prevent escape of the virus into the environment.
†Work with the virus can be carried out at BSL-3, but special precautions are required for inoculation of natural reservoir rodents.

Table 9   Contacts and Surveillance

1. Casual contact: Person who had remote contact with ill patient (e.g., same plane, same hotel)—*no special surveillance needed.*
2. Close contact: Household contact, patient providers, laboratory handlers, shaking hands, hugging.
   Surveillance: Temperature twice daily for 3 wk with immediate reporting of fever or symptom to surveillance team.
3. High-risk contact: Mucous membrane contact (kissing, intercourse, penetrating injury with patient's excretions, secretions or blood).
   Surveillance: Twice daily temperature as above. Isolation with fever and treat as viral hemorrhagic fever until diagnosis excluded by culture. Consider postexposure ribavirin prophylaxis, if sensitive virus—such as any Arenaviridae or Bunyaviridae (except hantavirus pulmonary syndrome).

Table 10   Autopsy and Handling of a Corpse

1. Handling of the body should be minimized, and the corpse should be wrapped in an airtight bag, then cremated or promptly buried in a sealed container.
2. Autopsy should be deferred or limited in scope using the same precautions described for clinicians with aerosol formation avoidance.

use is advised until body fluids are free of virus. All autopsy handling of a corpse should be minimized (Table 10).

Although increasing international travel increases the potential danger of an imported VHF, a good epidemiologic history coupled with heightened vigilance for clinical signs can permit early diagnosis and safe management of an index VHF case presenting in a community setting.

Contact Surveillance

Identification and surveillance of all patient contacts is essential to disease control. A contact is defined as a person who has been exposed to the secretions, excretions, or tissues of an index case within 3 weeks of illness. Contacts may be divided into three levels of risk (see Table 9). A team should be identified to cover a telephone hotline permitting 24-hour surveillance of contacts. Timely notification and education of the community about the presence of a VHF case can help to quell fears about disease transmission. Convalescent patients should be warned that VHF viruses can often be asymptomatically excreted for many weeks in semen and urine and remain infectious. Meticulous personal hygiene should be followed. Abstinence or condom

Suggested Reading

Centers for Disease Control and Prevention: Management of patients with suspected viral hemorrhagic fever, *MMWR* 37:1, 1988.

Centers for Disease Control and Prevention: Update: management of patients with suspected viral hemorrhagic fever—United States, *MMWR*, 44:475, 1995.

Feldmann H, Slenczka W, Klenk H-D: Emerging and reemerging of filoviruses, *Arch Virology* 11(suppl):77, 1996.

Lacy MD, Smego RA: Viral hemorrhagic fevers, *Adv Pediatr Infect Dis* 12:21, 1996.

McCormick JB, et al: Lassa fever: effective therapy with ribavirin, *N Engl J Med* 314:20, 1986.

Peters CJ, Jahrling PB, Khan AS: Patients infected with high-hazard viruses: scientific basis for infection control, *Arch Virology* 11(suppl):141, 1996.

Peters CJ, LeDuc JW, eds: Ebola: the virus and the disease, *J Infect Dis* 179(suppl):S1, 1999.

Robertson SE, et al: Yellow fever: a decade of reemergence, *JAMA* 276:1157, 1996.

HANTAVIRUS CARDIOPULMONARY SYNDROME

Howard Levy
Frederick Koster

Hantavirus cardiopulmonary syndrome (HCPS) is a distinctive but uncommon viral pneumonitis with a mortality rate of approximately 45%. HCPS occurs through most of the temperate and semiarid climates of the Americas. Since its description in 1993, more than 200 cases have been documented in both North and South America. HCPS is caused by one of several hantaviruses (family Bunyaviridae), small tripartite negative-strand RNA viruses. Sin Nombre virus is the most common hantavirus through most of North America, with rare infections caused by New York virus in the northeast United States, and Bayou virus and Black Creek Canal virus in the Southeast United States. In the Patagonian region of Argentina and Chile, Andes virus causes a severe form of HCPS in which renal involvement may be more common, and person-to-person transmission appears to have been documented. Most other regions of South America also have sporadic cases of HCPS. Related hantaviruses, particularly Hantaan virus in Asia, and Puumala virus in Europe, cause more than 100,000 cases annually of hemorrhagic fever renal syndrome.

Hantavirus infection is transmitted by infected aerosols contaminated by dried urine or feces from hantavirus-infected rodents, particularly the deer mouse in North America, and is therefore almost exclusively a rural disease. Following an incubation period of 7 to 30 days, the syndrome exhibits three distinct phases. The first phase is a febrile prodromal phase characterized by fever, chills, myalgias, headache, nausea, vomiting, and malaise. After 2 to 8 days of nonspecific flulike illness, there is an abrupt 6- to 24-hour transition into the cardiopulmonary phase characterized by oliguria and cardiogenic shock in approximately half of patients, and dry cough, dyspnea, and noncardiogenic pulmonary edema in all patients. Patients surviving the first 2 days of shock, the direct cause and interval of most of the mortality, will begin diuresing the accumulated pulmonary edema fluid after 3 to 5 days. Convalescence is characterized by fatigue, exercise intolerance, and a modest obstructive defect in the small airways.

■ EARLY DIAGNOSIS

Therapy is entirely supportive and requires the skills and technology of the intensive care unit (ICU), yet most infections occur in remote rural settings, providing challenges to transport the patient safely to an ICU. Because the initial phase of the illness is a nonspecific viral prodrome and the transition to shock and pulmonary edema occurs rapidly, special emphasis must be put on early presumptive diagnosis.

During the viral prodrome phase, the patient complains of day-by-day worsening of the fever, myalgias, and nausea, yet the physical examination is unremarkable. The presence of acute rhinitis, otitis, and sinusitis, and the occurrence of cough among the initial symptoms are *not* seen in HCPS. The only consistent laboratory finding in prodromal HCPS is thrombocytopenia. Serial platelet counts show the count declining rapidly by at least $40,000 \times mm^{-3}$ during a 24-hour period, and in almost all cases, the platelet count falls below $110,000 \times mm^{-3}$. Other nonspecific abnormalities include elevated lactate dehydrogenase (LDH), AST and ALT enzymes, and a metabolic (lactic) acidosis. During the transition into the cardiopulmonary phase, however, two distinctive cellular elements enter the blood. The triad of thrombocytopenia, left shift of the myeloid series with circulating myelocytes, and immunoblasts appearing as large atypical lymphocytes with azurophilic cytoplasm, is a relatively sensitive and specific presumptive diagnosis of HCPS. Definitive diagnosis relies on detecting antihantavirus IgM antibody in serum, already present during the prodrome IgG antibody persists for years after convalescence.

■ STABILIZATION AND TRANSPORT TO THE ICU

When sufficient suspicion of HCPS is aroused, the patient should be transported to a facility where cardiovascular and ventilation support is available. Initial fluid resuscitation should attempt to minimize crystalloid volume used because this may exacerbate pulmonary edema but can be administered as long as oxygenation can be maintained easily. When advanced pulmonary edema is present, even colloids may leak into the alveoli because the pulmonary capillary-endothelial barrier is so abnormal that all plasma proteins leak. Even if the patient is stable, dobutamine should be prepared and available for use in transport if the patient deteriorates. All drugs used in advanced cardiac life support should be available. High-flow oxygen masks should be used when desaturation occurs and the trachea intubated if they fail to provide adequate oxygen saturation.

■ CARDIOVASCULAR SUPPORT

Dobutamine is the best inotrope to support cardiac output and mean blood pressure as it allows afterload reduction, which is typically elevated, in the cardiogenic shock phase. A flow-directed pulmonary artery catheter should be placed even in milder presentations of the disease because the decrease in cardiac function is often underestimated. When dobutamine alone is insufficient to support cardiovascular function, dopamine and norepinephrine at high dosages should be used. When terminal shock supervenes, we have used epinephrine boluses of 0.5 to 1 mg every 3 to 5 minutes while instituting extracorporeal membrane oxygenator (ECMO) therapy. ECMO is used when cardiac output falls in the face of rapidly increased pressor therapy, cardiogenic shock (<2.2 L/min/m²), ventricular arrhythmias, particularly ventricular tachycardia or fibrillation, or electromechanical dissociation. Venoarterial ECMO allows the provision of up to 6 L/min cardiac output and has been applied successfully in some moribund patients.

■ RESPIRATORY SUPPORT

Tracheal intubation is used when intractable hypoxemia occurs. We use high inspired oxygen concentrations and positive end-expiratory pressure (PEEP) at levels above 12 cm H_2O, which may minimize pulmonary edema fluid production. Pressure-control ventilation with paralysis is preferred, usually without inverse-ratio ventilation. Inhaled nitric oxide therapy has been used in one surviving case but cannot be recommended until further use substantiates its efficacy and safety.

■ ADJUNCTIVE THERAPY

There is no available antiviral therapy approved for use by the FDA, although a randomized, placebo-controlled trial of ribavirin is currently under way in the United States and Canada. High-dose corticosteroids are administered for HCPS caused by Andes virus infection in Argentina and Chile, with anecdotal evidence supporting their use. Glucocorticoids were studied in small randomized trials for the related hantaviral illness hemorrhagic fever with renal syndrome in Korea. Improvements in survival during the shock and oliguria phases were offset by increases in nosocomial infection-related mortality during the recovery phase.

Suggested Reading

Crowley MR, et al: Successful treatment of adults with severe Hantavirus pulmonary syndrome with extracorporeal membrane oxygenation, *Crit Care Med* 26:409, 1998.

Duchin JS, et al: Hantavirus pulmonary syndrome: a clinical description of 17 patients with a newly recognized disease, *N Engl J Med* 330:949, 1994.

Hallin GW, et al: Hantavirus pulmonary syndrome: experience at the University of New Mexico hospital, *Crit Care Med* 24:252, 1996.

Koster FT, Jenison SA: Hantaviruses. In Gorbach SL, Bartlett JG, Blacklow NR, eds: *Infectious diseases*, ed 2, Philadelphia, 1998, Saunders.

Levy H, Simpson SQ: Hantavirus pulmonary syndrome, *Am J Respir Crit Care Med* 149:1710, 1994.

RABIES

Geetika Sharma

Rabies is a viral infection transmitted in the saliva of infected animals. The infection is widespread in some animal species and occasionally is transmitted to humans. Over the last 50 years, the incidence of rabies has declined significantly in the industrialized world, although developing nations still have a high case rate. The geographic distribution of human cases generally follows the distribution of animal cases, but persons returning from endemic areas may import the disease to nonendemic areas. As rabies in domestic animals is better controlled, human cases resulting from wild animal exposure have become relatively more common. Bat rabies has become an important source of exposure in the United States.

■ PATHOGENESIS AND IMMUNITY

The rabies virus is highly neurotropic and is restricted to the nervous tissue during most of the course of infection. There is no viremia in rabies. After inoculation, the virus may enter the peripheral nerves immediately, but usually there is an incubation period during which the virus is amplified. The virus then crosses the myoneural junction and enters the nervous system through the unmyelinated sensory and motor axons. Rabies can be prevented only by postexposure immunization during this incubation period and before the virus enters the central nervous system (CNS). The virus then moves rapidly through the axons until it reaches the spinal ganglion. At this time, the first symptoms of the disease process (i.e., pain and paresthesia at the wound site) may appear. The virus then disseminates rapidly in the CNS, causing a rapidly progressive encephalitis that is almost always fatal.

■ CLINICAL PRESENTATION

The clinical course in humans is acute, usually progressing from initial symptoms to death within 2 to 3 weeks even with intensive supportive care. The incubation period of rabies can vary from a few days to several years. The length of the incubation period varies with the infecting strain and is thought to be inversely related to the size of the inoculum and the proximity of the bite to the central nervous system. Subsequent clinical course can be described in three stages. In the prodromal stage, symptoms include fever, anorexia, nausea, vomiting, and generalized malaise. Approximately half of the patients develop pain or paresthesias at the wound site. Within a few days, neurologic manifestations such as anxiety, agitation, irritability, and insomnia may manifest. Acute neurologic stage follows with objective signs of CNS involvement. Most patients have furious rabies characterized by marked hyperactivity, disorientation, hallucination, or bizarre behavior. This hyperactivity later becomes intermittent and may be spontaneous or precipitated by tactile, auditory, or visual stimuli. Hydrophobia (spasm of the pharynx and larynx provoked by drinking or the sight of water) or aerophobia (similar effect produced by blowing air on the face of the patient) are considered hallmarks of the disease. Seizures may also occur during this stage, as can dysfunction of the autonomic nervous system. A few patients die during this stage, but most go on to develop progressive paralysis and eventually coma. In some patients, the paralytic state dominates the entire clinical picture. Paralysis or paresis involves the proximal muscles and can be accompanied by constipation, urinary retention, and respiratory failure. In patients receiving intensive supportive care, the average duration of illness between onset of paralysis and death is 7 days. Once neurologic symptoms have developed, survival is rare. The only survivors recorded so far had received postexposure prophylaxis or had previously been vaccinated.

DIAGNOSIS

Although human rabies in the United States is rare, it is underdiagnosed. The differential diagnosis can be difficult if a history of animal exposure is not obtained. Hydrophobia and aerophobia are pathognomic when present but may be absent in some cases. Rabies should be considered in the differential diagnosis of any rapidly progressive encephalitis even if a history of bite is not available. Tetanus, Guillain-Barré syndrome, transverse myelitis, and toxic ingestions should be considered in the differential diagnosis. It is also important to exclude other treatable encehalitides such as herpes encephalitis.

Routine laboratory tests and diagnostic studies are of little value in the diagnosis of rabies. Examination of the cerebrospinal fluid (CSF) may show leucocytosis, but protein and glucose assays are often normal. Computed tomography (CT) scan and magnetic resonance imaging (MRI) may be normal even in the presence of advanced rabies encephalitis. Therefore specific diagnostic tests are necessary for diagnosis and include virus antigen detection, serologic studies, virus culture, and histopathologic examination. Virus antigen can be detected when a 6-mm punch biopsy of the skin from the nape of the neck is taken and sent for immunofluorescent rabies antibody staining. This detects rabies antigen in sensory nerve endings at the base of hair follicles. This test is positive in 50% of patients in the first week of illness and more thereafter. Immunofluorescent antibody staining of the epithelial cells of cornea in the corneal impression test can also help with diagnosis. Seroconversion, in unvaccinated individuals, usually happens in the second week of illness, although it can be delayed by several days. In individuals who have been vaccinated, it is difficult to distinguish serologically between infection and

vaccination, but measurable spinal fluid levels and very high serum antibody titers suggest infection. Rabies virus can also be cultured from saliva, throat, tracheal secretions, CSF, or brain biopsy specimens but the yield is low. Postmortem examination of the brain shows perivascular inflammation of the gray matter, neuronal degeneration, and the characteristic cytoplasmic inclusions called the *Negri bodies*.

TREATMENT

Specific treatment for rabies is not available. Therefore treatment efforts are concentrated on preventing and treating complications of established infection and protecting those who come in contact with the patient from virus exposure. Neither vaccine nor rabies immunoglobulin increases survival in symptomatic patients and should be avoided. Steroids should also be avoided in the treatment of cerebral edema if it develops. Universal precautions should be followed by hospital staff, and respiratory precautions are recommended for suctioning. Postexposure prophylaxis is recommended for contacts who were bitten or had clear contamination of mucous membranes to the patient's saliva, urine, or other body tissue.

PREVENTION

Because rabies is almost invariably fatal, emphasis should be placed on preventing human infection. Preventive measures include control of rabies in animals, especially domestic animals, preexposure prophylaxis for those at increased risk of being exposed to the virus, and postexposure prophylaxis to persons who have been exposed.

PREEXPOSURE PROPHYLAXIS

Preexposure prophylaxis should be offered to persons at high risk for exposure to rabies. Three rabies vaccines are currently available in the United States. These include human diploid cell vaccine (HDCV), rabies vaccine adsorbed (RVA), and purified chick embryo cell vaccine (PCEC). A regimen of three 1.0-ml injections of HDCV, RVA, or PCEC is given intramuscularly (IM) in the deltoid region on days 0, 7, and 21 or 28, respectively. HDCV is also approved for intradermal injections in a dose of 0.1 ml to be given in three doses on days 0, 7, and 21 or 28 for preexposure prophylaxis. It comes packaged for reconstitution just before administration. Persons who work with rabies virus in research laboratories or vaccine-production facilities are at highest risk for exposure and should have rabies antibody titers checked every 6 months. Other laboratory workers (e.g., those performing rabies diagnostic testing), spelunkers, veterinarians and staff, and animal-control and wildlife officers in areas where animal rabies is enzootic should also have antibody measurements done every 2 years. Booster doses (IM or intradermal [ID]) of vaccine should be administered to maintain an adequate serum titer. The immunization practices advisory committee (ACIP) recommends three preexposure doses of the HDCV vaccine given IM or ID at 0, 7, and 21 or 28 days. This ensures both seroconversion and adequate duration of protective antibody. Routine serologic testing after vaccination is not needed as seroconversion has been uniform. Patients who are immunosuppressed or taking medications such as chloroquine phosphate, which may interfere with antibody response to the vaccine, should postpone preexposure vaccinations and consider avoiding activities for which rabies preexposure prophylaxis is indicated. When this is not possible, they should be vaccinated and their antibody titers checked. In these cases, failures to seroconvert after the third dose should be managed in consultation with appropriate public health officials.

■ POSTEXPOSURE PROPHYLAXIS

The following factors should be considered before initiating specific antirabies prophylaxis.

Evaluation of Involved Animal Species

Raccoons, skunks, foxes, and coyotes are the wild animals most often infected with the rabies virus. Patients exposed to these animals should receive postexposure prophylaxis as soon as possible. Table 1 provides a postexposure prophylaxis schedule. Bats have been increasingly implicated as important wildlife reservoirs of rabies. Recent data suggest that transmission of rabies virus can occur from minor, even unrecognized bites from bats. Therefore rabies postexposure prophylaxis is recommended for all persons with bite, scratch, or mucous membrane exposure to a bat and should be considered if the history indicates that a bat was physically present, even if the person is unable to reliably report contact that could have resulted in a bite. Such a situation may arise when a bat bite causes an insignificant wound or the circumstances do not allow recognition of contact, such as when a bat is found in the room of a sleeping person or near a previously unattended child. In recent years, a significant number of rabies cases have been attributable to bats. This presumably reflects a greater likelihood that exposure to bats may be ignored or go unnoticed. The likelihood of rabies in domestic animals such as dogs, cats, cattle, and ferrets varies in different regions of the United States and is reported most commonly along the U.S.-Mexico border.

If the animal has been vaccinated, it is unlikely to be infected; if not vaccinated but otherwise healthy, the animal should be confined and observed for 10 days. Any illness during this time should be evaluated by a veterinarian and the public health department. Vaccination can be withheld if the animal remains healthy during this time. Although uncommon in the United States, dog bites remain a common cause of rabies in the developing world, especially India and China. Small rodents (e.g., squirrels, hamsters, guinea pigs, gerbils, chipmunks, rats, mice) and lagomorphs (including rabbits and hares) are almost never infected with the rabies virus and have not been known to transmit rabies to humans. Large rodents such as woodchucks are sometimes found to be infected. Therefore, in cases involving rodent exposure, the state or local health department should be consulted before initiating prophylaxis.

Type of Exposure

Rabies is transmitted when the virus in the saliva of infected animals is introduced into bite wounds or open cuts in skin or mucous membranes. Any penetration of the skin by teeth represents a potential risk of rabies transmission. Nonbite exposures of highest risk appear to be among persons who were exposed to a large amount of aerosolized virus in caves containing millions of bats. Contamination of open wounds, abrasions, or mucous membranes with saliva or other infectious material such as neural tissue also constitutes a nonbite exposure. As noted, bites from bats may be minor and can go unnoticed. Human-to-human transmission has been documented in recipients of corneal transplants when the donors had died of an illness compatible with or proved to be rabies. Bite or nonbite exposure to infected humans theoretically can transmit rabies though there has been no documented example of this. Health care workers who had exposure of mucous membranes or nonintact skin to potentially infectious material (e.g., saliva) should receive postexposure prophylaxis.

Circumstances of Exposure

An unprovoked attack by a domestic animal is more likely than a provoked attack to indicate that the animal is rabid.

Postexposure therapy for rabies is highly effective, and no failures have been recorded in patients who have received all three arms of treatment. Failures have occurred outside the United States when some deviation was made from the recommended protocol. Preventive therapy should be

Table 1 Rabies Postexposure Prophylaxis Schedule

VACCINATION STATUS	TREATMENT	COMMENTS
Unvaccinated	Wound cleaning	Soap and water and, if available, povidone-iodine solution
	HRIG	20 IU/kg body weight infiltrated into and around the wound completely if possible, and remainder into gluteal area
	Vaccine; HDCV, RVA	1.0 ml IM (deltoid) on day 0, 3, 7, 14, and 28
		Do not give vaccine and HR1G in the same syringe or same site
Previously vaccinated	Wound cleaning	With soap and water and, if possible, with povidone-iodine
	HRIG	HRIG should not be given
	Vaccine; HDCV, RVA	1.0 ml IM (deltoid) on days 0 and 3

HRIG, Human rabies immunoglobulin; *HDCV,* human diploid cell vaccine; *RVA,* rabies vaccine absorbed.

instituted as soon as possible after a potential rabies exposure. Before beginning therapy, every effort should be made to ascertain risk of infection, but unnecessary delay should be avoided because it can increase the likelihood of vaccine failure. Therapy should include the following measures (see Table 1).

Local Wound Treatment

Wounds should be washed thoroughly with 20% soap solution and, if available, a virucidal agent such as povidone-iodine. Tetanus prophylaxis and antibiotics may be necessary to prevent secondary infection. Local wound treatment should also include infiltrating the wound with rabies immune globulin.

Rabies Immunoglobulin Administration

A single dose of 20 IU/kg of human rabies immunoglobulin (HRIG) should be given at the beginning of antirabies prophylaxis. HRIG provides protection for the first 2 weeks before the vaccine elicits an antibody response. It should be given to all patients except those who have previously received a cell culture vaccine as preexposure or postexposure prophylaxis or have documented rabies antibody titers after receiving another vaccine. HRIG should be given even if there is a significant delay between exposure and initiation of postexposure prophylaxis. If not given when the vaccination was begun, it can be given up to the seventh day of vaccine administration, after which the vaccine should have elicited an antibody response.

If anatomically possible, the full dose of HRIG should be infiltrated into the wound. Any remaining volume should be administered IM at a site distant from the vaccine site. It should never be administered in the same syringe as the vaccine.

Vaccine Administration

Rabies vaccines induce an active immune response that includes the production of neutralizing antibodies. This antibody response requires approximately 7 to 10 days to develop and usually persists for greater than or equal to 2 years. Any one of the three vaccine preparations, HDCV, RVA, or PCEC can be administered in a 1-ml dose given IM in the deltoid area. In children, it may be given in the anterolateral area of the thigh. The vaccine should never be given in the gluteal area because of a lower antibody response and possibility of failure. The dose is given as soon as possible (day 0) and then repeated on days 3, 7, 14, and 28. Postexposure therapy for previously vaccinated individuals should include only two IM doses, one immediately and one after 3 days. Previously vaccinated individuals are those who have received a complete preexposure or postexposure regimen with HDCV, RVA, or PCEC, or those who have received another vaccine and had a documented rabies antibody titer. These individuals also should not be given RIG.

Adverse reactions to the current vaccines have been noted and include local reactions such as pain, erythema, swelling, or itching at the injection site. Mild systemic reactions such as headaches, nausea, and abdominal pain have also been reported. A small percentage of patients experience immune complex reactions characterized by generalized urticaria, arthralgias, arthritis, angioedema, nausea, vomiting, fever, and malaise. This typically develops 2 to 21 days after administration of the booster dose of HDCV. These reactions have been attributed to the presence of betapropiolactone-altered human albumin in the HDCV. Local reactions can usually be managed with antiinflammatory agents. Steroids should not be used because they can interfere with the development of immunity after vaccination. When a person has a serious hypersensitivity reaction to the vaccine, revaccination should be supervised carefully and undertaken only after careful consideration of the risk of acquiring rabies. Epinephrine should be readily available to counteract anaphylactic reactions. RIG can also cause pain and low-grade fever. There have been no specific reported adverse reactions to HRIG, although immunoglobulin itself has been associated with angioneurotic edema, nephrotic syndrome, and anaphylaxis. Many developing countries use inactivated nerve tissue vaccines made from the brains of adult animals or suckling mice. Nerve tissue vaccine (NTV) is reported to induce neuroparalytic reactions among approximately 1 per 200 to 1 per 2000 persons vaccinated; suckling mouse brain vaccine (SMBV) causes reactions in approximately 1 per 8000 persons vaccinated. The vaccines HDCV and PCEC are cell culture–derived and not of nerve tissue origin. In addition, unpurified antirabies serum of equine origin might still be used in some countries where neither RIG nor ERIG is available. The use of this antirabies serum is associated with higher rates of serious adverse reactions, including anaphylaxis. Pregnancy is not considered a contraindication for postexposure prophylaxis.

■ RABIES IN TRAVELERS

Rabies vaccination is not a requirement for entry into any country; however, travelers to rabies-endemic countries should be warned about the risk of acquiring rabies outside the United States. Dogs are the main reservoir of the disease in many developing countries, but other animals may carry the virus; therefore all animal bites should be evaluated. Travelers bitten by an animal should notify local health authorities immediately to assess the need for rabies postexposure prophylaxis. Upon returning to the United States, travelers who have been bitten should contact their physician or state health department as soon as possible. Additional treatment may be necessary if the patients had received an inadequate regimen or vaccines of nerve tissue origin. Preexposure vaccination should be considered for international travelers likely to come in contact with animals in areas where rabies is present and where immediate access to appropriate medical care, including biologics, may be difficult. Thus the need for preexposure rabies vaccinations depends both on the destination of the traveler and on the traveler's anticipated activities. Preexposure vaccination greatly simplifies but does not eliminate the need for postexposure treatment. For international travelers, preexposure vaccination can be given in three doses over 3 to 4 weeks before travel. The vaccination series should be initiated early enough to allow all three doses to be completed before departure. Travelers who will also be taking mefloquine or chloroquine for malaria prevention should complete their three-dose rabies vaccination series *before* beginning these medications, which may interfere with the antibody response to rabies vaccine. Thus, if the rabies series is given intradermally, it should be initiated at least 1 month before travel. If this timing is not possible, the rabies vaccine should be given intramuscularly because this dose/route provides a sufficient margin of safety for persons who must also take antimalarial drugs.

Suggested Reading

Noah DL, et al: Epidemiology of human rabies in the United States, 1980 to 1996, *Ann Intern Med* 128:922, 1998.

Recommendations of the Advisory Committee on Immunization Practices (ACIP), *MMWR* 48(RR-1):1, 1999.

Strady A, et al: Antibody persistence following preexposure regimens of cell-culture rabies vaccines: 10-year follow-up and proposal for a new booster policy, *J Infect Dis* 177:1290, 1998.

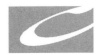
SYPHILIS AND OTHER TREPONEMATOSES

Adaora A. Adimora

Treponemes are members of the family Spirochaetaceae, which also contains *Borrelia* and *Leptospira*. Although most treponemes do not cause disease in human beings, a few cause substantial morbidity. This chapter briefly reviews the clinical manifestations and treatment of syphilis in adults and the nonvenereal treponematoses, yaws, pinta, and bejel.

■ SYPHILIS

Clinical Manifestations

Like other treponemal diseases, the clinical manifestations of syphilis are divided into early and late stages. Early syphilis is further divided into primary, secondary, and early latent stages. During the latent syphilis stage, patients have positive serologic tests for syphilis but no other signs of disease. The Centers for Disease Control and Prevention (CDC) classifies patients in the latent stage as having early syphilis if they acquired infection during the preceding year. Otherwise, persons with latent disease are classified as having either late latent syphilis or latent syphilis of unknown duration. Although clinical staging is useful for diagnosis and treatment, it is also imprecise; overlap between stages is relatively common.

Primary and Secondary Syphilis

Treponema pallidum, the causative agent of syphilis, usually enters the body through breaks in the epithelium that occur during sexual contact. Some organisms persist at the site of entry, while others disseminate via the lymphatic system throughout the body, proliferating and stimulating an immune response. The incubation period of primary syphilis is usually about 21 days, although extremes of 10 to 90 days have been noted.

The first clinical manifestation is usually a chancre at the site of genital trauma. The chancre begins as a red macule that subsequently becomes papular and then ulcerates. The lesion is painless and has a well-defined margin and thickened, rubbery base. If untreated, the chancre persists for 3 to 6 weeks and then heals. Nontender regional lymphadenopathy also develops.

In untreated individuals, *T. pallidum* disseminates throughout the body, and secondary syphilis develops about 3 to 6 weeks after the chancre's onset. Common symptoms include malaise, headaches, sore throat, fever, musculoskeletal pains, and weight loss. Physical examination reveals rash in 75% to 100%, regional or generalized lymphadenopathy in 50% to 85%, and mucosal ulceration in 5% to 30% of persons with secondary syphilis. The appearance of the rash can vary greatly, but lesions are often maculopapular or papulosquamous and often involve the entire body, including the palms and soles. Broad, flat lesions, known as *condylomata lata,* may develop in warm, moist areas, such as the scrotum, vulva, or perianal regions. Patchy alopecia and shallow painless mucosa ulcerations, called *mucous patches,* may also be seen. Like the chancre, these manifestations of secondary syphilis resolve spontaneously with or without therapy. A small proportion of patients develop complications, such as hepatitis, syphilitic glomerulonephritis with nephrotic syndrome, anterior uveitis, choroiditis, arthritis, bursitis, or osteitis. A wide variety of neurologic complications, including meningitis, cranial nerve palsies, transverse myelitis, nerve deafness, and cerebral artery thrombosis, can occur.

Neurosyphilis

T. pallidum often invades the meninges during the course of secondary syphilis. Inadequately treated infection may spontaneously resolve or may result in either asymptomatic meningeal involvement or symptomatic acute meningitis. Further progression of infection causes persistent asymptomatic neurosyphilis or a variety of neurologic syndromes, such as meningovascular syphilis, tabes, or paresis.

Syphilitic meningitis most commonly occurs during the first year of infection. Most patients do not have a rash of secondary syphilis when they present with syphilitic meningitis, and meningitis is sometimes the first manifestation of syphilis. The clinical picture may suggest a viral aseptic meningitis, as patients may present with headache, fever, stiff neck, photophobia, and a mild cerebrospinal fluid (CSF) lymphocytic pleocytosis. Differential diagnosis includes meningitis caused by enteroviruses and other viruses, tuberculosis, cryptococcus, and Lyme disease. Cerebral involvement may result in seizures or hemiplegia. Cranial nerve palsies are especially common. Characteristic CSF findings include a lymphocytic pleocytosis, increased protein, and hypoglycorrhachia in slightly less than half of cases. Nontreponemal serologic testing is positive in blood and CSF. Penicillin yields a prompt response.

Meningovascular syphilis usually occurs about 5 to 12 years after infection in patients between the ages of 30 and 50 years and may involve the cerebrum, brainstem, or spinal cord. The pathophysiology involves chronic meningitis and infarction due to syphilitic endarteritis. In cerebrovascular syphilis, the middle cerebral artery is most commonly involved, and hemiparesis, aphasia, and seizures commonly occur. CSF usually reveals a lymphocytic pleocytosis with increased protein and a positive CSF Venereal Disease Research Laboratory (VDRL) test. Spinal syphilis, a relatively uncommon entity, may present as meningomyelitis or transverse myelitis.

The major parenchymatous forms of neurosyphilis are general paresis and tabes dorsalis, which tend to occur 15 to 20 and 20 to 25 years, respectively, after initial infection. Both are now uncommon diseases.

General paresis is a chronic meningoencephalitis that results from direct invasion of the brain by *T. pallidum* and combines both psychiatric and neurologic manifestations. Early symptoms, such as irritability, memory loss, headache, and personality changes, may evolve into emotional lability, paranoia, and confusion. Pupillary abnormalities occur in more than half of patients with general paresis. Abnormal reflexes, slurred speech, and tremors are also common. In untreated patients, the interval between onset of symptoms and death can range from a few months to about 5 years.

Serum nontreponemal serologic tests are reactive in 95% to 100% of patients with generalized paresis. CSF VDRL is usually positive, but a negative result alone does not exclude the diagnosis. Differential diagnosis includes Alzheimer's disease, chronic alcoholism, and multiple sclerosis.

Tabes dorsalis is characterized by lightning pains and various combinations of other neurologic signs and symptoms, such as ataxia; bladder disturbances; pupillary abnormalities; absent ankle or knee reflexes; Romberg's sign; impaired vibratory and position sense; and development of extremely large, unstable, painless joints known as Charcot's joints. Lightning pains are paroxysms of severe stabbing pains, which usually occur in the legs. Although most patients have positive serum VDRL tests, 10% of patients with tabes have nonreactive serum VDRL serology. CSF may be normal or may reveal lymphocytic pleocytosis and elevated protein.

Nonneurologic Manifestations of Tertiary Syphilis

Syphilitic heart disease, now an uncommon cause of cardiovascular disease, occurs 15 to 30 years after initial infection. During the early phases of infection, *T. pallidum* organisms disseminate to the heart and lodge in the aortic wall, where they may cause endarteritis of the vasa vasorum of the aorta with resultant scarring and destruction of the vessel's wall. Major cardiac manifestations include thoracic aneurysm, aortic regurgitation (without associated aortic stenosis), and coronary ostial stenosis.

Late benign syphilis is another now uncommon form of tertiary syphilis. It results from the chronic inflammatory response to *T. pallidum* and the formation of a granulomatous type of lesion called a *gumma*. Gummas may be ulcerative, nodular, or noduloulcerative and most commonly occur in the skin and bones but may also invade the viscera, muscles, and other structures.

Laboratory Tests
Direct Microscopic Examination
Direct microscopic examination can provide immediate diagnosis of primary and secondary syphilis. Darkfield microscopy must be used because *T. pallidum's* narrow width

(0.15 μm), renders the organism below the level of resolution of light microscopy. Wet preparations can be made from the skin or mucous membrane lesions of primary or secondary syphilis; examination reveals tightly coiled organisms 6 to 14 μm long and 0.25 to 0.30 μm wide, with corkscrew motility. When examination of specimens must be delayed or oral lesions evaluated, direct fluorescent antibody testing can be useful. This test specifically detects *T. pallidum* and eliminates confusion with oral treponemal saprophytes whose morphology is similar to *T. pallidum*.

Serologic Tests
Serologic tests for syphilis measure either nonspecific nontreponemal antibody or specific treponemal antibody.

Nontreponemal antibody tests measure IgG and IgM antibodies formed by the host against lipid from *T. pallidum's* cell surfaces. These tests are used to screen for disease and disease activity; titers fall progressively over time and should decrease in response to therapy. The following nontreponemal tests are commonly used: VDRL test, rapid plasma reagin (RPR), automated reagin screen test (ART), unheated serum reagin test (USR), and the reagin screen test (RST). False-positive nontreponemal test results occur in 1% to 2% of the general population, but false-positive titers are usually less than 1:8. False-negative results may be seen in 10% to 20% of primary, latent, and late syphilis.

Specific treponemal antibody tests are usually used to confirm a current or past diagnosis of syphilis. These tests detect antibodies formed in response to treponemal antigens. Treponemal tests usually remain reactive after treatment, but a small proportion of infected persons become seronegative. Commonly used treponemal tests include the fluorescent antibody absorption (FTA-ABS), microhemagglutination assay for antibodies to *T. pallidum* (MHA-TP), and the hemagglutination treponemal test for syphilis (HATTS).

Cerebrospinal Fluid Evaluation
CSF should be examined in all syphilis patients with neurologic signs or symptoms and those with latent syphilis if any of the following are present: eye involvement, other evidence of active syphilis, human immunodeficiency virus (HIV) infection, or treatment failure. CSF of patients with latent syphilis should also be examined when duration of infection is known to be less than 1 year if nonpenicillin therapy is planned or the serum RPR or VDRL is greater than 1:32.

When CSF specimens are free of blood contamination, a positive CSF VDRL test almost always indicates neurosyphilis. Diagnosis is unclear, however, in patients with negative CSF serology, a positive blood serologic test, increased CSF protein levels, and slight pleocytosis. Although such patients may have asymptomatic neurosyphilis, other diagnoses should be considered.

Treatment and Follow-Up
Treatment and follow-up are outlined in Tables 1 and 2.

Syphilis in Persons with HIV Infection
Because syphilis and HIV infection share means of transmission and other risk factors, both infections often coexist. Moreover, increasing evidence suggests that syphilis, like

Table 1   Management of Syphilis in Nonpregnant Adults Without Known HIV Infection

PRIMARY AND SECONDARY SYPHILIS
Treatment
   Benzathine penicillin G, 2.4 million U IM once
   If penicillin allergy:
      Doxycycline, 100 mg PO bid for 2 wk *or* tetracycline, 500 mg PO qid for 2 wk
      Alternative if compliance is certain:
         Erythromycin, 500 mg PO qid for 2 wk
Management and follow-up
   HIV testing
   If evidence of neurologic disease, evaluate for neurosyphilis
   If evidence of eye disease, do slit-lamp examination
   Repeat serology and clinical examination at 6 and 12 mo
   If symptoms persist or recur, or if four-fold increase in RPR or VDRL titer occurs, repeat HIV testing and re-treat
   If RPR or VDRL titers do not fall four-fold within 6 mo of treatment, repeat HIV testing and consider LP

LATENT SYPHILIS
Treatment
   Early latent syphilis (duration <1 yr)
      Benzathine penicillin G, 2.4 million U IM once
      If penicillin allergy:
         Doxycycline, 100 mg PO bid for 2 wk *or* tetracycline, 500 mg PO qid for 2 wk
   Late latent syphilis or latent syphilis of unknown duration
      Benzathine penicillin G, 2.4 million U IM qwk, for 3 wk
      If penicillin allergy:
         Doxycycline, 100 mg PO bid for 4 wk *or* tetracycline, 500 mg PO qid for 4 wk
Management and follow-up
   HIV testing
   Clinical evaluation for evidence of tertiary disease (e.g., aortitis, neurosyphilis, gumma, iritis)
   Examine CSF before treatment if any of the following are present:
      Neurologic or ophthalmic signs or symptoms
      Other evidence of active tertiary syphilis
      Treatment failure
      HIV infection with late latent syphilis or syphilis of unknown duration
   Repeat quantitative VDRL or RPR at 6, 12, and 24 mo
      Evaluate for neurosyphilis and retreat if:
         Serologic titers increase four-fold or
         An initially high titer (≥1:32) fails to fall at least four-fold within 12-24 mo or
         Patient develops signs or symptoms consistent with syphilis

LATE SYPHILIS (GUMMA OR CARDIOVASCULAR SYPHILIS)
Treatment
   Benzathine penicillin G, 2.4 million U IM weekly for 3 wk
   If penicillin allergy, use treatment for late latent syphilis
Management
   Examine CSF

NEUROSYPHILIS
Treatment
   Aqueous crystalline penicillin G, 3 million to 4 million U IV q4h for 10-14 days; follow with benzathine penicillin G, 2.4 million U IM
   Alternative (if compliance is certain):
      Procaine penicillin, 2.4 million U IM qd for 14 days, plus probenecid, 500 mg PO qid for 14 days; follow with benzathine penicillin G, 2.4 million U IM
Management
   HIV testing
   Repeat CSF examination every 6 mo until CSF cell count is normal
   Consider re-treatment if cell count has not decreased after 6 mo or if CSF is not normal after 2 yr

HIV, Human immunodeficiency virus; *RPR,* rapid plasma reagin; *VDRL,* Venereal Disease Research Laboratory test; *LP,* lumbar puncture; *CSF,* cerebrospinal fluid.

other genital ulcer diseases, facilitates HIV transmission. The clinical impact of HIV infection on the course of syphilis remains poorly defined and controversial. Clinical observation and case reports suggest that HIV-infected patients may experience a more aggressive course of syphilis, and neurosyphilis is common. The prevalence of CSF abnor- malities among HIV-positive patients with asymptomatic syphilis appears to be high. Concerns have been raised about the adequacy of single-dose benzathine penicillin G for treatment of early syphilis in HIV-positive patients because some investigators have isolated *T. pallidum* and identified CSF abnormalities in HIV-infected patients with secondary

Table 2   Treatment of HIV-Positive Patients with Syphilis

PRIMARY AND SECONDARY SYPHILIS

Treatment

Benzathine penicillin G, 2.4 million U IM once

Alternative: benzathine penicillin G, 2.4 million U IM weekly × 3 wk

If penicillin allergy: manage according to recommendations for HIV-negative patients with primary and secondary syphilis (see Table 1).

Management

Clinical and serologic evaluation 3, 6, 9, 12, and 24 mo after therapy

Examine CSF if RPR or VDRL titers fail to show four-fold decrease by 4 mo or there is other evidence of treatment failure

If CSF normal, re-treat with penicillin G, 2.4 million U IM weekly × 3 wk

If CSF suggests neurosyphilis, treat for neurosyphilis as in Table 1

EARLY LATENT SYPHILIS

Manage and treat according to recommendations for HIV-negative patients with primary and secondary syphilis (see Table 1)

LATE LATENT SYPHILIS OR LATENT SYPHILIS OF UNKNOWN DURATION

Examine CSF

If CSF normal, give benzathine penicillin G, 2.4 million U IM weekly × 3 wk

If CSF suggests neurosyphilis, treat for neurosyphilis as in Table 1

Management

Clinical and serologic evaluation 6, 12, 18, and 24 mo after therapy

Examine CSF and re-treat accordingly if:

Clinical symptoms develop or RPR or VDRL titers rise four-fold at any time or RPR or VDRL titer fails to fall fourfold between 12 and 24 months

NEUROSYPHILIS

Treatment and management as in Table 1

CSF, Cerebrospinal fluid; *RPR,* rapid plasma reagin; *VDRL,* Venereal Disease Research Laboratory test; *HIV,* human immunodeficiency virus.

syphilis after this regimen. However, a randomized, controlled trial suggests that current treatment recommendations are adequate for most HIV-infected patients with early syphilis and that the presence of *T. pallidum* in CSF before treatment does not predict treatment failure. Thus the limited prospective data available suggest that HIV infection does not significantly change the presentation, clinical course, or response to treatment of syphilis.

Nevertheless, several points remain virtually uncontested. Careful evaluation and follow-up of all HIV-positive patients with syphilis are essential. CSF should be evaluated to exclude central nervous system (CNS) involvement in all HIV-infected syphilis patients with latent syphilis or neurologic signs or symptoms. Vigilant follow-up is essential to document resolution of infection and allow prompt evaluation and retreatment if relapse, reinfection, or other complications occur. HIV-positive patients with syphilis should be treated with penicillin if at all possible; those with a history of hypersensitivity should undergo desensitization.

■ NONVENEREAL TREPONEMATOSES

Yaws, pinta, and bejel (endemic syphilis) are caused respectively by *T. pallidum,* subspecies *pertenue; T. carateum;* and *T. pallidum,* subspecies *endemicum.* These diseases, seen mainly in tropical and subtropical regions, are transmitted by direct contact with infected skin lesions and not primarily by sexual contact. Like venereal syphilis, these diseases have self-limited primary and secondary stages, a latent stage, and a late stage with destructive lesions. The causative agents are morphologically indistinguishable from *T. pallidum,* sub-

species *pallidum,* and the serologic responses they elicit are identical to those of venereal syphilis. Diagnosis can be made by darkfield examination of lesions or serologic testing. Long-acting penicillin G, the treatment of choice, has dramatically decreased the incidence of these diseases in endemic regions.

Yaws occurs in the tropical regions of Africa, Southeast Asia, South America, and Oceania. About 3 to 5 weeks after infection, papules develop, which enlarge, erode, and then spontaneously heal. A generalized secondary eruption of similar lesions occurs weeks to months later, sometimes associated with osteitis or periostitis. In the late stage, infected persons may develop hyperkeratoses on the palms and soles; plaques, nodules, and ulcers of the skin; and gummatous bone lesions.

Pinta occurs in remote parts of Mexico, Central America, and Colombia. About 7 to 21 days after infection, small, red, pruritic papules develop, which enlarge, become squamous, and merge with other primary lesions. These lesions eventually heal, but residual hypopigmentation persists. Three to twelve months after the appearance of the primary lesions, small scaly papules known as *pintids* appear. These may eventually become brown, gray, or blue and may recur as long as 10 years after initial infection. Depigmented lesions develop in the late stage.

Bejel occurs in Africa and western Asia. Unlike yaws and pinta, bejel is spread not only by direct contact but also by eating and drinking utensils. Primary lesions are seldom seen. Secondary manifestations include mucous patches, condylomata lata, split papules at the angles of the mouth, and lymphadenopathy. Gummatous lesions of the skin, nasopharynx, and bones are common in the late stage.

Suggested Reading

Centers for Disease Control and Prevention: 1998 Sexually transmitted disease treatment guidelines, *MMWR* 147(No. RR-1):28, 1998.

Chulay JD: *Treponema* species (yaws, pinta, bejel). In Mandell GL, Bennett JE, Dolin R, eds: *Principles and practice of infectious diseases,* ed 5, New York, 2000, Churchill Livingstone.

Gordon SM, et al: The response of symptomatic neurosyphilis to high-dose intravenous penicillin G in patients with human immunodeficiency virus infection, *N Engl J Med* 331:1469, 1994.

Gourevitch MN, et al: Effects of HIV infection on the serologic manifestations and response to treatment of syphilis in intravenous drug users, *Ann Intern Med* 118:350, 1993.

Hook EW III, Marra C: Acquired syphilis in adults, *N Engl J Med* 326:1060, 1992.

Musher DM: Early syphilis. Holmes KK, Mardh PA, et al, eds: In *Sexually transmitted diseases,* ed 3, New York, 1999, McGraw-Hill.

Rolfs RT, et al: A randomized trial of enhanced therapy for early syphilis in patients with and without human immunodeficiency virus infection, *N Engl J Med* 337:307, 1997.

Swartz MN, Musher DM, Healy BP: Late syphilis. In Holmes KK, Mardh PA, et al, eds: *Sexually transmitted diseases,* ed 3, New York, 1999, McGraw-Hill.

LYME DISEASE

Janine Evans
Stephen E. Malawista

Lyme disease, a systemic illness caused by the spirochete *Borrelia burgdorferi,* is the most common tickborne disease in the United States. In 1997, 47 states reported 12,801 cases of Lyme disease using the Council of State and Territorial Epidemiologists (CTSE)/Centers for Disease Control and Prevention (CDC) surveillance case definition. Since the original discovery of Lyme arthritis in the mid 1970s, the clinical spectrum has expanded to include a wide variety of organ systems, primarily the skin, joints, nervous system, and heart. Protean symptoms, uncertainty in diagnosis because of the lack of definitive testing methods, and public fear of late sequela of disease often lead to overdiagnosis and overtreatment. Although optimal therapy of many of the clinical features of Lyme disease is unclear, better understanding of the natural history, epidemiology, and pathogenesis of Lyme disease help in the often confusing and difficult decisions related to diagnosis and treatment.

B. burgdorferi has been isolated from blood, skin, cerebrospinal fluid specimens, and (rarely) other specimens from infected patients although, with the exception of skin biopsy specimens, culture of *B. burgdorferi* from sites of infection is a low-yield procedure. *B. burgdorferi* displays phenotypic and genotypic diversity and has been classified into three separate genospecies: species I, which includes all strains studied thus far from the United States and some European and Asian strains, are termed *Borrelia burgdorferi sensu stricto:* species II, *Borrelia garinii;* and species III, *Borrelia afzelli,* are found in Europe and Asia. *B. afzelii* seems primarily associated with a chronic skin lesion, acrodermatitis chronica atrophicans, rare in the United States.

Lyme disease occurs in three principal foci in the United States: the Northeast, the upper Midwest, and the Pacific Coast. These areas correspond to the distribution of the predominant tick vectors of Lyme disease in the United States, *Ixodes scapularis* in the East and Midwest, and *Ixodes pacificus* in northern California. Lyme disease also occurs widely in Europe, where it is transmitted by the sheep tick, *Ixodes ricinus. I. scapularis* have a three-stage, 2-year life cycle. Transovarial passage of *B. burgdorferi* occurs at a low rate. Ticks become infected with spirochetes by feeding on a spirochetemic animal, typically small mammals, during larval and nymphal stages. In highly endemic areas, from 20% to more than 60% of *I. scapularis* carry *B. burgdorferi.* Man is only an incidental host of the tick; contact is typically made in areas of underbrush or high grasses but may occur in well-mown lawns in endemic areas. Lyme disease occurs predominantly during May through July, when nymphal *I. scapularis* feed. Animal models show that transmission is unlikely to occur before a minimum of 36 hours of tick attachment and feeding.

■ CLINICAL MANIFESTATIONS

Clinical features of Lyme disease are typically divided into three general stages, termed *early localized, early disseminated,* and *late persistent* infection. These stages may overlap, and most patients do not exhibit all stages. Direct invasion of the organism with a resultant vigorous inflammatory reaction has been demonstrated to be responsible for many of the clinical manifestations associated with Lyme disease, so the manifestations respond to antibiotic therapy. Some features, such as late neurologic deficits and chronic arthritis, may respond poorly to treatment. It is not absolutely clear that live organisms are responsible for these later symptoms. Seroconversion can occur in asymptomatic individuals but is rare with strict surveillance.

Early Localized Disease

Erythema migrans (EM), the hallmark of Lyme disease, begins at the site of a deer tick bite after 3 to 32 days. It is reported by 60% to 80% of patients, appearing as a centrifugally expanding erythematous macule or papule, often with central clearing. The thigh, groin, and axilla are common sites. The lesion may be warm, pruritic, and painful, but it is often asymptomatic and easily missed if out of sight. Occasionally, these lesions may develop blistering or scabbing in the center; remain an even, intense red without clearing; or develop a bluish discoloration. Spirochetes are present in the EM lesion and can be readily cultured from the expanding edge. Mild musculoskeletal flulike symptoms, such as a low-grade fever, chills, malaise, headache, fatigue, arthralgias, and myalgias, may accompany EM lesions. Theoretically, such symptoms can occur without dissemination of the organism, via local generation of cytokines. Untreated EM resolves after several weeks, and treated lesions clear within several days.

Early Disseminated

In some patients, the spirochete disseminates hematogenously to multiple sites, causing characteristic clinical features. Secondary annular lesions, sites of metastatic foci of *Borrelia* in the skin, develop within days of onset of EM in about half of U.S. patients. They are similar in appearance to EM but are generally smaller, migrate less, and lack indurated centers. In addition to musculoskeletal flulike symptoms, mild hepatitis, splenomegaly, sore throat, nonproductive cough, testicular swelling, conjunctivitis, and regional and generalized lymphadenopathy may sometimes occur during early stages.

Diagnosis of early localized and early disseminated Lyme disease is based on clinical presentation because serologic confirmation is often lacking and culture is not readily available. EM is diagnostic of Lyme disease, although atypical lesions and rashes mimicking EM may be confusing. A history of a tick bite and residence or travel in an endemic area should be sought in patients presenting with rashes compatible with EM or a flulike illness in summer. Specific IgM antibody responses against *B. burgdorferi* develop 2 to 6 weeks after the onset of EM. IgG antibody levels appear approximately 6 weeks after disease onset but may not peak until months or even years into the illness. The highest titers occur during arthritis. Antibodies are typically detected using indirect immunofluorescence, enzyme-linked immunosorbent assay (ELISA), and immunoblotting (Western blot). Antibody responses may persist for months to years after infection.

Late Disease

Late manifestations of Lyme disease typically occur months to years after the initial infection. In the United States, arthritis is the dominant feature of late Lyme disease, reported in approximately 60% of untreated individuals. Less often, individuals develop late chronic neurologic disease. Another late finding (years) associated with this infection is a chronic skin lesion, acrodermatitis chronica atrophicans, well known in Europe but still rare in the United States. These late manifestations are discussed next.

■ THERAPY

Early Lyme Disease

The symptoms of early Lyme disease resolve spontaneously in most cases; therefore the goals of therapy for early localized and mild early disseminated Lyme disease are to shorten the duration of symptoms and reduce the risk of

developing serious late manifestations of infection. Treatment of these stages with oral antibiotics is adequate in the majority of patients (Table 1). In patients with acute disseminated Lyme disease but without meningitis, oral doxycycline appears to be equally as effective as parenteral ceftriaxone in preventing the late manifestations of disease. Initial studies of treatment for early Lyme disease reported therapy

---

Table 1 Treament of Lyme Disease

Early Lyme disease[a]
  Amoxicillin, 500 mg tid for 21 days[b]
  Doxycyclin, 100 mg bid for 21 days
  Cefuroxime axetil, 500 mg bid for 21 days
  Azithromycin, 500 mg daily for 7 days[c] (less effective than other regimens)
Neurologic manifestations
  Bell's-like palsy (no other neurologic abnormalities)
    Oral regimens for early disease suffice
  Meningitis (with or without radiculoneuropathy or encephalitis)[d]
    Ceftriaxone, 2 g daily for 14-28 days
    Penicillin G, 20 million units daily for 14-28 days
    Doxycycline, 100 mg bid PO or IV for 14-28 days[e]
    Chloramphenicol, 1 g qid for 14-28 days
Arthritis[f]
  Amoxicillin and probenecid, 500 mg qid for 30 days[g]
  Doxycycline, 100 mg bid for 30 days
  Ceftriaxone, 2 g daily for 14-28 days
  Penicillin G, 20 million units daily for 14-28 days
Carditis
  Ceftriaxone, 2 g daily for 14 days
  Penicillin G, 20 million units daily for 14 days
  Doxycycline, 100 mg orally bid for 21 days[h]
  Amoxicillin, 500 mg 3 tid for 21 days[h]
Pregnancy
  Localized early disease
    Amoxicillin, 500 mg tid for 21 days
  Any manifestation of disseminated disease
    Penicillin G, 20 million units daily for 14-28 days
  Asymptomatic seropositivity
    No treatment necessary

From Rahn DW, Malawista SE: Treatment of Lyme disease. In *The year book of medicine,* St Louis, 1994, Mosby.
[a]Without neurologic, cardiac, or joint involvement. For early Lyme disease limited to single erythema migrans lesion, 10 days is sufficient.
[b]Some experts advise addition of probenecid, 500 mg three times daily.
[c]Experience with this agent is limited; optimal duration of therapy is unclear.
[d]Optimal duration of therapy has not been established. There are no controlled trials of therapy longer than 4 weeks for any manifestation of Lyme disease.
[e]No published experience in the United States.
[f]An oral regimen should be selected only if there is no neurologic involvement.
[g]Amoxicillin is generally administered three times daily, but the only trial of this agent for Lyme arthritis used a four-times-daily regimen.
[h]Oral regimens have been reserved for mild carditis limited to first-degree heart block with PR ≥0.30 seconds and normal ventricular function.

with phenoxymethyl penicillin, erythromycin, and tetracycline, at dosages of 250 mg four times a day for 10 to 20 days, shortened the duration of symptoms of early Lyme disease. Phenoxymethyl penicillin and tetracycline were superior to erythromycin in preventing serious late manifestations of disease. Subsequent clinical trials have proved amoxicillin and doxycycline to be equally efficacious. Amoxicillin has largely replaced use of penicillin because of greater in vitro activity against *B. burgdorferi*. Concomitant use of probenecid has not been definitively shown to improve clinical outcome and is associated with a higher incidence of side effects. Doxycycline is usually preferred over tetracycline because of its twice-daily dose schedule, increased gastrointestinal absorption and tolerability, and greater central nervous system penetration. Doxycycline is effective in treating the agent of human granulocytic ehrlichiosis, an organism also transmitted by *Ixodes scapularis* ticks; amoxicillin is not. Cefuroxime axetil, an oral second-generation cephalosporin, has recently been shown to be about as effective as amoxicillin and doxycycline in treating early Lyme disease; azithromycin, an azilide analog of erythromycin, is somewhat less so. Long-term follow-up of patients treated during early stages of Lyme disease support the current dosing regimens. Patients who received a 14- to 21-day course of a recommended antibiotic rarely developed late manifestations of illness. Jarisch-Herxheimer–like reactions, an increased discomfort in skin lesions and temperature elevation occurring within hours after the start of antibiotic treatment, have been encountered in 14% of patients treated for early Lyme disease. They typically occur within 2 to 4 hours of starting therapy, are more common in severe disease, and presumably result from rapid killing of a large number of spirochetes.

Minor symptoms, including arthralgia, fatigue, headaches, and transient facial palsy, are common after treatment and generally resolve over a 6-month period. Patients with disseminated disease are most likely to experience persistent symptoms. These symptoms may be caused by retained antigen rather than by ongoing infection with *B. burgdorferi* because longer courses of antibiotics have not been shown to shorten their duration. Prolonged courses of antibiotics should be reserved for those patients with evidence of persistent infection with *B. burgdorferi*.

Lyme Carditis

Cardiac involvement occurs in up to 10% of untreated patients. Transient and varying degrees of atrioventricular block several weeks to months after a tick bite are the most common manifestations. Other features are pericarditis, myocarditis, ventricular tachycardia, and in rare occasions, a dilated cardiomyopathy; valvular disease is not seen. Carditis is typically mild and self-limited, although patients may present quite dramatically in complete heart block, and some require the insertion of a temporary pacemaker. In most cases, carditis resolves completely, even without treatment with antibiotics. Recent studies examining endomyocardial biopsy specimens from patients with Lyme carditis have indicated that direct invasion of *B. burgdorferi* into myocardium and an associated inflammatory reaction are responsible for the clinical events. Although optimal treatment of carditis is unknown, oral therapy for mild forms of

cardiac involvement is usually sufficient. Intravenous antibiotics and cardiac monitoring are recommended for patients with varying, high-degree heart block and more serious cardiac involvement. There is no evidence of long-term cardiac abnormalities occurring in patients treated for carditis.

Dilated cardiomyopathy is a rare complication of Lyme disease reported in Europe but not yet in the United States. Most patients were from endemic areas for Lyme disease, had other clinical features of disease, and were seropositive for anti–*B. burgdorferi* antibodies. Their myopathy was cured by antibiotic treatment.

Early Neurologic Disease

Early neurologic involvement occurs in 15% to 20% of untreated patients and appears within 2 to 8 weeks after the onset of disease. Manifestations include cranial nerve palsies, meningitis or meningoencephalitis, and peripheral neuritis or radiculoneuritis. Unilateral or bilateral seventh nerve palsies are the most common neurologic abnormalities. Presenting symptoms depend on the area of the nervous system involved: patients with meningitis present with fever, headache, and a stiff neck; those with Bannwarth's syndrome (primarily in Europe) develop severe and migrating radicular pain, lasting weeks to several months; and those with encephalitis have concentration deficits, emotional lability, and fatigue. In patients with early central nervous system involvement analysis of cerebrospinal fluid typically reveals a lymphocytic pleocytosis. Specific antibodies against *B. burgdorferi* may also be present and concentrated in the cerebrospinal fluid relative to the serum concentration; they are useful to confirm disease.

Intravenous antibiotics are recommended for all cases of neuroborreliosis except isolated seventh nerve palsy. Patients presenting with a Bell's-like palsy who have features that suggest possible central nervous system involvement, such as high fever, headache, or stiff neck, should undergo a lumber puncture looking for evidence of more extensive disease. The most experience in the treatment of central nervous system Lyme disease has been with aqueous penicillin and third-generation cephalosporins. Although optimal duration of therapy is unknown, it is recommended that patients be treated for 2 to 4 weeks. Ceftriaxone, at dosages of 1 to 2 g/day, is the agent of choice because of better central nervous system penetration and ease of administration. Patients with persistent symptoms after recommended antibiotic therapy pose a particular management problem. It is often unclear whether these symptoms are caused by resolving inflammation or ongoing infection. Meningitis and sensory symptoms usually resolve within days to weeks; other features may take months to improve. In most cases, it is not necessary to continue antibiotic therapy until complete recovery.

Late Manifestations
Arthritis

Arthritis is the dominant feature of late Lyme disease and occurs in up to 60% of untreated patients days to years after initial infection (mean of 6 months). The initial pattern of involvement may be migratory arthralgias (early) followed in 60% of patients by intermittent attacks of arthritis lasting from days to months. Large joints, particularly the knee, are most commonly involved. Swelling is often prominent, with large effusions and Baker's cysts. Serologic testing in patients presenting with arthritis is positive in almost all cases.

Lyme arthritis has been treated successfully with oral and intravenous antibiotics. In early studies examining response to intravenous benzathine penicillin, 2.4 million units intramuscularly weekly for 3 weeks, 7 of 20 patients responded compared with 0 of 20 in the control group. Intravenous ceftriaxone, 2 to 4 g daily for 2 to 4 weeks, has been thought to be superior to benzathine penicillin. Oral regimens using doxycycline, 100 mg twice a day for 4 weeks, and amoxicillin plus probenecid, 500 mg of each orally four times a day for 4 weeks, have reported success in 18 of 20 patients and 16 of 18 patients, respectively. Response to antibiotics is typically excellent, but effusions may take months to resolve completely.

A small subgroup of patients with Lyme arthritis develop a chronic, potentially erosive arthritis unresponsive to antibiotics. These patients often have major histocompatability class II gene products, HLA DR4 accompanied by strong serum IgG responses to *Borrelia* outer surface proteins A or B (OspA or OspB). Repeated courses of antibiotics have not been shown to improve clinical outcome. Surgical synovectomy has cured a number of such patients.

Late Neurologic Lyme Disease

Chronic neurologic syndromes, which are relatively uncommon, may occur months to years after initial infection. Cognitive dysfunction, affective changes, seizures, ataxia, peripheral neuropathies, and chronic fatigue have all been reported. Because these complaints are often nonspecific and may be associated with post-Lyme syndromes, it is important to look for and document evidence of ongoing *B. burgdorferi* infection. Lymphocytic pleocytosis is uncommon in late neurologic disease, but increased intrathecal *B. burgdorferi*–specific antibodies may be present. Careful evaluation with neuropsychologic testing can help distinguish cognitive abnormalities in Lyme disease from those associated with chronic fatigue states and depression. Chronic neurologic dysfunction usually improves with antibiotics but may not completely reverse. Late neurologic manifestations of Lyme disease are treated with intravenous antibiotics. Agents with demonstrated efficacy are aqueous penicillin and third-generation cephalosporins. Doxycyline, both oral and intravenous forms, have been reported to be successful in treating late central nervous system Lyme disease in Europe.

Ocular Disease

Ocular lesions in Lyme disease are rare but have involved every portion of the eye and vary depending on the stage of the disease. The most common ophthalmic presentations in early disease include conjunctivitis, photophobia, and neuroophthalmologic manifestations from cranial nerve palsies. The most severe ocular manifestations occur in late stages; they include episcleritis, symblepharon, keratitis, iritis, chorioditis, panuveitis, and retinal vasculitis. Serologic testing in these patients is typically positive.

Experience treating late ocular lesions in Lyme disease is scanty. The most success has been with the use of intravenous ceftriaxone at dosages of 2 to 4 g daily for 10 to 14 days.

Pregnancy

Intrauterine transmission of *B. burgdorferi* is uncommon, usually occurring in cases of obvious disseminated infection during pregnancy. No uniform pattern of congenital anomaly has been reported. Prenatal exposure to Lyme disease has not been found to be associated with an increased risk of adverse pregnancy outcome. Optimal treatment of the pregnant patient with Lyme disease is unknown, but the recommended regimens have not been associated with adverse outcomes. Oral antibiotics for early localized disease is sufficient, and intravenous antibiotics are recommended for patients with symptoms suggesting disseminated disease.

Tick Bites

The risk of infection from a deer tick bite in a Lyme disease–endemic area is low. In mice, infected ticks have been attached for more than a 36-hour period before significant risk of developing Lyme disease occurred. In a controlled, double-blind study in patients with tick bites, no patient asymptomatically seroconverted, no treated patient developed EM, and the 2 of 182 untreated patients who did develop EM were treated successfully with oral antibiotics. These results support marking and watching a tick bite and, should EM develop, treating it early, when antibiotics are most effective.

Seropositive Patient with Nonspecific Symptoms

Patients with nonspecific symptoms such as myalgias, arthralgias, concentration difficulties, and fatigue are often tested for Lyme disease. Some patients, especially those from endemic areas, test positively and are treated for presumed Lyme disease, often without improvement in their symptoms. In several studies, more than 50% of patients reporting to Lyme disease clinics did not have evidence of Lyme disease, and the reason for a lack of response to antibiotics was an incorrect diagnosis. Objective clinical evidence in support of the diagnosis of Lyme disease should be sought before initiating antibiotics, treatment should be given for the recommended duration and then discontinued, and the patient observed for resolution of symptoms.

■ PREVENTION

Recommended personal protective measures against tick bites include wearing light-colored clothing, long-sleeve shirts, and long pants; tucking pant legs into socks; using a tick repellent on clothing and exposed skin; and performing regular body checks for ticks, strategies that require significant self-motivation.

Public interest in human and veterinary vaccines have prompted researchers to develop a safe and effective vaccine for the prevention of Lyme disease. The results of two large safety and efficacy trials using recombinant OspA preparations have been reported. Recipients were given three injections of either 30 μg of OspA lipoprotein or saline; the first two injections were given 1 month apart in the spring, and a booster dose followed 12 months later. Efficacy during the first year was 49% in one study and 68% in the other. Vaccine efficacy increased after the third injection in both trials to 76% and 92%, respectively. In view of differences in case ascertainment and the wide confidence limits of the estimates, it is likely that the two vaccines are equally efficacious. Vaccine-related side effects were mild to moderate in severity and were typically self-limited.

■ COMMENTS

Antibiotic regimens are recommended according to results of clinical trials and evolving clinical judgments and depend on the stage of infection and the organ system involved. Successful eradication of the infecting organism, *B. burgdorferi,* appears to occur in most patients with Lyme disease using these treatment guidelines. Patients with persistent symptoms after antibiotic therapy, particularly those with previous evidence of disseminated disease, pose a difficult management problem. Most persistent symptoms are likely caused by retained antigens or by noninfectious sequelae such as fibromyalgia, and are not indicative of persistent infection. In the former patients, resolution of symptoms occurs over the course of weeks to months and does not require prolonged courses of antibiotics; in the latter, treatment is that of the associated syndrome. Rarely, persistent or recurrent symptoms result from continued or recurrent infection and require additional courses of antibiotics. Such patients require careful diagnostic evaluation to determine the need for additional treatment.

Suggested Reading

Dattwyler RJ, et al: Ceftriaxone compared with doxycycline for the treatment of acute disseminated Lyme disease, *N Engl J Med* 337:289, 1997.

Halperin J, Volkman D, We P: Central nervous system abnormalities in Lyme neuroborreliosis, *Neurology* 41:1571, 1991.

Logigian EL, Kaplan RF, Steere AC: Chronic neurologic manifestations of Lyme disease, *N Engl J Med* 323:1438, 1990.

Rahn DW, Evans J, eds: *Lyme disease,* Philadelphia, 1998, American College of Physicians.

Rahn DW, Malawista SE: Treatment of Lyme disease. In *The year book of medicine,* St Louis, 1994, Mosby.

Sigal LH, et al: The recombinant outer-surface protein A Lyme disease Vaccine Consortium: a vaccine consisting of recombinant *Borrelia burgdorferi* outer-surface protein A to prevent Lyme disease, *N Engl J Med* 339:216, 1998.

Steere AC, Levin RE, Molloy PJ: Treatment of Lyme arthritis, *Arth Rheum* 6:878, 1994.

Steere AC, et al, and the Lyme Disease Vaccine Study Group: Vaccination against Lyme disease with recombinant *Borrelia burgdorferi* outer-surface lipoprotein A with adjuvant, *N Engl J Med* 339:209, 1998.

LEPTOSPIROSIS

William A. Petri, Jr.
Christopher D. Huston

Leptospirosis is an infection with spirochetes from the genus *Leptospira.* Humans become infected via exposure to animal urine or urine-contaminated water and soil. *Leptospira* penetrate intact mucous membranes and abraded skin and disseminate widely via the bloodstream. Symptoms develop 7 to 12 days after exposure. Most patients have an abrupt onset of a self-limited, 4- to 7-day anicteric illness characterized by fever, headache, myalgias, chills, cough, chest pain, neck stiffness, and/or prostration (Table 1). An estimated 10% of patients will present with jaundice, hemorrhage, renal failure, and/or neurologic dysfunction (Weil's disease). The major clinical manifestations of disease result from infection of capillary endothelial cells leading to vasculitis (Table 2).

Classically, leptospirosis has been considered a biphasic illness, although many patients with mild disease will not have symptoms of the secondary "immune" phase of illness. Patients with very severe disease will have a relentless progression from onset of illness to jaundice, renal failure, hemorrhage, hypotension, and coma. Overall, about half of the patients with leptospirosis will have a relapse 1 week after resolution of the initial febrile illness. A late manifestation is anterior uveitis, seen in up to 10% of patients months to years after convalescence. Leptospirosis in pregnancy is associated with spontaneous abortion but children with congenitally acquired leptospirosis have not been described to have congenital anomalies.

Case fatality rates for leptospirosis are less than 1%, and the illness is usually self-limited. Liver and renal dysfunction are for the most part reversible, with return to normal function over 1 to 2 months. The mortality rate for icteric disease has been reported in different studies to be 2.4% to 11.3%, with deaths resulting from renal failure, gastrointestinal and pulmonary hemorrhage, and the adult respiratory distress syndrome.

■ DIAGNOSIS

It is important to ask about exposure to animal urine in a patient with a flulike illness, respiratory illness, aseptic meningitis, acute hepatitis, acute renal failure, pericarditis, atrioventricular block, or anterior uveitis (Table 3). In some developing countries, leptospirosis is more common than hepatitis A as a cause of acute hepatitis. Useful means to distinguish icteric leptospirosis from acute viral hepatitis include the prominent myalgias, conjunctival suffusion, elevatd serum creatine phosphokinase (CPK), and the only twofold to threefold elevations in transaminases seen in

Table 1 Symptoms and Signs of Leptospirosis	
Abrupt onset (70%-100%)	Splenomegaly (5%-25%)
Fever, chills, rigors (98%)	Meningeal signs (12%-44%)
Headache (93%-97%)	Mental status changes
Myalgias, muscle tenderness	(7%-21%)
(40%-80%)	Oliguria (10%)
Vomiting, diarrhea, abdominal	Cough (10%-20%)
pain (30%-95%)	Chest pain (11%)
Conjunctival suffusion	Skin rash (9%-18%)
(33%-100%)	Jaundice (1.5%-6%)
Hepatomegaly (5%-22%; 80%	
of icteric cases)	

Table 2   Pathogenesis of Leptospirosis
Infectious vasculitis with damage to capillary endothelial cells resulting in the following:
Renal tubular dysfunction
Hepatocellular dysfunction
Pulmonary hemorrhage
Muscle focal necrosis
Coronary arteritis
Extravascular fluid shifts

Table 3   Epidemiology of Leptospirosis
Leptospira are excreted in animal urine and survive in the environment for up to 6 mo.
Disease is more common in the tropics, in young adult males, and in summer and fall.
Incubation period ranges from days up to 4 wk after exposure (mean 10-12 days).
Recreational exposures include windsurfing, kayaking, and swimming.
Occupational exposures:
New Zealand dairy farmers (incidence of 1.1 infections/10 person-years), Glasgow sewer workers (3.7/10 person-years), and U.S. Army soldiers undergoing jungle warfare training in Panama (4.1/10 person-years)
Veterinarians, abbatoir workers, and others with exposure to rat urine/bites (homeless people, rodent control workers)
Outbreaks seen after floods.

Table 4   Laboratory Findings of Leptospirosis
Renal failure—acute interstitial nephritis (15%-70%)
Jaundice with only twofold to threefold elevations in transaminases and alkaline phosphatases, conjugated bilirubinemia (2%-60%)
Myositis with elevated creatine phosphokinase (MM band) (20%-62%)
Thrombocytopenia (50%)
Cerebrospinal fluid pleiocytosis (80%-90%)—<300 cells/ml, lymphocyte predominance
Abnormal chest radiographs (20%-70%) patchy alveolar pattern in lower lobes with or without interstitial/ alveolar hemorrhage
Electrocardiogram abnormalities: sinus tachycardia, myocarditis, first-degree atrioventricular block
Microagglutination test (MAT) test for leptospirosis antibodies positive within first 1-2 wk of illness

Table 5   Treatment of Leptospirosis
Doxycycline, 100 mg PO bid for 7 days in adults (outpatient treatment)
or
Penicillin, 2.4-3.6 million U IV qd (severe infection requiring hospitalization)
Chemoprophylaxis—200 mg doxycycline once a week
Jarisch-Herxheimer reaction rare

leptospirosis (Table 4). The diagnosis is usually made retrospectively by a fourfold rise in agglutinating antibody titer. Agglutinins characteristically appear within the first 1 to 2 weeks of illness and peak at 3 to 4 weeks. It is possible in some cases to grow the organism from blood, urine, or cerebrospinal (CSF) collected during the first 1 to 2 weeks of illness.

■ THERAPY

Antibiotic treatment is most beneficial when started within 4 days of illness. Doxycycline, 100 mg orally twice daily for 7 days, started within 48 hours of illness decreased the duration of illness by 2 days in one study. Penicillin at a dosage of 2.4 to 3.6 million units per day has also been successful early treatment (Table 5). A benefit of antibiotic therapy given later in the disease course has not been uniformly seen. Jarish-Herxheimer reactions (fever, rigors, hypotension, and tachycardia) rarely occur upon initiation of antibiotic therapy. Supportive care and treatment of the hypotension, renal failure (including dialysis), and hemorrhage that can complicate leptospirosis are crucial for a good outcome.

Suggested Reading

Anon: Leptospirosis and unexplained acute febrile illness among athletes participating in triathlons—Illinois and Wisconsin, 1998, *MMWR* 47: 673, 1998.

Lecour H, Miranda M, Magro C: Human leptospirosis—a review of 50 cases, *Infection* 17:8, 1989.

McClain JBL, et al: Doxycycline therapy for leptospirosis, *Ann Intern Med* 100:696, 1984.

Watt G, et al: Placebo-controlled trial of intravenous penicillin for severe and late leptospirosis, *Lancet* i:433, 1988.

BORRELIOSIS

Joseph J. Burrascano, Jr.

Borrelia are spirochetes transmitted by arthropod vectors to humans. They are responsible for two important illnesses: Lyme disease, covered elsewhere, and the relapsing fevers.

■ THE RELAPSING FEVERS

The relapsing fevers are a group of illnesses caused by various species and strains of Borrelia. Relapsing fever can be louseborne or tickborne, and these two types differ in geographic distribution and severity, the former the more severe. It is difficult to separate the many Borrelia into individual serotypes because of this organisms's propensity to adapt to its current host, and thus express different surface antigens. Therefore they are grouped together and known collectively as the relapsing fevers.

Clinical Features

The illness begins 3 to 12 days after infection and is characterized by recurrent episodes of spirochetemia causing acute systemic symptoms and fever lasting on the average 1 week, separated by several days to weeks of asymptomatic or minimally symptomatic periods. The severity of presentation depends on host resistance, as well as by germ load, which can be estimated directly from thick blood smears. Manifestations are protean, and tissue damage occurs primarily as the result of a vasculitic process often associated with disseminated intravascular coagulation (DIC). Fever, headache, nausea and vomiting, myalgias, and arthralgias are associated with fleeting erythematous patches, hepatosplenomegaly with abnormal liver function tests, and various manifestations of the bleeding diathesis. These periods end by crisis, with a rapid rise and then fall of temperature, pulse rate, peripheral vascular resistance, and blood pressure. Acute myocardial insufficiency may result, and fatalities can occur, especially in compromised hosts. Acute episodes are terminated by a vigorous antibody response; relapses are caused by the organism's unique ability to undergo antigenic shifts that allow these mutant strains to proliferate until a new antibody response can be mounted. Over time, relapses diminish in severity and eventually disappear.

Relapsing fever Borrelia can be found in the central nervous system in animal and human hosts, and lymphocytic meningitis and cranial nerve palsy have been reported. In addition, chronic forms of this illness do exist. In utero transmission is possible, presenting as neonatal sepsis with jaundice and a high fatality rate.

Diagnosis

Diagnosis is made by darkfield examination of thick film peripheral blood smears obtained during an acute episode.

Convalescent specific antibody titers are often elevated, as are nonspecific febrile agglutinins. However, serologies can cross-react with Borrelia burgdorferi, the agent of Lyme disease, and Western blotting can be performed to differentiate the two. This can be important because both illnesses may exist in the same geographic area and certain Ixodid ticks (I. persulcatus) may contain both types of Borrelia. Xenodiagnosis with mouse inoculation can also be performed.

Treatment

Treatment is twofold and includes antibiotics (Table 1) and supportive measures (Table 2). Jarisch-Herxheimer (J-H) reactions are common within several hours after the onset of therapy and confirm the diagnosis. These result from lysis of spirochetes, liberating endotoxin-like compounds, and other antigens. Mediated by leucokines, J-H reactions can be particularly severe if antibiotics are initiated during an acute attack, especially in the louseborne type. Clinically, this resembles a typical crisis, with rigors, a rapid temperature spike, a rise in respiratory and pulse rate, and often a fall in blood pressure. Abdominal pain, nausea, and vomiting occur and are accompanied by leukopenia and thrombocytopenia. Supportive measures include correction of hypovolemia, control of pyrexia, and administration of vitamins K and B_6. Pretreatment with aspirin, acetaminophen, or even corticosteroids does not ameliorate this reaction.

Table 1 Treatment of Relapsing Fever

ANTIBIOTIC	ADULT'S DOSAGE	CHILDREN'S DOSAGE
PREFERRED		
Doxycycline	100 mg bid	Not recommended
Tetracycline	500 mg qid	Not recommended
ALTERNATIVE THERAPY		
Erythromycin	500 mg qid	40 mg/kg/day in 4 doses
Penicillin V	500 mg qid	50 mg/kg/day in 4 doses
Amoxicillin	500 mg tid	50 mg/kg/day in 3 doses
Chloramphenicol	500 mg qid	50 mg/kg/day in 4 doses
PARENTERAL THERAPY		
Penicillin G	25 million U/day	50,000 U/kg q8-12h
Ampicillin	500 mg q6h	50 mg/kg q6h (maximum 2g/day)
Ceftriaxone	2 g/day	50 mg/kg q24h
Erythromycin	500 mg q6h	20-50 mg/kg/day in 4 equal doses
Doxycycline	200 mg/day	Not recommended
Chloramphenicol	500 mg q6h	50 mg/kg/day in 2-4 equal doses

Table 2 Supportive Therapy as Needed

Acetaminophen, tepid baths, analgesics
Blood and volume replacement
Vitamin K, 30 mg IM
B-complex tablets, 50 mg each one daily, or B6, 50 mg IM
Specific treatment for disseminated intravascular coagulation
Bed rest the first 24 hr

For acute infection, antibiotics are given for a minimum of 10 days. Repeated or more prolonged courses are occasionally needed for subacute infections, late relapses, and the chronic forms, and the agent chosen and dosage should be sufficient to penetrate the central nervous system. Because treatment failures with the penicillins have been reported, the tetracyclines are the drugs of choice if not contraindicated (children, pregnancy). Other choices include chloramphenicol and erythromycin. Parenteral antibiotics can be given to those unable to tolerate oral dosing (see Table 1).

Worldwide, relapsing fevers are most prevalent in areas of poor living conditions and especially after natural or other disasters when personal hygiene and adequate housing are lacking. Therefore it is imperative that a search be made for concurrent illnesses and nutritional deficiencies likely to be present in this setting.

Suggested Reading

Cadavid D, Barbour AG: Neuroborreliosis during relapsing fever: review of the clinical manifestations, pathology, and treatment of infections in humans and experimental animals, *Clin Infect Dis* 26:151, 1998.

Felsenfeld O: *Borrelia*, St Louis, 1971, Warren H. Green.

LaVoie PC: *Borrelia hermseii*, the inciting agent in a case of juvenile polyarthritis? (abstract) IV International Conference on Lyme Borreliosis, June 18-21, 1990.

Negussie Y: Detection of plasma tumor necrosis factor, interleukins 6 and 8 during the Jarisch-Herxheimer reaction of relapsing fever, *J Exp Med* 175:1207, 1992.

Ras NM, et al: Phylogenesis of relapsing fever *Borrelia* spp, *Int J Syst Bacteriol* 46:859, 1996.

Schwann TG: Analysis of relapsing fever spirochetes from the Western United States, *J Spirochetal Tick Borne Dis* 2:3, 1995.

RICKETTSIAL INFECTIONS

Paul D. Holtom
John M. Leedom

Organisms belonging to the order Rickettsiales are gram-negative obligately intracellular bacteria. Rickettsial diseases are generally classified and grouped by antigenic relationships, vectors, and clinical manifestations. The pathogenesis of illness caused by both the spotted fever and typhus groups of organisms is vasculitis. The rickettsiae proliferate in the endothelial lining cells of small arteries, capillaries, and veins. Q fever, caused by *Coxiella burnetti*, is an exception, in that illness eventuates when organisms are inhaled into the alveoli, proliferate in the lungs, and cause inflammation and rickettsemia with seeding of organism in other organs, particularly the liver.

All the important rickettsial infections except Q fever are vectorborne. Q fever can be tickborne, although most cases result from the inhalation of dust contaminated by the birth fluids of domestic ungulates. Table 1 summarizes the epidemiologic and clinical features of the major rickettsioses.

In any discussion of the treatment of rickettsioses, it is important to stress that proper treatment cannot be given unless the diagnosis is suspected. Confirmation of diagnosis is almost always delayed. The arthropodborne rickettsioses are diseases of the spring and summer in temperate climates. Q fever can occur at any season if exposure to aerosols of the organism occurs. Given an appropriate geographic, temporal, and/or occupational history, the triad of fever, headache

and rash, characteristic for all the rickettsioses except Q fever, should cause the physician to suspect a rickettsial disease. As early treatment is deemed important in preventing fatalities, particularly in Rocky Mountain spotted fever (RMSF), therapy should be instituted when the diagnosis is suspected.

Confirmations of diagnoses are almost always serologic and thus usually retrospective, because antibodies occur no earlier than the second week of illness in any of the rickettsioses. The Weil-Felix reaction, which depends on the development of agglutinating antibodies to the heterologous antigens of *Proteus* OX-2, OX19, and OX-K, is no longer considered specific enough by the Centers for Disease Control and Prevention to diagnose RMSF. Patients with positive results by the Weil-Felix test are considered only probable cases at present. The more specific complement fixation and indirect immunofluorescent tests are used. In RMSF, a direct immunofluorescence test can confirm the presence of organisms in skin biopsies once rash appears. Polymerase chain reaction (PCR) has been used to diagnose acute infection with *Rickettsia prowazekii*, but its overall utility in clinical diagnosis of rickettsioses is not yet established.

■ ROCKY MOUNTAIN SPOTTED FEVER

RMSF was first described in the late 1800s in the Bitterroot Valley of Idaho. Although originally recognized only in the western United States, it now has a higher documented prevalence in the South Atlantic states and in the south-central region. The causative agent is *Rickettsia rickettsii*, a member of the spotted fever group of rickettsial infections.

R. rickettsii is transmitted to humans by the bite of an infected tick. Ticks are both the vectors and the main reservoirs of this agent. The specific tick responsible for transmission varies from area to area. In the eastern United

Table 1   Synopsis of Certain Epidemiologic and Clinical Features of Selected Rickettsioses

DISEASE	ORGANISM	GEOGRAPHIC AREA	HOSTS ARTHROPODS	HOSTS VERTEBRATES	RASH DISTRIBUTION
Spotted fever group					
Rocky Mountain spotted fever	*Rickettsia rickettsii*	Western hemisphere	Ticks	Wild rodents, dogs	Extremities to trunk
Boutonneuse	*Rickettsia conorii*	Africa, Mediterranean, India	Ticks	Wild rodents, dogs	Trunk, extremities, face
Queensland tick typhus	*Rickettsia australis*	Australia	Ticks	Wild rodents, marsupials	Trunk, extremities, face
North Asian tick typhus	*Rickettsia sibirica*	Siberia, Mongolia	Ticks	Wild rodents	Trunk, extremities, face
Rickettsialpox	*Rickettsia akari*	United States, former Soviet Union, Korea, Africa	Mites	Mice	Vesicular; trunk, extremities, face
Typhus group					
Epidemic	*Rickettsia prowazekii*	Highland areas of South America, Africa, Asia, ? United States	Body lice	Humans, flying squirrels	Trunk to extremities
Brill-Zinsser	*R. prowazekii*	Worldwide based on immigration	None	Humans (recurrence years after primary attack)	Trunk to extremities (may be absent)
Murine	*Rickettsia typhi*	Worldwide in pockets	Fleas	Small rodents	Trunk to extremities
Scrub	*Rickettsia tsutsugamushi*	South Pacific, Asia, Australia	Mites	Wild rodents	Trunk to extremities
Other					
Q fever	*Coxiella burnetii*	Worldwide	? Ticks	Cattle, sheep, goats, cats (inhalation of organism)	None

Adapted from Saah AJ, et al: Rickettsiosis. In Mandell GL, Bennett JE, Dolin R, eds: *Mandell, Douglas and Bennett's principles and practice of infectious diseases,* ed 4, New York, 1995, Churchill Livingstone.

States the vector is *Dermacentor variabilis,* the American dog tick, and in the western United States it is *Dermacentor andersoni,* the Rocky Mountain wood tick. The adult tick transmits the disease to humans during feeding, releasing *R. rickettsii* from the salivary glands after feeding for 6 to 10 hours. Humans can also be infected by exposure to an infected tick hemolymph, which may occur during the removal of ticks from persons or domestic animals, especially when the tick is crushed.

The incubation of RMSF ranges from 2 to 14 days, with a median of 7 days. Virtually all patients have fever, usually greater than 38.9° C (102° F). Other common symptoms include headache, myalgias, and gastrointestinal complaints such as nausea, vomiting, and severe abdominal pain. The major diagnostic sign is the rash, which occurs in approximately 90% of patients overall, usually 3 to 5 days after the onset of fever. Fewer than half of the patients show the rash during the first 3 days of illness. The rash typically starts around the wrists and ankles but may be diffuse at onset. Although involvement of the palms is considered characteristic, it does not occur in all patients and often occurs late in the course of the disease.

Complications of RMSF include meningismus, meningitis, renal failure, pulmonary involvement, hepatic dysfunction with development of jaundice, splenomegaly, myo-carditis, and thrombocytopenia. Although in the early reports the case fatality rate was 20%, in recent series of patients death occurs in 4% to 8% of cases. In patients with fulminant RMSF, death occurs within the first 5 days, often before the rash becomes apparent. In patients with classic RMSF, death occurs 8 to 15 days after the onset of symptoms.

Treatment of RMSF requires the administration of an effective antibiotic for 7 days, continuing for 2 days after the patient has become afebrile. Antibiotics shown to be effective against *R. rickettsii* by in vitro testing are chloramphenicol, tetracycline, rifampin, and some of the quinolone agents. *R. rickettsii* is resistant to beta-lactam antibiotics, aminoglycosides, erythromycin, and trimethoprim-sulfamethoxazole (TMP-SMX). The antibiotic of choice is oral doxycycline, 100 mg every 12 hours. Tetracycline, 25 to 50 mg/kg/day divided in four doses, is also effective. In pregnant patients and in young children, for whom staining of the teeth by a tetracycline compound is a concern, chloramphenicol, 50 to 75 mg/kg/day, is an alternative. Quinolones (ciprofloxacin, 500 mg twice a day, or levofloxacin, 500 mg/day) may be used in patients unable to take doxycycline or chloramphenicol. Glucocorticosteroids have been given to severely ill patients in the past, but there is no documentation of their efficacy.

■ RICKETTSIALPOX

Rickettsialpox, a nonfatal disease caused by *Rickettsia akari*, was first reported in 1946 in New York but is rarely diagnosed, although a series was reported from New York in 1994. It has been reported in other urban areas in the United States and in parts of Russia, South Africa, and Korea. The reservoir for this infection is the house mouse, *Mus musculus*, and the vector for transmission to humans is the mouse mite *Allodermanyssus sanguineus*. A painless papule that ulcerates and forms an eschar occurs at the site of the mite bite some 3 to 7 days before the onset of symptoms in most cases. Manifestations include chills, fever, headache, myalgia, backache, and photophobia. Rigors and profuse diaphoresis may be seen. Within 2 to 3 days after onset, a generalized papulovesicular rash occurs. The rash begins as red papules 2 to 10 mm wide that vesiculate and heal by crusting. The disease is benign. Death and complications are very rare. Tetracycline, 15 mg/kg/day in divided doses for 3 to 5 days, has been reported to be effective.

■ OTHER SPOTTED FEVER GROUP RICKETTSIOSES

At least eight other members of the spotted fever group seem to be pathogenic for humans; the most important are listed in Table 1. Successful treatment for them has been reported using doxycycline, 200 mg a day; tetracycline, 25 mg/kg/day; or chloramphenicol, 50 to 75 mg/kg/day. Alternatively, ciprofloxacin, 1.5 g/day, may be given for 5 to 7 days. The tetracyclines and quinolones should not be given to children.

■ EPIDEMIC, OR LOUSEBORNE, TYPHUS

Epidemic typhus is a classic plague of humanity caused by *Rickettsia prowazekii* and transmitted by the body louse *Pediculus humanus corporis*. The bacteria may remain latent in humans for many years after the initial infection. The infection can relapse clinically, with rickettsemia, when persons are stressed by other disease or deprivations. Thus, classically during war and refugee exodus, when persons are stressed and deprived and poor hygiene promotes the spread of lice, a rickettsemic person may initiate the cycle and cause an epidemic. This relapsing disease is generally milder than an initial attack, presumably because it occurs in a person with some established immunity. This recrudescent typhus is Brill-Zinsser disease.

It has recently been learned that *R. prowazekii* is not an obligate human pathogen but can be carried by the flying squirrel, *Glaucomys volans*, which is distributed over the entire eastern United States. Serologically confirmed human cases have occurred in persons with varying degrees of contact with the squirrels, but the exact method of transmission to humans is unknown, although fleas and mites from the squirrels are suspected.

The characteristic incubation period is about a week. The onset is usually abrupt, with intense headache, chills, fever, and myalgia. Fever progresses and becomes unremitting.

Rash begins on about the fifth day of illness, usually on the axillary folds and upper trunk, and spreads centrifugally. The rash begins as pink macules that fade on pressure but progresses to become maculopapular, darker, petechial, and nonfading on pressure. The rash may become confluent and involve the entire body, but the face, palms, and soles are spared. Indigenously acquired typhus related to flying squirrel exposure is a similar but milder illness.

The established therapy for epidemic typhus is tetracycline or chloramphenicol. Tetracycline is given in four equally divided oral doses of 25 mg/kg/day. Chloramphenicol is given at 50 mg/kg/day, also divided into four equal doses. If oral intake is impossible, the drugs should be given in the same doses intravenously. If renal function is impaired, doxycycline, 100 mg twice a day, or chloramphenicol, 50 mg/kg/day, should be used. Treatment should be continued until the patient has been afebrile for 2 or 3 days. For louseborne typhus only, a single dose of 100 mg of doxycycline has been reported to be curative. Indigenously acquired *R. prowazekii* requires conventional multidose therapy. If patients are treated within 48 hours of onset of symptoms, relapse may occur and require a second course of antimicrobials.

■ MURINE TYPHUS

Murine typhus, caused by *Rickettsia typhi*, has worldwide distribution with special prevalence in seaboard regions in the temperate areas and in the subtropics. It infects endothelial cells in mammalian hosts and midgut epithelial cells in fleas. Its most important reservoirs are *Rattus* species. The classic vector spreading the organisms from rats to people is the flea *Xenopsylla cheopis*.

The disease is clinically less severe than epidemic typhus, with reported case fatality ratios of 1% to 4%. The pathology is basically a vasculitis, as in the other rickettsioses. Illness begins 1 to 2 weeks after a bite from an infected flea. At first, it is quite nonspecific, with fever, headache, chills, myalgia, and nausea. Rash is seen in about 20% of patients at presentation and in about 50% at some time during the illness. The lesions are macular or maculopapular. The trunk is most often involved, but the extremities are involved in about half the patients who develop rash. The rash may also be seen on the palms and soles. The rash is often salmon colored and evanescent, and frank hemorrhagic vasculitic rash may develop. Occasional patients develop central nervous system (CNS) abnormalities, hepatic or renal failure, respiratory failure, or hematemesis.

The initial diagnosis, as with all the other rickettsioses, must be made on clinical and epidemiologic grounds. Most cases are confirmed by serologic methods such as indirect fluorescent or latex agglutination antibody rises. A solid-phase immunoassay is available in some laboratories. Immunologic methods for demonstrating the organism in tissues as well as PCR amplification have also been recently advocated.

R. typhi is treated with tetracycline, doxycycline, or chloramphenicol. Tetracycline is given at 25 to 50 mg/kg/day in four equally divided doses. The dosage of doxycycline is 100 mg twice a day. Chloramphenicol is recommended at 50 to

75 mg/kg/day in four equally divided doses. Antimicrobial therapy should be continued for 2 to 3 days after defervescence.

■ SCRUB TYPHUS

Scrub typhus eventuates when a larval-stage trombiculid mite (chigger) infected with *Rickettsia tsutsugamushi (Rickettsia orientalis)* bites a susceptible human host. The infection occurs from Korea to Australia to Japan to India and Pakistan.

A susceptible host is inoculated when an infected chigger feeds. There is local multiplication of *R. tsutsugamushi* at the site of the bite. A papule forms, and later, an eschar. There is regional lymphadenopathy, with generalized adenopathy appearing within the next 4 to 5 days. Rickettsemia antedates the onset of symptoms. Some 6 to 18 days after the chigger bite, the patient develops fever, severe headache, and myalgia. Fever may reach 40° to 40.6° C (104° to 105° F). Temperature-pulse dissociation may occur early in the illness, with an inappropriately slow pulse. Conjunctival injection, ocular pain, nonproductive cough, and apathy are also seen. The severity of the signs and symptoms is widely variable, depending on the virulence of the responsible strain and the degree of susceptibility of the host. After about 5 days, rash, sometimes evanescent, occurs. It begins on the trunk and spreads to the extremities. At first it is macular, but it may become papular. Splenomegaly and generalized adenopathy are also seen.

Complications include pneumonia, heart failure, respiratory failure, and renal failure. Some patients develop CNS signs and symptoms during the second week of illness. These manifestations may include nuchal rigidity, nervousness, slurred speech, tremors, delirium, and deafness. The cerebrospinal fluid is normal or has a mild mononuclear cell elevation. Case fatality rates as high as 30% in untreated patients have been reported. Treatment shortens the duration of illness and essentially eliminates fatalities.

Because of its simplicity, the Weil-Felix slide agglutination test still retains some utility for diagnosis in the less developed portions of the world, where most cases of scrub typhus occur. About 50% of patients with scrub typhus develop antibodies to *Proteus* OXK during the second week of illness. Positive tests are usually recorded as a single determination of 1:320 or greater or a fourfold rise in titer. Cross-reactions may be encountered in patients with leptospirosis. Indirect fluorescent antibody titers are more sensitive and more specific. PCR has been studied extensively and successfully in the diagnosis of scrub typhus. It has also been used in studies assessing therapeutic response.

Tetracycline and chloramphenicol are the established treatments. The dose of tetracycline is 25 mg/kg/day in four equally divided doses. Chloramphenicol is given as 50 mg/kg/day in four equally divided doses. There are reports of successful treatment with ciprofloxacin. Scrub typhus has a notorious tendency to relapse, particularly if treatment is begun before the forth or fifth day of illness or is terminated early. For this reason all patients should be treated for at least 2 weeks. Some authors have reported that 200 mg of doxycycline given at diagnosis was almost as effective in treatment and preventing relapse as two doses of doxycycline given at days 1 and 7 or conventional therapy with tetracycline for 7 days. However, at this time, it is not standard treatment.

■ Q FEVER

Q fever is an infection caused by the organism *C. burnetii*. It can present as an acute infection with an influenza-like illness, fever, and pulmonary and hepatic involvement, or can develop into a chronic form with endocarditis and chronic hepatitis.

C. burnetii is an extremely infectious organism. In fact, a single inhaled organism is sufficient to initiate infection. It is endemic worldwide except in New Zealand. *C. burnetii* infects many species of animals, and in animals the infection usually results in long-lasting parasitism. Mammals both wild and domestic, birds, fish, and arthropods have been infected with the organism. Q fever in humans is usually caused by the inhalation of aerosolized particles from infected domestic animals, which can be airborne even over long distances.

The clinical presentation of Q fever can resemble that of nearly any infectious disease. Many people who are infected with *C. burnetti* are asymptomatic. Those with clinical illness most commonly have an acute febrile systemic illness, pneumonia, hepatitis, or meningoencephalitis. Patients can go on to develop a chronic illness characterized by endocarditis and granulomatous hepatitis.

The incubation period for Q fever can be as short as 4 to 5 days, but it typically ranges from 9 to 39 days. Fever is the most common symptom, occurring in almost all patients, and the temperature often spikes to 40° to 40.5° C (104° to 105° F). Other signs and symptoms include chills, headache (often severe), retrobulbar pain, myalgias and arthralgias, neck pain and stiffness, pleuritic chest pain, cough, nausea and vomiting, diarrhea, jaundice, hepatomegaly, and splenomegaly. Unlike the other rickettsial diseases, Q fever does not usually present with a rash, although a transient erythematous macular rash has been noted in about 4% of patients. The manifestations of Q fever usually resolve within 2 to 4 weeks, although some patients have had fever as long as 9 weeks. Case fatality rates from acute Q fever are very low (none in most series), but in a recent French series of 323 hospitalized patients the case fatality rate was 2.4%.

Chronic Q fever is usually manifested by endocarditis, although other manifestations include chronic hepatitis, infections of vascular prostheses and aneurysms, osteomyelitis, and interstitial pulmonary fibrosis. Q fever endocarditis is usually accompanied by liver involvement and is a rare, severe, and often fatal complication of *C. burnetii* infection. The incidence of Q fever endocarditis appears to be increasing, but this may reflect improved diagnosis rather than a true change in epidemiology. Most patients have preexisting valvular heart disease, often a prosthetic valve. The illness evolves slowly, manifesting any time from 1 to 20 years after the acute infection, and presents clinically as a culture-negative endocarditis, although fever is often absent in Q fever endocarditis.

Most acute Q fever infections resolve spontaneously, and symptoms respond to nonspecific therapy such as antipyretics and hydration. However, because of the concern about the development of chronic Q fever and because some studies suggest that therapy shortens the duration of fever, we recommend specific antimicrobial therapy for acute Q fever. Tetracycline and its analogs are the mainstay of therapy. Tetracycline for 2 weeks at 25 mg/kg/day in four divided doses, or doxycycline at 100 mg twice a day for 15 to 21 days is recommended for adults.

The treatment of chronic Q fever has never been the subject of controlled studies. No antibiotics have been found to be bactericidal for *C. burnetti*, although several, including tetracycline, doxycycline, TMP-SMX, rifampin, and ciprofloxacin, have been shown to be bacteriostatic. We recommend rifampin plus either doxycycline or TMP-SMX for the treatment of Q fever endocarditis. The ideal duration of therapy is also unknown; recommended periods range from 12 months to an indefinite term. Valve replacement surgery in Q fever endocarditis is indicated only for significant hemodynamic problems.

■ PREVENTION

There are no human vaccines for any of the rickettsioses except epidemic typhus. Vaccine is recommended for persons who live, work, and visit in areas of poor hygiene where typhus is prevalent and who have close contact with the indigenous populace, medical personnel who provide care for patients in foreign areas where typhus occurs, and laboratory personnel working with the organism.

Unfortunately, *C. burnetti* infection in domestic ungulates in the United States is so widespread that persons engaged in animal husbandry can hardly prevent exposure. For example, sheep are widely used in research laboratories in medical centers, and several sheepborne outbreaks of Q fever in such facilities have been reported.

Suggested Reading

Didier R, Drancourt M: Antimicrobial therapy of rickettsial diseases, *Antimicrob Agents Chemother* 35:2457, 1991.

Olson JG, McDade JE: *Rickettsia* and *Coxiella*. In Murray PR, et al, eds: *Manual of clinical microbiology*, ed 6, Washington, DC, 1995, ASM Press.

Saah AJ, et al: Rickettsiosis. In Mandell GL, Bennett JE, Dolin R, eds: *Mandell, Douglas and Bennett's principles and practice of infectious diseases*, ed 5, New York, 2000, Churchill Livingstone.

MYCOPLASMA

Ken B. Waites

Mycoplasmas are the smallest free-living organisms and are unique among prokaryotes in that they lack a cell wall, a feature that is largely responsible for their biologic properties and lack of susceptibility to many commonly prescribed antimicrobial agents. Mycoplasmas are usually mucosally associated, residing primarily in the respiratory and urogenital tracts and rarely penetrating the submucosa, except in the case of immunosuppression or instrumentation when they may invade the bloodstream and disseminate to many different organs and tissues throughout the body.

Although there have been at least sixteen species of mycoplasmas isolated from humans, three species are responsible for most clinically significant infections that may come to the attention of the practicing physician. These species are *Mycoplasma pneumoniae*, *Mycoplasma hominis*, and *Ureaplasma* species, and they will be the focus of the following discussion of diseases and treatment alternatives.

■ *MYCOPLASMA PNEUMONIAE* RESPIRATORY DISEASE

M. pneumoniae occurs endemically and occasionally epidemically in persons of all age groups, most commonly in school-age children, adolescents, and young adults. The common misconception that *M. pneumoniae* disease is rare among the very young and among older adults has sometimes led to failure of physicians to consider this organism in differential diagnoses of respiratory infections in these age groups. *M. pneumoniae* is perhaps best known as the primary cause of "walking" or atypical pneumonia, but in fact the most common clinical syndrome is that of tracheobronchitis or bronchiolitis, often accompanied by upper respiratory tract symptomatology. Typical complaints can persist for weeks to months and include hoarseness; fever; cough, which is initially nonproductive but later may yield small to moderate amounts of nonbloody sputum; sore throat; headache; chills; coryza; and general malaise. The throat may be inflamed but cervical adenopathy is uncommon. Myringitis sometimes occurs. Bronchopneumonia, involving one or more lobes develops in 3% to 10% of infected persons, accounting for 20% or more of community-acquired pneumonias overall. The incubation period is generally 1 to 3 weeks and spread throughout households often occurs. Hospitalization may be necessary in about 10% of children and adults, but recovery is almost always complete without sequelae. Some people may experience extrapulmonary complications at variable time periods after onset of or even in the absence of respiratory illness. Such complications most commonly include skin rashes, pericarditis, hemolytic anemia, arthritis, meningoencephalitis, peripheral neuropathy, and pericarditis. Other nonspecific manifestations include nausea, vomiting, and diarrhea. Acute mycoplasmal infection may also be associated with exacerbations of chronic bronchitis and asthma.

Autoimmune reaction is thought to be responsible for many of the extrapulmonary complications associated with mycoplasmal infection. However, because *M. pneumoniae* has been isolated from extrapulmonary sites such as synovial fluid and cerebrospinal fluid (CSF), pericardial fluid, and skin lesions, direct invasion must always be considered. The frequency of direct invasion of these sites is unknown because the organism is rarely sought.

The hemogram is often normal, but about one fourth of patients may develop leukocytosis and one third may demonstrate an elevated erythrocyte sedimentation rate. The cellular response of the sputum is mononuclear, with no bacteria visible by Gram stain. In about 50% of patients, a cold agglutinin titer of 1:32 or greater may develop by the second week of illness, disappearing by 6 to 8 weeks. This is not a specific test for *M. pneumoniae* because other microorganisms may induce similar reactions. Several viruses, *Chlamydia pneumoniae*, *Streptococcus pneumoniae*, *Haemophilus influenzae*, *Moraxella catarrhalis*, *Legionella* species, and even some mycobacteria or fungi can produce infections that are clinically indistinguishable and that may occur simultaneously with mycoplasmal infection.

Abnormalities on chest radiographs often appear more severe than the clinical condition of the patient would predict. True lobar consolidation is uncommon, but pleural effusion may develop in about 25% of cases. Diffuse reticulonodular or interstitial infiltrates involving the lower lobes, appearing as streaks radiating from the hilus to the base, are the most common radiographic abnormalities. Lung involvement tends to be unilateral but can be bilateral.

Because of a widespread lack of diagnostic services, length of time needed to obtain results, impracticality of obtaining diagnostic specimens, and similarity of clinical syndromes caused by different microorganisms, clinicians often do not attempt to obtain a microbiologic diagnosis in mild to moderately ill outpatients and elect to treat empirically. If mycoplasmal respiratory infection is to be confirmed, culture, molecular-based, and/or serologic tests are necessary. Clinical laboratories may offer culture service through a reference laboratory familiar with the complex cultivation requirements of mycoplasmas. Respiratory tract specimens suitable for culture include throat swabs, sputum, tracheal aspirates, bronchial lavage fluid, pleural fluid, or lung biopsy tissue according to the patient's clinical condition. Care should be taken in specimen collection; inoculation into a suitable transport medium, such as SP4 broth, should be done at bedside when possible, without allowing desiccation. Freezing at −70° C is advised if specimens cannot be transported to the diagnostic laboratory immediately after collection. Growth in culture is slow, requiring 3 weeks or more in some cases.

Serology is most commonly used to confirm *M. pneumoniae* infection. Enzyme-linked immunosorbent assays are now preferred over the older, less sensitive complement fixation assays. Because primary infection does not guarantee protective immunity against future infections and residual antibody may remain from earlier encounters with the organism, there has been a great impetus to develop sensitive and specific tests that can differentiate between acute or remote infection. Definitive diagnosis requires seroconversion documented by paired specimens obtained 2 to 4 weeks apart. Although single-titer IgM or IgA assays purported to detect current infection have recently become available, it is not clear how long IgM persists after acute infection, and as many as 50% of adults may not mount a detectable IgM response. Conversely, some children may not mount a measurable IgG response. Therefore reliance on a single serologic test can be clinically misleading and paired assays for both IgM and IgG are recommended for optimum diagnosis.

Molecular-based systems for detection of *M. pneumoniae* using the polymerase chain reaction (PCR) have been developed for research purposes, and limited information is available describing the application of this methodology in a clinical setting. However, at present, there are no commercially available rapid diagnostic methods for detecting *M. pneumoniae* in clinical specimens to assist the practicing physician on a routine basis. The rapid advances in molecular diagnostic techniques may one day result in nucleic acid amplification tests such as the PCR becoming the tests of choice for detection of slow-growing, fastidious organisms such as *M. pneumoniae*. The possibility of multiplex PCR tests to detect mycoplasmas simultaneously with other atypical etiologic agents of community-acquired pneumonias such as chlamydia and legionellae may eventually prove useful for screening purposes.

■ THERAPY OF *MYCOPLASMA PNEUMONIAE* INFECTIONS

Formerly, it was believed that mycoplasmal respiratory infections were entirely self-limited and no antimicrobial treatment was indicated. More recently, it has been shown that appropriate antimicrobial therapy will shorten the symptomatic period and hasten radiologic resolution of pneumonia and recovery, even though organisms may be shed for several weeks. In general, the clinical efficacy of antimicrobial therapy is correlated with severity of pneumonia and elapsed time of illness before treatment is begun.

M. pneumoniae has remained predictably susceptible to macrolides, lincosamides, and teracyclines, so in vitro susceptibility testing to guide therapy is not indicated. Oral erythromycin has long been the drug of choice for mycoplasmal respiratory infections. Tetracycline and its analogs are also effective in vivo and in vitro but should not be used in children because of potential bone and tooth toxicity. Clindamycin is effective in vitro, but limited reports suggest it may not be active in vivo and should not be considered a first-line treatment. None of the beta-lactams, sulfonamides, or trimethoprim are effective in vitro or in vivo against *M. pneumoniae.*

Clarithromycin and azithromycin are broad-spectrum macrolides used primarily for treatment of community-acquired respiratory infections caused by a wide array of bacteria. Both agents are effective in vitro against *M. pneumoniae* at concentrations equivalent to or lower than those of erythromycin, and both have proved clinical efficacy against this organism. These drugs have the advantages of better tolerability, fewer gastrointestinal side effects, and longer half-life than erythromycin, allowing less frequent dosage. However, their drawback is increased cost, amounting to several times that of erythromycin. As with erythromycin, administration of clarithromycin may cause an increase in serum theophylline concentrations. Both drugs are now available as pediatric oral suspensions, and azithromycin is also available as an intravenous formulation. Neither should be used in pregnant women if there is any other available treatment.

The newer fluoroquinolones, including levofloxacin, sparfloxacin, moxifloxacin, and gatifloxacin, exhibit antimycoplasmal activity but are less potent in vitro than the macrolides against *M. pneumoniae.* Development of new quinolones with documented clinical efficacy and approved indications for treating *M. pneumoniae* has been driven largely by the need for therapeutic alternatives for beta-lactam and macrolide-resistant *S. pneumoniae,* and the desire for agents that can be used as empiric monotherapy for respiratory infections due to other typical and atypical organisms, including chlamydiae, legionellae, *H. influenzae,* and *M. catarrhalis.* At present, quinolones are not approved for use in persons younger than 18 years of age, but these drugs are rapidly achieving widespread use for treatment of respiratory infections in adults, mainly in the ambulatory setting, and represent reasonable alternative therapies for *M. pneumoniae* disease.

Mycoplasmas are slow-growing organisms; thus one would logically expect respiratory infections to respond better to longer treatment courses than might be offered for other types of infections. Although most treatment regimens are prescribed for 7 to 14 days, a 14- to 21-day course of oral therapy with most agents is also appropriate. A 5-day course of oral azithromycin is approved for treatment of community-acquired pneumonia due to *M. pneumoniae.* Clinical data indicate this duration of treatment is of comparable efficacy to a 10-day course of erythromycin.

In addition to the administration of antimicrobials for management of *M. pneumoniae* infections, other measures such as cough suppressants, antipyretics, and analgesics should be given as needed to relieve the headaches and other systemic symptoms. Because most extrapulmonary manifestations are diagnosed late in the course of disease, the benefit of early treatment is unknown.

Fortunately, the treatments of choice for *M. pneumoniae* are appropriate for many of the other microbial agents responsible for community-acquired respiratory infections. This is especially important in view of the fact that in the major proportion of ambulatory patients seeking medical care, the identity of their infectious organism is never determined. Standard and alternative drugs and their recommended dosages for use in mycoplasmal respiratory, genitourinary, and other systemic infections are listed in Table 1.

■ *MYCOPLASMA HOMINIS* AND *UREAPLASMA UREALYTICUM* INFECTIONS

Ureplasma species and *M. hominis* can be isolated from the lower genital tract in most sexually active women; their occurrence is somewhat less common in men. The presence of genital mycoplasmas in asymptomatic persons has made it difficult to prove their pathogenic potential, but in recent years, conditions such as urethritis have been proven unequivocally to be caused by ureaplasmas in some instances. Only a subgroup of otherwise healthy adult men and women who are colonized will develop clinically significant genitourinary disease from mycoplasmas or ureaplasmas, but the risk factors are poorly understood. Colonized women may transmit genital mycoplasmas to their offspring either in utero or at delivery. Superficial mucosal colonization in the newborn period tends to be transient and without sequelae, but neonates, especially those born preterm, have been shown to be susceptible to development of various systemic conditions resulting from either *M. hominis* or *Ureaplasma* species, the most significant being pneumonia, bacteremia, and meningitis.

Extragenital infection with *M. hominis* and/or *Ureaplasma* species is usually associated with some degree of immunocompromise such as congenital hypogammaglobulinemia or iatrogenic immunosuppression following solid organ transplantation or with invasive procedures such as instrumentation of the urinary tract. In fact, ureaplasmas are the most common etiologic agents of septic arthritis in the setting of congenital antibody deficiencies and should be considered early when attempting to diagnose these conditions. A summary of diseases caused by *M. hominis* and/or *Ureaplasma* species in the urogenital tracts and extragenital sites of men and women as well as neonatal infections due to these organisms is provided in Table 2.

Both *M. hominis* and *Ureaplasma* species grow more rapidly than *M. pneumoniae* and can therefore be detected in cultures of appropriate specimens within 2 to 5 days. Proper handling and bedside inoculation of 10B or SP4 transport broth as described for *M. pneumoniae* are recommended to enhance recovery of these organisms. Urethral or wound swabs, cervicovaginal or prostatic secretions, urine, respiratory specimens such as those described for *M. pneumoniae,* CSF, blood, or other body fluids or tissues are appropriate for culture, depending on the clinical setting. Cultures are available mainly through reference laboratories. At present, there are no commercial serologic assays or rapid-detection tests available for routine diagnostic studies.

Genitourinary or extragenital diseases known to be caused by or associated with mycoplasmas warrant appropriate diagnostic tests when available and treatment if infection is confirmed. This is particularly important if the organisms are recovered in the absence of other possible microbial etiologies and if the infection is present in a normally sterile site such as blood, synovial fluid, or CSF.

Table 1   Treatment of Infections Caused by *Mycoplasma pneumoniae*, *Mycoplasma hominis*, and *Ureaplasma* Species

DRUG	ROUTE	DOSAGE/24 HR*		COMMENTS
		PEDIATRIC	ADULT	
STANDARD TREATMENTS				
Doxycycline	PO	4 mg/kg loading dose day 1, then 2-4 mg/kg/day in 1-2 doses	200 mg loading dose day 1, then 100 mg q12h	Contraindicated in pregnant women and children <8 yr of age unless no other alternative
	IV	Same as PO	Same as PO	If giving IV, infuse over 60 min to prevent thrombophlebitis; activity inhibited in some strains of genital mycoplasmas possessing *tetM*
Tetracycline	PO	25-50 mg/kg/day in 4 doses	250-500 mg q6h	Same comments as for doxycycline
	IV	10-20 mg/kg/day in 2-4 doses	125-500 mg q6-12h	
Erythromycin	PO	20-50 mg/kg/day in 3-4 doses	250-500 mg q6h	Not useful for *M. hominis*
	IV	25-40 mg/kg/day in 4 doses	Same as PO	Infuse over 60 min to prevent thrombophlebitis and minimize risk of cardiac toxicity; may cause elevation of serum theophylline levels
Clindamycin	PO	10-25 mg/kg/day in 3-4 doses	150-450 mg q6h	Not useful for *Ureaplasma* species or *M. pneumoniae*
	IV	10-40 mg/kg/day in 3-4 doses For neonates do not exceed 15-20 mg/kg/day in 3-4 doses	150-900 mg q6-8h	
ALTERNATIVE TREATMENTS				
Chloramphenicol	PO	Not recommended	Not recommended	Frequent monitoring of hematologic parameters and blood levels of the antibiotic are necessary; may be useful for treatment of meningitis caused by *M. hominis* or *Ureaplasma* species
	IV	50-100 mg/kg/day in 4 doses For neonates up to 2 wk of age, use 25 mg/kg/day in 1 dose, thereafter 50 mg/kg/day in 1 dose	25 mg/kg q6h	
Azithromycin	PO	10 mg/kg/day on day 1, then 5 mg/kg/day for respiratory infections	1 g single dose for urogenital infections† 500 mg day 1, then 250 mg/day for respiratory infections	Not useful for *M. hominis*; no clinical data for neonates
	IV	Not recommended	500 mg/day IV × 2 days, then 500 mg PO qd	
Clarithromycin	PO	15 mg/kg/day in 2 doses	250-500 mg q12h	Not useful for *M. hominis*; may cause elevation in serum theophylline levels; not approved for use in urogenital infections; no clinical data for neonates
	IV	Not available	Not available	
Ofloxacin	PO	Not recommended	200-400 mg q12h for urogenital infections, including pelvic inflammatory disease	Active against *Ureaplasma* species and *M. hominis*; not approved for use in persons <18 yr of age or pregnant women
	IV	Not recommended	Same as PO	

*Dosages shown are for persons with normal renal and hepatic function. For some agents, dosage adjustments may be indicated in the setting of renal or hepatic dysfunction, depending on the route of drug metabolism and excretion.
†Data are based on patients with urethritis caused by *C. trachomatis* and not specifically for ureaplasmas.

Practitioners will usually have to rely on familiarity with clinical syndromes typically caused by genital mycoplasmas and treat empirically if facilities for laboratory diagnosis are not readily available. Many of the conditions associated with a mycoplasmal etiology can also be caused by many microbial agents, and some conditions, such as pelvic inflammatory disease, can be polymicrobial. Therefore the selection of drugs must take into account multiple causes.

■ THERAPY OF *MYCOPLASMA HOMINIS* AND *UREAPLASMA UREALYTICUM* INFECTIONS

Oral tetracyclines, given for at least 7 days, have historically been the drugs of choice for use against urogenital infections caused by *M. hominis,* but resistance now occurs in 20% to 40% of isolates and in 10% to 15% of *Ureaplasma* species,

Table 1 Treatment of Infections Caused by *Mycoplasma pneumoniae, Mycoplasma hominis,* and *Ureaplasma* Species—cont'd

| DRUG | ROUTE | DOSAGE/24 HR* | | COMMENTS |
		PEDIATRIC	ADULT	
ALTERNATIVE TREATMENTS—cont'd				
Levofloxacin	PO	Not recommended	250 mg/day for urogenital infections,† including acute pyelonephritis 500 mg/day for respiratory infections	Not approved for use in persons <18 yr of age or pregnant women
	IV	Not recommended	Same as PO	
Sparfloxacin	PO	Not recommended	400 mg day 1, then 200 mg/day	Phototoxicity limits usefulness as alternative for respiratory infections; not approved for use in persons <18 yr of age or pregnant women; sparfloxacin is contraindicated in persons who are receiving concomitant therapy with class 1A or class III antiarrhythmic agents or in persons with known QT prolongation on electrocardiogram
	IV	Not available	Not available	
Gatifloxacin	PO	Not recommended	400 mg qd for respiratory infections	Not approved for use in persons <18 yr of age or in pregnant women; gatifloxacin should not be taken concurrently with class 1A and class III antiarrhythmics or in persons with uncorrected hypokalemia or known prolongation of QT intervals on electrocardiogram
	IV	Not recommended	Same as PO	
Moxifloxacin	PO	Not recommended	400 mg qd for respiratory infections	Not approved for use in persons <18 yr of age or in pregnant women; moxifloxacin should not be taken concurrently with class 1A and class III antiarrhythmics or in persons with uncorrected hypokalemia or known prolongation of QT intervals on electrocardiogram
	IV	Not available	Not available	

indicating that the susceptibility of these organisms can no longer be assumed. The degree of resistance may vary according to geographic area, type of patient population, and previous exposure to antimicrobial agents. Alternative agents must be considered in the event of treatment failures if tetracyclines are relied on as first-line drugs. In vitro susceptibility testing is sometimes indicated for mycoplasmas recovered from a normally sterile body site, from immunocompromised hosts, and/or from persons who have not responded to an initial treatment. Susceptibility testing can be accomplished in 3 to 5 days by a reference laboratory once the organism is isolated. Clindamycin is one alternative treatment for tetracycline-resistant *M. hominis,* but it is much less active against ureaplasmas. Erythromycin or tetracyclines are the drugs of choice for *Ureaplasma* infections. Although tetracycline resistance has been described in *Ureaplasma* species, high-level erythromycin resistance is exceedingly rare, if indeed it occurs at all. A single dose of azithromycin is approved for treatment of urethritis caused by *Chlamydia trachomatis* and has been shown to work as well clinically as doxycycline in persons with urethritis caused by *Ureaplasma* species, reflecting its in vitro activity against this organism. Clarithromycin, although active against *Ureaplasma* species in vitro at concentrations comparable to or lower than erythromycin, has not been approved for use in treatment of urogenital infections. *M. hominis* is resistant to erythromycin, azithromycin, and clarithromycin. Despite apparent in vitro susceptibility, tetracycline or erythromycin treatment of vaginal mycoplasmas in women is not always successful.

Fluoroquinolones have now become useful alternatives for treatment of certain infections caused by *M. hominis* or *Ureaplasma* species within the urogenital tract and in some extragenital locations. Activity of quinolones is not affected

Table 2 Association of *Mycoplasma hominis* and *Ureaplasma* Species with Specific Pathologic Conditions

DISEASE	M. HOMINIS	UREAPLASMA SPECIES
MEN		
Urethritis	−	+
Prostatitis	+/−	+/−
Epididymitis	−	+/−
WOMEN		
Acute urethral syndrome	−	+/−
Pelvic inflammatory disease	+	+/−
Bacterial vaginosis	+	+/−
Chorioamnionitis	+/−	+
Spontaneous abortion/ stillbirth	+/−	+/−
Postpartum/postabortal fever/endometritis	+	+
MEN OR WOMEN		
Pyelonephritis	+	+/−
Cystitis	−	+/−
Urinary calculi	−	+
Extragenital diseases*		
Septic arthritis	+	+
Osteomyelitis	+	+
Bacteremia	+	+
Soft tissue abscesses	+	+
Wound infections	+	−
Peritonitis	+	−
Meningitis/brain abscess	+	−
Pneumonia	+	+
Pericarditis/endocarditis	+	+
NEONATES		
Prematurity	−	+
Congenital/neonatal pneumonia	+	+
Chronic lung disease of prematurity	−	+/−
Bacteremia	+	+
Soft tissue abscesses	+	+
Meningitis	+	+

−, No association or causal role demonstrated; +, causal role; +/−, association, but causal role not proved.

*Invasive extragenital diseases caused by either *M. hominis* or *Ureaplasma* species are almost always associated with genitourinary manipulation or trauma, hypogammaglobulinemia, or other immunocompromised state when they occur beyond the neonatal period. The true incidence of such infections in susceptible persons is unknown because mycoplasmas are rarely sought.

by tetracycline resistance caused by the *tetM* transposon, making these drugs attractive alternatives for tetracycline-resistant *M. hominis* or *U. urealyticum* infections. Ciprofloxacin and ofloxacin are generally less active in vitro against either species than newer agents such as levofloxacin, gatifloxacin, moxifloxacin, and sparfloxacin. In general, *M. hominis* is more susceptible than *Ureaplasma* species to quinolones in vitro based on minimal inhibitory concentrations. Most clinical trials of quinolones for treatment of genitourinary infections have focused primarily on other pathogens such as *C. trachomatis* and *Neisseria gonorrhoeae*. Very few studies have included microbiologic data specific for genital mycoplasmas, and there have been no systematic comparative evaluations of treatment regimens for extragenital infections in adults or for neonatal infections. Thus treatment recommendations, including dosages and duration, are based largely on in vitro susceptibility data, outcomes of treatment trials evaluating clinical response to syndromes such as pelvic inflammatory disease and urethritis that may be caused by genital mycoplasmas, and individual case reports. For infections such as urethritis that may be venereally transmitted, sexual contacts of the index case should also receive treatment.

Experience with mycoplasmal or ureaplasmal infections in immunocompromised patients, especially those with hypogammaglobulinemia who have been the best studied, demonstrate that even though mycoplasmas are primarily noninvasive mucosal pathogens in the normal host, they have the capacity to produce destructive and progressive disease. Infections may be caused by resistant organisms refractory to antimicrobial therapy and require prolonged administration of a combination of intravenous antimicrobials, intravenous immunoglobulin, and/or antisera prepared specifically against the infecting species. Even with aggressive therapy, relapses are still likely to occur. Repeat cultures of affected sites may be necessary to gauge in vivo response to treatment.

Isolation of *M. hominis* or *Ureaplasma* species from CSF in neonates with pleocytosis, progressive hydrocephalus or other neurologic abnormality, pericardial fluid, pleural fluid, tracheal aspirate in association with respiratory disease, abscess material, or blood are justification for specific treatment in critically ill neonates when no other verifiable microbiologic etiologies of the clinical condition are apparent. Whether treatment should be given for a positive CSF culture when inflammation or other evidence of clinical illness is not observed should be handled on a case-by-case basis. It may be pertinent to monitor the patient, repeat lumbar puncture, and reexamine for inflammation and organisms prior to initiating treatment because some cases may spontaneously resolve without intervention.

Parenteral tetracyclines have been used most often to treat neonatal meningitis caused by either *M. hominis* or *Ureaplasma* species despite contraindications, but erythromycin for *Ureaplasma* species, clindamycin for *M. hominis*, or chloramphenicol for either organism are alternatives. No single drug has been successful in every instance in eradication of these organisms from CSF of neonates. There have been no reports demonstrating efficacy of aminoglycosides against genital mycoplasmas. There has been little clinical experience with the new-generation macrolides in treatment of neonatal ureaplasmal infections, and currently neither of these agents is approved for general use in this population.

Overall, treatment guidelines for neonates are the same as for urogenital and systemic mycoplasmal infections in adults with appropriate dosage modifications based on weight, except that the intravenous route should be used for serious systemic infections. Duration of treatment and drug dosages for neonatal mycoplasmal infections have not been critically evaluated, but a minimum of 10 to 14 days of therapy is suggested based on experience in individual cases where microbiologic follow-up has been assessed.

■ OTHER MYCOPLASMAL SPECIES

Other mycoplasmal species, such as *M. fermentans* and *M. genitalium,* are known to occur in the human respiratory and/or urogenital tracts and may be associated with disease. *M. fermentans* has been detected in throat cultures of children with pneumonia, in some cases when no other etiologic agent was identified, but the frequency of its occurrence in healthy children is not known. This mycoplasma has also been detected in adults with an acute, influenza-like illness and in bronchoalveolar lavage specimens from patients with the acquired immunodeficiency syndrome and pneumonia. Thanks to the availability of PCR as a diagnostic tool, it is now clear that *M. genitalium,* perhaps even more so than *Ureaplasma* species, is an etiologic agent of nongonococcal, nonchlamydial urethritis.

Because of the difficulty in cultivation of *M. fermentans* and *M. genitalium* and the absence of clinical experience with antimicrobial chemotherapy for treating infections associated with these organisms, it is impossible to make specific recommendations regarding diagnosis or treatment alternatives. However, based on in vitro studies of small numbers of isolates, the susceptibilities of *M. fermentans* are generally similar to those of *M. hominis,* whereas those of *M. genitalium* approximate those for *M. pneumoniae.* Thus empiric treatments must be deduced from these in vitro data.

Suggested Reading

Cassell GH, Waites KB, Crouse DT: Mycoplasmal infections. In Remington JS, Klein JO, eds: *Infectious diseases of the fetus and newborn infant,* ed 4, Philadelphia, 1994, WB Saunders.

Cassell GH, et al: Efficacy of clarithromycin against *Mycoplasma pneumoniae,* J Antimicrob Chemother 27(suppl A):47, 1991.

Cherry JD: Mycoplasma and ureaplasma infections. In Feigin RD, Cherry JD, eds: *Textbook of pediatric infectious diseases,* vol 2, ed 3, Philadelphia, 1992, WB Saunders.

Furr PM, Taylor-Robinson, Webster ADB: Mycoplasmas and ureaplasmas in patients with hypogammaglobulinemia and their role in arthritis: microbiological observations over twenty years, Ann Rheum 53:183, 1994.

Waites KB, Crouse DT, Cassell GH: Therapeutic considerations for *Ureaplasma urealyticum* infections in neonates, Clin Infect Dis 17(suppl 1):S208, 1993.

Waites KB, et al: Serum concentrations of erythromycin after intravenous infusion in preterm neonates treated for *Ureaplasma urealyticum* infection, Pediatr Infect Dis J 13:287, 1994.

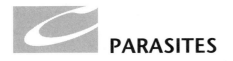 **PARASITES**

INTESTINAL ROUNDWORMS

Ramya Gopinath

Jay S. Keystone

Nematodes are the most common parasites infecting humans worldwide, with millions of people harboring more than one species of helminth. The severity of disease caused by helminths is related to the intensity of infection; however, heavy and recurrent infections occur in only a small segment of the population. People with heavy infections who manifest signs and symptoms or develop complications generally require treatment. Individuals with light infections often have few or no abnormal findings; they usually do not require treatment, as complications are rare and adult nematodes die within a few years in the absence of recurrent infection. Helminths do not multiply in the human host; the natural history of infection is a decrease in worm burden over time. The exception to this general rule is infection with *Strongyloides stercoralis,* in which low-level persistent infection is maintained for the lifetime of the host by autoinfection. Untreated persons are in danger of progression to parasite hyperinfection and dissemination should they become immunocompromised. This chapter focuses on seven important human nematodes and emphasizes clinical and laboratory diagnosis, and treatment.

■ *ASCARIS*

Ascaris lumbricoides, the largest intestinal nematode, infects more than 1 billion people worldwide. This may be attributed to the prodigious output of eggs by each adult female and the ability of these eggs to survive in a range of environmental conditions. Eggs are passed in human feces and require a soil maturation phase of 2 weeks to several months before becoming infective. Infection is acquired by ingestion of eggs containing second-stage larvae. These larvae hatch in the jejunum, penetrate the intestinal wall, and migrate to the right side of the heart, the pulmonary circulation, and the alveoli. They then ascend to the pharynx, are swallowed, and develop into adults in the distal small intestine. The life span of the adult is about 1 year.

Most infected persons are asymptomatic. However, the tissue or pulmonary phase may be marked by urticaria, eosinophilia, and Loeffler's syndrome—pulmonary hypersensitivity and eosinophilic inflammation, which may manifest as cough, shortness of breath, wheezing, and pulmonary infiltrates. The intestinal phase is generally asymptomatic. Any complications are usually caused by obstruction of the terminal ileum by a bolus of worms or migration of a single adult worm into the bile duct, pancreatic duct, or appendix with resultant obstruction or abscess formation. The diagnosis of ascariasis is made by stool examination, in which eggs are readily found. Occasionally, worms may be outlined by contrast medium during a barium meal procedure. Because of the danger of worm migration, all infections, whether symptomatic or not, should be treated. When more than one parasite infection is being treated, *Ascaris* should always be treated first, since medications may stimulate worms to migrate. Recommended regimens are summarized in Table 1.

■ HOOKWORM

Globally, human hookworm disease caused by *Necator americanus* and *Ancylostoma duodenale* is almost as prevalent as ascariasis. The hallmark of disease is iron deficiency anemia due to chronic blood loss. Hookworm ova are passed in feces and develop in soil, where under optimal conditions they hatch in 1 to 2 days, releasing rhabditiform larvae that develop over 3 to 7 days into the infective filariform stage. After penetrating the unbroken skin of bare feet, larvae migrate via veins or lymphatics to the heart. They then pass through the alveoli, migrate up to the pharynx, are swallowed, and develop further in the gut. Adults attach to the mucosa of the small intestine; egg production begins about 5 weeks after larval invasion of the skin. The life span of *A. duodenale* is about 6 to 7 years, and that of *N. americanus* is 5 to 6 years; however, worm burden begins to fall within 1 to 3 years in the absence of reinfection.

Clinical features correspond to the life cycle of the organism and intensity of infection. Skin penetration by filariform larvae can produce intense pruritus (ground itch or dew itch) followed by erythematous papules, vesiculation, and local edema; this can last for up to 2 weeks and may be complicated by secondary bacterial infection. The pulmonary phase may be characterized by cough, wheezing, or Loeffler's syndrome, but in general, symptoms are relatively mild. Epigastric pain suggestive of peptic ulcer disease, flatulence, and abdominal tenderness may occur early in the intestinal phase of infection. Rarely, young children with heavy primary infection may develop bloody diarrhea or severe gastrointestinal hemorrhage. Chronic iron deficiency anemia, the most common presentation, results from blood loss at the site of attachment of the adult as well as ingestion of blood by the worm. The development and severity of anemia depend on the intensity of infection, the iron reserves of the host, and the availability of iron in the diet;

Table 1   Treatment Regimens for Selected Helminth Infections*

INFECTION	DRUG	DOSAGE	EFFICACY (%)
Ascaris†	**Mebendazole**	500 mg once or 100 mg bid ×3 days	84-100
	Albendazole	400 mg once	>90
	Pyrantel pamoate	11 mg/kg once (maximum 1 g/dose)	90
	Piperazine	75 mg/kg once daily ×2 days	
Hookworm†	**Mebendazole**	100 mg bid ×3 days	76-95
	Albendazole	400 mg once	
	Pyrantel pamoate	11 mg/kg once daily ×3 days (maximum 1 g/day)	88
Trichuris†	Oxantel pamoate	15 mg/kg once	88
	Mebendazole	100 mg bid ×3 days	60-80
	Albendazole	600 mg once (repeat in heavy infection)	60
Enterobius†	**Pyrantel**	11 mg/kg once (maximum 1 g/dose) (repeat in 2 wk)	90-100
	Pyrvinium pamoate	5 mg/kg once; repeat in 2 wk	90-100
	Mebendazole	100 mg once; repeat in 2 wk	90-100
	Albendazole	400 mg once; repeat in 2 wk	90-100
Trichostrongylus†	**Pyrantel pamoate**	11 mg/kg (maximum 1 g/dose)	
	Albendazole	400 mg once	
	Mebendazole	100 mg bid ×3 days	
Strongyloides†	Ivermectin	100-200 µg/kg once daily ×2 days	85-100
	Albendazole‡	400 mg/day ×3 days	60-70
	Thiabendazole	25 mg/kg bid ×2-3 days	60-70
Anisakis	Mebendazole	200 mg bid ×3 days	
	Removal by surgery or endoscopy		

*Drugs of choice are shown in boldface.
†Benzimidazole derivatives (thiabendazole, mebendazole, albendazole) are contraindicated in pregnancy.
‡Treatment failures should be treated with 400 mg bid for 7 days.

therefore hookworm anemia is mostly seen in the Third World, where a hemoglobin of 3 to 8 g/dl is not unusual. Complications of severe anemia, including weakness, fatigue, and high-output cardiac failure, are common. Laboratory findings include hypochromic microcytic anemia, a low reticulocyte count, low serum ferritin and iron levels, and elevated transferrin. Eosinophilia is common in hookworm disease. Hypoalbuminemia may be due to protein-losing enteropathy. The diagnosis is made by finding hookworm ova in the stool, either by direct examination or after concentration techniques. Occasionally, rhabditiform larvae may be present in stool and must be differentiated morphologically from those of *Strongyloides*. Regimens for the treatment of hookworm infection are summarized in Table 1. Asymptomatic light infections in well-nourished hosts need not be treated.

■ *TRICHURIS*

Infection with *Trichuris trichiura* (whipworm), as with *Enterobius vermicularis* (pinworm), is confined to the gastrointestinal tract without a preceding tissue phase. Its global distribution parallels that of *Ascaris*. Infection is acquired by ingestion of embryonated eggs. The 3- to 5-cm adult worm burrows its whiplike anterior end into the mucosa of the cecum and may survive for years. Eggs are passed in feces and require a soil maturation period of 10 to 14 days. Most infected persons have a mild to moderate worm burden and are asymptomatic. Heavy infections are also generally asymptomatic but may manifest with abdominal pain, chronic diarrhea, or rarely in children, rectal prolapse,

growth stunting, and poor school performance. The diagnosis of trichuriasis is made by finding the characteristic barrel-shaped eggs in stool. Eosinophilia is unusual. In light asymptomatic infections, treatment is not mandatory because complications are virtually nonexistent. Treatment regimens are summarized in Table 1.

■ *ENTEROBIUS*

E. vermicularis (pinworm) is distributed worldwide and is the most prevalent helminth infection in the United States and Western Europe. Unlike other helminth infections, pinworms are found in children of all socioeconomic classes, and transmission within families is common. Eggs ingested from fecally contaminated hands or food hatch in the upper small intestine. Development occurs in the small intestine, and gravid adult females settle in the cecum, appendix, or adjacent ascending colon, where they live for about 13 weeks. Adults migrate out through the anus, mostly at night, to deposit eggs in the perianal and perineal skin. The resulting pruritus ani, the most common clinical manifestation, leads to scratching, contamination of fingers, subsequent ingestion of eggs from soiled hands, and further spread to the environment. Complications include perianal eczematoid dermatitis with secondary bacterial infection, perianal granuloma, and occasionally vulvovaginitis in girls.

A diagnosis of enterobiasis can be made by identifying the adult worm or eggs. The most reliable approach is the transparent adhesive tape (cellulose acetate tape, or Scotch tape) test to demonstrate eggs on perianal skin. A wooden tongue depressor draped with tape with the sticky side out is firmly pressed against the perianal skin immediately on waking in the morning before defecation or bathing. The tape is removed in the laboratory, placed sticky side down on a slide and examined under low power for eggs. Ninety percent of infections can be detected with three swabs on three consecutive mornings, and seven tests detect 100% of infections. By contrast, routine stool examination for ova and parasites is positive in only 10% to 15% of infected persons.

The treatment of enterobiasis is summarized in Table 1. In the absence of reinfection or autoinfection, a primary infection will clear without treatment in 30 to 45 days. Abdominal pain or diarrhea should prompt a search for *Dientamoeba fragilis,* since the coinfection rate with *E. vermicularis* may be as high as 50%. Because intrafamilial transmission is common, treatment of the entire family is usually recommended. Specific hygienic measures such as careful handwashing, weekly laundering of bedclothes, wearing of underwear and pajamas at night, daily change of underwear, and daily morning bathing are important for eradication of infection. Repeat treatment of the whole family after an interval of 2 weeks is recommended, as drugs are relatively ineffective against developing larvae and newly ingested eggs. Recurring infections should be treated at least four times at 2-week intervals.

■ *TRICHOSTRONGYLUS*

Trichostrongylus species, primarily parasites of herbivorous animals such as sheep, cattle, and goats, are most prevalent in the Middle East and Asia. Humans are accidental hosts who are usually infected by ingestion of food or water contaminated by the feces of infected animals or humans, although the larvae can penetrate skin. Ova hatch in soil within 1 to 2 days and pass through three free-living stages before becoming infective. There is no tissue phase, and adults reside in the duodenum or upper jejunum. Little is known about the pathology of human trichostrongyliasis. Most human infections are mild and asymptomatic, but diarrhea, flatulence, and epigastric pain may occur. Diagnosis depends on identification in stool of ova, which are often difficult to differentiate from hookworm ova; eosinophilia is present in a minority of infected persons. Treatment regimens are summarized in Table 1.

■ *ANISAKIS*

Anisakiasis (herring worm, or codworm disease), caused by infection with the third-stage larvae of *Anisakis simplex* or *Pseudoterranova decipiens,* is acquired by consumption of raw or inadequately cooked marine fish or squid. It is most prevalent in Japan and less frequent in Hawaii and the coastal areas of North America and Northern Europe. The primary hosts of *Anisakis* are dolphins, porpoises, and whales. Free-swimming second-stage larvae are ingested by small marine crustacea and develop to third-stage larvae that are transferred to squid or fish by the predatory food chain. Herring, salmon, mackerel, cod, squid, and many other fish harbor third-stage larvae in their muscles and are

important infectious sources for human anisakiasis. When raw or inadequately cooked fish is consumed by humans, larvae invade the submucosa of the stomach or intestine. The resulting local inflammation and hemorrhage generally last about 10 days, until death of the larvae. Clinical manifestations of gastric anisakiasis, which usually occur 1 to 7 hours after ingestion of infected food, consist of severe epigastric pain, nausea, and vomiting. Acute symptoms subside in a few days, but intermittent nausea, vomiting, and vague abdominal pain may persist for weeks to months. Symptoms of intestinal anisakiasis develop 1 to 5 days after the infecting meal and are due to invasion of the distal ileum. Abdominal pain, nausea, vomiting, and mild leukocytosis occur; complications include peritonitis and pleurisy caused by a worm that has burrowed through the intestinal wall.

A history of consumption of inadequately cooked fish or squid shortly before the onset of symptoms is essential to the diagnosis of anisakiasis, which can be most easily confirmed by endoscopy. Intestinal anisakiasis is difficult to differentiate from other causes of acute abdomen, and patients often undergo laparotomy. Serologic diagnosis may be helpful but is not readily available. Treatment is removal of the worm, although even untreated infection subsides in a few days. Intestinal anisakiasis should be treated conservatively, with fluids and supportive care. Although mebendazole has been tried, effective chemotherapy of human anisakiasis is not well established; it is best to prevent infection by not eating raw or undercooked fish or squid.

■ *STRONGYLOIDES*

S. stercoralis (threadworm) is nearly unique among helminths for its ability to autoinfect and maintain persistent infection for years, often for the lifetime of the infected person. It is endemic in Southeast Asia, South America, sub-Saharan Africa, eastern Europe, and the southern United States. Several features set this helminth apart from the others: adult females are parthenogenetic and live and lay their eggs in the mucosa of the small bowel. Because eggs hatch immediately there, neither adults nor eggs are found in stool samples. Strongyloides has a complex life cycle (Figure 1); rhabditiform larvae can mature directly to invasive filariform larvae in the human host, and thus infection is maintained for years without further exposure to exogenous infective larvae. The ability of *Strongyloides* to live and multiply outside the host (heterogonic development) and its ability to overwhelm the immunocompromised host during autoinfection are other well-recognized and unique features of this parasite.

Most infected persons have low worm burdens and are asymptomatic. Any symptoms occur irregularly, with long asymptomatic periods. Chronic infection with *Strongyloides* may present with episodic creeping urticaria (larva currens), epigastric pain mimicking peptic ulcer disease, or abdominal pain and diarrhea, which may persist for years after exposure. Bloating, distention, or frank malabsorption may also occur. Filariform larvae passing through the lung may produce Loeffler's pneumonitis, and peripheral eosinophilia is very common. Steroids, chemotherapeutic agents,

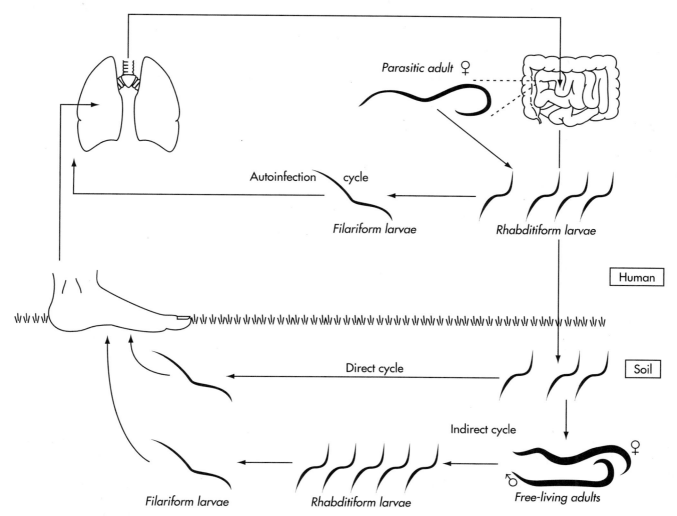

Figure 1

Alternative life cycles of *Strongyloides stercoralis*. Infective filariform larvae invade the skin or mucous membranes and then migrate via the circulation and lungs to the proximal intestine, where maturation occurs. First-stage rhabditiform larvae may develop into free-living adult worms in the soil, which give rise to a second generation of rhabditiform and filariform larvae. Rhabditiform larvae also can transform directly into infective filariform larvae in the soil or within the host intestine in the latter pathway. The filariform larvae enter the circulation or perianal skin, establishing repeated cycles of internal reinfection known as *autoinfection*. *(From Liu LX, Weller PF: Infect Dis Clin North Am 7:655, 1993.)*

hematologic malignancies, organ transplants, malnutrition, chronic alcoholism, and coinfection with HTLV-1 are the most common predisposing conditions for the hyperinfection syndrome; prior infection with human immuno-deficiency virus does not seem to consistently increase susceptibility to this complication. Hyperinfection may set in insidiously, with abdominal pain, nausea, vomiting, anorexia, or diarrhea eventually leading to steatorrhea, protein-losing enteropathy, or paralytic ileus. Cough, wheezing, or hemoptysis associated with diffuse pulmonary infiltrates may occur, and filariform larvae can be identified in sputum or bronchial washings. In uncontrolled hyperinfection, filariform larvae penetrate organs not normally involved in the life cycle, including the urinary tract, liver,

and brain. Bacterial superinfection often complicates the picture; gram-negative bacilli are carried through the intestinal wall to cause bacteremia, peritonitis, or meningitis. Eosinophilia in this situation is rare.

The diagnosis of stronglyoidiasis is difficult, requiring a high index of suspicion. Clinical features are nonspecific, and larval output in stool is minimal and irregular. Examination of a single stool specimen has a sensitivity of only 20% to 30%, whereas multiple samples increase the sensitivity to 60% to 70%. The Baermann stool and agar plate concentration techniques increase yield further, as does examination of duodenal fluid by aspiration or the string test. Eosinophilia (>5%) is present in 40% to 80% of patients with intestinal strongyloidiasis, but in fewer than

20% of patients with the hyperinfection syndrome. Specific serology for *Strongyloides,* available at the Centers for Disease Control and Prevention in Atlanta, has a sensitivity of 85% to 90%; titres decline within 6 months after successful treatment. False-positive results have been observed with filariasis and acute schistosomiasis. Treatment of strongyloidiasis is difficult and may require repeated attempts. Recommended regimens are summarized in Table 1.

Suggested Reading

Grencis RK, Cooper ES: Enterobius, trichuris, capillaria, and hookworm including *Ancylostoma caninum, Gastro Clin North Am* 35:579, 1996.
Khuroo MS: Ascariasis, *Gastroentero Clin North Am* 35:553, 1996.
Liu LX, Weller PF: Strongyloidiasis and other intestinal nematode infections, *Infect Dis Clin North Am* 7:655, 1993.

TISSUE NEMATODES

Thomas A. Moore
Theodore E. Nash

Tissue-dwelling helminths include a large number of nematodes, cestodes, and trematodes that cause many clinical manifestations. IgE elevations tend to accompany eosinophilia caused by helminth infections, but a normal level does not eliminate parasitic disease. The diagnostic considerations can be narrowed through an understanding of the various parasites, specifically the geographic distribution, the likelihood of exposure in endemic areas, incubation periods, and knowledge of the common manifestations of infection. Serologic tests are sometimes helpful, but panels of helminth serologic tests are most likely to be unrewarding if not confusing. Treatment strategies must be tailored to the individual parasitic disease.

■ TRICHINOSIS

Trichinosis develops when raw or inadequately cooked meat containing the encysted larvae of *Trichinella* species is eaten. The larvae are released from the cysts and attach to the mucosa of the small intestinal villi, where they develop into male and female adult worms. The infective newborn larvae invade striated muscle, where they encyst within individual muscle fibers.

Trichinosis has a worldwide distribution, occurring in temperate and tropical climates. In the United States, most cases of trichinosis are acquired domestically from infected pork products, although the meat of other animals, such as game, is becoming more common as a source of infection. Among U.S. travelers, most cases of trichinosis have been associated with consumption of wild pigs, especially the bush pig and warthog. However, meat from other sources can result in trichinosis as well, and outbreaks of the disease have been associated with consumption of meat from bears, walruses, and horses. Most reported travel-related infections have been associated with visits to Mexico, southeast Asia, and sub-Saharan Africa.

The severity of symptoms depends on the absolute number of ingested larvae. Because most infections result from ingestion of a small number of larvae, most infected persons are asymptomatic. The adult worm in the small intestine may cause gastrointestinal symptoms within a week of infection. Symptoms include abdominal discomfort, vomiting, and diarrhea, which may evolve into a fulminant enteritis in unusually heavy infections. However, most clinical manifestations are related to systemic invasion by larvae, and they usually begin in the second week after infection, peak over a week's time, then slowly subside. These symptoms include fever and myositis with pain, swelling, and weakness. Myositis usually begins in the extraocular muscles and progresses to involve the masseters, neck muscles, and limb flexors. Other symptoms include headache, cough, and dysphagia. Occasionally, subconjunctival or subungual splinter hemorrhages develop. A petechial or macular rash is sometimes seen. In fulminant infections myocarditis, pneumonia, and encephalitis occasionally lead to death.

Fever and eosinophilia associated with periorbital edema and myositis are the cardinal features of trichinosis. Eosinophilia begins about 10 days after infection and may be quite high. The erythrocyte sedimentation rate is usually normal. Elevated creatine phosphokinase and lactate dehydrogenase levels reflect extensive muscle involvement.

Serologic testing is available from the Centers for Disease Control and Prevention (CDC), but antibodies are not detectable until at least 3 weeks after infection. Although muscle biopsy may confirm the diagnosis, it is usually unnecessary.

Therapy

The mainstays of treatment are supportive. A number of drugs, including thiabendazole and albendazole, have been used successfully in animal models, but there is no clinical evidence of efficacy in symptomatic humans. Corticosteroids have been used in critically ill patients, with equivocal results. Persons who are known to have recently eaten trichinous meat should be given an 8-day course of albendazole, 400 mg orally twice daily, to eliminate the intestinal infection. A 7-day course of thiabendazole, 25 mg/kg/day (to a maximum of 3 g/day), can be given as an alternative.

■ FILARIASIS

Of the eight filarial species capable of infecting humans, the four that cause the most disease worldwide are *Brugia malayi, Wuchereria bancrofti, Onchocerca volvulus,* and *Loa loa.* Because only a small proportion of insect bites are infective, the disease generally occurs only after long exposure in an endemic area. The clinical manifestations of filariasis depend in part on the immune response of the host. Generally, the response to the parasite in endemic populations is dampened, and a large parasite burden is common. In contrast, individuals who have grown up outside of endemic regions and who move or travel to these regions and become infected manifest prominent signs and symptoms of inflammatory reactions to the parasites and usually have a low parasite burden. Treatment of the filarial infections is summarized in Table 1.

To diagnose filarial organisms properly, it is critical that blood is filtered during the period of peak microfilaremia, which differs among organisms.

Lymphatic Filariasis

Lymphatic filariasis is caused by infection with one of the lymph-dwelling filariae, *W. bancrofti, B. malayi,* or *Brugia timori.* The bite of an infected mosquito deposits larvae in the subcutaneous tissue. Over time, they mature into adult worms. These threadlike adults reside in afferent lymphatic channels or sinuses of lymph nodes.

W. bancrofti, found in tropical and subtropical regions throughout the world, is the most widely distributed of the human filariae. In most of the world, the parasite is nocturnally periodic, meaning that microfilariae are scarce in peripheral blood during the day but increase at night. In the Pacific Islands, however, the microfilariae are subperiodic; microfilaremia is seen throughout the day, reaching maximal levels in the afternoon. Brugian filariasis occurs throughout Asia and the Far East, including India and the Philippines. This form of filariasis is nocturnally periodic, except in forested areas, where it is subperiodic.

Among endemic populations, the common manifestations of lymphatic filariasis include asymptomatic microfilaremia, filarial fevers, and lymphatic obstruction. Most infected individuals are clinically well and have an asymptomatic condition associated with microfilaremia. More than half of these patients have hematuria, proteinuria, or both. Filarial fevers are acute episodes of high fever and chills accompanied by signs of lymphatic inflammation (lymphangitis and lymphadenitis) and transient lymphedema. The episodes spontaneously abate after a week to 10 days but can recur. Importantly, the lymphangitis develops in a descending fashion, opposite the direction seen in cellulitis. Regional lymphadenopathy is often present and thrombophlebitis can also develop. Both upper and lower extremities may be involved but genital involvement, which may manifest as epididymitis, funiculitis, and scrotal pain and tenderness, is found exclusively with *W. bancrofti.*

Damage to the lymphatics, which may result in obstruction or lymphatic dysfunction, manifests early as pitting edema. The edema may progress with time, eventually resulting in the characteristic features of elephantiasis, which include thickening of subcutaneous tissues, hyperkeratosis, and fissuring of the skin. Lymphedema alone renders the patient susceptible to recurrent bacterial and fungal infections. Hydrocele formation is the most common manifestation of lymphatic filariasis, and scrotal lymphedema may also develop. If the retroperitoneal lymphatics are obstructed, chyluria develops.

Persons new to endemic areas (expatriates, transmigrants) who acquire lymphatic filariasis usually develop symptoms and signs of acute lymphatic inflammation such as lymphangitis, lymphadenitis, and in the case of *W. bancrofti,* genital pain, but they may also develop allergylike problems such as hives, urticaria, and eosinophilia.

Definitive diagnosis can be made only by finding the parasites. Unless microfilariae are detected in the peripheral blood or other body fluid, the diagnosis must be established on clinical grounds because the adult worms in lymphatics are generally inaccessible and excisional biopsies are unhelpful. Detection of microfilariae in the blood is most efficiently performed by filtering 1 ml or more of blood through a polycarbonate filter with 3-μm pores or examining the sediment from a Knott's prep (1 ml of blood with 10 ml of 2% formalin). Filtration of blood for nocturnally periodic microfilariae must be performed between 10 PM and 4 AM. It is important to note that a 10- to 14-day period is required for microfilarial periodicity to adjust to the local time zone.

Data supporting filarial infection include eosinophilia, elevated serum IgE levels, and antifilarial antibodies in the serum. Serologic studies have greater diagnostic value in persons new to endemic areas. A negative or low antibody level effectively rules out active infection in this population. However, interpretation of serologic findings may be problematic because of extensive cross-reactivity between filarial antigens and antigens of other helminths, such as *Strongyloides stercoralis.* For individuals from endemic areas who are likely to have antifilarial antibodies, infection with *W. bancrofti* can be established by identifying circulating antigens in the serum. This is most easily done using an antigen card assay, which can rapidly identify infected individuals with low or absent microfilaremia.

Table 1	Recommended Treatment for Filarial Infections
INFECTION AND ORGANISM	**TREATMENT**
Lymphatic filariasis *Wuchereria bancrofti* *Brugia malayi* *Brugia timori*	DEC, 6-8 mg/kg/day ×14 days
Tropical pulmonary eosinophilia *W. bancrofti* *Brugia malayi*	DEC, 6-8 mg/kg/day ×21 days
Loaiasis *Loa loa*	DEC, 8-10 mg/kg/day ×21 days
Onchocerciasis *Onchocerca volvulus*	Ivermectin, 150 μg/kg once
Other filariases	
Mansonella streptocerca	DEC, 6 mg/kg/day ×21 days
Mansonella perstans	DEC, 10 mg/kg/day ×21 days
Mansonella ozzardi	Ivermectin, 150 μg/kg once

DEC, Diethylcarbamazine.

Additional supportive data can be obtained with the use of lymphoscintigraphy, which (in early infections) will demonstrate a paradoxically brisk lymphatic flow on the affected side. Ultrasound of the scrotum using a high-frequency (7.5 to 10 MHz) transducer with Doppler may also demonstrate the motile adult worm in the lymphatic channel.

Therapy

The mainstay of treatment for lymphatic filariasis remains diethylcarbamazine (DEC), 6 to 8 mg/kg/day in either single or divided doses for 14 days. DEC, an orphan drug, can be obtained from the CDC drug service (telephone 404-639-3670). Although extended treatment is usually necessary to kill the adults, the drug rapidly kills microfilariae. The severity of adverse reactions correlates with the pretreatment level of microfilaremia. Usually, the reactions, which include fevers, headache, lethargy, arthralgias, and myalgias, can be managed easily with antipyretics and analgesics. Side effects are minimized by initiating treatment with a small dose of DEC (e.g., a single 50-mg tablet) and premedicating the patient with corticosteroids 0.5 to 1 mg/kg/day. A note of caution: the geographic distribution of onchocerciasis and loiasis overlap with lymphatic filariasis and coinfection occurs. Because treatment of onchocerciasis and loiasis with DEC can result in severe adverse effects, it is imperative that the clinician exclude the possibility of coinfection with organisms before giving DEC to patients with lymphatic filariasis.

Because adult worms may survive the initial treatment, symptoms can recur within a few months after therapy, and re-treatment is recommended for such patients. Some individuals have suggested treating such patients with DEC at the standard dosage of 6 to 8 mg/kg/day for 1 week each month for 6 to 12 months. Combination therapy with DEC and either albendazole or ivermectin has been tried in populations for mass chemotherapy of filariasis and other helminths, with good success; however, the use of these combination regimens to treat individual patients cannot be recommended at this time.

The optimal treatment of acute lymphatic inflammation is unknown, and these attacks usually resolve in 5 to 7 days without therapy. Treatment of chronic lymphatic obstruction is problematic. If the infection is recognized early, some signs of lymphatic obstruction can be reversed. In severely damaged lymphatics, however, only supportive measures may be helpful. These include elevation of the infected limb, use of elastic stockings, and good foot care with use of antifungal topical ointments and antibacterial antiseptics containing iodine. Prophylactic antibiotics should be considered for prevention of recurrent bacteremia and cellulitis. Hydroceles can be managed surgically, and surgical decompression with a nodovenous shunt may provide relief for severely affected limbs. No treatment has proved satisfactory for chyluria. DEC is useful for prophylaxis, but the optimal dosage and frequency have not been established.

Tropical Pulmonary Eosinophilia

Tropical pulmonary eosinophilia (TPE) is a distinct syndrome caused by immunologic hyperresponsiveness to *W. bancrofti* or *B. malayi*. The syndrome affects men four times as often as women, often in the third decade of life. Most cases have been reported from Pakistan, India, Sri Lanka, Southeast Asia, and Brazil.

TPE has been hypothesized to be caused by the trapping of microfilariae in the pulmonary vasculature, where they incite intense eosinophilic alveolitis. The clinical entity is characterized by paroxysmal cough and wheezing that is usually nocturnal and probably related to the nocturnal periodicity of the microfilariae, anorexia, and low-grade fever. Extreme eosinophilia (>3000/µl), high polyclonal IgE levels, marked elevations of specific antifilarial antibodies, and a therapeutic response to DEC are required for the diagnosis.

Therapy

DEC is recommended at 4 to 6 mg/kg/day for 14 days. Symptoms usually dramatically resolve within the first week of therapy. Most patients with this syndrome are already being treated with corticosteroids, and these can be readily tapered as the clinical situation warrants. Relapse occurs in 12% to 25% of treated patients and requires retreatment.

Loiasis

Also known as *African eyeworm*, loiasis results from infection with *Loa loa* acquired in the rain forests of West and Central Africa. After the bite of an infected tabanid (horse) fly, the parasites are inoculated into the subcutaneous tissue, where they mature and mate. Although the adults reside in the subcutaneous tissue, they migrate widely over the body. The microfilariae released into the blood by the adult female exhibit diurnal periodicity.

Clinical manifestations, mostly resulting from the host's response to the migrating adult worm, differ between natives to endemic areas and newcomers. In the indigenous population, microfilaremia generally is asymptomatic, remaining subclinical until the adult migrates through the subconjunctival tissues of the eye or causes Calabar swellings, which are angioedematous lesions that develop in response to proteins excreted by the migrating adult worm and are most often noted in the extremities. Nephropathy, encephalopathy, and cardiomyopathy are rare. In nonresidents, allergic or hypersensitivity responses are predominant and microfilaremia is rare, but Calabar swellings occur more often and are more debilitating. Peripheral blood eosinophilia, parasite-specific IgG, and vigorous lymphocyte proliferation to parasite antigens are typical.

Definitive diagnosis requires the identification of either microfilariae in peripheral blood or isolation of the adult worm. The microfilariae can be identified with the technique described for lymphatic filariasis. However, because the microfilariae of *Loa loa* exhibit diurnal periodicity, blood must be filtered between noon and 4 PM after the patient has been in the local time zone for 10 to 14 days. The adult worm is difficult to find unless it crawls across the eye. Calabar swellings develop after the adult worm has migrated through the tissue, so biopsy of the lesion is fruitless. In amicrofilaremic patients, the diagnosis must be based on a characteristic history and clinical presentation, blood eosinophilia, and elevated levels of antifilarial antibodies.

Therapy

The drug of choice to treat loaiasis is DEC, which is effective against both the adult worm and microfilariae. It is dosed as 8 to 10 mg/kg/day (divided into three doses) for 21 days. It is not unusual for treated patients to develop localized inflammatory reactions such as subcutaneous papules or vermiform hives. These reactions, which are distinct from Calabar swellings, are a response to dying adult worms. The adult worms can be extracted surgically from these lesions, but removal is usually unnecessary.

Greater caution is warranted in patients who have microfilaremia. Treatment of such individuals with standard dosages of DEC has resulted in severe neurologic complications and even death caused by microfilariae in the central nervous system (CNS). To reduce the risk of developing treatment-induced encephalopathy, some experts have tried to reduce the microfilarial burden by performing apheresis of the blood before initiating treatment with DEC. In addition, gradual institution and escalation of DEC dosages has been tried with apparent success. In this regimen, DEC should be gradually instituted, giving 0.5 mg/kg for the first dose and then doubling it every 8 hours until the full dose of 8 to 10 mg/kg/day (divided into three doses) is achieved. Prednisone (1 mg/kg/day) should be used during the first 3 to 6 days of treatment, and the first dose of prednisone should be given at least 6 hours before the first dose of DEC. Because onchocerciasis occurs in the same geographic areas as loiasis and treatment of onchocerciasis with DEC can result in severe adverse effects, the clinician must rule out coinfection with onchocerciasis.

Other side effects of treatment are pruritus, fever, anorexia, light-headedness, and hypertension. These symptoms usually resolve after the first few doses. A single course of DEC cures roughly half of those treated, and additional courses are often necessary to achieve cure. A few individuals who failed to respond to multiple courses of DEC were cured with albendazole (400 mg/day), a benzimidazole derivative effective against the adult parasites. The decision to re-treat must be made on clinical grounds because no objective laboratory data can predict treatment failures.

Once an individual has developed loiasis, serious consideration should be given to providing prophylaxis if that person is planning on returning to an endemic area. Although once-weekly treatment with DEC has been shown to be effective prophylaxis, the drug is difficult to come by in tropical countries because it is now manufactured only in the United States. Instead, albendazole, 400 mg/day once weekly, is an acceptable alternative, although the efficacy of this regimen is not clearly established.

Onchocerciasis

Infection with *O. volvulus*, is the second leading infectious cause of blindness worldwide. Onchocerciasis occurs mainly in equatorial Africa, stretches from the Atlantic to the Red Sea, and is found in savannah and rain forest. It is also found scattered throughout Central and South America. Areas of transmission are focal because the *Simulium* blackfly vector flies only within a few kilometers of the streams where it breeds.

After the bite of an infected blackfly, larvae penetrate the skin and migrate into the subcutaneous tissue, where they mature into adults. About 7 to 36 months after infection, the gravid female releases microfilariae, which migrate throughout the skin and concentrate in the dermis. There they can be ingested by female blackflies during their feeding to complete the life cycle.

Most of the symptoms of onchocerciasis result from the effects of microfilariae migrating through host tissues, primarily the skin, lymph nodes, and eyes. As with the other filariases, clinical presentations differ between individuals from endemic and nonendemic areas. However, pruritus is the most common manifestation of onchocerciasis in all individuals. An itchy, erythematous, papular rash prominent early in the infection is also seen. With chronic infection, there is epidermal atrophy, loss of elasticity with exaggerated wrinkling, and loose, redundant skin. The pigmentary changes have led to the term *leopard skin*. Lymph node involvement, usually found in persons from endemic areas, presents as inguinal and femoral lymphadenopathy that may lead to enlargement of lymph nodes, which hang down (so-called hanging groin).

The most serious result of infection is blindness. It usually affects only individuals with moderate to heavy infections. These individuals are overwhelmingly persons from endemic areas. Lesions may be found anywhere in the eye, and the most common early finding is conjunctivitis with photophobia. In the cornea, microfilariae in the anterior chamber of the eye elicit an inflammatory reaction resulting in punctate keratitis with "snowflake" opacities. In Africa, sclerosing keratitis, which may develop later, is the most common cause of blindness. Anterior uveitis and iridocyclitis occur in about 5% of infected Africans. In the Americas, secondary glaucoma may result from damage to the anterior uveal tract. Chorioretinal lesions, constriction of the visual fields, and frank optic atrophy may also develop.

Laboratory findings differ between persons from endemic and nonendemic areas. Eosinophilia and elevated polyclonal IgE are prominent findings in infected individuals. Eosinophilia and IgE levels are greater in natives of endemic areas, a finding that is contrary to the findings in the other filariases.

Like the other filariases, definitive diagnosis rests on the detection of an adult worm in an excised nodule or, more commonly, microfilariae in a skin snip. Skin snips are easily and bloodlessly obtained by sampling the most superficial skin layers using a corneoscleral punch. However, a 25-gauge needle may also be used to carefully tent up the skin while a scalpel is used to excise the most superficial layers of skin. The sample is incubated in saline or tissue culture medium on a glass slide or in a flat-bottomed microtiter plate at 37° C (98.6° F) for at least 2 hours.

Therapy

Ivermectin (Stromectol) is the drug of choice for treating onchocerciasis. Given as a single dose of 150 μg/kg on an empty stomach, it is available in 6-mg tablets. It is generally available to most pharmacies in the United States. Treatment with this agent is contraindicated in children younger than 5 years of age, pregnant or breast-feeding women, and patients with CNS disorders that may increase the penetration of ivermectin into the CNS.

Because ivermectin does not kill adult worms, the effect of the drug may last only 6 months. Re-treatment is generally required either yearly or semiannually. It is advisable to try to remove any subcutaneous nodules. Suramin, the only effective drug to kill adult worms, is rarely indicated. It is available only from the CDC drug service (telephone 404-639-3670).

Other Filarial Infections

Humans can harbor infections with other filariae, most notably *Mansonella* species: *M. streptocerca, M. perstans,* and *M. ozzardi.* Most of these organisms are discovered incidentally, but occasionally, infected persons develop clinical manifestations of illness.

M. streptocerca, found in central Africa, is transmitted by biting midges. The major clinical manifestations, which are limited to the skin, are analogous to onchocerciasis, with pruritus, papular rashes, pigmentation changes, and occasionally inguinal adenopathy. The diagnosis is made by finding the characteristic unsheathed microfilariae in skin snips. DEC, 6 mg/kg/day (in three divided doses) for 21 days, is the recommended therapy.

M. perstans, also transmitted by biting midges, is found in both central Africa and South America. The clinical manifestations, which are poorly defined, may resemble loiasis, with pruritus and transient angioedema, fever, headache, and arthralgias. Occasionally, pericarditis and hepatitis occur. The diagnosis is established by the demonstration of typical microfilariae in blood or serosal effusion. As with other filariases, eosinophilia and antifilarial antibodies are often seen. Although no therapy is conclusively effective, DEC, 8 to 10 mg/kg/day for 21 days, is recommended.

M. ozzardi is found only in Central and South America and the Caribbean. No clear picture of infection with this organism has been established. Diagnosis relies on finding the microfilariae, which circulate in the peripheral blood without periodicity. Although a single case report describes successful treatment with ivermectin, no broader studies of efficacy have been performed.

Humans are accidental hosts for various filariae that primarily infect small mammals. The parasite never completely develops, and the worms are usually found incidentally. The canine heartworm *Dirofilaria immitis* occurs mainly in the southeastern United States. The bite of an infected mosquito deposits the parasite, which develops in the subcutaneous tissues, then migrates to the pulmonary vasculature, where it is trapped and dies. It usually presents as a solitary pulmonary nodule that cannot be easily differentiated from other nonparasitic causes of pulmonary nodules. Eosinophilia is seen in fewer than 15% of infected persons and is seen only in the early stages of the lesion. Other *Dirofilaria* can cause discrete subcutaneous nodules. *Brugia* of small mammals can cause isolated lymph node enlargement in humans, but eosinophilia and antifilarial antibodies are uncommon. These zoonotic infections are diagnosed and cured by excisional biopsy.

■ DRACUNCULIASIS

Also known as *guinea worm infection,* dracunculiasis is an uncommon infection distributed unevenly throughout the tropics, usually in arid regions where populations bathe or wade in water used for drinking. The infection develops after the consumption of water contaminated with water fleas infested with *Dracunculus medinensis* larvae. The larvae are released in the stomach, pass into the small intestine, and penetrate the mucosa, ultimately reaching the retroperitoneum, where they mature and mate. The infection remains largely asymptomatic until about a year later, when the female worm migrates to the subcutaneous tissues, usually in the legs. A tender papule forms and is occasionally associated with a generalized reaction that may include urticaria, dyspnea, nausea, and vomiting. The lesion develops into a vesicle that eventually ruptures and ulcerates, exposing a portion of the gravid worm. On contact with water, large numbers of larvae are released to be ingested by crustaceans to complete the life cycle.

Therapy

Although the recommended drugs have no effect on the worm itself, metronidazole (750 mg/day in three divided doses for 10 days) or thiabendazole (35 mg/kg twice daily for 3 days) gradually resolves the inflammation, allowing removal of the worm over the course of a week by progressively winding it around a small stick by a few centimeters a day.

■ UNUSUAL TISSUE HELMINTH INFECTIONS

Toxocariasis

Infections with *Toxocara canis* from dogs and, less commonly, *Toxocara cati* from cats may produce the syndromes of visceral or ocular larva migrans. Because these nematodes are normally parasitic for other host species, the larvae do not develop into adult worms and elicit eosinophilic inflammation as they migrate through host tissues. Visceral larva migrans is seen mainly among preschool children, but most infections remain subclinical.

Humans acquire toxocariasis mainly by eating soil contaminated with the infective eggs shed in the stool of the host animal. Visceral larva migrans (VLM) is also usually asymptomatic, but those who seek medical attention present with fever, malaise, anorexia, weight loss, cough, wheezing, and rashes. Eosinophilia, the hallmark feature of VLM, may be strikingly elevated. Hepatomegaly is typical, but splenomegaly is seen in only a minority of those infected. Neurologic involvement is uncommon, and death, which is even rarer, results from severe brain, lung, or heart involvement. Serum antibodies to *Toxocara* larvae are a useful adjunct in establishing the diagnosis, but elevated titers are also found in patients without VLM.

Ocular larva migrans (OLM) is occasionally associated with clinically recognized VLM but is usually unaccompanied by systemic symptoms or signs. Children are most often affected; they usually present with a unilateral posterior or peripheral inflammatory mass that mimics retinoblastoma. Serum antibodies to *Toxocara* larvae may be present, but because many patients with OLM have low or negative titers, they are unhelpful unless compared with titers in vitreous and aqueous humor, which are generally higher in affected patients.

Therapy

There is no established therapy for either VLM or OLM, although many antihelminthic agents, including albendazole (400 mg twice daily for 3 to 5 days), mebendazole (100 to 200 mg twice daily for 5 days), and DEC (2 mg/kg three times daily for 7 to 10 days) have been tried.

Infection with the raccoon ascarid *Balyisascaris procyonis* uncommonly causes a severe form of VLM usually associated with severe brain involvement and/or characteristic eye findings termed *diffuse unilateral subacute neuroretinitis* (DUSN). The developing worm can sometimes be found in the retina and killed by laser treatment. Albendazole treatment may be tried in persons with systemic disease or if the larval worm cannot be found.

Cutaneous Larva Migrans (Creeping Eruption)
Infection with *Ancylostoma braziliense* or *Ancylostoma caninum* (hookworms of dogs and cats) results in cutaneous larva migrans, although other animal hookworms may cause the syndrome as well. As with human hookworms, the infection starts when the worm enters the skin from contaminated soil that is protected from desiccation and temperature extremes, such as on beaches and under houses. As in toxocariasis, the worm cannot complete the infective cycle, so it continues to burrow through the subcutaneous tissues, resulting in the characteristic serpiginous, erythematous, elevated, and pruritic skin lesion. The pruritus is sometimes incapacitating. The infection is often seen in travelers who have walked barefoot on beaches frequented by roaming cats and dogs. Systemic symptoms and eosinophilia are rare.

Therapy
Without treatment, the lesions resolve spontaneously over 4 weeks, although the patients are often miserable with pruritus. Treatment with a single dose of ivermectin (150 to 200 μg/kg on an empty stomach) or a 3-day course of albendazole (400 mg daily) has been shown to resolve the infection within 1 week.

Eosinophilic Meningitis Caused by Helminths
Eosinophilic meningitis caused by infection with helminths is most often caused by the rat lungworm *Angiostrongylus cantonensis,* followed by the nematode *Gnathostoma spinigerum* and the raccoon ascarid *Baylisascaris procyonis.* However, the condition has been reported to be a consequence of infection with other helminths, specifically *Schistosoma japonicum, Paragonimus* species, and *Taenia solium* cysticerci. Eosinophilic meningitis occurs widely throughout Southeast Asia and the Pacific, including Hawaii, but is focally distributed in many other tropical areas worldwide.

Humans acquire angiostrongyliasis incidentally by eating raw infected mollusks, vegetables contaminated with mollusk slime, or marine fauna that have eaten the infected mollusks themselves, such as crabs and freshwater shrimp. Although nausea, vomiting, and abdominal discomfort may occur soon after eating the larvae, most patients have no symptoms until after an incubation period that ranges from 2 to 30 days (average about 2 weeks). At that time, patients develop an intermittent excruciating headache that may either be insidious or abrupt. Peripheral blood eosinophilia is prominent and lasts for about 3 months. Typical CSF findings consist of an elevated initial pressure, turbid fluid showing a pleocytosis with at least 10% eosinophilia, and elevated protein content but normal glucose. Diagnosis is based on the clinical findings because recovery of the larvae from CSF or ocular fluids is rare. Treatment is mostly supportive. The headache responds poorly to analgesics and sedatives, but removal of CSF affords symptomatic relief and may be repeated as necessary. Corticosteroids have been tried in severe cases with some benefit. Because clinical deterioration and death can result from the inflammatory reaction to dying worms, antihelminthic therapy is likely contraindicated.

Gnathostoma spinigerum, an intestinal parasite of dogs and cats, has been found to cause human infections most commonly in Southeast Asia, although other foci of gnathostomiasis have recently been reported in Mexico and East Africa. Humans usually acquire the parasite by eating undercooked freshwater fish that harbor the encysted larvae. Gnathostomiasis is always associated with leukocytosis and hypereosinophilia. Intermittent subcutaneous swelling associated with edema and pruritus is the most common manifestation. It often occurs in one eyelid, mimicking the Calabar swelling of loiasis. However, the most feared complication of gnathostomiasis is eosinophilic myeloencephalitis, which can be fatal. This neurologic condition begins as intense radicular pain and is followed by paralysis of the lower extremities and urinary retention. Sudden onset of severe headache followed by coma and death may occur. The diagnosis of gnathostomiasis is usually established clinically. The only serologic test available is performed in Bangkok, Thailand and samples can be sent via the CDC. Albendazole (400 mg twice daily for 28 days) is the mainstay of treatment. Occasionally, the worm will erupt from the skin shortly after treatment is initiated. Removal of the worm is both diagnostic and curative. Adjunctive treatment should include corticosteroids and adequate analgesia when indicated.

Suggested Reading
Burnham G: Onchocerciasis, *Lancet* 351:1341, 1998.

Caumes E, et al: A randomized trial of ivermectin versus albendazole for the treatment of cutaneous larva migrans, *Am J Trop Med Hyg* 49:641, 1993.

Hopkins DR, Ruiz-Tiben E, Ruebush TK: Dracunculiasis eradicaiton: almost a reality, *Am J Trop Med Hyg* 57:252, 1997.

Klion AD, et al: Loiasis in endemic and nonendemic populations: immunologically mediated differences in clinical presentation, *J Infect Dis* 163:1318, 1991.

McCarthy JS, et al: Onchocerciasis in endemic and nonendemic populations: differences in clinical presentation and immunologic findings, *J Infect Dis* 170:736, 1994.

Moore TA, Nutman TB: Eosinophilia in the returning traveler, *Infect Dis Clin North Am* 12:503, 1998.

Moore TA, et al: Diethylcarbamazine-induced reversal of early lymphatic dysfunction in a patient with bancroftian filariasis: assessment with use of lymphoscintigraphy, *Clin Infect Dis* 23:1007, 1996.

Moorhead A, et al: Trichinellosis in the United States, 1991-1996: declining but not gone, *Am J Trop Med Hyg* 60:66, 1999.

Ong RK, Doyle RL: Tropical pulmonary eosinophilia, *Chest* 13:1673, 1998.

Ottesen EA: Filariasis now, *Am J Trop Med Hyg* 41:9, 1989.

Punyagupta S, Bunnag T, Juttijudata P: Eosinophilic meningitis in Thailand: clinical and epidemiological characteristics of 162 patients with myeloencephalitis probably caused by *Gnathostoma spinigerum, J Neurol Sci* 96:241, 1990.

Schantz PM, Meyer D, Glickman LT: Clinical, serologic, and epidemiologic characteristics of ocular toxocariasis, *Am J Trop Med Hyg* 28:24, 1979.

Worley G, Green JA, Frothingham TE: *Toxocara canis* infection: clinical and epidemiological associations with seropositivity in kindergarten children, *J Infect Dis* 149:591, 1984.

Yii CY: Clinical observations on eosinophilic meningitis and meningoencephalitis caused by *Angiostrongylus cantonensis* in Taiwan, *Am J Trop Med Hyg* 25:233, 1976.

SCHISTOSOMES AND OTHER TREMATODES

James H. Maguire

The trematode flatworms that infect human beings include the schistosomes, which live in venules of the gastrointestinal or genitourinary tract, and other flukes that inhabit the bile ducts, intestines, or bronchi. The geographic distribution of each species of trematode parallels the distribution of the specific freshwater snail that serves as its intermediate host (Table 1). Schistosomes infect as many as 200 million persons worldwide; infections caused by the other flukes are more limited in distribution and number. Most trematode infections are subclinical, and in general only the small proportion of persons who have heavy worm burdens develop severe disease.

■ SCHISTOSOMIASIS

Clinical Presentation

A history of contact with possibly infested freshwater in an endemic area should prompt an evaluation for schistosomiasis, even in the absence of symptoms. Clinical manifestations that suggest the diagnosis vary according to the stage of infection. Some persons complain of intense pruritus or rash shortly after the infective cercariae penetrate the skin. Previously uninfected visitors to endemic areas may develop acute schistosomiasis, or Katayama fever, 2 to 6 weeks after exposure, as the immune system begins to respond to maturing worms and eggs. Symptoms range from mild malaise to a serum sickness–like syndrome that lasts for weeks and may be life-threatening. Common features include fever, headache, abdominal pain, myalgia, arthralgia, dry cough, diarrhea, hepatosplenomegaly, lymphadenopathy, urticaria, and marked eosinophilia.

Chronic infections with schistosomes usually are asymptomatic and often are accompanied by a slight or moderate eosinophilia. Long-term residents of endemic areas may harbor heavy infections for long periods and thus are more likely than transient visitors to have symptoms. Disease is the consequence of egg deposition in tissues and the ensuing inflammatory and fibrotic response. In infections of the *Schistosoma* species, *S. mansoni, S. japonicum,* and *S. mekongi,* involvement of the bowel and liver leads to mucosal polyps, strictures, bloody diarrhea, periportal fibrosis, portal hypertension, hepatosplenomegaly, and esophageal varices. Hematuria and dysuria are the first symptoms of chronic infection by *Schistosoma haematobium;* later, fibrosis of the bladder and lower ureters results in hydroureter and hydronephrosis. Ectopic deposition of eggs in other organs occurs during both the acute and chronic stages of infection with all species of schistosomes. Transverse myelitis, seizures, and other serious sequelae result from eggs in the central nervous system.

Table 1 Geographic Distribution of Important Trematodes*†

SCHISTOSTOSOMES	
Schistosoma mansoni	South America, Caribbean, Middle East, Africa
Schistosoma japonicum	China, Philippines, Indonesia, Thailand
Schistosoma mekongi	Cambodia, Laos
Schistosoma haematobium	Africa, Middle East
BILIARY AND LIVER FLUKES	
Clonorchis sinensis	China, Taiwan, Korea, Japan, Vietnam
Opisthorchis viverrini	Thailand, Laos, Cambodia
Opisthorchis felineus	Eastern Europe, former Soviet Union
Fasciola hepatica	Europe, North Africa, Asia, western Pacific, Latin America
Fasciola gigantica	Africa, western Pacific, Hawaii
LUNG FLUKES	
Paragonimus westermani and other species	Far East, South Asia, Philippines, Central and South America, West Africa
INTESTINAL FLUKES	
Fasciolopsis buski	Far East
Heterophyes heterophyes	Far East, Egypt, Middle East
Metagonimus yokogawai	Far East
Nanophyetus salmincola	Pacific Northwest

*Parasites may be limited to certain countries in the regions listed and certain foci within these countries.
†Many less common trematodes that infect human beings are not listed here.

Diagnosis

The most direct method of diagnosis is microscopic examination of stool or urine for schistosome eggs. Because egg output is low in light infections, concentration techniques and examination of several specimens obtained on different days should be routine. Egg counts should be measured to estimate the intensity of infection and to monitor the response to therapy. Counts above 400 eggs per gram of feces or 10 ml of urine are considered heavy and are associated with an increased risk of complications. Microscopic examination of snips of rectal mucosa obtained at proctoscopy may reveal eggs when stool examination is negative.

Serologic tests for antibodies to schistosomes are available at several commercial laboratories in the United States and at the Centers for Disease Control and Prevention (CDC) in Atlanta. The CDC uses a sensitive and specific Falcon assay screening test–enzyme-linked immunosorbent assay (FAST-ELISA) for screening and a highly specific immunoblot for confirmation and species determination. These tests cannot distinguish active from past infections but are useful for the diagnosis of acute schistosomiasis before eggs are shed in the stool. Serologic tests may be used to screen previously unexposed travelers and expatriates to determine whether stool or urine examination is necessary. In such persons a positive serologic test is presumptive evidence of infection when microscopy is negative.

Persons with confirmed schistosomiasis should be evaluated for evidence of disease. Urinalysis, urine culture, serum creatinine determination, and an ultrasound are indicated

Table 2 Treatment of Trematode Infections

PARASITE	DRUG	DOSAGE
*Schistosoma mansoni,** *Schistosoma haematobium,*	Praziquantel	40 mg/kg/day in 2 doses ×1 day
Schistosoma japonicum, *Schistosoma mekongi*	Praziquantel	60 mg/kg/day in 3 doses ×1 day
Clonorchis sinensis, *Opisthorchis* spp.	Praziquantel	75 mg/kg/day in 3 doses ×1 day
Fasciola hepatica,† *Fasciola gigantica*	Bithionol	30-50 mg/kg on alternate days ×10-15 doses
Paragonimus spp.	Praziquantel	75 mg/kg/day in 3 doses ×2 days
Fasciolopsis buski, Heterophyes heterophyes, *Metagonimus yokogawai*	Praziquantel	75 mg/kg/day in 3 doses ×1 day
Nanophyetus salmincola	Praziquantel	60 mg/kg/day in 3 doses ×1 day

Regimens are from Drugs for parasitic infections (author anonymous), *Med Lett Drugs Ther* 40:1, 1998. With permission.
*S. mansoni infections acquired in Africa should be treated with praziquantel, 30 mg/kg/day for 2 days. Oxamniquine, 15 mg/kg/day in one dose, is an alternative to praziquantel for *S. mansoni* infections. Metrifonate, an alternative to praziquantel for *S. haematobium* infections, is not available in the United States.
†Triclabendazole, 10 mg/kg ×1, not yet available in the United States, but will probably become the drug of choice.

for persons with *S. haematobium* infection. Ultrasonography detects complications such as hydronephrosis, polyps, stones, and carcinoma of the bladder. Evaluation of infections due to the intestinal schistosomes includes measurement of liver function tests and tests for chronic hepatitis B and C to rule out concomitant hepatocellular disease. Heavy infection or evidence of liver disease should prompt an ultrasound to document periportal fibrosis and signs of portal hypertension. Esophageal varices are visualized by barium swallow or endoscopy.

Therapy

All persons with schistosomiasis should receive treatment. Eradication of infection is desirable because even a single pair of worms may deposit eggs in the central nervous system. In endemic areas where reinfection is inevitable, the goal is to reduce worm burdens to levels that are unlikely to produce disease. Successful treatment not only prevents complications but also may cause regression of polyps and fibrotic lesions. Fortunately, available drugs are safe and highly effective after one or a few oral doses.

The drug of choice for treating all species of schistosomes is praziquantel (Table 2). Praziquantel causes an influx of calcium ions across the tegument of the adult worm, leading to a tetanic contraction and vacuolization of the tegument that makes the parasite susceptible to immune destruction. Cure rates range from 70% to 100%, and in persons not cured, egg excretion is reduced by more than 90%. A few reports suggest that resistance to praziquantel may be developing. Adverse effects, which are usually mild and last less than 24 hours, may be caused by reactions to dying worms rather than drug toxicity. Patients occasionally report malaise, headache, dizziness, or abdominal discomfort. Nausea, vomiting, diarrhea, bloody stools, fever, and urticaria are uncommon. Pregnant women should take praziquantel only if absolutely necessary, and breast-feeding should be suspended during treatment and for 72 hours afterward. Persons with known or suspected cysticercosis should remain under observation during therapy because of the risk of seizures or other neurologic consequences of dying cysti-

cerci. Praziquantel is metabolized in the liver, and the dosage need not be reduced because of renal insufficiency.

Oxamniquine, an alternative for treatment of *S. mansoni* infections, has an unknown mechanism of action. It is as effective as praziquantel for infections acquired in the western hemisphere, but higher doses are needed for African strains. Drug resistance has been documented. Side effects include transient dizziness, drowsiness, headache, and in persons with a history of epilepsy, seizures. Metrifonate, an inhibitor of acetylcholinesterase, is effective only against urinary schistosomes. Cholinergic side effects are infrequent and transient. A requirement for three doses 2 weeks apart offsets the advantage of its low cost.

Severely ill persons with acute schistosomiasis should receive corticosteroids as well as antischistosomal drugs. Treatment of acute infection should not be delayed, even though maturing schistosomes are less susceptible to chemotherapy than adult worms.

Because antischistosomal drugs may temporarily inhibit egg laying by adult worms, stool and urine should be examined 3 and 6 months after completion of therapy. Eosinophilia, hematuria, and other symptoms that persist beyond this time should prompt repeat parasitologic studies and evaluation for causes other than schistosomiasis. Serologic tests may remain positive for years after successful treatment, so they play no role in the assessment of cure.

■ OTHER TREMATODE INFECTIONS

More than 65 species of trematodes other than schistosomes cause human infections. Most are parasites of wild and domestic animals. Human beings accidentally become infected by ingestion of metacercariae encysted in freshwater fish, crustacea, and plants, the second intermediate hosts.

Clonorchiasis and Opisthorchiasis

The oriental liver flukes *Clonorchis sinensis, Opisthorchis viverrini,* and *Opisthorchis felineus* inhabit the biliary tree of persons who ingest infected carp without proper cooking.

Most patients are asymptomatic, but eosinophilia is possible. An acute illness resembling Katayama fever occasionally occurs 2 to 3 weeks after initial exposure. Persons with heavy infections for many years develop symptoms due to irritation and inflammation of biliary epithelium. Patients complain of right upper quadrant discomfort, anorexia, and weight loss. On physical examination the liver is palpable and firm. Cholangitis, pancreatitis, and cholangiocarcinoma are infrequent.

Diagnosis is made by finding eggs in the stool or identifying adult worms during surgery for complications. Ultrasonography or computed tomography (CT) is useful in symptomatic cases for demonstrating dilation and stricture of bile ducts, thickening of the gallbladder wall, and stones. A single course of praziquantel eradicates infection in more than 85% of cases.

Fascioliasis

Infection with the sheep liver fluke *Fasciola hepatica* and the closely related *Fasciola gigantica* results from ingestion of uncooked watercress or other fresh aquatic vegetation from sheep- and cattle-raising parts of the world. After excysting in the duodenum, immature worms invade the liver and burrow through the parenchyma to the bile ducts. This migration provokes an acute syndrome of fever, nausea, tender hepatomegaly, eosinophilia, and urticaria that lasts for weeks to months. Aberrant migration may produce nodules in the skin or painful inflammation of the intestinal wall. Chronic fascioliasis is usually subclinical, but some persons have symptoms due to inflammation and obstruction of bile ducts.

The definitive diagnosis is made by demonstrating eggs in samples of stool, bile, or duodenal aspirates or by recovering worms at surgery. Serologic tests are useful during acute infection because symptoms develop 1 to 2 months before eggs are detectable in the stool. Ultrasonography and cholangiography may demonstrate adult worms and biliary pathology, and CT shows hypodense lesions in the liver.

Unlike infections with other flukes, fascioliasis responds poorly to praziquantel. In the United States, bithionol, a compound closely related to hexachlorophene, is available through the CDC for treatment of fascioliasis. Side effects, which include photosensitivity reactions, abdominal pain, hepatitis, and urticaria, are caused in part by a reaction to degenerating worms. Outside of the United States the veterinary drug triclabendazole is the drug of choice for fascioliasis.

Paragonimiasis

Infection with *Paragonimus westermani*, the oriental lung fluke, and less commonly, other species of *Paragonimus*, follows ingestion of raw or poorly cooked freshwater crabs or crayfish. An acute phase with fever, abdominal and chest pain, cough, and eosinophilia corresponds to migration of immature parasites through the bowel wall, diaphragm, and pleura en route to the lungs. The inflammatory reaction to adults encapsulated in the lungs and the shedding of eggs into the bronchial tree are responsible for chronic symptoms. Patients complain of cough, rusty or golden sputum, hemoptysis, vague chest pains, and dyspnea on exertion. Radiographs of the chest show poorly defined infiltrates,

cysts, nodules, cavities, calcified lesions, and pleural effusions that on aspiration are seen to contain eosinophils. The findings may suggest tuberculosis. Bronchiectasis, bacterial pneumonia, or empyema complicates heavy infections. Extrapulmonary migration of flukes is common, and it gives rise to migratory subcutaneous nodules, involvement of abdominal viscera, or focal lesions of the central nervous system. Cerebral paragonimiasis is characterized by headache, seizures, focal neurologic deficits, cerebrospinal fluid eosinophilia, and cystic lesions on radiographs and scans.

The diagnosis of paragonimiasis is established by identifying expectorated eggs in the sputum, swallowed eggs in the feces, or worms and eggs in biopsy specimens. Several examinations of stool and sputum may be necessary. Serologic tests, such as the immunoblot offered by the CDC, are useful for diagnosis of light infections and extrapulmonary infections.

The treatment of choice for paragonimiasis is praziquantel. The alternative, bithionol, has more frequent side effects. Because an inflammatory reaction to dying worms may precipitate seizures or other neurologic complications, corticosteroids should be used simultaneously with praziquantel for cerebral paragonimiasis.

Intestinal Fluke Infections

Adult intestinal flukes live attached to the mucosa of the duodenum and jejunum, where they cause local inflammation and ulceration. Of the dozens of species that infect human beings, *Fasciolopsis buski*, the giant intestinal fluke, is the best known. Infection is acquired by eating uncooked aquatic plants, such as water caltrop, water chestnut, and watercress. Heavily infected persons develop hunger pains that suggest peptic ulcer disease, diarrhea with mucus, and in extremes cases, malabsorption, ascites, anasarca, and intestinal obstruction. Eosinophilia is common.

Other important intestinal flukes include *Heterophyes heterophyes* and *Metagonimus yokogawai*, both of which are acquired by ingestion of raw or undercooked freshwater fish. Symptoms caused by these parasites resemble those produced by *Fasciolopsis*, but embolization of eggs that enter the circulation may cause severe myocarditis or cerebral hemorrhage. The source of infection with *Nanophyetus salmincola* is raw or poorly cooked salmon or trout. Manifestations include abdominal pain, watery diarrhea, and eosinophilia.

The diagnosis of all intestinal fluke infections is made by demonstrating eggs in the feces. Because the number of eggs excreted may be low, concentration techniques and repeated examinations are recommended. Praziquantel is the drug of choice.

Suggested Reading

Blair D, Xu ZB, Agatsuma T: Paragonimiasis and the genus, *Paragonimus Adv Parasitol* 42:113, 1998.

Jordan P, Webbe G, Sturrock RF: *Human schistosomiasis*, Wallingford, UK, 1993, CAB International.

MacLean JD, Cross J, Siddhartha M: Liver, lung, and intestinal fluke infections. In Guerrant RL, Walker DH, Weller PF, eds. *Tropical infectious diseases: principles, pathogens, and practice*, Philadelphia, 1999, Churchill Livingstone.

Strickland GT, Ramirez BL: Schistosomiasis. In Strickland GT, ed. *Hunter's tropical medicine and emerging infectious diseases*, ed 8, Philadelphia, 2000, WB Saunders.

TAPEWORMS (CESTODES)

Zbigniew S. Pawlowski

Cestodes cause intestinal (taeniasis, hymenolepiasis) and/ or tissue parasitoses (cysticercosis, echinococcosis). Most intestinal tapeworm infections are meatborne or insect-borne zoonoses, whereas tissue infections with larval cestodes are fecalborne, acquired mainly through ingestion of the tapeworm eggs from human, dog, or fox feces.

■ *TAENIA SAGINATA* TAENIASIS

Taenia saginata, the beef tapeworm, sometimes more than 5 meters long, may live up to 30 years in the small intestine. Humans are infected by ingestion of the cysticercus, a bladder worm less than 1 cm in diameter, in raw or undercooked beef.

T. saginata infections can spread easily because of the fecundity of the tapeworm (>500,000 eggs produced daily for years), wide and long-term contamination of the environment with eggs, bovine cysticercosis that often escapes routine meat inspection because of a low intensity of infection, and finally, common consumption of raw beef. More than 10% of nomads are infected in East Africa; in Europe the annual incidence in urban populations is around 0.1%; in the United States and Canada *T. saginata* taeniasis is uncommon and is seen mainly among migrants from Latin America.

T. saginata infection is suspected in well-nourished middle-age patients who eat raw beef. Complaints include vague abdominal pains, nausea, weight loss or gain, and some perianal discomfort, caused by gravid proglottids (about six per day) crawling out of the anus. Sometimes, the patient passes a long part of tapeworm strobila; in that case, the expulsion of proglottids may stop for weeks. The diagnosis is confirmed by macroscopical examination of fresh proglottids of the tapeworm. *Taenia* eggs are found more often on anal swabs than in feces. Tests detecting parasite antigen in feces—not yet commercially available—may detect early infections before proglottids or eggs are expelled.

Treatment of *T. saginata* taeniasis with praziquantel or niclosamide is safe and effective in 95% and 80% of cases, respectively. Praziquantel is given orally in a single dose of 5 to 10 mg/kg an hour after a light breakfast. Niclosamide is preferred for children younger than 4 years of age and for pregnant women. Niclosamide (use only original products recently manufactured) should be chewed thoroughly on an empty stomach in a single dose of 2 g by adults, 1 g by children 10 to 35 kg and 0.5 g by smaller children. Adverse effects, such as abdominal discomfort, headache, and dizziness, are rare and transient. Tapeworm is usually expelled in fragments within a few hours; the scolex, indicating elimination of the entire worm, is often difficult to find. Therefore successful therapy can be confirmed only when no proglottids reappear for 4 months after treatment.

■ *TAENIA SOLIUM* TAENIASIS AND CYSTICERCOSIS

Taenia solium (pork tapeworm) infection is common in Latin American countries, West and South Africa, India, Indonesia, and China. Intestinal infection is acquired by eating undercooked pork. Cysticercosis, cystic forms developed in the tissues, is acquired by ingesting *T. solium* eggs present in contaminated food or water or on hands spoiled with feces (autoinfections or family infections are not uncommon). Sporadic cases of human cysticercosis are seen in the United States, having been acquired from immigrants infected with *T. solium* tapeworm.

The pork tapeworm is smaller than *T. saginata*, and its proglottids are usually expelled with feces, starting 2 months after ingestion of infected pork. Clinical symptoms and signs of taeniasis are not characteristic. The diagnosis is made by examination of the expelled proglottids, or by finding *Taenia* eggs (*T. solium* eggs are morphologically indistinguishable from those of *T. saginata*) or *Taenia* coproantigens. Proglottids and feces should be handled with care because *T. solium* eggs are infective for humans. Because of the danger of cysticercosis, treatment is mandatory as soon as possible in both diagnosed and suspected cases of intestinal taeniasis.

Treatment of the intestinal infection is the same as for *T. saginata* taeniasis; on rare occasions, praziquantel may aggravate symptoms of concomitant cysticercosis. Evaluation of treatment is by frequent fecal examination for *Taenia* eggs for 3 months after the anthelmintic therapy.

In cysticercosis, *T. solium* cysticerci may be localized in muscle and subcutaneous tissues without much symptomatology; the clinically important syndromes are neurocysticercosis, ocular cysticercosis, and heart cysticercosis. Neurocysticercosis is suspected when epileptiform seizures, intracranial hypertension, or psychiatric disturbances occur, especially in adolescents and adults having contact with endemic areas or with a *T. solium* carrier. Final diagnosis can be made by biopsy of subcutaneous nodules containing *T. solium* cysticerci, if present. Most often, cysticerci are suspected by the inflammatory reaction and edema around the parasite, or by ventricular dilation, as seen on computed axial tomography (CAT) or magnetic resonance imaging (MRI) scans; less often they are suspected on the basis of ultrasound scanning and x-ray examination, particularly if calcifications are present. Positive serologic tests, especially enzyme immunoassay (EIA) and EITB assays, support the clinical diagnosis.

Neurocysticercosis is often asymptomatic; in such cases, indications for treatment must be considered carefully. Symptomatic cases, which may be active or inactive, call for antihelminthic therapy plus surgery, corticosteroids, and symptomatic treatment in selected patients. Antihelminthic therapy with praziquantel or albendazole is indicated in active cysticercosis with several parenchymal cysts or with clinical signs of vasculitis, encephalitis, and arachnoiditis. Traditionally, praziquantel is given orally in a daily dose of

50 mg/kg for 14 days, but a shorter regimen with a higher dose has been recently proposed. Albendazole is given orally in a daily dose of 15 mg/kg for 8 days. For parenchymal brain cysticerci, the efficacy is about 60% for praziquantel and 85% for albendazole. Damage to cysticerci, caused by both of the drugs, may result in a local inflammatory reaction and edema, which necessitates a concomitant additional corticosteroid or antihistaminic drugs therapy.

Surgical extirpation is indicated mainly for single parenchymal, intraventricular, spinal, and ocular cysticerci and with focal symptoms (e.g., cranial nerve dysfunction). A ventricular shunt is indicated in hydrocephalus. Corticosteroids and immunosuppressants may control vasculitis and encephalitis. Antiepileptic drugs are used mainly in inactive cysticercosis with granulomatous or calcified lesions. The mortality from neurocysticercosis is still considerable.

■ *HYMENOLEPIS NANA* INFECTIONS

Hymenolepsis nana, the dwarf tapeworm, 15 to 40 mm long, lives only up to 3 months in human small intestine. Some of the tapeworm eggs are expelled with feces and constitute a source of autoinfection or infection for other people. The other eggs hatch in the human intestine and within a month develop into cysticercoids in intestinal villi and later on into the next generation of adult tapeworms. Such a cycle facilitates spread of infection in close communities (day-care centers, schools, psychiatric institutions) and permits intensive infections of thousands of tapeworms in malnourished or immunodeficient individuals. Developing immunity regulates the intensity and duration of infection, which occurs mainly in children and often clears spontaneously in adolescence. Hymenolepiasis is very common in regions with a hot, dry climate; it is rare in developed countries with appropriate sanitation.

Intensive infections may cause diarrhea, abdominal pains, and general symptoms such as weight loss, pallor, and weakness. Diagnosis is made by finding characteristic *H. nana* eggs in feces. Treatment with a single dose of praziquantel, 15 to 25 mg/kg, is highly effective; in intensive infections treatment must be repeated after 3 weeks. Niclosamide is much less effective and requires repeated courses of 7 days with the same daily doses as for *T. saginata* taeniasis. Successful treatment has to be confirmed by negative fecal examination every 2 weeks for 2 months after therapy.

■ OTHER INTESTINAL CESTODIASES

Diphyllobothriasis, caused by the fish tapeworms, *Diphylobothrium latum* and *Diphyllobothrium pacificum,* is now rare; it still occurs around unpolluted large lakes in moderate climates (Great Lakes in the United States and Canada, lakes in Finland) and along the Pacific Coast in South America, respectively. An uncommon clinical complication of diphyllobothriasis is vitamin B_{12} deficiency. Diagnosis is made by finding characteristic eggs on fecal examination. Treatment is a single dose of praziquantel, 15 to 25 mg/kg. Evaluation of successful therapy is by repeated fecal examination.

Hymenolepis diminuta (rat tapeworm) and *Dipylidium caninum* (dog tapeworm) infections occur accidentally in humans and are usually asymptomatic. They are diagnosed by fecal examination and can be easily treated by a single dose of praziquantel 15 mg/kg.

■ CYSTIC ECHINOCOCCOSIS (HYDATID DISEASE)

Echinococcus granulosus is a tiny tapeworm living in the small intestine of some carnivores, mainly dogs. *E. granulosus* eggs, excreted in dog feces and contaminating an environment, are the source of cystic echinococcosis in herbivorous animals, mainly sheep, and accidentally in humans. Echinococcosis is common in sheep-breeding regions of southern South America, Mediterranean countries, Central Asia, and China. Small enzoonotic foci are found in Alaska, California, southern Utah and northern Arizona.

Echinococcus cysts develop mainly in the liver (about 65%) or lungs (about 25%), but they can invade any tissue, including the brain, kidney, spleen, heart, and bone. Clinical manifestations are diverse, depending on location, size, and number of cysts as well as the complications resulting from a cyst's rupture and communication with biliary or bronchial systems or with adjacent body cavities. Bacterial infection of the cysts and secondary peritoneal echinococcosis are not uncommon. Clinical diagnosis is confirmed by imaging techniques (sonography, CT, MRI, x-ray examination) and serologic tests (sensitive enzyme-linked immunosorbent assay [ELISA] followed by more specific immunodiffusion or immunoblot tests). In some cases the clinical picture, imaging, and serology are not conclusive, and the final diagnosis is made by finding parasite hooks, protoscoleces, or cyst wall fragments in sputum or in biopsy, surgical, or necropsy samples.

The echinococcus cysts may be sterile or fertile (with protoscoleces), simple or multiple, small or large, asymptomatic or symptomatic, active and inactive, complicated or noncomplicated. The choices of management are surgery, chemotherapy, PAIR (puncture, aspiration, injection, and reaspiration), or observation without any intervention. Major indications for surgery are large, active, superficially located and easy-to-rupture liver cysts, and most of the brain, spinal, heart, and bone cysts. Surgery can be radical (removal of the whole intact cyst) or conservative (cystectomy and removal of the parasite but not the host pericyst). Surgery brings a risk of complications such as secondary echinococcosis (2% to 21%) or death (0.5% to 4%).

Chemotherapy is used more widely, mainly but not exclusively in inoperable cases. An important indication for chemotherapy before a surgery or a puncture is prevention of secondary echinococcosis due to unintentional spillage of a cyst's contents. The drug used are mebendazole, 40 to 50 mg/kg daily for at least 3 months, or albendazole, 10 to 15 mg/kg daily for at least 1 month. Chemotherapy with both drugs brings a risk of embriotoxicity in early pregnancy. Careful clinical monitoring can prevent hepatotoxicity, neutropenia, and thrombocytopenia but not alopecia.

In some specialized centers, cyst puncture with a fine needle guided by sonography and performed under the cover of albendazole is used in cases of inconclusive diagnosis. PAIR (puncture with injection of a protoscolicide) is used for therapy rather than to diagnosis. Unfortunately, no protoscolicide is both effective and safe; widely used now are 75% to 95% ethanol, 20% hypertonic sodium chloride solution, and 0.5% cetrimide. Formalin solution is no longer in use, as it can provoke sclerotic cholangitis.

■ ALVEOLAR AND POLYCYSTIC ECHINOCOCCOSES

Echinococcus multilocularis tapeworms develop in the intestine of some carnivores, mainly foxes; the intermediate hosts are rodents such as voles, lemurs, and mice. Natural enzoonotic foci of alveolar echinococcosis are the Alps of central Europe (France, Germany, Switzerland, Austria), Siberia, northern Japan, Alaska, and northwest Canada. Humans are infected accidentally by *E. multilocularis* eggs on fox or dog hair or in fecally polluted natural environment (water, soil, berries).

E. multilocularis lesions, composed of clusters of tiny vesicles, usually begin in the liver, grow slowly in a tumorlike pattern, and metastasize to lungs and brain. The early clinical manifestations are usually vague; the advanced disease is invariably symptomatic due to liver lesions or lung or brain metastases. Diagnosis is based on imaging techniques and serologic tests; the latter (e.g., Em2$^+$ and/or Em18) are highly specific. Treatment is by radical surgical resection of liver lesions followed by at least 2 years of chemotherapy. Recurrent or nonresectable lesions require lifelong chemotherapy with mebendazole or albendazole, which are parasitostatic rather than parasitocidal. The treatment has to be performed in specialized centers because of various and frequently severe complications, which may need another surgery or liver transplantation.

Polycystic echinococcosis occurs in humans in Latin America and is caused by *Echinococcus vogeli* and *E. oligarthrus,* the parasites of wild mammals. The numerous small cystic lesions can be found in the liver, lungs, abdominal cavity, stomach, heart, and orbit. The clinical course is similar to alveolar echinococcosis. Polycystic echinococcosis frequently requires surgery and responds well to albendazole.

Suggested Reading

Ammann RW, Eckert J: Cestodes. Echinococcus. Parasitic diseases of the liver and intestines, *Gastroenterol Clin North Am* 25:655, 1996.

Arriagada C, Nogales-Gaete J, Apt W, eds: *Neurocysticercosis,* Santiago, Chile, 1997, Arrynog Editiones.

Morris DL, Richards KS: *Hydatid disease: current medical and surgical management,* Oxford, 1992, Botterworth-Heineman.

Pawlowski ZS: Taeniasis and cysticercosis. In Hue YH, et al, eds: *Foodborne disease handbook,* vol 2, New York, 1994, Marcel Dekker.

Schantz PM, Wilkins PP, Tsang VCW: Immigrants, imaging, and immunoblots: the emergence of neurocysticercosis as a significant public health problem. In Scheld WM, Craig WA, Hughes JM, eds: *Emerging infections,* vol 2, Washington, DC, 1998, American Society for Microbiology Press, p. 213.

TOXOPLASMA

Maye Berroya

Julie Antique

Benjamin J. Luft

Toxoplasmosis, caused by the obligate intracellular parasite *Toxoplasma gondii,* is responsible for significant morbidity and mortality throughout the world. Although it has long been recognized as a serious congenital disease, it is only with the advent of the acquired immunodeficiency syndrome (AIDS) and the increased use of immunosuppressive therapy that toxoplasmosis has reached epidemic proportions.

Humans are incidental hosts in the life cycle of *T. gondii.* Acute infection occurs via ingestion of meats or beverages contaminated with tissue cysts or tachyzoites or by handling cats, the definitive host. Once the human host develops an adequate immune response, tissue cysts are formed and a chronic or latent infection ensues. Antibodies against *T. gondii* will be present in serum for life. When a chronically infected person becomes immunocompromised, particularly with defects in cell-mediated immunity, devastating reactivation of the latent infection may occur.

■ CLINICAL MANIFESTATIONS AND DIAGNOSIS

Toxoplasmosis in the AIDS patient is most commonly manifested by toxoplasmic encephalitis (TE), usually alone but sometimes as part of a multiorgan infection. Isolated organ involvement without central nervous system (CNS) disease is uncommon. In most cases, TE develops when the CD4 lymphocyte count falls below 100/mm^3, although the risk of developing overt infection begins when CD4 counts fall below 200/mm^3. The clinical manifestations of TE are protean, including signs and symptoms of focal or generalized neurologic dysfunction or more commonly both, depending on the number, size, and location of the lesions. Cerebral edema, vasculitis, and hemorrhage, which can accompany active infection, also contribute to the disease process. TE most commonly presents with a subacute onset of focal neurologic deficits with or without evidence of generalized cerebral dysfunction. Less often, seizures are the initial manifestation. Occasionally, signs and symptoms of generalized cerebral dysfunction dominate the presentation, and patients develop focal deficits as the infection progresses. The clinical presentation varies from an insidious process evolving over several weeks to a more acute or even fulminant course. Headaches may be focal or generalized and unremitting.

Serologic tests for diagnosis of toxoplasmosis in AIDS patients are useful only to identify human immunodeficiency virus (HIV)-infected individuals at risk for development of TE and as support for the diagnosis in AIDS patients with focal brain lesions. The Sabin-Feldman dye test is the accepted standard for measurement of IgG antibodies, which have been shown to be higher in AIDS patients with TE than in those without TE. The immunofluorescent assay (IFA), which is used more commonly, measures the same IgG antibodies as the dye test. Almost all AIDS patients with TE have detectable IgG. The absence of these antibodies strongly suggests another cause of the neurologic signs and symptoms.

The standard of care allows for the treatment of TE to be initiated upon presumptive diagnosis when a neuroradiographic abnormality is noted on computed tomography (CT) or magnetic resonance imaging (MRI). MRI is more sensitive than CT in the demonstration of focal CNS lesions. The clinical diagnosis is a result of clinical and radiographic response to specific therapy because patients may have similar symptoms resulting from lesions of other causes. The practice of presumptive therapy for patients with a characteristic finding on CT or MRI and positive serology for *Toxoplasma* is widely accepted. With the use of these criteria, the predictive value has been estimated at 80%. However, for patients such as intravenous drug abusers in whom other CNS processes are more prevalent, the predictive value of a positive serology for *Toxoplasma* is reduced, and the widespread use of prophylaxis may further reduce it. TE is predominantly intraaxial, so significant meningeal involvement is uncommon. Examination of cerebrospinal fluid (CSF) was used to exclude other diseases. However, detection of *T. gondii* DNA by polymerase chain reaction (PCR) in CSF has shown to be a promising tool in the definitive diagnosis of TE in AIDS patients with focal lesions.

The lungs are the second most common site of infection in AIDS patients. The clinical manifestations of toxoplasma pneumonia are nonspecific, similar to those seen with *Pneumocystis carinii* pneumonia (PCP). Most patients have fever, a nonproductive cough, dyspnea, and occasionally hemoptysis. However, the onset of disease tends to be faster than with PCP. The chest roentgenogram typically reveals bilateral interstitial infiltrates, although multiple nodular infiltrates, single nodules, isolated cavitary disease, lobar infiltrates, pleural effusions, and hilar adenopathy may occur. Pneumothorax complicating toxoplasmic pneumonia has been reported, as well as adult respiratory distress syndrome (ARDS). The diagnosis relies on a high index of suspicion and the demonstration of *T. gondii* from bronchoalveolar lavage (BAL) fluid or biopsy specimens, given nonspecific nature of both clinical and radiologic manifestations in most cases.

After cytomegalovirus (CMV) retinitis, ocular toxoplasmosis is the most common retinal infection in patients with AIDS. It is rarely reported, and the exact incidence of ocular toxoplasmosis is unknown. Patients usually present with decreased visual acuity and, less often, eye pain. Ocular toxoplasmosis may be the sole manifestation of infection or may accompany TE or disseminated disease. At times, ocular toxoplasmosis is a harbinger of TE. A CT scan of the head should be obtained to assess presence of concomitant TE. Funduscopic findings are consistent with a necrotizing chorioretinitis. The lesions, which may be single or multiple and bilateral and are usually nonhemorrhagic, are yellow-white areas of retinal necrosis with ill-defined fluffy borders. They occur at the posterior pole and may be associated with a moderate to severe inflammatory response in the vitreous and anterior chamber. These characteristics help in the differential diagnosis with CMV retinitis. Fluorescein angiography may also be helpful. Dye leakage tends to occur along the edge of the lesions in toxoplasmosis and to be more prominent in the center of lesions in CMV retinitis. Ocular toxoplasmosis should be suspected if the AIDS patient is seropositive for *T. gondii* and has changes in visual acuity with accompanying funduscopic changes. A prompt response to specific therapy should also be expected. Definitive diagnosis has been made by demonstrating the organism in retinal biopsy specimens or isolation of *T. gondii* from vitreal fluid.

■ THERAPY

Immunocompetent Host

Most infections in immunocompetent hosts are asymptomatic and do not require therapy. Lymphadenopathy, the most common manifestation, is self-limited and usually resolves within 1 to 3 weeks. Treatment should be considered only if systemic symptoms are severe or long lasting or in the rare event of visceral involvement (encephalitis, myocarditis, pneumonitis). Acute infection as a result of laboratory accidents or transfusions may be severe and should be treated. The treatment regimen of choice consists of a combination of pyrimethamine (Daraprim) and sulfadiazine or trisulfapyrimidine (a mixture of equal parts of sulfamethazine, sulfamerazine, and sulfadiazine) given for 2 to 4 weeks with folinic acid (leucovorin) (Table 1). In the event of pyrimethamine-induced hematologic toxicity, the dosage of folinic acid can be increased to 20 to 50 mg/day. For patients allergic to sulfa, clindamycin in combination with pyrimethamine and folinic acid has been used successfully (see Table 1).

For ocular toxoplasmosis, the drugs of choice are pyrimethamine and sulfadiazine or trisulfapyrimidine with folinic acid in the same dosages as described earlier. Therapy is given for 4 weeks and repeated as needed. Treatment is required to prevent relapse with the risk of progressive vision loss and other complications such as glaucoma. Adjunctive therapy with systemic corticosteroids (prednisone, 80 to 120 mg/day, or an equivalent) is indicated if the macula, optic nerve, or papillomacular bundle is involved.

Immunocompromised Host

For TE, the combination of pyrimethamine, 200 mg loading dose in two divided doses followed by 50 to 75 mg/day

Table 1 Drugs for Treatment of Toxoplasmic Encephalitis and Extraneural Toxoplasmosis

ANTIMICROBIAL	MODE OF ACTION	METABOLISM	ADVERSE EFFECTS	RECOMMENDED DOSAGE (IMMUNOCOMPROMISED)	RECOMMENDED DOSAGE (IMMUNOCOMPETENT)
Pyrimethamine (Daraprim) oral	Inhibits folic acid synthesis	Readily absorbed by gut; hepatic metabolism, lipid soluble	Cytopenias, rash, GI intolerance	Acute: loading dose 100-200 mg; 50-75 mg daily, 3-6 wk; with oral folinic acid (leucovorin) 10-20 mg/day. Maintenance: 25-50 mg/day with oral folinic acid 10-20 mg/day	Loading dose 2 mg/kg/day (maximum 100-200 mg) for 2 days, then 25-50 mg daily for 2-4 wk with oral folinic acid 10-20 mg/day
Sulfadiazine*† or trisulfapyrimidine† oral	Inhibits folic acid synthesis; acts synergistically and sequentially with pyrimethamine	Readily absorbed by gut; penetrates blood-brain barrier; some hepatic metabolism	GI intolerance, rash (Stevens-Johnson syndrome), cytopenias, nephrolithiasis, crystalluria, interstitial nephritis, encephalopathy	Acute: 4-6 g/day, 3-6 wk. Maintenance: 2-4 g/day in 4 divided doses	100 mg/kg/day (maximum 4-8 g/day) in 4 divided doses, 2-4 wk
Clindamycin† oral and IV	Unknown; possibly inhibition of protein synthesis	Readily absorbed by gut; excellent tissue penetration	GI intolerance, rash, pseudomembranous colitis	Acute: 600 mg q6h, 3-6 wk. Maintenance: same as acute	300 mg q6h, 4 wk, repeat as needed

GI, Gastrointestinal.

*Sulfadiazine is available in the United States through Eon Labs Manufacturing, Inc. 227-15 North Conduit Avenue, Laurelton, NY 11413; 800-336-1595, 718-276-8607.

†Used in combination with pyrimethamine.

Table 2 Alternative Drugs for Treatment of Toxoplasmosis in Immunocompromised Patients*

DRUG	MODE OF ACTION	METABOLISM	ADVERSE EFFECTS	RECOMMENDED DOSAGES
Atovaquone oral	Uncoupling electron bio-synthesis; inhibition of de novo pyrimidine biosynthesis	Suspension has better bio-availability than old tablet formulation; improved absorption if taken with food, particularly fatty foods	Rash, elevated liver function tests	Acute: suspension 1500 mg bid; 3-6 wk Maintenance: same
Azithromycin oral	Unknown; possibly inhibition of protein synthesis	Readily absorbed by gut; high intracellular levels	GI intolerance	Acute: 1250-1500 mg/day; 3-6 wk Maintenance: same
Clarithromycin oral	Unknown; possibly inhibition of protein synthesis	Readily absorbed by gut; high tissue levels	GI intolerance, hearing loss, elevated liver function tests	Acute: 500 mg bid, 3-6 wk Maintenance: same

GI, Gastrointestinal.
*Used in combination with pyrimethamine.

orally, plus sulfadiazine, 4 to 6 g/day by mouth in four divided doses, remains the mainstay of treatment (see Table 1). Oral folinic acid is added to preclude the hematologic toxicities associated with antifolate agents. Therapy is given for at least 3 weeks; 6 weeks or more is indicated in severely ill patients and when a complete clinical and radiographic response has not been achieved. Patients who cannot tolerate sulfas can be given clindamycin in combination with pyrimethamine as described. Prophylactic use of anticonvulsants is not recommended. Corticosteroids should not be used routinely but are indicated it there is evidence of increased intracranial pressure. In one study, 70% of AIDS patients treated for TE had a quantifiable clinical improvement by day 7 of therapy. Conversely, patients not responding to empiric therapy had evidence of progressive disease within the first 10 days. Ninety percent of patients had improvement on neuroradiographic studies within 6 weeks of starting therapy.

The same chemotherapeutic regimens are used for extraneural toxoplasmosis; however, there are limited data available on the optimal length and outcome of treatment. As a rule, ocular toxoplasmosis responds favorably to therapy, and treatment of pulmonary infection has been reported to be successful in 50% to 77% of patients.

Intravenous trimethoprim-sulfamethoxazole (TMP-SMX, Bactrim, Septra) at 5 mg/kg/day trimethoprim component has been used when oral therapy is contraindicated. Although TMP-SMX is available for oral use, response rates have been lower than standard regimens. Recently, trials have shown higher initial response rates when the dose was increased (6.6 to 10 mg/kg body weight [BW] per day—trimethoprim).

The drugs described thus far are active only against the tachyzoite form of *T. gondii*. Surviving tissue cysts can reinitiate TE and other manifestations of reactivated latent disease if treatment is discontinued. Therefore it is necessary to give long-term suppressive therapy. Pyrimethamine, 25 to 50 mg/day, and sulfadiazine, 2 to 4 g/day orally in four divided doses, with 10 mg/day of oral folinic acid is recommended because of the low relapse rate associated with this combination. Clindamycin is used in cases of sulfa allergy.

Primary chemoprophylaxis is a very attractive therapeutic option for patients known to be at risk for toxoplasmosis (i.e., those with CD4 counts <100/mm³ and seropositive for anti–*T. gondii* antibodies). Retrospective data suggest that oral TMP-SMX 1 double-strength tablet per day is efficacious. Neither dapsone nor pyrimethamine, when used as single agents are consistently effective. However, the combination of pyrimethamine, 50 mg/wk, plus dapsone, 50 mg/day, plus folinic acid has been a useful alternative. In patients with a sulfa allergy, desensitization is also an option.

Drug regimens being studied for their usefulness as initial and maintenance therapy (Table 2) include atovaquone (Mepron). A recent ACTG trial evaluating the efficacy of atovaquone-containing regimens (either in combination with pyrimethamine or sulfadiazine) shows encouraging results, with greater than 80%, initial response to therapy (unpublished data). As salvage therapy, atovaquone alone induced initial clinical response in 50% of study patients. The response to therapy with atovaquone has been directly correlated with serum drug levels achieved. The newest formulation of atovaquone is administered as an oral suspension 1.5 g twice daily with food, preferably fatty foods, to increase the bioavailability. The new macrolide antibiotics azithromycin (Zithromax) and clarithromycin (Biaxin) in combination with pyrimethamine have limited utility as alternative agents.

Pregnancy

Women who acquire toxoplasmosis during pregnancy expose their fetuses to risk of infection. Infection of the fetus may result in stillbirth, spontaneous abortion, or birth of a symptomatic or an asymptomatic infant. Rarely, transmission has been reported in cases where the mother contracts acute toxoplasmosis 6 to 8 weeks before conception. Fetal infection is less common when the mother is treated during pregnancy. Early diagnosis, through serology, amniotic sampling, and fetal ultrasonography, is important in further management (antibiotics or therapeutic abortion).

Pyrimethamine plus a sulfonamide or spiramycin, a macrolide antibiotic available in Western Europe, Mexico, and

Table 3 Drugs Used in Treatment of Toxoplasmosis in Pregnant Women

ANTIMICROBIAL	ADVERSE EFFECTS	RECOMMENDED DOSAGE	
		FIRST TRIMESTER	SECOND AND THIRD TRIMESTER
Spiramycin*	Nausea, vomiting	30-50 mg/kg/day PO in 3 divided doses	30-50 mg/kg/day PO in 3 divided doses; if fetal infection is suspected or confirmed then pyrimethamine and sulfadiazine may be superior for treatment of the fetus
Pyrimethamine (Daraprim)	Cytopenias, rash, GI intolerance	Teratogenic; not recommended	Loading dose, 100 mg/day for 2 days, then 50 mg/day with folinic acid 10 mg PO, with sulfadiazine or trisulfapyrimidine
Sulfadiazine, trisulfapyrimidine	GI intolerance, rash (Stevens-Johnson syndrome), cytopenias, nephrolithiasis, crystalluria, interstitial nephritis, encephalopathy	50-100 mg/kg/day in 2 divided doses alone	50-100 mg/kg/day in 2 divided doses with pyrimethamine

GI, Gastrointestinal.
From Remington JS, McLeod R, Desmonts G: Toxoplasmosis. In Remington JS, Klein JO, editors: *Infectious diseases of the fetus and newborn infant,* ed 4, Philadelphia, 1995, Saunders.
*Spiramycin is available upon request from U.S. Food and Drug Administration (301-443-9553).

Canada and through the Food and Drug Administration of the United States (301-443-9553), appears to decrease the incidence of congenital toxoplasmic infection when given to women who acquire *T. gondii* during pregnancy (Table 3). Pyrimethamine is teratogenic and should not be used until after the first trimester. There is no optimal medical therapy in the United States for treatment of women who become infected during the first trimester. However, sulfadiazine or trisulfapyrimidines should be used during the first trimester because sulfonamides alone have been shown to be effective in acute toxoplasmosis in animal models. If spiramycin can be obtained, pregnant women acutely infected in the first trimester may be treated until term with 30 to 50 mg/kg/day in three divided doses until fetal infection is confirmed or excluded. Treatment with spiramycin alone decreases the incidence of transmission but not the severity of established congenital infection. If fetal infection is suspected or confirmed after the first trimester, pyrimethamine and sulfadiazine plus folinic acid should be used to treat the maternal infection.

Suggested Reading

Luft BJ, et al: Toxoplasmic encephalitis in patients with the acquired immunodeficiency syndrome, *N Engl J Med* 324:995, 1993.

Mariuz P, Bosler EM, Luft BJ: Toxoplamosis in individuals with AIDS, *Infect Dis Clin North Am* 365, 1994.

Novati R, et al: Polymerase chain reaction for toxoplasma gondii DNA in the cerebrospinal fluid of AIDS patients with focal brain lesions, *AIDS* 8:1691, 1994.

Pomeroy C, Felice GA: Pulmonary toxoplasmosis: a review, *Clin Infect Dis* 14:863, 1992.

Porter SB, Sande M: Toxoplasmosis of the central nervous system in the acquired immunodeficiency syndrome, *N Engl J Med* 327:1643, 1992.

Remington JS, et al: Toxoplasmosis. In Remington JS, Klein JO, eds: *Infectious diseases of the fetus and newborn infant,* ed 4, Philadelphia, 1995, Saunders.

Torre D, et al: Randomized trial of trimethoprim-sulfamethoxazole vs. Pyrimethamine-sulfadiazine for therapy of toxoplasmic encephalitis in patients with AIDS, *Antimicrob Agent Chemother* 42:1346, 1998.

Torres R, et al: Atovaquone for salvage treatment and suppression of toxoplasmic encephalitis in patients with AIDS, *CID* 24:422, 1997.

Wong SY, Remington JS: Toxoplasmosis in pregnancy, *Clin Infect Dis* 18:853, 1994.

MALARIA—TREATMENT AND PROPHYLAXIS

Phyllis E. Kozarsky
Jay S. Keystone

Malaria is one of the most common causes of fever in a returned traveler or recent immigrant from a malarious endemic area. Because death from malaria can occur within several days of the onset of symptoms, it is necessary to consider a febrile illness in a patient from a malarious endemic area to be a medical emergency. This is particularly so when symptoms begin within the first 2 months of arrival because more than 90% of those with malaria caused by *Plasmodium falciparum* present within this time frame. Those infected with other species, such as *Plasmodium vivax,* usually become symptomatic within a year of arrival from the tropics. An additional clue to the likely species of malaria is the area from which a traveler returns. For example, 85% of those with imported *P. falciparum* malaria acquire the infection in Africa, whereas *P. vivax* malaria is most commonly acquired in South Asia.

The standard approach to diagnosing malaria is the examination of thick and thin blood films, but many laboratories do not have the expertise to examine the former. Thick films are five to six times as sensitive as thin films, but thin films are better for determining the species of malaria. If the expertise to examine thick films is not available, as is usually the case in the middle of the night, thin blood films are better than none at all. Although the diagnosis may be missed on a thin blood film, a negative result will rule out a life-threatening infection, which is always associated with high parasitemia. If the initial blood films are negative, they should be repeated two or three times at 12-hour intervals.

Becton-Dickinson, Optimal, and PATH have developed rapid diagnostic kits for malaria using monoclonal antibody on a dipstick or pad to detect malaria antigen. These tests are not yet commercially available but are being used primarily in parts of the developing world. They have a high degree of sensitivity and specificity for falciparum malaria and are probably equivalent to think and thin smears.

Treating malaria appropriately requires knowledge of the infecting species, the likely location the infection was acquired, the geographic patterns of drug resistance, and the percent parasitemia in the case of *P. falciparum* malaria. Figure 1 shows the worldwide distribution of malaria. When there is any doubt about the infecting species, the clinician should treat for the worst-case scenario, chloroquine-resistant *P. falciparum* (CRPF) malaria. Malaria caused by *P. vivax* and *Plasmodium ovale* may leave dormant forms, hypnozoites, in the liver after the blood phase has been eradicated. Thus treatment of these two infections requires eradication of the erythrocytic phase followed by a second drug, primaquine, to eradicate the liver phase.

Treatment of malaria has been increasingly complicated in recent years by the rapid spread of drug-resistant strains. No longer do clinicians have to be concerned only with CRPF malaria, but also with chloroquine-resistant and primaquine-resistant *P. vivax* malaria. Drug resistance has not been established in *P. ovale* or *P. malariae.* Drug regimens for treatment are provided in Table 1.

■ THERAPY

P. vivax Malaria

P. vivax malaria, which has very low mortality, is the most commonly imported malaria. The erythrocytic phase of *P. vivax* malaria is usually effectively treated with chloroquine; primaquine is then used to eradicate hepatic hypnozoites. Because primaquine is one of the most potent oxidizing agents known, a glucose-6-phosphate dehydrogenase (G6PD) level must be determined before primaquine therapy is initiated.

Chloroquine-resistant *P. vivax* malaria was first described in Indonesia in 1989. Since then, it has been shown to be highly endemic in Irian Jaya, Papua New Guinea, the Amazon basin of Brazil, Columbia, and Guyana. Malaria caused by chloroquine-resistant *P. vivax* should be suspected when the illness recurs within 28 days after a patient has received standard therapy with chloroquine and primaquine. Although studies from Indonesia suggested that a standard course of chloroquine combined with high-dose primaquine (2.5 mg/kg over 48 hours) would be effective therapy for drug-resistant *P. vivax* malaria, the regimen was not effective in strains from Guyana. Both mefloquine and halofantrine are effective, although the latter is not available in North America.

When a relapse of *P. vivax* occurs more than 28 days after treatment with chloroquine and primaquine, primaquine resistance should be considered. Primaquine-resistant *P. vivax* malaria is often reported from Papua New Guinea, Irian Jaya, other parts of Southeast Asia and Somalia, and less commonly, Colombia. Patients who fail the usual course of primaquine should receive two times the standard dose over 14 days, or a total dose of 6 mg/kg, to prevent further relapses.

P. ovale Malaria

Malaria caused by *P. ovale,* which is found mostly in Africa, is managed as is that caused by chloroquine-sensitive *P. vivax.* No drug-resistant strains of *P. ovale* have been documented.

Plasmodium malariae and Uncomplicated Chloroquine-Sensitive P. falciparum Malaria

Chloroquine-sensitive *P. falciparum* malaria is confined to Central America north of Panama, Haiti, parts of North Africa, and the Middle East. Chloroquine in standard doses should be used to treat *P. falciparum* from these areas and *P. malariae* infections from any part of the world. Chloroquine does not eradicate the gametocytes of *P. falciparum* malaria, which circulate harmlessly for several months after the other erythrocytic forms of the parasite have been eradicated.

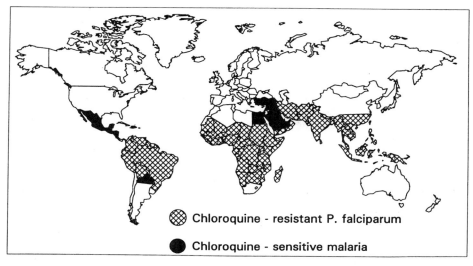

Figure 1
Distribution of malaria and chloroquine-resistant *Plasmodium falciparum*, 1998.

Table 1 Treatment of Malaria		
DRUG	**ADULT DOSAGE**	**PEDIATRIC DOSAGE**
CHLOROQUINE-SENSITIVE MALARIA (ALL SPECIES)		
Chloroquine phosphate 1 tablet (150 mg base = 250 mg salt)	600 mg base (1 g) 300 mg in 6 hr, then 300 mg daily ×2 days	10 mg/kg (maximum 600 mg) 5 mg/kg in 6 hr, then 5 mg/kg ×2 days
	plus in *P. vivax* and *P. ovale* only:	
Primaquine phosphate	15 mg base/day ×14 days	0.3 mg base/kg/day ×14 days
CHLOROQUINE-RESISTANT *P. VIVAX*		
Mefloquine	1-1.5 g (base) in single or divided dose over 12 hr	15 mg/kg in individual dose over 12 hr
Chloroquine as above plus primaquine	10 mg base/kg total over 14 days or 2.5 mg base/kg total over 48 hr	Same as for adults
UNCOMPLICATED CHLOROQUINE-RESISTANT *P. FALCIPARUM*		
Quinine sulfate plus	650 mg tid ×3 days +	24 mg/kg (base)/day in 3 doses ×3 days
Pyrimethamine-sulfadoxine (Fansidar) 25 mg/500 mg or	3 tablets in a single dose	2-11 mo, ¼ tab 1-3 yr, ½ tab 4-8 yr, 1 tab 9-14 yr, 2 tab >14 yr, adult dose
Doxycycline	100 mg bid ×7 days	5 mg/kg qid ×7 days
Clindamycin	900 mg tid ×3 days	20-40 mg/kg/day in 3 doses ×3 days
Mefloquine	1-1.5 g (base) in a single or divided dose over 12 hr	15 mg/kg in a single or divided dose over 12 hr
TREATMENT OF SEVERE ILLNESS, PARENTERAL DOSE FOR ALL SPECIES		
Quinine loading	20 mg/kg (salt) [1 mg salt = 0.83 mg base] in 300 ml normal saline IV over 2-4 hr Maintenance, 10 mg/kg q8h	Same as for adults
Quinidine loading	24 mg/kg (salt) in 300 ml of normal saline IV over 2-4 hr Maintenance: 12 mg/kg q8h or 10 mg/kg (salt) IV over 1-2 hr, then constant infusion of 0.02 mg/kg/min by infusion pump	Same as for adults

*Double initial dose if parasitemia ≥1%.
†Seven days if CRPF acquired in southeast Asia.

Uncomplicated Chloroquine-Resistant *P. falciparum* Malaria

With the exception of the regions where chloroquine-sensitive *P. falciparum* malaria remains, malaria caused by *P. falciparum* should be considered chloroquine resistant. Quinine sulfate remains the drug of choice for treatment of CRPF malaria in combination with a second agent such as pyrimethamine-sulfadoxine (Fansidar), a tetracycline derivative, or clindamycin. Pyrimethamine-sulfadoxine should not be used for treatment of strains acquired along the Thai-Cambodian or Thai-Myanmar borders or in the Amazon basin of Brazil, where multidrug-resistant strains occur. Clindamycin is usually reserved for pregnant women and for young children, in whom no tetracycline derivative is generally used. Because these second agents tend to be slower acting, it is important to institute quinine therapy as soon as the diagnosis is confirmed. Virtually everyone who takes quinine will suffer from cinchonism, and complaints of tinnitus, dizziness, headache, and possibly temporary hearing loss are common. If the parasitemia is 1% or greater, strong consideration should be given to the use of a loading dose of quinine (doubling the initial dose).

Mefloquine alone is a very effective therapy for uncomplicated CRPF malaria. Along the Thai borders the treatment dose must be increased from 15 to 25 mg/kg because of multidrug resistance. Unfortunately, data confirm the development of cross-resistance among mefloquine, halofantrine, and quinine because of their chemical relatedness. Major concerns about the use of mefloquine for treatment of malaria are the severe neuropsychiatric adverse reactions (psychosis, convulsions), which occur 10 to 60 times as often as when the drug is used for prophylaxis; these complications are estimated to occur in 1:215 to 1:1700 users. In an attempt to decrease the gastrointestinal side effects of mefloquine, the dose may be split and administered over 12 hours.

Halofantrine is widely used in malarious areas throughout the world. In standard doses, however, it is not very effective along the borders of Thailand. Studies have documented cardiotoxicity with halofantrine, particularly in those who have taken the drug with food, as drug absorption increases sixfold with a fatty meal. Halofantrine should be taken on an empty stomach. It is contraindicated in those with a family history of prolonged QT interval or conduction disturbances or when any other QT-prolonging agent such as mefloquine or quinine has been administered. An electrocardiogram is recommended before halofantrine administration.

Malarone, a combination of atovaquone (250 mg) and proguanil (100 mg), has been shown to be highly effective for the treatment of *P. falciparum* malaria infections, even in multidrug-resistant areas of Thailand. It is available in Europe and in Canada. The 3-day course of therapy is generally well tolerated, with a small percentage of individuals suffering from gastrointestinal upset. Dividing the dose twice daily may reduce this problem.

Increasingly in Southeast Asia and more recently in Africa, malaria is being treated with the oral artemisinin derivative artesunate. This drug is well tolerated, and it leads to a rapid reduction in parasitemia and fever; however, monotherapy is associated with a high rate of recrudescence. The combination of a second agent such as mefloquine or tetracycline with artesunate is necessary to ensure cure of the infection. If travelers or expatriates need to be treated with artemisinin derivatives because of treatment failures with quinine and mefloquine, therapy should be conducted under expert supervision. Artesunate is available in parenteral, oral, and suppository forms.

Complicated *P. falciparum* Malaria

When *P. falciparum* parasitemia reaches 5% or more, complications such as cerebral malaria, renal failure, adult respiratory distress syndrome (ARDS), and massive hemolysis may occur. It is not uncommon for these serious complications to occur on the third to fourth day of treatment while the parasitemia is dropping. The mortality of even appropriately treated severe *P. falciparum* malaria ranges from 10% to 20%. Patients with complicated malaria, and those who cannot tolerate oral quinine because of vomiting, require parenteral therapy with quinine or quinidine. Because parenteral quinine preparations are not readily available in most centers, quinidine should be used. However, because of its potential for cardiotoxicity, continuous electrocardiographic monitoring should be undertaken. Because both quinine and quinidine cause insulin to be released from the pancreas, it is important to monitor for hypoglycemia, a common complication of severe malaria, especially in pregnant women and children. Fluid balance should be corrected judiciously with the aim of avoiding fluid overload because of the risk of ARDS. Lactic acidosis, a common complication of severe malaria, indicates a poor prognosis. For parasitemias above 10%, particularly when other complications are present, exchange transfusion with at least four units of blood or red cell pheresis may be lifesaving. When patients present with severe *P. falciparum* malaria, it is prudent to rule out other concomitant infections such as meningitis in those who are comatose and septicemia in those who are hypotensive.

■ PROPHYLAXIS

The primary goal of prophylaxis is to prevent *P. falciparum* infection in nonimmune travelers because almost all fatal cases are associated with illness caused by this species. For decades, chloroquine was widely effective in the prevention and treatment of all species of malaria. However, with the spread of chloroquine resistance, recommendations for antimalarial chemoprophylaxis have become more complicated and often controversial. Figure 2 is an algorithm for determining an appropriate antimalarial chemoprophylactic regimen.

Areas within a country may differ with respect to risk. For example, travel in most areas in Kenya places travelers at risk for acquisition of chloroquine-resistant *P. falciparum*. The risk is highest near Lake Victoria, intermediate on the coast, and lowest in the game parks. However, if the traveler will be staying only in Nairobi, the capital, where there is no malaria, prophylaxis is not necessary.

Mefloquine is the agent of choice for the prevention of chloroquine-resistant *P. falciparum* infections. It is contraindicated for those with a history of seizure disorder, neuropsychiatric problems, or cardiac conduction defects. Meflo-

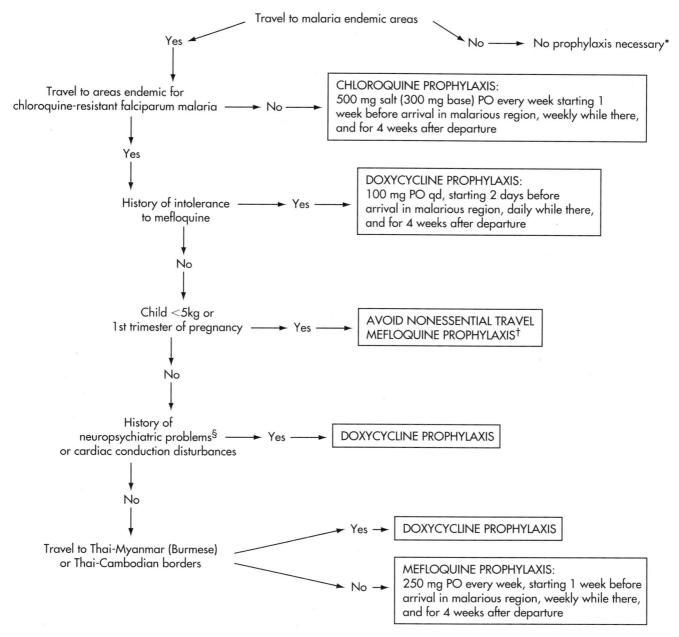

Travel to malaria endemic areas

Yes → No → No prophylaxis necessary*

Travel to areas endemic for chloroquine-resistant falciparum malaria → No →

CHLOROQUINE PROPHYLAXIS:
500 mg salt (300 mg base) PO every week starting 1 week before arrival in malarious region, weekly while there, and for 4 weeks after departure

Yes

History of intolerance to mefloquine → Yes →

DOXYCYCLINE PROPHYLAXIS:
100 mg PO qd, starting 2 days before arrival in malarious region, daily while there, and for 4 weeks after departure

No

Child <5kg or 1st trimester of pregnancy → Yes →

AVOID NONESSENTIAL TRAVEL
MEFLOQUINE PROPHYLAXIS†

No

History of neuropsychiatric problems§ or cardiac conduction disturbances → Yes → DOXYCYCLINE PROPHYLAXIS

No

Travel to Thai-Myanmar (Burmese) or Thai-Cambodian borders → Yes → DOXYCYCLINE PROPHYLAXIS

→ No →

MEFLOQUINE PROPHYLAXIS:
250 mg PO every week, starting 1 week before arrival in malarious region, weekly while there, and for 4 weeks after departure

* Malaria in many countries is confined to rural areas or regions not on usual tourist itineraries.

† Data collected suggest there is no significant increase in spontaneous abortions or congenital malformations when mefloquine taken during 1st trimester; inadvertent use *not* a reason for abortion.

§ Seizures, psychoses, depression, anxiety reactions.

Figure 2
Algorithm for the chemoprophylaxis of malaria. Dosages given are for adults.

quine may be used during pregnancy, and dosage regimens are available for children of all ages.

Disabling neuropsychiatric side effects (anxiety, depression, headaches, nightmares, and irritability) occur in approximately 1 in 200 users and more often in women. Dividing the dose twice weekly may reduce these effects. If

mefloquine and doxycycline cannot be used, consultation with a travel medicine specialist is appropriate.

Prolonged exposure to malaria in areas intensely endemic for *P. vivax* (for example, Central America, Northwest Africa, South Asia, Oceania) warrants terminal malaria prophylaxis with primaquine phosphate to eradicate the hepatic hypnozoites and prevent relapsing malaria. As noted, G6PD levels should be checked before prescribing this drug. Primaquine is usually taken after completing chloroquine, mefloquine, or doxycycline therapy and is contraindicated during pregnancy. The adult dose is 15 mg base/day for 14 days.

Because no antimalarial regimen is 100% effective, all travelers to malarious regions need to be meticulous about personal protection measures. Between dusk and dawn, when the *Anopheles* mosquitoes bite, travelers should wear permethrin-impregnated protective clothing (long sleeves, pants), use mosquito repellents and sleep under permethrin-impregnated netting or in screened or air-conditioned rooms. Insect repellents that contain 35% or less diethyltoluamide (DEET) are very effective. Repellents containing 5% to 10% deet should be used on young children to prevent toxicity. Knock-down sprays should be used indoors and in infected areas before bedtime.

Because there is no worldwide consensus concerning malaria chemoprophylaxis, travelers should be advised to listen with great caution to antimalarial advice received from fellow travelers and overseas health care providers. Also, travelers should be advised to seek medical attention immediately in the event of fever during or soon after travel; they should tell the health care provider to check them for malaria with blood smears, and have them repeated several times.

Physicians who are responsible for preventing and treating malaria will have to keep abreast of the global spread of drug resistance and the new agents being developed to combat this problem. Assistance may be sought from the Centers for Disease Control and Prevention by calling toll free 877-FYI-TRIP (394-8747) or through their website www.cdc.gov/travel.

Suggested Reading

Anonymous: Artemisinin, *Trans R Soc Trop Med Hyg* 88(suppl 1):1, 1994.

Centers for Disease Control and Prevention: Health information for international travel 1999-2000, DHHS, Atlana.

Lobel H, Kozarsky PE: Update on prevention of malaria for travelers, *JAMA*, 278:1767, 1997.

Phillips P, Nantel S, Benny WB: Exchange transfusion as an adjunct to the treatment of severe falciparum malaria: case report and review, *Rev Infect Dis* 12:1100, 1990.

World Health Organization: Severe and complicated malaria, *Trans R Soc Top Med Hyg* 84(suppl 2):1, 1990.

World Health Organization: A rapid dipstick antigen capture assay for the diagnosis of falciparum malaria, *Bull WHO* 74:47, 1996.

BABESIOSIS

Jeffrey A. Gelfand

Debra Poutsiaka

Babesiosis is a disease caused by a malaria-like parasite in man. The first case of human babesiosis was described by Skrabalo in 1957. Initial case descriptions were in splenectomized individuals. However, in 1969, human babesiosis in a patient with a functioning spleen was reported from the island of Nantucket off the coast of Massachusetts. Since then, more than 100 cases of human babesiosis have been reported. The disease has been described in the eastern, central, and western regions of the United States, Europe, and Asia. The rodent strain *Babesia microti* has been implicated in the United States, whereas the cattle strains *B. divergens* and *B. bovis* have been associated with human disease in Europe. Previously unknown *Babesia* strains or *Babesia*-like organisms infecting humans have been recently described.

■ THE ORGANISM

The taxonomy of babesias was recently reviewed by Telford and associates as phylum Apicomplexa, class Aconoidasida, order Piroplasmidora, family Babesdiidae, and genus *Babesia*. Only a few species are known to cause disease in humans. The organisms are intracellular parasites, which are piriform, round, or oval, depending on the species. *B. microti*, whose host is normally rodents, measures 2.0 by 1.5 microns. These organisms are often mistaken for *Plasmodium falciparum*, one of the agent that causes malaria, because of their intracellular ring forms and the peripheral location of the parasite in the erythrocyte. However, in contrast to the appearance of the developing intraerythrocytic *Plasmodium*, intraerythrocytic *Babesia* contain no hemoglobin-derived pigment. The appearance of the tetrad form of *B. microti*, the result of division by budding rather than schizogeny, is diagnostic of babesiosis (Figure 1).

■ THE TICK VECTOR

Babesiosis, a zoonotic disease, requires the transmission from an animal reservoir to the human host via a tick vector. In 1976, Spielman described studies identifying the tick *Ixodes dammini*, the northern deer tick, as the vector of

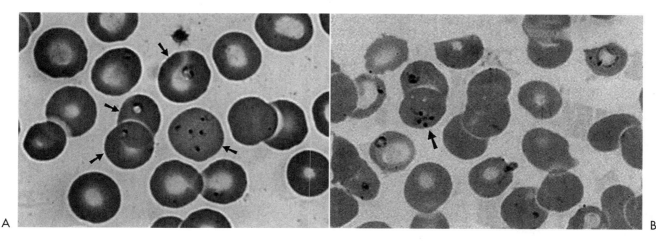

Figure 1
A, Thin blood smear, Giemsa-stained, from a patient with *B. microti.* One erythrocyte has five merozoites; the other erythrocytes contain ring-form merozoites, with central pallor, distinctive from *P. falciparum.* **B,** Thin blood smear, Giemsa-stained. Four mature merozoites, dividing asexually, forming a tetrad that appears to be a "maltese cross," pathognomonic for Babesiosis.

babesiosis on Nantucket Island. *I. dammini* is thought to be the same as *I. scapularis.* The cattle tick *Ixodes ricinus,* in its larval form, is the vector for *B. divergens.*

Three developmental forms of ticks exist: the larval, nymph, and adult forms. The larval and nymph forms of *I. scapularis* feed mainly on *Peromyscus leucopus,* the white-footed deer mouse, but have been found on other hosts such as rats, other mice, rabbits, deer, dogs, and humans. The adult forms feeds mainly on deer. Interestingly, deer do not become infected with *B. microti.* It is thought that the reintroduction of the deer to Nantucket Island in the 1930s after decimation of herds as a result of hunting, with the subsequent growth of the deer population, is responsible for the spread of *I. scapularis.* The tick requires a blood meal to progress to the next developmental stage. While feeding on the deer, the adult female tick becomes impregnated and produces up to 20,000 eggs.

Almost 80% of white-footed deer mice sampled during a 1976 survey on Nantucket Island were infected with *B. microti.* While feeding on an infected mouse, the tick larvae become infected with *B. microti.* After infection of the nymphal form, the nymph obtains another blood meal and in the process, infects the host. The host is usually a rodent. Infestation of a human by a nymph is difficult to detect because the nymph is small (1.5 to 2.5 mm long). The three development forms of *I. scapularis* feed on humans, but the nymph is the main vector of babesiosis. The three forms also feed on deer, which do not become infected. Thus deer are an important link in the life cycle of *B. microti* because they sustain the adult form of the arthropod vector. A convergence of all three organisms—deer, mouse, and tick—is necessary to create the conditions favoring the infection of humans, as incidental hosts, with *B. microti.* For *B. divergens* and *B. bovis,* the convergence of cattle and ticks is necessary to create conditions favoring the infection of humans in Europe.

During the final hours of attachment of the tick to the host, thousands of sporozoites are deposited into the skin. The direct invasion of sporozoites into mammalian host erythrocytes has not been demonstrated for *B. microti,* and the process by which sporozoites transform into merozoites is not understood. Via asynchronous budding, two to four merozoites are formed. The rare but diagnostic tetramere seen with light microscopy of erythrocytes parasitized by *B. microti* is a representation of four merozoites within the parental babesia (see Figure 1). The erythrocyte membrane is damaged, with perforations, protrusions, and inclusions, as the merozoites leave the cell, ultimately resulting in hemolysis. Because there is no synchronous schizogony, as with *Plasmodium* species, massive hemolysis does not occur.

■ INJURY TO THE HOST

There are three known mechanisms by which infection with *Babesia* species causes injury to the host: hemolysis and resultant anemia, increased cytoadherance of erythrocytes within the vasculature, and the release of harmful mediators. A newly identified strain of *Babesia,* strain WA-1, recently isolated from a patient in Washington State, was noted to cause profound intravascular stasis within several organs in infected hamsters. Aggregates of inflammatory cells occluded blood vessels. Thrombosis and coagulation necrosis were described. It is possible that *Babesia* also elicit the production of cytokines by host cells and that cytokines might be responsible for some of the observed injury, in much the same manner as postulated for malaria.

■ EPIDEMIOLOGY

Well over 100 cases of human babesiosis have been reported, with new reports now arising frequently. Human infections with *Babesia* species have been documented from several continents. Most human cases of babesiosis have been reported from the United States, particularly from the northeastern part of the country. *B. microti* is responsible for almost all of the American cases. However, recent reports document infection by newly identified species of *Babesia* in California, Missouri, and Washington State. The emergence of human babesiosis in the United States, where most of the epidemiologic studies on this disease have been conducted, appears to be related to the increase in the deer population. In Europe, reports of infection, usually with *B. divergens*, have come from the former Yugoslavia, France, Russia, Ireland, Scotland, Sweden, and the Canary Islands. Most European cases have occurred in splenectomized individuals. In addition, several cases of babesiosis in Asia, Central America, and South Africa have been reported.

A group with an increased likelihood of seropositivity for *B. microti* is persons with a history of infection by *Borrelia burgdorferi*, the causative agent of Lyme disease. Positive *B. microti* serologies have been found in 9.5% to 66% of adults with positive serologies for *B. burdorferi*. Similar findings occur in children. The explanation for this is the transmission of each agent by the same vector, *I. scapularis*. Coinfection with *Ehrlichia*, which is also transmitted by *I. scapularis*, has been documented in persons infected with *Babesia* and/or *Borrelia*. The phenomenon of coinfection might be more than a mere curiosity because there is evidence that persons coinfected with *B. burgdorferi* and *B. microti* exhibit more severe and prolonged symptoms.

Although transmission of human babesiosis occurs in most cases through a tick bite, there are other modes of transmission. Infectious parasites have been retrieved from *B. microti*–infected blood stored at 4° C (39.2° F) for up to 21 days, under conditions that are replicated during blood banking. Not surprisingly, acquisition of babesiosis through blood transfusion has been well documented. Almost all reports have concerned the transmission of *B. microti*. However, there is a recent case report of transmission of the WA1-type parasite by transfusion in Washington State in the United States. A comparison between *B. microti*–seronegative and *B. microti*–seropositive blood donors in Massachusetts identified no differences that would enable the identification of high-risk donors. Despite this, the risk of acquiring babesiosis from a blood transfusion obtained from a donor residing in an endemic area is very low.

■ CLINICAL FEATURES

European and North American cases of human babesiosis differ markedly in clinical manifestations. Human babesiosis in North America is usually caused by the rodent strain *B. microti*. The infection is often subclinical, and symptomatic disease is usually less severe than the European form, even in splenectomized individuals. The incubation period is usually from 1 to 3 weeks, although periods as long as 6 weeks have been observed. Most patients do not recall a tick bite, most likely because of the small size (2 mm) of the engorged nymph. Approximately 70% of patients infected with *B. microti* have intact spleens. Almost all of the more than 120 patients with babesiosis caused by *B. microti* have survived. Those individuals with intact spleens who have

developed serious clinical illness usually have been 50 years of age or older, suggesting that age is a risk factor for more severe disease. Patients with splenectomies who have contracted babesiosis tend to be younger than previously healthy persons who develop the infection.

Clinical manifestations of *B. microti* infection are nonspecific and of gradual onset. Fever is common and may reach levels of 40° C (104° F) and be sustained or intermittent. Common symptoms are malaise, fatigue, anorexia, rigors, headache, myalgias, arthralgias, nausea, vomiting, abdominal pain, and dark urine. Other symptoms include photophobia, conjunctival injection, sore throat, depression, emotional lability, and cough.

Physical findings in addition to fever are few, if any. Splenomegaly is probably the most common finding. Hepatomegaly also occurs. Skin changes have been noted and include splinter hemorrhages, petechiae, ecchymoses, purpura, and palor. In addition, a rash resembling erythema chronicum migrans (ECM) has been observed but this most likely represents patients with intercurrent Lyme disease. Other findings include icteric sclerae and jaundice. Lymphadenopathy has not been noted.

Patients may become critically ill when infected with *B. microti*. In one series, hospital stay for 17 patients averaged 19 days, with the duration of convalescence lasting up to 18 months. Adult respiratory distress syndrome is a complication of babesiosis. Fatalities, although unusual, have occurred.

Hemolytic anemia, occasionally severe, is common, as are associated findings of decreased haptoglobin and increased reticulocyte count. The leukocyte count may be normal or somewhat decreased. Thrombocytopenia is common, observed in two thirds of patients in one series. The erythrocyte sedimentation rate can be elevated and the direct Coombs' test can react positively. Renal function can be disturbed, as manifested by hemoglobinuria, proteinuria, and elevated blood urea nitrogen and creatinine. Elevations of bilirubin, alkaline phosphatase, serum aspartate aminotransferase, serum alanine aminotransferase, and lactic dehydrogenase have been observed. In a few cases in which bone marrow examination has been performed, hemophagocytosis has been noted, although it is not invariably present.

Severe infections with newly identified *Babesia* organisms have occurred in the United States. In Washington State, the WA1 strain of *Babesia* was identified from a man with an intact spleen who suffered moderately severe disease. Subsequently, four asplenic patients from Northern California were infected with a similar if not identical organism and suffered severe disease, with two fatalities. The infecting organism was more closely related to the canine strain *B. gibsoni* than to *B. microti*. Finally, a fatal infection with an organism closely related to *B. divergens* occurred in an 73-year-old asplenic man in the state of Missouri.

Certain groups of patients might be at more risk for severe disease. There is some evidence that those with concurrent Lyme disease and babesiosis have more severe and prolonged symptomatology. Thus intercurrent Lyme disease should be investigated in any patient with known or suspected babesiosis. Advanced age might be a risk factor for more severe disease. Underlying medical illness, including splenectomy, might predispose to severe disease. One underlying illness, human immunodeficiency virus (HIV) infection, is associated with severe *B. microti* infections, which can be prolonged and chronic.

Most cases (84%) in Europe have occurred in splenectomized individuals in whom the infecting organism is usually bovine *Babesia* species, particularly *B. bovis* and *B. divergens*. Of the 19 cases reviewed by Telford, more than half died. Mortality among splenectomized individuals was greater than 70%. The infection is fulminant, with sudden onset accompanied by hemoglobinuria, jaundice, and fever. Renal failure is a common complication. This usually results from intravascular hemolysis, which can be severe.

■ LABORATORY DIAGNOSIS

The usual method in diagnosing babesiosis is by microscopic examination of Giemsa- or Wright-stained thick and thin smears of the blood. Most studies have been in reports of humans infected with *B. microti*. However, differentiation between species on morphologic grounds is unreliable. Usually 1% to 10% of erythrocytes are parasitized in patients with clinical disease. However, the range is from less than 1% to 85%. More than one ring form can be present in an individual erythrocyte. The ring forms of *Plasmodium falciparum* are very similar to the predominant forms of *Babesia* seen within the erythrocyte, making differentiation difficult. The babesial forms can have one or more chromatin masses or dots. In heavy infestation, trophozoites can be seen outside erythrocytes. Several morphologic features enable distinction between *Babesia* and *P. falciparum*: (1) older stages of *P. falciparum* contain hemozoin, which are brownish pigment deposits not found in babesial forms; (2) *Babesia* forms lack the synchronous stages, schizonts and gametocytes, found with *Plasmodium* species; (3) a rare but pathognomonic feature of *Babesia* infection is the presence of tetrads of merozoites (see Figure 1), which are not present in malaria; (4) in *Babesia* infection, larger ring forms can contain a central white vacuole which is not present in malaria.

Serologic testing for *B. microti* using an indirect immunofluorescence test is available though the Centers for Disease Control and Prevention (CDC). Cross-reaction among species of *Babesia*, as well as among species of *Plasmodium*, occur. Usually, persons with active infection have titers of 1:1024 or greater, which fall over time to 1:256 or less. A titer of 1:256 is diagnostic of *B. microti* infection. Titers of 1:32 or greater are indicative of past infection. Some consider a titer as low as 1:16 as positive. An IgM indirect immunofluorescent antibody test was found useful for the rapid diagnosis of acute babesiosis in a research setting.

Diagnosis by polymerase chain reaction holds promise as a sensitive and specific method for the diagnosis of *B. microti*.

■ CLINICAL MANAGEMENT

Most patients infected with *B. microti* develop mild or subclinical illness and recover without specific therapy. In severely ill patients, clindamycin (900 to 1200 mg intravenously every 12 hours) and oral quinine (25 mg/kg/day in children, 650 mg every 6 to 8 hours) for 7 to 10 days appear effective. Failure of this regimen has occurred. Other promising agents include atovaquone and azithromycin in combination. Atovaquone, often used in the treatment of toxoplasma encephalitis in patients with acquired immunodeficiency syndrome (AIDS), is a promising agent for the treatment of babesiosis. Atovaquone (750 mg every 12 hours) and azithromycin (500 mg on day one, then 250 mg daily thereafter) together may be as effective (and relatively nontoxic) as clindamycin and quinine.

European babesiosis, particularly disease caused by *B. divergens*, is a potentially explosive disease, particularly in splenectomized individuals. Thus supportive measures and specific antiparasitic treatment should be instituted rapidly. Most sources recommend treatment with quinine (650 mg administered orally three times per day) and clindamycin (600 mg intravenously administered three to four times per day) for 7 to 10 days, often with erythrocyte exchange transfusion as adjunctive therapy. Pentamidine and cotrimoxazole were used to successfully treat one patient with babesiosis caused by *B. divergens*. Novel approaches to the treatment of European babesiosis currently under study include the use of the 3-hydroxy-3-methylglutaryl coenzyme-A reductase inhibitors lovastatin and simvastatin, which inhibit the intraerythrocytic development of *B. divergens*, and the use of the lipophilic folate analoges piritrexam and trimetrexate, which inhibited the growth of *B. bovis*. in vitro.

Erythrocyte exchange transfusions are useful in severely ill patients with high levels of parasitemia and hemolysis. When used in conjunction with chemotherapy, the level of parasitemia is reduced. In addition, toxic factors produced by the parasites or of host origin might be removed.

Persons infected with *B. microti* should receive therapy for early infection with *B. burgdorferi* because of the well-documented cotransmission of these two pathogens by *I. scapularis*. Effective regimens include doxycycline, 100 mg twice daily; amoxicillin, 500 mg four times daily (50 mg/kg/day in children); or cefuroxime axetil, 500 mg twice daily. Unless there is evidence of disseminated Lyme disease, a 10-day course should be sufficient.

■ PREVENTION AND CONTROL

Prevention of human babesiosis relies on avoidance of exposure to the tick vectors. For *I. scapularis*, the months of May through September represent times of greatest activity. In endemic areas, avoidance of grassy areas and brush is advisable. Splenectomized individuals and those who are immunocompromised in other ways should avoid areas of endemicity during times of high tick activity. Clothing should cover the body, especially the lower portion, through wearing long-sleeved shirts and long pants with socks. Tucking pant legs into socks is effective in preventing ticks from crawling up the legs. Ticks are more obvious if light-colored clothing is worn. Insect repellents such as diethyltoluamide (DEET) applied to the skin or clothing, or permethrin applied to clothing only, might be effective. Children and pets should be inspected carefully for ticks. If a tick is found, it should be removed expediently. The tick is grasped below the mouth at the site of attachment to the skin with forceps or tweezers and pulled off steadily. Vaccines against human babesiosis are not available.

Although transfusion-associated babesiosis is rare, this form of transmission can potentially be reduced by discouraging blood donors from endemic areas during times of the year characterized by increased tick activity. Donors with fever within 2 months before donation should be avoided. Screening of blood for babesiosis is unlikely to be adopted, so the possibility of transfusion-associated babesiosis will remain.

Suggested Reading

Dammin GJ: Babesiosis. In Weinstein L, Fields B, eds: *Seminars in infectious disease,* New York, 1978, Stratton.

Krause PJ, et al: Concurrent Lyme disease and babesiosis. Evidence for increased severity and duration of illness, *JAMA* 275:1657, 1996.

Krause PJ, et al: Treatment of babesiosis: Comparison of atovaquone and azithromycin with clindamycin and quinine. In *Program and Abstracts of the 46th Annual Meeting of the American Society of Tropical Medicine and Hygiene* (abstract), Lake Buena Vista, Florida.

Persing DH, et al: Infection with a *Babesia*-like organism in northern California, *N Engl J Med* 332:298, 1995.

Telford S, et al: Babesiosis. In Kreier J, ed: *Parasitic protozoa,* vol 5, New York, 1993, Academic Press.

PNEUMOCYSTIS CARINII

Walter T. Hughes

The diffuse bilateral pneumonitis caused by *Pneumocystis carinii* occurs almost exclusively in immunocompromised patients with cancer, organ transplantation, congenital immunodeficiency disorders, and the acquired immunodeficiency syndrome (AIDS). The organism is known to cause pneumonitis occasionally in patients without underlying immunodeficiency.

■ CLINICAL FEATURES

The clinical manifestations of *P. carinii* pneumonitis are fever, cough, tachypnea, and dyspnea progressing to cyanosis. The onset may be abrupt or subtle.

With an abrupt onset, fever, marked increase in respiratory rate, and severe dyspnea occur within 24 to 48 hours. The disease progresses rapidly with marked decrease in arterial oxygen tension (Pao_2) and increase in alveolar-arterial oxygen gradient. The chest radiograph shows bilateral diffuse alveolar disease with an air bronchogram. Without treatment, the disease worsens and within a month all patients will have died. Even in fatal cases and even in the most severely compromised host, the organism and the disease remain localized to the lung, with rare exception. When specific and supportive treatment is introduced early in the disease, the mortality rate can be reduced to around 10% in most medical centers. Abrupt onset tends to occur in patients with cancer, organ transplantation, and AIDS.

With a subtle onset, an increase in respiratory rate occurs, with or without fever. No abnormality may be found by chest radiograph early in the course, although computed

tomography (CT) scans may show perihilar infiltrates. The disease slowly progresses over 1 to 2 weeks to the more severe and life-threatening disease described above for abrupt onset presentation. The subtle pattern is seen in some AIDS patients, rarely in cancer and transplant patients, and usually in the infantile epidemic form of the pneumonitis. In the immunocompromised host, the subtle form progresses to a fatal outcome if untreated. However, during the outbreaks of infantile plasma cell pneumonitis caused by *P. carinii,* approximately half of the patients will eventually recover without treatment.

■ DIAGNOSIS

A definitive diagnosis of *P. carinii* pneumonitis requires the identification of the organism in tissue or secretions from the lung. Specimens are usually obtained by bronchoalveolar lavage (BAL). Induced sputum samples may contain the organism but less often than BAL. Open lung or transbronchial lung biopsy is the most sensitive source for diagnostic material. Specimens from BAL, induced sputum and biopsy are processed with Gomori-Grocott methenamine silver, Giemsa and fluorscein-labeled antibody stains. No serologic method is of diagnostic use and the polymerase chain reaction (PCR) amplification of *P. carinii* DNA sequences have not been adequately studied as diagnostic tests.

■ THERAPY

Trimethoprim-sulfamethoxazole (TMP-SMX) is the drug of first choice for treatment. Moderately and severely ill patients should receive 15 mg TMP and 75 mg SMX/kg intravenously per day in four doses 6 hours apart. Patients with mild pneumonitis, who can take oral medication may be treated with 20 mg TMP and 100 mg SMX/kg/day in four divided doses by mouth. Usually, 21 days of therapy is required, and most patients who qualify for prophylaxis will continue taking the drug at one-fifth the therapeutic dose for life or until no longer at risk for recurrence or reinfection. Adverse reactions are uncommon in non-AIDS patients, but about 40% of those with AIDS have significant reactions to TMP-SMX. Rash, neutropenia, and fever are the most common treatment-limiting events. Some patients can tolerate mild reactions while TMP-SMX is continued. Rare but life-threatening reactions include Stevens-Johnson syndrome, hepatic necrosis, aplastic anemia, agranulocytosis, and allergic reactions. Leucovorin is not used routinely with TMP-SMX therapy.

Patients who cannot tolerate or who fail to respond to TMP-SMX may be changed to other effective drugs. (See the chapter *Prophylaxis of Opportunistic Infections in HIV Disease.*) These include atovaquone, pentamidine isethionate, and trimetrexate with leucovorin, which have been approved by the Food and Drug Administration (FDA). Other effective drugs with proved efficacy, but not FDA approved, are dapsone-trimethoprim and clindamycin plus primaquine. The drug of second choice is usually pentamidine isethionate, but recent studies indicate that atovaquone is equally effective and less toxic. Trimetrexate plus leucovorin is effective but has been less extensively studied.

Pentamidine isethionate, 4 mg/kg/day as a single intravenous dose, may be used for *P. carinii* pneumonitis of any severity. This drug is similar in efficacy to TMP-SMX, but more than 50% of patients, including patients without AIDS, have significant adverse effects. These include nephrotoxicity, leukopenia, hypoglycemia, hypotension, thrombocytopenia, hypocalcemia, and Stevens-Johnson syndrome. Pentamidine can be given intramuscularly, but serious injection site reactions are common. Aerosolized pentamidine has only limited therapeutic effect but is relatively safe. There is no oral preparation of pentamidine.

Atovaquone is available in only a suspension formulation (750 mg/5 ml). The adult dosage is 750 mg three times daily by mouth (total adult dose is 2250 mg/day). Children should be given 30 mg/kg/day in three divided doses. It is important for each dose to be given after a meal high in fat to achieve maximal absorption. Clinical experience with atovaquone for the treatment of *P. carinii* pneumonitis has been limited to patients with mild and moderate disease, (A-a)Do$_2$ of 45 mm Hg or less. No serious adverse effects or toxic dose have been reported. The most common adverse effects are diarrhea, headache, rash, and nausea.

Trimetrexate glucuronate, 45 mg/m^2, is given as a single infusion over 60 to 90 minutes plus leukovorin, 20 mg/m^2 over 5 to 10 minutes every 6 hours (total daily dose, 80 mg/m^2). Leukovorin, but not trimetrexate, may be given orally in the same dosage. This regimen is an alternative therapy for moderate and severe cases of *P. carinii* pneumonia.

Dapsone, 100 mg (total dose) per day, plus trimethoprim, 5 mg/kg of body weight three times a day, is efficacious but the drugs are available only by the oral route. Adverse events include anemia, methemoglobinemia, and rash. About one third of the patients intolerant to TMP-SMX may also be intolerant to dapsone-trimethoprim.

The combination of clindamycin, 600 mg every 6 hours and primaquine, 30 mg base per day orally for 21 days, is another regimen shown efficacious in limited studies.

Supportive therapy for patients with a Pao$_2$ of 70 mm Hg or less, or arterial-alveolar gradient of 35 mm Hg or greater includes the administration of a corticosteroid, such as prednisolone, 40 mg twice a day on days 1 to 5, 40 mg daily on days 6 to 10, and 20 mg a day on days 11 to 21.

■ PREVENTION

P. carinii pneumonitis can be effectively prevented with chemoprophylaxis. Indications for prophylaxis include the following:

- Human immunodeficiency virus (HIV)-infected adults and children 6 years of age and older, with CD4+ T-lymphocyte counts (%) of 200 cells/μl (15%) or less
- Immunocompromised patients who have recovered from one or more episodes of *P. carinii* pneumonitis
- Infants born of HIV-infected mothers, beginning at 4 to 6 weeks of age; once HIV infection has been excluded, the prophylaxis can be stopped; infected infants are continued on the drug
- HIV-infected infants ages 1 to 5 years of age with CD4+ T-lymphocyte counts of 500 cells/μl (15%) or less
- Certain high-risk patients with cancer, organ transplantation, and congenital immune deficiency disorders

TMP-SMX is the preferred drug with any of the following schedules: 160 mg TMP + 800 mg SMX once or twice a day to adults, either daily or 3 days a week. Some evidence suggests 80 mg TMP + 400 mg SMX is also effective in adults. Infants and children should receive 5 mg TMP + 25 mg SMX per kilogram daily or 3 days a week, but not to exceed the adult doses.

For patients who cannot tolerate TMP-SMX, atovaquone, dapsone with or without pyrimethamine, or aerosolized pentamidine may be used in the following dosages: atovaquone, 750 mg twice daily for adults and 30 mg/kg/day for infants and children; dapsone, 100 mg as a single or divided dose daily; or dapsone, 50 mg/day, plus pyrimethamine, 50 mg, and leucovorin, 25 mg/wk (also provides prophylaxis for *Toxoplasma gondii* encephalitis); or dapsone, 200 mg, plus pyrimethamine, 75 mg, plus leucovorin, 25 mg once a week. Alternatively, aerosolized pentamidine, 300 mg delivered by nebulizer once a month, may be used. (Refer also to the chapter *Prophylaxis of Opportunistic Infections in HIV Disease.*)

Suggested Reading

Centers for Disease Control and Prevention: 1997 USPHS/IDSA guidelines for prevention of opportunistic infections in persons infected with human immunodeficiency virus, *MMWR* 46(No. RR-12):1, 1997.

El-Sadir WM, et al: Atovaquone compared with dapsone for the prevention of *Pneumocystis carinii* pneumonia in patients with HIV infection who cannot tolerate trimethoprim, sulfonamides, or both, N Engl J Med 339:1889, 1998.

Hughes WT: Use of dapsone in the prevention and treatment of *Pneumocystis carinii* pneumonia: a review, *Clin Infect Dis* 27:191, 1998.

TRYPANOSOMIASIS AND LEISHMANIASIS

Richard D. Pearson
Susan M. Lareau

American trypanosomiasis (Chagas' disease), African trypanosomiasis (sleeping sickness), and leishmaniasis are caused by protozoa of the family Trypanosomatidae, order Kinetoplastida (Table 1). They have a unique mitochondrial structure: the kinetoplast. They are transmitted by various insect vectors and exist in multiple morphologic forms, some of which are flagellated. They are important causes of morbidity and mortality in developing areas of the world, Chagas' disease in South and Central America, sleeping sickness in sub-Saharan Africa, and leishmaniasis in scattered areas on every continent except Australia and Antarctica. They are rarely encountered in North America but may be diagnosed in immigrants, returning travelers, or military personnel.

Most of the drugs used to treat these diseases have been available for decades. Unfortunately, they are often associated with serious side effects and must be administered over prolonged periods. With the exception of amphotericin B deoxycholate, liposomal amphotericin B, and pentamidine isethionate, they have not been approved for use by the U.S. Food and Drug Administration (FDA) and are considered investigational. Several can be obtained from the Centers for Disease Control and Prevention (CDC) Drug Service, Atlanta, Georgia, 404-639-3670 during normal work hours and 404-939-2888 during evenings, weekends, and holidays, along with detailed information about their administration and side effects.

Because these diseases occur primarily in impoverished areas, there has been little incentive for pharmaceutical companies to pursue improved forms of therapy. Recent efforts in the scientific community have yielded new insights into their immunobiology and pathophysiology. Hopefully, more effective, less toxic forms of chemotherapy and protective vaccines will become available in the future.

■ AMERICAN TRYPANOSOMIASIS (CHAGAS' DISEASE)

Chagas' disease, which is caused by *Trypanosoma cruzi*, is transmitted by reduviid bugs that reside in adobe buildings in rural areas of Latin America. *T. cruzi* can infect a large number of animal species as well as humans. The parasite develops in the intestine of the reduviid bug and is passed in feces at the time it takes a blood meal. When infective metacyclic trypomastigotes enter a bite site in the skin, they invade cells and elicit a local inflammatory nodule, or chagoma. When parasites invade through the conjunctiva, unilateral, painless, periorbital edema (Romaña's sign) may develop. After a period of local multiplication, trypomastigotes disseminate through the bloodstream producing fever, constitutional symptoms, carditis, and rarely meningoencephalitis. Acute Chagas' disease can result in death, but it typically resolves spontaneously over 4 to 8 weeks as immunity develops. Acute infections may be mild or asymptomatic. Those infected then enter the indeterminate phase. They are asymptomatic but continue to have low-grade parasitemia. Years later, 10% to 30% of infected individuals progress to chronic Chagas' cardiac or intestinal disease (megadisease). Progressive disseminated Chagas' disease with carditis and/or brain abscesses has been reported in some patients with acquired immunodeficiency syndrome (AIDS) and other immunocompromising conditions.

The diagnosis of acute Chagas' disease is often made by identifying the parasite in blood or tissue. Several serologic assays are available to detect IgG antitrypanosomal antibodies in persons with indeterminate phase or chronic Chagas' disease. The tests differ in their sensitivity and specificity. Polymerase chain reaction (PCR)-based assays using species-specific gene probes are under development.

Two drugs are used for the treatment of Chagas' disease: nifurtimox and benznidazole. Nifurtimox is the only drug available in the United States. Although production has stopped, supplies are still available from the CDC Drug Service. Benznidazole is the mainstay of therapy in Brazil and other Latin American countries. It is likely that it will eventually replace nifurtimox for use in the United States as well. Untoward effects are common with both drugs and may necessitate premature discontinuation of therapy.

Nifurtimox (Lampit, Bayer) is typically given for 90 to 120 days (Table 2). The drug is better tolerated in children and adolescents than adults; higher dosages per kilogram of

Table 1   Diseases Caused by Protozoa of the Family Trypanosomatidae

DISEASE	CAUSATIVE AGENT	GEOGRAPHIC DISTRIBUTION	VECTOR	RESERVOIR
American trypanosomiasis (Chagas' disease)	*Trypanosoma cruzi*	Latin America	Reduviid bugs	Multiple species of animals
African trypanosomiasis (sleeping sickness)	*Trypanosoma brucei gambiense*	West and Central Africa and Uganda	Tsetse flies (*Glossina* species)	Humans
	Trypanosoma brucei rhodesiense	East Africa and Uganda		Large game animals, occasionally humans
Leishmaniasis (visceral, cutaneous, mucosal)	*Leishmania* species	Worldwide	Sand flies (*Phlebotomus* species and *Lutzomyia* species)	Rodents, canines (dogs, foxes), or humans

body weight are used in those groups. Neurologic and gastrointestinal side effects are common. They include sleep disturbances, restlessness, tremor, memory loss, paresthesias, weakness, polyneuritis, and rarely seizures, as well as anorexia, nausea, vomiting, abdominal pain, and weight loss. Other, rare side effects include fever, pulmonary infiltrates, and effusions.

Benznidazole (Rochagan, Roche) is usually administered for 60 days. Higher dosages are used in children. Side effects are common and include gastrointestinal disturbances, psychiatric manifestations, dose-dependent polyneuropathy, and cutaneous hypersensitivity reactions. On rare occasions, there may be hepatitis or neutropenia.

Treatment with nifurtimox or benznidazole reduces mortality and morbidity in patients with acute Chagas' disease. Recent experience in Brazil suggests that treatment of persons in the indeterminate phase results in parasitologic cure in approximately half. Many experts now recommend treatment, particularly in children and young adults, for those with indeterminate phase infection. Once the chronic manifestations of Chagas' disease develop, neither drug appears to alter the outcome. Supportive therapy includes cardiotropic drugs for congestive heart failure, pacemaker placement for heart block, and palliative endoscopic or surgical procedures for intestinal disease. Nifurtimox has been used to prevent disseminated infection in a small group of persons who have undergone cardiac transplantation for chagasic cardiomyopathy in the United States.

■ AFRICAN TRYPANOSOMIASIS (SLEEPING SICKNESS)

African trypanosomasis is caused by *Trypanosoma brucei gambiense,* which is endemic in West and Central Africa, and *Trypanosoma brucei rhodesiense* in East Africa. Uganda is the only country where both are found. The African trypanosomes are transmitted by tsetse flies. Humans are the primary reservoir of *T. brucei gambiense. T. brucei rhodesiense* is found primarily in large game animals in East Africa, but humans can serve as a reservoir.

An indurated chancre may develop at the site of parasite inoculation. In *T. brucei gambiense* infection, the early (hemolymphatic) stage is characterized by recurrent bouts of fever, constitutional symptoms, and lymphadenopathy. Trypanosomes are found in blood and lymph nodes. After a

Table 2   Treatment of American and African Trypanosomiasis and Leishmaniasis

DISEASE	TREATMENT	PEDIATRIC DOSAGE AND NOTES
American trypanosomiasis (Chagas' disease)	Nifurtimox, 8-10 mg/kg/day in 4 doses for 90-120 days	Ages 1-10: 15-20 mg/kg/day in 4 doses for 90 days Ages 11-16: 12.5-15 mg/kg/day in 4 doses for 90 days
	or	
African trypanosomiasis (sleeping sickness)	Benznidazole, 5 mg/kg/day for 60 days	Ages 1-11: 10 mg/kg/day in 2 doses for 60 days
Hemolympathic disease	Eflornithine (*T. b. gambiense*), 400 mg/kg/day IV in 4 divided doses for 14 days	Supplies very limited; same as adult dose
	or	
	Suramin sodium, 1-1.5 g on days 1, 3, 7, 14, and 21 following test dose of 100-200 mg	Children: 20 mg/kg on days 1, 3, 7, 14, and 21 following test dose
	or	
	Pentamidine isethionate, 4 mg/kg/day IM or IV for 10 days	4 mg/kg/day for 10 days
Late disease in central nervous system	Eflornithine (*T. b. gambiense*), 400 mg/kg/day IV only in 4 divided doses for 14 days	Supplies very limited; same as adult dose
	or	
	Melarsoprol, 2-3.6 mg/kg/day IV for 3 days; after 1 week, 3.6 mg/kg/day for 3 days; repeat after 10-21 days	Children: initial dose of 0.36 mg/kg IV, increasing gradually to maximum 3.6 mg/kg at intervals of 1-5 days for total of 9-10 doses; total of 18-25 mg/kg, over 1-mo period
Leishmaniasis		
Visceral	Immunocompetent: Liposomal amphotericin B, 3 mg/kg IV on days 1-5, 14, and 21 Immunocompromised: 4 mg/kg on days 1-5, 10, 17, 24, 31, and 38	Same as adult dose
	or	
	Pentostam or Glucantime, 20 mg/kg/day (Sb^V) IV or IM for 28 days	Same as adult dose
Cutaneous	Pentostam or Glucantime, 20 mg/kg/day (Sb^V) IV or IM for 20 days	Same as adult dose Treatment may not be necessary for inconspicuous or healing lesions caused by *Leishmania* species that do not cause mucosal disease
Mucosal leishmaniasis (*L. [V.] braziliensis*)	Pentostam or Glucantime, 20 mg/kg/day (Sb^V) IV or IM for 28 days or longer	Same as adult dose

period of months to more than a year, they invade the central nervous system, producing meningoencephalitis. Symptoms and findings include severe headache, personality changes, memory loss, and eventually obtundation and coma.

In *T. brucei rhodesiense* infection symptoms begin a few days to several weeks after the tsetse fly bites. Fever, headache, malaise, and rash are common. There is usually little distinction between the early and late stages of disease with *T. brucei rhodesiense*. Death can occur within weeks if treatment is not initiated.

Eflornithine, which has been called the "resurrection drug," is highly effective in the treatment of hemolymphatic and central nervous system disease caused by *T. brucei gambiense*. Unfortunately, it was relatively expensive, and the original manufacturer stopped production. Supplies are now very limited, but attempts continue to find a new manufacturer. Different treatment regimens have been used; a 14-day course administered intravenously (IV) is effective (see Table 2). Eflornithine is not active against *T. brucei rhodesiense*.

Persons with hemolymphatic disease caused by *T. brucei rhodesiense* and those with *T. brucei gambiense* when eflornithine is not available should be treated with either pentamidine isethionate or suramin sodium (Bayer, Germany). Pentamidine may be somewhat better for *T. brucei gambiense* and suramin for *T. brucei rhodesiense*.

After a test of suramin, treatment doses are given IV on days 1, 3, 7, 14, and 21. Toxicity is common and includes gastrointestinal disturbances such as nausea and vomiting; neurologic effects such as photophobia, hyperesthesias, and peripheral neuropathy; and urticaria and pruritus. Administration of the drug is occasionally associated with shock, renal toxicity, optic atrophy, or blood dyscrasias.

Pentamidine isethionate is administered daily, intramuscularly (IM) or IV, for 10 days. If infused too rapidly, intravenous pentamidine can produce hypotension and shock. Gastrointestinal disturbances, pain at the injection site when the drug is given IM, liver enzyme abnormalities, and nephrotoxicity are other side effects. Some patients develop life-threatening hypoglycemia as a result of pancreatic beta cell injury and insulin release; insulin-dependent diabetes may follow. Rare side effects include acute pancreatitis, hyperkalemia, anaphylaxis, and ventricular arrhythmias.

When the central nervous system is involved, eflornithine is the drug of choice for *T. brucei gambiense*. Persons infected with *T. brucei rhodesiense* or with *T. brucei gambiense* when eflornithine is not available are treated with melarsoprol (Arsobal, Rhone-Poulenc Rorer) given IV daily for 3 days with the course repeated after 1 week and again after another 10 to 21 days (see Table 2). Reduced dosages have been used in cachectic patients. Untoward effects are common. In addition to encephalopathy, which occurs in as many as 18% of cases and is fatal in 4% to 6%, recipients often experience nausea, vomiting, abdominal pain, peripheral neuropathy, hypertension, allergic reactions, and rarely shock. Administration of prednisolone, 1 mg/kg/day, appears to reduce the severity of arsenical encephalopathy and the risk of death by approximately half.

■ LEISHMANIASIS (CUTANEOUS, MUCOSAL AND VISCERAL)

Leishmaniasis refers to the broad spectrum of disease caused by the more than 20 *Leishmania* species that infect humans. Leishmania are transmitted by sand flies. In most sites, leishmaniasis is a zoonosis with dogs, other canines, or rodents serving as reservoirs and humans becoming infected when they venture into endemic habitats. In some cases, such as visceral leishmaniasis in India, humans serve as the reservoir. The manifestations of disease depend on complex and only partially understood interactions between the virulence characteristics of the infecting *Leishmania* species and the genetically determined cell-mediated immune responses of its human host.

In persons with cutaneous leishmaniasis, parasites multiply in macrophages at the site where they are inoculated. In the typical case, a nodule develops and then ulcerates. Lesions may be single or multiple, and they vary in morphology. Some have a pizzalike appearance with a raised, erythematous, outer border, a central area of granulation tissue, and a yellowish or brown overlying crust. In mucosal leishmaniasis caused by *Leishmania (Viannia) braziliensis* and related species in Latin America, mucosal lesions of the nose, oral pharynx, and rarely other sites develop months to years after the initial skin lesion heals.

Most persons infected with *Leishmania (Leishmania) donovani* or other species associated with visceral leishmaniasis are asymptomatic or have mild manifestations of infection that resolve spontaneously. In the subset who develop progressive visceral leishmaniasis, known as *kala-azar*, leishmania amastigotes disseminate throughout the reticuloendothelial system and are found within macrophages in the liver, spleen, bone marrow, and occasionally other organs. Patients typically present with massive splenomegaly, hepatomegaly, fever, weight loss, constitutional symptoms, and hypergammaglobulinemia. Visceral leishmaniasis has emerged in Spain, southern France, Italy, and elsewhere in the Mediterranean littoral as a major opportunistic infection in persons with AIDS. Persons with concurrent infections may present in the classical manner, but splenomegaly may be absent, and gastrointestinal and pulmonary involvement are more common.

The diagnosis of cutaneous or visceral leishmaniasis is suggested by a history of exposure in an endemic region and the clinical findings. It is confirmed by identifying leishmania amastigotes or growing promastigotes in cultures of blood, splenic aspirates, or tissue in patients with visceral leishmaniasis, or in biopsies of skin lesions in those with cutaneous leishmaniasis. Antileishmanial antibodies are present at high titer in persons with visceral leishmaniasis, but they are not always present in those with AIDS. Several assays are available; an enzyme-linked immunosorbent assay (ELISA) using a recombinant 39-kD kinesin-like antigen appears to be the most sensitive and specific for visceral leishmaniasis. Serologic assays are of little diagnostic value in cutaneous leishmaniasis. Antileishmanial antibodies are variably present and at low titer in that condition. The leishmanin (Montenegro) skin test is not available in the United States. It is negative in patients with visceral leishmaniasis and typically positive in those with simple cutaneous or mucosal disease.

All patients with clinically apparent visceral leishmaniasis should be treated. Liposomal amphotericin B (AmBisome, Fugisawa) recently became the first drug licensed in the United States for that indication. It is as effective as traditional pentavalent antimony therapy or amphotericin B deoxycholate, and less toxic. The regimen is detailed in Table 2. Liposomal amphotericin B is now considered the drug of choice for the treatment of visceral leishmaniasis in the United States and other industrialized countries.

Sodium stibogluconate (Pentostam, Glaxo-Wellcome) and meglumine antimonate (Glucantime, Rhone-Poulenc Rorer), both pentavalent antimony compounds, have been used for decades to treat leishmaniasis in many areas of the world. Pentostam is available through the CDC Drug Service in the United States. These drugs are dosed on the basis of their pentavalent antimony content; Pentostam contains 100 mg of pentavalent antimony/ml and Glucantime contains 85 mg/ml. They remain the treatment of choice for visceral leishmaniasis in many areas, but antimony resistance and treatment failures have been increasingly reported from India and some other sites. In South America, the Sudan, and other areas where pentavalent antimony failures are uncommon, Glucantime or Pentostam are given at a dosage of 20 mg of pentavalent antimony/kg body weight/day IV or IM for 28 days. In areas with a high frequency of antimony failure, longer durations of therapy, multiple courses of antimony, or alternative drugs such as amphotericin B or pentamidine are used. Recombinant interferon-γ has been used in combination with Pentostam or Glucantime to successfully treat persons who fail to respond to antimony alone. A number of other compounds and combinations have been tried with variable success.

When relapses occur in persons treated with pentavalent antimony, they are usually observed within the first 6 months. They can be treated with a second course of antimony or an alternative therapeutic regiment. Relapses are particularly common after therapy with either pentavalent antimony or liposomal amphotericin in persons with AIDS. Suppressive antileishmanial therapy is probably advisable in that setting, but there have been no controlled trials to suggest the optimal drug or regiment. Many persons with visceral leishmaniasis in the developing world are severely wasted when they present and die from secondary bacterial or viral infections. Attention should focus on addressing their nutritional needs and treating secondary infections with appropriate antibiotics.

Cutaneous leishmaniasis eventually undergoes spontaneous resolution in most cases. If lesions are small, cosmetically inconsequential, or show evidence of spontaneous healing, treatment may not be necessary. For lesions that are large, cosmetically significant, or caused by *L. (V.) braziliensis* or related species associated with mucosal leishmaniasis, treatment is advisable with either Pentostam or Glucantime, 20 mg of pentavalent antimony/kg/day for 20 days. Cutaneous leishmaniasis responds slowly, and lesions are often only partially healed at the completion of therapy.

In geographic areas where antimony failures are common, amphotericin B and pentamidine are alternatives. Topical administration of paromomycin (15%) and methylbenzethonium chloride (12%) in white paraffin has been effective in persons with localized disease caused by *Leishmania (Leishmania) major*. Local instillation of pentavalent antimony has also been reported to be effective in treating cutaneous leishmaniasis caused by species that are not associated with mucosal involvement. Ketoconazole and itraconazole are also considerations, but they are variably effective.

Persons with mucosal leishmaniasis are usually treated initially with Pentostam or Glucantime, 20 mg of pentavalent antimony/kg/day for 28 days; failures and relapses are common. Alternatives include amphotericin B, pentamidine isethionate, or possibly interferon-γ administered concurrently with a penatavalent antimony. The activity of liposomal amphotericin B in the treatment of mucosal or cutaneous leishmaniasis has not yet been systematically assessed. Plastic surgical repairs should be delayed for 12 months because grafts may be lost if a relapse occurs after surgery.

Selected Reading

Berman JD: Human leishmaniasis: clinical, diagnostic, and chemotherapeutic developments in the last 10 years, *Clin Infect Dis* 24:684, 1997.

Drugs for parasitic infections: *Med Lett Drugs Ther* 40:1, 1998.

Herwaldt BL, Berman JD: Recommendations for treating leishmaniasis with sodium stibogluconate (Pentostam) and review of pertinent clinical studies, *Am J Trop Med Hyg* 46:296, 1992.

Kirchhoff LV: American trypanosomiasis (Chagas' disease). In Guerrant RL, Walker DH, Weller PF, eds: *Tropical infectious diseases, principles, pathogens and practice*, Philadelphia, 1999, Churchill Livingstone, p. 785.

Pepin J, Donelson JE: African trypanosomiasis (sleeping sickness). In Guerrant RL, Walker DH, Weller PF, eds: *Tropical infectious diseases, principles, pathogens and practice*, Philadelphia, 1999, Churchill Livingstone, p. 774.

INTESTINAL PROTOZOA

Paul Kelly
Michael J.G. Farthing

Intestinal protozoal infection produces substantial morbidity and mortality in people of all ages, particularly in tropical and subtropical parts of the world. Amebiasis, giardiasis, cryptosporidiosis, and those infections associated with acquired immunodeficiency syndrome (AIDS) are important problems for health in many parts of the world, but some protozoa found in the human digestive system do not cause disease. Vaccines are not yet available for protection against these infections, and many are difficult to treat. The intestinal protozoa that produce important human infections are summarized in Table 1.

■ ENTAMEBA HISTOLYTICA

Entameba histolytica causes dysentery, chronic colonic amebiasis, and hepatic amebiasis. The last is dealt with in the chapter *Extraintestinal Amoebic Infection*. Amoebic dysentery is a syndrome of bloody diarrhea caused by invasion of the colonic wall by trophozoites of *E. histolytica*. It is common in many parts of the world, especially West and Southern Africa, Central America, and South Asia. In the United States, 3000 to 4000 cases are reported each year. There is now consensus that the species formerly recognized as *E. histolytica* in fact comprises two species: *E. histolytica* and *E. dispar*. The first is the pathogenic protozoan long associated with human invasive disease and with hepatic amebiasis, and the latter is a morphologically identical nonpathogenic protozoan first recognized as the nonpathogenic zymodeme of *E. histolytica*. The latter does not require treatment, but it cannot be differentiated from *E. histolytica* morphologically. Diagnosis of invasive amebiasis is achieved by the identification of hematophagous trophozoites in very fresh stool smears or in colonic biopsies. Serologic testing using an immunofluorescent antibody test (IFAT) is now an important contribution to the diagnosis of a seriously ill patient, particularly in distinguishing colonic dilation resulting from amebiasis from that caused by ulcerative colitis.

Treatment of invasive amebiasis is shown in Table 2. Treatment can be divided into two stages: (1) eradication of tissue forms with metronidazole, tinidazole, dehydroemetine, or chloroquine, and (2) eradication of luminal carriage with diloxanide furoate or iodoquinol. Dehydroemetine and iodoquinol are toxic and no longer used.

Intestinal amebiasis may be complicated by acute toxic colitis, presenting in a similar manner to the dilation of acute severe ulcerative colitis. The patient will be febrile and unwell, sometimes with signs of peritoneal irritation, and a plain abdominal radiograph will indicate dilation. Intravenous fluids must be given, the patient starved, and metroni-

Table 1	Intestinal Protozoa	
The sarcodina (amoebae)	Pathogenic	*Entamoeba histolytica*
	Nonpathogenic	*Entamoeba dispar*
		Entamoeba moshkovskii
		Entamoeba chattoni
		Endolimax nana
		Iodamoeba butschlii
		Dientamoeba fragilis
The mastigophora (flagellates)	Pathogenic	*Giardia intestinalis*
	Nonpathogenic	*Trichomonas hominis*
		Chilomastix mesnili
		Embadomonas intestinalis
		Enteromonas hominis
The ciliophora		*Balantidium coli*
The coccidia		*Cryptosporidium parvum*
		Isospora belli
		Sarcocystis species
		Cyclospora cayetanensis
The microspora		*Enterocytozoon bieneusi*
		Encephalitozoon intestinalis
Uncertain classification, uncertain pathogenicity		*Blastocystis hominis*

dazole and a third-generation cephalosporin given intravenously. Worsening dilation of the colon or perforation will necessitate surgery, but in the event of perforation, the outcome is poor. If treatment with metronidazole is aggressive in patients with severe amoebic colitis, medical management should nearly always suffice, but surgery should not be delayed if perforation is impending.

Chronic amebiasis may be difficult to distinguish from intestinal tuberculosis or Crohn's disease, but responds to metronidazole and diloxanide as above. Surgery is sometimes necessary because stricturing may persist.

■ GIARDIA INTESTINALIS

Giardia intestinalis infection, first recognized by Van Leeuwenhoek in 1681, is a cause of acute and persistent diarrhea and possibly malnutrition in children in many tropical and subtropical countries and is a well-recognized cause of traveler's diarrhea. In many cases it is self-limiting, but the course may be prolonged in immunoglobulin deficiencies. Asymptomatic infection is common. Diagnosis is by stool microscopy, although when this is negative and the clinical suspicion is strong, trophozoites may be detected in small intestinal aspirates by endoscopy. Fecal enzyme linked immunosorbent assay (ELISA) for *Giardia* antigens and DNA-based tests have been tried but are not yet in general use.

Treatment of giardiasis is unsatisfactory with currently available drugs because of a high failure rate and because the available drugs cannot be regarded as safe in pregnancy. Five classes of chemotherapy are available (Table 3): nitroimida-

Table 2   Drug Treatment of Amebiasis

		ADULT DOSAGE	CHILD DOSAGE
TISSUE INFECTION			
First choice	Metronidazole*	750 mg tid for 10 days	50 mg/kg/day for 10 days†
	Tinidazole*	2 g/day for 3 days	60 mg/kg/day for 3 days
Second choice	Paromomycin	30 mg/kg/day for 10 days†	30 mg/kg/day for 10 days†
LUMINAL CARRIAGE			
First choice	Diloxanide furoate	500 mg tid for 10 days	20 mg/kg/day for 10 days†
Second choice	Paromomycin	30 mg/kg/day for 10 days†	30 mg/kg/day for 10 days†

*Must be followed by eradication of luminal carriage.
†Divided in three doses.

Table 3   Drug Treatment of Giardiasis

DRUG	ADULT DOSAGE	CHILD DOSAGE	EFFICACY
Metronidazole	2 g daily for 3 days	15 mg/kg/day for 10 days (maximum 750 mg daily)	>90%
Tinidazole	2 g single dose	75 mg/kg single dose	>90%
Mepacrine (quinacrine)	100 mg tid for 7 days	2 mg/kg tid for 7 days	>90%
Furazolidone	100 mg qid for 10 days	2 mg/kg tid for 10 days	>80%

Table 4   Treatment of Ciliophora, Coccidia, and Microsporidia

ORGANISM	DRUG REGIMEN
CILIOPHORA	
Balantidium coli	Tetracycline, 500 mg qid for 10 days
COCCIDIA	
Cryptosporidium parvum	Paromomycin, 30 mg/kg/day in 3 divided doses
	Nitazoxanide, 1 g twice daily for 14 days
Isospora belli	Trimethoprim-sulfamethoxazole, 960 mg qid for 7 days
	Prophylaxis: 960 mg daily
Sarcocystis species	As for *I. belli*
Cyclospora cayetanensis	Trimethoprim-sulphamethoxazole, 960 mg qid for 7 days
MICROSPORA	
Enterocytozoon bieneusi	Albendazole, 400 mg bid for 28 days
Encephalitozoon intestinalis	As for *E. bieneusi*
BLASTOCYSTIS HOMINIS	
	The status of this organism as a pathogen is still the subject of controversy, and so it is uncertain whether it requires treatment. It is our practice to attempt eradication with metronidazole, 750 mg tid for 10 days, when there are gastrointestinal symptoms and no other cause is apparent.

zoles (metronidazole and tinidazole), acridine dyes such as mepacrine (quinacrine), nitrofurans (furazolidone), paromomycin, and benzimidazoles, particularly albendazole. If single agents fail repeatedly, combination therapy may be tried, but there are few controlled data to guide drug choice, dose, or duration.

■ *BALANTIDIUM COLI*

Balantidium coli infection manifests as a severe, sometimes life-threatening, colitis indistinguishable from amoebic dysentery. It is uncommon but occurs in Central and South America, Iran, Papua New Guinea, and the Philippines. Diagnosis is made by identification of the large trophozoites

in feces or in rectal biopsies. Treatment is with tetracycline, 500 mg four times daily for 10 days (Table 4). Metronidazole and paromomycin are alternatives.

■ CRYPTOSPORIDIOSIS

Infection with *Cryptosporidium parvum* is likely to present as acute, self-limiting watery diarrhea in children, or in travelers or as a waterborne epidemic. Most episodes require no specific therapy, but attention to fluid and electrolyte balance is important. Cryptosporidiosis is associated with persistent diarrhea, even in apparently immunocompetent children, and in human immunodeficiency virus (HIV)-infected individuals often persists until death. Cryptosporidiosis is common in malnourished children in the tropics. In patients with HIV-related diarrhea, cryptosporidiosis can be found in 10% to 30% of cases in industrialized countries and 10% to 40% of cases in tropical populations. Diagnosis is usually made by microscopy of fecal smears using a modified Ziehl-Neelsen stain, which reveals the red-staining 5-μm oocysts.

Although many drugs have been tried, only two have been shown to have any value in controlled trials: paromomycin and nitazoxanide. Hyperimmune bovine colostrum is a form of passive immunotherapy but is not in clinical use. Paromomycin (30 mg/kg/day in three divided doses) has been found to be of moderate efficacy, and it appears to ameliorate diarrhea by reduction of the intensity of infection. Nitazoxanide (1 g twice daily for 14 days) has been demonstrated to be effective in African AIDS patients in an open study and in Mexican patients in a placebo-controlled trial.

◼ *ISOSPORA BELLI*

Isospora belli is uncommon in industrialized countries but may be found in up to 40% of patients with HIV-related diarrhea in Africa. In HIV-infected individuals it causes a clinical syndrome of persistent diarrhea and wasting, which is indistinguishable from that attributed to other intracellular enteropathogenic protozoa (*C. parvum,* microsporidia). There were reports of isosporasis before HIV infection appeared. Diagnosis rests on the identification in fecal smears of elongated, large sporocysts, which appear red with the modified Ziehl-Neelsen stain.

Trimethoprim-sulfamethoxazole (TMP-SMX) has been reported to be effective at a dosage of 160/800 mg four times daily for 10 days. In patients with AIDS, this needs to be followed with the same drug in a dose of 160/800 mg three times weekly indefinitely as prophylaxis against recurrence. Otherwise, recurrence is seen in 50% of patients with HIV infection at 2 months. An alternative drug is sulfadoxine-pyrimethamine (500/25 mg weekly) as secondary prophylaxis. Patients intolerant of sulfonamides could be given diclazuril, but only anecdotal evidence of its efficacy is available.

◼ *SARCOCYSTIS* SPECIES

Sarcocystis infection, which may give rise to a persistent diarrhea, is treated in the same way as *I. belli.* This infection is uncommon.

◼ *DIENTAMOEBA FRAGILIS*

Most infections with *Dientamoeba fragilis* are asymptomatic and do not require treatment. When required, treatment is as for amebiasis.

◼ *CYCLOSPORA CAYETANENSIS*

Cyclospora cayetanensis is a newly recognized enteropathogen that causes traveler's diarrhea (especially in travelers to South America and Nepal) and foodborne outbreaks. In fecal smears, the oocysts resemble those of *C. parvum* in taking up carbol fuchsin in the modified Ziehl-Neelsen stain, but the oocysts are larger than *C. parvum* at 8-10 μm and they autofluoresce. Eradication is achieved using TMP-SMX (160/800 mg twice daily) for 7 days.

◼ MICROSPORIDIA

Two microsporidia are pathogenic in the human gastrointestinal tract: *Enterocytozoon bieneusi* and *Encephalitozoon intestinalis* (formerly termed *Septata intestinalis*). These organisms have only recently been described and are representatives of a phylum of primitive protozoa. They are intracellular parasites, which generally infect severely immunocompromised individuals. The most common manifestation is a persistent diarrhea associated with weight loss, but a syndrome of sclerosing cholangitis is also described. Diagnosis relies on either electron microscopy of small bowel biopsies (usually distal duodenal) or on the finding of the spores in the feces using a variety of stains. *Encephalitozoon intestinalis* may cause a disseminated infection with renal spore excretion.

Treatment is with albendazole. The usual regimen is 400 mg twice daily for 1 month, but maintenance suppression may be needed if relapse occurs following the cessation of therapy. Albendazole in this dose often leads to temporary suppression of *E. bieneusi* infection, but *E. intestinalis* infection may be completely eradicated in a proportion of patients. Albendazole can be used in higher doses, but its efficacy in human microsporidiosis when used in these doses is not fully established. Metronidazole is not effective for this infection.

Suggested Reading

Farthing MJG, Cevallos AM, Kelly P: Intestinal protozoa. In Cook GC, ed: *Manson's tropical diseases,* ed 7, London, 1995, WB Saunders.

Fayer R, ed: *Cryptosporidium and cryptosporidiosis,* Boca Raton, FL, 1997, CRC Press.

Tannich E: *Entamoeba histolytica* and *E. dispar:* comparison of molecules considered important for host tissue destruction, *Trans Roy Soc Trop Med Hyg* 92:593, 1998.

EXTRAINTESTINAL AMOEBIC INFECTION

Samuel L. Stanley, Jr.

Extraintestinal disease is the most dangerous manifestation of *Entamoeba histolytica* infection. Approximately 10% of individuals with intestinal amoebiasis will develop extraintestinal disease, most commonly amoebic liver abscess. Amoebic liver abscess is almost invariably fatal if not treated, and kills approximately 50,000 individuals every year. However, when medical therapy is promptly initiated, more than 97% of infected individuals are cured. Rarer extraintestinal manifestations of amoebiasis include entities such as pleuropulmonary amoebiasis and amoebic pericarditis (Table 1). The cornerstone of therapy for all of these conditions is metronidazole, but there are differences in the therapeutic approach to each of these diseases that will be discussed below.

■ AMOEBIC LIVER ABSCESS

Amoebic liver abscess arises when *E. histolytica* trophozoites invade through the colonic wall, reach the portal circulation, and lodge in the liver. Amoebic liver abscesses consist of a well-circumscribed cavity of dead hepatocytes and tissue debris, surrounded by a thin wall of fibroblasts, macrophages, lymphocytes, and rare neutrophils. Given the extent of the damage, remarkably few amoebic trophozoites are seen, and most of these are within the wall of the cavity. Recent studies in a murine model of disease suggest that some of the hepatocyte death may arise by amoebic-induced apoptosis of liver cells. Liver abscess formation can occur in association with amoebic dysentery but more often occurs with asymptomatic *E. histolytica* intestinal infection. Such patients may give no history of an antecedent diarrheal disease. In addition, amoebic liver abscess may not develop or be recognized until years after an individual has left an area endemic for amoebiasis, hence a high index of suspicion and a detailed history may be required to make the correct diagnosis. Most cases of amoebic liver abscess are seen in individuals between 20 and 50 years of age. The prevalence of intestinal infection with *E. histolytica* may be

slightly higher in women, but men are 3 to 10 times more likely to develop amoebic liver abscess than women.

The diagnosis of amoebic liver abscess is based on the triad of clinical findings of fever, abdominal pain, and liver tenderness, radiographic findings of a space-occupying lesion in the liver, and a positive serologic test for amoebiasis. The white blood cell count is usually elevated in individuals with amoebic liver abscess, and abnormal liver function tests are seen in approximately half of affected patients. Examination of stool reveals amoebic trophozoites or cysts in less than one third of the patients with amoebic liver abscess and therefore is useful in confirming, but not excluding, the diagnosis. Amoebic liver abscesses are visualized by computed tomography (CT) scanning of the abdomen or right upper quadrant ultrasound as space-occupying lesions within the liver. They are often solitary, are usually located in the right lobe of the liver, and can be large, occupying more than 50% of the liver in some cases. Multiple amoebic liver abscesses can be seen as well, and may be associated with more severe systemic symptoms and a more complicated course. The differential diagnosis includes pyogenic (bacterial) liver abscesses developing from an intraabdominal or biliary source, or from hematogenous seeding of the liver, metastatic disease, echinococcal cysts, and primary liver tumors. Amoebic serology represents the best test to establish the diagnosis of amoebic liver abscess and should be performed in all patients with a suspicious lesion. Essentially all individuals with amoebic liver abscess develop antibodies to *E. histolytica,* and negative serologic tests are seen only when they are obtained very early in infection, before an antibody response to *E. histolytica* can develop. In those rare cases in which the clinical suspicion for amoebic liver abscess is high but serologic tests were negative, repeating the serologic study 1 to 2 weeks later may provide the correct diagnosis.

Most individuals with amoebic liver abscess can be cured by medical therapy alone, without percutaneous or open drainage of the abscess. The drug of choice for the treatment of amoebic liver abscess is metronidazole (Table 2). Metronidazole is effective in relatively short courses, and the 5- to 7-day regimen probably cures more than 90% of patients with amoebic liver abscess. Strikingly, therapy is so effective that the related nitroimidazole compound tinidazole has been used as single-dose therapy for amoebic liver abscess in South Africa with 90% cure rates. Although failure of both of these regimens is seen occasionally, clear evidence for *E. histolytica* resistance to metronidazole has not been found. This may change in the future, given the relatively widespread and inappropriate use of metronidazole in many parts of the world, and the development of metronidazole resistance in the metabolically similar protozoan *Giardia lamblia.* For patients unable to take oral medications, metronidazole can be give intravenously with equivalent efficacy. Metronidazole is also the drug of choice in children and in pregnant women with amoebic liver abscess. Side effects of metronidazole can be seen and are usually dose related (see Table 2).

A clinical response to metronidazole is usually seen within 72 hours of beginning therapy, evident by a decrease in fever, improvement in abdominal pain, and a normalization of the white blood cell count. This is not always

Table 1	Extraintestinal Amebiasis

Amoebic liver abscess
  Pleuropulmonary amebiasis
  Amoebic pericarditis
  Amoebic peritonitis
Amoebic brain abscess
Genitourinary amebiasis

Table 2 Treatment of Amoebic Liver Abscess

DRUG OF CHOICE	ADULT DOSAGE	PEDIATRIC DOSAGE	SIDE EFFECTS
Metronidazole	750 mg PO tid ×5 to 10 days or 2.4 g PO day (single dose) ×2 days	30-50 mg/kg/day ×5-10 days in three divided doses; not to exceed 2250 mg/day	Common: nausea, headache, metallic taste Occasional: ataxia, confusion, insomnia paresthesias, neuropathy Disulfiram effect (nausea, vomiting) with alcohol ingestion
	In patients unable to take PO medications, give metronidazole IV 750 mg q8h ×5-10 days	IV dose same as PO dose	
SECOND-LINE AGENTS Dehydroemetine* (mebadin)	1-1.5 mg/kg/day IM ×5 days (maximum 90 mg/day)	1-1.5 mg/kg/day IM ×5 days (maximum 90 mg/day)	Common: nausea, vomiting, myalgias Occasional: hypotension, chest pain, tachycardia, ECG abnormalities (T wave inversions, prolonged QT interval) Toxicity is related to cumulative dose
Chloroquine (aralen) (Used only as an adjunct to metronidazole therapy)	600 mg base/day ×2 days then 300 mg base/day ×14 days	10 mg/kg base/day (maximum 300 mg/day) ×14 days	Pruritus, headache, nausea

ECG, Electrocardiogram.
*Available only from the Centers for Disease Control and Prevention. Approval required from the Parasitology Branch: 770-488-7775. Drug control phone number: 404-639-3670.

associated with radiographic evidence for a decrease in abscess size, and it is well recognized that abscesses can actually increase in size early on in treatment. This should not be construed as a therapeutic failure. Resolution of the liver abscess by radiographic criteria takes months but is usually complete 1 year after successful therapy.

The use of second-line agents as supplements to metronidazole therapy is controversial. Emetine, and its less toxic derivative dehydroemetine, represent effective agents against *E. histolytica* in amoebic liver abscess but have more serious side effects than metronidazole (see Table 2). Some authorities recommend adding dehydroemetine therapy to metronidazole in gravely ill patients with amoebic liver abscess or individuals who seem to be responding slowly to metronidazole therapy. There are theoretic reasons to believe that adding dehydroemetine could be beneficial because of its rapid amoebicidal action, but there are no controlled studies indicating that the combination of metronidazole and dehydroemetine is associated with better outcomes (improved mortality or more rapid resolution of symptoms) than metronidazole alone. Chloroquine also has been used in combination with metronidazole for the treatment of patients with amoebic liver abscess. It is probably a less potent antiamoebic agent than either metronidazole or dehydroemetine, and again, there are no controlled studies indicating that the addition of chloroquine to metronidazole improves outcomes in individuals with amoebic liver abscess.

Once therapy with metronidazole is completed, individuals with amoebic liver abscess and all other patients with extraintestinal disease should receive treatment with a luminal agent to eliminate any residual intestinal infection. This should be performed in all individuals with extraintestinal disease, even if stool microscopy is negative. Patients should receive paromomycin (adult dosage is 30 mg/kg/day administered in three divided doses for 7 days; pediatric dosage is 25 mg/kg/day administered in three divided doses for 7 days, not to exceed 2 g/day). This regimen is 85% to 90% effective in eliminating intestinal carriage of *E. histolytica*.

Although most patients with amoebic liver abscess will respond to medical therapy alone, certain patients may benefit from percutaneous drainage of the liver abscess under radiographic visualization. Open drainage is rarely, if ever, indicated for amoebic liver abscess. In seriously ill patients in whom the diagnostic considerations are amoebic liver abscess versus pyogenic abscess and serologic results are not immediately available, percutaneous aspiration for diagnostic purposes (culture and Gram stain) may be indicated. In individuals with amoebic liver abscess who do not show a clinical response to metronidazole over a 3- to 5-day period and in whom possible abscess rupture is a concern (expanding abscess at the liver periphery) percutaneous aspiration and temporary drain placement may have a therapeutic benefit. Finally, large abscesses in the left lobe of the liver should be considered for aspiration and percutaneous drainage because of the risk of abscess extension into the pericardium.

■ PLEUROPULMONARY AMOEBIASIS

Pleuropulmonary amoebiasis almost always arises as a complication of amoebic liver abscess, with extension of disease from the right lobe of the liver into the right pleural space and right lower lobe of the lung. Disease may be manifest as empyema, right lower lobe pneumonia or lung abscess formation, and hepatobronchial fistula. A right-sided pleural effusion, often accompanying right lower lobe atelectesis, is not uncommon in amoebic liver abscess. These effusions are usually asymptomatic and resolve rapidly with treatment of the amoebic liver abscess. Amoebic empyema is associated with a pleural effusion, right-sided pleuritic pain, shortness of breath, and persistent fever. Effective treatment requires drainage of the empyema with insertion of a chest tube and medical therapy with metronidazole, using the same regimen recommended for amoebic liver abscess. In some cases, decortication and open drainage have been required for cure. Amoebic pneumonia and lung abscess can be managed by medical therapy with metronidazole. Patients who develop a hepatobronchial fistula literally "cough up" their amoebic liver abscesses, with the production of abundant amounts of thick brown sputum containing necrotic material. Examination of this sputum will reveal amoebic trophozoites in about 30% of affected patients. These patients respond well to medical management with metronidazole, and surgical intervention is almost never required.

■ AMOEBIC PERICARDITIS

Amoebic pericarditis is a rare, potentially fatal complication of amoebic liver abscess, arising from rupture of an amoebic liver abscess into the pericardium. When rupture occurs acutely, patients present with sudden shortness of breath, chest pain, and hypotension. Death can occur within hours. More subacute presentations can occur, with gradual leakage of abscess contents into the pericardium, and are associated with increasing symptoms of tamponade such as dyspnea and hypotension. Treatment requires immediate pericardiocentesis with closed drainage. If pericardial fluid is loculated, and adequate drainage cannot be achieved from a percutaneous approach, open drainage may be required. Medical therapy is with metronidazole (at dosages used for amoebic liver abscess).

■ AMOEBIC PERITONITIS

Amoebic peritonitis is an unusual complication of disease, occurring in approximately 2% of patients with amoebic liver abscess by rupture of abscess contents into the peritoneum, and in approximately 2% of amoebic colitis patients by perforation of the colon. Colonic perforation is the more deadly form of disease because of soilage of the peritoneal cavity by colonic bacteria. Effective medical therapy requires the addition of antibiotics effective against colonic flora (enteric gram-negative rods, enterococcus, and anaerobes) to antiamoebic therapy. Ampicillin, gentamicin, and metronidazole, or alternatively, ampicillin-sulbactam, and metronidazole are reasonable initial antibiotic regimens. Therapy may be prolonged in cases of colonic perforation, and repeated percutaneous drainage of collections under radiographic visualization may be necessary for cure. In cases of liver abscess rupture into the peritoneum, medical therapy is with metronidazole alone, and early surgical intervention, with drainage of any collections, may be beneficial.

■ AMOEBIC BRAIN ABSCESS

Amoebic brain abscesses are extraordinarily rare, occurring in fewer than 1 in 2000 individuals with amoebic liver abscess. Children may be more susceptible to this complication than adults. Symptoms of mental status changes, headache, and any focal neurologic findings should suggest the possibility of amoebic brain abscesses. Diagnosis is based on seeing a space-occupying lesion in the brain, in association with known amoebiasis. Abscesses are often multiple, and their CT scan appearance early in infection may be that of circumscribed areas of low attenuation, without definitive rims or enhancement. The drug of choice for treatment of amoebic brain abscess is metronidazole, which reaches much better levels in the central nervous system than any of the second-line agents. The dosage should be the same as that used for amoebic liver abscess, but courses may be more prolonged (≥21 days), and the response to therapy followed clinically and radiographically.

■ GENITOURINARY AMOEBIASIS

There are case reports of amoebic involvement of the kidney and upper urinary tract, with the development of amoebic perinephric abscesses. Percutaneous aspiration of the perinephric collection, and medical therapy with metronidazole, are the optimal therapeutic approach. Rarely, individuals with colitis will develop genital lesions, generally because of secondary spread of rectal disease to mucous membranes or skin. These lesions respond to metronidazole, in doses used for the treatment of amoebic liver abscess.

Suggested Reading

Adams EB, MacLeod IN: Invasive amoebiasis II. Amoebic liver abscess and its complications, *Medicine* 56:325, 1977.

Li E, Stanley SL Jr: Protozoa: amoebiasis, *Gastro Clin North Am* 25:471, 1996.

Reed SL, Braude AI: Extraintestinal amoebiasis. In Ravdin JI, ed: Amoebiasis. Human infection by *Entamoeba histolytica*, New York, 1988, John Wiley & Sons.

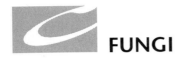

FUNGI

CANDIDIASIS*

Christopher F. Carpenter

Janine R. Maenza

*C*andida species are common causes of disease ranging from superficial cutaneous and mucocutaneous infections to candidemia and disseminated candidiasis. The most common clinical isolate is *Candida albicans*; other encountered pathogens include *C. tropicalis, C. parapsilosis, C. glabrata* (formerly *Torulopsis glabrata*), *C. krusei, C. kefyr* (formerly *pseudotropicalis*), *C. lusitaniae, C. dubliniensis,* and *C. guilliermondii*. Less-commonly isolated species with medical significance include *C. lipolytica, C. famata, C. rugosa, C. viswanathii, C. haemulonii, C. norvegensis, C. catenulata, C. ciferri, C. intermedia, C. utilis, C. lambica, C. pulcherrima,* and *C. zeylanoides*. Most species are commensal organisms, colonizing the skin, gastrointestinal tract, and vagina, and they become opportunistic pathogens only when the host has compromised immunologic or mechanical defenses or when there are changes in the host's normal flora, such as those triggered by broad-spectrum antibiotic use.

Diagnosis of *Candida* infections is primarily via culture, although the insensitivity, and at times protracted nature, of contemporary culture methods for yeast have prompted the development of rapid and sensitive nonculture diagnostic methods such as polymerase chain reaction (PCR) and antigen detection. Once diagnosed, only a small number of antifungals are available to treat the candidal infection, some with significant toxicities (please see Antimicrobial Agent Table C, Antifungal Agents). Certain *Candida* species have intrinsic resistance to antifungal agents. Furthermore, as with bacterial and viral pathogens, the increased use of antifungal agents has also led to increasing levels of resistance of *Candida* species to the currently available antifungals agents (Table 1). Resistance testing for amphotericin B remains the most problematic but fortunately resistance is much less common.

*The authors would like to acknowledge the helpful and insightful review of this chapter provided by John E. Bennett, M.D., and William G. Merz, Ph.D.

■ INFECTIOUS SYNDROMES AND TREATMENT/PROPHYLAXIS

Mucocutaneous *Candida* Syndromes
Cutaneous Candidiasis

Primary cutaneous candidiasis is commonly seen in normal hosts manifesting as diaper dermatitis and intertriginous infections. Other manifestations include balanitis, vulvitis, paronychia, onychia, and folliculitis. Cutaneous candidiasis most commonly presents in skin areas that are moist and/or occluded, although other areas where altered local skin immunity has occurred, such as burn sites, are susceptible to infection. Patients who are systemically immunocompromised, including patients with diabetes mellitus, are also at increased risk. The diagnosis is usually made on clinical grounds. Findings may include an erythematous rash of intertriginous areas, such as the inguinal region, with satellite lesions, or lesions may be papular, pustular, or ulcerated. Microscopic examination of skin scrapings revealing budding yeast cells and hyphae may be used to confirm the diagnosis. Positive cultures for *Candida* species may also assist with diagnosis; however, false-positive results may occur because of colonization or contamination. Bacterial superinfection may also occur with cutaneous candidiasis. Superinfection may also be detected by culture and necessitates concomitant antibacterial treatment. Nonantimicrobial methods are important in both prophylaxis and treatment of cutaneous candidiasis. These include maintenance of a dry skin surface, frequent diaper changes, and control of hyperglycemia in diabetics. Topical antifungals, such as nystatin cream or an imidazole cream, applied twice daily, are effective. Systemic treatment for paronychia or onychia with fluconazole or itraconazole may be required.

Chronic Mucocutaneous Candidiasis

Individuals with chronic mucocutaneous candidiasis suffer from persistent and recurrent *Candida* infections of the skin, nails, and mucous membranes. The disease is a complex disorder that may manifest as one of many different syndromes with variable severity. It can occur at any age but is most commonly recognized in children younger than 3 years of age. T-cell dysfunction is the primary immune abnormality associated with chronic mucocutaneous candidiasis, although deficits in humoral immunity, neutrophil function, and complement activity are also often found. The disorder may also be associated with abnormal function of the thyroid, parathyroid, and/or adrenal glands, as well as with diabetes mellitus, thymoma, and interstitial keratitis. Other opportunistic bacterial or viral infections may also occur. Other than esophagitis, deeply invasive infections are rarely encountered. Systemic antifungal therapy with azoles or amphotericin B leads to improvement in chronic mucocuta-

Table 1   Typical in Vitro Susceptibility Patterns for Select Antifungal Agents Against Commonly Isolated *Candida* Species*

CANDIDA SPECIES	ANTIFUNGAL AGENTS			
	FLUCONAZOLE	ITRACONAZOLE	VORICONAZOLE†	AMPHOTERICIN B
C. albicans	++	++	++	+++
C. tropicalis	++	++	++	++
C. parapsilosis	++	++	++	++
C. lusitaniae	++	+	++	+/–
C. glabrata‡	–	+/–	++	++
C. krusei	––	+/–	++	++/+
C. kefyr§	++	++	++	++
C. guilliermondii	+	+	++	–

+++, Always susceptible; ++, usually susceptible, consider resistance testing; +, occasionally susceptible, perform resistance testing, consider dose escalation; –, usually resistant; ––, always resistant.
*Clinical correlation of in vitro susceptibility patterns is not firmly established for most species, especially for systemic *Candida* infections.
†Currently undergoing phase III clinical trials.
‡Previously *Torulopsis glabrata*.
§Previously *C. pseudotropicalis*.

neous candidiasis; topical nystatin or imidazole therapy can be used for local treatment. The underlying immunodeficiency, however, often leads to frequent relapses, and the patient may require long-term treatment or prophylaxis. When possible, attempts at reversing the immunodeficiency should be pursued.

Oropharyngeal and Esophageal Candidiasis

As normal members of the gastrointestinal tract flora, *Candida* species become pathogenic in the oropharynx and esophagus in patients with various risk factors, including impaired cell-mediated immunity (e.g., human immunodeficiency virus [HIV] infection, chronic mucocutaneous candidiasis, bone marrow and solid organ transplant recipients), diabetes mellitus, extremes of age, esophageal achalasia or reflux, or the use of progesterones, broad-spectrum antibiotics, or immunosuppressive medications such as corticosteroids.

Oral candidiasis most commonly presents as thrush: painless white pseudomembranous plaques on the surfaces of the oropharynx that can be removed by scraping with a tongue blade. It may also present in more symptomatic forms as erythematous mucosal patches without the pseudomembranous plaques (erythematous candidiasis), rough plaques that cannot be removed by scraping (*Candida* leukoplakia or hyperplastic candidiasis), and cracking and erythema at the corners of the lips (angular chelitis). As with cutaneous candidiasis, the diagnosis is usually made clinically, although microscopic examination of scrapings can confirm diagnosis (culture is not helpful because colonization commonly occurs). Empiric therapy with a topical antifungal should be initiated for oral thrush, unless it is associated with esophageal candidiasis (in which case systemic therapy is usually required). Nystatin suspension or clotrimazole troches are common first-line agents for oropharyngeal candidiasis; both require frequent administration. Amphotericin B suspension is an alternative, and refractory oropharyngeal candidiasis may require systemic fluconazole, itraconazole, or ketoconazole. Particularly severe cases, or those with decreased susceptibility to azoles,

may require systemic amphotericin B. Angular chelitis may be treated with topical imidazole creams or nystatin. Maintenance therapy in patients with chronic immunosuppression may be necessary, although this may lead to infection with resistant *Candida* species. In patients with HIV, reversal of immune deficits with antiretroviral therapy is often beneficial for improving or resolving oral candidiasis.

Esophageal candidiasis often presents as a sense of obstruction and/or pain (retrosternal, subxiphoid, or rarely cervical) and can be mimicked by or coincide with cytomegalovirus esophagitis, herpes simplex virus esophagitis, or esophageal aphthous ulcers. Patients may be asymptomatic; the infection ranges from superficial to erosive. Empiric therapy is usually initiated with a systemic azole antifungal; in some cases, amphotericin B treatment may be required. In refractory situations, esophagoscopy with mucosal brushings or biopsy may be necessary to establish the diagnosis, test for antifungal resistance, and evaluate for other potential concomitant pathogens.

Vulvovaginal Candidiasis

Vaginal candidiasis is a common infection in women of childbearing age and although pregnancy, oral contraceptive use, antibiotic use, and diabetes mellitus can be identified as predisposing host risk factors, often no precipitating factor can be found. In a small percentage of women, repeatedly recurrent episodes occur. It remains unclear by what mechanism this often-commensal, asymptomatic colonization transforms into symptomatic vaginitis. Vaginal candidiasis often occurs with vulvar candidiasis. The clinical manifestations of vulvovaginal candidiasis usually include acute vulvar pruritus and vaginal discharge, although these symptoms are neither sensitive nor specific. Signs include erythema and edema of the vulva with erythema of the vagina. Often, there will be no or minimal vaginal discharge of variable consistency. Diagnosis is usually made by a wet mount or 10% KOH preparation or Gram stain of vaginal secretions revealing yeast and hyphal forms with few neutrophils; concurrent evaluation for other pathogens is also important. Multiple topical azole and polyene agents are available for treatment of vaginal and vulvovaginal candidiasis. Formulations include creams, lotions, tablets, and suppositories, with application required from 3 to 7 days—single-dose regimens may be less effective and more irritating. Of note, clinical and mycologic cure rates are higher with the azoles than with polyenes. Patient preference usually should dictate choice of administration. Oral azoles also have demonstrated high clinical and mycologic cure rates and are an appropriate alternative to the topical agents; fluconazole at 150 mg as a single dose is commonly used. Patients with immunosuppression may require a longer course of the selected topical or systemic antifungal. Refractory or repeatedly recurrent cases of vaginal candidiasis may require long-term use of topical or systemic antifungals, such as 6-month prophylactic regimens of oral ketoconazole, 100 mg daily, or fluconazole, 150 mg weekly.

Candidemia and Disseminated Candidiasis
Candidemia

Candida species are the fourth most common cause of nosocomial bloodstream infection in the United States (from 5% to 10% of all bloodstream isolates, affecting 15,000 to 30,000 patients per year). Crude mortality is at least 40%, and attributable mortality, initially considered low, is now believed to be at least 25%. Excess hospital stay in candidemia survivors approaches 1 month. Candidemia is defined as the isolation, from at least one blood culture, of a pathogenic *Candida* species. Candidemia is often catheter related (especially in the immunocompetent patient), and when possible, all vascular access devices should be changed when candidemia is suspected or diagnosed (see also the chapter *Intravascular Catheter-Related Infection*). Furthermore, it is important to determine the extent of the infection to define both the prognosis as well as treatment course. Dissemination to areas such as the eye, liver, spleen, kidney, heart, skin and soft tissues, bone, central nervous system (CNS), and gastrointestinal tract may occur more commonly in the immunosuppressed patient. These organs/systems often (approaching 50% of all deep infections) may also be infected without culture evidence of candidemia, and their management is outlined next.

In patients with isolated candidemia, it is impossible to accurately differentiate those who may respond to catheter removal alone from those who need antifungal treatment. Given this information and the high attributable morbidity and mortality of candidemia, all patients with candidemia should be treated aggressively. In nonneutropenic patients, treatment should be initiated early with either fluconazole or conventional amphotericin B or, when indicated, one of the alternative formulations of amphotericin B. Fluconazole should be considered for initial therapy in patients who are stable and who have a low likelihood of infection with *C. krusei* (intrinsically resistant to fluconazole) or another resistant *Candida* species. Patients with *C. krusei* infection or azole-resistant infections require amphotericin B. Although *Candida* species become rapidly resistant to 5-fluorocytosine when it is used as monotherapy, it may provide benefit in combination with amphotericin B and it should be considered in the unstable patient. Amphotericin B can be initiated at 0.5 to 0.7 mg/kg/day and fluconazole at 400 mg/day; higher dosages of both may be required in the

deteriorating patient and for certain *Candida* species (see Table 1). Dosing of the alternative "lipid" formulations of amphotericin B is less established, and a suggested starting point is between 3 and 5 mg/kg/day. Treatment should be continued for an additional 2 weeks after the last positive blood culture was obtained. Vigilance for late complications of candidemia, such as endophthalmitis, osteomyelitis, endocarditis, and chronic disseminated candidiasis (also known as hepatosplenic candidiasis), should be continued for at least 3 months after the acute illness.

Neutropenic patients are at higher risk for candidemia and its complications. In general, management is similar to that for nonneutropenic patients with candidemia, although higher dosages of fluconazole (≥800 mg/day) and/or amphotericin B (0.7 to 1.5 mg/kg/day) may be indicated. In addition, concomitant use of 5-fluorocytosine is much more likely to be associated with bone marrow suppression. Furthermore, amphotericin should be strongly considered as the initial regimen for candidemia in a neutropenic patient in view of the overall poorer prognosis in this patient population, the potentially more rapid response to amphotericin B compared with azoles, possible prior azole prophylaxis, delayed availability of *Candida* speciation and resistance pattern results, and insufficient evidence of azole efficacy in the current literature.

Urinary Tract Infections (See Also the Chapter Candiduria)

The isolation of *Candida* in the urine is common in hospitalized or nursing home patients, especially in those with indwelling urinary catheters. It is often difficult to distinguish patients with asymptomatic candiduria from those with true *Candida* urinary tract infections. Infections are more common and potentially more serious in patients who are taking broad-spectrum antibiotics or immunosuppressive agents, in patients with diabetes mellitus, and in patients with genitourinary abnormalities (including obstructive uropathy and postrenal transplant). The diagnosis is problematic; high colony count is not a strong indicator of infection. Pyuria in this setting should suggest the diagnosis; however, clinical suspicion combined with culture results postremoval of the catheter may be all that is available for the clinician. In most episodes of candiduria, catheter removal is often all that is required. Higher-risk patients (e.g., those with genitourinary abnormalities) or those with a high clinical suspicion of infection may be managed with oral fluconazole, 100 mg/day. Amphotericin B is an alternative for cystitis and may be administered as a bladder washing, 50 mg in 1 L of sterile water daily for 5 days. Upper tract disease requires systemic antifungal therapy, and if a prosthetic device such as a stent is present, it may need to be removed to achieve eradication.

Ocular Infections

Up to 15% of patients with candidemia have retinal lesions, often visible within 1 week of the onset of illness. All patients with candidemia should be screened for endophthalmitis by an ophthalmologist; white lesions on the retina with ill-defined borders with possible vitreal extension are characteristic. Symptoms may include bulbar pain, scotomas, and blurred vision. Management involves the early use of systemic antifungals as well as pars plana vitrectomy and intravitreal amphotericin B, when required. Small, uncomplicated lesions in stable, low-risk patients may initially be managed with fluconazole alone; any suggestion of progression or an absence of response should prompt a change to amphotericin B and 5-fluorocytosine as well as the consideration of pars plana vitrectomy (see also the chapter *Endophthalmitis*).

Endocarditis

Patients with *Candida* endocarditis and patients with bacterial endocarditis share both risk factors (intravenous drug use, cardiac surgery, prosthetic heart valves, abnormal native heart valves, and central venous catheters) and clinical presentation (fevers, nonspecific signs and symptoms, cardiac murmur, and congestive heart failure). Mycotic emboli to major arteries are more common in *Candida* endocarditis, and blood cultures are often negative. The diagnosis should be considered in all patients with candidemia. Evidence of a valvular vegetation by transthoracic, or the more sensitive transesophageal echocardiogram, establishes the diagnosis. Definitive treatment requires surgical resection of the infected valve (histopathologic examination and culture of the valvular material should be obtained for confirmation and resistance testing) and administration of amphotericin B (at least 0.7 mg/kg/day), with or without 5-fluorocytosine, for at least 6 weeks postoperatively. Some experts would consider subsequent suppressive therapy with fluconazole.

Chronic Disseminated Candidiasis

Chronic disseminated candidiasis (formerly *hepatosplenic candidiasis*) is an indolent process most commonly found in patients with severe persistent neutropenia (e.g., in patients with acute leukemia or post–bone marrow or stem cell transplant) that usually becomes apparent when the neutrophil count is recovering. It typically involves the liver and/or spleen, although other organs such as the kidney or lung may be involved. Computed tomography (CT) or magnetic resonance imaging studies are more than 90% sensitive later in the disease course. Typically, multiple small hepatic and splenic abscesses are present. Patients may be afebrile before their marrow recovery and may have right upper quadrant tenderness, elevated transaminases, and hepatosplenomegaly; no symptoms or signs are particularly sensitive or specific. Blood cultures are often negative, and biopsy may be required to confirm the diagnosis. Often, fluconazole may be used in the initial management of nonneutropenic patients with the course of treatment determined by follow-up CT scans. In neutropenic patients or in patients with a suboptimal response to azole therapy and/or infected with a fluconazole-resistant *Candida* species, amphotericin B, with or without 5-fluorocytosine, should be instituted. Notably, in patients who receive repeated courses of antineoplastic therapy or who persistently remain immunosuppressed, long-term (6 months or more) suppressive therapy may be required.

Central Nervous System Infections

Meningitis is the most common form of CNS candidiasis. Other forms of infection include mycotic aneurysms and cerebral abscesses. Low-birth-weight or premature infants and immunosuppressed hosts are at risk for *Candida* meningitis. Other risk factors include thermal burns, recent neurosurgery, and the presence of ventricular shunts and drains. Signs and symptoms are similar, yet often more subtle, when compared with other forms of meningitis, and typically there is a more indolent and chronic course. Cerebrospinal fluid (CSF) analysis reveals a monocyte or neutrophil pleocytosis, elevated protein, and either normal or depressed glucose. Repeated cultures of the CSF may be required to establish a diagnosis. Treatment should be with amphotericin B, with or without 5-fluorocytosine. In appropriate patients, fluconazole may have a role. The duration of therapy is usually at least 6 weeks. Removal of any ventricular shunt or drain is usually required to achieve eradication.

Gastrointestinal Candidiasis

Candida peritonitis may develop in patients on peritoneal dialysis, after gastrointestinal surgery, as a complication of candidemia, or as an extension of local organ or tissue infection. In addition, gastric and duodenal mucosal infections may develop in patients with peptic ulcer disease or mucosal neoplasm. Diagnosis is made by paracentesis or by endoscopic, percutaneous, or open biopsy. Therapy is with systemic amphotericin B or fluconazole, as well as surgical exploration and drainage of the infection when indicated. In patients receiving chronic ambulatory peritoneal dialysis, systemic antifungals should be administered, as intraperitoneal amphotericin B may lead to adhesions, complicating future attempts at peritoneal dialysis. The catheter should be removed.

Bone and Soft-Tissue Infections

Bone and soft-tissue infections, rare complications of *Candida* dissemination or direct extension of a local *Candida* infection, are diagnosed by needle aspiration or via surgical debridement. Treatment usually requires a combination of surgical debridement and systemic antifungals, and both amphotericin B and high-dose fluconazole have been used successfully as adjuncts to surgery.

Suggested Reading

Edwards JE Jr, et al: International Conference for the Development of a Consensus on the Management and Prevention of Severe Candidal Infections, *Clin Infect Dis* 25:43, 1997.

Rex JH, et al: A randomized trial comparing fluconazole with amphotericin B for the treatment of candidemia in patients without neutropenia, *N Engl J Med* 331:1325, 1994.

Swerdloff JN, Filler SG, Edwards JE Jr: Severe candidal infections in neutropenic patients, *Clin Infect Dis* 17(suppl 2):S457, 1993.

Walsh TJ, et al: Liposomal amphotericin B for empirical therapy in patients with persistent fever and neutropenia. National Institute of Allergy and Infectious Diseases Mycoses Study Group, *N Engl J Med* 340:764, 1999.

ASPERGILLOSIS

Sanjay Ram

Stuart M. Levitz

*A*spergillus is readily isolated from samples of soil, decaying vegetation, water, and air worldwide. The *Aspergillus* species *A. fumigatus,* followed by *A. flavus* and *A. niger,* are the most common species that cause human disease. Aspergillosis follows exposure of a susceptible host to the ubiquitous conidia (spores). Germinating conidia form hyphae, the invasive form of the fungus. *Aspergillus* hyphae average 2 to 4 microns in diameter and are septate, with dichotomous (Y-shaped) branching. The spectrum of diseases caused by aspergilli is wide and profoundly influenced by the underlying immune status of the host.

■ INVASIVE ASPERGILLOSIS

Although inhalation of conidia is common, invasive disease is relatively rare. Most affected patients are severely immunosuppressed either from profound, prolonged neutropenia, usually secondary to cytotoxic agents, or from high-dose corticosteroid therapy such as might occur after organ transplantation. Patients with chronic granulomatous disease (CGD) are also predisposed to *Aspergillus* infections. Invasive pulmonary aspergillosis with or without dissemination is the most common form of disease in high-risk patients. Signs and symptoms of invasive aspergillosis are nonspecific. Fever is almost always present. Radiographic features include patchy densities or well-defined nodules that may be single or multifocal and can progress to cavitation or consolidation. Invasive aspergillosis must be strongly suspected in any high-risk patient with fever unresponsive to broad-spectrum antibiotics, and empiric antifungal therapy should be considered. Although *Aspergillus* can be a laboratory contaminant, a positive culture for *Aspergillus* in a high-risk patient is highly predictive of invasive disease. *Aspergillus* sinusitis is the second most common manifestation. Its clinical features include fever, head or sinus pain, proptosis, and monocular blindness. Less common manifestations include cutaneous aspergillosis, which may be seen at the insertion sites of intravenous catheters in neutropenic patients, as invasive fungal dermatitis in premature neonates and children with acquired immunodeficiency syndrome (AIDS), or at sites of burn wounds in immunocompromised persons. Cerebral aspergillosis occurs in 10% to 20% of all cases of invasive aspergillosis. Involvement of the epiglottis, larynx, liver, cardiac valves, thyroid, kidneys, pericardium, and peritoneum has also been reported.

Currently, the only two Food and Drug Administration (FDA)-approved agents with efficacy against *Aspergillus* are amphotericin B and itraconazole. Clinical experience indicates that amphotericin B is the drug of choice for treatment of invasive aspergillosis, although the optimal daily dosage remains controversial. Following a test dose of 1 mg, dosages ranging from 0.5 to 1.2 mg/kg/day are generally recommended, with the higher dosages reserved for those patients who are severely ill and/or profoundly immunosuppressed. Fevers, chills, and rigors, observed in a significant number of patients treated with amphotericin B, may be alleviated by premedication with acetaminophen, meperidine (25 to 50 mg given intravenously), or the addition of 25 to 50 mg of hydrocortisone sodium succinate to the infusion solution. Amphotericin nephrotoxicity has been associated with sodium-depleted states and may be reduced by the avoidance of diuretics and by giving 1 L of normal saline a day to patients with no contraindications to volume expansion. Because amphotericin B causes renal tubular losses of potassium and magnesium, their levels should be monitored closely and supplementation provided as needed. The dosage of amphotericin B must be individualized depending on factors such as the expected duration and degree of immunosuppression and the extent of the disease.

In an effort to reduce the toxicity associated with the conventional amphotericin B preparation, lipid-associated formulations have been developed. Currently available formulations include amphotericin B lipid complex (ABLC), amphotericin B colloidal dispersion (ABCD), and a liposomal preparation of amphotericin B (AmBisome). Comparisons between the different formulations of amphotericin B are difficult to make because of the lack of well-designed randomized trials. However, at the usual daily dosages recommended for the treatment of invasive aspergillosis (4 to 5 mg/kg/day), the lipid formulations appear to be equally efficacious as amphotericin B deoxycholate, but not more so. The lipid formulations are less nephrotoxic than the conventional preparation, but because of their considerably greater cost, their use at present probably should be limited to patients who cannot tolerate amphotericin B. Although amphotericin B has been used in combination with other agents, including flucytosine, rifampin, and tetracycline, there are no controlled data and we do not recommend their use routinely.

Although fluconazole and ketoconazole do not have any useful clinical activity against *Aspergillus,* the synthetic triazole derivative, itraconazole, does. Randomized trials directly comparing itraconazole and amphotericin B have not been performed, but based on historical controls, the rates of clinical response are similar with the two drugs. Currently, two oral formulations are available: capsules and an oral aqueous acidified solution in 5% hydroxypropyl-β-cyclodextrin. Absorption of the capsular form is best in an acidic environment and in the presence of a meal. H_2-blockers and antacids may interfere with absorption. In contrast, the oral aqueous hydroxypropyl-β-cyclodextrin solution should be taken without food. This preparation has an absolute bioavailability of 55% and achieves peak serum concentrations about 60% higher than the capsules. Drugs that induce hepatic microsomal enzymes (e.g., rifampin, isoniazid, phenytoin, phenobarbital, carbamazepine) may significantly reduce serum itraconazole levels. Itraconazole itself slows hepatic drug metabolism and may increase the toxicity of phenytoin, oral hypoglycemics, digoxin, warfarin, and cyclosporin. Loading doses of 200 mg thrice daily for

3 days followed by maintenance doses of 200 mg twice daily are recommended. One of the metabolites of itraconazole, hydroxy-itraconazole, has antifungal activity in vitro that is comparable with the parent compound. Given the variable absorption of itraconazole, the lack of a parenteral preparation, and the numerous drug interactions, we recommend amphotericin B as first-line therapy in seriously ill patients with invasive aspergillosis. Itraconazole seems a reasonable alternative in patients with indolent or slowly progressive disease, and those unable or unwilling to tolerate amphotericin provided they have good intestinal function and are not concomitantly on drugs that induce the metabolism of cytochrome P450. Indications for monitoring drug levels during itraconazole therapy include patients with life-threatening infections in whom erratic absorption and drug interactions frequently occur and in cases of treatment failure or relapse. Plasma concentrations should be measured 1 to 2 weeks after starting therapy when steady state levels have been reached. Although not established, levels of 250 μg/ml or greater of unmetabolized itraconazole or 750 to 1000 μg/ml or more of itraconazole plus hydroxy-itraconazole may provide useful guidelines for dosing.

Terbinafine, an allylamine derivative that is available in the United States, has been tried successfully in select non-immunocompromised patients with bronchopulmonary or chronic necrotizing invasive aspergillosis refractory to the conventional agents. Several novel agents, including azoles and echinocandins, are undergoing clinical evaluation. The azole voriconazole has shown good clinical efficacy and tolerability among immunocompromised patients with invasive aspergillosis.

Enhancement of host defenses may prove important in the treatment of invasive aspergillosis because even with aggressive antifungal therapy poor outcomes are common in patients who have prolonged neutropenia or other forms of immunosuppression. In suitable patients, recombinant human cytokines such as granulocyte colony-stimulating factor (G-CSF) and granulocyte-macrophage colony-stimulating factor (GM-CSF) decrease the duration of neutropenia and may increase the fungicidal action of phagocytes.

Given the high mortality associated with established disease, strategies for the prevention of invasive aspergillosis have been advocated and are summarized in Table 1.

■ ASPERGILLOSIS IN PATIENTS WITH AIDS

Invasive aspergillosis is being seen with increasing frequency in AIDS patients because of the prolonged survival of profoundly immunosuppressed patients. Most patients have a CD4 count of less than 100/μl. Classical risk factors, including neutropenia and corticosteroid therapy, are seen in more than half the patients. In addition to clinical and radiographic features similar to those seen in non-AIDS patients, AIDS patients are predisposed to ulcerative or pseudomembranous tracheobronchitis, and a more non-invasive form called *obstructing bronchial aspergillosis*. Cough, fever, wheezing, hypoxemia, and hemoptysis are the main clinical features. Bronchoscopy helps confirm the diagnosis.

The response to antifungal therapy of AIDS patients is considerably inferior to that observed in patients without AIDS, probably reflecting the advanced stage of the disease and the presence of intercurrent infections or tumors. Optimal therapy in this group of patients is not yet defined. Amphotericin B is recommended, with titration of dosages according to clinical response and toxicity. Itraconazole may be considered in patients with less serious forms of disease, in patients unable to tolerate amphotericin B, or in patients who are not candidates for long-term intravenous access. Patients with AIDS tend to have lower serum levels of itraconazole, which may reflect decreased absorption of the drug secondary to achlorhydria or human immunodeficiency virus (HIV)-related enteropathy. Didanosine (ddI) contains a buffer that can interfere with itraconazole

Table 1 Prevention of Invasive Aspergillosis	
PREVENTIVE STRATEGY	**COMMENTS**
1. Avoidance of exposure to *Aspergillus* conidia	
Avoidance of environmental exposure	Heavily contaminated areas include compost heaps, grain silos, moldy hay, and marijuana
High-efficiency particulate air (HEPA) filters or laminar air flow (LAF)	Although expensive, HEPA and LAF may be considered for patients at very high risk of invasive aspergillosis
2. Prophylaxis (administration of low-dose amphotericin B or itraconazole to high-risk patients)	Efficacy data are conflicting but may be considered in very-high-risk groups
3. Administration of colony-stimulating factors to neutropenic patients	Expensive; may be considered as part of an overall strategy to reduce infections in selected patients
4. Empiric administration of amphotericin B to neutropenic patients with persistent or recurrent fevers despite broad-spectrum antibacterial agents	Strongly recommended; has been shown to reduce mortality from fungal infections; amphotericin B at dosages of 0.6 mg/kg/day are recommended*
5. Secondary prophylaxis (antifungal treatment to prevent recrudescence of proven invasive aspergillosis that was treated during a prior episode of immunosuppression)	Relapse rates greater than 50%; amphotericin B, 0.6 to 1.0 mg/kg/day, should be given at the onset of chemotherapy or neutropenia; consider surgical resection of localized disease*

*Oral itraconazole may be considered in patients with good gastrointestinal function and not concomitantly on drugs that could have clinically significant interactions.

absorption, resulting in undetectable itraconazole levels when the two drugs are administered simultaneously. Care must be taken to stagger the interval by at least 2 hours if a patient is to receive both drugs. Significant interactions can also occur with protease inhibitors, and patients should be observed closely. Lifelong maintenance therapy is usually required in persons with aspergillosis and AIDS.

The value of prophylaxis remains uncertain, but it may be worthwhile to use itraconazole in the subgroup of patients with positive sputum cultures for *Aspergillus* especially if they have one or more of the classic risk factors.

◼ ASPERGILLOMAS

Pulmonary aspergillomas are the result of saprophytic colonization of *Aspergillus* within preexisting lung cavities. The diagnosis is most often made by chest radiography, where a round to oval intracavitary mass partially surrounded by a radiolucent crescent of air is seen. Serum precipitins and sputum cultures for *Aspergillus* are positive in about 90% and 50% of cases, respectively. Hemoptysis is the most common symptom and in most cases is mild and self-limited.

Therapy for aspergillomas must be individualized according to the pulmonary and immunologic status of the host, but in most cases a conservative approach with close clinical follow-up is recommended. Systemic antifungal agents have not proved superior to pulmonary toilet alone. Resection generally is reserved for those with life-threatening hemoptysis. Bronchial artery embolization can be tried as a temporizing measure for massive hemoptysis in patients at a high operative risk.

A subset of patients with aspergillomas tend to be chronically ill, with fever, weight loss, pulmonary symptoms, and leukocytosis. This entity, termed *chronic necrotizing pulmonary aspergillosis*, or "semi-invasive" aspergillosis, is seen in patients with chronic pulmonary disorders and mild systemic immunocompromise such as occurs in diabetes mellitus, alcoholism, low-dose corticosteroid use, or malnutrition. When possible, host defenses should be strengthened by diminishing factors responsible for immunosuppression. In some cases, dramatic clinical response has been observed following a course of intravenous or intracavitary amphotericin B. Itraconazole has also been used with some success. Resection may be considered in the small subset of patients with focal disease whose pulmonary function and underlying disease do not preclude surgery.

◼ ALLERGIC MANIFESTATIONS OF *ASPERGILLUS*

Extrinsic allergic alveolitis occurs in nonatopic individuals who are exposed to *Aspergillus conidia*, as in "malt-workers lung" or "farmers lung," following their exposure to moldy grain or hay. Spontaneous recovery usually occurs over several weeks, without the need for corticosteroids. Exposure to *Aspergillus* in individuals with asthma can result in an exacerbation of their disease (extrinsic asthma).

Some atopic individuals develop allergic bronchopulmonary aspergillosis (ABPA), a syndrome characterized by episodic bronchial asthma, pulmonary infiltrates, peripheral eosinophilia, in association with immediate wheal-and-flare skin response to *Aspergillus* antigens, serum precipitins against *Aspergillus* antigens, elevated serum IgE concentrations, and elevated serum IgG and IgE antibodies specific to *A. fumigatus.*

Prednisone in daily doses of 1 mg/kg followed by a gradual taper over a 3- to 6-month period remains the primary treatment. High dosages of inhaled beclomethasone may be useful in some patients and allow reduction in the dose of oral corticosteroids. Limited data suggest that itraconazole at dosages of 200 mg twice daily for prolonged periods may be used in selected patients who would benefit significantly from reductions in corticosteroid doses. However, prompt recolonization of the airways with *Aspergillus* invariably occurs following discontinuation of the drug.

Allergic aspergillus sinusitis usually responds to surgical debridement and drainage. Recurrences after surgery may be prevented by the use of intranasal steroid sprays or systemic corticosteroids in selected cases.

Saprophytic colonization of the paranasal sinuses and external auditory canal in immunocompetent patients must be distinguished from allergic and invasive forms of the disease. Surgical debridement and drainage of the sinuses and treatment of the chronic otitis are usually curative. Antifungal therapy in the absence of tissue invasion generally is not indicated.

Suggested Reading

Denning DW: Invasive aspergillosis, *Clin Infect Dis* 26:781, 1998.

Fink JN: Therapy of allergic bronchopulmonary aspergillosis, *Immunol Allergy Clin North Am,* 18:655, 1998.

Levitz SM: Aspergillosis, *Infect Dis Clin North Am* 3:1, 1989.

Mylonakis E, et al: Pulmonary aspergillosis and invasive disease in AIDS. Review of 342 cases, *Chest* 114:251, 1998.

Wong-Beringer A, Jacobs RA, Guglielmo JB: Lipid formulations of amphotericin B: clinical efficacy and toxicities, *Clin Infect Dis* 27:603, 1998.

MUCORMYCOSIS (ZYGOMYCOSIS)

Scott F. Davies

The term *mucormycosis* refers to a group of highly lethal fungal infections caused by the members of the order Mucorales, which include various species of the genera *Rhizopus, Absidia,* and *Mucor* (all from the family Mucoraceae). Most infections are caused by *Rhizopus* species. It is incorrect to use the term *mucormycosis* to refer only to infections caused by members of the genus *Mucor,* which are among the least common causes of mucormycosis. An even broader term—*zygomycosis*—is increasingly preferred because it encompasses not only the entire order Mucorales (which includes infections due to *Cunninghamella* species) but also the order Entomophthorales, including *Conidiobolus* species, which have on rare occasions caused pulmonary mucormycosis in profoundly immunosupressed patients. Figure 1, gives an overview of the taxonomy of the causitive organisms.

The causative agents of mucormycosis are found throughout the world, associated with decaying organic matter. The grow as a mycelium (broad nonseptate hyphae with short stubby right-angle branches) in nature and in infected mammalian tissue.

■ PATHOGENESIS

Airborne spores of the fungi settle on the skin or are inhaled into the nose, the pharynx, and the lung. The organism has little chance of invading healthy tissue defended by neutrophils. Because *Rhizopus* organisms grow best at acid pH in a high-glucose environment, diabetic ketoacidosis provides a favorable opportunity for the fungus to locally invade tissues of the upper airway, resulting in the fulminant rhinocerebral form of mucormycosis. Once established the fungus is angioinvasive, leading to infarction of tissues and wider areas of necrosis, in which the fungus thrives. The tissue response to the fungus includes pyogenic inflammation, but there is little tendency for granuloma formation. A second form of mucormycosis is pulmonary mucormycosis, in which infection occurs in the lung or less commonly in proximal airways. The disease resembles invasive pulmonary aspergillosis and occurs, although much less commonly, in the same substrate—that is, patients with profound neutropenia and patients in whom phagocyte function is depressed by high-dose glucocorticoid therapy. Like *Aspergillus* species, agents of mucormycosis are angioinvasive in the lung, leading to tissue necrosis and eventually to pyemic spread to distant sites, including the skin, kidney, and brain. Rare forms of mucormycosis include a direct cutaneous infection that can complicate severe burns and a gastrointestinal form of the illness, associated with profound protein malnutrition (usually in infants), in which organisms directly invade the bowel wall, causing hemorrhage, bowel infarction, peritonitis, and death.

■ CLINICAL MANIFESTATIONS

Rhinocerebral mucormycosis is an extremely fulminant infection. Infection begins in the nose, sometimes manifested by dark, blood-tinged discharge from one or both nostrils. Necrosis of the nasal septum and turbinates then follow, with spread to the paranasal sinuses. In sequence, the disease accelerates with ulceration and necrosis of sinus walls, periorbital cellulitis, and direct invasion of the orbit, eye, cavernous sinuses, and brain. Arterial thrombosis adds to the extent of tissue destruction. Early clinical findings include eye pain, decreased visual acuity, and cranial nerve palsies. These may be followed by seizures and progressive decrease in level of consciousness. Death may occur in 1 week.

Pulmonary mucormycosis is acquired by inhalation. It presents as an acute or subacute pneumonia, with fever, cough, and purulent sputum. Some patients have pleuritic pain and hemoptysis from superimposed pulmonary infarction caused by invasion of pulmonary vessels. The most characteristic finding on chest radiograph is a wedge-shaped area of dense infiltrate in the lung periphery. The spectrum of radiographic abnormalities also includes large masses (even to 6 to 10 cm in size), multiple nodules, and multiple peripheral infiltrates. Focal areas of consolidation often cavitate as the infection progresses. Metastatic abscesses may develop in the brain, liver, spleen, kidney, and skin. Metastatic skin lesions often show extensive necrosis (ecthyma gangrenosum) and offer easy diagnosis with a simple punch biopsy. Clinically, the illness cannot easily be distinguished from invasive aspergillosis. Most cases occur in patients with hematologic malignancy who have prolonged neutropenia. Cases of pulmonary mucormycosis also occur in organ transplant recipients, in patients receiving long courses of high-dose glucocorticoid therapy for malignant or nonmalignant disorders, and even in diabetic patients. Desferoxamine therapy, used for chelation in some patients receiving long-term dialysis and in other iron-overloaded states, is also a risk factor for mucormycosis because it mobilizes iron from peripheral storage sites and makes it more available to the fungus as a growth factor.

Endobronchial mucormycosis is a rarer form of pulmonary mucormycosis that occurs in similar types of patients. Patients have irritative cough, purulent sputum, and often hemoptysis. Physical findings may include a localized wheeze. The chest radiograph may be normal or may show segmental or even lobar infiltrates with significant volume loss beyond the obstructed airway.

Pulmonary mucormycosis is a rare complication of AIDS. Several other unusual forms of mucormycosis also have been reported in this population. Isolated renal mucormycosis has been described in AIDS patients who abuse drugs intravenously or have long-term intravascular access catheters for various therapeutics. Nodular skin lesions have also been reported in AIDS patients who abuse drugs intravenously. Intravenous drug abusers have been described with cerebral mucormycosis of the basal ganglia.

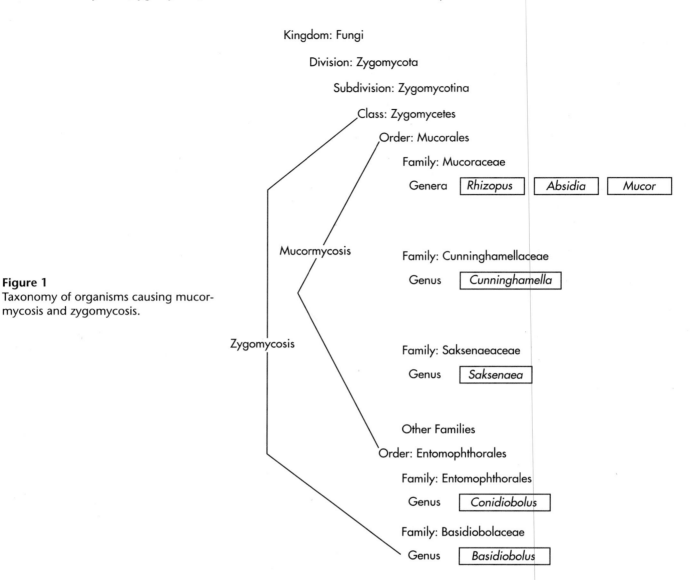

Figure 1
Taxonomy of organisms causing mucor-mycosis and zygomycosis.

■ DIAGNOSIS

The diagnosis of rhinocerebral mucormycosis can often be strongly suspected based on the setting of diabetic ketoaci-dosis and the clinical features of the illness. High suspicion and early recognition are important. Specific diagnosis usu-ally depends on histopathologic demonstration of charac-teristic broad nonseptate hyphae in biopsies of diseased tissue. Positive cultures are confirmatory and the only way to define the exact species causing the infection. Positive cul-tures for causative organisms of mucormycosis must be interpreted cautiously and in clinical context because the organisms are ubiquitous in the environment and occasion-ally can be recovered from the skin, pharynx, and sputum of patients without disease. No useful skin tests or serologic tests are available.

■ TREATMENT

Rhinocerebral mucormycosis has a very high mortality, probably beyond 80% of all cases. Successful therapy is most likely if the diagnosis is made early and based entirely on clinical findings. There are three aspects to the treatment. First, the diabetic ketoacidosis must be controlled. Second and most importantly, aggressive surgical debridement of all necrotic tissue must be done. Sometimes, a sequence of several procedures are needed as the limits of the diseased tissue become more apparent. Finally, full doses of ampho-tericin B (daily doses up to 1.0 to 1.5 mg/kg, as tolerated) must be given quickly. Amphotericin B likely contributes to successful outcome but is not sufficient in itself without metabolic control and surgical debridement.

Pulmonary mucormycosis is also highly lethal. Once there is spread to distant sites and particularly to the brain, fatal outcome is nearly certain. Localized pulmonary disease can sometimes be managed successfully. Again, a three-pronged approach is necessary. First, the predisposing causes must be reversed. This means return of neutrophils (either spontaneously or aided by colony-stimulating fac-tors) and/or rapid taper of glucocorticoid therapy to the extent it is possible. Second, amphotericin B should be started and escalated quickly to full dosages of up to 1.0 to 1.5 mg/kg/day, again as tolerated. Third, if the patient stabilizes, strong consideration should be given to surgical resection of necrotic lung tissue; if the lung disease is localized, the risk of thoracotomy is reasonably low, and the decision to operate is appropriate in the context of the patient's underlying disease. There are anecdotal reports of successful treatment of pulmonary mucormycosis by surgical resection alone. In most cases, the preoperative diagnosis was uncertain, total excision of all involved lung was accomplished, the diagnosis was established by histopathology of the resected tissue, and the patient recovered fully without other therapy.

When possible, isolated renal mucormycosis in patients with AIDS should be treated with nephrectomy combined with amphotericin B. When nephrectomy is either not possible or is not a reasonable option given the overall condition of the patient, then amphotericin B alone should be used. There are some anecdotal successes using amphotericin B without surgery.

Unfortunately, amphotericin B is not highly effective for mucormycosis. The high dosages recommended are nephrotoxic, particularly in some of the patients most at risk who may have underlying renal dysfunction and are often receiving other nephrotoxic drugs, including aminoglycosides and other antibacterial agents, antiviral agents such as ganciclovir, and immunosuppressives including cyclosporin. Alternative amphotericin preparations, including liposomal formulations, reduce renal toxicity greatly. Although less toxic, they are more expensive and are not proved to be more effective. The dosage is 5 mg/kg/day (or even higher in some cases) and is usually tolerated without renal embarrassment. One large series summarizing the emergency use of amphotericin B lipid complex (ABLC) for all indications includes 24 cases of mucormycosis with 17 partial or complete responses. A similar publication summarizing compassionate use of liposomal AMB (Ambisome) for all indications (from the United Kingdom) includes only three cases of mucormycosis—two rhinocerebral cases that were successfully treated, and one pulmonary case that died within 3 days of onset of treatment. There have also been a few anecdotal reports detailing the successful use of either ABLC or liposomal AMB for various forms of mucormycosis. In toto, these reports suggest some promise for the newer forms of AMB. Further experience will have to be gained before the exact role for these agents is determined.

Finally, hyperbaric oxygen therapy has been proposed as an adjunctive therapy for mucormycosis, based on limited and anecdotal reports. Most published experience has been with the rhinocerebral form of the illness. Although successes have been reported, this therapy is not standard and does not reduce the need for early diagnosis, metabolic control, debridement of all necrotic tissue, and rapid escalation to full doses of either standard or newer lipid-based forms of amphotericin B.

Suggested Reading

Boelaeret JR, et al: The role of desferoxamine in dialysis-associated mucormycosis: report of three cases and review of the literature, *Clin Nephrol* 29:261, 1988.

Couch L, Theilen F, Mader JT: Rhinocerebral mucormycosis with cerebral extension successfully treated with adjunctive hyperbaric oxygen therapy, *Arch Otolaryngol Head Neck Surg* 114;791, 1988.

Ferguson BJ, et al: Adjunctive hyperbaric oxygen for treatment of rhinocerebral mucormycosis, *Rev Inf Dis* 10:551, 1988.

Ng TT, Denning DW: Liposomal amphotericin B (Ambisome) therapy in invasive fungal infections. Evaluation of United Kingdom compassionate use data, *Arch Int Med* 155;1093, 1995.

Walsh TJ, et al: Amphotericin B lipid complex for invasive fungal infectuions: analysis of safety and efficacy in 556 cases, *Clin Inf Dis* 26;1383, 1998.

Walsh TJ, Rinaldi MR, Pizzo PA: Zygomycosis of the respiratory tract. In Sarosi GA, Davies SF, eds: *Fungal diseases of the lung,* New York, 1993, Raven Press.

SPOROTRICHOSIS

Ronald A. Greenfield
E. Nan Scott

Sporotrichosis is a subacute or chronic fungal infection caused by *Sporothrix schenckii*. It occurs most commonly in cutaneous or lymphocutaneous form resulting from direct inoculation of the pathogen but also occurs in various extracutaneous forms. Among the extracutaneous forms, a primary sporotrichotic pneumonia, presumably acquired by inhalation, occurs rarely. More commonly, musculoskeletal or osteoarticular sporotrichosis occurs, either as a result of direct inoculation into tendons, bursae, and joints or as a result of hematogenous dissemination. Hematogenous dissemination may result in disseminated cutaneous sporotrichosis, or infection of a variety of unusual sites, including the meninges.

■ EPIDEMIOLOGY

S. schenckii is widely distributed in nature. It grows on plant debris in soil and on the bark of trees, shrubs, and garden plants. The fungus and the disease occur in much of the world, primarily in the tropical and temperate zones. The abundance of the organism and the reported incidence of the disease shows great geographic variation. The penetrating trauma that introduces the fungal conidia into the human host is most commonly accomplished by splinters, thorns, or woody fragments of plants, but any contact with plants or plant products (e.g., sphagnum peat moss, mulch, hay, timber) accompanying minor skin trauma may initiate infection. Activities most commonly associated with acquisition of sporotrichosis include gardening (particularly rose gardening), landscaping, farming, berry-picking, horticulture, and carpentry. Skin test and serologic surveys demonstrate that most *S. schenckii* inoculations promote the development of resistance without clinically apparent infection. Zoonotic transmission can also occur from infected animals (usually cats or horses with extensive skin lesions) to animal handlers. Both pulmonary and disseminated sporotrichosis appear to occur more commonly in patients with a history of alcoholism.

Patients with immunosuppression from human immunodeficiency virus (HIV) infection and the acquired immunodeficiency syndrome (AIDS) appear to develop disseminated cutaneous sporotrichosis and hematogenously disseminated sporotrichosis, including sporotrichotic meningitis, more often than immunocompetent hosts. Although the incidence of HIV- or AIDS-associated sporotrichosis is not precisely known, the incidence of disseminated sporotrichosis in patients living with AIDS appears to be less than that of other endemic mycoses.

■ LABORATORY DIAGNOSIS

Definitive diagnosis of sporotrichosis requires the isolation of *S. schenckii* in culture specimens from a normally sterile body site. Occasionally, the organism can be visualized in biopsied tissue specimens stained with periodic acid–Schiff, Gomori methenamine silver, or immunochemical stains. The organism can be recovered by fungal culture from sputum; pus, synovial fluid, bone drainage, and surgical specimens. Concentrations of organisms in joint fluid and particularly cerebrospinal fluid (CSF) may be relatively low. Therefore repetitive large-volume cultures may be required for diagnosis. Serologic techniques for measurement of antibody are available but may demonstrate significant interlaboratory variability in sensitivity and specificity; they are best used to suggest the need for more aggressive attempts at definitive diagnosis.

■ CLINICAL MANIFESTATIONS

Cutaneous Sporotrichosis

The primary lesion develops at the site in the skin, 20 to 90 days after inoculation, most typically distally in the upper extremities. Over a few weeks, the initial small nodule enlarges, reddens, becomes pustular, and ulcerates, releasing purulent material from which the organism is readily cultured. Patients are typically afebrile and not systemically ill. In the lymphocutaneous form of the disease, an ascending chain of nodules develops along lymphatic channels of the skin, with the older distal lesions ulcerating and draining and the younger, more proximal lesions forming subcutaneous nodules that attach to the skin as they age and begin to ulcerate. The lesions are usually minimally painful, but extensive disease may result in functional impairment. Some patients exhibit no lymphangitic spread, and the disease presents as an indolent ulcerating plaque that persists for years if untreated. Patients often have received courses of antibacterial therapy without benefit before the process is recognized as sporotrichosis. The lymphocutaneous form of sporotrichosis can be mimicked by *Nocardia, Mycobacterium marinum, Leishmania,* and *Francisella tularensis.*

Pulmonary Sporotrichosis

Pulmonary sporotrichosis is a subacute or chronic pneumonitis with cavitation, usually in the upper lobes, clinically indistinguishable from mycobacterial infection or chronic pulmonary histoplasmosis. Most patients have underlying chronic obstructive pulmonary disease. They present with productive cough with few constitutional symptoms. Diagnosis requires isolation of *S. schenckii* from sputum cultures or its histopathologic recognition in biopsy specimens.

Osteoarticular Sporotrichosis

Lesions of deeper tissues may occur in almost any organ, but there is a distinct predilection for the joints, particularly of the extremities, and the long bones adjacent to these joints. The resulting chronic arthritis is often confused with rheumatoid or other chronic inflammatory arthritis, sometimes for 10 years or more, until destruction of adjacent bone or development of draining fistulae encourage efforts to establish the microbial etiology of the chronic osteomyelitis by culture. Cutaneous or lymphocutaneous lesions are not prominent in these patients. The process generally begins in a single joint, but additional joints may be involved successively. The patient usually has pain on motion, and the involved areas may be warm and red. Functional impairment resulting from osteoarticular sporotrichosis can become very severe.

Disseminated Sporotrichosis

Sporotrichotic lesions occur infrequently in many other organs such as the eye, the prostate, the oral mucosa, and the larynx, and the clinical manifestations in these patients depend on the organ involved. Involvement of the central nervous system (CNS) and meninges, which was distinctly rare in the pre-AIDS era, has become more common but is still rare in patients living with AIDS. Patients may present with subtle changes in mental status as the only symptom, and are found to have a chronic lymphocytic meningitis. Recovery of the fungus from extracutaneous lesions may be difficult, particularly in CNS disease. Elevated serum and often CSF antibody titers are often detectable in these patients and should be measured in all patients with unexplained chronic lymphocytic meningitis; this finding should encourage repeated culture attempts.

■ THERAPY

Spontaneous healing of the cutaneous forms of sporotrichosis has been reported, but without treatment, the lesions usually progress slowly with draining and scarring. Therapy is therefore indicated (Table 1). Historically, cutaneous and lymphocutaneous sporotrichosis have been treated with SSKI, although the mechanism of action and response rate have not been precisely determined. An initial dose of 5 to 10 drops diluted in liquid, preferably fruit juice, is given three times daily after meals and increased dropwise to 120 drops/day or the maximum tolerated by the individual patient (often <60 drops/day). Although relatively inexpensive, this form of therapy is poorly accepted by many patients because of the adverse effects, including increased lacrimation, increased salivation, metallic taste perversion, salivary gland swelling, gastrointestinal upset, and frequent rash. Therefore the orally available azole antifungals have become the therapy of choice for cutaneous or lymphocutaneous sporotrichosis in the developed world. Ketoconazole, 200 to 800 mg orally daily, has been used, but by historical comparison, it is less effective than itraconazole or fluconazole and therefore is no longer indicated. Itraconazole has become the treatment of choice for lymphocutaneous sporotrichosis. Response rates of 89% to 100% have been demonstrated for treatment of cutaneous or lymphocutaneous sporotrichosis with itraconazole, 100 to 200 mg orally daily for 3 to 12 months. Treatment with fluconazole, 200 to 400 mg orally daily, was less effective (71% response rate) than itraconazole by historical comparison. Whether higher dosages of fluconazole may be more effective is speculative. Nonetheless, there is a role for fluconazole therapy for patients who cannot tolerate itraconazole because of adverse effects or drug-drug interactions. Terbinafine shows activity

Table 1 Treatment of Sporotrichosis

FORM OF SPOROTRICHOSIS	PREFERRED TREATMENT	ALTERNATIVE AGENTS
Cutaneous or lymphocutaneous	Itraconazole	SSKI, fluconazole, amphotericin B, ? terbinafine
Pulmonary	Itraconazole	Amphotericin B
Osteoarticular or musculoskeletal	Itraconazole	Fluconazole, amphotericin B
Disseminated	Amphotericin B	Amphotericin B plus flucytosine, ? itraconazole, ? fluconazole

in treatment of lymphocutaneous sporotrichosis, but such therapy cannot be recommended based on limited available data. Treatment for lymphocutaneous sporotrichosis should be continued for 1 month beyond complete healing of all lesions. Because many strains of *S. schenckii* that cause lymphocutaneous disease grow poorly in the laboratory at 37° C (98.5° F), local application of heat may be an effective adjunct to antifungal therapy.

Pulmonary sporotrichosis should be treated with either itraconazole, 200 mg orally twice daily, for patients with non–life-threatening infection or amphotericin B in patients with life-threatening or extensive pulmonary infection. For the latter patients who have the lung capacity to tolerate such a procedure, amphotericin B with subsequent surgical resection of involved lung areas may be the best therapy.

Itraconazole, 200 mg orally twice daily, should be initial therapy for patients with osteoarticular sporotrichosis. As with other joint and bone infections, drainage and debridement are important surgical adjuncts to antimicrobial therapy. Amphotericin B therapy appears to be approximately as effective as itraconazole but is less convenient and associated generally with more common adverse reactions; therefore it is generally used only after failed itraconazole therapy. Fluconazole has been used with only modest success in osteoarticular sporotrichosis. It should therefore be used only when itraconazole and amphotericin B are not tolerated or have failed; in such cases, the minimum dosage should be 800 mg orally daily. Azole treatment should generally be continued for 12 months, therapy with conventional amphotericin B to a total dose of 1 to 2 g or for 6 to 10 weeks.

Sporotrichotic meningitis should be treated with amphotericin B, based on limited numbers of anecdotally reported cases. Based on possible in vitro synergy and anecdotal reports, the addition of flucytosine may be beneficial for patients with recalcitrant meningitis. Itraconazole and fluconazole are inadequately studied to be recommended for this form of sporotrichosis.

Based on anecdotal experience, amphotericin B should be considered initial therapy for patients with disseminated sporotrichosis and AIDS. Itraconazole might be used for non–life-threatening infection and in cases in which CNS involvement has been actively excluded. Itraconazole may also play a role in lifelong suppressive therapy for patients with disseminated sporotrichosis and AIDS after initial induction therapy with amphotericin B.

Suggested Reading

Kauffman CA, Hajjeh R, Chapman SW: Guidelines for the management of patients with sporotrichosis, *Clin Infect Dis* (in press).

Kauffman CA, et al: Treatment of lymphocutaneous and visceral sporotrichosis with fluconazole, *Clin Infect Dis* 22:46, 1996.

Rotz LD, et al: Disseminated sporotrichosis with meningitis in a patient with AIDS, *Infect Dis Clin Practice* 5:566, 1996.

Sharkey-Mathis PK, et al: Treatment of sporotrichosis with itraconazole, *Am J Med* 95:279, 1993.

Winn RE: A contemporary view of sporotrichosis, *Curr Top Med Mycol* 6:73, 1995.

CRYPTOCOCCUS

Woraphot Tantisiriwat
William G. Powderly

Prior to the 1980s, infection with the fungus *Cryptococcus neoformans* was rare, occurring mainly among persons with impaired cell-mediated immunity. Up to half of cases of cryptococcal disease were associated with lymphomas, and many other patients with cryptococcosis received corticosteroid therapy before the onset of the infection. However, since the beginning of the acquired immunodeficiency syndrome (AIDS) epidemic, cryptococcosis has emerged as a major cause of morbidity and mortality in persons infected with the human immunodeficiency virus (HIV), affecting between 5% and 10% of all AIDS patients in the United States, and as one of the most common causes of meningitis in many urban institutions in the United States. With the use of highly active antiretroviral therapy (HAART) for the treatment of HIV infection and the widespread use of the azole antifungals, the incidence of invasive cryptococcosis in the HIV-infected population has declined but has not disappeared.

■ PRESENTATION AND DIAGNOSIS

The most common manifestation of cryptococcal infection is meningitis. Most patients develop insidious features of a subacute meningitis or meningoencephalitis, with fever, malaise, and headache, and are generally symptomatic for at least 2 to 4 weeks before presentation. In patients with a more subacute or chronic course, mental status changes such as forgetfulness and coma can also be seen. Classic meningeal symptoms and signs such as stiff neck and photophobia occur in only about a quarter to a third of all patients and generally are less likely to occur in HIV-positive patients. The typical pattern in the cerebrospinal fluid (CSF) is chronic meningitis with a lymphocytic pleocytosis. However, the CSF may appear normal in HIV-positive patients with cryptococcal meningitis because the usual response to infection is usually markedly blunted. In fact, fewer than half of HIV-positive patients with cryptococcal meningitis have an elevated protein level, only about one-third have hypoglycorrhachea, and only about 20% have more than 20 white blood cells per cubic millimeter of CSF. The opening pressure is usually elevated in patients with cryptococcal meningitis (up to 70% of patients present with pressures greater than 20 cm H_2O) and is an important issue associated with therapy. India ink stain of the CSF is positive, showing encapsulated yeast, in about 75% of cases, and the cryptococcal antigen titer in the CSF is almost invariably positive with sensitivity of 93% to 100% and specificity of 93% to 98%. Serum cryptococcal antigen (sCRAG) is elevated in 95% of patients with meningitis. A positive sCRAG with titer above 1:8 suggests disseminated cryptococcosis. Such patients should be evaluated for possible meningeal involvement. False-positive sCRAG can happen secondary to infection with *Trichosporon beigelii* and secondary to residual disinfectant on laboratory test slides. Culture of *C. neoformans* from any body site should also be regarded as an indication for further evaluation and initiation of therapy. However, colonization of *Cryptococcus* can be found in the respiratory system, and therapy might not be necessary in immunocompetent patients with no symptoms and negative sCRAG.

C. neoformans can invade sites other than the meninges. Isolated pulmonary disease has been well described. It usually presents as a solitary nodule in the absence of other symptoms. Cryptococcus pneumonia has also been described. In immunocompromised patients, especially those with AIDS, disseminated disease is common. About half of HIV-positive patients with cryptococcal meningitis have evidence of pulmonary involvement at presentation, with clinical symptoms such as cough or dyspnea and abnormal chest radiographs. The chest radiographic finding is usually diffuse interstitial infiltrates in immunocompromised patients or focal lesions in immunocompetent patients. Concomitant opportunistic infections, especially with *Pneumocystis carinii,* occur in about 15% to 35% of patients. Cutaneous involvement is common and with this presentation suggests disseminated disease. The most common skin involvement resembles that of molluscum contagiosum. As many as three quarters of patients with cryptococcal meningitis have positive blood cultures. Infection of bone, eye, adrenal glands, prostate, and urinary tract has also been described. The prostate gland represents a reservoir of infection and potential source of reinfection after completion of therapy.

■ THERAPY

Management of cryptococcal infection depends on the extent of disease and the patient's immune status. A solitary pulmonary nodule in a normal host may not need treatment, provided the patient has careful follow-up. The advent of relatively safe antifungals such as fluconazole permits a short course of therapy for most patients with localized disease. Extrapulmonary disease is generally managed in the same way as meningitis. A search for the underlying problems should be initiated in patients who are not known to be immunosuppressed, including an HIV antibody test and CD4 lymphocyte count, because cryptococcal infections have been described as one of manifestations of so-called isolated CD4 T cell lymphocytopenia. Drugs generally used in the treatment of cryptococcal infection are summarized in Table 1.

Cryptococcal Infection in Normal Hosts

Before the AIDS era, the standard treatment for cryptococcal meningitis had been the combination of amphotericin B and flucytosine (5-FC). The National Institute of Allergy and Infectious Disease (NIAID)-sponsored Mycosis Study Group (MSG) showed that amphotericin B, 0.3 mg/kg, plus 5-FC for 6 weeks was effective and less nephrotoxic than amphotericin B, 0.4 mg/kg, given alone for 10 weeks. A subsequent study compared 4 weeks of combination therapy with a 6-week course. That study was designed to randomize patients at the end of a uniform 4-week course of combination therapy. Only 91 of 181 patients initially treated were randomized. Of these 91 patients, cure or improvement was seen in 75% of those receiving 4 weeks of therapy compared with 85% of patients in the 6-week cohort. There was no difference in toxicity between the two regimens. Furthermore, 31 of the 80 nonrandomized patients died, giving an overall acute mortality of 17% with this treatment. This study concluded that 4 weeks of combination therapy was acceptable for patients who did not have risk factors that correlated with a high frequency of relapse. The factors predicting relapse are shown in Table 2. The MSG

Table 1   Drugs Used in the Treatment of Cryptococcal Infection

DRUGS	DOSAGE	SIDE EFFECTS	DRUG INTERACTIONS	COMMENTS
Amphotericin B	0.7-1.0 mg/kg/day 3-6 mg/kg/day (liposomal) 5 mg/kg/day (lipid complex)	Immediate hypersensitivity reaction, fever, hypotension, nausea and vomiting during administration, hypokalemia, and nephrotoxicity	Nephrotoxic drugs (e.g., aminoglycosides, pentamidine, foscarnet, cidofovir)	Liposomal or lipid complex formulation should be considered in patients with renal dysfunction
Flucytosine (5-FC)	25 mg/kg q6h	Gastrointestinal, bone marrow suppression	Nephrotoxic drugs	Dosage must be reduced in patients with renal dysfunction; drug level should be monitored
Fluconazole	400 mg/day (acute therapy), 200 mg/day (suppressive therapy)	Nausea, rash, and hepatitis	Rifabutin (increased rifabutin levels); rifampin (decreased fluconazole levels)	Dosage may need to be adjusted in renal dysfunction
Itraconazole	200-400 mg bid	Nausea, abdominal pain, rash, headache, edema, and hypokalemia	Rifamycins, ritonavir, phenobarbitol, phenytoin all decrease itraconazole levels The effect of nevirapine is unknown; the drug should not be used concomitantly with terfenadine or astemizole Antacids, H_2-blockers decrease itraconazole absorption Itraconazole itself acts as a moderate inhibitor of cytochrome P450 system and can increase levels of indinavir, cyclosporin, digoxin, and phenytoin	Absorption of itraconazole is dependent on food and gastric acid and may be erratic; the newer solution is better absorbed

Table 2 Factors Predicting Relapse of Cryptococcal Meningitis
Immunosuppression
Presentation with neurologic abnormalities
CSF leukocyte count <20 cells/mm^3
CSF antigen titer >1:32
Positive India ink stain after 4 wk of treatment
CSF antigen titer greater than 1:8 after 4 wk of treatment

CSF, Cerebrospinal fluid.

Table 3 Factors at Baseline Predictive of a Poor Outcome in AIDS Patients with Cryptococcal Meningitis
Decreased mental status at diagnosis
CSF leukocyte count <20 cells/mm^3
High titer of CSF cryptococcal antigen
Positive blood culture for *C. neoformans*
Age <35 yr
Hyponatremia

CSF, Cerebrospinal fluid.

investigators suggested that patients at risk of relapse were candidates for longer therapy.

Untreated cryptococcal meningitis is uniformly fatal, so all patients with meningitis must be treated. The issue that arises when reviewing the previous NIAID/MSG studies is the dosage of the amphotericin B. Since these studies were conducted, clinicians have become much more familiar with amphotericin B and its toxicities. The use of saline loading (i.e., giving a bolus of 250 to 500 ml of normal saline before amphotericin B infusions) appears to minimize nephrotoxicity. Our preference is to administer higher dosages of amphotericin B (0.7 mg/kg) as treatment for cryptococcal meningitis. Although it is unclear whether 5-FC is necessary with higher dosages of amphotericin B, we recommend its use at a dosage of 37.5 mg/kg four times daily. Levels must be measured to minimize toxicity (especially bone marrow suppression), and dosages must be adjusted for renal insufficiency.

It is clear that normal subjects with no evident risk factors for a poor outcome respond well to 4 weeks of combination therapy, and this is often curative. Azole therapy (i.e., fluconazole, 400 mg orally daily) for 3 to 6 months is likely to be effective in such patients but has not been well studied. Pulmonary cryptococcosis without meningeal involvement can be treated initially with fluconazole. However, for meningitis, there is no controlled trial of fluconazole, especially comparing initial azole therapy with an amphotericin B–based regimen. With current available data, we still recommend amphotericin B plus 5-FC as standard therapy for cryptococcal meningitis. Fluconazole can be used to treat patients (or to complete a course of treatment) who cannot tolerate amphotericin B or patients without neural involvement. Immunocompetent patients probably do not require any long-term suppressive therapy.

Cryptococcal Infection in AIDS

In early reports, the experience with treatment with amphotericin B and 5-FC regimens in patients with AIDS was not favorable, and the acute mortality was reported to be 10% to 25%. In addition, the regimen was thought to be too toxic for patients with AIDS. Multiple clinical factors have been identified in studies as predictors of a poor outcome, as summarized in Table 3. These initial poor outcomes led to a search for more effective treatment strategies.

The availability of the orally active antifungal triazoles fluconazole and itraconazole led to a number of controlled comparative trials. In each trial, the azole antifungals were effective in about 50% of patients. Similarly, in a study

directly comparing fluconazole and itraconazole, fewer than 50% of patients responded to either drug. Thus at least 50% of patients treated initially with azole antifungals will fail to respond. Most studies of amphotericin B report response rates of 70% to 80% or more. The lowest response rates with amphotericin B occurred in the NIAID randomized prospective trial comparing fluconazole with amphotericin B. Fewer than 50% of patients had complete clinical and mycologic responses. Although there was no significant difference in the overall mortality between the two groups, mortality was higher during the first 2 weeks of therapy with fluconazole. As with some other trials, the dosage of amphotericin B may have been too low with the median dosage of 0.4 mg/kg.

Given this experience, the NIAID/MSG and the AIDS Clinical Trials Group (ACTG) investigated a strategy of induction amphotericin B (for 2 weeks) followed by azole treatment. Patients with cryptococcal meningitis were randomized to receive 2 weeks of amphotericin B (0.7 mg/kg/day) with either 5-FC (25 mg/kg every 6 hours) or matching placebo. The study was designed to address two questions: (1) Does adding 5-FC to amphotericin B as induction therapy for cryptococcal meningitis improve 2- or 10-week survival compared with induction with amphotericin B alone, and (2) is itraconazole as effective as fluconazole in suppressing relapse of cryptococcal meningitis during the maintenance phrase of treatment? At the end of 2 weeks, patients who were stable or improved were again randomized to receive either fluconazole, 400 mg per day, or itraconazole, 200 mg twice daily. The acute mortality with this regimen was 6%. The addition of 5-FC to amphotericin B did not improve the mortality and clinical course. However, 5-FC was well tolerated. Furthermore, the use of 5-FC as initial therapy has been associated with a decreased risk of later relapse of cryptococcal meningitis. There was no significant difference in clinical symptoms, response rate, or mortality among patients randomized to either fluconazole or itraconazole. In light of these data, we recommend this approach as a standard one for the treatment of acute cryptococcal meningitis in AIDS (Figure 1).

The availability of the alternative formulations of amphotericin B raises the issue of their use in cryptococcal meningitis. A randomized study comparing amphotericin B lipid complex with amphotericin B deoxycholate in 55 HIV-positive patients with cryptococcal meningitis noted less hematologic toxicity and nephrotoxicity in the lipid complex arm. There was no difference in mycologic outcome. Small randomized studies of liposomal amphotericin

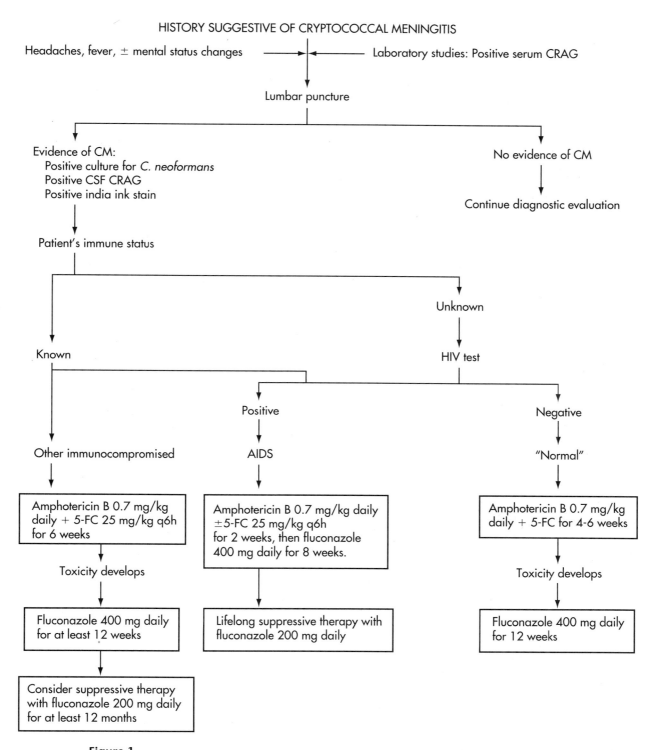

Figure 1
Algorithm for the diagnosis and treatment of cryptococcal meningitis (CM). *AIDS,* Acquired immunodeficiency syndrome; *CRAG,* cryptococcal antigen; *CSF,* cerebrospinal fluid; *5-FC,* flucytosine; *HIV,* human immunodeficiency virus.

B (4 mg/kg) compared with conventional amphotericin B (0.7 mg/kg) noted an earlier CSF sterilization rate in patients in the liposomal preparation arm with also less nephrotoxicity. Thus the role of lipid preparations of amphotericin B remains uncertain, although they may be useful in patients with impaired renal function.

There remains some interest in oral therapy. Initial experience with combination of fluconazole (400 mg/day) with 5-FC (150 mg/kg/day) showed that 75% of CSF culture were negative with median time of 23 days, which was less than previously reported times with either drug alone. Almost 30% of patients had to discontinue 5-FC because of dose-limiting adverse effects. Another study suggests that combination of 5-FC with high dosages of fluconazole (800 to 2000 mg/day) is associated with initial response rate of more than 70%. A small number of patients have also been treated successfully with the combination of itraconazole and 5-FC. Further studies should determine the value of these combination therapies. The combination of amphotericin B with azoles is also worth further study; an initial trial comparing amphotericin B combined with itraconazole had a better outcome compared with amphotericin B alone.

An important aspect of management of acute cryptococcal meningitis in AIDS is the recognition that clinical deterioration may be caused by increased intracranial pressure (ICP), which may not respond rapidly to antifungal therapy. Analyses have shown a relationship between baseline opening pressure and long-term outcome, with the median survival in patients with the highest pressures being significantly less than that in patients whose pressure were normal. We believe that all patients with cryptococcal meningitis should have opening pressure measured when a lumbar puncture is performed and strong consideration should be given to reducing such pressure if the opening pressure is high (>25 cm H_2O). Lumbar puncture with removal of 30 ml of spinal fluid daily is often effective. If elevated opening pressure persists with neurologic symptoms despite serial lumbar puncture, lumbar drainage should be considered. Some patients have required placement of lumbar peritoneal shunts for persistently elevated ICP despite successful antifungal therapy. The role of corticosteroids in this situation is not known and we do not recommend their use.

Lifelong maintenance therapy is required in AIDS patients with cryptococcal infection to prevent relapse of infection. Relapse rates of 50% to 60% and a shorter life expectancy have been reported in patients who did not receive long-term suppressive therapy. Fluconazole, 200 mg daily, is the drug of choice. Routine monitoring by measurement of sCRAG has not been shown to predict relapse, although elevations of antigen in the CSF may predict recurrence.

Cryptococcal Infection in Other Immunocompromised Hosts

Management of cryptococcal meningitis in the setting of organ transplantation or lymphoma is also uncertain. The MSG found patients with underlying immunosuppression to have poor outcomes when treated with amphotericin B and 5-FC and to be likely to relapse. Furthermore, amphotericin B nephrotoxocity complicates the use of immunosuppressives such as cyclosporin in such patients. However, there is very little published experience with the use of fluconazole or itraconazole or fluconazole plus 5-FC in this setting, and these agents are also associated with significant drug interactions. We recommend an approach similar to that used with AIDS patients (i.e., an initial period of treatment with amphotericin B plus 5-flucytosine followed by fluconazole). An area of considerable uncertainty is the duration of fluconazole therapy after acute therapy. We currently recommend suppressive antifungal therapy for at least 1 year after the completion of acute treatment.

Suggested Reading

Aberg JA, Powderly WG: Cryptococcal disease: implications of recent clinical trials on treatment and management, *AIDS Clin Rev* 1997/1998: 229, 1998.

Dismukes WE, et al: Treatment of cryptococcal meningitis with combination of amphotericin B and flucytosine for 4 as compared with 6 weeks, *N Engl J Med* 317:334, 1987.

Mundy LM, Powderly WG: Invasive fungal infections: cryptococcosis, *Sem Respir Crit Care Med* 18:249, 1997.

Powderly WG: Recent advances in the management of cryptococcal meningitis in patients with AIDS, *Clin Infect Dis* 22(suppl 2):S119, 1996.

Saag MS, et al: Comparison of amphotericin B with fluconazole in the treatment of acute AIDS-associated cryptococcal meningitis, NEJM 326:83, 1992.

Van Der Horst CM, et al: Treatment of cryptococcal meningitis associated with the acquired immunodeficiency syndrome, *N Engl J Med* 337:15, 1997.

HISTOPLASMOSIS

Mitchell Goldman
George A. Sarosi

Histoplasmosis is the illness caused by the thermal dimorphic fungus *Histoplasma capsulatum.* The spectrum of histoplasmosis ranges from asymptomatic skin test conversion to a rapidly fatal pulmonary or widely disseminated illness.

The epidemiology of histoplasmosis is well understood. The fungus is a soil-dwelling organism that requires large amounts of organic nitrogen for growth. This growth requirement explains the common occurrence of histoplasmosis in association with chicken coops, bat caves, and bird roosts. In nature, the organism grows as a mycelium, producing small infective particles 2 to 5 μm in size. When the site harboring the fungus is disturbed, these infecting spores become airborne and an infectious aerosol is produced.

The inhaled spores reach the alveoli, where they convert to the tissue-invasive form, a small yeast. Multiplication of the yeast is by binary fission. Nonimmune phagocytosis cannot kill these yeasts, and during the preimmune phase of the illness, they spread to organs rich in cells of the reticuloendothelial (RE) system. After development of adequate cell-mediated immunity (CMI), the armed macrophages kill the fungi, ending the infection.

Most normal individuals develop adequate CMI; thus recovery from acute histoplasmosis is the rule. In occasional patients with an overwhelming infection or in individuals whose CMI is faulty, progressive dissemination ensues.

■ CLINICAL MANIFESTATIONS

Most infected individuals do not develop clinical illness. The only evidence of the infection is the conversion of the histoplasmin skin test to positive. A small minority of patients who inhale infecting particles develop acute illness. The illness is influenza-like, with rapid onset of fever and chills and a brassy, nonproductive cough. Erythema multiforme or erythema nodosum often occurs simultaneously. These symptoms develop approximately 14 days after the exposure, and the disease usually runs its course in 2 weeks or so. Occasional patients in whom the infective dose is exceptionally high may develop an acute, fulminant pneumonitis with life-threatening hypoxia. Unless it is recognized and treated quickly, respiratory insufficiency may cause death.

The chest radiograph commonly shows single or multiple areas of pneumonitis, often with involvement of the ipsilateral hilar lymph nodes. When the inhaled dose is unusually large, the chest radiograph shows large numbers of nodular lesions. In patients with abnormal lungs, such as smokers with centrilobular emphysema, the acute infection may involve the upper lung zones. In these instances the infiltrate outlines preexisting air spaces, mimicking reinfection tuberculosis. Even so, most of these infections will clear completely.

The pulmonary lesions of histoplasmosis are slow to heal. Although many disappear completely, often healing occurs by rounding off of the infiltrate. These areas undergo fibrosis, producing the characteristic coin lesion seen in so many patients in the endemic area. When these lesions calcify, they produce a highly characteristic lesion in which central calcification is surrounded by layers of thinner calcification. In the absence of these telltale signs of their benign nature, the lesions cannot be readily distinguished from malignant neoplasms.

Even though most patients with primary pulmonary histoplasmosis recover completely, often there is residual local disease within the thorax. In addition to the coin lesion, mediastinal lymph nodes may be enlarged, causing diagnostic concern. Perhaps the most feared late complication of healing histoplasmosis is mediastinal fibrosis. In this instance, exuberant fibroblastic proliferation entraps vital mediastinal structures, leading to superior vena cava syndrome.

■ PROGRESSIVE DISSEMINATED HISTOPLASMOSIS

During the preimmune phase of the infection, the fungus gains access to the circulation via the hilar lymph nodes, usually traveling within macrophages. It is highly likely that fungemia occurs in all infected patients. The circulating yeasts of *H. capsulatum* are taken out of the circulation by cells of the RE system, where they multiply. After development of adequate CMI, the cells of the RE system destroy the fungus, leading to granuloma formation and eventual fibrosis. In patients with faulty CMI, this process does not occur, and progressive multiplication of the fungus leads to death of the host.

Clinically, progressive disseminated histoplasmosis (PDH) is a severe systemic illness. Although the tempo of the disease varies from patient to patient, most individuals develop a rapidly progressive wasting systemic illness. Fever and cough may be present, and the cough is usually nonproductive. Physical examination often shows only signs of recent weight loss. Occasionally, patients show either cutaneous ulcers or ulcers in the mucocutaneous junctions, such as in the buccal cavity, teeming with the fungus. Hepatosplenomegaly is frequently present. The laboratory evaluation is not diagnostic, although pancytopenia resulting from bone marrow involvement is common. The chest radiograph is quite variable. Some individuals have negative chest radiographs, but most often the disease appears as a diffuse reticulonodular infiltrate involving both lungs.

Histopathologic examination of involved tissues shows two distinct histopathologic types, the so-called infantile form originally described in children, with which there is virtually no attempt at granuloma formation, and the adult form, with well-formed granulomas. Special stains usually show numerous organisms in the infantile form, while the organisms are difficult to find in the adult form.

Table 1   Treatment of Histoplasmosis

TYPE OF INFECTION	MILD TO MODERATE SEVERITY	SEVERE ILLNESS
Acute pulmonary	Observe; if no improvement after 1 month, ITRA, 200 mg/day for 12 wk	AMB, 0.7 mg/kg/day until stable, then ITRA, 400 mg/day to complete 12 wk; consider adjunctive corticosteroids
Cavitary	ITRA, 400 mg/day for 12-24 mo, or AMB, 35 mg/kg total dose over 12 wk	AMB, 0.7 mg/kg/day until improvement noted, then ITRA, 200-400 mg/day to complete 12-24 mo, or AMB, 35 mg/kg total dose over 12 wk
Progressive disseminated Non-AIDS	ITRA, 200-400 mg/day for 6 to 18 mo	AMB, 0.7 mg/kg/day until stable, then ITRA, 200-400 mg/day for 6-18 mo
Progressive disseminated AIDS	ITRA, 200-400 mg/day for life	AMB, 0.7 mg/kg/day until stable, then ITRA, 200-400 mg/day for life

AMB, Amphotericin B; *ITRA,* itraconazole; *AIDS,* acquired immunodeficiency syndrome.

Before the widespread use of glucocorticoids and cytotoxic chemotherapy, most patients recognized with PDH had diseases known to depress CMI, such as Hodgkin's disease. This group of patients is still at risk, but at present, human immunodeficiency virus (HIV)-infected individuals are at greatest risk for PDH.

In endemic areas, PDH is an opportunistic infection complicating the course of HIV disease. It is a rapidly progressive, chronic wasting disease, and although eventually all patients have an abnormal chest radiograph, often it is negative at the time of presentation.

■ DIAGNOSIS

The gold standard for diagnosis is the recovery of fungus in culture from biologic material. Although recovery of the organism in a mycology laboratory is not difficult, it is time-consuming, often requiring 30 days. In addition, sputum or other respiratory secretions are seldom obtained from patients with acute pulmonary histoplasmosis.

For that reason, serodiagnosis is the cornerstone of diagnosis in histoplasmosis. The time-honored complement fixation (CF) test becomes positive 3 weeks after the onset of infection, and by 6 weeks diagnostic titer may be obtained in as many as three quarters of the patients. The immunodiffusion test lacks both specificity and sensitivity. A histoplasma polysaccharide antigen test is extremely useful in the diagnosis of histoplasmosis in HIV-infected patients, whose burden of organisms is high. The test lacks adequate sensitivity for patients with a low infecting dose.

Histopathologic examination of biologic material such as is obtained from a cutaneous ulcer, bronchoalveolar lavage, or bone marrow examination should be examined with special stains. Most laboratories use one of the modifications of the silver stain, but we prefer the periodic acid–Schiff stain. The recent development of the lysis centrifugation blood culture system has improved diagnostic accuracy, especially in patients with a high burden of organisms. The blood culture becomes positive in 3 to 5 days, significantly shortening the time required for diagnosis.

■ THERAPY

The overwhelming majority of acutely infected individuals have self-limited infections and require no treatment. Treatment with oral itraconazole, 200 mg once or twice daily for 12 weeks, should be considered for those with localized pulmonary histoplasmosis who show no clinical improvement after 1 month of observation. In patients who develop overwhelming pulmonary infection and manifest severe gas exchange problems, intravenous amphotericin B should be started promptly. We recommend daily amphotericin B at 0.7 mg/kg/day until the patient is clinically stable, then a switch to oral itraconazole, 200 mg twice daily. Because the inflammatory response may contribute to the pathogenesis of the respiratory compromise in immunocompetent patients with acute overwhelming histoplasmosis, corticosteroids can be helpful. Although the use of corticosteroids for these patients has not been tested, prednisone as adjunctive therapy, administered at 60 mg daily for 2 weeks, could be considered (Table 1).

Progressive upper lobe histoplasmosis can be treated adequately with oral itraconazole, 200 once or twice daily, or if cost is a major consideration, oral ketoconazole, 400 to 800 mg daily, can be used. For patients who are severely ill, initial treatment with intravenous amphotericin B at a dosage of 0.7 mg/kg/day is recommended, followed by oral itraconazole. In individuals whose upper lobe cavitary histoplasmosis fails to respond to oral azole therapy, amphotericin B at a total dose of 35 mg/kg over 12 to 16 weeks should be administered. The likelihood of clinical response for this condition is high, and frequency of relapse if low.

Patients who are severely ill with progressive disseminated histoplasmosis should initially be treated with intravenous amphotericin B at a dosage of 0.7 to 1.0 mg/kg/day. After clinical improvement, a switch to oral itraconazole at a dosage of 200 to 400 mg daily is recommended. For patients with progressive disseminated histoplasmosis with mild to moderate severity of illness, consideration of initiating therapy with oral itraconazole at 200 to 400 mg daily is appropriate. In patients whose immunosuppressive state is transient, a total dose of 40 mg/kg of amphotericin B or completing 6 to 18 months of therapy with itraconazole is likely to be adequate. In patients whose immunocompromised state cannot be improved, such as patients with acquired immunodeficiency syndrome (AIDS), lifelong suppression with itraconazole, 200 mg daily, is recommended.

Suggested Reading

Davies SF: Serodiagnosis of histoplasmosis, *Semin Respir Infect* 1:9, 1986.

Goodwin RA Jr, DesPrez RM: Histoplasmosis: state of the art, *Am Rev Respir Dis* 117:929, 1978.

Goodwin RA Jr, et al: Disseminated histoplasmosis: clinical and pathologic correlations, *Medicine* 59:1, 1980.

Sarosi GA, Davies SF: Therapy for fungal infections, *Mayo Clin Proc* 69:1111, 1994.

Wheat J. Histoplasmosis: experience during outbreaks in Indianapolis and review of the literature. *Medicine* 76:339, 1997.

BLASTOMYCOSIS

Peter G. Pappas

Blastomycosis is a systemic pyogranulomatous disease caused by the thermally dimorphic fungus *Blastomyces dermatitidis*. The disease is endemic to parts of the midwestern and south central United States and Canada, although blastomycosis has been reported worldwide, including isolated reports from Africa and Central and South America. Within the United States and Canada, the disease is concentrated in areas along the Mississippi and Ohio River basins and the Great Lakes. In endemic areas, small point-source outbreaks of blastomycosis have been associated with recreational and occupational activities occurring in wooded areas along waterways. Current evidence indicates that *B. dermatitidis* exists in warm moist soil enriched by organic debris, including decaying vegetation and wood.

Most infections with *B. dermatitidis* occur through inhalation of aerosolized spores, although infection through direct inoculation has been reported rarely. Primary infections are usually asymptomatic or may result in a self-limited flulike illness. Hematogenous dissemination of organisms from the lung can result in extrapulmonary manifestations.

Blastomycosis is usually recognized as a chronic, indolent systemic fungal infection associated with various pulmonary and extrapulmonary manifestations. Pulmonary blastomycosis usually manifests as a chronic pneumonia syndrome characterized by productive cough, chest pain, hemoptysis, weight-loss, and low-grade fever. There are no distinguishing radiologic features of pulmonary blastomycosis, although one or more fibronodular infiltrates or mass lesions with or without cavitation are common, often mimicking other granulomatous diseases or bronchogenic carcinoma. Hilar adenopathy and pleural effusions are uncommon. Rarely, diffuse pulmonary infiltrates consistent with adult respiratory distress syndrome may occur secondary to blastomycosis. The skin is involved in 40% to 80% of cases, and multiple organ involvement occurs in approximately 50% to 60% of cases. After lung and skin disease, bone and joint disease is most common, followed by disease of the male genitourinary tract (especially the prostate and epididymis). Central nervous system (CNS) involvement is uncommon but may present as either granulomatous meningitis or an intracerebral mass lesion. *B. dermatitidis* is an uncommon opportunistic pathogen but may cause overwhelming disease in the immunocompromised host. Among patients with predisposing factors, chronic glucocorticosteroid use, solid organ transplant recipients, and advanced human immunodeficiency virus (HIV) disease are the most common underlying conditions.

◼ DIAGNOSIS

The definitive diagnosis of blastomycosis requires a positive culture for *B. dermatitidis* from clinical specimens. A presumptive diagnosis is based on the finding of broad-based budding yeasts with doubly refractile cell walls compatible with *B. dermatitidis* on histopathologic examination of clinical specimens. Ten percent KOH is used to prepare wet specimens for examination, whereas fixed specimens are usually stained with hematoxylin and eosin, periodic acid–Schiff (PAS), or Giomori's methenamine silver (GMS) reagents. Serologic assays are of limited value in the diagnosis of blastomycosis. The complement fixation assay for serum antibody is highly cross-reactive and of little diagnostic value. Recent studies suggest that immunodiffusion or enzyme immunoassay tests for A antigen of *B. dermatitidis* or antibody to more purified antigens have potential as serologic markers of disease. The blastomycin skin test antigen lacks sufficient sensitivity and specificity and should not be used as a diagnostic test.

◼ TREATMENT

Presently, three drugs are approved for the treatment of blastomycosis: amphotericin B, itraconazole, and ketoconazole. Traditionally, amphotericin B has been the mainstay of therapy for all forms of blastomycosis, but studies and experience gained over the last 15 years indicate that ketoconazole, itraconazole, and fluconazole are highly effective alternative oral therapies, particularly in patients with chronic indolent disease without involvement of the CNS. Although no comparative trials have been performed, itraconazole appears to have greater efficacy and less toxicity than either fluconazole or ketoconazole and therefore is the oral agent of choice. In a recently published trial, 95% of patients with non–life-threatening, non-CNS blastomycosis were treated successfully with itraconazole, 200 to 400 mg daily for 2 to 6 months. This approximates the observed efficacy seen with amphotericin B. Clinical data regarding the use of ketoconazole and fluconazole suggests similar efficacy of these two agents, with at least 80% of patients responding to 400 to 800 mg daily for 6 months. Most patients with blastomycosis can be started on oral itraconazole, 200 mg daily and advanced by 100-mg increments at monthly intervals to a maximum of 400 mg daily in patients with persistent or progressive disease. In patients with more aggressive disease, an initial dose of 400 mg is appropriate. Ketoconazole and fluconazole are usually initiated at a dose of 400 mg daily and advanced by 200-mg increments monthly to 800 mg daily in patients with persistent or progressive disease. Therapy with any of the azoles should be given for a minimum of 6 months. Among the azoles, ketoconazole is the least well tolerated, but it is considerably less expensive than either itraconazole or fluconazole.

Amphotericin B should be reserved for patients with overwhelming life-threatening or CNS disease, patients who are immunocompromised, and those in whom oral therapy has failed. A total dose of 1.5 to 2.5 g is sufficient therapy for most patients. In selected patients, an induction dose of amphotericin B (totaling about 500 mg) for a rapid fungicidal effect to gain control of the disease may be useful, followed by oral therapy with itraconazole for at least 6 months. For patients with CNS involvement, several reports suggest that fluconazole, the only azole with significant CNS penetration, may have potential as a therapeutic agent among individuals who have had an initial favorable response to amphotericin B. There is only limited experience and few published data concerning the use of the lipid formulation of amphotericin B in the treatment of blastomycosis. There are no data to suggest superior efficacy of these agents compared with conventional (deoxycholate) amphotericin B, and their use should probably be restricted to patients with preexisting renal disease and in whom renal or other dose-limiting toxicities occur while receiving amphotericin B.

The treatment of acute pulmonary blastomycosis remains controversial. Many investigators suggest close observation without therapy in patients who are not immunocompromised. Available data suggest that most cases resolve spontaneously without therapy, although careful long-term evaluation of these untreated patients is important to monitor for evidence of active disease.

All patients with chronic blastomycosis should receive antifungal therapy. Cure rates of at least 90% should be expected, with relapse rates of less than 10%. A few patients, especially chronically immunocompromised individuals such as solid organ transplant recipients, patients receiving chronic glucocorticosteroid treatment, and patients with acquired immunodeficiency syndrome (AIDS), require long-term suppressive therapy to prevent relapse.

Suggested Reading

Bradsher RW: Blastomycosis, *Infect Dis Clin North Am* 2:877, 1988.

Chapman SW, et al: Guidelines for the management of patients with blastomycosis, *Clin Infect Dis* (in press).

Dismukes WE, et al: Treatment of blastomycosis and histoplasmosis with ketoconazole: results of a prospective randomized clinical trial, *Ann Intern Med* 103:861, 1985.

Dismukes WE, et al: Itraconazole therapy for blastomycosis and histoplasmosis, *Am J Med* 93:489, 1992.

Meyer KC, McManus EJ, Maki DG: Overwhelming pulmonary blastomycosis associated with the adult respiratory distress syndrome, *N Engl J Med* 329:1231, 1993.

Pappas PG, et al: Blastomycosis in immunocompromised patients, *Medicine* 72:311, 1993.

Pappas PG, et al: Treatment of blastomycosis with higher dose fluconazole, *Clin Infect Dis* 25:200, 1997.

Sarosi GA, Davies SF, Phillips JR: Self-limited blastomycosis: a report of 39 cases, *Semin Resp Infect* 1:40, 1986.

COCCIDIOIDOMYCOSIS

Stanley C. Deresinski

■ BACKGROUND

Coccidioidomycosis, first described just more than a century ago by Alejandro Posada, is a disease of protean manifestations endemic to portions of the Lower Sonoran Life Zone of the southwestern United States and northern Mexico, and scattered areas in Central and South America. The etiologic agent, *Coccidioides immitis*, is a dimorphic fungus that exists in its soil reservoir in the mycelial phase. Under appropriate conditions, arthroconidia disarticulate from the mycelia and are carried airborne and inhaled, reaching the alveoli of the unfortunate host. There the organism converts to the spherule phase, which then reproduces by endosporulation. Infection may be controlled locally at the site of alveolar implantation or may spread, both within the lungs and distantly, via the bloodstream. Disseminated infection, especially when it involves the meninges, carries with it a potentially high mortality rate.

After an incubation period of 10 to 21 days, approximately 40% of acutely infected individuals develop symptoms of fever, cough, myalgias, and arthralgias, which may last for several weeks. Some of these patients may develop a diffuse erythematous macular skin eruption, erythema nodosum, or less commonly, erythema multiforme. These lesions are the result of hypersensitivity reactions to the fungus, possibly with immune complex formation, as is a self-limited arthritis ("desert rheumatism"), which may also occur. Of patients, 5% to 10% develop persisting pulmonary nodules or cavities. Clinically important dissemination of the infection is fortunately uncommon, occurring in fewer than 1% of those infected.

Certain characteristics define individuals or groups with an increased risk of dissemination (Table 1) or progressive pneumonitis. These include those who are pregnant (especially in the third trimester) or in the immediate postpartum state, the presence of immunocompromising disease or therapies, and being Filipino. African-Americans and Hispanics also appear to be at increased risk of dissemination. Pregnant patients who develop erythema nodosum appear to have a low risk of an adverse outcome of infection.

Skin lesions are the most commonly recognized evidence of extrapulmonary dissemination. These lesions may take a variety of forms, including verrucous papules, plaques, and pustules. Other sites of clinically important dissemination include bone and joints, lymph nodes, liver, spleen, genitourinary tract, peritoneum, retina, thyroid, and the meninges.

C. immitis causes a chronic granulomatous meningitis with typical findings of a predominantly mononuclear pleocytosis with high cerebrospinal fluid (CSF) protein and low glucose concentration. Hydrocephalus develops commonly, even in the face of treatment.

The diagnosis of coccidioidomycosis is best made by direct examination of tissues or secretions and by culture, which requires 2 to 6 days for recovery of the organism. Skin testing with coccidiodal antigens is not useful diagnostically. Serologic tests, on the other hand, are both sensitive (except in some severely immunocompromised patients, such as those with advanced human immunodeficiency virus [HIV]-related disease) and specific. Furthermore, the height of the complement-fixing antibody titer correlates with the extent of the disease so that most patients with dissemination have titers of 1:16 or greater. Patients with dissemination only to the meninges often have relatively low titers. Culture of CSF in coccidiodal meningitis yields the organism in only a minority, but antibodies to the organism can be detected in the fluid in more than 90% of cases.

■ TREATMENT

When treatment is indicated, the choice is between amphotericin B and the azoles. Table 2 summarizes treatment recommendations. Many clinicians continue to prefer amphotericin B for initial therapy of life-threatening, rapidly progressive infection, with substitution of azole therapy after stabilization. Insufficient data exist with regard to the use of lipid-associated amphotericin B in the treatment of patients with coccidioidomycosis. Whether an azole is used initially or in later replacement of amphotericin B, either fluconazole or itraconazole may be safely chosen. Itraconazole was compared with fluconazole in the treatment of 191 patients with coccidioidomycosis, including 70 with pulmonary, 71 with soft-tissue, and 50 with bone/joint infection. The response (50% improvement by 8 months) rates in the total group were 50% in the fluconazole and 63% in those assigned itraconazole ($p = .07$). There was also a trend toward statistical significance in those with bone/joint infection, with response rates of 26% in the fluconazole and 52% in the itraconazole group ($p = .06$).

There is a tendency to use increasingly higher dosages of azoles. To ensure adequate bioavailability, patients treated with orally administered itraconazole should have assessment of blood levels of this drug and, preferably, its active metabolite, hydroxyitraconazole.

■ PRIMARY PULMONARY INFECTION

In most cases, primary infection with *C. immitis* is self-limited, and no controlled studies evaluating the efficacy of treatment of patients without evidence of disseminated or

Table 1   Risk Factors for Dissemination
Ethnicity: Filipino > African-American > Hispanic
Pregnancy
Immunodeficiency states, including acquired immunodeficiency syndrome

---

Table 2   Summary of Treatment Recommendations

PRIMARY PULMONARY

No dissemination risk: observe or treat with fluconazole, 400 mg daily, or itraconazole, 200 mg bid for approximately 3-6 mo or for 3 mo after resolution of clinical infection.

Dissemination risk or progressive pulmonary: fluconazole, ≥400 mg daily, or itraconazole, ≥200 mg bid for approximately 3-6 mo, including for 3 mo after resolution of clinical infection.

PULMONARY CAVITY (UNCOMPLICATED) OR FIBRONODULAR DISEASE

Fluconazole, 400 mg daily for 6-12 mo.

PROGRESSIVE PULMONARY OR DISSEMINATED (NONMENINGEAL):

Immediately life-threatening: amphotericin B, 0.6-1.0 mg/kg/day to approximate total of 2000 mg; consideration given to switching to fluconazole or itraconazole when disease under control. Alternatively, fluconazole, ≥400 mg daily, or itraconazole, ≥200 mg bid. The duration of therapy is usually at least 1 yr; some patients may require lifelong therapy.

Slowly progressive or stable: fluconazole, ≥400 mg daily, or itraconazole, ≥200 mg bid. The duration of therapy is usually at least 1 yr; some patients may require lifelong therapy.

Meningitis

Fluconazole, ≥400 mg daily, or itracoazole, ≥200 mg bid.

or

Amphotericin B directly into cerebrospinal fluid together with systemic therapy followed by oral fluconazole.

HIV-infected patients

All HIV-infected patients with coccidioidomycosis should receive, after control of the infection with amphotericin B (or, in the case of mild disease in low risk patients, an azole), lifelong suppressive therapy with fluconazole or itraconazole.

Pregnant patients

Amphotericin B, 0.6-1.0 mg/kg/day.

HIV, Human immunodeficiency virus.

---

progressive disease have been performed. For this reason, many clinicians do not treat such patients unless they fall into one of the described groups at higher risk of dissemination. Nonetheless, despite the lack of solid evidence that therapy shortens the duration of symptoms or prevents dissemination, it is reasonable to consider treatment of at least some low-risk patients, especially those most acutely ill. The presence of a high complement-fixing antibody titer and/or the absence of a delayed hypersensitivity reaction to antigens of *C. immitis* in a patient who otherwise appears to be at low risk for dissemination adds weight to the argument for the potential benefits of treatment.

Patients with apparently uncomplicated primary pulmonary infection who fall into any of the risks groups described earlier should also be treated, most often with an azole. Pregnant patients should be treated with amphotericin B. The required duration of treatment is uncertain but should probably be at least 3 months or for 3 months after resolution of clinically apparent disease. Patients in categories with a high risk of dissemination who also have high titers of complement-fixing antibody may benefit from even more prolonged therapy.

■ DISSEMINATED (NONMENINGEAL) OR PROGRESSIVE PULMONARY INFECTION

Treatment with an azole agent is effective in most cases of this form of infection. Nonetheless, some clinicians still consider amphotericin B to be the treatment of choice in cases of progressive pulmonary or disseminated coccidioidomycosis, which are immediately life-threatening. The role of various lipid-associated preparations of amphotericin B is unclear at this time. Nonmeningeal coccidioidomycosis that is progressing at a more indolent pace may be treated with an orally administered azole.

Ketoconazole, administered at a dosage of 400 mg once daily, is effective in many cases but may have somewhat erratic absorption, possibly accounting for relatively low response rates reported in some studies. This, at least in part, results from a requirement of gastric acid for its absorption from the gastrointestinal tract. However, higher dosages of the drug do not appear to significantly improve response rates. Ketoconazole interferes with synthesis of testosterone and cortisol and may result in decreased libido and gynecomastia in men and, rarely, in adrenal insufficiency. As with all the azoles, hepatotoxicity may occur.

Itraconazole, at the commonly used dosage of 200 mg twice daily with food, appears to be similarly effective but also requires gastric acid for absorption. An oral suspension of itraconazole, formulated with cyclodextrin, has improved bioavailability. Both ketoconazole and itraconazole, which are metabolized by the hepatic P450 enzyme system, may also participate in a number of important pharmacokinetic interactions with other drugs. The drugs with which interactions may occur include diphenylhydantoin, carbamazepine, cyclosporin, rifampin, isoniazid, terfenadine, astemizole, HIV-1 protease inhibitors and nonnucleoside reverse transcriptase inhibitors, and coumarin anticoagulants.

Fluconazole, at dosages of 400 mg or more daily, is also effective. Its absorption, which does not depend on the presence of gastric acid, is more reliable than that of ketoconazole and itraconazole, and it does not affect human sterol synthesis to an important extent. Although it may interact with other drugs, such as those listed above for the other azoles, most such interactions tend to be of limited significance. Recent evidence in acquired immunodeficiency syndrome (AIDS) patients indicates that fluconazole interacts with clarithromycin and with rifabutin.

Treatment of nonmeningeal disseminated or progressive pulmonary coccidioidomycosis should continue for at least 6 months after the infection appears to have been controlled and is inactive. Nonetheless, relapses may occur despite prolonged treatment. Negative serial coccidioidin skin tests and a peak complement fixing antibody titer of 1:256 have been identified as independent predictors of relapse. Patients with severe and persisting immunodeficiency should be treated for longer durations. Those with AIDS should be maintained on therapy for life.

■ MENINGITIS

A multicenter study demonstrated a response (defined as elimination of ≥40% of baseline abnormalities) rate of 79%

with a daily dose of fluconazole of 400 mg given for a median duration of 37 months in the treatment of coccidioidal meningitis. Daily doses of fluconazole of 800 mg or more may be associated with an improved early response to therapy but also with a greater incidence of adverse reactions. Itraconazole, at dosages of 400 mg or more daily, may be similarly effective. In either case, relapse after discontinuation of drug administration is sufficiently frequent that lifelong suppressive therapy may be necessary.

Treatment of coccidioidal meningitis previously invarably involved the administration of amphotericin B directly into the CSF, and this method of therapy continues to be recommended for the initial control of infection by some clinicians. This may be accomplished by lumbar, lateral cervical, or cisternal injection by direct puncture or via implanted devices such as the Ommaya reservoir. Amphotericin may also be administered into the lateral ventricles by use of such a device. CSF flow patterns should be defined by radionuclide studies when these routes are used because flow patterns may be disturbed and some sites may be loculated.

When administered by the lumbar intrathecal route, some clinicians prefer to do so using a "hyperbaric" technique that delivers the drug in high concentration to the basal cisterns, where the major evidence of infection is ordinarily present. Furthermore, its rapid removal from the lumbar area may theoretically decrease the likelihood of some of the local complications of this procedure, such as radiculitis, myelitis, arachnoiditis, and spinal artery thrombosis. Treatment is initiated with a dose of 0.01 to 0.05 mg and escalated, initially on a daily basis, as tolerated until a maximum dose of 0.75 to 1.5 mg is reached, when the frequency of administration is decreased. Once laboratory and clinical improvement is achieved and stabilized at a desirable level, the interval between doses may be progressively prolonged. The amphotericin B is mixed with sterile, preservative-free 10% dextrose in water and administered by barbotage. Immediately after administration, the patient is placed in a 30 degree head-down position for approximately 45 minutes. It has been suggested that a dosage of at least 0.75 mg three times weekly with rapid escalation to a cumulative dose of 20 mg is associated with better survival than less aggressive approaches.

Concomitant azole therapy may decrease the total amount of amphotericin B necessary to achieve a stable response to therapy. The use of fluconazole or itraconazole may obviate the need for direct administration of amphotericin B into CSF.

Blockage to CSF flow and the development of hydrocephalus is a common complication of coccidioidal meningitis. This should be suspected when the patient's neurologic status deteriorates or if the CSF protein concentration increases to high levels. Hydrocephalus should be managed by the placement of a CSF shunting device.

■ OTHER INFECTIONS

In the absence of immunosuppressive disease or therapy, antifungal therapy is not required in the treatment of a solitary pulmonary nodule caused by *C. immitis.* Airway coccidioidomycosis may be treated with an azole.

Chronic pulmonary cavities respond poorly to antifungal therapy and, if asymptomatic, may be best left untreated. Complications include bacterial superinfection, which is amenable to antibacterial therapy, and hemoptysis. On occasion, hemoptysis may be the result of the development of a fungus ball, most often caused by *Aspergillus* species but occasionally caused by *C. immitis* itself. Cavitation may be progressive despite chemotherapy. All of these complications are potential indications for surgical intervention. An alternative approach to the management of pulmonary mycetoma in the patient who is a poor surgical candidate, is intracavitary instillation of amphotericin B. Rarely, a coccidioidal cavity may rupture into the pleural cavity, resulting in pyopneumothorax. This complication should be managed surgically with concomitant administration of an antifungal agent.

Chronic fibrocavitary pneumonia requires prolonged antifungal therapy, usually with an azole; surgical resection may be of value in some cases.

The musculoskeletal system is a common site of involvement in cases of disseminated infection. In addition to antifungal chemotherapy, surgical debridement may be warranted in some cases of osteomyelitis. The role of synovectomy in chronic coccidiodal arthritis remains unproved.

■ PATIENTS WITH AIDS

Many clinicians prefer that patients with AIDS who develop coccidioidomycosis be initially treated with amphotericin B. If the disease improves or stabilizes, therapy can be switched to fluconazole or possibly itraconazole. However, many patients with AIDS have reduced gastric acidity and as a result may absorb the latter drug poorly. Patients with lower $CD4^+$ lymphocyte counts and severe disease should also be initially treated with amphotericin B, whereas those with less severe disease may initially be given azole therapy. Suppressive therapy should then be administered for life.

Suggested Reading

Dewsnup DH, et al: Is it ever safe to stop azole therapy for *Coccidioides immitis* meningitis? *Ann Intern Med* 124:305, 1996.

Fish DG, et al: Coccidioidomycosis during human immunodeficiency virus infection. A review of 77 patients, *Medicine* 69:384, 1990.

Galgiani JN, et al: Fluconazole therapy for coccidioidal meningitis: the NIAID-Mycoses Study Group, *Ann Intern Med* 119:28, 1993.

Galgiani JN, et al: Fluconazole vs. itraconazole for coccidioidomycosis: randomized, multicenter, double-blinded trial in nonmeningeal progressive infection. Abstracts of the 1998 Annual IDSA Meeting, (abstract #100), *Clin Infect Dis* 27:939, 1998.

Graybill JR, et al: Itraconazole treatment of coccidioidomycosis. NIAID Mycoses Study Group, *Am J Med* 89:282, 1990.

Labadie EL, Hamilton RH: Survival improvement in coccidioidal meningitis by high-dose intrathecal amphotericin B, *Arch Intern Med* 146:2013, 1986.

Tucker RM, et al: Itraconazole therapy for chronic coccidioidal meningitis, *Ann Intern Med* 112:108, 1990.

MISCELLANEOUS FUNGI AND ALGAE

George A. Pankey
Donald L. Greer

Many species of fungi and algae may cause disease among the increasing population of individuals at risk. These microorganisms, loosely called *opportunistic agents,* cannot cause disease unless two major criteria are met: (1) the patient suffers from some predisposing factor that has mechanically (e.g., trauma) or immunologically (e.g., organ transplantation) decreased the capacity to resist infection; (2) the infecting agent can survive and multiply at body temperature (37° C [98.6° F]). At present, the number of these opportunistic agents reported to cause infection exceeds 200.

Although some opportunistic fungal infections are noteworthy for specific predisposing factors (e.g., ketoacidosis, zygomycete infection), neutropenia or a defect in cell-mediated immunity is the usual predisposing factor. However, any trauma, disease state, or pharmacologic insult to host defenses increases the chance of fungal invasion, even from a patient's own normal flora.

The microorganisms considered in this chapter (Table 1) are ubiquitous but are uncommon causes of disease in humans. Therefore the diagnosis is usually made when a patient has an infectious disease that does not respond to antibacterial therapy, when the microbiology laboratory reports the isolation of one of these agents, or when the pathologist identifies a fungus or alga on histopathology.

A high degree of suspicion of an opportunistic agent is necessary for appropriate clinical specimens to be sent to the pathology department. Any material may be examined for fungi and algae, but the laboratory cannot guess the clinical diagnosis, and it is essential that the physician indicates the suspected pathogens and informs the laboratory. For example, to maximize the yield from blood cultures, a lysis centrifugation of cultured blood should be requested.

Many of the pathogens considered in this chapter require special media or conditions for culture. However, the challenge is not isolating the agent once it is suspected but the relevance of the isolate to the clinical picture. Mere isolation of a ubiquitous agent does not indicate pathogenesis. For causation to be proved, the culture must be confirmed either by tissue invasion as seen on biopsy or by repeatedly positive cultures from a usually sterile body fluid. The appearance of these agents in tissue is extremely variable (see Table 1). A culture is imperative for specific identification.

Virtually all of these species grow rapidly at 25° to 30° C (77° to 86° F). Most of the common contaminants, or opportunistic fungi, can be identified to genus in a clinical microbiology laboratory; however, a mycology expert is usually needed to identify the species. Fortunately, treatment of all species within the genus is typically the same. There are no reliable serologic tests, and direct microscopy using Gram, potassium hydroxide, India ink, and Papanicolau preparations of lesion scrapings and sputum is often not helpful.

Table 1   Opportunistic Fungi and Algae
HYALOHYPHOMYCOSES
Long septate hyphae in tissue
Fusarium species
Penicillium marneffei
Scedosporium apiospermum (Pseudallescheria boydii)
PHAEOHYPHOMYCOSES (DEMATIACEAE)
Short septate hyphae, pseudohyphae, and/or yeast with melanin in cell walls identified by Fontana-Mason stain
Alternaria
Bipolaris
Cladosporium
Curvularia
Dactylaria (Ochroconis)
Exophiala
Exserohilum
Phialophora
Wangiella
OPPORTUNISTIC YEAST OR YEASTLIKE FUNGI
Hansenula species; only yeast in tissue
Malassezia (Pityrosporum) furfur: yeast only in deep tissue; "meatballs and spaghetti" in stratum corneum (tinea versicolor)
Rhodotorula: "red yeast"
Trichosporon beigelii: yeast, pseudohyphae, arthroconidia, true hyphae
PROTOTHECOSIS
Achlorophyllic unicellular algae produce spherical cells that multiply by cytoplasmic cleavage, forming a morula in tissue
Prototheca wickerhamii
Prototheca zopfii

■ THERAPY

Therapy is often unsatisfactory without total surgical excision. This is a result both of the severity of the patient's underlying disease and the lack of effective drugs. It is unlikely that there will ever enough cases to conduct double-blind therapeutic trials, even if the pharmaceutical industry develops new drugs. At present, these opportunistic agents are tested in vitro against antifungal agents developed primarily to treat fungi that more commonly produce disease in immunocompromised patients, such as *Candida* and *Cryptococcus.* Therefore only anecdotal case reports and small series are available in the literature. In addition, antifungal susceptibility testing in general is still in its infancy, with few laboratories even attempting it. Variations in susceptibility occur with these organisms, just as they do with bacteria, but the information is less readily available. Therefore, when these fungi are isolated, they should be sent to a reference laboratory for susceptibility testing, including

Table 2 Therapy of Infections by Opportunistic Fungi and Algae

PATHOGEN	CHARACTERISTICS	THERAPY	COMMENTS
Fusarium species	Blood culture positive in patient with fever and bone marrow transplant; extensive burn; taking high-dose corticosteroids; or receiving cytotoxic chemotherapy Multiple purpuric cutaneous nodules with central necrosis	Correct neutropenia Amphotericin B, 1-1.5 mg/kg/day, or liposomal amphotericin B, 5-7 mg/kg/day, plus 5-flucytosine, 25 mg/kg q6h for nonresponders Consider GM-CSF	Little correlation between the clinical results and in vitro susceptibility to agents used Reversal of neutropenia necessary for recovery
Penicillium marneffei	Pneumonia; adenitis; skin lesions; osteomyelitis	Amphotericin B, 0.6 mg/kg/day, or itraconazole, 400 mg/day orally	Fluconazole not effective AIDS-defining opportunistic infection in Southeast Asia
Scedosporium (*Pseudallescheria boydii*)	Mycetoma; sinusitis; pneumonia; endocarditis; meningitis; osteomyelitis; arthritis	Surgical removal if possible Miconazole, 600 mg q6h IV, usually best initial treatment for seriously ill patients Itraconazole or voriconazole (Pfizer) for nonresponsive patients	Amphotericin B not effective Cannot be distinguished from *Aspergillus* by histopathology
Dematiaceae (Phaeohyphomycosis):	Skin and subcutaneous tissue; occasional dissemination	Itraconazole, 400 mg/day orally for 6 mo	
Trichosporon beigelii	Fungemia in neutropenic patients; nodular skin lesions containing the organism; pneumonia	Correct neutropenia Amphotericin B, 1-1.5 mg/kg/day, or liposomal amphotericin B, 5-7 mg/kg/day, plus 5-flucytosine, 25 mg/kg q6h, and/or fluconazole, up to 2 g/day Itraconazole or voriconazole for nonresponsive patients	Use better-absorbed cyclodextrin suspension formulation if possible False-positive reaction with cryptococcal latex agglutination
Malassezia (*Pityrosporum*)	Usually associated with lipid infusions, folliculitis in AIDS patients; tinea versicolor	Remove any intravascular catheter Fluconazole, 1 g IV qd if fungemia persists Treat folliculitis with ketoconazole or itraconazole	Amphotericin B is not very active in vitro
Hansenula species	Intravascular fungemia	Remove intravascular catheter Amphotericin B, 1-1.5 mg/kg/day, or liposomal amphotericin B, 5-7 mg/kg/day Voriconazole for nonresponsive patients	
Rhodotorula species	Intravascular fungemia; meningitis; peritonitis	Remove intravascular catheter Amphotericin B, 1-1.5 mg/kg/day, or liposomal amphotericin B, 5-7 mg/kg/day	Indwelling vascular catheter in immuno-compromised patient is risk factor
Prototheca	Skin and soft-tissue; occasional dissemination	Amphotericin B, 1-1.5 mg/kg/day, or liposomal amphotericin B, 5-7 mg/kg/day Fluconazole for nonresponsive patient	

AIDS, Acquired immunodeficiency syndrome; GM-CSF, granulocyte-macrophage colony-stimulating factor.

synergy studies, with the hope of obtaining helpful information for a specific patient.

Failure of response to antifungal drugs occurs because (1) the drug is fungistatic (most drugs) rather than fungicidal (amphotericin B), (2) combination therapy was not used, (3) the drug has no in vitro activity, (4) neutropenia was not reversed, (5) ketoconazole or itraconazole (oral) was given with antacid therapy, or (6) the dosage is too low. For example, very high dosages of fluconazole (up to 2 g/day) may be more effective than lower dosages, and liposomal formulations of amphotericin B clearly allow much higher dosages without increasing toxicity.

The initial therapeutic approach in adults for infection caused by these microorganisms reflects our personal experience and information from the literature. An infectious disease consultation should be obtained for all patients for advice regarding length and modifications of therapy. Optimal therapies with the agents discussed in this chapter (Table 2) remain controversial at best. Clearly, surgical excision of localized skin and subcutaneous lesions is critical. Pharmaceutical companies evaluating antifungal agents may make them available for compassionate use for patients failing or intolerant to Food and Drug Administration (FDA)-approved agents. Examples include Bristol-Myers Squibb (triazole), Merck (echinocandin), Pfizer (voriconazole), and Schering (triazole).

Correction of the immunosuppression, if possible, is the major approach to the hospitalized patient with neutropenia or other immunosuppression. When this cannot be accomplished, prolonged antifungal therapy will be necessary, although the morbidity and mortality will remain high.

■ PREVENTION

It is important that immunocompromised patients be educated about the possibility of acquiring fungal infection from the environment. Prompt recognition by patient and physician of the possibility of these pathogens in infected skin lesions following trauma is necessary to avoid surgery or dissemination. Proper intravascular catheter care and prevention of neutropenia are critical for the hospitalized patient.

Suggested Reading

Boutati EI, Anaissie EJ: *Fusarium,* a significant emerging pathogen in patients with hematologic malignancy: ten years' experience at a cancer center and implications for management, *Blood* 90(s):999-8, 1997.

Boyd AS, Langley M, King LE Jr: Cutaneous manifestations of *Prototheca* infections, *J Am Acad Dermatol* 32:758, 1995.

Hazen KC: New and emerging yeast pathogens, *Clin Microbiol Rev* 8:462, 1995.

Kamberi P, et al: Efficacy of amphotericin B and azoles alone and in combination against disseminated trichosporonosis in neutropenic mice, *Chemotherapy* 44:55, 1998.

Kim ST, et al: Successful treatment with fluconazole of prothecosis developing at the site of an intralesional corticosteroid injection, *Br J Dermatol* 135:803, 1996.

Kremery V, et al: Hematogenous trichosporonosis in cancer patients: report of 12 cases including 5 during prophylaxis with itraconazole, *Support Care Cancer* 7:39, 1999.

Nelson KE, Kaufman L, Cooper CR, Merz WG: Penicillum *marneffei*: an AIDS-related illness from southeast Asia, *Infect Med* 16(2):118, 1999.

Odds FC, et al: Evaluation of possible correlations between antifungal susceptibilities of filamentous fungi in vitro and antifungal treatment outcomes in animal infection models, *Antimicrob Agents Chemother* 42:282, 1998.

Sharkey PK, et al: Itraconazole treatment of phaeohyphomycosis, *J Am Acad Dermatol* 23:577, 1990.

Sheehan DJ, Hitchcock CA, Sibley CM: Current and emerging azole antifungal agents, *Clin Microbiol Rev* 12:40, 1999.

Singh N, et al: Infections due to dematiaceous fungi in organ transplant recipients: case report and review, *Clin Infect Dis* 24:369, 1997.

Vartivarian SE, Anaisse EJ, Bodey GP: Emerging fungal pathogens in immunocompromised patients: classification, diagnosis and management, *Clin Infect Dis* 17(suppl 2):S487, 1993.

GENERAL THERAPEUTIC CONSIDERATIONS

PRINCIPLES OF ANTIBIOTIC THERAPY

Richard A. Gleckman
Sharat Narayanan

The introduction of antibacterial agents in the 1930s and 1940s was heralded as a historic milestone in the treatment of infectious diseases. The 1950s and 1960s witnessed the development of newer, more broad-spectrum antibacterial agents, as well as the improvement/refinement of the existing beta-lactam antibiotics. The 1970s and 1980s can be characterized as a time when patients and physicians were rather blasé, and there was often inappropriate, frivolous, and excessive administration of antibiotics. As we approach the next millennium, however, the concern is increasingly antibiotic-resistant gram-positive bacteria (specifically penicillin, cephalosporin, and macrolide-resistant *Streptococcus pneumoniae*, and ampicillin, vancomycin-resistant *Enterococcus faecium*), and *Staphylococcus aureus* with decreased susceptibility to vancomycin. Unfortunately, only a few novel compounds, such as oxazolidinones (linezolid) and quinupristin/dalfopristin, are active against these organisms and are undergoing rapid clinical development.

Antimicrobial agents are prescribed to prevent infection (medical and perioperative prophylaxis), to manage established infections, and to treat presumptive infections (those occasions when the clinician cannot readily exclude the possibility of infection and the patient's clinical situation demands empiric treatment). It is important to underscore, however, that successful eradication of an infection often requires adjunctive measures, such as relief of an obstruction, drainage of an abscess and repeated debridement, and management of the underlying medical disorders.

■ PHARMACOKINETICS AND PHARMACODYNAMICS

The absorption of most oral antibiotics occurs by passive diffusion in the small intestine. Some antibiotics, including vancomycin, aminoglycosides, and aztreonam, are not adequately absorbed when given orally. Others, such as cefpodoxime proxetel, are administered as prodrugs to facilitate absorption. Food interferes with the absorption of some antimicrobials, such as penicillin, ampicillin cephalexin, tetracycline, azithromycin, and lomefloxacin.

A fundamental concept is that the antibiotic must achieve therapeutic concentrations at the tissue (extravascular) source of the infection. A number of factors influence the distribution of antibiotics from the plasma to extravascular sites: the nature of the capillary bed (those fenestrated by small pores versus those unfenestrated capillaries of the brain, leptomeninges, and vitreous humor), the lipid solubility, the degree of protein binding (as only unbound drug is antibacterially active and capable of diffusing across capillaries), and the presence of active transport pumps (located in the choroid plexus of the brain, retina, kidneys, and biliary ducts).

The aminoglycosides are classified as concentration-dependent antibacterials and are currently usually administered as once-daily dosing, taking advantage of the observation that the ratio of maximum peak drug concentration to organism minimum inhibitory concentration (MIC) (8 to 12) correlates with clinical response. Alternatively, for the beta-lactam antibiotics (concentration-independent compounds) the percentage of time the drug concentration exceeds the MIC generally correlates with enhanced bacteriologic cure.

The development of new oral antimicrobials that can be prescribed as infrequently as once per day or twice per day achieves enhanced compliance. These include cefprozil and cefpodoxime (cephalosporins), loracarbef (carbacephem), azithromycin and clarithromycin (macrolides), enoxacin, trovafloxacin, grepafloxacin, sparfloxacin, levofloxacin, maxifloxacin, and gatifloxacin (fluoroquinolones).

Antibacterial agents are eliminated from the body through hepatic and biliary excretion (cefperozone, ceftriaxone), hepatic metabolism (clindamycin, chloramphenicol, metronidazole, erythromycin, sulfonamides, some tetracyclines, isoniazid, rifampin), and predominantly renal excretion (most penicillins and cephalosporins, imipenem, aminoglycosides, nitrofurantoin, ofloxacin, most tetracyclines, vancomycin, trimethoprim-sulfamethoxazole). It is essential that the clinician be aware of renal compromise (e.g., from congestive heart failure, hypertension, diabetes, medication, physiologic alteration with age) because this will mandate a dosage reduction for those compounds predominantly eliminated by renal excretion. The creatinine clearance determination has been traditionally used to assess drug doses for antimicrobials eliminated primarily by renal excretion.

Table 1   Selection of Therapy

HOST FACTOR	SPECIAL ANTIBIOTIC CONCERN
Drug allergy	Track record
Site of infection	Most likely organism(s) and susceptibility
Pregnancy	Bactericidal/bacteriostatic
Epidemiologic information	Penetration into privileged sites (central nervous system, endocardium)
Renal function	Potential to cause major untoward event
Recent antibiotic exposure	
Infection acquisition (community/nursing home/hospital)	
Concomitant medication	

Table 2   Combination Therapy

Tuberculosis
Disseminated *Mycobacterium avium* complex
Helicobacter pylori
Endocarditis (alpha-hemolytic streptococcus, enterococcal)
Vancomycin-resistant enterococcal disease
Life-threatening infection caused by *Pseudomonas aeruginosa*
Empiric treatment (pneumococcal meningitis; febrile, severely neutropenic host; polymicrobial infection; life-threatening infection with inapparent source)

■ SELECTION OF THERAPY

Table 1 lists some of the more important host and drug features that influence antibacterial selection. Additional concerns relate to adherence to the program and cost of the medication.

Antibiotic combinations are used to manage selective infections (Table 2). There are potential disadvantages to the administration of antibiotic combinations, however, such as increased untoward events, heightened costs, and suprainfection.

The optimal duration of antibacterial treatment has not been defined by rigorous controlled studies. Recommended duration of antibacterial therapy has predominantly evolved from clinical experience. Treatment duration is influenced by a number of factors, including the immune competence of the host, the nature of the organism(s), and the site of the infection. As a general statement, patients with cellulitis, an exacerbation of chronic bronchitis, community-acquired sinusitis/pharyngitis, and uncomplicated urinary tract infections are candidates for a treatment course of approximately 10 days. Alternatively, patients with bacterial osteomyelitis, chronic bacterial prostatitis, endocarditis, and *Legionella* pneumonia require antibacterial treatment for 3 weeks to 3 months. For some infections (e.g., *Pneumocystis carinii* pneumonia [PCP], *Mycobacterium avium* complex [MAC]) in human immunodeficiency virus (HIV)-infected patients, antimicrobial treatment is continued for life, unless highly active antiretroviral therapy restores considerable immunocompetence.

Special Populations

Physiologic changes in the urinary tract and complications of parturition predispose the pregnant woman to urinary tract infections, as well as chorioamnionitis and endometritis. Antibiotic selection for the pregnant woman must take into consideration the potential for drug-induced toxicity for both the woman and her developing fetus. Animal studies and epidemiologic data generated from pregnant women who were exposed to antibacterial agents because of clinical need suggest that the penicillins, including those in combination with a beta-lactamase inhibitor, cephalosporins, aztreonam, erythromycin, azithromycin, clindamycin, and metronidazole have not demonstrated human fetal risk. Sulfonamides should be avoided in late pregnancy because of the potential for the development of neonatal kernicterus. Chloramphenicol should not be administered to the mother near term because of the risk for accumulation in the neonate and the resulting "gray baby" syndrome. The aminoglycosides gentamicin, tobramycin, and amikacin should not be administered to pregnant women, particularly pre-eclamptic women, unless there is a compelling reason. If they are prescribed, serum concentrations must be monitored carefully.

The fluoroquinolones are not recommended for use in pregnancy because of their adverse effects on developing cartilage. Tetracyclines are contraindicated in pregnant women because these compounds can cause interference with normal development of teeth and bones and have caused hepatorenal failure and death, particularly when administered intravenously to treat pyelonephritis.

There are a number of unique concerns when a clinician prescribes an antibacterial agent to an elderly patient. Noncompliance with an oral antibiotic program has been confirmed repeatedly in elderly patients. The physiologic decline in kidney function that occurs in many older patients, particularly when accompanied by the added adverse renal effects exerted by diabetes mellitus, hypertension, and congestive heart failure, will influence the excretion of numerous antibiotics, such as the aminoglycosides and vancomycin, and predispose the patient to antibiotic-related adverse events.

Elderly patients appear to experience adverse drug reactions from antibacterial compounds more often than younger patients (Table 3).

Route of Administration

Antibiotics are administered intravenously when the patient has hypotension, has bacterial infection at a unique site (e.g., leptomeninges, endocardium, a deep neck infection, epiglottitis, endophthalmitis, fasciitis, myopericarditis, me-

Table 3 Adverse Drug Reaction	
DRUG	**UNTOWARD EVENT**
Aminoglycoside	Nephrotoxicity, ototoxicity
Amoxicillin-clavulanic acid (chronic administration)	Hepatotoxicity
Trimethoprim-sulfamethoxazole	Blood dyscrasia; hyperkalemia
Fluoroquinolone	Seizure
Doxycycline	Esophageal ulcer/stricture
Nitrofurantoin (chronic administration)	Pulmonary fibrosis, hepatitis, agranulocytosis

Table 4 Penicillin Member-Specific Adverse Event	
COMPOUND	**ADVERSE REACTION**
Ampicillin	*C. difficile* colitis; diarrhea
Amoxicillin	Rash (chronic lymphocytic leukemia)
Amoxicillin-clavulanate	
Nafcillin	Neutropenia
Ticarcillin	Hypokalemia; fluid overload
Ampicillin	Interstitial nephritis
Ticarcillin	Platelet-mediated bleeding
Piperacillin	

diastinitis, septic thrombophlebitis), has an infection that is imminently life-endangering (e.g., meningococcemia, Rocky Mountain spotted fever, plague, bacteremia), has an infection that would preclude oral administration because of the presence of nausea/vomiting or impaired function of the intestinal tract (e.g., peritonitis, appendicitis, ascending cholangitis, pancreatic abscess), or has an infection that cannot be managed with an oral antibacterial compound (disease caused by methicillin-resistant *S. aureus* or vancomycin-resistant *Enterococcus faecium*). Traditionally, physicians would elect to prescribe an intravenous antibiotic simply because a patient was admitted to the hospital. However, it is apparent that meeting the threshold of being hospitalized does not automatically dictate that the antibacterial agent be administered intravenously. Unless one of the indications previously listed are present, some patients can be managed successfully by the oral administration of an antibacterial agent (the patient with uncomplicated pyelonephritis; the patient with an exacerbation of chronic bronchitis or uncomplicated community-acquired pneumonia; the patient with infectious bacterial enterocolitis; and the patient with a traditional cellulitis, one that was not precipitated by a unique exposure).

Adverse Reactions

Adverse antibiotic-induced reactions are a concern not only because they cause host injury but also because they interrupt and complicate therapy and often necessitate alternative, more-expensive agents that have the ability to foster the emergence and spread of drug-resistant organisms. Adverse antibiotic-related effects can also contribute to excess medical costs and serve as a source of litigation.

Adverse events attributed to antibiotics are usually caused by three mechanisms: exaggerated response to the known pharmacologic effects of the drug, immunologic reactions to the drug or its metabolites, and toxic effects of the compound or its metabolites. Most antibiotic-related adverse events are precipitated by an extension of the drug's normal pharmacology and are often avoided by appropriate dosage adjustment.

In addition to the direct influence of the antibiotic, however, numerous host factors (genetic constitution, integrity of drug elimination mechanisms, concomitant medical disorders) can affect the frequency and severity of antibiotic-related adverse events. A prime example is the HIV-infected patient. There are numerous reports of oxacillin-induced hepatitis and cutaneous reactions occurring in HIV-infected

Table 5 Cephalosporin Member-Specific Adverse Event	
COMPOUND	**ADVERSE REACTION**
Ceftriaxone	Diarrhea
Cefixime	
Ceftibuten	
Cefdinir	
Cefoperazone	
Ceftriaxone	Reversible biliary sludge
Cefoperazone	Hypoprothrombinemic bleeding
Cefotetan	
Cefamandole	
Ceftazidime	Alteration of hepatic function
Cefoperazone	Disulfiram-like reactions
Cefonicid	
Cefamandole	

patients who have received trimethoprim-sulfamethoxazole or aminopenicillins. Moreover, trimethoprim-sulfamethoxazole causes more non–dose-related gastrointestinal intolerance, fever, and altered liver function in patients with acquired immunodeficiency syndrome (AIDS), than in non–HIV-infected patients.

The penicillin family of drugs are usually well tolerated, but they have been associated with a wide range of hypersensitivity reactions, including fever, rash (maculopapular and urticarial), anaphylaxis, exfoliative dermatitis, erythema multiforme, serum sickness, and hemolytic anemia. When administered intravenously at high dosages, particularly to patients with renal impairment, they have the potential to cause central nervous system toxicity, manifested by myoclonic jerks, seizures, or coma. Table 4 lists specific family members.

The cephalosporins have proved to be very safe compounds, and this is one explanation for their wide appeal. Untoward events attributed to the cephalosporins have included diarrhea, pseudomembranous colitis, and rarely, hypersensitivity reactions. Table 5 lists specific family members.

Imipenem-cilastatin and aztreonam have caused phlebitis, gastrointestinal untoward events, and rash. A particular concern is the development of seizures attributed to imipenem-cilastatin.

The most notorious side effects of clindamycin are diarrhea and *C. difficile*–related colitits. This drug has rarely caused drug fever, rash, blood dyscrasias, and hepatotoxicity.

Doxycycline has been associated with diarrhea and, occasionally, photosensitivity, rash, hepatitis, and particularly in elderly patients, esophageal ulcerations or strictures. Uncommon untoward events attributed to vancomycin include rash, fever, nephrotoxoicity, ototoxicity, and reversible, transient hematopoietic toxicity. The most dramatic side effect is the red man syndrome, a nonimmunologically mediated reaction consisting of pruritus and erythema with/without hypotension, which appears to be dependent on dose, frequency of administration, and rate of infusion.

Concerns regarding administration of the aminoglycosides include nephrotoxicity, specifically nonoliguric acute renal failure, ototoxicity, both the auditory and vestibular components, and neuromuscular blockade, a rare event that has developed in patients with myasthenia gravis, renal disease, hypocalcemia, or hypermagnesemia. Factors contributing to nephrotoxicity include duration of therapy, older age, liver disease, shock, and the coadministration of drugs that have the potential to cause nephrotoxicity. Factors contributing to ototoxicity include hypovolemia, total dose administered, renal impairment, liver dysfunction, and elevated serum trough concentrations.

Rash, fever, and gastrointestinal adverse reactions are the most common side effects precipitated by trimethoprim-sulfamethoxazole. Additional rare untoward events include nephrotoxicity, hyperkalemia, hematologic derangements (neutropenia, thrombocytopenia, agranulocytosis, aplastic anemia, megaloblastic anemia), hepatitis, pancreatitis, pseudomembranous colitis, and adverse central nervous system events (headache, insomnia, vertigo, ataxia, and aseptic meningitis).

Adverse events attributed to the macrolides have included nausea, vomiting, abdominal pain, diarrhea, and, rarely, antibiotic-associated colitis, pancreatitis, cholestatic jaundice, acute hepatitis, abnormal taste (clarithromycin), and reversible ototoxicity. Clarithromycin and azithromycin cause less gastrointestinal adverse events than erythromycin.

The most common adverse events attributed to the fluoroquinolones are gastrointestinal symptoms, nervous system complaints (headache, dizziness, insomnia, agitation, hallucinations), and allergic reactions (rash, pruritus). Rare adverse effects include seizures, elevations of liver enzymes, and tendinopathy. Photosensitivity has been a concern with lomefloxacin and sparfloxacin, and very rarely with trovafloxacin. Patients receiving trovafloxacin are at risk to develop hepatotoxicity, which can be fatal, as well as dizziness, and they should not drive a car, operate machinery, or engage in activity that requires mental alertness. Grepafloxacin, moxifloxacin, and sparfloxacin should not be used in patients with known Qt$_c$ prolongation or in patients receiving Qt$_c$ prolonging drugs.

Hypersensitivity Reactions

IgE-mediated hypersensitivity reactions are the most feared adverse events attributed to the penicllins, imipenem-cilastatin, and cephalosporins. These reactions are manifested by urticaria, pruritus, hypotension, bronchospasm, and laryngeal edema. "Late" or delayed hypersensitivity events comprise severe cutaneous reactions such as Stevens-Johnson syndrome, toxic epidermal necrolysis, exfoliative dermatitis, and small vessel vasculitis. Classically sulfonamides have been associated with these dermatologic reactions, but penicillins, cephalosporins, fluoroquinolones, and vancomycin have been implicated as well. (This subject is presented in the Chapter *Hypersensitivity to Antibiotics*).

Drug-Drug Interactions

Drug interactions can be subtle, or alternatively, life-endangering, and they occur when one drug modifies the pharmacokinetics (absorption, distribution, metabolism, or excretion) or pharmacodynamics of another drug. Magnesium antacid reduces the absorption of nitrofurantoin, food reduces the absorption of azithromycin, and antacids, sucralfate, ferrous sulfate, and zinc alter the bioavailability of oral tetracyclines and quinolones. The newly released angiotensin-converting enzyme inhibitor quinapril has a high concentration of magnesium and can impede the absorption of the oral fluoroquinolones. Suppression by oral tetracycline, erythromycin, or trimethoprim-sulfamethoxozole of upper intestinal bacteria that inactivate digoxin can result in digoxin-induced toxicity. Alcohol ingestion in patients receiving metronidazole or cefoperazone can produce a disulfiram reaction, and caution should be used when prescribing metronidazole to patients receiving zalcitabine, didanosine, or stavudine because there is the potential for additive peripheral neuropathy.

Drug-drug interactions have not been a major concern for patients receiving the penicillins, aztreonam, and the cephalosporins. Theophylline and cyclosporine may reduce the threshold for seizures in patients receiving imipenem. There is the potential for enhanced aminoglycoside-induced nephrotoxicity and/or ototoxicity when patients receive vancomycin, amphotericin B, cyclosporine, cisplatin, and ethacrynic acid.

Ciprofloxacin and, to a greater extent, enoxacin have the potential to inhibit the metabolism of theophylline (through their effect on the enzymes of the cytochrome P450 system) and cause theophylline toxicity. Coadministration of cimetidine can aggravate this interaction. The newer fluoroquinolones (sparfloxacin, grepafloxacin) have the potential to cause life-endangering rhythms when coadministered with antiarrhythmic compounds (disopyramide, amiodarone, quinidine, procainamide, sotalol hydrochloride, bepridil hydrochloride). Macrolide antibiotics bind to and inhibit cytochrome P450 isoforms, especially CYP3A4, and there is the potential for numerous and life-threatening drug-drug interactions (Table 6). Inhibition of P450 enzymes is greatest with erythromycin and less with clarithromycin. Azithromycin and dirithromycin do not bind CYP3A4 and are associated with the fewest adverse interactions. Because clarithro-

Table 6	Drugs with Potential Interaction with Macrolides
Astemizole	Ergot alkaloids
Benzodiazepines	Felodipine
Buspirone	Pinozide
Carbamazepine	Simvastatin
Cisapride	Tacrolimus
Clozapine	Theophylline
Cyclosporin	Warfarin
Digoxin	

mycin is an inhibitor of CYP3A4 isoenzyme, it can precipitate rifabutin-related uveitis in the HIV-infected patient receiving prophylaxis to prevent disseminated MAC infection.

The absorption of doxycycline is diminished when there is coadministration of antacids, ferrous sulfate, and cimetidine. Administration of doxycycline has been associated with failure of oral contraceptive preparations.

Coadministration of trimethoprim-sulfamethoxazole with phenytoin, glipizide, methotrexate, and thiazide diuretics has resulted in phenytoid toxicity, enhanced hypoglycemia, bone marrow suppression, and severe hyponatremia, respectively. Trimethoprim-sulfamethoxazole can enhance warfarin-induced anticoagulation and ganciclovir-induced bone marrow suppression and can diminish cyclosporin concentrations, resulting in transplant rejection. Neutropenia and thrombocytopenia can occur in renal allograft recipients who receive azathioprine and more than 3 weeks treatment with trimethoprim-sulfamethoxazole. Trimethoprim-sulfamethoxazole has caused hyperkalemia when prescribed to patients receiving a potassium-sparing diuretic.

Drug Monitoring

Monitoring the adequacy of antibiotic treatment involves assessing the patient's response, as determined by the resolution of the systemic and local manifestations of inflammation, supplemented by results obtained from x-ray, imaging, and microbiologic studies. Antibiotic concentrations in blood are not routinely measured. Aminoglycoside antibiotics are an exception, however, because serum concentrations of these compounds are performed to reduce the risk of nephrotoxicity and ototoxicity and to ensure the attainment of recommended therapeutic levels. The serum bactericidal test has been used to predict clinical cure for patients with osteomyelitis or gram-negative bacillary bacteremia. This test does not predict the clinical outcome for patients with infective endocarditis.

Outpatient Parenteral Antibiotic Therapy

More than 250,000 Americans receive outpatient parenteral antibiotic therapy each year. This form of treatment is designed to either avoid hospitalization or to continue treatment initiated in the hospital. The primary goal of outpatient parenteral antibiotic therapy is to provide care that is equivalent in quality to the inpatient setting while enhancing the patient's quality of life. Outpatient parenteral antimicrobial therapy provides a safe and effective modality of treatment, which offers cost savings and patient satisfaction.

The decision to offer a patient outpatient parenteral antimicrobial therapy would be influenced by the following factors: the patient's clinical status and acceptance of this form of treatment, the need for additional treatments, the home environment and support systems, the potential for treatment plan compliance, and the reimbursement status.

Outpatient parenteral antimicrobial therapy has been successfully and safely used to treat patients with a wide array of infectious disorders, such as pneumonia, complicated urinary tract infections, pelvic inflammatory disease, endocarditis, Lyme disease, visceral abscesses, and most commonly, skin infections and osteomyelitis. Antibiotics

that lend themselves to infrequent dosing include ceftriaxone, vancomycin, and aminoglycosides. Patients who are to receive aminoglycosides should be informed of the risks of hearing impairment and vestibular toxicity and advised to report dizziness and reduced hearing. Consideration should be given to performing serial measurements of serum creatinine and aminoglycoside concentrations, as well as serial audiograms specifically for patients with renal insufficiency. In addition to antibiotic-related adverse events, there is a risk of infectious complications (access-related) when patients undergo outpatient parenteral antimicrobial therapy.

Switch ("Step Down") Therapy

The last 10 years has witnessed the development of safe and effective oral antimicrobials (cephalosporins, loracarbef, clarithromycin, azithromycin, fluoroquinolones) that are well absorbed, can be administered infrequently, and have a proven track record for the management of many infections, including disorders previously treated exclusively by intravenous antibiotics. These compounds, as well as doxycycline, have emerged as appropriate therapy (switch or step down) for the patient, hospitalized for the management of uncomplicated community-acquired pneumonia, who has stabilized, appears to be turning the corner (afebrile, improved appetite and strength), has no concomitant disorder requiring a continued hospitalization, and no longer requires parenteral antimicrobial therapy. This switch therapy frees the patient from the inconvenience, discomfort, and risks (thrombophlebitis, infectious) of intravenous infusions of antibiotics, can result in considerable cost savings, and can often be achieved within 48 to 72 hours of the patient's admission to the hospital. The success of switch therapy depends upon patient compliance and adequate intestinal absorption of the antimicrobial prescribed.

Antibacterial Prophylaxis

Appropriately administered antibiotic prophylaxis (in which the agent causes minimal untoward events, does not select for virulent organisms, achieves adequate local tissue levels, is relatively inexpensive, demonstrates inhibitory activity for the bacteria anticipated to cause postoperative infection, and is prescribed within 30 minutes of the surgical incision) is the standard of care for patients who are to be subjected to selective surgical procedures.

In addition to their indication for the prevention of postoperative infections, antibacterial agents have been effective in the prevention (primary/secondary) of a number of nonsurgical related disorders, including rheumatic fever, syphilis, travelers' diarrhea, tuberculosis, invasive meningococcal disease, pertussis, diphtheria, plague, and recurrent cystitis in women. Although no definitive studies have confirmed that antibiotic prophylaxis provides protection against the development of endocarditis during bacteremia-inducing procedures, it is currently recommended that patients with moderate- to high-risk cardiac conditions receive antibiotic prophylaxis when subjected to selective dental, respiratory tract, gastrointestinal tract, and genitourinary tract bacteremia-producing procedures. Antibacterial agents are also indicated for the prevention of PCP, toxoplasmic encephalitis, tuberculosis, and disseminated MAC in specific HIV-infected patients.

Inappropriate Administration

Antibacterial agents are not a substitute for a thorough medical history, physical examination, and diagnostic evaluation, and they have no role in the management of the patient with rhinitis, nonbacterial pharyngitis, acute bronchitis, or asymptomatic bacteriuria (unless the latter patient is pregnant or immunocompromised).

Prolonged antibacterial therapy is not indicated for the patient, not obviously infected, with persistent unexplained fever. This patient merits a comprehensive diagnostic evaluation. Perioperative prophylactic antibiotic administration should be restricted to 48 hours.

All too often there is the failure to administer specific treatment, and to replace it with multiple empiric drug therapy, when the cause of the infection and susceptibility profile is known. Often, this occurs because the patient has demonstrated clinical improvement with the multidrug empiric antibacterial program. Multiple drug treatments can be more expensive, can promote the emergence of resistant pathogens, and enhance the possibility for the development of drug-drug interactions and drug-induced untoward events.

When making decisions regarding antibiotic selection, physicians should avoid undue reliance on published guidelines developed by prestigious committees. These guidelines are recommendations based on clinical experience, consensus opinions, and evidence-based medicine. However, even though antibacterial agents have been available for more than 60 years, there are major gaps in our knowledge and the practice guidelines often exclude specific segments of the population and are subject to revision as new data are developed.

Antimicrobial Failure

When the patient is not responding to an antibiotic, there is a temptation to administer an alternative antimicrobial agent with an extended spectrum of inhibitory activity. On occasion, this approach is valid, particularly for the seriously ill patient. In general, however, it is preferable for the clinician to establish the accuracy of the diagnosis (gout, thrombophlebitis, and Lyme disease resemble bacterial cellulitis; Charcot's joint in the foot of the diabetic simulates osteomyelitis; pulmonary infarction, lung cancer, adult respiratory distress syndrome [ARDS], aspiration of gastric contents, and congestive heart failure can imitate bacterial pneumonia), to search for those features that could compromise the host (such as obstruction, necrotic tissue, abscess, prosthetic device), to identify those infections arising in "privileged" sites (meningitis, endocarditis, chronic bacterial prostatitis) that require antimicrobials with unique penetration properties, and to recognize the polymicrobic nature of selective infections.

It is also essential for the clinician to confirm drug compliance, appropriate drug dosage, and susceptibility reports, and to recognize those infections (life-threatening infections in the granulocytopenic host, endocarditis, gram-negative bacillary meningitis) that require a bactericidal antibiotic.

Suggested Reading

Andes D, Craig WA: Pharmacokinetics and pharmacodynamics of outpatient intravenous antimicrobial therapy, *Infect Dis Clin North Am* 12:849, 1998.

Borrego F, Gleckman R: Preventing antibiotic treatment failure, *Contemp Intern Med* 8:9, 1996.

Borrego F, Gleckman R: Principles of antibiotic prescribing in the elderly, *Drug Therapy* 11:7, 1997.

Gregg CR: Drug interactions and anti-infective therapies *Am J Med* 106: 2270, 1999.

Thompson RL, Wright AJ: General principles of antimicrobial therapy, *Mayo Clin Proc* 73:995, 1998.

ANTIFUNGAL THERAPY

Sofia Perea
Thomas F. Patterson

This chapter focuses on the use of drugs that treat systemic mycoses (Table 1). Treatment of cutaneous fungal infections is discussed in the chapter *Superficial Fungal Infection*.

■ AMPHOTERICIN B

Amphotericin B (AmB), a polyene antifungal synthesized by *Streptomyces nodosus*, remains the standard therapy for many invasive mycoses, particularly in critically ill patients. Its chemical structure confers it with amphoteric properties that are essential for the drug's ability to form channels through the cytoplasmatic membrane. The pores formed from preferential binding of amphotericin B to ergosterol, the primary fungal cell sterol, results in an increase in membrane permeability, leading to a loss of essential elements such as potassium and other molecules, that impairs fungal viability. Amphotericin B binds with less affinity to cholesterol, the primary cell sterol of mammalian cells, which are therefore less affected by amphotericin B than the fungal target.

Amphotericin B is commercially available as a complex with sodium deoxycholate: commercial vials contain amphotericin B, 50 mg; sodium deoxycholate, 41 mg; and a sodium phosphate buffer, 25.2 mg, being insoluble in water at physiologic pH. The clinical pharmacology of amphotericin B is characterized by extensive binding to plasma proteins (>90%) and wide distribution to the peripheral compartment with preferential accumulation in liver and spleen,

Table 1 Antifungal Agents: Therapeutic Options

DISEASE	THERAPY	
	PRIMARY	**ALTERNATIVE**
Aspergillosis: Invasive	AmB, 1.0-1.5 mg/kg/day IV to total dose of 2.0-2.5 g, *or* Initial AmB followed by itraconazole, 200-400 mg/day PO long-term in severe infection/immunosuppressed patient	Liposomal formulations of AmB (see Table 3 for dosage)
Blastomycosis	Itraconazole, 200-400 mg/day PO for 6 mo; *or* AmB, 0.5 mg/kg/day to a total dose of ≥1.5 g for critically ill patients	Fluconazole, 400-800 mg/day for at least 6 mo
Candidiasis		
Candidemia	Fluconazole, 400 mg/day IV ×7 days then PO for 7+ days to complete 14-day course after last positive blood culture, *or* AmB, 0.5-0.6 mg/kg/day IV for 14-day course If neutropenic, AmB, 0.6-1.0 mg/kg/day, or fluconazole, 400-800 mg/day ×7 day IV then PO (if no prior azole therapy) until neutropenia resolved	In patients who fail to respond or deteriorate, higher dosages may be used (AmB, 0.8-1.0 mg/kg/day IV, or fluconazole, 800 mg/day PO) Avoid fluconazole if patient recently was taking fluconazole or if *C. krusei* likely
Hepatosplenic candidiasis	AmB, 0.8-1.0 mg/kg/day IV, ± 5-FC, 37.5 mg/kg PO q6h, *or* Fluconazole, 800 mg/day IV	AmB lipid complex (ABLC), 5 mg/kg/day
Coccidiomycosis		
Nonmeningeal (AIDS and non-AIDS)	Fluconazole, 400-800 mg/day PO for 12-18 mo	Itraconazole, 200 mg bid PO ×12-18 mo, *or* AmB, 0.6-1.0 /kg/day IV; total dose, ≥2.5 g In AIDS patients, lifetime suppressive treatment with fluconazole, 200-400 mg/day PO, or itraconazole, 200-400 mg/day PO
Meningeal (AIDS and non-AIDS)	Fluconazole, 400-600 mg/day PO indefinitely	AmB IV as for nonmeningeal
Cryptococcosis		
Nonmeningeal (non-AIDS)	AmB, 0.7 mg/kg/day IV until response, then fluconazole, 400 mg/day PO for 8-10 wk, *or* Fluconazole, 400 mg/day IV or PO for 8 wk	AmB, 0.5 mg/kg/day ± fluconazole, 25 mg/kg qid PO ×6 wk
Meningeal (non-AIDS)	AmB, 0.7 mg/kg/day IV ± 5-FC, 25 mg/kg q6h PO for 2 wk, then fluconazole, 400 mg/day PO 8-10 wk, *or* Fluconazole, 400 mg/day PO ×8-10 wk (for less severely ill patients)	
HIV+/AIDS (usually meningitis)	AmB, 0.7 mg/kg/day IV, ± 5-FC, 25 mg/kg q6h PO for 2 wk or until clinically stable, then fluconazole, 400 mg/day PO for 10 wk total, then 200 mg/day (suppressive treatment) indefinitely	Fluconazole, 400 mg/day PO ×6-10 wk, then suppressive treatment, *or* lipid AmB IV, 5 mg/kg/day ×2 wk, followed by fluconazole, 400 mg/day PO ×8-10 wk
Histoplasmosis		
Non-AIDS	Itraconazole, 200 mg/day PO for 9 mo; if life-threatening, AmB, 0.7-1.0 mg/kg/day IV ×14 days, followed by itraconazole, 400 mg/day ×8-10 wk if clinical response	
Disseminated, AIDS	AmB, 0.7-1.0 mg/kg/day IV ×14 days, followed by itraconazole, 400 mg/day ×8-10 wk, then begin suppressive treatment with itraconazole 200 mg/day PO	Itraconazole, 300 mg bid PO ×3 days, then 200 mg bid PO ×12 wk, *or* 400 mg/day ×12 wk, then 200 mg/day PO
Zygomycosis	Surgery plus AmB, 0.8-1.5 mg/kg/day IV; when improvement, then qod; total dose, 2.5-3 g	No role for azoles
Sporotrichosis		
Lymphocutaneous	Itraconazole, 200 mg/day PO ×6 mo	Potassium iodide solution (SSKI), 10-15 gtt tid ×6-12 wk
Extracutaneous	AmB, 1.5-3.0 g (may require adjunctive intraarticular therapy or surgery)	Itraconazole, 200-300 mg PO bid ×6 mo, then 200 mg PO bid long term

Note: Dosages and duration of therapy given are approximations based on clinical response and underlying condition in the host. Individual responses and therapeutic requirements may vary.
AIDS, Acquired immunodeficiency syndrome; *AmB,* amphotericin B; *5-FC,* flucytosine.

with lesser amounts in kidney and lung. Intravenous administration of therapeutic doses results in peak plasma levels of 1.0 to 1.5 µg/ml falling to 0.5 to 1.0 µg/ml 24 hours later. At therapeutic doses, less than 5% of the drug each dose is excreted in the urine. The elimination of the amphotericin B is not altered in patients with renal or liver dysfunction and does not require dose adjustment in patients who are anephric or undergoing hemodyalisis. Cerebrospinal fluid (CSF) levels are low, although higher concentrations occur in brain tissue. Amphotericin B also diffuses poorly into other body fluids such as saliva, amniotic fluid, aqueous humor, and vitreous humor. However, drug concentrations in inflamed pleura, peritoneum, aqueous humor, and joint spaces are roughly two thirds of the trough plasma concentration.

For clinical administration, amphotericin B is diluted in 5% dextrose (at a concentration of ≤0.1 mg of amphotericin B per ml of diluent) and infused intravenously over 2 to 4 hours at dosages of 0.5 to 1.5 mg/kg/day. The most common side effects of amphotericin B treatment are acute infusion-related reaction and nephrotoxicity. The acute infusion-related reaction consists of a syndrome of chills, fever, and tachypnea that typically occurs 30 to 45 minutes after beginning the first infusion and may last for 2 to 4 hours. Premedication with acetaminophen (650 mg given orally or rectally), hydrocortisone (25 to 50 mg given intravenously or mixed with the amphotericin B infusion solution), and diphenhydramine (50 mg given orally or rectally) can diminish the frequency and severity of these reactions. Chills may be terminated by the administration of meperidine (50 mg given intravenously). The acute symptoms associated with amphotericin B infusion can be serious, including life-threatening anaphylaxis. Occurrence of these symptoms has led physicians to infuse a "test dose" of a small volume containing 1 mg of the prepared amphotericin B solution over 20 to 30 minutes, followed by the full dose 2 hours later. If the test dose is poorly tolerated, traditionally small doses (e.g., 5 mg) have been administered the first day with daily increments until the target dose is achieved. The benefit of a test dose remains controversial, and it is clear that critically ill patients who have life-threatening mycoses should receive the full therapeutic doses of amphotericin B within the first 24 hours of therapy so that the use of an incremental daily dosing of amphotericin B is rarely, if ever, currently indicated. The occurrence of severe infusion reactions have been considered indications for use of lipid-associated amphotericin B preparations (see the following), which may be better tolerated in some patients.

The other major side effect of amphotericin B is the development of nephrotoxicity, which occurs through a dose-dependent decrease in the glomerular filtrate rate as a result of a direct vasoconstrictive effect on afferent renal arterioles, reducing glomerular and renal tubular blood flow. The nephrotoxicity may be exacerbated by other nephrotoxic agents (Table 2). There is evidence that renal vasoconstriction is partially reversible by salt loading with 500 to 1000 ml of normal saline before each infusion. Other renal effects include potassium and bicarbonate wasting and decreased erythropoietin production. Permanent loss of renal function can occur if the drug is continued in the setting of worsening renal function. Other chronic toxicities include nausea and vomiting, anorexia, normocytic normochronic anemia (with the hematocrit rarely falling below 20% to 25%), and rarely thrombocytopenia, leukopenia, and peripheral vein phlebitis.

Amphotericin B is active against most fungal pathogens that cause systemic or deep-seated infections. Despite its significant dose-limiting toxicities, amphotericin B remains the gold standard for many mycoses because of its broad spectrum of activity and rapid fungicidal activity. Recommendations for appropriate dosages of amphotericin B and for duration of therapy remain poorly defined for most infections. In the past, total doses of 1 to 2 g for serious infections (which is approximately 15 to 30 mg/kg over a 6-week period) were usually recommended. However, the dosage and duration of amphotericin B depend largely on response of infection to therapy and resolution of underlying host immunodeficiency (e.g., resolution of neutropenia). Increasingly, a therapeutic approach that includes aggressive "induction" courses of amphotericin B followed by "consolidation" therapy with an azole, which can be administered orally, is used. This strategy has been evaluated most thoroughly in cryptococcal meningitis, but clinical reports have documented success of sequential amphotericin B to azole therapy in candidemia (using oral fluconazole), invasive aspergillosis (with oral itraconazole), and endemic fungi (coccidioidomycosis and histoplasmosis with fluconazole and itraconazole, respectively). Generally, a 2-week course of amphotericin B (or until signs of infection have resolved or significantly improved) can be followed by azole therapy.

Local instillation is rarely indicated. Historically, itrathecal amphotericin B was a mainstay of therapy for coccidioidal meningitis, but the use of intrathecal amphotericin B is associated with substantial toxicity; consequently, that approach is now usually reserved for patients in whom systemic therapy, including high dosages of an azole, fails. In other cases, local instillation of amphotericin B into the bladder via a Foley catheter has been used for urinary tract candidiasis, but systemic azole therapy, usually with fluconazole, is well tolerated and effective for that indication.

New liposomal preparations of amphotericin B have been developed, in an attempt to reduce the nephrotoxicity of the conventional form of amphotericin B deoxycholate. The administration of such liposomal forms modifies the pharmacologic and toxicologic properties of amphotericin B. Characteristics of the commercially available lipid amphotericin B preparations, amphotericin B lipid complex (ABLC, Abelcet), amphotericin B colloidal dispersion (ABCD), and liposomal amphotericin B (AmBisome) are shown in Table 3. The antifungal activities of these preparations in vitro are comparable to those of standard amphotericin B. Serum levels of the liposomal amphotericin B are higher than those achieved with standard amphotericin B, but serum levels of amphotericin B lipid complex and amphotericin B colloidal dispersion are similar to amphotericin B deoxycholate. The advantage of the administration of amphotericin B in lipid complexes or in liposomes is the reduced rate of nephrotoxicity, allowing the delivery of larger amounts of the drug. Although few direct comparisons of the preparations have been performed, the fewest infusion reactions appear to occur with liposomal amphotericin B (AmBisome) with slightly more reactions, including chills and fevers, associated with amphotericin B lipid complex. The highest incidence of infusion-related toxici-

Table 2 Antifungal Drug-Drug Interaction

ANTIFUNGAL AGENT (A)			OTHER DRUG (B)	EFFECT	SIGNIFICANCE/ CERTAINTY
Amphotericin B/Amphotericin B Lipid Formulations			Antineoplastic drugs	↑ Nephrotoxicity risk	+
			Foscarnet	↑ Nephrotoxicity risk	+
			Corticosteroids and adrenocorticotropic hormone	May potentiate hypokalemia	+
			Digitalis	↑ Toxicity of B if K^+ ↓	+
			Flucytosine	Possible ↑ toxicity of A	±
			Nephrotoxic drugs: aminoglycosides, cidofovir, cyclosporin, foscarnet, pentamidine	↑ Nephrotoxicity of A	++
Fluconazole	Itraconazole	Ketoconazole			
−	+	+	Isoniazid	↓ Levels of A	+
+	+	+	Rifampin/rifabutin	↑ Levels of B, ↓ serum levels of A	+
+	+	+	Theophyllines	↑ Levels of B with toxicity	+
+	−	?	Zidovudine	↑ Levels of B	+
?	+	+	Didanosine	↓ Absorption of A	+
	+	+	Indinavir	↑ Levels of B	+
	+	+	Nelfinavir	↑ Levels of B	+
	+	+	Saquinavir	↑ Levels of B	+
+	+	+	Cyclosporin, tacrolimus	↑ Levels of B	+
+	+	+	Antihistamines	↑ Levels of B (cardiac arrhythmias)	++
−	+	+	Proton pump inhibitors	↓ Absorption of A	+
−	+	+	H_2-blockers, antacids, sucralfate	↓ Absorption of A	+
+	+	+	Cisapride	↑ Levels of B (arrhythmias, ↑ QT interval)	++
+	+	+	Midazolam/triazolam	↑ Levels of B	++
+	?	?	Amytriptyline	↑ Levels of B	+
+	+	+	Hydantoins	↑ Levels of B, ↓ levels of A	++
−	+	−	Carbamazepine	↓ Levels of A	+
+	+	+	Oral anticoagulants	↑ Levels of B	++
+	+	?	Oral hypoglycemics	↑ Levels of B	++
?	+	?	Lovastatin/simvastatin	Rhabdomyolysis reported	+

Data from Gilbert DN, Moellering RC, Jr, Sande MA, eds: *The Sanford guide to antimicrobial therapy,* ed 28, Hyde Park, VT, 1999, Antimicrobial Therapy. and Kwon-Chung KJ, Bennett JE: *Medical mycology,* Philadelphia, 1992, Lea & Febiger.

ties, including hypoxia, have been reported with amphotericin B colloidal dispersion.

The clinical indications for use of these preparations remain controversial largely because of their high cost. Very limited evaluation of these preparations in comparison with amphotericin B or with each other has been performed. The lipid amphotericin B formulations have shown efficacy in many indications, including their use as salvage therapy for patients who fail amphotericin B deoxycholate or who are intolerant to it. In addition, liposomal amphotericin B was shown to have fewer adverse events and to reduce proved emergent fungal infections when used as empiric therapy for persistent fever in febrile neutropenic patients, although no change in overall outcome was noted. However, despite the improved therapeutic index of these amphotericin B formulations as compared with amphotericin B deoxycholate, they have not been shown superior in efficacy. Although it has not been confirmed in prospective clinical trials, it appears that the selective use of these preparations in patients with severe fungal infection who have baseline renal insufficiency or who are at very high risk for nephrotoxicity (e.g., allo-

genic bone marrow transplant recipients receiving nephrotoxic medications) may be justified. In addition, in patients who have infections that respond poorly to amphotericin B, including infections caused by Zygomycetes, *Fusarium,* and other invasive moulds such as *Aspergillus,* it is possible that high dosages of lipid formulations of amphotericin B will improve outcome. Other liposomal polyene preparations, including liposomal nystatin (Nyrontan), are undergoing clinical evaluation but are not commercially available.

■ AZOLES

The principal azoles used in the treatment of invasive mycosis are ketoconazole (keto), itraconazole (Itra), and fluconazole (Flu).

Ketoconazole, an early azole still used for limited indications for systemic infection, is available in only an oral formulation. Itraconazole, a triazole similar to ketoconazole, has been available only in an oral preparation, although an intravenous preparation was recently approved for use in the

Table 3   Amphotericin B Lipid Formulations

AMPHOTERICIN B LIPID FORMULATIONS	STRUCTURE	INDICATIONS	DOSAGES
Amphotericin B lipid complex (ABLC) (Abelcet)	Ribbonlike structures of a bilayered membrane formed by combining a 7:3 mixture of dimyristoyl-phosphatidylcholine and dimyristoylphosphatidylglycerol with amphotericin B (drug/lipid ratio of 1:1)	Invasive fungal infections in patients refractory or intolerant to amphotericin B deoxycholate	5 mg/kg/day as single infusion
Amphotericin B cholesteryl sulfate complex colloidal dispersion (ABCD), (Amphotec)	Disklike structures of cholesterol sulfate complexed with amphotericin B in equimolar concentration	Treatment of patients who either failed or are intolerant to amphotericin B deoxycholate	3-4 mg/kg/day (up to 6 mg/kg/day)
Liposomal amphotericin B (Ambisome)	Small unilamellar liposomes about 55-75 nm in diameter made up of a bilayer membrane of hydrogenated soy phosphatidylcholine and distearoylphosphatidylglycerol stabilized by cholesterol and combined with amphotericin B in a 2:0.8:1:0.4 ratio	Empirical treatment for presumed fungal infection in febrile neutropenic patients; treatment of patients with *Aspergillus* species, *Candida* species, and/or *Cryptococcus* species infection refractory to amphotericin B deoxycholate, or in patients in whom renal impairment or toxicity precludes the use of amphotericin B deoxycholate	3-5 mg/kg/day as single infusion

Data from Hiemenz JW, Walsh TJ: Lipid formulations of amphotericin B: recent progress and future directions, *Clin Infect Dis* 22(suppl 2):5133, 1996.

United States. Fluconazole, another triazole, is commercially available in both an oral and an intravenous preparation. Fluconazole is well absorbed independently of the fasting state or gastric pH. However, the absorption of both ketoconazole and itraconazole is greatly influenced by gastric pH and the fasting state. Ketoconazole is a weak base and requires a low gastric pH for absorption. On the other hand, the absorption of itraconazole is enhanced when administered with food.

The most common dosages of these agents are shown in Table 1. Ketoconazole and itraconazole do not require dosage adjustment in patients with renal dysfunction. These agents are highly lipophilic and do not diffuse to the CSF even in presence of meningeal inflammation. Ketoconazole is not indicated in patients with meningeal or central nervous systemic infection. However, despite low CSF levels, itraconazole has been used successfully in patients with fungal meningitis, including coccidioidal meningitis and cryptococcosis. In contrast to the other azoles, fluconazole has a wide tissues distribution and extensively diffuses to the CSF (concentrations in CSF and urine are 70% to 90% of peak plasma concentrations). Fluconazole is mainly excreted in urine, and the dosages need to be adjusted in case of renal failure.

The side effects of the azoles are generally mild, consisting of nausea, vomiting, headache, dizziness, rash, pruritus, and anorexia. These effects occur in fewer than 5% of patients and are often dose related. All azoles can cause significant hepatitis (estimates of toxicity range from 1 in every 10,000 to 50,000 patients after a mean of 4 weeks of therapy). Typically, the liver dysfunction is characterized by asymptomatic elevation of transaminases in the range of two to three times the upper limit of normal. Mild, asymptomatic transaminase elevations can be managed without drug discontinuation and close follow up. Symptomatic liver dysfunction, however, requires discontinuation of treatment. Enzyme elevations are reversible but may take months to normalize. Drug interaction also occur because of inhibition of cytochrome P450 pathways. Fluconazole has the least toxicity and fewest drug interactions (Table 2). Ketoconazole can inhibit steroidogenesis at dosages at or above 400 mg/day and may cause gynecomastia, adrenal insufficiency, and decreased libido. Likewise, itraconazole at dosages greater than 400 mg/day can cause hypokalemia, hypertension, and pedal edema. Such side effects have not been observed with fluconazole. Coadministration of drugs that interact with hepatic microsomal enzymes may cause subtherapeutic plasma drug levels or systemic toxicity (see Table 2). When possible, monitoring levels of coadministered drugs is advisable, particularly if associated with a narrow therapeutic index.

Fluconazole has been used extensively in the treatment of systemic yeast infections, including primary therapy for candidemia, particularly that caused by *C. albicans* but also other yeasts, including *C. tropicalis, C. parapsilosis,* and *C. glabrata.* Only *C. krusei* is inherently resistant to fluconazole, although resistance may develop to fluconazole and other azoles in *C. glabrata.* Fluconazole is also effective in the therapy of cryptococcal infections, including meningitis, with most use for consolidation therapy after initial therapy with amphotericin B and for long-term suppressive therapy in immunosuppressed patients, including those with acquired immunodeficiency syndrome (AIDS). Fluconazole is an alternative, when appropriate, to amphotericin B in the management of *C. immitis* meningitis. In addition, fluconazole is indicated for the prophylaxis of yeast infection in patients with chemotherapy-induced neutropenia.

Itraconazole is indicated for the therapy of endemic mycoses, including histoplasmosis, blastomycosis, and sporotricosis, usually used after amphotericin B in severely ill patients or as primary therapy in patients with less extensive infection. For aspergillosis, itraconazole is indicated in patients not responding to or tolerant of amphotericin B. It is used for sequential therapy following initial amphotericin B in invasive aspergillosis and as primary therapy in less immunosuppressed patients with less extensive infection. In addition, itraconazole is effective in cutaneous and systemic infection resulting from dematiacious fungi, including *Exophiala* species and *Bipolaris* species.

The indications for ketoconazole for systemic mycoses are limited. Most use for more serious infection has been replaced by the newer azoles itraconazole or fluconazole. Ketoconazole is used for chronic mucocutaneous candidiasis, but its use for systemic mycoses is reduced by poor oral absorption in critically ill patients and lack of an intravenous formulation.

■ FLUCYTOSINE

The clinical usefulness of flucytosine (5-FC) is limited by its narrow spectrum of activity, frequent emergence of resistance, and toxicity. 5-FC is usually administered at a dosage of 150 mg/kg/day in four divided doses, although 100 mg/kg/day in four divided doses may be used in combination with amphotericin B for cryptococcal meningitis. More than 90% of the drug is excreted unchanged in the urine, and patients with renal insufficiency require dosage reduction. As an approximation, the total daily dose should be reduced to 75 mg/kg with a creatinine clearance of 26 to 50 ml/min and to 37 mg/kg when the creatinine clearance is 13 to 25 ml/min. In azotemic patients, blood levels should be measured and dosage should be adjusted so that serum levels do not exceed 50 to 100 μg/ml. The drug readily diffuses to the CSF and achieves concentrations of about 74% of serum. 5-FC is usually well tolerated and results in minor and uncommon adverse effects, such as rash, diarrhea, and mild hypertransaminasemia. The presence of azotemia or the concomitant use of amphotericin B might exacerbate the toxicity, resulting in severe leukopenia, thrombocytopenia, and enterocolitits. These complications seem to occur in many, but not all, patients with blood levels exceeding 100 μg/ml.

5-FC has been used extensively to treat chromomycosis. It is not used alone because of the rapid development of resistance and the availability of other less toxic agents, although it has activity in candidiasis and cryptococcosis. Importantly, 5-FC has been shown to have synergistic effects in combination with amphotericin B against most isolates of *Candida, Cryptococcus neoformans,* and possibly *Aspergillus.* The combination of amphotericin B and 5-FC has been proved useful in the treatment of cryptococcal meningitis in terms of more rapid sterilization of CSF and possibly in reducing rate of relapse. 5-FC has been used with amphotericin B for invasive aspergillus infections as well as in the therapy of refractory candidemia, although its benefit in these infections has not been shown in controlled trials. Flucytosine has also been used in combination with fluconazole in both cryptococcal infections and against *Candida.*

■ NEW THERAPIES

Investigational Azoles

A number of new azoles are in various stages of development, such as voriconazole (UK-109,496), posaconazole (SCH-56592), and ravuconazole (BMS-207,147). Less advanced in clinical development include other azoles such as T-8581, D0870, UR-9746, and UR-9751. Only voriconazole and posaconazole are currently undergoing clinical trials with initial human trials just beginning with ravuconazole. Voriconazole has shown to have a broad-spectrum activity that includes filamentous fungi, particularly *Aspergillus* as well as *Candida albicans* and fluconazole-resistant *Candida* species. In the case of posaconazole, it has shown to be active against *Candida* species, *Cryptococcus neoformans, Aspergillus fumigatus,* and many other opportunistic yeasts and moulds. A similar broad spectrum of activity in vitro has been demonstrated by ravuconazole. Of these agents, only voriconazole has a intravenous formulation used in the clinical setting, although prodrug formulations of both posaconazole and ravuconazole have been developed, which may allow the intravenous administration of those compounds as well.

Echincocandins and Pneumocandins

The echinocandins are cyclic lipopeptide fungicidal antifungals that prevent cell-wall synthesis by noncompetitive inhibition of 1,3-β-glucan synthase, an enzyme that is absent in mammalian cells. Echinocandins and pneumocandins that are currently in various stages of development include cancidas (MK-991), LY 303366, and FK-463. These agents have activity against *Candida* species and *Aspergillus* species and appear to have very limited nephrotoxicity while retaining significant fungicidal activity against many fungi.

Pradimicins

The pradimicins, such as BMS-181184, are antifungal compounds that bind to cell-wall mannoproteins in a calcium-dependent manner that causes osmotic-sensitive lysis, causing leakage of intracellular potassium. They are active against *Aspergillus* species, *Candida* species, and *C. neoformans.* While this class of agent is not currently in active clinical development because of toxicities of the prototype compounds, they represent an important new antifungal target.

Nykkomycins

These compounds are potent chitin-synthase inhibitors, which are necessary for cell-wall synthesis. Nikkomycin Z has shown activity against *C. immitis* and *B. dermatitidis* alone and against *Candida* species, *C. neoformans,* and *Aspergillus fumigatus* in combination with azoles.

Sordarins

This new class of antifungals in early preclinical development inhibits protein synthesis through the binding to elongation factor 2. These compounds have shown to have activity against a wide range of fungi, including *Candida* species, *C. neoformans, P. carinii,* and some filamentous fungi as well as emerging invasive fungal pathogens.

■ FUTURE DIRECTIONS

Despite the increasing number of antifungal agents, treatment of fungal diseases still remains unsatisfactory. In many cases, host factors such as neutropenia associated with cytotoxic chemotherapy or other causes of underlying immunosuppression play a pivotal role as important risk factors for the acquisition of fungal infections as well as for response to therapy. Future research efforts should be aimed at reducing risk of acquiring fungal infections as well as improving host defenses against these opportunistic pathogens. The use of recombinant hematopoietic growth factors, such as recombinant cytokine granulocyte-colony-stimulating factor (G-CSF) and granulocyte-macrophage colony-stimulating factor (GM-CSF) has been demonstrated to shorten the duration of neutropenia in patients undergoing cyototoxic chemotherapy. These growth factors may be useful in reducing risk for opportunistic mycoses as well as improving host responses in these infections. In addition, as more antifungal agents for systemic disease become clinically available, the role of combinations of agents, particularly using agents that target distinct fungal targets, may be a means for improving overall outcome of antifungal therapy in these infections. These future research efforts are essential in improving clinical responses of antifungal agents in the therapy of systemic mycoses in severely immunosuppressed hosts.

Suggested Reading

Denning DW: Invasive aspergillosis, *Clin Infect Dis* 26:781, 1998.

Edwards JE Jr et al: International conference for the development of a consensus on the management and prevention of severe candidal infections, *Clin Infect Dis* 25:43, 1997.

Gallis HA, Drew RH, Pickard WW: Amphotericin B: 30 years of clinical experience, *Rev Infect Dis* 12:308, 1990.

Gilbert DN, Moellering RC Jr, Sande MA, eds: *The Sanford guide to antimicrobial therapy,* ed 28, Hyde Park, VT, 1999, Antimicrobial Therapy.

Graybill JR: The future of antifungal therapy, *Clin Infect Dis* 22(suppl 2):S166, 1996.

Groll AH, Piscitelli SC, Walsh TJ: Clinical pharmacology of systemic antifungal agents: a comprehensive review of agents in clinical use, current investigational compounds, and putative targets for antifungal drug development, *Adv Pharmacol* 44:343, 1998.

Hiemenz JW, Walsh TJ: Lipid formulations of amphotericin B: recent progress and future directions, *Clin Infect Dis* 22(suppl 2):S133, 1996.

Kwon-Chung KJ, Bennett JE: *Medical mycology,* Philadelphia, 1992, Lea & Febiger.

Patterson TF: Editorial response: approaches to the therapy of invasive mycoses—the role of amphotericin B, *Clin Infect Dis* 26:339, 1998.

Walsh TJ, et al: Amphotericin B lipid complex for invasive fungal infections: analysis of safety and efficacy in 556 cases, *Clin Infect Dis* 26:1383, 1998.

ANTIVIRAL THERAPY

Sankar Swaminathan
Roger J. Pomerantz

Successful antiviral therapy remains one of the most difficult challenges facing the physician today. The reasons stem from some intrinsic characteristics of the major human viral pathogens. Because all viruses parasitize host cell enzymes and structures to varying degrees, designing or discovering drugs that specifically target the virus without toxicity is difficult. Second, many viruses establish a latent infection in the host, during which they are essentially quiescent. Elimination of such latent viruses from the host has so far remained an elusive goal. Some of the most serious viral infections today stem from the reactivation of latent viruses during periods of impaired cell-mediated immunity.

Most of the currently available antiviral agents target the virus by exploiting differences in the viral and host replication machinery. Many viruses have their own specific DNA polymerases, which are more susceptible to inhibition by specific drugs than the cellular DNA replication enzymes. Thus many antiviral agents are nucleoside analogs. In addition, some of these compounds accumulate preferentially in virus-infected cells or are activated by virus-encoded enzymes, increasing their specificity. Nevertheless, unlike many antibacterial agents, most antiviral agents remain far from being "magic bullets" and can have considerable dose-related toxicities.

This chapter describes the Food and Drug Administration (FDA)-approved antiviral drugs available in the United States, their primary uses, and the major toxicities associated with their administration. Since the last edition of this book, there have been dramatic changes in the approach to the therapy of human immunodeficiency virus type 1 (HIV-1). These changes and the available antiretroviral drugs are discussed in the chapter *HIV Infection: Antiretroviral Therapy.* There have also been additions to the armamentarium against other viruses and some new uses discovered for old drugs. New viral diseases and syndromes continue to emerge and promise to remain a major challenge to all practicing physicians, emphasizing the need for continued research aimed at developing new and effective antiviral agents.

■ ACYCLOVIR

Acyclovir (9-[2-hydroxy-ethoxy)methyl) guanine sodium, a guanine derivative has in vitro activity against herpes simplex virus (HSV), varicella-zoster virus (VZV), Epstein-Barr virus (EBV), and cytomegalovirus (CMV), but it is used primarily in HSV and VZV infections. Acyclovir inhibits viral DNA polymerase and causes DNA chain termination when incorporated into replicating DNA. Acyclovir is preferentially taken up by HSV-infected cells and is phosphorylated by HSV thymidine kinase, which is necessary for conversion to the active triphosphate form.

Acyclovir may be used in primary episodes of genital herpes to reduce the time of viral shedding and time to healing at 200 mg orally five times per day for 10 days. Acyclovir can be used as chronic suppressive therapy to decrease the incidence of recurrent genital herpes at 400 mg orally twice daily. Therapy should be evaluated periodically to reassess the need for chronic suppression. In some patients, preemptive therapy with 200 mg five times a day for 5 days at the first sign of a recurrence is enough to prevent its development. An ointment is available for primary herpes genitalis, but its impact on the natural course of the infection is marginal.

Acyclovir reduces mortality in HSV encephalitis and should be used at high dosages (10 mg/kg IV every 8 hours). Severe mucosal and cutaneous infections in immunocompromised patients may require IV therapy (5 mg/kg every 8 hours). HIV-1–infected patients often require oral suppression to prevent recurrences. Refractoriness to therapy in such patients may indicate the development of acyclovir resistance.

Acyclovir is also active against VZV, but treatment of VZV infections requires higher dosages than treatment of uncomplicated HSV infections. Acyclovir at 10 mg/kg every 8 hours for 7 days should be used in immunocompromised patients with herpes zoster (shingles) to prevent dissemination. Oral acyclovir, 400 mg five times a day, or IV therapy is effective in preventing mucocutaneous HSV infections in transplant patients and may be given longer term (6 months) to decrease the incidence of VZV infections in bone marrow transplant recipients. Acyclovir may also be used in the treatment of zoster in immunocompetent patients (800 mg orally five times daily for 7 days), in whom it shortens the time to healing. Such treatment does not convincingly alter the subsequent development of postherpetic neuralgia, however. Ophthalmic zoster, involving the first branch of the trigeminal nerve, warrants evaluation by an ophthalmologist and immediate therapy, which may be given orally. VZV has also been associated with the syndrome of acute retinal necrosis, which should be treated promptly.

Acyclovir is effective in the treatment of primary varicella or chickenpox, shortening the duration and severity of illness when begun within 24 hours after the onset of rash. Whether such treatment of children affects long-term immunity or the subsequent incidence of zoster remains to be demonstrated. Chickenpox in pregnant women may be life-threatening, particularly when varicella pneumonia develops. It is our practice to treat all adults with clinical varicella pneumonia with IV acyclovir. Acyclovir

treatment of neonates with VZV or HSV infection is also indicated.

Acyclovir may be of some benefit in EBV-induced lymphoproliferative disease in immunocompromised patients, but it is not clinically useful in EBV disease such as mononucleosis. Incidentally, acyclovir is of no utility in the treatment of chronic fatigue because this syndrome has no causal association with EBV infection. Acyclovir is active and has been clinically useful against *Herpesvirus simiae,* or B virus, an endemic herpesvirus of certain primate species, which, when transmitted to humans has resulted in severe neurologic disease and death.

Pharmacokinetics

Acyclovir is excreted renally. The serum half-life is 2.5 to 3 hours. Acyclovir has good tissue distribution.

Major Toxicities

Central nervous system (CNS) effects range from confusion to seizures and coma, especially in the setting of renal insufficiency, underlying altered mental status and old age. Renal failure may occur from precipitation in the renal tubules. Acyclovir is potentially teratogenic but inadvertent or therapeutic administration during pregnancy has occurred without obvious adverse effects.

■ FAMCICLOVIR

Famciclovir, a diacetyl 6-deoxy analog of penciclovir (9-[4-hydroxy-3-hydroxymethylbut-1-yl] guanine), is a nucleoside analog that has a spectrum of activity similar to that of acyclovir. Famiciclovir is an inactive prodrug of penciclovir. After oral administration, famciclovir is rapidly metabolized to active penciclovir, which is phosphorylated by viral thymidine kinase and has a mechanism of action similar to acyclovir. Famciclovir is more bioavailable than acyclovir and has a prolonged intracellular half-life, which permits thrice-daily dosing. Famciclovir is approved for treatment of herpes zoster (500 mg three times daily for 7 days) and is similar to acyclovir in ameliorating the course of the acute attack. It is also claimed, on the basis of two studies, that famciclovir shortens the duration of postherpetic neuralgia.

Pharmacokinetics

Famciclovir is excreted renally. The serum half-life is 2.5 to 3 hours, but the intracellular half-life is 10 to 20 times longer.

Major Toxicities

In clinical trials, no major adverse effects have been reported to date. It should be noted that famciclovir, like acyclovir, has potentially teratogenic effects. Testicular toxicity was observed in animal models and decreased fertility was observed in male rats after 10 weeks of administration at 1.9 times the human dosage.

Drug Interactions

Probenecid may lead to increased famciclovir levels. Famciclovir may lead to increased digoxin levels.

VALACYCLOVIR

Valacyclovir is a valyl ester of acyclovir that is metabolized to acyclovir after oral administration, resulting in plasma levels of acyclovir similar to those achieved with IV acyclovir. However, such higher bioavailability is expected to be dependent on factors such as gastrointestinal absorption and hepatic function. Valacyclovir given at a dosage of 1 g three times daily has been shown to reduce time to healing and postherpetic neuralgia in herpes zoster and to do so more effectively than acyclovir. Valacyclovir may also be used in primary and recurrent genital herpes when given twice daily. In most respects, valacyclovir is appropriate when oral acyclovir is used and may be a potential substitute for IV acyclovir. However, the exact situations in which oral valacyclovir may be safely substituted for IV acyclovir, especially in the immunosuppressed patient, remain to be defined.

Major Toxicities

The major toxicities are similar to those of acyclovir. In addition, thrombotic thrombocytopenic purpura (TTP) has been reported in immunosuppressed patients receiving valacyclovir for extended periods. The overall risk of such complications, especially in the general population, is undefined.

PENCICLOVIR

Penciclovir is a nucleoside analog similar to ganciclovir in structure. It has activity similar to that of acyclovir and is available only as a topical preparation for recurrent herpes labialis. In clinical trials, it shortened the duration of symptoms by half a day if applied within 1 hour of the beginning of symptoms and again every 2 hours while awake. Thus its unimpressive performance is similar to that of all topical preparations available for the treatment of herpes infections other than in the eye.

GANCICLOVIR

Ganciclovir (DHPG, 9-(1,3-dihydroxy-2-propoxymethyl) guanine, a guanine derivative) is the major antiviral agent used against cytomegalovirus (CMV). Ganciclovir is phosphorylated by viral and then cellular kinases and preferentially accumulates in CMV-infected cells. It competitively inhibits viral DNA polymerase and is incorporated into DNA, acting as a chain terminator. Ganciclovir is used primarily in acquired immunodeficiency syndrome (AIDS)-associated CMV retinitis, colitis, pneumonitis, and disseminated disease. Efficacy in AIDS is clearly established only for retinitis, in which it slows progression and is not curative. Retinitis is treated with an induction phase (5 mg/kg every 12 hours for 14 to 21 days) followed by maintenance at the same dose once a day. Maintenance may also be given orally as 1000 mg three times daily with food. Patients who fail while receiving maintenance therapy may be "reinduced" or changed to foscarnet (see the following). Ganciclovir prevents CMV disease in high-risk transplant patients when given for 7 to 14 days at the same dosages as for induction

therapy. The duration of maintenance therapy depends on the intensity of immunosuppression and should be given for at least 100 days after the transplant in the case of marrow transplant patients. Treatment of established CMV pneumonia in bone marrow transplant patients is effective when combined with intravenous immunoglobulin.

Recently, an intravitreal ganciclovir implant for the treatment of CMV retinitis has become available. Because such local therapy does not prevent the development of CMV disease elsewhere, most importantly in the contralateral eye (see also "Fomivirsen," following), combination therapy with systemic ganciclovir has been studied. A recently completed large-scale study demonstrated that oral ganciclovir, albeit at a dosage of 4.5 g/day, prevented the development of retinitis in the unaffected eye almost as well as intravenous ganciclovir. CMV retinitis is much less common since the advent of highly active antiretroviral therapy (HAART), and prophylaxis may be unnecessary in those patients achieving immune reconstitution. However, CMV retinitis often occurs in patients in whom antiretroviral therapy has already failed. The role of intravitreal and prophylactic ganciclovir in the setting of HAART and earlier antiretroviral therapy for HIV-1 will thus undoubtedly be further defined in the future.

Pharmacokinetics, Major Toxicities, and Drug Interactions

Ganciclovir is excreted renally and crosses the blood-brain barrier. The major toxicity of ganciclovir is hematologic, leading to neutropenia and thrombocytopenia. Ganciclovir may cause renal impairment and is carcinogenic and teratogenic. All cytotoxic drugs that inhibit cell replication have the potential to significantly increase the marrow toxicity of ganciclovir. These include chemotherapeutic agents, trimethoprim-sulfamethoxasole, dapsone, and other nucleoside analogs. Cyclosporin, amphotericin B, and other nephrotoxic agents should be used with caution because of the increased risk of combined nephrotoxicity. Probenecid may lead to increased ganciclovir levels.

FOSCARNET

Foscarnet (phosphonoformic acid) binds to pyrophosphate binding sites on viral DNA polymerases and reverse transcriptases. This compound does not bind to cellular DNA polymerases at virus-inhibitory concentrations. Foscarnet is active against all herpesviruses and has some direct activity in vitro against HIV-1. Foscarnet is used in AIDS patients with CMV retinitis who cannot tolerate or worsen on ganciclovir. Foscarnet is not curative but delays progression to greater than 3 months versus less than 1 month without therapy. Induction treatment is given at 60 mg/kg IV every 8 hours for 2 to 3 weeks, followed by maintenance therapy at 90 mg/kg once daily. Foscarnet is also used in resistant VZV and HSV infections in AIDS patients.

Pharmacokinetics

Foscarnet is excreted renally. Its half-life is variable and highly dependent on renal function which is invariably impaired by foscarnet. Thus close monitoring of renal function with dosage adjustment is mandatory in all patients.

Major Toxicities

The major toxicity of foscarnet is impairment of renal function. In addition, hypocalcemia, hypophosphatemia, hyperphosphatemia, hypomagnesemia, and hypokalemia may occur.

Drug Interactions

Foscarnet may interact with pentamidine, increasing the risk of fatal hypocalcemia and may have additive effects on anemia due to zidovudine.

■ CIDOFOVIR

Cidofovir is an acyclic nucleoside derivative with antiviral activity. Cidofovir was designed to minimize the resistance that develops in response to nucleoside analogs that require phosphorylation by viral enzymes such as acyclovir and ganciclovir. Although cidofovir must be diphosphorylated to become active, it does not require phosphorylation by viral kinases. Rather, cidofovir is activated by cellular enzymes. Cidofovir is more active against herpesvirus DNA polymerases than cellular DNA polymerases and thus has selective antiviral activity.

Cidofovir is primarily used for the treatment of CMV retinitis in AIDS patients and has been FDA approved for this indication in adults. Its use in other CMV infections and in other immunocompromised patients has not been adequately evaluated. Cidofovir has been effective in delaying the progression of CMV retinitis in AIDS patients, including those who have failed ganciclovir or foscarnet therapy. Ganciclovir-resistant strains of CMV, which carry mutations in the UL97 phosphokinase gene, generally remain susceptible to cidofovir. However, other ganciclovir-resistant mutants, especially those carrying mutations in the DNA polymerase gene may be cross-resistant to cidofovir. CMV strains resistant to ganciclovir, foscarnet, and cidofovir have also been described.

IV cidofovir is administered with probenecid to prevent rapid secretion of the drug by the renal tubules. Creatinine clearance should be estimated by calculation or directly measured before initiating therapy with cidofovir. The nephrotoxic potential of cidofovir is such that a creatinine clearance less than 55 ml/min, a serum creatinine greater than 1.5 mg/dl, or 2+ proteinuria are contraindications to its use. Induction therapy with cidofovir is initiated at a dosage of 5 mg/kg once weekly for 2 weeks, followed by the same dose once every 2 weeks as maintenance therapy. IV saline prehydration with 1 L of normal saline immediately before cidofovir infusion is mandatory to prevent nephrotoxicity. If possible, an additional liter of saline should be administered with and after cidofovir over a 1- to 3-hour period. In addition, great care should be paid to monitoring renal function with both urine and serum measurements, and the importance of taking the probenecid should be emphasized. Probenecid is administered as follows: 2 g 3 hours before infusion and 1 g at 2 and 8 hours after infusion.

Pharmacokinetics

Approximately 70% of cidofovir is eliminated unchanged by the kidneys. Its plasma half-life is approximately 2.5 hours, but it has a long-lasting antiviral effect. The latter is the result of the intracellular persistence of its active phosphorylated metabolite.

Major Toxicities

As described, the major toxicity of cidofovir is its nephrotoxicity. Neutropenia has occurred in approximately 20% of cidofovir recipients in clinical trials.

Drug Interactions

The most important drug interactions in general are those leading to additional nephrotoxicity. Additive or synergistic nephrotoxic effects with other drugs known to result in nephrotoxicity, such as aminoglycosides or amphotericin B, have not been studied. In addition, the potential for probenecid effects on the metabolism and disposition of other drugs must be considered.

■ FOMIVIRSEN

Fomivirsen, a novel agent active against CMV, is a prototype of an "antisense" approach to antiviral therapy. Fomivirsen has engendered much excitement as a possible forerunner of a class of agents targeted against specific molecular targets in the genome of bacterial and viral pathogens. Fomivirsen consists of a synthetic oligonucleotide with a DNA sequence complementary to the messenger RNA of the immediate early transcriptional unit IE2 of human CMV. Its presumed mechanism of action is to bind to and inactivate CMV messenger RNA. Interestingly, however, fomivirsen-resistant mutant strains of CMV derived in the laboratory carry mutations outside of the gene targeted by fomivirsen, leaving open the possibility that its mechanism of action may be unrelated to its ability to bind to its intended RNA target. Fomivirsen is administered by intravitreal injection. Fomivirsen injection may be considered in situations in which conventional therapy, including systemic or intravitreal ganciclovir, foscarnet, or cidofovir, has failed or is contraindicated. Induction therapy consists of 330 μg by intravitreal injection every other week for two doses followed by maintenance therapy once every 4 weeks. Response is usually seen within days, with a reported median time to response of 8 days. Intravitreal injection of fomivirsen, as might be expected does not provide any systemic anti-CMV treatment.

Pharmacokinetics

Systemic absorption after intravitreal injection is thought to be minimal. Metabolism is via exonucleases and catabolism of the resultant mononucleotides.

Major Toxicities

Transient increases in intraocular pressure and inflammation have been reported. Retinal toxicity has been noted with injection of amounts above the recommended dosage. Systemic toxicity or interactions with other drugs have not been reported.

■ AMANTADINE

Amantadine is an anti-Parkinson's and antiviral agent that prevents uncoating of influenza A virus after host cell entry.

It is indicated for the prophylaxis of unimmunized high-risk patients in the presence of a documented outbreak of influenza A. It is also useful in those high-risk patients who have had an anaphylactic reaction to egg proteins or prior influenza vaccination. Amantadine does not impair antibody response and so may be used concurrently with vaccine to protect till development of immunity. Treatment of influenza A with amantadine may be useful if instituted early in disease (<48 hours after onset). Dosage is 200 mg/day, which may be given as two 100-mg doses. Prophylaxis should be given for at least 10 days after exposure. It may be given for 90 days when the vaccine is contraindicated. Drug-resistant strains develop rapidly and may limit its usage in children, who shed virus for longer periods of time.

Pharmacokinetics, Major Toxicities, and Drug Interactions

Amantadine is excreted renally. Its major toxicities are related to the central nervous system (CNS): dizziness, confusion, and seizures. Anticholinergic drugs and amantadine used concurrently may lead to unacceptable atropine-like effects. Hydrochlorothiazide and triamterene used with amantadine have led to increased amantadine levels.

■ RIMANTADINE

Rimantadine is a structural analog of amantidine. It has essentially the same indications as amantadine and the dosage is the same. It is associated with fewer CNS side effects, however. Unlike amantadine, rimantadine undergoes extensive metabolism and dosage may need to be adjusted in those with either hepatic or renal insufficiency.

Drug Interactions

Aspirin and acetaminophen reduce plasma levels of rimantadine slightly, whereas cimetidine may lead to increased levels.

■ RIBAVIRIN

Ribavirin is a synthetic nucleoside that interferes with viral RNA transcription, but its complete mechanism of action may be more complex. Ribavirin has a broad spectrum of activity against RNA viruses, including respiratory syncytial virus (RSV), hepatitis C, measles virus, Lassa fever virus, and hantaviruses.

A major new use for ribavirin is as combination therapy with interferon alfa against chronic hepatitis C. Oral ribavirin combined with injected interferon alfa (see the following) has been shown to produce a sustained virologic response when used either as initial therapy or after relapse in patients previously treated with interferon alfa alone. Oral dosage is based on the patient's body weight and is 400 mg in the morning and 600 mg in the evening daily for those weighing less than 75 kg. For those weighing more than 75 kg, the dosage is 600 mg twice a day. For previously untreated patients, treatment should be administered for 24 to 48 weeks. Discontinuation of therapy should be considered in those who have not responded by 24 weeks. For patients who have relapsed after interferon therapy, the recommended duration is 24 weeks. There are no safety and efficacy data beyond this period, but these recommendations may change based on future studies. The combination may be effective in interferon nonresponders, but its utility in this setting or in liver transplantation has not been established. It is commonly necessary to adjust the dosage based on adverse effects in individual patients. The need for close monitoring and dosage modification based on parameters such as white blood cell count and hemoglobin is emphasized.

Ribavirin is administered as an aerosol for confirmed, severe, lower respiratory (RSV) infection in infants or the immunosuppressed adult host. Because ribavirin has in vitro activity against Lassa fever virus and hantaviruses, it has been used intravenously in Lassa fever cases, in hemorrhagic fevers, and in the recent hantavirus pulmonary syndrome outbreak in the United States. Management of these rare and often fatal infections mandates contact with the Centers for Disease Control and Prevention (Atlanta, Georgia).

Pharmacokinetics

The elimination half-life of ribavirin is more than 300 hours after multiple dosing. Ribavirin thus accumulates over the long term in vivo. Aerosolized ribavirin is absorbed systemically with a plasma half-life greater than 9 hours.

Major Toxicities

Ribavirin is potentially mutagenic, teratogenic, and embryotoxic. Documentation that the female patient is not pregnant and two methods of contraception while receiving therapy and for 6 months after treatment is therefore recommended. It is also recommended that similar precautions be observed if the male partner is being treated. Hematologic side effects, principally anemia, are common, and the recommendations for dosage adjustment and discontinuation vary depending on whether the patient has known cardiac disease. Ribavirin by the aerosol route may lead to respiratory failure in chronic obstructive pulmonary disease (COPD) and asthma. The drug may precipitate in the mechanical ventilator and lead to an inability to ventilate the patient.

■ INTERFERONS

Interferons are naturally occurring glycoproteins with antiviral, antitumor (antiproliferative), and immunomodulatory activities. They are induced by viral infection, especially double-stranded RNA viruses. Alpha-interferon is primarily synthesized by B lymphocytes and beta-interferon by fibroblasts and other cells. Alpha-interferon and beta-interferon are closely related. Alpha-interferon is actually a heterogeneous family of proteins encoded by multiple similar genes. Gamma-interferon is produced by T lymphocytes and is induced by mitogenic stimuli such as antigen-presenting cells and antigen. Gamma-interferon also has macrophage-activating functions and other interleukin activities, modulating the function of other lymphocytes. Recently, a form of interferon termed *interferon alfacon-1* was introduced. Interferon alfacon-1 is not found in nature, but its structure was derived by combining the sequences of various naturally occurring interferons and produced by recombinant DNA technology.

The mechanism(s) of action of interferons is varied. Their antiviral effect is partly mediated by inducing cellular enzymes that lead to a shutdown of protein synthesis in virus-infected cells as well as activating RNA degradation.

Route of Administration and Major Toxicities

Administration is subcutaneous, intramuscular (IM), or intralesional. Major toxicities commonly observed are flu-like symptoms, fever (in almost all patients treated), myalgias, fatigue, and alopecia. Exacerbation of some autoimmune diseases and psoriasis with interferon have been observed. Depression has been associated with administration of some interferons. Ophthalmologic side effects such as retinal hemorrhages have been rarely reported concomitantly with interferon therapy.

■ INTERFERON ALFA-2a

Interferon alfa-2a (recombinant human protein made in *Escherichia coli*) may be used in the treatment of the following conditions: (1) AIDS-associated Kaposi's sarcoma—the response correlates with extent of HIV-1 progression more than the severity of Kaposi's sarcoma, and (2) chronic hepatitis C—see the following section.

■ INTERFERON ALFA-2b

Interferon alfa-2b (recombinant human protein made in *E. coli*) is used in the treatment of the following conditions:

· Condyloma acuminata: Interferon alfa-2b is injected intralesionally for the treatment of condyloma acuminata. Injection of 1 million units per lesion is performed with a tuberculin syringe on alternate days, three times a week for 3 weeks. The product literature should be consulted for other details regarding administration and dosage.
· AIDS-associated Kaposi's sarcoma: The dosage is 30 million units/m^2 three times a week, administered intramuscularly (IM) or subcutaneously. If tolerated, treatment may be continued until resolution of tumors.
· Chronic hepatitis C: Interferon treatment decreases transaminase levels and may lead to sustained virologic response. The benefit extends beyond period of therapy. Relapse may be treated with combination ribavirin-interferon therapy. Interferon-naive patients may also be treated with combination therapy. The dosage is 3 million units subcutaneously three times weekly. The optimal duration of therapy in different situations remains to be defined.
· Chronic hepatitis B: A virologic response with loss of eAg (and sAg in some patients) and improved transaminases may occur. Lasting remission may also be occasionally obtained. Interferon alfa-2b has been administered as 5 million units daily or 10 million units three times a week for this indication.

■ INTERFERON ALFA-n3

Interferon alfa-n3 is a purified natural human leukocyte interferon. It is produced by infecting human leukocytes with Sendai virus and purifying the induced interferon. It is used intralesionally for condyloma acuminata.

■ INTERFERON ALFACON-1

Interferon alfacon-1 is used in the treatment of chronic hepatitis C. A dose of 9 µg is administered subcutaneously three times a week for 24 weeks.

■ LAMIVUDINE (3TC)

Lamivudine is a pyrimidine analog most commonly used as part of combination regimens for treatment of HIV-1 infection. Lamivudine also inhibits hepatitis B DNA polymerase and may be used as treatment for chronic hepatitis B infection. Treatment with 100 mg daily has been shown to result in serologic conversion, virologic response, and histologic improvement. Treatment has been associated with the development of lamivudine-resistant mutants. Treatment of HIV-1–positive patients with lamivudine alone is not recommended because it is likely to result in rapid appearance of lamivudine-resistant HIV-1 strains. Lactic acidosis with severe hepatomegaly with steatosis are rare side effects of lamivudine. The majority of lamivudine is excreted unchanged in the urine.

■ PALIVIZUMAB

Palivizumab is a monoclonal antibody directed against the F protein of RSV. It is used for the prevention of RSV infection in high-risk pediatric patients by passive immunization. Palivizumab is a "humanized" monoclonal antibody. It is produced in vitro and was developed using recombinant technology. It is genetically composed of 95% human and 5% murine sequences. It is administered as an IM injection at a dose of 15 mg/kg of body weight. Its efficacy has been demonstrated in children with bronchopulmonary dysplasia (BPD) and premature infants born at less than 35 weeks' gestation. Use of the monoclonal antibody resulted in a 55% decrease in the rate of hospitalization due to RSV infections. The severity of infection occurring despite prophylaxis did not appear to be significantly affected, however.

Pharmacokinetics and Major Toxicities

The mean half-life in pediatric patients was 20 days. Although no major toxicities have been observed, the potential for local and anaphylactic reactions may exist with this preparation as with all protein injections.

■ TRIFLURIDINE

Trifluridine (Trifluorothymidine) is a fluorinated pyrimidine analog that interferes with DNA synthesis and is used topically for the treatment of HSV keratitis. Trifluridine may cause local irritation and palpebral edema.

■ VIDARABINE

Vidarabine (Ara-A, adenine arabinoside) is a purine analog made from *Streptomyces antibioticus* that inhibits viral DNA polymerases. It has been supplanted by acyclovir because of the greater efficacy and lower toxicity of acyclovir in HSV and VZV infections. It was the first agent used against HSV encephalitis but has been made almost obsolete by acyclovir. Acyclovir-resistant strains of HSV and VZV are currently treated with foscarnet. Vidarabine is currently only used as an ointment for the treatment of herpetic keratitis caused by HSV-1 and HSV-2.

■ IMIQUIMOD

Imiquimod is a topical agent that may be used for the treatment of condyloma acuminata. Its mode of action is unknown but may act as an immune response modifier. It has no direct antiviral activity. Systemic absorption appears to be minimal, and local reactions appear to be the major toxicity. However, its long-term effects and safety have not been evaluated.

The FDA has recently approved two new agents against influenza A and B. They represent nevraminidase inhibitors (i.e., oseltramavir, oral; and zanamivir, topical).

Suggested Reading

Balfour HH Jr: Antiviral drugs, *N Engl J Med* 1999, 340:1255, 1999.

Hayden FG, Douglas RG: Antiviral agents. In Mandell GL, Dolin R, eds: *Principles and practice of infectious diseases*, New York, 1994, Churchill Livingstone.

HYPERSENSITIVITY TO ANTIBIOTICS

R. Stokes Peebles, Jr.
N. Franklin Adkinson, Jr.

One would hope that accurately diagnosing the microbiology and extent of disease would be the most difficult aspect of treating an infection; however, treatment complications and determining alternative therapeutic options can add a great deal of complexity to an already difficult clinical situation. Unexpected adverse reactions to an antimicrobial agent may be worse than the original infection for which the treatment was instituted, even leading to the patient's death. However, a careful review of a patient's previous adverse medication reactions, an understanding of the types of reactions that can occur, an accurately assessment of a patient's risk for a future reaction, early recognition of an severe reaction, and institution of appropriate immediate treatment can minimize therapeutic misadventures with antiinfective agents.

Adverse reactions to medications can take many different clinical forms and can result from many mechanisms. Toxic reactions are the dose-related direct pharmacologic adverse effects of a medication. The severity of a toxic reaction for a particular dose of a drug varies among individuals, but everyone will eventually suffer toxic drug effects as doses are increased. Examples of toxic reactions include nephrotoxicity from aminoglycosides, and nausea and headaches from theophylline. Drug hypersensitivity reactions, on the other hand, are restricted to a vulnerable subset of the population, who are, for various reasons, predisposed. Drug hypersensitivity can be divided into three broad categories: drug intolerance, idiosyncratic reactions, and immunologic drug reactions.

Drug intolerance is a predictable pharmacologic response to medication at a dosage usually tolerated by most patients. Genetic or metabolic factors may be responsible, and some patients are intolerant of multiple drugs. An example is tinnitus occurring after two aspirin tablets. This is a known toxic effect of salicylates but usually occurs only at much higher dosages. Idiosyncratic responses to a medication are unexpected reactions that do not have any relationship to the known pharmacologic or toxic properties of the drug. These reactions are often produced by normal doses and can occur on first exposure to the drug. Mechanisms for idiosyncratic reactions vary; most are unknown. An example of an idiosyncratic reaction is the irreversible aplastic anemia that occurs in 1 in every 25,000 to 40,000 exposures to chloramphenicol. This idiosyncratic reaction has occurred with all routes and doses of chloramphenicol, even by ocular exposure to the drug. This idiosyncratic reaction can be contrasted to the toxic, dose-related, reversible bone marrow suppression that commonly occurs at maximal recommended doses of chloramphenicol.

Table 1 Gell and Coombs' Classification of Immunologically Mediated Reactions

CLASS	MECHANISM	IMMUNE ELEMENTS	CLINICAL REACTIONS
I	Anaphylactic	IgE	Rhinorrhea, urticaria, bronchospasm, angioedema, anaphylaxis
II	Cytotoxic	IgM, IgG, complement	Hemolytic anemia, drug-induced nephritis
III	Immune complex	IgG, complement	Serum sickness, fever
IV	Delayed	T lymphocytes	Contact dermatitis, probably maculopapular eruptions, exfoliative dermatitis
V	Obscure	Unknown	Isolated eosinophilia, toxic epidermal necrolysis, erythema multiforme (Stevens-Johnson)

Adapted from Weiss ME, Adkinson NF: *Clin Allergy* 18:515, 1988.

■ IMMUNOLOGIC DRUG REACTIONS

Immunologic drug reactions, which are the primary focus of this chapter, are those mediated by a specific immune response. For many allergic drug reactions, the mechanism of the immunopathologic response is readily defined; for others, the exact immunologic mechanism remains obscure. Gell and Coombs have proposed a useful scheme for delineating known immunopathologic mechanisms (Table 1). Type I reactions are initiated by IgE-dependent activation of mast cells and basophils. Prior drug exposure produces IgE antibodies with specificities for the drug itself, or for a neoantigen formed by covalent binding of a drug or metabolite to a native protein. In the latter case, the drug behaves as a hapten, and the process of covalent drug binding to the native protein is known as haptenation. Most drugs are too small (usual molecular weight <600) to be immunologic by themselves and must be complexed polyvalently with a native protein to trigger immune recognition or immunopathology. When the drug is readministered to a sensitized patient, cross-linking of IgE on basophils and mast cells occurs, leading to degranulation of these cells and release of their inflammatory mediators. Systemic reactions that ensue as a result of this IgE cross-linking event are termed *anaphylaxis.* The anaphylactic syndrome is a continuum of pathologic responses ranging from mild allergic responses confined to nasal congestion and coryza, conjunctivitis, and/or pruritus as the primary features, to more severe consequences of mediator release including generalized urticaria, laryngeal edema, bronchospasm, cardiovascular collapse, and death. Anaphylactic reactions usually start within 20 to 30 minutes after first-dose drug exposure but can be delayed in onset (up to 4 to 6 hours after exposure), and biphasic reactions have been described. Anaphylactoid or pseudo-allergic reactions are clinically indistinguishable from IgE-mediated anaphylaxis and also result from mast cell and basophil mediator release, but cell activation occurs by a nonimmunologic mechanism. Examples include opiate-induced urticaria (direct histamine release) and radiocontrast media reactions (hyperosmolarity).

Type II hypersensitivity reactions to a medication result from the formation of a drug-specific cytotoxic antibody, either IgG or IgM, which binds to cells haptenated by the sensitizing drug. Beta-lactam drugs provide the best-studied examples of this mechanism. High and prolonged dosages of these drugs may produce drug-induced anemias and thrombocytopenias, as well as interstitial nephritis. Type III hypersensitivity results from antibody-antigen complexes, which may then be deposited in body tissues, leading to serum-sickness–like syndromes, or simple cutaneous vasculitis. Accelerated type II and type III reactions can occur within 6 to 24 hours after reexposure in highly sensitive patients. Type IV reactions (e.g., contact dermatitis) are T cell mediated and are characterized by pruritic papular eruptions, although eczematoid dermatitis, erythema multiforme, and erythema nodosum may also occur. Maculopapular rashes and many cases of exfoliative dermatitis increasingly appear to be T cell mediated and therefore type IV. In type IV reactions, T cells that recognize the drug in context with an antigen-presenting cell produce cytokines and other mediators that lead to recruitment of macrophages, monocytes, and other lymphocytes to the site of drug. Reactions that are believed to be immunologic but for which a clear mechanism has not be delineated have been classified as type V reactions. Such reactions include Stevens-Johnson syndrome and toxic epidermal necrolysis. Table 2 categorizes commonly used antibiotics for their risk for producing immunologic reactions.

■ DIAGNOSIS

Accurate diagnosis of antibiotic hypersensitivity requires careful history and physical examination and sometimes in vivo and in vitro diagnostic tests. Important historical data include the timing of the reaction in relation to the onset of drug administration, whether the clinical reaction observed is a known complication of the drug taken, whether the suspect drug is known to be intrinsically allergenic, whether the patient has previously taken the drug and the course the patient experienced during prior administration, and whether the patient has ever experienced similar side effects to medications that may be cross-reactive with the suspect drug. Other important questions include what other drugs are currently being taken by the patient as well as what other coexisting medical conditions might be present. Patients with systemic lupus erythematosus (SLE) may be more likely to have a rash when treated with beta-lactams, sulfonamides, or erythromycin. As another example, cystic fibrosis patients may be at higher risk for immunologic reactions to aztreonam than the general population because of their greater exposure to other beta-lactam antibiotics.

Human immunodeficiency virus (HIV) infected patients present many special dilemmas to the physicians who care

Table 2 Risk of Immunologic Drug Reaction with Commonly Used Antibiotics

ANTIBIOTIC (OR ITS CLASS)	RISK OF INDUCING AN IMMUNOLOGIC REACTION[1]
Aztreonam	Rare
Aminoglycosides	Rare[2]
Amphotericin B	Rare[3]
Bacitracin	Intermediate
Cephalosporins	Intermediate[4]
Chloramphenicol	Rare
Clindamycin	Rare
Fluconazole	Rare
Flucytosine	Rare[5]
Griseofulvin	Rare
Imipenem	Intermediate
Itraconazole	Intermediate[6]
Ketoconazole	Rare[7]
Macrolides	Rare
Miconazole	Intermediate[8]
Polymyxin	Rare
Tetracyclines	Rare
Penicillins	Common
Quinolones	Intermediate
Spectinomycin	Rare
Sulfonamides	Common
Vancomycin	Rare[9]

Adapted from Weiss ME, Adkinson NF: *Clin Allergy* 18:515, 1988.
[1]Rare reactions are those that have an incidence less than 1%. Intermediate reactions have an incidence of 1% to 5%. Common reactions have an incidence of greater than 5%.
[2]Contact dermatitis can occur with streptomycin.
[3]Anaphylactoid reactions can occur.
[4]Serum sickness reactions have been most frequently reported with cefaclor.
[5]Has been reported in a patient with acquired immunodeficiency syndrome.
[6]Occurs more often in immunocompromised patients.
[7]Idiosyncratic reactions reported to occur in some patients after the first dose.
[8]Miconazole is administered in polyoxyl 35 castor-oil containing vehicle and anaphylactic reactions have been reported with the parenteral administration of other drugs in this same vehicle.
[9]Anaphylactoid reactions generally occur during rapid infusion of the drug.

for them, including a seemingly high rate of adverse medication reactions. Hypersensitivity reactions to drugs have been estimated to occur up to 100 times more often in the HIV-positive population compared with either immunocompetent or HIV-negative immunodeficient patients. The drugs most commonly associated with hypersensitivity reactions in HIV-positive patients include sulfonamides, sulfadiazine, pentamidine, and dapsone, and hypersensitivity reactions have been reported to the reverse transcriptase inhibitors nevirapine and delaviridine. The reason for the high rate of adverse medication reactions in HIV-positive patients is not totally clear but could be related to altered drug metabolism, coexisting infection with cytomegalovirus or Epstein-Barr virus, or the longer courses and higher dosages of medication required for management of infectious diseases in AIDS patients.

In vitro laboratory tests that are helpful in diagnosing drug hypersensitivity reactions include a complete blood count with differential and chemistry panel. The presence of an anemia and/or thrombocytopenia may indicate the presence of a type II hypersensitivity reaction. This can be further evaluated with a Coombs' test or the presence of IgG and IgM antibodies specific for the drug in question. Tests are available to determine the presence of antigen-antibody complexes; however, the presence of such complexes does not necessarily indicate that they are pathogenic in a type III reaction. Eosinophilia may be helpful in evaluating the presence of a drug-induced interstitial nephritis, drug fever, or serum sickness. The radioallergosorbent testing (RAST) can detect drug-specific IgE antibodies in serum. RAST is less sensitive than skin testing and if negative does not exclude significant type I drug allergy.

Intradermal skin testing has proved to be the most reliable indicator of drug-specific IgE and thereby the risk for anaphylaxis. At this time the only group of antibiotics for which skin testing has been validated for its predictive value is the beta-lactams. Beta-lactams are numerous, widely used, and the most common source of allergic drug reactions. IgE-dependent allergic reactions to penicillins occur during 0.7% to 2.0% of treatment courses and fatalities occur with a frequency of 1 per 50,000 to 100,000 treatment courses. Evaluation by skin testing can be very helpful in the evaluation of patients with a history of beta-lactam allergies.

Skin testing for penicillin allergy should ideally be performed in all patients with histories of type I penicillin allergy convincing enough to deny them further treatment. In addition, penicillin skin testing can also be helpful when the patient has a history compatible with a type II or III reaction to ensure that IgE sensitization has not taken place. Skin testing is not indicated for patients who have experienced maculopapular eruptions, exfoliative dermatitis, or Stevens-Johnson from a beta-lactam antibiotic. The reagents used for skin testing include benzylpenicilloyl polylysine (the major determinant reagent), a mixture of minor determinants (commonly made up of benzylpenicillin, benzylpenilloate, and benzylpenicilloate), and histamine and saline controls. Skin testing must be performed with both the major determinant and minor determinant mixture as false-negative results caused by incomplete testing can have serious sequelae, especially in patients with a history of anaphylaxis. Most type I allergic reactions to penicillin are urticarial and are associated with IgE antibodies against the major determinant. Some severe anaphylactic reactions have been associated with minor determinant IgE alone. Unfortunately, only the major determinant skin test reagent is available commercially (PREPEN, Bayer) at this time in the United States. Minor determinant reagents are still unlicensed orphan drugs and are generally available only at major medical centers, especially those with Allergy/Immunology training programs. Macy and colleagues have recently published results of a new penicillin minor determinant preparative method, which when used as a skin test reagent with the major determinant mixture and oral amoxicillin challenge, proved to have clinical safety and efficacy. Penicillin G (10,000 IU/ml) has been suggested as an acceptable substitute for the minor determinant mixture, when the latter is not available. About 80% of minor determinant

Table 3   Oral Desensitization Protocol

STEP*	PHENOXYMETHYL PENICILLIN (U/ml)	AMOUNT (ml)	DOSE (U)	CUMULATIVE DOSAGE (U)
1	1,000	0.1	100	100
2	1,000	0.2	200	300
3	1,000	0.4	400	700
4	1,000	0.8	800	1,500
5	1,000	1.6	1,600	3,100
6	1,000	3.2	3,200	6,300
7	1,000	6.4	6,400	12,700
8	10,000	1.2	12,000	24,700
9	10,000	2.4	24,000	48,700
10	10,000	4.8	48,000	96,700
11	80,000	1.0	80,000	176,700
12	80,000	2.0	160,000	336,700
13	80,000	4.0	320,000	656,700
14	80,000	8.0	640,000	1,296,700
Observe patient for 30 minutes.				
Change to benzylpenicillin G IV (slow intravenous drip over 15 minutes).				
15	500,000 U/ml	0.25	125,000	
16	500,000	0.50	250,000	
17	500,000	1.00	500,000	
18	500,000	2.25	1,125,000	

Adapted from Sullivan TJ: Penicillin allergy. In *Current therapy in allergy,* St Louis, 1985, Mosby.
*Fifteen-minute interval between steps

mixture reactors will have a positive skin test with penicillin G. Among those missed by penicillin G major and minor determinant mixtures, yet have reactions when challenged with amoxicillin. Cystic fibrosis patients may also have allergy to selective semisynthetic penicillins after repeated courses of therapy. Therefore it may be useful to consider skin testing with semisynthetic penicillin drugs in selected cases where side chain-specific reactions are suspected.

Cross-reactivity among the beta-lactam antibiotics, most notably between the penicillins and the cephalosporins, is a justifiable concern. Cross-reactivity between semisynthetic penicillins is virtually complete. Cephalosporin treatment produces reactions (including potentially life-threatening and fatal reactions) in 10% to 20% of penicillin-allergic patients, but determining which patients are cross-sensitive to a particular cephalosporin is a complex and difficult task. Because appropriate skin testing reagents are not commonly available, we recommend first performing penicillin skin testing. If this is positive, the patient should be considered at risk for acute allergic reactions to any beta-lactam and should be given any cephalosporin in an intensively monitored situation using a modified desensitization protocol if no alternative antibiotic is acceptable. Imipenem is a member of the carbapenem family of beta-lactam antibiotics and has cross-reactivity to penicillins comparable to cephalosporins. Aztreonam, a monobactam, has very little cross-reactivity with the standard beta-lactams both in vitro and clinically. Aztreonam has been safely used in many patients who are highly penicillin allergic. However, aztreonam should be administered with caution to cystic fibrosis patients who have allergy to other beta-lactam antibiotics because aztreonam may have allergenic potential with repeated use.

■ DESENSITIZATION

On rare occasions, a drug-allergic patient may require an antibiotic for which there is no acceptable non–cross-reactive alternative. In this circumstance, drug desensitization may allow the drug to be safely administered. Desensitization is a procedure by which a small amount of drug is given by incremental doses as tolerated until the patient has achieved the desired therapeutic dose. The medication may then given at a regular therapeutic dosing interval with care to avoid lapses in therapy. Should the patient stop the medication for even a short time, perhaps as little as 2 days, the entire desensitization protocol may have to be repeated to ensure safe full dose administration of the drug. Desensitization should be performed in a controlled medical setting where the patient is under constant monitoring. The medical care of the patient should be optimized before the initiation of the procedure, especially for patients suffering from asthma or cardiac disease. In addition, beta-adrenergic antagonists should be discontinued because they will exaggerate anaphylactic events should they occur.

Two widely accepted protocols for penicillin desensitization are shown in Tables 3 and 4. Table 3 outlines an oral desensitization protocol that is putatively safer because few deaths have occurred with oral as opposed to parenteral medication. This protocol should not be used when there is concern about the patient's ability to adequately absorb substances through the gastrointestinal tract. It has been previously reported that approximately one third of patients will experience a transient allergic reaction either during the course or after desensitization while the patient is still receiving the drug. Most of the reactions are very mild and resolve without treatment. Parenteral desensitiza-

Table 4 Parenteral Desensitization Protocol*

INJECTION NO.	BENZYLPENICILLIN CONCENTRATION (U/ml)	VOLUME/ROUTE† (ml)
1	100	0.1 ID
2	100	0.2 SC
3	100	0.4 SC
4	100	0.8 SC
5	1,000	0.1 ID
6	1,000	0.3 SC
7	1,000	0.6 SC
8	10,000	0.1 ID
9	10,000	0.2 SC
10	10,000	0.4 SC
11	10,000	0.8 SC
12	100,000	0.1 ID
13	100,000	0.3 SC
14	100,000	0.6 SC
15	1,000,000	0.1 ID
16	1,000,000	0.2 SC
17	1,000,000	0.2 IM
18	1,000,000	0.4 IM
19	continuous IV infusion (1,000,000 U/hr)	

Adapted from Weiss ME, Adkinson NF: *Clin Allergy* 18:515, 1988.
ID, Intradermal; *SC,* subcutaneous; *IM,* intramuscular; *IV,* intravenous.
*Doses are administered at 20-minute intervals.
†Observe skin wheal and flare response to intradermal doses.

Table 5 One-Day Trimethoprim-Sulfamethoxazole (TMP-SMX)-Graded Challenge*

DOSE	TMP-SMX (μg)	DOSE	TMP-SMX (mg)
1	1/0.2	7	1/0.2
2	3/0.6	8	3/0.6
3	9/1.8	9	9/1.8
4	30/6	10	30/6
5	90/18	11	90/18
6	300/60	12	300/60

From Demoly P, et al: *J Allergy Clin Immunol* 102:1033, 1998.
*Doses given orally (pediatric suspension) at 30-minute intervals.

tion to penicillin, as described in Table 4, may be used when oral desensitization is not possible, and has also been proved to be safe when performed in the appropriate surroundings. The mechanism of desensitization is unclear, but one accepted hypothesis is that the antigen threshold for mast cell and basophil mediator release is increased by giving the patient small incremental doses of the medication.

Generally, desensitization is not rationally used for hypersensitivity reactions other than type I. Treatment of infections with medications that have caused type II or III reactions can be attempted when the drug is intended for short courses with moderate doses; however, it is advisable to closely monitor the parameters that formerly indicated the presence of the type II or III reaction (e.g., complete blood count for anemia, thrombocytopenia, or eosinophilia). Maculopapular eruptions that occur with beta-lactams (particularly those that occur with ampicillin or amoxicillin during infection with Epstein-Barr virus) are not a contraindication for future therapy with these drugs. In this situation, patient risk on retreatment is similar to the general population who have previously never had an adverse reaction to these diamino penicillins. Patients who experience contact dermatitis to a topical exposure of an antibiotic usually tolerate oral or parenteral administration of the same drug without adverse consequences. However, a desquamative rash consistent with Stevens-Johnson syndrome or toxic epidermal necrolysis is a nearly absolute contraindication for retreatment as there are no valid predictive tests for recurrence of these drug reactions.

Desensitization may have a role in preventing drug adverse reactions that do not appear to be IgE mediated in HIV-positive patients. Recently, a 6-hour incremental dose protocol for sulfonamide was reported to be well tolerated in HIV-infected patients (Table 5). In this report, 44 patients who had a history of hypersensitivity manifested as pruritus, maculopapular eruption, and/or fever that was so severe to have caused discontinuation of the drug were evaluated. The patients underwent the 6-hour trimethoprim-sulfamethoxasole–graded challenge and were advised to "treat through" all nonbullous cutaneous adverse reactions that occurred in 11 of 44 patients. After a follow-up of 10 months, 95% of the patients were taking trimethoprim-sulfamethoxazole without any adverse reaction. Desensitization protocols have also been recently reported for zidovudine and nelfinavir.

Adverse reactions to antibiotics will continue to be a significant clinical problem, particularly when the offensive antibiotic is deemed the treatment of choice. These guidelines for diagnosis of different types of reactions and for strategies that can be taken to minimize potentially life-threatening sequelae from antibiotics will allow most patients with drug allergy history to receive safe and effective antibiotic therapy.

Suggested Reading

Coleman JW, Blanca M: Mechanisms of drug allergy, *Immunol Today* 19:196, 1998.

Demoly P, et al: Six-hour trimethoprim-sulfamethoxasole-graded challenge in HIV-infected patients, *J Allergy Clin Immunol* 102:1033, 1998.

Macy E, et al: Skin testing with penicilloate and penilloate prepared by an improved method: amoxicillin oral challenge in patients with negative skin test responses to penicillin reagents, *J Allergy Clin Immunol* 100:586, 1997.

Middleton E, et al, eds. Drug allergy. In *Allergy principles and practice*, ed 5, St Louis, 1998, Mosby.

Pichler WJ, Schnyder B, Zanni MP: Role of T cells in drug allergies, *Allergy* 53:225, 1998.

ANTIMICROBIAL AGENT TABLES

Rosalie Pepe
David Schlossberg

Table 1   Antibacterial Agents

NAME		USUAL DOSE		COST (PER DAY)*	CHANGE IN ABSORPTION WITH FOOD	PREGNANCY CLASS†
GENERIC	BRAND	ADULT	PEDIATRIC			
Amikacin‖	Amikin	15 mg/kg/day; divide q8-12h IV	15 mg/kg/day; divide q8-12h	$130.00		D
Amoxicillin	Amoxil	0.25-0.5 g q8h PO	6.6-13.3 mg/kg PO q8h	$0.82	Decreased	B
Amoxicillin-clavulanate	Augmentin	0.25-0.5 g q8h PO	6.6-13.3 mg/kg q8h PO	$5.60	Decreased	B
Ampicillin	Ampen, Omnipen	0.5-1 g q8h PO; 1-2 g q4-6h IV	12.5-25 mg/kg q8h PO 6.25-25 mg/kg q8h IV	$0.53 PO $12.40 IV	Decreased	B
Ampicillin-sulbactam	Unasyn	1.5-3 g q6h IV	25-50 mg/kg q6h IV	$22.90 1.5 g $40.70 3.0 g		B
Azithromycin	Zithromax	5 g day 1; 0.25 g days 2-5 PO	§	$6.55 $39.30/5 day course	Decreased	B
Azlocillin	Azlin	2-4 g q4-6h IV	75 mg/kg q6h IV	Not available		B
Aztreonam	Azactam	1-2 g q6-8h IV	30-50 mg/kg q6-12h (N.A.)	$104.00		B
Bacampicillin	Spectrobid	0.4-0.8 g q12h PO	12.5-25 mg/kg q12h PO	Not available		B
Carbenicillin indanyl sodium	Geocillin	1-2 0.382 g tabs q6h PO	7.5-12.5 mg/kg q6h PO	$8.09	Decreased	B
Carbenicillin	Geopen	5-6.5 g q4-6h IV	25-100 mg/kg q4-6h IV	Not available		B
Cefaclor	Ceclor	0.25-0.5 q8h PO	20-40 mg/kg/day; divide q8h PO	$6.72	Decreased	B
Cefadroxil	Duricef	0.5-1 g q 12-24h PO	30 mg/kg/day; divide q12h PO	$7.99	Decreased	B
Cefamandole	Mandol	0.5-2 g q4-8h IV	50-150 mg/kg/day; divide q4-8h IV	$36.25 (1 g q6h)		B

CRCI, Creatinine clearance ml/min; HD, hemodialysis; PD, peritoneal dialysis; CNS, central nervous system; GI, gastrointestinal; pHD, post-
*Average wholesale price according to the 1999 Red Book.
†FDA pregnancy categories: A, adequate studies in pregnant women, no risk; B, animal studies no risk, human studies inadequate, or animal benefit may outweigh risk; X, fetal abnormalities in humans, risk exceeds benefit.
‡Use in breast-feeding: limited data are available. Because all drugs are probably excreted in small amounts into breast milk, the potential for continued during treatment based on information available at present. "Avoid if possible" indicates that an alternative drug should be chosen or
§Insufficient information available to make a recommendation.
‖Aminoglycoside dosing may be modified after obtaining serum levels. The generally desired peak and trough concentrations are as follows: for kanamycin, peak 15-30 µg/ml, trough <5-10 µg/ml. "Once-daily" administration of aminoglycosides is gaining acceptance. The usual regimen is blockade. Dosage may be modified according to creatinine clearance or by following serum levels (see Nicolau et al. in "Suggested Reading").

USE IN BREASTFEEDING‡	DOSE INTERVAL ADJUSTMENT FOR REDUCED CRCL			SUPPLEMENTAL DOSE IN DIALYSIS		MAJOR TOXICITY
	>50	10-50	<10	HD	PD	
Avoid if possible	q8-12h	q12-48h	>48 hr	2.5-3.75 mg/kg pHD	2.5 mg/kg/day IV or 3-4 mg/2 L dialysate removed	Renal toxicity, vestibular or auditory toxicity, CNS reactions, neuromuscular blockade (rare)
Probably safe	q8h	q8-12h	q16-24h	0.25-0.5 g	0.25 g q12h	Allergic reactions (rare: anaphylactic), rash, diarrhea, nausea, vomiting
Probably safe	q8h	q12h	q12-24h	0.25 g PO	§	Allergic reactions (rare: anaphylactic), diarrhea, nausea, vomiting, cholestatic hepatitis
Probably safe	q4-6h	q8h	q12-24h	0.5-2 g	0.25 g q12h PO or 1-4 g q24h IV	Allergic reactions (rare: anaphylactic), diarrhea, nausea, vomiting
Probably safe	q6-8h	q8-12h	q24h	2 g ampicillin pHD	§	Allergic reactions (rare: anaphylactic), diarrhea, nausea, vomiting
Probably safe	Usual	Usual	Usual	§	§	GI disturbance, headache
Probably safe	q4-6h	q8h	q12h	3 g pHD	§	Allergic reactions (rare: anaphylactic), diarrhea, nausea, vomiting
Probably safe	q6-8h	q12-18h	q24h	⅛ first dose (60-250 mg) pHD	Usual dose (1-2 g) then ¼ usual dose at usual intervals	Rash, diarrhea, nausea, vomiting, elevated AST/ALT
Probably safe	q12h	q12h	§	§	§	Allergic reactions (rare: anaphylactic), diarrhea, nausea, vomiting
Probably safe	§	§	§	§	§	Allergic reactions (rare: anaphylactic), diarrhea, nausea, vomiting
Probably safe	q4h	2-3 g q6h	N.R.	0.75-2 g pHD	2 g q6-12h	Allergic reactions (rare: anaphylactic), diarrhea, nausea, vomiting
Probably safe	q8h	q8h	q8h	0.25-0.5 g	§	Allergic reactions, GI disturbance, arthritis, serum sickness
Probably safe	q12-24h	0.5 g q12-24 h	0.5 g q36h	0.5-1 g	§	Allergic reactions, GI disturbance
Probably safe	q4-8h	q8h	0.5-1 g q12h	0.5-1 g	§	Thrombophlebitis with IV infusion, allergic reactions, GI disturbance

hemodialysis; *N.A.,* not approved; *AST,* aspartate aminotransferase; *ALT,* alanine aminotransferase; *N.R.,* not recommended; *IT,* intrathecal.

toxicity, human studies no risk; *C,* animal studies show toxicity, human studies inadequate but benefit may exceed risk; *D,* evidence of human risk,

adverse reactions in the infant must be considered, although few have been reported. "Probably safe" indicates that breast-feeding can be consideration given to discontinuing breast-feeding.

gentamicin and tobramycin, peak 6-12 μg/ml and trough <2 μg/ml; for netilmicin, peak 6-10 μg/ml, trough <2 μg/ml; for amikacin and 5-7 mg/kg q24h for gentamicin and tobramycin, 15 mg/kg q24h for amikacin. The dose is infused over 60 minutes to avoid neuromuscular

Continued

748   Antimicrobial Agent Tables

Table 1   Antibacterial Agents—cont'd

NAME		USUAL DOSE		COST (PER DAY)*	CHANGE IN ABSORPTION WITH FOOD	PREGNANCY CLASS†
GENERIC	BRAND	ADULT	PEDIATRIC			
Cefazolin	Ancef, Kefzol	0.5-2 g q8h IV	25-100 mg/kg/day; divide q6-8h IV	$15.99 (1 g q8h)		B
Cefepime	Maxipime	0.5-2 g q12h IV	50 mg/kg q8h IV (N.A.)	$63.76		B
Cefixime	Suprax	0.4 g q24h PO	8 mg/kg/day; divide q24h PO	$6.96	Decreased	B
Cefmetazole	Zefazone	2 g q6-12h IV	§	Not available		B
Cefonicid	Monocid	0.5-2 g q24h IV	§	$26.10		B
Cefoperazone	Cefobid	1-2 g q6-12h IV	25-100 mg/kg q12h IV (N.A.)	$35.10		B
Cefotaxime	Claforan	0.5-2 g q8-12h IV 3 g q6h for CNS	50-200 mg/kg/day; divide q4-8h IV	$90.39 2 g q6h		B
Cefotetan	Cefotan	1-2 g q12h IV	40-60 mg/kg/day; divide q12h IV (N.A.)	$46.04		B
Cefoxitin	Mefoxin	1-2 g IV q6-8h IV	80-160 mg/kg/day; divide q4-8h IV	$83.60		B
Cefpodoxime	Vantin	0.1-0.4 g q12h PO	5 mg/kg q12h PO	$5.94	Increased	B
Cefprozil	Cefzil	0.25-0.5 g q12-24h PO	15 mg/kg q12h PO	$6.34		B
Ceftazidime	Fortaz, Tazicef, Tazidime	1-2 g q8-12h IV	25-50 mg/kg q8h IV	$86.80 2g q8h		B
Ceftizoxime	Cefizox	1-3 g q6-8h IV	33-50 mg/kg q6-8h IV	$36.90		B
Cetriaxone	Rocephin	0.5-2 g q12-24h IV	50-100 mg/kg/day; divide q12-24h IV	$81.60 2 g q24h		B
Cefuroxime	Zinacef, Kefurox	0.75-1.5 g q8h IV	50-100 mg/kg/day divide q6-8h IV	$20.29		B
Cefuroxime axetil	Ceftin	0.125-0.5 g q12h PO	0.125-0.25 g q12h PO	$7.34	Decreased	B
Cephalexin	Keflex, Biocef, Keftab	0.25-1 g q6h PO	25-100 mg/kg/day; divide q6h PO	$5.03 generic $11.94 trade	Unchanged	B
Cephalothin	Keflin	0.5-2 g q4-6h IV	80-160 mg/kg/day; divide q6h IV	$43.20		B
Cephapirin	Cefadyl	0.5-2 g q4-6h IV	40-80 mg/kg/day divide q6h IV	$6.56		B

CRCl, Creatinine clearance ml/min; *HD,* hemodialysis; *PD,* peritoneal dialysis; *CNS,* central nervous system; *GI,* gastrointestinal; *pHD,* post-
*Average wholesale price according to the 1999 Red Book.
†FDA pregnancy categories: *A,* adequate studies in pregnant women, no risk; *B,* animal studies no risk, human studies inadequate, or animal benefit may outweigh risk; *X,* fetal abnormalities in humans, risk exceeds benefit.
‡Use in breast-feeding: limited data are available. Because all drugs are probably excreted in small amounts into breast milk, the potential for continued during treatment based on information available at present. "Avoid if possible" indicates that an alternative drug should be chosen or
§Insufficient information available to make a recommendation.
‖Aminoglycoside dosing may be modified after obtaining serum levels. The generally desired peak and trough concentrations are as follows: for kanamycin, peak 15-30 µg/ml, trough <5-10 µg/ml. "Once-daily" administration of aminoglycosides is gaining acceptance. The usual regimen is ockade. Dosage may be modified according to creatinine clearance or by following serum levels (see Nicolau et al. in "Suggested Reading").

USE IN BREASTFEEDING‡	DOSE INTERVAL ADJUSTMENT FOR REDUCED CRCL			SUPPLEMENTAL DOSE IN DIALYSIS		MAJOR TOXICITY
	>50	10-50	<10	HD	PD	
Probably safe	q8h	0.5-1 g q8-12h	0.5-1 g q24h	0.25-0.5 g	§	Allergic reactions, GI disturbance, diarrhea
Probably safe	0.5-2 g q12h IV	q24h	0.25-0.5 g q24h	dose pHD	0.5-2 g q48h	Nausea, diarrhea, vomiting, rash, phlebitis
Probably safe	q24h	0.3 g q24h	q48h	None	§	Thrombophlebitis, allergic reactions, GI disturbance
Probably safe	q6-12h	q16-24h	q48h	§	§	Thrombophlebitis, allergic reactions, GI disturbance
Probably safe	q24h	4-15 mg/kg q24-48h	4-15	None	§	Allergic reactions, GI disturbance, hypoprothrombinemia or hemorrhage
Probably safe	q6-12h	q6-12h	q6-12h	Dose after HD	§	Thrombophlebitis, allergic reactions, GI disturbance
Probably safe	q8-12h	q12-24h	0.5 g q24-48h	0.5-2 g	§	Thrombophlebitis, allergic reactions, GI disturbance
Probably safe	q12h	q24h	q48h	25% dose nonHD days, 50% HD	§	Thrombophlebitis, allergic reactions, GI disturbance, hypoprothrombinemia, hemorrhage
Probably safe	q6-8h	q12-24h	0.5-1 g q12-24h	1-2 g	§	Thrombophlebitis, allergic reactions, GI disturbance
Probably safe	q12h	q24h	q24h	Dose 3× wk	§	Allergic reactions, GI disturbance
Probably safe	q12-24h	50% dose q12-24h	50% dose q12-24h	§	§	Allergic reactions, GI disturbance
Probably safe	q8-12h	q12-24h	q24-48h	1 g load then 1 gpHD	0.5 g q24h IV or 250 mg/2 L dialysate	Thrombophlebitis, allergic reactions, GI disturbance
Probably safe	q6-8h	0.25-1 g q12h	0.5 g q24h	Dose pHD	3 g q48h	Thrombophlebitis, allergic reactions, GI disturbance
Probably safe	q12-24h	q12-24h	q12-24h	None	§	Thrombophlebitis, allergic reactions, GI disturbance, cholelithiasis
Probably safe	q8h	q8-12h	0.75 g q24h	0.75 g	15 mg/kg aftr dialysis	Thrombophlebitis, allergic reactions, GI disturbance
Probably safe	q12h	q12h	0.25 g q24h	§	§	Allergic reactions, GI disturbance
Probably safe	q6h	q8-12h	q24-48h	0.25-1 g	§	Allergic reactions, GI disturbance
Probably safe	q4-6h	1-1.5 g q6h	0.5 g q8h	0.5-2 g	Add up to 6 mg/kg to dialysate	Thrombophlebitis with IV infusion, allergic reactions, GI disturbance
Probably safe	q4-6h	q8h	q12h	7.5-15 mg/kg pHD then q12h	§	Thrombophlebitis, allergic reactions, GI disturbance

hemodialysis; *N.A.,* not approved; *AST,* aspartate aminotransferase; *ALT,* alanine aminotransferase; *N.R.,* not recommended; *IT,* intrathecal.

toxicity, human studies no risk; *C,* animal studies show toxicity, human studies inadequate but benefit may exceed risk; *D,* evidence of human risk,

adverse reactions in the infant must be considered, although few have been reported. "Probably safe" indicates that breast-feeding can be consideration given to discontinuing breast-feeding.

gentamicin and tobramycin, peak 6-12 μg/ml and trough <2 μg/ml; for netilmicin, peak 6-10 μg/ml, trough <2 μg/ml; for amikacin and 5-7 mg/kg q24h for gentamicin and tobramycin, 15 mg/kg q24h for amikacin. The dose is infused over 60 minutes to avoid neuromuscular

Continued

Table 1   Antibacterial Agents—cont'd

NAME		USUAL DOSE		COST (PER DAY)*	CHANGE IN ABSORPTION WITH FOOD	PREGNANCY CLASS†
GENERIC	BRAND	ADULT	PEDIATRIC			
Cephradine	Velosef	0.25-1 g q6h PO 0.5-2 g q4-6h IV	25-100 mg/kg/day; divide q6-12h PO 50-100 mg/kg divide q6h IV	$3.30 PO	Decreased	B
Chloram-phenicol	Chloromycetin	0.25-0.75 g q6h PO 0.25-1 g q6h IV	50-100 mg/kg/day; divide q6h PO, IV	$5.01 PO $16.59 IV	No data	C
Cinoxacin	Cinobac	0.25 g q6h, 0.5 g q12h PO	N.R.	$4.44	No data	C
Ciprofloxacin	Cipro	0.25-0.75 g q12h PO 0.2-0.4 g q12h IV	N.R.	$7.98 PO $57.62 IV	Decreased	C
Clarithromycin	Biaxin	0.25-0.5 g q12h PO	7.5 mg/kg q12h (N.A.)	$6.90	Increased or unchanged	B
Clindamycin	Cleocin	0.15-0.3 g q6h PO 0.3-0.9 g q6-8h IV	8-25 mg/kg/day; divide q6-8h PO 15-40 mg/kg/day; divide q6-8h IV	$13.55 PO $33.53 IV	Unchanged	B
Cloxacillin	Tegopen	0.5-1 g q6h PO	12.5-25 mg/kg q6h PO	$2.71	Decreased	B
Colistin		5-15 mg/kg/day q8h PO 2.5-5 mg/kg/day q6-12h IV	5-15 mg/kg/day; divide q8h PO 2.5-5 mg/kg/day; divide q6-12h IV	Not available		Not established
Dapsone		0.05-0.1 g q24h PO	1-2 mg/kg/day; divide q24h	$0.34		C
Dicloxacillin	Dynapen	0.25-0.5 g q6h PO	3.125-6.25 mg/kg q6h PO	$10.68	Decreased	Not established
Doxycycline	Vibramycin	0.1 g q12h PO, IV	2.2 mg/kg q12-24h PO, IV	$1.04 PO generic $6.86 PO trade	Decreased with milk, antacids	D
Enoxacin	Penetrex	0.4 g q12h PO, IV	N.R.	$3.23	Decreased	C
Erythromycin base	EryC, PCE, Emycin, Erytab	0.25-0.5 g q6h PO	30-50 mg/kg/day; divide q6h	$1.00 PO	Decreased	B

CRCI, Creatinine clearance ml/min; *HD,* hemodialysis; *PD,* peritoneal dialysis; *CNS,* central nervous system; *GI,* gastrointestinal; *pHD,* post-
*Average wholesale price according to the 1999 Red Book.
†FDA pregnancy categories: *A,* adequate studies in pregnant women, no risk; *B,* animal studies no risk, human studies inadequate, or animal benefit may outweigh risk; *X,* fetal abnormalities in humans, risk exceeds benefit.
‡Use in breast-feeding: limited data are available. Because all drugs are probably excreted in small amounts into breast milk, the potential for continued during treatment based on information available at present. "Avoid if possible" indicates that an alternative drug should be chosen or §Insufficient information available to make a recommendation.
‖Aminoglycoside dosing may be modified after obtaining serum levels. The generally desired peak and trough concentrations are as follows: for kanamycin, peak 15-30 µg/ml, trough <5-10 µg/ml. "Once-daily" administration of aminoglycosides is gaining acceptance. The usual regimen is blockade. Dosage may be modified according to creatinine clearance or by following serum levels (see Nicolau et al. in "Suggested Reading").

USE IN BREASTFEEDING‡	DOSE INTERVAL ADJUSTMENT FOR REDUCED CRCL			SUPPLEMENTAL DOSE IN DIALYSIS		MAJOR TOXICITY
	>50	10-50	<10	HD	PD	
Probably safe	q6h	0.5 g q6h	0.25 g q12h	0.25 g before HD, then 12, 36, and 48 hr pHD	0.5 g q6h	Allergic reactions, GI disturbance
Avoid if possible	Usual	Usual	Usual	Dose pHD	Usual	Blood dyscrasias, gray baby syndrome, GI disturbance
Avoid if possible	q6h	0.25 g q12-24h	N.R.	§	§	Nausea, vomiting, dizziness, headache, tremors, confusion
Avoid if possible	q12h	0.25-0.5 g q12h PO, q12-24h IV	0.25-0.5 g q18h PO, q18-24h IV	0.25-0.5 g q24h, pHD on HD days	0.25-0.5 g q24h	Nausea, vomiting, dizziness, headache, tremors, confusion
Probably safe	q12h	q12-24h	q24h	§	§	GI disturbance, abnormal taste, headache
Avoid if possible	Usual	Usual	Usual	Usual	Usual	Diarrhea, including pseudomembranous colitis, allergic reactions
Probably safe	q6h	q6h	q6h	Usual	Usual	Allergic reactions (rare: anaphylactic), diarrhea, nausea, vomiting
§	q6-12h	2.5 mg/kg/day q12-24h	1.5 mg/kg q36h	§	§	Nephrotoxicity, CNS side effects including confusion, coma, seizures
Avoid if possible	q24h	q24h	q24h	§	§	Rash, headache, GI irritation, infectious mono-like syndrome
Probably safe	q6h	q6h	q6h	Usual	Usual	Allergic reactions (rare: anaphylactic), diarrhea, nausea, vomiting
Avoid if possible	q12h	q12h	q12h	Usual	Usual	GI disturbance, photosensitivity reactions, hepatic toxicity, esophageal ulcers
Avoid if possible	q12h	0.1-0.2 g q12h	0.1-0.2 g q12h	§	§	Nausea, vomiting, dizziness, headache, tremors, confusion
Probably safe	q6h	q6h	q6h	Usual	Usual	GI disturbance; rare: allergic reactions, hepatic dysfunction, hearing loss

hemodialysis; *N.A.,* not approved; *AST,* aspartate aminotransferase; *ALT,* alanine aminotransferase; *N.R.,* not recommended; *IT,* intrathecal.

toxicity, human studies no risk; *C,* animal studies show toxicity, human studies inadequate but benefit may exceed risk; *D,* evidence of human risk,

adverse reactions in the infant must be considered, although few have been reported. "Probably safe" indicates that breast-feeding can be consideration given to discontinuing breast-feeding.

gentamicin and tobramycin, peak 6-12 μg/ml and trough <2 μg/ml; for netilmicin, peak 6-10 μg/ml, trough <2 μg/ml; for amikacin and 5-7 mg/kg q24h for gentamicin and tobramycin, 15 mg/kg q24h for amikacin. The dose is infused over 60 minutes to avoid neuromuscular

Continued

Table 1   Antibacterial Agents—cont'd

NAME		USUAL DOSE		COST (PER DAY)*	CHANGE IN ABSORPTION WITH FOOD	PREGNANCY CLASS†
GENERIC	**BRAND**	**ADULT**	**PEDIATRIC**			
Erythromycin estolate	Ilosone	0.25-0.5 g q6h PO	3-50 mg/kg/day; divide q6h	$3.05	Decreased	B
Erythromycin ethyl succinate	EES, eryPed	0.4 g q8h PO	30-50 mg/kg/day divide q8h PO	$0.98		B
Erythromycin lactobionate	Erythrocin	0.5-1 g q6h IV	15-20 mg/kg/day; divide q6h IV	$41.20 IV		B
Gentamicin‖	Garamycin	3-5 mg/kg/day; divide q8h IV 4-8 mg/day IT	3-7.5 mg/kg/day; divide q8h IV	$32.11		C
Imipenem	Primaxin	0.5-1 g q6h IV	15-25 mg/kg q6h IV (N.A.)	$88.08		C
Kanamycin‖	Kantrex	15 mg/kg/day; divide q8-12h IV	15 mg/kg/day; divide q8-12h IV	$13.56		D
Levofloxacin	Levaquin	0.25 0.5 g/day PO or IV	§	$6.94	Unchanged	C
Lincomycin	Lincocin	0.5 g q6-8h PO 0.6-1 g q8-12 IV	30-60 mg/kg/day; divide q6-8h PO 10-20 mg/kg/day; divide q6h IV	$6.04 PO $45.18 IV		Not established
Lomefloxacin	Maxaquin	0.4 g q24h PO	N.R.	$6.93	No data	C
Loracarbef	Lorabid	0.2-0.4 g q12-24h PO	15-30 mg/kg/day; q12h	$6.30	Decreased	B
Meropenem	Merrem	0.5-1 g q8h IV	20-40 mg/kg q8h IV	$155.52		B
Metronidazole	Flagyl	0.25-0.5 g q6-12h PO 0.5 g q6-8h IV	15 mg/kg/day; divide tid (N.A.)	$2.48 PO generic $8.18 PO trade $59.90 IV	Unchanged	B
Mezlocillin	Mezlin	3-4 g q4-6h IV	50 mg/kg q4-6h IV	$75.36 4 g q6h		B
Minocycline	Minocin, Dynacin	0.1 g q12h PO, IV	2 mg/kg q12h PO, IV	$6.65 PO $79.60 IV	Decreased with milk, antacids	D

CRCI, Creatinine clearance ml/min; *HD,* hemodialysis; *PD,* peritoneal dialysis; *CNS,* central nervous system; *GI,* gastrointestinal; *pHD,* post-
*Average wholesale price according to the 1999 Red Book.
†FDA pregnancy categories: *A,* adequate studies in pregnant women, no risk; *B,* animal studies no risk, human studies inadequate, or animal benefit may outweigh risk; *X,* fetal abnormalities in humans, risk exceeds benefit.
‡Use in breast-feeding: limited data are available. Because all drugs are probably excreted in small amounts into breast milk, the potential for continued during treatment based on information available at present. "Avoid if possible" indicates that an alternative drug should be chosen or
§Insufficient information available to make a recommendation.
‖Aminoglycoside dosing may be modified after obtaining serum levels. The generally desired peak and trough concentrations are as follows: for kanamycin, peak 15-30 µg/ml, trough <5-10 µg/ml. "Once-daily" administration of aminoglycosides is gaining acceptance. The usual regimen is blockade. Dosage may be modified according to creatinine clearance or by following serum levels (see Nicolau et al. in "Suggested Reading").

USE IN BREASTFEEDING‡	DOSE INTERVAL ADJUSTMENT FOR REDUCED CRCL			SUPPLEMENTAL DOSE IN DIALYSIS		MAJOR TOXICITY
	>50	10-50	<10	HD	PD	
Probably safe	Usual	Usual	Usual	No change	No change	Cholestatic hepatitis, hearing loss or tinnitus, GI disturbance, hypersensitivity reactions
Probably safe	Usual	Usual	Usual	Usual	Usual	GI disturbance; rare: allergic reactions, hepatic dysfunction
Probably safe	Usual	Usual	Usual	Usual	Usual	GI disturbance; rare: allergic reactions, hepatic dysfunction, hearing loss
Avoid if possible	q8-12h	q12-48h	>48 hr	1-1.7 mg/kg pHD	1 mg/2 L dialysate removed	Renal toxicity, vestibular and auditory toxicity, CNS reactions, neuromuscular blockade (rare)
Probably safe	q6h	0.5 q8-12h	0.25-0.5 g q12h	0.25-0.5 pHD then q12h	§	Fever, rash, nausea, vomiting, diarrhea, seizures (rare)
Avoid if possible	q8-12h	q12-48h	>48 hr	4-5 mg/kg pHD	3.75 mg/kg/day	Cranial nerve VIII and renal damage
Avoid if possible	Usual	0.25 q24-48h	0.25 q48h	0.25 q48h	0.25 q48h	Diarrhea, nausea, headache
Avoid if possible	Usual	Usual	Usual	§	§	Diarrhea, including pseudomembranous colitis, allergic reactions
Avoid if possible	q24h	0.2 g q24h	0.2 g q24h	0.4 g load, then 0.2 g q24h	§	Nausea, vomiting, dizziness, headache, tremors, confusion, photosensitivity
Probably safe	q12-24h	q24-48h	q3-5 days	Dose after HD	§	Allergic reactions, GI disturbance
Probably safe	0.5-1 g q8h IV	q12h	0.25-0.5 q24h	§	§	Nausea, diarrhea, vomiting, rash
Avoid if possible	Usual	Usual	Usual	Usual	Usual	Nausea, headache, metallic taste
Probably safe	q4-6h	q8h	q8h	2-3 g then 3-4 g q12h	3 g q12h	Allergic reactions (rare: anaphylactic), diarrhea, nausea, vomiting
Avoid if possible	q12h	q12h	q12h	Usual	Usual	GI disturbance, photosensitivity, hepatic toxicity, esophageal ulcers, vestibular toxicity; tooth discoloration

hemodialysis; *N.A.,* not approved; *AST,* aspartate aminotransferase; *ALT,* alanine aminotransferase; *N.R.,* not recommended; *IT,* intrathecal.

toxicity, human studies no risk; *C,* animal studies show toxicity, human studies inadequate but benefit may exceed risk; *D,* evidence of human risk,

adverse reactions in the infant must be considered, although few have been reported. "Probably safe" indicates that breast-feeding can be consideration given to discontinuing breast-feeding.

gentamicin and tobramycin, peak 6-12 µg/ml and trough <2 µg/ml; for netilmicin, peak 6-10 µg/ml, trough <2 µg/ml; for amikacin and 5-7 mg/kg q24h for gentamicin and tobramycin, 15 mg/kg q24h for amikacin. The dose is infused over 60 minutes to avoid neuromuscular

Continued

Table 1   Antibacterial Agents—cont'd

NAME		USUAL DOSE		COST (PER DAY)*	CHANGE IN ABSORPTION WITH FOOD	PREGNANCY CLASS†
GENERIC	BRAND	ADULT	PEDIATRIC			
Nafcillin	Nallpen, Unipen	0.5-2 g q4-6h IV	150 mg/kg/day; divide q4-6h IV	$18.00 2 g q6h		B
Neomycin	Neo-tabs	50 mg/kg/day; divide q6h PO	§	$0.72	Not established	Not established
Netilmycin‖	Netromycin	4-6.5 mg/kg/day; divide q8-12h IV	3-7.5 mg/kg/day; divide q8-12h IV	$15.70		D
Norfloxacin	Noroxin	0.4 g q12h PO	N.R.	$6.79	Decreased	C
Ofloxacin	Floxin	0.2-0.4 g q12h PO, IV	N.R.	$7.50 PO $52.80 IV	Decreased	C
Oxacillin	Bactocil	0.5-1 g q4-6h IV	37.5-50 mg/kg q6h IV	$2.10 PO $10.72 IV	Decreased	B
Penicillin V	Pen-VeeK, Pen-V	0.25-0.5 g q6h PO	6.25-12.5 mg/kg q6h PO	$0.49	Decreased	B
Penicillin G benzathine	Bicillin	600,000-2,400,000 units IM × 1	600,000 units IM × 1	$33.07 2.4 million units		B
Penicillin G		0.5-1 g q6h PO 1-4 million units q4-6h IV	25,000-90,000 units/kg/day; divide q4-8h PO 25,000-400,000 units/kg/day; divide q4-6h IV	$0.77 PO $10.16 IV	Decreased	B
Piperacillin	Pipracil	3-4 g q4-6h IV	50 mg/kg q4-6h IV (N.A.)	$99.29 4 g q6h		B
Piperacillin-tazobactam	Zosyn	3.375 g q6-8h IV		$48.42		B
Polymyxin B	Aerosporin, Neosporin	15,000-25,000 units/kg/day q12h IV	15,000-25,000 units/kg/day q12h IV	$28.80		Not established
Procaine penicillin G	Wycillin	0.6-1.2 million units q12h IM	25,000-50,000 units/kg q12-24h IM	$5.79		B
Quinupristin-dalfopristin	Synercid	7.5 mg/kg IV q8h	§	$309.40		§

CRCI, Creatinine clearance ml/min; *HD,* hemodialysis; *PD,* peritoneal dialysis; *CNS,* central nervous system; *GI,* gastrointestinal; *pHD,* post-
*Average wholesale price according to the 1999 Red Book.
†FDA pregnancy categories: *A,* adequate studies in pregnant women, no risk; *B,* animal studies no risk, human studies inadequate, or animal benefit may outweigh risk; *X,* fetal abnormalities in humans, risk exceeds benefit.
‡Use in breast-feeding: limited data are available. Because all drugs are probably excreted in small amounts into breast milk, the potential for continued during treatment based on information available at present. "Avoid if possible" indicates that an alternative drug should be chosen or
§Insufficient information available to make a recommendation.
‖Aminoglycoside dosing may be modified after obtaining serum levels. The generally desired peak and trough concentrations are as follows: for kanamycin, peak 15-30 μg/ml, trough <5-10 μg/ml. "Once-daily" administration of aminoglycosides is gaining acceptance. The usual regimen is blockade. Dosage may be modified according to creatinine clearance or by following serum levels (see Nicolau et al. in "Suggested Reading").

USE IN BREASTFEEDING‡	DOSE INTERVAL ADJUSTMENT FOR REDUCED CRCL			SUPPLEMENTAL DOSE IN DIALYSIS		MAJOR TOXICITY
	>50	10-50	<10	HD	PD	
Probably safe	q4-6h	q4-6h	q4-6h	Usual	Usual	Allergic reactions (rare: anaphylactic), diarrhea, nausea, vomiting; platelet dysfunction with high doses
Probably safe	§	§	§	§	§	Cranial nerve VIII and renal damage
Avoid if possible	q8-12h	q12-48h	>48 hr	2 mg/kg pHD	§	Renal toxicity vestibular and auditory toxicity, CNS reactions, neuromuscular blockade (rare)
Avoid if possible	q12h	q24h	q24h	§	§	Nausea, vomiting, dizziness, headache, tremors, confusion
Avoid if possible	q12h	q24h	0.1-0.2 g q24h	0.2 g load; then 0.1 g q24h	§	Nausea, vomiting, dizziness, headache, tremors, confusion
Probably safe	q4-6h	q4-6h	q4-6h	Usual	Usual	Allergic reactions (rare: anaphylactic), diarrhea, nausea, vomiting
Probably safe	q6h	q6h	q6h	250 mg	§	Allergic reactions (rare: anaphylactic), diarrhea, nausea, vomiting
Probably safe	Usual	Usual	Usual	Usual	Usual	Allergic reactions (rare: anaphylactic), diarrhea, nausea, vomiting
Probably safe	q4-6h	q4-6h	25-50% of standard dose q4-6h	500,000 U	§	Allergic reactions (rare: anaphylactic), diarrhea, nausea, vomiting
Probably safe	q4-6h	q6-8h	q8-12h	1 g pHD, then 2 g q8h IV	§	Allergic reactions (rare: anaphylactic), diarrhea, nausea, vomiting; platelet dysfunction with high doses
Probably safe	q6-8h	2.25 g q6h	2.25 g q8h	§	§	Allergic reactions (rare: anaphylactic), diarrhea, nausea, vomiting
§	q12h	q12h	2250-3750 U/kg/day; divide q12h	§	§	Nephrotoxicity, flushing; CNS effects: confusion, seizures; allergic reactions
Probably safe	q12h	q12h	q12h	§	§	Allergic reactions (rare: anaphylactic), diarrhea, nausea, vomiting
§	Usual	Usual	Usual	§	§	Pain at infusion site Thrombophlebitis, arthralgia, myalgia

hemodialysis; *N.A.,* not approved; *AST,* aspartate aminotransferase; *ALT,* alanine aminotransferase; *N.R.,* not recommended; *IT,* intrathecal.

toxicity, human studies no risk; *C,* animal studies show toxicity, human studies inadequate but benefit may exceed risk; *D,* evidence of human risk,

adverse reactions in the infant must be considered, although few have been reported. "Probably safe" indicates that breast-feeding can be consideration given to discontinuing breast-feeding.

gentamicin and tobramycin, peak 6-12 µg/ml and trough <2 µg/ml; for netilmicin, peak 6-10 µg/ml, trough <2 µg/ml; for amikacin and 5-7 mg/kg q24h for gentamicin and tobramycin, 15 mg/kg q24h for amikacin. The dose is infused over 60 minutes to avoid neuromuscular

Continued

Table 1 Antibacterial Agents—cont'd

NAME		USUAL DOSE		COST (PER DAY)*	CHANGE IN ABSORPTION WITH FOOD	PREGNANCY CLASS†
GENERIC	BRAND	ADULT	PEDIATRIC			
Sparfloxacin	Zagam	0.4 g PO ×1 day then 0.2 g/day	§	$6.68	Unchanged	C
Spectinomycin	Trobicin	2 g qd IM	§	$24.69		B
Streptomycin		0.5-1 g q12h IV or IM	20-40 mg/kg/day; divide q6-12h IV or IM	$11.90		D
Sulfadiazine	Microsulfon	2-4 g/day; q4-8h PO	120-150 mg/kg/day; divide q4-6h PO	$2.02	Decreased	C
Sulfamethoxazole	Gantanol, Urobac	1 g q8-12h PO	50-60 mg/kg/day; divide q12h PO	$3.18	Decreased	C
Sulfisoxazole	Gantrisin	0.5-1 g q6h PO 25 mg/kg/q6h IV	120-150 mg/kg/day; divide q4-6h PO	$1.98 PO	Decreased	C
Teichoplanin		0.2-0.4 g q24h IV	10 mg/kg q24h IV	Not available		Not established
Tetracycline	Achromycin	0.25-0.5 g q6h PO	25-50 mg/kg/day; divide q6-12h	$0.25	Decreased with milk, antacids	D
Ticarcillin	Ticar	3 g q4-6h	50 mg/kg q4-6h	$51.15		B
Ticarcillin-clavulanate	Timentin	3.1 q4-8h IV	50 mg/kg q4-6h IV	$45.36		B
Tobramycin‖	Nebcin	3-5 mg/kg/day; divide q8h IV 4-8 mg/day IT	3-6 mg/kg/day; divide q8h IV	$34.13		D
Trimethoprim-sulfamethox-azole	Bactrim, Septra	0.16-0.8 g q12-24h PO 3-5 mg/kg q6-8h IV trimetho-prim	6-12 mg/kg/day; divide q6-12h PO IV	$2.56 PO $32.80 IV	Decreased	C
Trimethoprim	Proloprim	0.1 g q12h PO	4 mg/kg/day; divide q12h PO	$2.06	No data	C
Trovafloxacin	Trovan	0.2-0.2 g/day PO 0.2-0.3 g day IV	§	$6.03 PO $36.88 IV	Unchanged	C
Vancomycin	Vancocin	0.5-2 g q6-8h PO 1 g q12h IV IT: 5-10 mg q48-72h	40 mg/kg/day; divide q6-8h PO 40 mg/kg/day; divide q6-12h IV	$31.20 IV $8.40 oral solution $17.20 pulvules	Not absorbed	B

CRCI, Creatinine clearance ml/min; *HD*, hemodialysis; *PD*, peritoneal dialysis; *CNS*, central nervous system; *GI*, gastrointestinal; *pHD*, post-
*Average wholesale price according to the 1999 Red Book.
†FDA pregnancy categories: *A*, adequate studies in pregnant women, no risk; *B*, animal studies no risk, human studies inadequate, or animal benefit may outweigh risk; *X*, fetal abnormalities in humans, risk exceeds benefit.
‡Use in breast-feeding: limited data are available. Because all drugs are probably excreted in small amounts into breast milk, the potential for continued during treatment based on information available at present. "Avoid if possible" indicates that an alternative drug should be chosen or §Insufficient information available to make a recommendation.
‖Aminoglycoside dosing may be modified after obtaining serum levels. The generally desired peak and trough concentrations are as follows: for kanamycin, peak 15-30 μg/ml, trough <5-10 μg/ml. "Once-daily" administration of aminoglycosides is gaining acceptance. The usual regimen is blockade. Dosage may be modified according to creatinine clearance or by following serum levels (see Nicolau et al. in "Suggested Reading").

USE IN BREASTFEEDING‡	DOSE INTERVAL ADJUSTMENT FOR REDUCED CRCL			SUPPLEMENTAL DOSE IN DIALYSIS		MAJOR TOXICITY
	>50	10-50	<10	HD	PD	
Avoid if possible	Usual	0.2 q48h	0.2 q48h	§	§	Photosensitivity, diarrhea, nausea, headaches, cardiac arrhythmias in patients taking antiarrhythmic drugs
§	q24h	q24h	q24h	§	§	Pain at injection site, nausea, allergic reactions
Avoid if possible	q12h	7.5 mg/kg q24h	7.5 mg/kg q72-96h	0.5 g pHD	§	Cranial nerve VIII damage, paresthesias, rash, fever, renal toxicity, neuromuscular blockade, optic neuritis
Avoid if possible	§	§	§	§	§	Rash, photosensitivity, drug fever
Avoid if possible	§	§	§	§	§	Rash, photosensitivity, drug fever
Avoid if possible	q6h	q8-12h	q12-24h	§	§	Rash, photosensitivity, drug fever
§	q24h	q48h	q72h	§	§	Ototoxicity
Avoid if possible	q6h	Use doxycycline	Use doxycycline	500 mg pHD	§	GI disturbance, photosensitivity, hepatic toxicity, esophageal ulcers
Probably safe	q4-6h	q6-8h	2 g q12h	3 g pHD; then 2 g q12h	3 g q12h	Allergic reactions (rare: anaphylactic), diarrhea, nausea, vomiting
Probably safe	q4-6h	q6-8h	2 g q12h IV	3.1 g	3.1 g q12h	Allergic reactions (rare: anaphylactic), diarrhea, nausea, vomiting
Avoid if possible	q8-12h	q12-48h	>48 hr	1 mg/kg pHD	1 mg/2 L dialysate removed	Renal toxicity, vestibular and auditory toxicity, CNS reactions, neuromuscular blockade (rare)
Avoid if possible	q6-12h	q24h	Avoid	4-5 mg/kg pHD	0.16-0.8 g q48h	Rash, nausea, vomiting
Probably safe	q12h	q18-24h	Avoid	§	§	Nausea, vomiting
Avoid if possible	Usual	Usual	Usual	§	§	Hepatoxicity, including severe liver failure, dizziness, nausea, headache
Probably safe	Levels vary; use serum assays and manufacturer's nomogram to guide dosage	Levels vary; use serum assays and manufacturer's nomogram to guide dosage	Levels vary; use serum assays and manufacturer's nomogram to guide dosage	None needed	None needed	Thrombophlebitis, fever, chills, rash, cranial nerve VIII toxicity

hemodialysis; *N.A.,* not approved; *AST,* aspartate aminotransferase; *ALT,* alanine aminotransferase; *N.R.,* not recommended; *IT,* intrathecal.

toxicity, human studies no risk; *C,* animal studies show toxicity, human studies inadequate but benefit may exceed risk; *D,* evidence of human risk,

adverse reactions in the infant must be considered, although few have been reported. "Probably safe" indicates that breast-feeding can be consideration given to discontinuing breast-feeding.

gentamicin and tobramycin, peak 6-12 µg/ml and trough <2 µg/ml; for netilmicin, peak 6-10 µg/ml, trough <2 µg/ml; for amikacin and 5-7 mg/kg q24h for gentamicin and tobramycin, 15 mg/kg q24h for amikacin. The dose is infused over 60 minutes to avoid neuromuscular

Table 2 Antimycobacterial Agents

NAME		USUAL DOSE		COST (PER DAY)*	CHANGE IN ABSORPTION WITH FOOD	PREGNANCY CLASS†
GENERIC	BRAND	ADULT	PEDIATRIC			
Capreomycin	Capastat	1 g IM q24h	10-20 mg/kg q24h (N.A.)	$24.33		C
Clofazimine	Lamprene	0.1 g q24h PO	§	$0.32	Increased	C
Cycloserine	Seromycin	0.25-0.5 g q12h PO	10-20 mg/kg q12h (N.A.)	$7.65	No data	C
Ethambutol	Myambutol	15-25 mg/kg q24h PO	10-15 mg/kg q24h (N.R.)	$5.67	Unchanged	B
Ethionamide	Trecator	0.25-0.5 g q12h PO	15-20 mg/kg q24h (N.A.)	$4.39	No data	C
INH + RIF + PZA	Rifater	6 tabs/day		$10.80	Decreased	As with individual drugs
INH + RIF	Rifamate	2 tabs/day		$4.86	Decreased	As with individual drugs
Isoniazid		0.3 g q24h PO, IM	10-20 mg/kg/day; divide q12-24h PO, IM	$0.12	Decreased	C
Paraamino salicylic acid	PAS	150 mg/kg q6-12h	150-360 mg/kg/day; divide q6-8h	Not available	Decreased but advised	C
Pyrazinamide		15-30 mg/kg q24h PO	30 mg/kg/day; divide q12-24h (N.A.)	$3.54	No data	C
Rifabutin (ansamycin)	Mycobutin	0.3 g q24h PO	§	$9.18	Unchanged	C
Rifampin	Rifadin, Rimactane	0.6 g q24h PO, IV	10-20 mg/kg/day; divide q12-24h PO, IV	$3.21 PO $79.38 IV	Decreased	B
Rifapentine	Priftin	4 tabs 2×/wk	§	$11.00	Increased	C
Streptomycin		1 g q24h IM	20-40 mg/kg q24h IM	$11.90		D

CRCI, Creatinine clearance ml/min; *HD,* hemodialysis; *PD,* peritoneal dialysis; *N.A.,* not approved; *GI,* gastrointestinal; *N.R.,* not recommended;
*Average wholesale price according to the 1999 Red Book.
†FDA pregnancy categories: *A,* adequate studies in pregnant women, no risk; *B,* animal studies no risk, human studies inadequate, or animal benefit may outweigh risk; *X,* fetal abnormalities in humans, risk exceeds benefit.
‡Use in breast-feeding: limited data are available. Because all drugs are probably excreted in small amounts into breast milk, the potential for continued during treatment based on information available at present. "Avoid if possible" indicates that an alternative drug should be chosen or
§Insufficient information available to make a recommendation.

USE IN BREASTFEEDING‡	DOSE INTERVAL ADJUSTMENT FOR REDUCED CRCL			SUPPLEMENTAL DOSE IN DIALYSIS		MAJOR TOXICITY
	>50	10-50	<10	HD	PD	
Probably safe	q24h	7.5 mg/kg q24-48h	7.5 mg/kg 2×/wk	§	§	Renal and cranial nerve VIII toxicity, hypokalemia, sterile abscesses at injection site
Avoid if possible	q24h	q24h	q24h	§	§	Hyperpigmentation, ichthyosis, dry eyes, GI disturbance
Avoid if possible	q12h	q24h	0.25 g q24h	§	§	Anxiety, depression, confusion, hallucinations, headache, peripheral neuropathy
§	q24h	q24-36h	q48h	15 mg/kg/day pHD	15 mg/kg/day	Optic neuritis, allergic reactions, GI disturbance, acute gout
§	q12h	q12h	5 mg/kg q24h	§	§	GI disturbance, liver toxicity, CNS disturbance
Avoid if possible	q24h	q24h	Avoid	§	§	As with individual drugs
Avoid if possible	q24h	q24h	Avoid	§	§	As with individual drugs
Probably safe	q24h	q24h	½ dose in slow acetylators	5 mg/kg pHD	Daily dose pPd	Peripheral neuropathy, liver toxicity (possibly fatal), glossitis, GI disturbance, fever
§	§	§	§	§	§	GI disturbance
Avoid if possible	q24h	q24h	12-20 mg/kg q24h	§	§	Arthralgia, hyperuricemia, liver toxicity, GI disturbance, rash
Avoid if possible	§	§	§	§	§	Uveitis, orange discoloration of urine, sweat, tears; liver toxicity, GI disturbance
Avoid if possible	q24h	q24h	q24h	§	§	Orange discoloration of urine, sweat, tears; liver toxicity, GI disturbance, flulike syndrome
Avoid if possible	§	§	§	§	§	Similar to rifampin
Avoid if possible	q24h	q24-72h	q72-96h	0.5 g pHD	§	Vestibular nerve damage, paresthesias, rash, fever, pruritus, renal toxicity

pHD, posthemodialysis; *pPD*, postperitoneal dialysis; *CNS*, central nervous system.

toxicity, human studies no risk; *C,* animal studies show toxicity, human studies inadequate but benefit may exceed risk; *D,* evidence of human risk,

adverse reactions in the infant must be considered, although few have been reported. "Probably safe" indicates that breast-feeding can be consideration given to discontinuing breast-feeding.

Table 3 Antifungal Agents

NAME		USUAL DOSE		COST (PER DAY)*	CHANGE IN ABSORPTION WITH FOOD	PREGNANCY CLASS†
GENERIC	BRAND	ADULT	PEDIATRIC			
Amphotericin B	Fungizone	0.25-1 mg/kg q24h IV	0.25-1 mg/kg q24-48h IV	$16.60		B
Amphotericin B liposomal formulations	Abelcet	5 mg/kg IV q24h	5 mg/kg IV q24h	$679		B
	AmBisome	3-5 g/kg IV q24h	3-5 g/kg, IV q24h	$791		B
	Amphotec	3-4 g/kg q24h	3-4 g/kg q24h	$448		B
Clotrimazole	Mycelex	10 mg PO 5×/day	§	$5.67	Not absorbed	C
Fluconazole	Diflucan	0.05-0.4 g q24h PO, IV	3-6 mg/kg qd (N.A.)	$6.10 PO $105.37 IV	Unchanged	C
Flucytosine	Ancobon	50-150 mg/kg/day; divide q6h PO	50-150 mg/kg/day; divide q6h PO	$29.44	Decreased	C
Griseofulvin	Grisactin, Grifulvin, Fulvicin	0.5-1 g q24h PO	15 mg/kg/day; q24h PO	$1.90	Increased	C
Itraconazole	Sporanox	0.2-0.4 g q24h PO 0.2 g q12h IV	§	$13.59 PO $320.00 IV	Increased	C
Ketoconazole	Nizoral	0.2-0.4 g q12-24h PO	5-10 mg/kg/day; divide q12-24h PO	$6.75	Increased	C
Miconazole	Monostat	0.4-1.2 g q8h IV	20-40 mg/kg/day; divide q8h IV	$230.82		C
Nystatin	Mycostatin	400,000-1,000,000 U q8h PO	400,000-600,000 U q6h PO	$3.13 (20 ml)	Not absorbed	C

CRCI, Creatinine clearance ml/min; *HD,* hemodialysis; *PD,* peritoneal dialysis; *N.A.,* not approved; *GI,* gastrointestinal; *N.R.,* not recommended;
*Average wholesale price according to the 1999 Red Book.
†FDA pregnancy categories: *A,* adequate studies in pregnant women, no risk; *B,* animal studies no risk, human studies inadequate, or animal benefit may outweigh risk; *X,* fetal abnormalities in humans, risk exceeds benefit.
‡Use in breast-feeding: limited data are available. Because all drugs are probably excreted in small amounts into breast milk, the potential for continued during treatment based on information available at present. "Avoid if possible" indicates that an alternative drug should be chosen or
§Insufficient information available to make a recommendation.

USE IN BREASTFEEDING‡	DOSE INTERVAL ADJUSTMENT FOR REDUCED CRCL			SUPPLEMENTAL DOSE IN DIALYSIS		MAJOR TOXICITY
	>50	10-50	<10	HD	PD	
Avoid if possible	q24h	q24h	q24h	Usual	Usual	Fever, chills, nausea with infusion; renal insufficiency, anemia
Avoid if possible	§	§	§	§	§	Fever, chills, renal insufficiency (less than non-liposomal amphotericin)
Avoid if possible	§	§	§	§	§	Fever, chills, renal insufficiency (less than non-liposomal amphotericin)
Avoid if possible	§	§	§	§	§	Fever, chills, renal insufficiency (less than non-liposomal amphotericin)
Probably safe	§	§	§	§	§	
Avoid if possible	q24h	50% dose q24h	25% dose q24h	§	§	Nausea, vomiting, rash, elevated liver enzymes
Avoid if possible	q6h	q12-24h	15-25 mg/kg q24h	20-37.5 mg/kg pHD	§	Leukopenia
§	q24h	q24h	q24h	§	§	GI disturbance, allergic and photosensitivity reactions, blood dyscrasias, liver toxicity, exacerbation of SLE and leprosy
Avoid if possible	q12-24h	§	§	§	§	Nausea, rash, headache, edema, hypokalemia, hepatotoxicity
Avoid if possible	q12-24h	Usual	Usual	Usual	Usual	Nausea, vomiting, gynecomastia, decreased testosterone synthesis, rash, hepatotoxicity, adrenal insufficiency
§	q8h	q8h	q8h	§	§	Phlebitis, thrombocytosis, pruritus, rash, blurred vision, anaphylaxis (rare)
Probably safe	q8h	q8h	q8h	§	§	GI disturbance, allergic reactions

pHD, posthemodialysis; *pPD,* postperitoneal dialysis; *CNS,* central nervous system.

toxicity, human studies no risk; *C,* animal studies show toxicity, human studies inadequate but benefit may exceed risk; *D,* evidence of human risk,

adverse reactions in the infant must be considered, although few have been reported. "Probably safe" indicates that breast-feeding can be consideration given to discontinuing breast-feeding.

Table 4   Antiviral Agents

NAME		USUAL DOSE		COST (PER DAY)*	CHANGE IN ABSORPTION WITH FOOD	PREGNANCY CLASS†
GENERIC	BRAND	ADULT	PEDIATRIC			
Abacavir	Ziagen	0.3 g PO q12h	8 mg/kg PO q12h	$11.66	Unchanged	§
Acyclovir	Zovirax	0.2-0.8 g 2-5× / day PO 5-12 mg/kg q8h IV	0.2 g 5×/day (HSV) PO 20 mg/kg q6h PO, max 800 mg q6h (VZV) 25-50 mg/kg/ day q8h IV	$6.46 PO (200 mg) $24.40 (800 mg) $119.02 IV (10 mg/kg dose)	Unchanged	C
Amantadine	Symmetrel	0.1 g q12h PO	2.2-4.4 mg/kg q12h PO	$1.81	No data	C
Amprenavir	Agenerase	1.2 g PO q12h	§	$21.15	Decreased with high-fat meal	§
Cidofovir	Vistide	5 mg/kg IV q wk ×2 wk, then 5 mg/kg q2wk	§	$108.85		C
Didanosine	Videx	0.167-0.2 g q12h PO	0.143-0.248 mg/m² divided q12h PO	$7.25	Decreased	B
Efavirenz	Sustiva	06.6 PO qhs	§	$13.14	Unchanged	C
Famciclovir	Famvir	0.125 g q12h PO (HSV) 0.5 g q8h PO (VZV)	§	$5.60 HSV $21.10 VZV	Unchanged	B
Foscarnet	Foscavir	60 mg/kg q8h IV × 14-21 days; then 90 mg/kg/day	§	$219.82		C
Ganciclovir	Cytovene	5 mg/kg q12h IV × 14-21 days; then 5 mg/kg/day or 1 g tid PO	5 mg/kg q12h IV	$71.34 IV $47.97 PO		C
Indinavir	Crixivan	800 mg PO q8h	§	$15.45	Decreased	C
Lamivudine	Epivir	150 mg PO q12h	4 mg/kg PO q12h	$8.66	Unchanged	C
Nelfinavir	Viracept	0.75 g PO tid or 1.25 g PO q12h	0.2-0.3 mg/kg q8h	$19.44	Increased	B
Nevirapine	Viramune	200 mg PO q24h × 14 days, then 200 mg PO q12h	§	$8.50	Unchanged	C
Oseltamivir	Tamiflu	75 mg PO bid × 5 days	§	$10.60		§
Ribavirin	Virazole	12-18 hr/day × 3 days via aerosol, PO, IV investigational	12-22 hr/day × 6 days via aerosol	Not available		X

CRCI, Creatinine clearance ml/min; HD, hemodialysis; PD, peritoneal dialysis; N.A., not approved; GI, gastrointestinal; N.R., not recommended;
*Average wholesale price according to the 1999 Red Book.
†FDA pregnancy categories: A, adequate studies in pregnant women, no risk; B, animal studies no risk, human studies inadequate, or animal benefit may outweigh risk; X, fetal abnormalities in humans, risk exceeds benefit.
‡Use in breast-feeding: limited data are available. Because all drugs are probably excreted in small amounts into breast milk, the potential for continued during treatment based on information available at present. "Avoid if possible" indicates that an alternative drug should be chosen or
§Insufficient information available to make a recommendation.

USE IN BREASTFEEDING‡	DOSE INTERVAL ADJUSTMENT FOR REDUCED CRCL			SUPPLEMENTAL DOSE IN DIALYSIS		MAJOR TOXICITY
	>50	10-50	<10	HD	PD	
Avoid	§	§	§	§	§	Nausea, hypersensitivity reaction with myalgias, fever, rash; anaphylaxis
Probably safe	2-5×/day PO q8h IV	2-5×/day PO q12-24h IV	0.2-0.8 g q24h PO 2.5-6 mg/kg q24h IV	0.5 g PO pHD	2-5 mg/kg/day	Headache, rash, renal toxicity, CNS symptoms (rare)
Avoid if possible	q12h	0.1-0.2 g 2-3×/wk	0.1-0.2 g qwk	§	§	Livedo reticularis, edema, insomnia, dizziness, lethargy
Avoid if possible	Usual	Usual	Usual	Usual	Usual	Nausea, diarrhea, rash
Avoid if possible	Check prescribing information	Check prescribing information	Check prescribing information	§	§	Proteinuria, renal insufficiency, neutropenia
Avoid if possible	q12h	q12-24h	100 mg q24h PO	Dose pHD	§	Diarrhea, nausea, vomiting, pancreatitis, peripheral neuropathy
Avoid if possible	Usual	Usual	Usual	Usual	Usual	Drowsiness, CNS side effects, rash
Avoid if possible	0.5g q8h 0.125 g q12h	0.5 g q12-24h 0.125 g q12-24h	0.25 g q48h 0.125 g q48h		ND	Headache, nausea
Probably safe	63-90 mg/ kg/day maintenance	78-63 mg/ kg/day maintenance	§	§	§	Renal dysfunction, anemia, nausea, disturbances of calcium, magnesium, phosphorus, potassium metabolism
Avoid if possible	q12h	2.5 mg/kg q24h	1.25 mg/kg q24h	1.25 mg/kg pHD	§	Neutropenia, thrombocytopenia
Avoid if possible	§	§	§	§	§	Nephrolithiasis, nausea, headache
Avoid if possible	150 mg PO q12h	100-150 g PO qd	25-50 mg PO qd	§	§	Headache, nausea, neutropenia, increased AST, ALT.
Avoid if possible	Usual	Usual	Usual	Usual	Usual	Diarrhea, nausea
Avoid if possible	§	§	§	§	§	Rash, including Stevens-Johnsons syndrome; hepatotoxicity
§	§	§	§	§	§	Nausea, vomiting and headache
Avoid if possible	§	§	§	§	§	Anemia, headache, hyperbilirubinemia, bronchospasm

pHD, posthemodialysis; *pD,* postperitoneal dialysis; *CNS,* central nervous system.

toxicity, human studies no risk; *C,* animal studies show toxicity, human studies inadequate but benefit may exceed risk; *D,* evidence of human risk,

adverse reactions in the infant must be considered, although few have been reported. "Probably safe" indicates that breast-feeding can be consideration given to discontinuing breast-feeding. *Continued*

Table 4 Antiviral Agents—cont'd

NAME		USUAL DOSE		COST (PER DAY)*	CHANGE IN ABSORPTION WITH FOOD	PREGNANCY CLASS†
GENERIC	BRAND	ADULT	PEDIATRIC			
Rimantadine	Flumadine	0.1 g q12h PO	§	$3.49	Unchanged	C
Ritonavir	Norvir	600 mg PO q12h	§	$22.26	Unchanged	B
Saquinavir hard gel	Invirase	0.4 g PO q12h with 0.4 g PO ritonavir		$8.67	Increased	B
Saquinavir soft gel	Fortovase	1.2 g PO tid		$19.59	Increased	B
Stavudine	Zerit	0.04 g q12h PO	§	$9.12	Unchanged	C
Valacyclovir	Valtrex	1 g PO tid (VZV) 0.5 g PO bid (HSV)	Unchanged	$11.95 VZV $3.98 HSV		
Vidarabine	Vira-A	10-15 mg/kg/day over 12 hr IV	10-15 mg/kg/day over 12 hr IV	Not available		Not established
Zalcitabine	Hivid	0.375-0.75 g q8h PO	0.75 g q8h PO (children >13 yr)	$7.07	Decreased	C
Zanamivir	Relenza	10 mg bid in half × 50	§	$8.88	§	§
Zidovudine	Retrovir	0.1 g q4h PO or 0.2 g q8h PO 1-2 mg/kg q4h IV	180 mg/m² q6h PO	$10.12	Decreased	C

*CRCI,*Creatinine clearance ml/min; *HD,* hemodialysis; *PD,* peritoneal dialysis; *N.A.,* not approved; *GI,* gastrointestinal; *N.R.,* not recommended;
*Average wholesale price according to the 1999 Red Book.
†FDA pregnancy categories: *A,* adequate studies in pregnant women, no risk; *B,* animal studies no risk, human studies inadequate, or animal benefit may outweigh risk; *X,* fetal abnormalities in humans, risk exceeds benefit.
‡Use in breast-feeding: limited data are available. Because all drugs are probably excreted in small amounts into breast milk, the potential for continued during treatment based on information available at present. "Avoid if possible" indicates that an alternative drug should be chosen or
§Insufficient information available to make a recommendation.

USE IN BREASTFEEDING‡	DOSE INTERVAL ADJUSTMENT FOR REDUCED CRCL			SUPPLEMENTAL DOSE IN DIALYSIS		MAJOR TOXICITY
	>50	10-50	<10	HD	PD	
Avoid if possible	q12h	q12h	q12h	§	§	Fewer CNS side effects than amantadine
Avoid if possible	Usual	Usual	Usual	Usual	Usual	Nausea, vomiting, diarrhea
Avoid if possible	Usual	Usual	Usual	Usual	Usual	Diarrhea, nausea
Avoid if possible	Usual	Usual	Usual	Usual	Usual	Diarrhea, nausea, headache
Avoid if possible	§	§	§	§	§	Peripheral neuropathy, liver toxicity
Probably safe	Usual	112-24 hr	0.5 g q24h	0.5 g q24h	0.5 g q24h	Nausea, headache; thrombotic thrombocytopenic purpura in immunocompromised pts.
§	Usual	Usual	10 mg/kg/ day over 12 hr	Usual dose pHD	§	GI disturbance, nausea, vomiting, thrombophlebitis
Avoid if possible	q8h	q12h	q24h	§	§	Peripheral neuropathy, stomatitis, esophageal ulcers, pancreatitis
§	§	§	§	§	§	Nasal and throat discomfort, headache and cough
Avoid if possible	q4h	q6h	q6-12h	100 mg pHD	100 mg q6-12h	Anemia, granulocytopenia, headache, nausea, insomnia, nail pigment changes

pHD, posthemodialysis; *pD*, postperitoneal dialysis; *CNS*, central nervous system.

toxicity, human studies no risk; *C,* animal studies show toxicity, human studies inadequate but benefit may exceed risk; *D,* evidence of human risk,

adverse reactions in the infant must be considered, although few have been reported. "Probably safe" indicates that breast-feeding can be consideration given to discontinuing breast-feeding.

Table 5   Antiparasitic Agents

NAME		USUAL DOSE		COST (PER DAY)*	CHANGE IN ABSORPTION WITH FOOD	PREGNANCY CLASS†
GENERIC	BRAND	ADULT	PEDIATRIC			
Albendazole‖	Zentel	15 mg/kg/day PO	§	Not listed		Not established
Artemisinin#		10 mg/kg/day ×5 days	Same as adult	Not listed		Not established
Atovoquone	Mepron	750 mg tid PO	§	$41.67	Increased	C
Benznidazole#		5 mg/kg bid PO 1-4 mo	§	Not listed		Not established
Bithionol¶	Bitin	30-50 mg/kg on alternate days ×10-15 days	Same as adult	Not listed		Not established
Chloroquine HCL	Aralen HCL	300 mg qwk PO (prophylaxis) 600 mg PO, then 300 mg after 6, 24, 48 hr 200 mg q6h IM (treatment)	5 mg/kg qwk PO (for prophylaxis) 10 mg/kg, then 5 mg/kg, same intervals as adult (treatment) IM treatment not recommended	$17.06 IM	Increased	C
Chloroquine phosphate	Aralen phosphate	500 mg qwk PO (prophylaxis) 1 g, then 500 mg after 6, 24, 48 hr (treatment)	8.3 mg/kg qwk PO (prophylaxis)	$21.65 (2-day treatment course)	Increased	C
Dehydroemetine†		1-1.5 mg/kg/day IM (maximum dose 90 mg)	1-1.5 mg/kg IM qd, divided in 2 doses	Not listed		Not established
Diethyl carbamazine‖	Hetrazan	Day 1: 50 mg PO Day 2: 50 mg tid Day 3: 50 mg tid Days 4-21: 6 mg/ kg/day divided tid	Day 1: 1 mg/kg PO Day 2: 1 mg/kg tid Day 3: 1-2 mg/kg tid Days 4-21: 6 mg/ kg/day divided tid	Not listed		Not established
Diloxanide furoate¶	Furamide	500 mg tid × 10 days	20 mg/kg/day divided tid × 10 days	Not listed		Not established
Eflornithine‖		400 mg/kg/day IV divided qid × 14 days then 300 mg/kg/ day ×3-4 wk PO	§	Not listed		Not established
Furazolidone	Furoxone	100 mg q6h PO	25-50 mg q6h PO	$10.60		Not established

*CRCI,*Creatinine clearance ml/min; *HD,* hemodialysis; *PD,* peritoneal dialysis; *AST,* aspartate aminotransaminase; *ALT,* alanine aminotransferase; meals; *CSF,* cerebrospinal fluid.
*Average wholesale price according to the 1999 Red Book.
†FDA pregnancy categories: *A,* adequate studies in pregnant women, no risk; *B,* animal studies no risk, human studies inadequate, or animal benefit may outweigh risk; *X,* fetal abnormalities in humans, risk exceeds benefit.
‡Use in breast-feeding: limited data are available. Because all drugs are probably excreted in small amounts into breast milk, the potential for continued during treatment based on information available at present. "Avoid if possible" indicates that an alternative drug should be chosen or
§Insufficient information available to make a recommendation.
‖Available in the United States only from the manufacturer.
¶Available from the Centers for Disease Control and Prevention drug service.
#Not available in the United States.

USE IN BREASTFEEDING‡	DOSE INTERVAL ADJUSTMENT FOR REDUCED CRCL			SUPPLEMENTAL DOSE IN DIALYSIS		MAJOR TOXICITY
	>50	10-50	<10	HD	PD	
§	§	§	§	§	§	Diarrhea, abdominal discomfort, elevated AST, ALT, bone marrow suppression, alopecia with high dose
§	§	§	§	§	§	Transient heart block, elevated AST, ALT, neutropenia, decreased reticulocyte count, abdominal pain, diarrhea, fever
Probably safe	§	§	§	§	§	Rash, GI disturbance, fever, headache
§	§	§	§	§	§	Peripheral neuropathy, rash, bone marrow suppression
§	§	§	§	§	§	
Avoid if possible	§	§	§	§	§	Blurred vision (retinopathy with prolonged use), GI effects, pruritus, hemolysis in patients with G6PD deficiency
Avoid if possible	§	§	§	§	§	Blurred vision (retinopathy with prolonged use), GI effects, pruritus, hemolysis in patients with G6PD deficiency
§	§	§	§	§	§	Diarrhea, nausea, vomiting, cardiac arrhythmias, tachycardia
§	§	§	§	§	§	Headache, malaise, arthralgia, nausea, vomiting, anorexia, pruritus, fever, hypotension, lymphadenitis, encephalopathy
§	§	§	§	§	§	Flatulence
§	§	§	§	§	§	Anemia, thrombocytopenia, leukopenia, nausea, vomiting, diarrhea, transient hearing loss
§	§	§	§	§	§	Nausea, vomiting, rash, fever, headache, hemolysis in patients with G6PD deficiency

GI, gastrointestinal; *G6PD,* glucose-6 phosphate dehydrogenase; *AIDS,* acquired immunodeficiency syndrome; *N.R.,* not recommended; *p.c.,* after

toxicity, human studies no risk; *C,* animal studies show toxicity, human studies inadequate but benefit may exceed risk; *D,* evidence of human risk,

adverse reactions in the infant must be considered, although few have been reported. "Probably safe" indicates that breast-feeding can be consideration given to discontinuing breast-feeding.   *Continued*

Table 5 Antiparasitic Agents—cont'd

NAME		USUAL DOSE		COST (PER DAY)*	CHANGE IN ABSORPTION WITH FOOD	PREGNANCY CLASS†
GENERIC	**BRAND**	**ADULT**	**PEDIATRIC**			
Halofantrine	Halfan	500 mg q6h PO ×3, repeat in 1 wk	8 mg/kg q6h PO ×3 (patient <40 kg), repeat in 1 wk	Not listed		Not established
Hydroxy-chloroquine	Plaquenil	400 mg qwk PO (prophylaxis) 800 mg, then 400 mg after 6, 24, 48 hr (treatment)	5 mg/kg/qwk PO (prophylaxis) 10 mg/kg, then 5 mg/kg at same intervals as adult (treatment)	$13.56 (2-day treatment course)		C
Iodoquinol	Yodoxin, Diquinol	650 mg tid PO	30-40 mg/kg/day; divide tid PO	$1.64	Minimally absorbed	Not established
Ivermectin¶	Mectizan	200 units/kg/day 0.15 mg/kg/day PO	§	Not listed		Not established
Mebendazole	Vermox	100-400 mg q8-24h PO depending on infection being treated	Same as adults	$5.68	Minimally absorbed	B
Mefloquine	Lariam	250 mg/wk (prophylaxis) 1250 mg ×1 (treatment)	25 mg/kg qwk PO (prophylaxis)	$8.20 prophylaxis $41.03 treatment		C
Meglumine antimonate	Glucantine	20 mg/kg IV ×2 days (850 mg/day limit)	§	Not listed		Not established
Melarsoprol B¶	Mel B, Arsobal	1.2 mg/kg tid IV ×3 days; repeat qwk ×2 wk	§	Not listed		Not established
Niclosamide	Niclocide	2 g qd PO	0.5-1.5 g/day PO	Not listed	Not absorbed	B
Nifurtimox¶	Lampit	3 mg/kg tid PO ×3 mo	§	Not listed		Not established
Niridazole	Ambilhar	§	§	Not listed		Not established
Oxamniquine	Vansil	12-60 mg/kg qd or divide bid	20-60 mg/kg divided bid	Not listed	Decreased	Not established

*CRCl,*Creatinine clearance ml/min; *HD,* hemodialysis; *PD,* peritoneal dialysis; *AST,* aspartate aminotransaminase; *ALT,* alanine aminotransferase; meals; *CSF,* cerebrospinal fluid.
*Average wholesale price according to the 1999 Red Book.
†FDA pregnancy categories: *A,* adequate studies in pregnant women, no risk; *B,* animal studies no risk, human studies inadequate, or animal benefit may outweigh risk; *X,* fetal abnormalities in humans, risk exceeds benefit.
‡Use in breast-feeding: limited data are available. Because all drugs are probably excreted in small amounts into breast milk, the potential for continued during treatment based on information available at present. "Avoid if possible" indicates that an alternative drug should be chosen or
§Insufficient information available to make a recommendation.
‖Available in the United States only from the manufacturer.
¶Available from the Centers for Disease Control and Prevention drug service.
#Not available in the United States.

USE IN BREASTFEEDING‡	DOSE INTERVAL ADJUSTMENT FOR REDUCED CRCL			SUPPLEMENTAL DOSE IN DIALYSIS		MAJOR TOXICITY
	>50	10-50	<10	HD	PD	
§	§	§	§	§	§	Abdominal pain, vomiting, diarrhea, headache, pruritus, rash
Avoid if possible	§	§	§	§	§	Blurred vision, GI effects, pruritus; rare: cardiomyopathy
§	§	§	§	§	§	Optic neuritis, peripheral neuropathy, anorexia, nausea, vomiting, diarrhea, skin reactions
§	§	§	§	§	§	Fever, pruritus, headache, edema
Probably safe	§	§	§	§	§	Diarrhea, nausea, vomiting, abdominal pain, fever, headache, neutropenia, thrombocytopenia
§	§	§	§	§	§	Nausea, dizziness, seizures, bradycardia, rash
§	§	§	§	§	§	
§	§	§	§	§	§	Fever, hypertension, abdominal pain, vomiting, arthralgia, encephalopathy, rash, hemolysis in patients with G6PD deficiency
Probably safe	§	§	§	§	§	Nausea, abdominal discomfort, diarrhea, drowsiness, dizziness, headache
§	§	§	§	§	§	Nausea, vomiting, abdominal pain, anorexia, weight loss, restlessness, insomnia, paresthesias, seizures, rash, neutropenia
§	§	§	§	§	§	
	§	§	§	§	§	Dizziness, drowsiness, headache, nausea, vomiting, abdominal pain, orange-red discoloration of urine

GI, gastrointestinal; *G6PD*, glucose-6 phosphate dehydrogenase; *AIDS*, acquired immunodeficiency syndrome; *N.R.*, not recommended; *p.c.*, after

toxicity, human studies no risk; *C*, animal studies show toxicity, human studies inadequate but benefit may exceed risk; *D*, evidence of human risk,

adverse reactions in the infant must be considered, although few have been reported. "Probably safe" indicates that breast-feeding can be consideration given to discontinuing breast-feeding.

Continued

Table 5   Antiparasitic Agents—cont'd

NAME		USUAL DOSE		COST (PER DAY)*	CHANGE IN ABSORPTION WITH FOOD	PREGNANCY CLASS†
GENERIC	BRAND	ADULT	PEDIATRIC			
Paromomycin	Humatin	25-35 mg/kg PO divided tid 2-3 g qd divided qid in AIDS	§	$20.99	Not absorbed	Not established
Pentamidine	Pentam, Nebupent	3-4 mg/kg/day IV 300 mg aerosol-ized qmo	3-4 mg/kg/day IV	$98.75 IV $98.75 aer		C
Piperazine citrate	Antepar	2-3.5 g/day PO	65-75 mg/kg qd PO	$0.26		Not established
Praziquantel	Bitricide	5-25 mg/kg ×1 (intestinal cestodiasis) 50-75 mg/kg/day, divided tid other infections	Not shown to be safe for children under 4	$35.70		B
Primaquine phosphate		26.3 mg/day PO × 14 days 29 mg qwk PO × 8 wk	0.5 mg/kg/day PO 1.5 mg/kg qwk PO	$1.21		Not established
Proguanil#	Paludrine	200 mg/day P0	<2 yr 50 mg qd PO 2-6 yr 100 mg PO 7-10 yr 150 mg PO >10 yr 200 mg PO	Not listed		Not established
Pyrantel pamoate	Antiminth	11 mg/kg (max 1 g/day) PO	11 mg/kg/day PO; not recom-mended for children <2 yr	Not listed		Not established
Pyrimethamine	Daraprim	25-75 mg/day PO	0.5-2 mg/kg PO, divide bid Contraindicated for children <2 yr	$1.30		C
Pyrimethamine + sulfadiazine	Fansidar	1 tab qwk PO (prophylaxis) 3 tabs PO ×1 (treatment)	½ tab PO 5-10 kg 1 tab 10-20 kg 1½ tab 21-30 kg 2 tabs 31-40 kg For children >2 yr	$3.45/wk (prophylaxis) $10.36 (treat-ment course)		C

CRCI, Creatinine clearance ml/min; HD, hemodialysis; PD, peritoneal dialysis; AST, aspartate aminotransaminase; ALT, alanine aminotransferase; meals; CSF, cerebrospinal fluid.

*Average wholesale price according to the 1999 Red Book.

†FDA pregnancy categories: A, adequate studies in pregnant women, no risk; B, animal studies no risk, human studies inadequate, or animal benefit may outweigh risk; X, fetal abnormalities in humans, risk exceeds benefit.

‡Use in breast-feeding: limited data are available. Because all drugs are probably excreted in small amounts into breast milk, the potential for continued during treatment based on information available at present. "Avoid if possible" indicates that an alternative drug should be chosen or

§Insufficient information available to make a recommendation.

‖Available in the United States only from the manufacturer.

¶Available from the Centers for Disease Control and Prevention drug service.

#Not available in the United States.

USE IN BREASTFEEDING‡	DOSE INTERVAL ADJUSTMENT FOR REDUCED CRCL			SUPPLEMENTAL DOSE IN DIALYSIS		MAJOR TOXICITY
	>50	10-50	<10	HD	PD	
Probably safe	§	§	§	§	§	Anorexia, nausea, vomiting, abdominal pain, diarrhea, malabsorption
Probably safe	§	§	§	§	§	Nephrotoxicity, hypotension, sterile abscess with IM injection, hypoglycemia or hyperglycemia, nausea, vomiting, abdominal pain, pancreatitis, hypocalcemia, cough and bronchospasm with inhalation
Probably safe	§	§	§	§	§	Nausea, vomiting, diarrhea, abdominal cramps, headache, dizziness, rash, hemolytic anemia, ataxia
Avoid if possible	Usual dose	N.R.	N.R.	§	§	Transient dizziness, headache, drowsiness, fatigue, seizures, CSF reaction syndrome with treatment of neurocysticercosis, abdominal pain, nausea, rash
Avoid if possible	§	§	§	§	§	Hemolytic anemia in patients with G6PD deficiency, nausea, vomiting, abdominal cramps, headache, pruritus
§	§	§	§	§	§	Rare hematologic toxicity
Probably safe	§	§	§	§	§	Nausea, vomiting, cramps, dizziness, drowsiness, headache
Probably safe	§	§	§	§	§	Bone marrow suppression with high doses, pulmonary eosinophilia, photosensitivity
Probably safe	§	§	§	§	§	Leukopenia, hemolysis in patients with G6PD deficiency, rash and hypersensitivity reactions including Stevens-Johnson syndrome, hepatitis, pulmonary hypersensitivity reactions

GI, gastrointestinal; *G6PD*, glucose-6 phosphate dehydrogenase; *AIDS*, acquired immunodeficiency syndrome; *N.R.*, not recommended; *p.c.*, after

toxicity, human studies no risk; *C,* animal studies show toxicity, human studies inadequate but benefit may exceed risk; *D,* evidence of human risk,

adverse reactions in the infant must be considered, although few have been reported. "Probably safe" indicates that breast-feeding can be consideration given to discontinuing breast-feeding.

Continued

Table 5 Antiparasitic Agents—cont'd

NAME		USUAL DOSE		COST (PER DAY)*	CHANGE IN ABSORPTION WITH FOOD	PREGNANCY CLASS†
GENERIC	BRAND	ADULT	PEDIATRIC			
Quinacrine HCl	Atabrine	100 mg tid PC ×5 days	6 mg/kg tid PC ×5 days (<50 kg)	Not listed		C
Quinidine		10 mg/kg load over 1-2 h, then 0.02 mg/ kg/min ×72 hr	Same as adult	$55.08		C
Quinine	Legatrin Quinamm	325-650 g PO bid-tid	25-30 mg/kg/day PO; divide tid	$10.80		X
Spiramycin#		3 g/day PO	§	Not listed		
Stibogluconate¶	Pentostam	20 mg/kg IV qd ×20 days (not to exceed 850 mg)	§	Not listed		Not estab- lished
Suramin¶	Germanin	1 g IV qwk ×5 wk (100-mg test dose)	§	Not listed		Not estab- lished
Thiabendazole	Mintizol	25 mg/kg PO bid (maximum 3 g/day)	22 mg/kg bid PO	$5.86		Not estab- lished
Trimetrexate	Neutrexin	45 mg/m²/day with leucovorin 20 mg/m² q6h; continue leu- covorin at least 72 hr after last dose	§	$150.00 + $66.00 leucovorin		Not established

CRCI, Creatinine clearance ml/min; *HD*, hemodialysis; *PD*, peritoneal dialysis; *AST*, aspartate aminotransaminase; *ALT*, alanine aminotransferase; meals; *CSF*, cerebrospinal fluid.

*Average wholesale price according to the 1999 Red Book.

†FDA pregnancy categories: *A*, adequate studies in pregnant women, no risk; *B*, animal studies no risk, human studies inadequate, or animal benefit may outweigh risk; *X*, fetal abnormalities in humans, risk exceeds benefit.

‡Use in breast-feeding: limited data are available. Because all drugs are probably excreted in small amounts into breast milk, the potential for continued during treatment based on information available at present. "Avoid if possible" indicates that an alternative drug should be chosen or

§Insufficient information available to make a recommendation.

‖Available in the United States only from the manufacturer.

¶Available from the Centers for Disease Control and Prevention drug service.

#Not available in the United States.

USE IN BREASTFEEDING‡	DOSE INTERVAL ADJUSTMENT FOR REDUCED CRCL			SUPPLEMENTAL DOSE IN DIALYSIS		MAJOR TOXICITY
	>50	10-50	<10	HD	PD	
§	§	§	§	§	§	Nausea, vomiting, headache, dizziness, yellow discoloration of skin and urine, rash, fever, psychosis
	§	§	§	§	§	Diarrhea, abdominal pain, hypersensitivity reactions, systemic lupus erythematosus like syndrome, elevated AST, elevated alkaline phosphatase, jaundice, cardiac arrhythmias
	§	§	§	§	§	Flushing, pruritus, rash, fever, tinnitus, headache, nausea, thrombocytopenia, hemolysis in patients with G6PD deficiency, hypoglycemia
	§	§	§	§	§	
§	§	§	§	§	§	Abdominal pain; nausea; vomiting; malaise; headache; elevated AST, ALT; nephrotoxicity; myalgia; arthralgia; fever; rash; cough
§	§	§	§	§	§	Nausea, vomiting, shock, loss of consciousness, death during administration; fever, rash, exfoliative dermatis, paresthesia, photophobia, renal insufficiency, diarrhea
§	§	§	§	§	§	Anorexia, nausea, vomiting, dizziness
§	§	§	§	§	§	Neutropenia (must be given with leucovorin); rash; elevated AST, ALT; reversible peripheral neuropathy

GI, gastrointestinal; *G6PD*, glucose-6 phosphate dehydrogenase; *AIDS*, acquired immunodeficiency syndrome; *N.R.*, not recommended; *p.c.*, after

toxicity, human studies no risk; *C*, animal studies show toxicity, human studies inadequate but benefit may exceed risk; *D*, evidence of human risk,

adverse reactions in the infant must be considered, although few have been reported. "Probably safe" indicates that breast-feeding can be consideration given to discontinuing breast-feeding.

Suggested Reading

American Academy of Pediatrics Committee on Drugs. Transfer of drugs and other chemicals into human milk, *Pediatrics* 84:924, 1989.

Drug Topics Red Book: Montvale, NJ, 1999, Medical Economics.

Fulton B, Moore L: The galactopharmacopedia antiinfectives in breastmilk. I: penicillins and cephalosporins, *J Human Lactation*, 1995, 8:157, 1992.

Fulton B, Moore L: The galactopharmacopedia antiinfectives in breastmilk. II: sulfonamides, tetracyclines, macrolides, aminoglycosides and antimalarials, *J Human Lactation* 8:221, 1992.

Fulton B, Moore L: The galactopharmacopedia antiinfectives in breastmilk. III: antituberculars, quinolones and urinary germicides, *J Human Lactation* 9:43, 1993.

Mandell GL, et al: *Mandell, Douglas, and Bennett's principles and practice of infectious diseases*, ed 4, New York, 1995, Churchill Livingstone.

McEvoy GK: *American hospital formulary service drug information 1999*, Bethesda, MD, 1999, American Society of Hospital Pharmacists.

Nicolau D, et al: Experience with a once daily aminolgycoside program administered to 2,184 adult patients, *Antimicrob Agents Chemother* 39:650, 1995.

INDEX

Page numbers in italics indicate illustrations;
t indicates tables.